T0205764

Lecture Notes in Statistics **220**

Edited by P. Bickel, P. Diggle, S.E. Fienberg, U. Gather, S. Zeger

More information about this series at http://www.springer.com/series/694

Dietrich von Rosen

Bilinear Regression Analysis

An Introduction

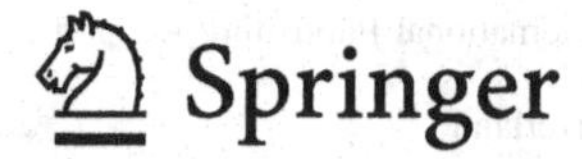

Dietrich von Rosen
Department of Energy and Technology
Swedish University of Agricultural Sciences
Uppsala, Sweden

ISSN 0930-0325 ISSN 2197-7186 (electronic)
Lecture Notes in Statistics
ISBN 978-3-319-78782-4 ISBN 978-3-319-78784-8 (eBook)
https://doi.org/10.1007/978-3-319-78784-8

Library of Congress Control Number: 2018943157

Mathematics Subject Classification (2010): 62H12, 62H15, 62H99, 62J20, 15A69, 15A03, 15A63

Printed on acid-free paper

This Springer imprint is published by the registered company Springer International Publishing AG part of Springer Nature
The registered company address is: Gewerbestrasse 11, 6330 Cham, Switzerland

To

Tatjana,

Alexander, Evelina, Michael,
Philip, Sophie

Preface

This book can be regarded as a textbook on bilinear regression analysis which could be used for a second course on classical multivariate analysis. The first course in such a series would deal with multivariate linear models, focusing, for example, on the estimation of parameters and the testing of hypotheses in such models. However, the book definitely does not require any knowledge of PCA, PCR, PLS, factor analysis, cluster analysis, multidimensional scaling, etc., since it does not treat any of these methods or any related methods. The most important prerequisite is some knowledge of linear models (univariate and/or multivariate models), and some knowledge of the basics of linear algebra would be helpful. The book has been written for PhD students in mathematical statistics or statistics, but researchers will probably also find some of the presented ideas and results to be of interest. The main purpose of writing this book was to present basic statistical theory for bilinear models, extending linear models theory, which from a theoretical point of view is a big and relevant step to take. For example, we mainly deal with non-linear estimators where the estimators of the mean parameters are not independent of the estimators of the dispersion parameters. Statistics goes hand in hand with data analysis. Therefore, one of the topics included in the book is the analysis of residuals, and it is emphasized that residuals are very important quantities to study. Moreover, the problem of the influence of observations is treated with some care. Generally speaking, a major part of the book includes tools that have been developed for handling bilinear regression models from a practical perspective.

One can view the approach adopted in the book as a combination of solid mathematics and illustrative and intuitive derivations, employing examples and pure data analysis, and to some extent, this reflects my view of statistical thinking. One of the cornerstones of the book is the definition of models which permit a clear mathematical treatment, including the estimation of unknown parameters, together with the presentation of methods for model validation against data.

It is worth noting that in several places in the book only the most enthusiastic reader will follow the details, and in fact, there are many places where the reader has to work out the details by themselves. For example, concerning several "moment calculations", only a few intermediate hints are presented together with the final result. The same can be said about the "matrix differentiation" which is performed. If all the details had been given, I believe the technical side of the material would have taken too much space. However, without any techniques it is difficult to derive new results. My intention has been that readers should be able to identify the ideas behind the different approaches presented in the book and should also be able to copy the included calculations.

The book is not meant to provide easy reading. However, if one is willing to devote time and effort to working with the material, one can expect to be rewarded. Students should perhaps read the book in a manner similar to jumping on a trampoline. One's first jump on a trampoline is not high, one's second jump is higher and then, in a short time, one approaches the maximum height. There are different thresholds to be crossed, but after a while readers will understand the logic and basic ideas used in the book. One can also compare reading the book to travelling on a safari which at the beginning takes one through a landscape filled with trees and bushes severely obstructing one's view, after which one reaches a savannah, with an open landscape offering an excellent view of numerous exciting animals.

The whole book can be studied within the framework of a two-semester course which also includes solving some of the suggested problems, which can very well be worked on in pairs. Note that some problems take quite a long time to solve. Another alternative is to use the material in the first three chapters for a course comprising, for example, 10 seminars, leading to knowledge about maximum likelihood estimation in bilinear regression models (BRM) and extended bilinear regression models. A third alternative is to consider only the BRM, i.e. the growth curve model (GMANOVA), in each of the eight chapters. This would probably lead to a course which takes a somewhat longer time to complete than one semester. If desired one could reduce the course length by omitting Chap. 8, or Chaps. 7 and 8.

The structure of the book deserves a few comments. In the main body of the text, few technical derivations are given if the results are available in the literature. Instead, the reader is referred to the appendices, where notations and technical results are presented. For proofs of many of the results, however, one is referred to other sources where detailed proofs can be found. Concerning the literature reviews at the end of each chapter, I have attempted to trace early references, and it is fascinating to see how much was accomplished and understood a long time ago. It is beyond my competence, from a statistics point of view, to provide a historical perspective on the material, but I hope that some readers will delve deeper into the early works, with a view to understanding the conceptual core of statistics and how to transmit achieved knowledge to the next generation of scientists. The problems that we face today can be solved better once we have apprehended how people were thinking in the pre-PC era. Moreover, I have tried to cite the literature which is directly connected to the content of this book, but I am convinced that I have omitted important references which I do not know of or have merely missed during the writing process. I would be happy to receive information about such omissions.

This book owes a great deal to many friends and colleagues. I am without doubt most indebted to my wife, Tatjana, who encouraged me to start this project and with whose blessing a large amount of my time has been invested in. It has been a long journey which has lasted for many years, and I am happy that it has come to an end. My colleagues and friends Kai-Tai Fang, Tõnu Kollo and Muni Srivastava have all been very important for my view of statistics in general and multivariate analysis in particular. I have learnt a great deal from our jointly written articles and a book written together with Tõnu Kollo. For example, some of the material in this book stems from our collaborative works on Edgeworth-type expansions and mean shift analysis, as well as influence analysis in general. Over the years, many PhD students have contributed to discussions which have helped me to understand various ideas implemented in this book. In particular, I have borrowed ideas and material produced by Jemila Hamid (on residual analysis) and Chengcheng Hao (on perturbation analysis). Furthermore, special thanks are extended to Martin Singull, with whom I have shared the supervision of several PhD students and have had numerous discussions on topics related to this book. I am grateful to Thomas Holgersson who unselfishly spent time reading a draft version of the book. Thanks also go to Katarzyna Filipiak and Augustyn Markiewicz for organizing and inviting me to a very interesting workshop series in Bedlewo, Poland (the Mathematical Research and Conference Center (MRCC) which is part of the Institute of Mathematics of the Polish Academy of Sciences). I have visited the workshops an uncountable number of times, and the stimulating discussions and the "free thinking environment" have had a great impact on this book. At the very end of this project, Paul McMillen made a complete linguistic revision and I am both thankful for and impressed by his improvement of the English of the manuscript. Finally, I would like to acknowledge gratefully all those (who are too many to be listed) who have helped me by providing references and shedding light on detailed concerns which I have had over the years.

I would be grateful to be informed of any errors which readers might find in the book. The responsibility for the errors is, of course, mine alone.

Uppsala, Sweden
November 2017

Dietrich von Rosen

Contents

Chapter 1
Introduction

1.1 What Is Statistics

Statistical science is about planning experiments, setting up models to analyse experiments and observational studies, and studying the properties of these models or the properties of some specific building blocks within these models, e.g. parameters and independence assumptions. Statistical science also concerns the validation of chosen models, often against data. Statistical application is about connecting statistical models to data.

The general statistical paradigm is based on the following steps:

1. setting up a model;
2. evaluating the model via simulations or comparisons with data;
3. if necessary, refining the model and restarting from step 2;
4. accepting and interpreting the model.

There is indeed also a step 0, namely determining the source of inspiration for setting up a statistical model. At least two cases can be identified: (i) the data-inspired model, i.e. depending on our experiences and what is seen in data, a model is formulated; (ii) the conceptually inspired model, i.e. someone has an idea about what the relevant components are and how these components should be included in the model of some process, for example.

It is obvious that when applying the paradigm, a number of decisions have to be made which unfortunately are all rather subjective. This should be taken into account when relying on statistics. Moreover, if statistics is to be useful, the model should be relevant for the problem under consideration, which is often relative to the information which can be derived from the data, and the final model should be interpretable. Statistics is instrumental, since, without expertise in the discipline in which it is applied, one usually cannot draw firm conclusions about the data which are used to evaluate the model. On the other hand, "data analysts", when applying statistics, need a solid knowledge of statistics to be able to perform efficient analysis.

D. von Rosen, *Bilinear Regression Analysis*, Lecture Notes in Statistics 220,
https://doi.org/10.1007/978-3-319-78784-8_1

The purpose of this book is to provide tools for the treatment of the so-called bilinear models. Bilinear models are models which are linear in two "directions". A typical example of something which is bilinear is the transformation of a matrix into another matrix, because one can transform the rows as well as the columns simultaneously. In practice rows and columns can, for example, represent a "spatial" direction and a "temporal" direction, respectively.

Basic ingredients in statistics are the concept of probability and the assumption about the underlying distributions. The distribution is a probability measure on the space of "random observations", i.e. observations of a phenomenon whose outcome cannot be stated in advance. However, what is a probability and what does a probability represent? Statistics uses the concept of probability as a measure of uncertainty. The probability measures used nowadays are well defined through their characterization via Kolmogorov's axioms. However, Kolmogorov's axioms tell us what a probability measure should fulfil, but not what it is. It is not even obvious that something like a probabilistic mechanism exists in real life (nature), but for statisticians this does not matter. The probability measure is part of a model and any model, of course, only describes reality approximatively.

1.2 What Is a Statistical Model

A statistical model is usually a class of distributions which is specified via functions of parameters (unknown quantities). The idea is to choose an appropriate model class according to the problem which is to be studied. Sometimes we know exactly what distribution should be used, but more often we have parameters which generate a model class, for example the class of multivariate normal distributions with an unknown mean and dispersion. Instead of distributions, it may be convenient, in particular for interpretations, to work with random variables which are representatives of the random phenomenon under study, although sometimes it is not obvious what kind of random variable corresponds to a distribution function. In Chap. 5 of this book, for example, some cases where this phenomenon occurs are dealt with. One problem with statistics (in most cases only a philosophical problem) is how to connect data to continuous random variables. In general it is advantageous to look upon data as realizations of random variables. However, since our data points have probability mass 0, we cannot directly couple, in a mathematical way, continuous random variables to data.

There exist several well-known schools of thought in statistics advocating different approaches to the connection of data to statistical models and these schools differ in the rigour of their method. Examples of these approaches are "distribution-free" methods, likelihood-based methods and Bayesian methods. Note that the fact that a method is distribution-free does not mean that there is no assumption made about the model. In a statistical model there are always some assumptions about randomness, for example concerning independence between random variables. Perhaps the best-known distribution-free method is the least squares approach.

Likelihood methods utilize classes of distributions which are generated by unknown parameters and the idea is to estimate these parameters. A consequence of this procedure is that we obtain the distribution which should be considered the true distribution, as well as acquiring information about the parameters which, if the model is appropriately specified, is interpretable. Concerning the normal distribution, usually the mean and variance act as parameters, although from an exponential family point of view, a more natural equivalent parametrization can be set up.

In Bayesian methods the basic idea is that everything unknown is modelled with the help of distributions, for instance, unknown parameters. One is avoiding some of the problems with the likelihood approach, such as connecting continuous data to a model, but instead one generates other problems; for example it is difficult to specify distributions for all the unknown elements. Moreover, in the Bayesian approach the concept of conditional independence is crucial, in contrast to the likelihood approach, where independence is used. Which method is to be preferred is a matter of taste.

This book is mainly likelihood-inspired, i.e. likelihood acts as a basis for the presentations. However, one should note that many statistical inference procedures are not purely frequentistic, Bayesian or likelihood procedures. For example, if one is dealing with normally distributed variables with unknown singular dispersion matrices, it is not clear which school of thought can be adopted when trying to follow the general statistical paradigm. Other deep discussions can concern the concept of confidence intervals and variable selection methods. General material of interest, including deliberations on deeper philosophical issues, are presented in Evans et al. (1986), Davison (2003), Berger and Molina (2004), Geisser (2006), Mayo and Cox (2006) and Cox (2006), for example.

In fact, in some way, restricting the inference procedures to one particular procedure is inconsistent with the statistical paradigm. The problem at hand should guide one's choice. Moreover, one has to decide if the conclusions and decision making should be based on probabilistic arguments, for example hypotheses testing. In this book we emphasize understanding the statistical model and the statistics under consideration. For example, in the case of an estimator or a hypothesis test, we want to understand what is really being estimated or tested. The basic problem is the difference between a statistical model and the corresponding estimated model, which is data-dependent, i.e. different data sets may lead to different interpretations and conclusions.

Example 1.1 In this example, several statistical approaches for evaluating a model are presented. Let

$$\boldsymbol{x}' = \boldsymbol{\beta}'\boldsymbol{C} + \boldsymbol{e}',$$

where $\boldsymbol{x} : n \times 1$, a random vector corresponding to the observations, $\boldsymbol{C} : k \times n$, is the design matrix, $\boldsymbol{\beta} : k \times 1$ is an unknown parameter vector which is to be estimated, and $\boldsymbol{e} \sim N_n(\boldsymbol{0}, \sigma^2\boldsymbol{I})$, which is considered to be the error term in the model and where σ^2 denotes the variance, which is supposed to be unknown. In this book the term "observation" is used in the sense of observed data which are thought to be realizations of some random process. In statistical theory the term "observation" often refers to a set of random variables. Let the projector $\boldsymbol{P}_{C'} = \boldsymbol{C}'(\boldsymbol{C}\boldsymbol{C}')^{-}\boldsymbol{C}$ be defined in Appendix A, Sect. A.7, where $(\bullet)^{-}$ denotes an arbitrary g-inverse (see Appendix A, Sect. A.6). Some useful results for projectors are presented in Appendix B, Theorem B.11.

The least squares approach works as follows. Let $\boldsymbol{x}_o$ be the observations of $\boldsymbol{x}$, and let us minimize, with respect to $\boldsymbol{\beta}$,

$$(\boldsymbol{x}_o' - E[\boldsymbol{x}'])(\boldsymbol{x}_o' - E[\boldsymbol{x}'])' = (\boldsymbol{x}_o' - \boldsymbol{\beta}'\boldsymbol{C})(\boldsymbol{x}_o' - \boldsymbol{\beta}'\boldsymbol{C})',$$

which yields

$$\widehat{\boldsymbol{\beta}}_o'\boldsymbol{C} = \boldsymbol{x}_o'\boldsymbol{P}_{C'}, \tag{1.1}$$

where $\widehat{\boldsymbol{\beta}}_o$ stands for the estimate of $\boldsymbol{\beta}$, i.e. an explicit numerical value of $\boldsymbol{\beta}$. Moreover, it follows that

$$(\boldsymbol{x}_o' - \boldsymbol{\beta}'\boldsymbol{C})(\boldsymbol{x}_o' - \boldsymbol{\beta}'\boldsymbol{C})' = \boldsymbol{x}_o'(\boldsymbol{I} - \boldsymbol{P}_{C'})\boldsymbol{x}_o + (\boldsymbol{x}_o'\boldsymbol{P}_{C'} - \boldsymbol{\beta}'\boldsymbol{C})()' \geq \boldsymbol{x}_o'(\boldsymbol{I} - \boldsymbol{P}_{C'})\boldsymbol{x}_o,$$

where $(\bullet)()'$ is used according to Appendix A, Sect. A.7, with equality if and only if (1.1) is true. In order to study properties of the estimate, $\boldsymbol{x}_o$ is replaced by $\boldsymbol{x}$, and when doing so, the estimator

$$\widehat{\boldsymbol{\beta}}'\boldsymbol{C} = \boldsymbol{x}'\boldsymbol{P}_{C'}$$

is obtained. Due to the linearity of the estimator

$$\widehat{\boldsymbol{\beta}}'\boldsymbol{C} \sim N_n(\boldsymbol{\beta}\boldsymbol{C}, \sigma^2\boldsymbol{P}_{C'});$$

i.e. $\widehat{\boldsymbol{\beta}}\boldsymbol{C}$ is unbiased and normally distributed with variance $\sigma^2\boldsymbol{P}_{C'}$. The variance parameter can be estimated as $n\widehat{\sigma}^2 = \boldsymbol{x}'(\boldsymbol{I} - \boldsymbol{P}_{C'})\boldsymbol{x}$. According to the statistical paradigm, models should be evaluated. The linear model in this example may, for instance, be evaluated via residuals, i.e. $\boldsymbol{x}_o'(\boldsymbol{I} - \boldsymbol{P}_{C'})$ and $\boldsymbol{x}'(\boldsymbol{I} - \boldsymbol{P}_{C'})$. For example, one should validate the model with respect to influential observations and outliers as well as the fit of the model to data. Moreover, specific properties such as the smallest variance properties of the $\boldsymbol{\beta}$-estimator can be shown or the "best quadratic" properties of the variance estimator.

An alternative estimation procedure is based on finding estimators which minimize the overall variance

$$E[(\boldsymbol{x}' - \boldsymbol{\beta}'\boldsymbol{C})(\boldsymbol{x}' - \boldsymbol{\beta}'\boldsymbol{C})'],$$

which can be rewritten in the following way:

$$E[(\boldsymbol{x}' - \boldsymbol{\beta}'\boldsymbol{C})(\boldsymbol{x}' - \boldsymbol{\beta}'\boldsymbol{C})']$$
$$= E[\boldsymbol{x}'(\boldsymbol{I} - \boldsymbol{P}_{C'})\boldsymbol{x}] + E[(\boldsymbol{x}'\boldsymbol{P}_{C'} - \boldsymbol{\beta}'\boldsymbol{C})(\boldsymbol{x}'\boldsymbol{P}_{C'} - \boldsymbol{\beta}'\boldsymbol{C})']. \qquad (1.2)$$

Thus, it follows that the estimator equals

$$\widehat{\boldsymbol{\beta}}'\boldsymbol{C} = \boldsymbol{x}'\boldsymbol{P}_{C'},$$

because in this case the second term in (1.2) equals 0. In order to verify the model via comparisons to data, the estimate

$$\widehat{\boldsymbol{\beta}}'_o\boldsymbol{C} = \boldsymbol{x}'_o\boldsymbol{P}_{C'},$$

is calculated. The expressions for the estimator and estimate are the same as the corresponding expressions in the least squares approach, although conceptually the methods differ to a great extent; i.e. for the least squares method we start with data, find an estimate and then construct an estimator by replacing the data, $\boldsymbol{x}_o$, by $\boldsymbol{x}$. For the minimization of the variance we started with $\boldsymbol{x}$, found an estimator and then constructed an estimate by replacing $\boldsymbol{x}$ by $\boldsymbol{x}_o$.

Now we turn to the likelihood approach. Here one starts with the likelihood, which nowadays, for continuous random variables, is the density of $\boldsymbol{x}$ evaluated at $\boldsymbol{x}_o$, i.e.

$$L(\boldsymbol{\beta}, \sigma^2) = (2\pi)^{-n/2}(\sigma^2)^{-n/2}\exp\{-\tfrac{\sigma^{-2}}{2}(\boldsymbol{x}'_o - \boldsymbol{\beta}'\boldsymbol{C})(\boldsymbol{x}'_o - \boldsymbol{\beta}'\boldsymbol{C})'\}.$$

This function is maximized with respect to σ^2 and $\boldsymbol{\beta}$ which gives

$$\widehat{\boldsymbol{\beta}}'_o\boldsymbol{C} = \boldsymbol{x}'_o\boldsymbol{C}'(\boldsymbol{C}\boldsymbol{C}')^{-}\boldsymbol{C} = \boldsymbol{x}'_o\boldsymbol{P}_{C'},$$
$$n\widehat{\sigma}^2_o = \boldsymbol{x}'_o(\boldsymbol{I} - \boldsymbol{C}'(\boldsymbol{C}\boldsymbol{C}')^{-}\boldsymbol{C})\boldsymbol{x}_o = \boldsymbol{x}'_o(\boldsymbol{I} - \boldsymbol{P}_{C'})\boldsymbol{x}_o.$$

In a second step of the likelihood approach $\widehat{\boldsymbol{\beta}}$ is constructed by replacing $\boldsymbol{x}_o$ by $\boldsymbol{x}$. Hence, we establish that the likelihood approach will lead to the same conclusion as the least squares and the minimum variance approaches.

□

Over the years many more estimation methods have been presented. For example, shrinkage methods, robust methods and Bayesian methods. We would also like to emphasize that models should be meaningful, i.e. that the parameters and their estimators should be understandable, and computations connected to the model should be fast. The past 20 years, with the arrival of increasingly powerful PCs and computer facilities, have witnessed an absurd use of algorithms and one can even see programs running for days and nights. The beauty of statistics, as well as its relation to mathematics, has been partly lost. This is serious, because mathematics helps us to examine the models and understand the analysis. Without mathematics it is easy to become trapped in too many ad hoc procedures. Intuition and ad hoc procedures should be basic ingredients in statistical model building, but they should also be possible to verify. This is the best way to create an end-product which can later be improved. Using too many simulation studies will result in an end-product which only with difficulty can be transmitted to the next generation of statisticians.

This book considers models which are called bilinear. Briefly speaking, the main difference between linear and bilinear models is that in the estimation process, the latter uses random weights when performing projections (due to an estimated inner product), whereas linear models generally use non-random projections. Another important fact is that under usual normality assumptions bilinear models do not belong to the exponential family.

1.3 The General Univariate Linear Model with a Known Dispersion

In this section the classical Gauss-Markov set-up is considered but we assume the dispersion matrix to be completely known. If the dispersion matrix is positive definite (p.d.), the model is just a minor extension of the model in Example 1.1. However, if the dispersion matrix is positive semi-definite (p.s.d.), other aspects related to the model will be introduced. In general, in the Gauss-Markov model the dispersion is proportional to an unknown constant, but this is immaterial for our presentation. The reason for investigating the model in some detail is that there has to be a close connection between the estimators based on models with a known dispersion and those based on models with an unknown dispersion. Indeed, if one assumes a known dispersion matrix, all our models can be reformulated as Gauss-Markov models. With additional information stating that the random variables are normally distributed, one can see from the likelihood equations that the maximum likelihood estimators (MLEs) of the mean parameters under the assumption of an unknown dispersion should approach the corresponding estimators under the assumption of a known dispersion. For example, the likelihood equation for the model $\boldsymbol{X} \sim N_{p,n}(\boldsymbol{ABC}, \boldsymbol{\Sigma}, \boldsymbol{I})$ which appears when differentiating with respect to $\boldsymbol{B}$ (see Appendix A, Sect. A.9 for definition of the matrix normal distribution and Chap. 1, Sect. 1.5 for a precise specification of the model) equals

$$\boldsymbol{A}'\boldsymbol{\Sigma}^{-1}(\boldsymbol{X} - \boldsymbol{ABC})\boldsymbol{C}' = \boldsymbol{0};$$

and for a large sample any maximum likelihood estimator of $\boldsymbol{B}$ has to satisfy this equation asymptotically, because we know that the MLE of $\boldsymbol{\Sigma}$ is a consistent estimator. For interested readers it can be worth studying generalized estimating equation (GEE) theory, for example see Shao (2003, pp. 359–367).

Now let us discuss the univariate linear model

$$\boldsymbol{x}' = \boldsymbol{\beta}'\boldsymbol{C} + \boldsymbol{e}', \qquad \boldsymbol{e} \sim N_n(\boldsymbol{0}, \boldsymbol{V}), \tag{1.3}$$

where $V : n \times n$ is p.d. and known, $x : n \times 1$, $C : k \times n$ and $\beta : k \times 1$ is to be estimated. Let x_o, as previously, denote the observations of x and let us use $V^{-1} = V^{-1}P_{C',V} + P_{(C')^o,V^{-1}}V^{-1}$ (see Appendix B, Theorem B.13), where $(C')^o$ is any matrix satisfying $\mathcal{C}((C')^o)^{\perp} = \mathcal{C}(C')$, where $\mathcal{C}(\bullet)$ denotes the column vector space (see Appendix A, Sect. A.8). Then the likelihood is maximized as follows:

$$\begin{aligned} L(\beta) &\propto |V|^{-1/2}\exp\{-1/2(x_o' - \beta'C)V^{-1}(x_o' - \beta'C)'\} \\ &= |V|^{-1/2}\exp\{-1/2(x_o'P_{C',V}' - \beta'C)V^{-1}()'\} \\ &\quad \times\exp\{-1/2(x_o'P_{(C')^o,V^{-1}}V^{-1}x_o)\} \\ &\leq |V|^{-1/2}\exp\{-1/2(x_o'P_{(C')^o,V^{-1}}V^{-1}x_o)\}, \end{aligned}$$

which is independent of any parameter, i.e. β, and the upper bound is attained if and only if

$$\widehat{\beta}_o'C = x_o'P_{C',V}',$$

where $\widehat{\beta}_o$ is the estimate of β. Thus, in order to estimate β a linear equation system has to be solved. The solution can be written as follows (see Appendix B, Theorem B.10 (i)):

$$\widehat{\beta}_o' = x_o'V^{-1}C'(CV^{-1}C')^{-} + z'(C)^{o'},$$

where z' stands for an arbitrary vector of a proper size.

Suppose that in model (1.3) there are restrictions (a priori information) on the mean vector given by

$$\beta'G = 0.$$

Then

$$\beta' = \theta'G^{o'},$$

where θ is a new unrestricted parameter. After inserting this relation in (1.3), the following model appears:

$$x' = \theta'G^{o'}C + e', \qquad e \sim N_n(0, V).$$

Thus, the above-presented calculations yield

$$\widehat{\beta}_o'C = x_o'P_{C'G^o,V}'$$

and from here, since this expression constitutes a consistent linear equation in $\widehat{\boldsymbol{\beta}}_o$, a general expression for $\widehat{\boldsymbol{\beta}}_o$ $(\boldsymbol{\beta})$ can be obtained explicitly.

If $\boldsymbol{V}$ is p.s.d the likelihood does not exist and the model consists of a continuous and a discrete part. Because $\boldsymbol{V}$ is p.s.d., there exists a semi-orthogonal matrix $\boldsymbol{H}$: $n \times r$, where $r = r(\boldsymbol{V})$ and $\boldsymbol{V} = \boldsymbol{H}\boldsymbol{H}'$ (see Appendix A, Sect. A.5), such that

$$\boldsymbol{H}^{o'}\boldsymbol{V} = \boldsymbol{0}.$$

Note that we do not lose any "information" if a one-to-one transformation of $\boldsymbol{x}$ takes place. Therefore the estimation of $\boldsymbol{\beta}$ in (1.3) can equivalently be carried out via $\boldsymbol{x}'(\boldsymbol{H} : \boldsymbol{H}^o)$, where $(\boldsymbol{H} : \boldsymbol{H}^o)$ denotes the partitioned matrix of $\boldsymbol{H}$ and $\boldsymbol{H}^o$ (see Appendix A, Sect. A.8). Hence, with probability 1

$$\boldsymbol{x}_o'\boldsymbol{H}^o = \boldsymbol{\beta}'\boldsymbol{C}\boldsymbol{H}^o \tag{1.4}$$

and therefore we assume (consistency assumption) $\boldsymbol{H}^{o'}\boldsymbol{x}_o \in \mathcal{C}(\boldsymbol{H}^{o'}\boldsymbol{C}')$, which is equivalent to $\boldsymbol{x}_o \in \mathcal{C}(\boldsymbol{C}' : \boldsymbol{V})$. Thus, the data put restrictions on $\boldsymbol{\beta}$, which is a new feature in comparison with the case when $\boldsymbol{V}$ is of full rank. The meaningfulness of this depends on the problem under consideration. Moreover,

$$\boldsymbol{x}'\boldsymbol{H} = \boldsymbol{\beta}'\boldsymbol{C}\boldsymbol{H} + \widetilde{\boldsymbol{e}}, \qquad \widetilde{\boldsymbol{e}} \sim N_r(\boldsymbol{0}, \boldsymbol{H}'\boldsymbol{V}\boldsymbol{H}). \tag{1.5}$$

Equation (1.4) is linear in $\boldsymbol{\beta}$ and because of consistency (see Appendix B, Theorem B.10 (i))

$$\boldsymbol{\beta}' = \boldsymbol{x}_o'\boldsymbol{H}^o(\boldsymbol{C}\boldsymbol{H}^o)^- + \boldsymbol{\theta}'(\boldsymbol{C}\boldsymbol{H}^o)^{o'},$$

where one can view the elements of $\boldsymbol{\theta}$ as a new set of unrestricted parameters. Inserting the solution into (1.5) yields

$$\boldsymbol{x}'\boldsymbol{H} = \boldsymbol{x}_o'\boldsymbol{H}^o(\boldsymbol{C}\boldsymbol{H}^o)^-\boldsymbol{C}\boldsymbol{H} + \boldsymbol{\theta}'(\boldsymbol{C}\boldsymbol{H}^o)^{o'}\boldsymbol{C}\boldsymbol{H} + \widetilde{\boldsymbol{e}}.$$

From earlier calculations we know that

$$\begin{aligned}\widehat{\boldsymbol{\theta}}_o' &= \boldsymbol{x}_o'(\boldsymbol{I} - \boldsymbol{H}^o(\boldsymbol{C}\boldsymbol{H}^o)^-\boldsymbol{C})\boldsymbol{H}\\ &\quad\times(\boldsymbol{H}'\boldsymbol{V}\boldsymbol{H})^{-1}\boldsymbol{H}'\boldsymbol{C}'(\boldsymbol{C}\boldsymbol{H}^o)^o((\boldsymbol{C}\boldsymbol{H}^o)^{o'}\boldsymbol{C}\boldsymbol{H}(\boldsymbol{H}'\boldsymbol{V}\boldsymbol{H})^{-1}\boldsymbol{H}'\boldsymbol{C}'(\boldsymbol{C}\boldsymbol{H}^o)^o)^-\\ &\quad+\boldsymbol{z}'((\boldsymbol{C}\boldsymbol{H}^o)^{o'}\boldsymbol{C}\boldsymbol{H})^{o'},\end{aligned} \tag{1.6}$$

where $\boldsymbol{z}$ is an arbitrary vector and then

$$\begin{aligned}\widehat{\boldsymbol{\beta}}_o' &= \boldsymbol{x}_o'\boldsymbol{H}^o(\boldsymbol{C}\boldsymbol{H}^o)^- + \boldsymbol{x}_o'(\boldsymbol{I} - \boldsymbol{H}^o(\boldsymbol{C}\boldsymbol{H}^o)^-\boldsymbol{C})\boldsymbol{H}\\ &\quad\times(\boldsymbol{H}'\boldsymbol{V}\boldsymbol{H})^{-1}\boldsymbol{H}'\boldsymbol{C}'(\boldsymbol{C}\boldsymbol{H}^o)^o((\boldsymbol{C}\boldsymbol{H}^o)^{o'}\boldsymbol{C}\boldsymbol{H}(\boldsymbol{H}'\boldsymbol{V}\boldsymbol{H})^{-1}\boldsymbol{H}'\boldsymbol{C}'(\boldsymbol{C}\boldsymbol{H}^o)^o)^-(\boldsymbol{C}\boldsymbol{H}^o)^{o'}\\ &\quad+\boldsymbol{z}'((\boldsymbol{C}\boldsymbol{H}^o)^{o'}\boldsymbol{C}\boldsymbol{H})^{o'}(\boldsymbol{C}\boldsymbol{H}^o)^{o'}.\end{aligned}$$

If we study the statistical properties of this estimate, we should consider the following (remember (1.4) and that $\boldsymbol{H}'\boldsymbol{H} = \boldsymbol{I}$):

$$\begin{aligned}
\widehat{\boldsymbol{\beta}}' &= \boldsymbol{\beta}'\boldsymbol{C}\boldsymbol{H}^o(\boldsymbol{C}\boldsymbol{H}^o)^- \\
&\quad -\boldsymbol{\beta}'\boldsymbol{C}\boldsymbol{H}^o(\boldsymbol{C}\boldsymbol{H}^o)^-\boldsymbol{C}\boldsymbol{H}\boldsymbol{H}'\boldsymbol{C}'(\boldsymbol{C}\boldsymbol{H}^o)^o((\boldsymbol{C}\boldsymbol{H}^o)^{o'}\boldsymbol{C}\boldsymbol{H}\boldsymbol{H}'\boldsymbol{C}'(\boldsymbol{C}\boldsymbol{H}^o)^o)^-(\boldsymbol{C}\boldsymbol{H}^o)^{o'} \\
&\quad +\boldsymbol{x}'\boldsymbol{H}\boldsymbol{H}'\boldsymbol{C}'(\boldsymbol{C}\boldsymbol{H}^o)^o((\boldsymbol{C}\boldsymbol{H}^o)^{o'}\boldsymbol{C}\boldsymbol{H}\boldsymbol{H}'\boldsymbol{C}'(\boldsymbol{C}\boldsymbol{H}^o)^o)^-(\boldsymbol{C}\boldsymbol{H}^o)^{o'} \\
&\quad +\boldsymbol{z}'((\boldsymbol{C}\boldsymbol{H}^o)^{o'}\boldsymbol{C}\boldsymbol{H})^{o'}(\boldsymbol{C}\boldsymbol{H}^o)^{o'}
\end{aligned}$$

and then assume some conditions (estimability conditions) so that for $\widehat{\boldsymbol{\beta}}'\boldsymbol{L}$, for some specific $\boldsymbol{L}$, the term including $\boldsymbol{z}$ will disappear. Moreover, in practice the condition $\boldsymbol{x}_o \in \mathcal{C}(\boldsymbol{C}' : \boldsymbol{V})$ may not be satisfied and then a pretreatment of data has to take place, for example a projection of data on the space $\mathcal{C}(\boldsymbol{C}' : \boldsymbol{V})$.

Example 1.2 Here the singular Gauss-Markov model is illustrated. In an experiment where the eating behaviour of n dairy cows was studied in connection with the administration of food, one could keep the total amount of food fixed (let us say t) over a 24 h day-and-night cycle. During the 24 h, a record was made of how much each of the n cows was eating. Due to breeding and local environmental conditions, the cows are correlated with a covariance matrix $\sigma^2\boldsymbol{V}$, where σ^2 is an unknown scaling parameter. Since the cows have been part of many feeding experiments, the correlation between the cows can be supposed to be known. The main idea is to relate the recorded values to various explanatory variables, such as lactation, the amount of produced milk and variables measuring the quality of the milk. If the measurements are denoted as x_{0i}, $i = 1, 2, \ldots, n$, and the other explanatory variables as $c_{1i}, c_{2i}, \ldots c_{ki}$, the following linear model can be set up:

$$x_i = \mu + \sum_{j=1}^{k} \beta_j c_{ji} + \epsilon_i, \qquad i = 1, 2, \ldots, n,$$

which in matrix notation equals

$$\boldsymbol{x}' = \boldsymbol{\beta}'\boldsymbol{C} + \boldsymbol{e}';$$

$\boldsymbol{C} = (\boldsymbol{1}_n, \boldsymbol{c}_1, \boldsymbol{c}_2, \ldots, \boldsymbol{c}_k)'$, $\boldsymbol{c}_j = (c_{ji})$, $\boldsymbol{e} \sim N_n(\boldsymbol{0}, \sigma^2\boldsymbol{V})$, and $\boldsymbol{\beta} = (\mu, \beta_1, \ldots, \beta_k)'$ and σ^2 are unknown parameters. As an estimator of σ^2 we can use

$$(n - k - 1)\widehat{\sigma}^2 = (\boldsymbol{x}' - \widehat{\boldsymbol{\beta}}'\boldsymbol{C})()',$$

for some estimator $\widehat{\boldsymbol{\beta}}$ of $\boldsymbol{\beta}$. Thus, if we are able to estimate $\boldsymbol{\beta}$, all the parameters can be estimated.

The technical treatment of the model proceeds as follows. Note that by making a one-to-one transformation of $\boldsymbol{x}$, there is no information loss. Thus, $\boldsymbol{x}$ will be pre-multiplied by $\mathbf{1}'$ and $\mathbf{1}^{o'}$. From the experimental assumptions it follows that $\boldsymbol{x}'\mathbf{1} = t$, which in turn implies $\boldsymbol{V}\mathbf{1} = \mathbf{0}$ and

$$\boldsymbol{\beta}'\boldsymbol{C}\mathbf{1} = \boldsymbol{x}'\mathbf{1} = t.$$

This means that, according to the model, we have an equation with no variation, and thus the equation can be treated as a deterministic equation which puts restrictions on $\boldsymbol{\beta}$. Solving this equation (see Appendix B, Theorem B.10 (i)) leads to

$$\boldsymbol{\beta}' = t(\boldsymbol{C}\mathbf{1})^{-} + \boldsymbol{\theta}(\boldsymbol{C}\mathbf{1})^{o'},$$

where $\boldsymbol{\theta}$ is an arbitrary vector of a proper size. Moreover,

$$\boldsymbol{x}'\mathbf{1}^{o} = t(\boldsymbol{C}\mathbf{1})^{-}\boldsymbol{C}\mathbf{1}^{o} + \boldsymbol{\theta}(\boldsymbol{C}\mathbf{1})^{o'}\boldsymbol{C}\mathbf{1}^{o} + \widetilde{\boldsymbol{e}},$$

where $\widetilde{\boldsymbol{e}} \sim N_n(\mathbf{0}, \mathbf{1}^{o'}\boldsymbol{V}\mathbf{1}^{o})$. In this model the MLE is obtained via

$$\widehat{\boldsymbol{\beta}}'\boldsymbol{C}\mathbf{1}^{o} = t(\boldsymbol{C}\mathbf{1})^{-}\boldsymbol{C}\mathbf{1}^{o} + \widehat{\boldsymbol{\theta}}(\boldsymbol{C}\mathbf{1})^{o'}\boldsymbol{C}\mathbf{1}^{o},$$

where

$$\begin{aligned}\widehat{\boldsymbol{\theta}}(\boldsymbol{C}\mathbf{1})^{o'}\boldsymbol{C}\mathbf{1}^{o} &= (\boldsymbol{x}' - t(\boldsymbol{C}\mathbf{1})^{-}\boldsymbol{C})\mathbf{1}^{o}(\mathbf{1}^{o'}\boldsymbol{V}\mathbf{1}^{o})^{-1}\mathbf{1}^{o'}\boldsymbol{C}'(\boldsymbol{C}\mathbf{1})^{o}\\ &\quad\times((\boldsymbol{C}\mathbf{1})^{o'}\boldsymbol{C}\mathbf{1}^{o}(\mathbf{1}^{o'}\boldsymbol{V}\mathbf{1}^{o})^{-1}\mathbf{1}^{o'}\boldsymbol{C}'(\boldsymbol{C}\mathbf{1})^{o})^{-}(\boldsymbol{C}\mathbf{1})^{o'}\boldsymbol{C}\mathbf{1}^{o}.\end{aligned}$$

from which $\widehat{\boldsymbol{\beta}}$ can be obtained under certain conditions on $\boldsymbol{C}$. □

In the example it was supposed that $\boldsymbol{x}'\mathbf{1} = t$, which implied that $\mathbf{1}'\boldsymbol{V} = \mathbf{0}$. However, as noted above, we can assume that we have models where $\boldsymbol{V}$ is singular without any exact restrictions on $\boldsymbol{x}$. When restrictions are put on the dispersion (covariance) matrix, we have restrictions on the random variable which only hold with probability 1. Therefore, it must in this case also be assumed that the data belong to a proper subspace, which may indeed be difficult to verify.

Moreover, for the linear model

$$\boldsymbol{x}' = \boldsymbol{\beta}'\boldsymbol{C} + \boldsymbol{e}', \qquad \boldsymbol{e} = (\mathbf{0}, \sigma^2\boldsymbol{V})$$

with restrictions

$$\boldsymbol{\beta}'\boldsymbol{K} = \boldsymbol{h};$$

the situation can be described via the following model:

$$(\boldsymbol{x}' : \boldsymbol{h}) = \boldsymbol{\beta}'(\boldsymbol{C} : \boldsymbol{K}) + \boldsymbol{e}', \qquad \boldsymbol{e} = (\mathbf{0}, \sigma^2\boldsymbol{W}),$$

where

$$W = \begin{pmatrix} V & 0 \\ 0 & 0 \end{pmatrix}.$$

This clearly shows how general the singular Gauss-Markov model is.

1.4 The General Multivariate Linear Model

In this book we study models which are based on an underlying multivariate normal distribution. The multivariate normal distribution is closely connected to linearity, since a linear function of a normal variable is also normally distributed. The theory around the normal distribution is well developed and one can, among other things, show that the general multivariate linear model under certain conditions belongs to the exponential family, which is very important. For example, for models which belong to the exponential family, there are complete and sufficient statistics, and all the moments and cumulants are at our disposal.

The general multivariate linear model equals

$$X = BC + E, \tag{1.7}$$

where $X : p \times n$ is a random matrix which corresponds to the observations, $B : p \times k$ is an unknown parameter matrix and $C : k \times n$ is a known design matrix. Furthermore, $E \sim N_{p,n}(0, \Sigma, I)$, where Σ is an unknown p.d. matrix. For a definition of the matrix normal distribution $N_{p,n}(\mu, \bullet, \bullet)$ see Appendix A, Sect. A.9. The model in (1.7) is also called the MANOVA model. According to the model specifications, the model consists of independently distributed columns. The design matrix C is also called a between-individuals design matrix. In order to be able to draw any conclusions from the model, we have to estimate the unknown parameters B and Σ. Following the statistical paradigm, we also have to verify the model and this usually takes place with the help of residuals.

If we examine the likelihood function, $L(B, \Sigma)$, we have

$$\begin{aligned} L(B, \Sigma) &\propto |\Sigma|^{n/2}\exp\{-1/2\mathrm{tr}\{\Sigma^{-1}(X_o - BC)()'\}\} \\ &= |\Sigma|^{n/2}\exp(-1/2\mathrm{tr}\{\Sigma^{-1}S_o + \Sigma^{-1}(X_oP_{C'} - BC)()'\}), \end{aligned}$$

where

$$S_o = X_o(I - P_{C'})X'_o.$$

Let S be as S_o, but with X_o replaced by X. From here it follows that the model belongs to the exponential family and that $XP_{C'}$ and S are sufficient statistics. It can be shown that the statistics also are complete. The MLEs for $\boldsymbol{B}$ and $\boldsymbol{\Sigma}$ are obtained from

$$\widehat{\boldsymbol{B}}_o\boldsymbol{C} = \boldsymbol{X}_o\boldsymbol{P}_{C'}, \tag{1.8}$$
$$n\widehat{\boldsymbol{\Sigma}}_o = \boldsymbol{S}_o,$$

since (1.8) constitutes a linear consistent equation system in $\boldsymbol{B}$. The likelihood is always smaller or equal to $(2\pi)^{-pn/2}|n^{-1}\boldsymbol{S}_o|^{-n/2}\exp\{-np/2\}$, where the upper bound is obtained when inserting $\widehat{\boldsymbol{B}}_o\boldsymbol{C}$ and $\widehat{\boldsymbol{\Sigma}}_o$.

Example 1.3 This is an example where several variables are to be modelled simultaneously. In environmental monitoring one can use many chemical biomarkers. For example, in Sweden, one monitors calcium, magnesium, sodium, potassium, sulphate, chloride, fluoride, nitrogen, phosphorus, conductivity and other substances/properties in lakes spread over the whole country. Observations are collected several times over the year. Imagine that we want to compare two regions for a specific year. Then one can select 20 lakes from each region and as response variables use the above-mentioned chemical variables, for which an average over the summer months can be used, for example. The model for the data with ten response variables and 40 observations equally divided between the two regions can be presented in the following way:

$$\boldsymbol{X} = \boldsymbol{B}\boldsymbol{C} + \boldsymbol{E},$$

where $\boldsymbol{X}$: 10×40, $\boldsymbol{B}$: 10×2 consists of the mean parameters, $\boldsymbol{E} \sim N_{10,40}(\boldsymbol{0}, \boldsymbol{\Sigma}, \boldsymbol{I})$, where $\boldsymbol{\Sigma}$: 10×10 is the unknown dispersion matrix, and

$$\boldsymbol{C} = \begin{pmatrix} \boldsymbol{1}'_{20} & \boldsymbol{0} \\ \boldsymbol{0} & \boldsymbol{1}'_{20} \end{pmatrix}.$$

□

Example 1.4 Now an example with repeated measurements with an unstructured mean is briefly presented. Another strategy for comparing regions than that presented in Example 1.3 is to focus on one of the chemical variables, for example nitrogen. Moreover, instead of averaging over the summer months as in Example 1.3, we can use the measurements from June, July and August. Thus we could set up the following model:

$$\boldsymbol{X} = \boldsymbol{B}\boldsymbol{C} + \boldsymbol{E},$$

where $\boldsymbol{X}$: 3×40, $\boldsymbol{B}$: 3×2 consists of the mean parameters, $\boldsymbol{E} \sim N_{3,40}(\boldsymbol{0}, \boldsymbol{\Sigma}, \boldsymbol{I})$, where $\boldsymbol{\Sigma}$: 3×3 is the unknown dispersion matrix, and the between-individuals design matrix $\boldsymbol{C}$ is as in Example 1.3. □

There are two natural follow-up questions concerning the models presented in Examples 1.3 and 1.4. The first concerns with the repeated measurements for nitrogen over the summer months. It would be of interest to use a linear model for these measurements, in particular if we were to include data from some more months. Then we would have a complete analogy with the analysis of growth curve data, but here, instead of growth, nitrogen over time would be studied. The second question is if we could analyse all ten chemical variables over time simultaneously. In that case we would have an analogy with a spatio-temporal model setting. Here, instead of geographic spatial information, we would be observing different chemical variables. Both these extensions would be outside the general multivariate linear model setting. However, under certain restrictions they could be analysed with bilinear regression models, since the mean structure, instead of being linear, would be bilinear. This would imply, among other things, that the models do not belong to the exponential family.

1.5 Bilinear Regression Models: An Introduction

Throughout the book BRM is used as an abbreviation for bilinear regression model. Other common names are the growth curve model or GMANOVA (generalized multivariate analysis of variance). At the end of the previous section, it was noted that even under normality assumptions, we have very natural models which do not belong to the exponential family. It was also noted in the previous section that if a model has a linear mean structure, the model belongs to the exponential family. In this section, it will be shown, among other things, that if a bilinear mean structure is assumed together with an arbitrary dispersion matrix, the model is not a member of the exponential family and instead belongs to the curved exponential family. Remember that if a matrix is pre- and post-multiplied by other matrices, we perform a bilinear transformation.

Often the mean structure $\boldsymbol{ABC}$ is considered, where the unknown parameter is given by $\boldsymbol{B}$. Hence, we have a bilinear model:

$$\boldsymbol{X} = \boldsymbol{ABC} + \boldsymbol{E}, \qquad (1.9)$$

where $\boldsymbol{X}$: $p \times n$, the unknown mean parameter matrix $\boldsymbol{B}$: $q \times k$, the two design matrices $\boldsymbol{A}$: $p \times q$ and $\boldsymbol{C}$: $k \times n$, and the error matrix $\boldsymbol{E}$ build up the model. Moreover, let $\boldsymbol{E}$ be normally distributed with independent columns, mean $\boldsymbol{0}$, and a positive definite dispersion matrix $\boldsymbol{\Sigma}$ for the elements within each column of $\boldsymbol{X}$. Then the density function for $\boldsymbol{X}$ is proportional to

$$|\boldsymbol{\Sigma}|^{-1/2n}\exp\{-1/2\mathrm{tr}\{\boldsymbol{\Sigma}^{-1}(\boldsymbol{X} - \boldsymbol{ABC})(\boldsymbol{X} - \boldsymbol{ABC})'\}\}$$

and after some manipulations it can be shown that this model belongs to the curved exponential family. For example, this can be shown through a reparametrization, i.e. according to Appendix B, Theorem B.1 (i), $\boldsymbol{A}$ can be factored as $\boldsymbol{A} = \boldsymbol{\Gamma}\binom{\boldsymbol{I}}{\boldsymbol{0}}\boldsymbol{T}$, where $\boldsymbol{\Gamma}$ is orthogonal and $\boldsymbol{T}$ is a non-singular matrix. Moreover, let $\boldsymbol{\Theta} = \boldsymbol{T}\boldsymbol{B}$, $\boldsymbol{\Psi} = \boldsymbol{\Gamma}'\boldsymbol{\Sigma}\boldsymbol{\Gamma}$, $\boldsymbol{Y} = \boldsymbol{\Gamma}'\boldsymbol{X}$, $\boldsymbol{Y}' = (\boldsymbol{Y}_1' : \boldsymbol{Y}_2')$ and

$$\boldsymbol{\Psi}^{-1} = \begin{pmatrix} \boldsymbol{\Psi}^{11} & \boldsymbol{\Psi}^{12} \\ \boldsymbol{\Psi}^{21} & \boldsymbol{\Psi}^{22} \end{pmatrix}.$$

Then the density function for the new variable $\boldsymbol{Y}$ is proportional to

$$|\boldsymbol{\Psi}^{-1}|^{n/2}\exp\{-1/2(\mathrm{tr}\{\boldsymbol{\Psi}^{-1}\boldsymbol{Y}(\boldsymbol{I} - \boldsymbol{P}_{\boldsymbol{C}'})\boldsymbol{Y}'\} - 2\mathrm{tr}\{\boldsymbol{Y}_1\boldsymbol{\Psi}^{11}\boldsymbol{\Theta}\boldsymbol{C}\} \\ -2\mathrm{tr}\{\boldsymbol{Y}_2\boldsymbol{\Psi}^{21}\boldsymbol{\Theta}\boldsymbol{C}\} + \mathrm{tr}\{\boldsymbol{\Psi}^{11}\boldsymbol{\Theta}\boldsymbol{C}\boldsymbol{C}'\boldsymbol{\Theta}'\})\},$$

which shows that the model belongs to the curved exponential family, since the number of "free" parameters, i.e. $\boldsymbol{\Psi}^{-1}$ and $\boldsymbol{\Psi}^{11}\boldsymbol{\Theta}$, is less than the number of functions including observations and parameters. Note that

$$\boldsymbol{\Psi}^{21}\boldsymbol{\Theta} = (\boldsymbol{I} : \boldsymbol{0})\boldsymbol{\Psi}^{-1}(\boldsymbol{0} : \boldsymbol{I})'((\boldsymbol{I} : \boldsymbol{0})\boldsymbol{\Psi}^{-1}(\boldsymbol{I} : \boldsymbol{0})')^{-1}\boldsymbol{\Psi}^{11}\boldsymbol{\Theta}.$$

The above-mentioned model is often termed the growth curve model and was introduced by Potthoff and Roy (1964), although very similar models had been considered earlier. The $\boldsymbol{A}$ matrix is often referred to as the within-individuals design matrix and $\boldsymbol{C}$, as in (1.7), is called the between-individuals design matrix.

A natural extension of the BRM is the following "sum of profiles" model

$$\boldsymbol{X} = \sum_{i=1}^{m} \boldsymbol{A}_i\boldsymbol{B}_i\boldsymbol{C}_i + \boldsymbol{E},$$

where $\boldsymbol{X}$: $p \times n$ is the sample matrix, the mean parameter matrices are $\boldsymbol{B}_i$: $q_i \times k_i$, the within-individual design matrices equal $\boldsymbol{A}_i$: $p \times q_i$ and the between-individual design matrices $\boldsymbol{C}_i$: $k_i \times n$, are such that

$$\mathcal{C}(\boldsymbol{C}_m') \subseteq \mathcal{C}(\boldsymbol{C}_{m-1}') \subseteq \cdots \subseteq \mathcal{C}(\boldsymbol{C}_1'). \tag{1.10}$$

Let $\boldsymbol{E}$ be matrix normally distributed with independent columns, mean $\boldsymbol{0}$, and a dispersion matrix $\boldsymbol{\Sigma}$ for the elements within each column of $\boldsymbol{E}$. Note that instead of (1.10), we can suppose that

$$\mathcal{C}(\boldsymbol{A}_m) \subseteq \mathcal{C}(\boldsymbol{A}_{m-1}) \subseteq \cdots \subseteq \mathcal{C}(\boldsymbol{A}_1). \tag{1.11}$$

The model is referred to herein as the extended bilinear regression model ($EBRM_\bullet^\bullet$) and in order to distinguish between (1.10) and (1.11), as well as indicate m in the profile expression, $EBRM_B^m$ and $EBRM_W^m$ are used, where the subscripts B and W stand for "between" and "within", respectively, and are used depending on whether (1.10) or (1.11) is assumed to hold. Sometimes the $EBRM^m_\bullet$ is called the extended growth curve model. The conditions in (1.10) or (1.11) are mathematically motivated since they lead to explicit MLEs. Concerning these conditions, there is an analogy with the Behrens-Fisher problem; i.e. the purpose is to compare two groups of size n_1 and n_2, respectively, for testing equality of the means with the additional assumption that random variables corresponding to the observations from different groups have different variances, i.e.

$$\boldsymbol{x}' = \boldsymbol{\mu}'\boldsymbol{C} + \boldsymbol{e}',$$

where $\boldsymbol{\mu}' = (\boldsymbol{\mu}_1' : \boldsymbol{\mu}_2')$,

$$\boldsymbol{C} = \left(\mathbf{1}_{n_1}' \otimes \begin{pmatrix} 1 \\ 0 \end{pmatrix} : \mathbf{1}_{n_2}' \otimes \begin{pmatrix} 0 \\ 1 \end{pmatrix}\right),$$

where $\otimes$ denotes the Kronecker product (see Appendix A, Sect. A.6) and

$$\boldsymbol{e}' \sim N_n(\mathbf{0}, \begin{pmatrix} \sigma_1^2 \boldsymbol{I}_{n_1} & 0 \\ 0 & \sigma_2^2 \boldsymbol{I}_{n_2} \end{pmatrix}), \qquad n = n_1 + n_2.$$

Comparing $\boldsymbol{\mu}_1$ and $\boldsymbol{\mu}_2$ will not give any precise answer about differences between groups, i.e. their distributions, unless σ_i^2 is taken into account. If (1.10) or (1.11) does not hold, we have, instead of a common mean and different variances (Behrens-Fisher case), different means and a common dispersion matrix. This situation is called seemingly unrelated regression (SUR) and has been extensively studied in a univariate setting (e.g. see Kariya and Kurata, 2004). An example of a univariate SUR model is the SUR model with two functionally independent regression lines, but correlated error terms. In the multivariate case it becomes more difficult to interpret results and there are reasons why one should avoid this type of model.

This section is concluded by giving some more examples.

Example 1.5 This example illustrates the use of the BRM to analyse Swedish liming data (see also Examples 1.3 and 1.4). For many years there has been a problem with the acidification of lakes in Sweden, and to help lakes to recover, one is liming them to stimulate the recovery process. Below we present a data set which covers ten lakes from each of two regions where the pH concentration has been measured at three different depths, 0.5, 5 and 10 m. Since the pH is highest close to the surface and thereafter decreases we can try to model the concentration with a linear model. The data are presented in Table 1.1. The following matrices are involved in the description of the data. The matrix $\boldsymbol{X}$ is the random matrix which corresponds to the data and $\boldsymbol{X} \sim N_{3,20}(\boldsymbol{ABC}, \boldsymbol{\Sigma}, \boldsymbol{I})$, where $\boldsymbol{B}$ is an unknown

Table 1.1 Selected data, with some minor modifications, from the integrated monitoring of the effects of liming project at the Swedish University of Agricultural Sciences; pH represents minus the decimal logarithm of the hydrogen ion activity

Lake	Depth	pH	Region	Lake	Depth	pH	Region
1	0.5	6.72	1	11	0.5	7.29	2
1	5.0	6.61	1	11	5.0	6.78	2
1	10.0	6.41	1	11	10.0	6.76	2
2	0.5	6.80	1	12	0.5	6.91	2
2	5.0	6.80	1	12	5.0	6.91	2
2	10.0	6.70	1	12	10.0	6.71	2
3	0.5	7.16	1	13	0.5	7.23	2
3	5.0	7.12	1	13	5.0	7.37	2
3	10.0	7.01	1	13	10.0	7.10	2
4	0.5	7.17	1	14	0.5	6.81	2
4	5.0	7.20	1	14	5.0	6.68	2
4	10.0	7.08	1	14	10.0	6.18	2
5	0.5	6.96	1	15	0.5	6.66	2
5	5.0	6.68	1	15	5.0	6.47	2
5	10.0	6.48	1	15	10.0	6.17	2
6	0.5	7.23	1	16	0.5	6.89	2
6	5.0	7.02	1	16	5.0	6.59	2
6	10.0	6.80	1	16	10.0	6.19	2
7	0.5	6.87	1	17	0.5	6.98	2
7	5.0	6.73	1	17	5.0	6.64	2
7	10.0	6.43	1	17	10.0	6.24	2
8	0.5	7.15	1	18	0.5	6.88	2
8	5.0	7.18	1	18	5.0	7.01	2
8	10.0	6.80	1	18	10.0	6.71	2
9	0.5	7.23	1	19	0.5	7.01	2
9	5.0	7.03	1	19	5.0	6.90	2
9	10.0	6.73	1	19	10.0	6.80	2
10	0.5	7.24	1	20	0.5	7.20	2
10	5.0	7.19	1	20	5.0	7.17	2
10	10.0	6.99	1	20	10.0	7.07	2

parameter matrix and $\boldsymbol{\Sigma}$ is p.d. but unstructured, and where

$$\boldsymbol{A} = \begin{pmatrix} 1 & 0.5 \\ 1 & 5 \\ 1 & 10 \end{pmatrix}, \qquad \boldsymbol{C} = \left(\mathbf{1}'_{10} \otimes \begin{pmatrix} 1 \\ 0 \end{pmatrix} : \mathbf{1}'_{10} \otimes \begin{pmatrix} 0 \\ 1 \end{pmatrix} \right). \qquad \square$$

Example 1.6 This example concerns the hormone melatonin and acute severe depression. More than 30 years ago, depression was already being studied concerning its relation to various hormones, in particular melatonin. Among other

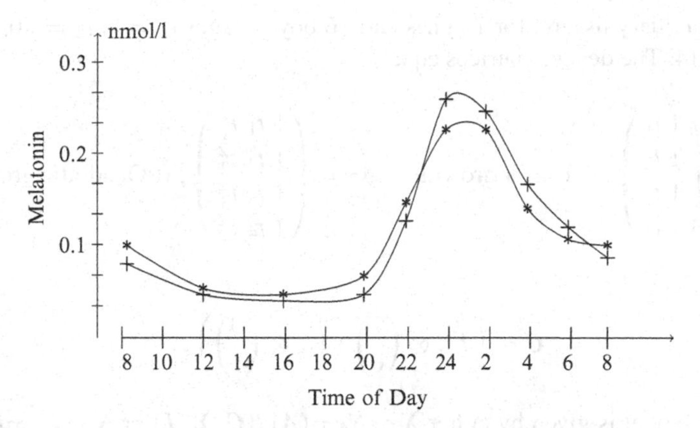

Fig. 1.1 Serum melatonin levels patients with acute depression (∗) and a control group of healthy individuals (+). Group-averaged sample means have been joined in the figure

discoveries, the melatonin peak level was found to be lowered in patients suffering from acute depression in comparison to the corresponding level in healthy subjects. The melatonin levels for these two groups are shown in Fig. 1.1. The peak levels remained low when these patients were re-examined during remission. Therefore, melatonin levels can be viewed as a bio-marker for depression. It is typical of melatonin, as well as some other hormones (e.g. cortisol), that they follow a day-and-night cycle.

If the data consist of ten repeated measurements over the day-and-night cycle, the following model can be used: $\boldsymbol{X} \sim N_{10,60}(\boldsymbol{ABC}, \boldsymbol{\Sigma}, \boldsymbol{I})$, where $(\omega = \pi/24)$

$$\boldsymbol{A} = \begin{pmatrix} 1 & \sin(\omega) & \cos(\omega) & \sin(2\omega) & \cos(2\omega) \\ 1 & \sin(4\omega) & \cos(4\omega) & \sin(4*2\omega) & \cos(4*2\omega) \\ 1 & \sin(8\omega) & \cos(8\omega) & \sin(8*2\omega) & \cos(8*2\omega) \\ 1 & \sin(12\omega) & \cos(12\omega) & \sin(12*2\omega) & \cos(12*2\omega) \\ 1 & \sin(14\omega) & \cos(14\omega) & \sin(14*2\omega) & \cos(14*2\omega) \\ 1 & \sin(16\omega) & \cos(16\omega) & \sin(16*2\omega) & \cos(16*2\omega) \\ 1 & \sin(18\omega) & \cos(18\omega) & \sin(18*2\omega) & \cos(18*2\omega) \\ 1 & \sin(20\omega) & \cos(20\omega) & \sin(20*2\omega) & \cos(20*2\omega) \\ 1 & \sin(22\omega) & \cos(22\omega) & \sin(22*2\omega) & \cos(22*2\omega) \\ 1 & \sin(24\omega) & \cos(24\omega) & \sin(24*2\omega) & \cos(24*2\omega) \end{pmatrix},$$

$$\boldsymbol{C} = \left(\mathbf{1}'_{28} \otimes \begin{pmatrix} 1 \\ 0 \end{pmatrix} : \mathbf{1}'_{32} \otimes \begin{pmatrix} 0 \\ 1 \end{pmatrix}\right),$$

i.e. there are two groups (28 patients and 32 healthy controls, which are supposed to follow the mean structure indicated in Fig. 1.1). □

Example 1.7 This is an additional example illustrating the application of the BRM, utilizing the classical dental data set of Potthoff and Roy (1964). The data consist of growth measurements, i.e. the distance in mm from the centre of the pituitary to the pterygomaxillary fissure, for 11 girls and 16 boys at ages $t_1 = 8$, $t_2 = 10$, $t_3 = 12$ and $t_4 = 14$. The design matrices equal

$$A_1 = \begin{pmatrix} 1 & t_1 \\ 1 & t_2 \\ 1 & t_3 \\ 1 & t_4 \end{pmatrix}, \quad \text{Linear growth;} \quad A_2 = \begin{pmatrix} 1 & t_1 & t_1^2 \\ 1 & t_2 & t_2^2 \\ 1 & t_3 & t_3^2 \\ 1 & t_4 & t_4^2 \end{pmatrix}, \quad \text{Quadratic growth;}$$

$$\boldsymbol{C} = \left(\mathbf{1}_{11}' \otimes \begin{pmatrix} 1 \\ 0 \end{pmatrix} : \mathbf{1}_{16}' \otimes \begin{pmatrix} 0 \\ 1 \end{pmatrix}\right).$$

Then, the model is given by either $\boldsymbol{X} \sim N_{4,27}(\boldsymbol{A}_1\boldsymbol{B}\boldsymbol{C}, \boldsymbol{\Sigma}, \boldsymbol{I})$ or $\boldsymbol{X} \sim N_{4,27}(\boldsymbol{A}_2\boldsymbol{B}\boldsymbol{C}, \boldsymbol{\Sigma}, \boldsymbol{I})$. The data are presented in Table 1.2 and illustrated in Fig. 1.2. One can observe that there is a difference between the boys and girls, and in subsequent sections we are going to investigate if there is a statistical model which can be used in the analyses, including a validation of the model, and where the difference between the genders can be tested. □

Table 1.2 Four repeated growth measurements were taken at ages $t_1 = 8$, $t_2 = 10$, $t_3 = 12$ and $t_4 = 14$ from 11 girls and 16 boys (by permission of Potthoff and Roy (1964) © Oxford University Press 1964)

Id	Gender	t_1	t_2	t_3	t_4	Id	Gender	t_1	t_2	t_3	t_4
1	F	21.0	20.0	21.5	23.0	12	M	26.0	25.0	29.0	31.0
2	F	21.0	21.5	24.0	25.5	13	M	21.5	22.5	23.0	26.5
3	F	20.5	24.0	24.5	26.0	14	M	23.0	22.5	24.0	27.5
4	F	23.5	24.5	25.0	26.5	15	M	25.5	27.5	26.5	27.0
5	F	21.5	23.0	22.5	23.5	16	M	20.0	23.5	22.5	26.0
6	F	20.0	21.0	21.0	22.5	17	M	24.5	25.5	27.0	28.5
7	F	21.5	22.5	23.0	25.0	18	M	22.0	22.0	24.5	26.5
8	F	23.0	23.0	23.5	24.0	19	M	24.0	21.5	24.5	25.5
9	F	20.0	21.0	22.0	21.5	20	M	23.0	20.5	31.0	26.0
10	F	16.5	19.0	19.0	19.5	21	M	27.5	28.0	31.0	31.5
11	F	24.5	25.0	28.0	28.0	22	M	23.0	23.0	23.5	25.0
						23	M	21.5	23.5	24.0	28.0
						24	M	17.0	24.5	26.0	29.5
						25	M	22.5	25.5	25.5	26.0
						26	M	23.0	24.5	26.0	30.0
						27	M	22.0	21.5	23.5	25.0

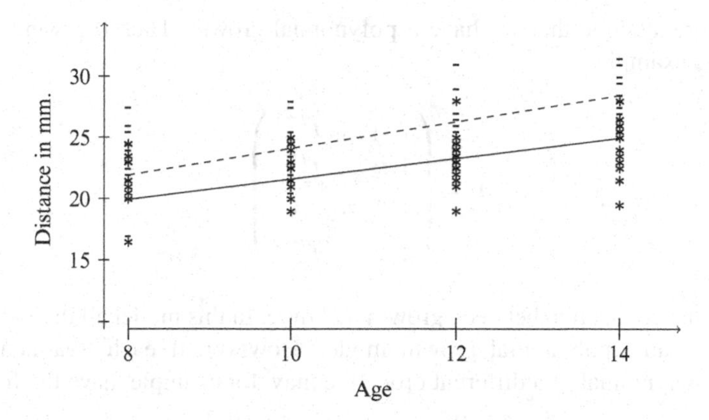

Fig. 1.2 The distance in mm from the centre of the pituitary to the pterygomaxillary fissure in girls (solid line) and boys (dashed line) at ages 8, 10, 12 and 14

Example 1.8 Now an example illustrating the applications of the $EBRM_B^3$ is presented. Let us start from the very beginning and suppose that we have a random vector $\boldsymbol{x}$ associated with observations which follow the model

$$\boldsymbol{x} = \boldsymbol{\mu} + \boldsymbol{e},$$

where $\boldsymbol{e} \sim N_p(\boldsymbol{0}, \boldsymbol{\Sigma})$. Assume that there exists a linear relation between the components in $\boldsymbol{\mu}$, i.e. $\boldsymbol{\mu} \in \mathcal{C}(\boldsymbol{A})$. Thus, $\boldsymbol{\mu} = \boldsymbol{A\beta}$ for some $\boldsymbol{\beta}$ (see Appendix B, Theorem B.3 (i)) and $\boldsymbol{x} = \boldsymbol{A\beta} + \boldsymbol{e}$. Moreover, suppose that we have n independent observations which all have the same within-individuals model $\boldsymbol{\mu} \in \mathcal{C}(\boldsymbol{A})$, and suppose that there additionally exists a linear model between the independent observations. For example, there are three groups of individuals one corresponding to a group receiving a placebo treatment and the others corresponding to groups receiving two different treatments. Thus we end up with the following model:

$$\boldsymbol{X} = \boldsymbol{ABC} + \boldsymbol{E},$$

where $\boldsymbol{X} = (\boldsymbol{x}_1, \boldsymbol{x}_2, \ldots, \boldsymbol{x}_n)$, $\boldsymbol{B} = (\boldsymbol{\beta}_1, \boldsymbol{\beta}_2, \boldsymbol{\beta}_3)$, $\boldsymbol{E} \sim N_{p,n}(\boldsymbol{0}, \boldsymbol{\Sigma}, \boldsymbol{I})$ and

$$\boldsymbol{C} = \begin{pmatrix} 1\,1 \ldots 1\,0\,0 \ldots 0\,0\,0 \ldots 0 \\ 0\,0 \ldots 0\,1\,1 \ldots 1\,0\,0 \ldots 0 \\ 0\,0 \ldots 0\,0\,0 \ldots 0\,1\,1 \ldots 1 \end{pmatrix}.$$

Furthermore, assume that we have a polynomial growth. Then the Vandermonde matrix, for example,

$$A = \begin{pmatrix} 1 & t_1 & \dots & t_1^{q-1} \\ 1 & t_2 & \dots & t_2^{q-1} \\ \vdots & \vdots & \ddots & \vdots \\ 1 & t_p & \dots & t_p^{q-1} \end{pmatrix}$$

describes the connection between growth and time. In this model all the individuals follow the same polynomial growth model. However, if each treatment group follows a polynomial of a different order, we may, for example, have the following model:

$$\boldsymbol{X} = \boldsymbol{A}_1\boldsymbol{B}_1\boldsymbol{C}_1 + \boldsymbol{A}_2\boldsymbol{B}_2\boldsymbol{C}_2 + \boldsymbol{A}_3\boldsymbol{B}_3\boldsymbol{C}_3 + \boldsymbol{E},$$

where

$$\boldsymbol{C}_1 = \begin{pmatrix} 1\,1\dots1\,0\,0\dots0\,0\,0\dots0 \\ 0\,0\dots0\,1\,1\dots1\,0\,0\dots0 \\ 0\,0\dots0\,0\,0\dots0\,1\,1\dots1 \end{pmatrix},$$

$$\boldsymbol{C}_2 = \begin{pmatrix} 1\,1\dots1\,0\,0\dots0\,0\,0\dots0 \\ 0\,0\dots0\,1\,1\dots1\,0\,0\dots0 \end{pmatrix},$$

$$\boldsymbol{C}_3 = \begin{pmatrix} 1\,1\dots1\,0\,0\dots0\,0\,0\dots0 \end{pmatrix},$$

$$\boldsymbol{A}_1 = \begin{pmatrix} 1 & t_1 & \dots & t_1^{q-3} \\ 1 & t_2 & \dots & t_2^{q-3} \\ \vdots & \vdots & \ddots & \vdots \\ 1 & t_p & \dots & t_p^{q-3} \end{pmatrix}, \qquad \boldsymbol{B}_1 = (\boldsymbol{\beta}_1, \boldsymbol{\beta}_2, \boldsymbol{\beta}_3),$$

$$\boldsymbol{A}_2' = \begin{pmatrix} t_1^{q-2} & t_2^{q-2} & \dots & t_p^{q-2} \end{pmatrix}, \qquad \boldsymbol{B}_2 = (\beta_3, \beta_4),$$

$$\boldsymbol{A}_3' = \begin{pmatrix} t_1^{q-1} & t_2^{q-1} & \dots & t_p^{q-1} \end{pmatrix}, \qquad \boldsymbol{B}_3 = \beta_5.$$

Note that $\mathcal{C}(\boldsymbol{C}_3') \subseteq \mathcal{C}(\boldsymbol{C}_2') \subseteq \mathcal{C}(\boldsymbol{C}_1')$. The above example implies, for instance, that the mean of the placebo group and that of the treatment groups, respectively, equal

$$\begin{aligned}
&\beta_{11} + \beta_{12}t + \cdots + \beta_{1(q-2)}t^{q-3},\\
&\beta_{21} + \beta_{22}t + \cdots + \beta_{2(q-2)}t^{q-3} + \beta_{2(q-1)}t^{q-2},\\
&\beta_{31} + \beta_{32}t + \cdots + \beta_{3(q-2)}t^{q-3} + \beta_{3(q-1)}t^{q-2} + \beta_{3q}t^{q-1}.
\end{aligned}$$

□

Example 1.9 In order to illustrate certain ideas, the "real" example presented as Example 1.6 is now extended to form Example 1.9. An additional purpose of this is to present the ingredients for performing simulation studies which, several times, will take place later in this book. Suppose that there are three treatment groups comprising 10, 15 and 20 patients. The groups are assumed to follow different models over the day-and-night cycle, according to a nested subspace assumption:

$$\begin{aligned}
\boldsymbol{X} &= \boldsymbol{A}_1\boldsymbol{B}_1\boldsymbol{C}_1 + \boldsymbol{A}_2\boldsymbol{B}_2\boldsymbol{C}_2 + \boldsymbol{A}_3\boldsymbol{B}_3\boldsymbol{C}_3 + \boldsymbol{E},\\
\boldsymbol{E} &\sim N_{p,n}(\boldsymbol{0}, \boldsymbol{\Sigma}, \boldsymbol{I}), \quad \mathcal{C}(\boldsymbol{C}_3') \subseteq \mathcal{C}(\boldsymbol{C}_2') \subseteq \mathcal{C}(\boldsymbol{C}_1'),
\end{aligned}$$

where ($\omega = \pi/24$),

$$\boldsymbol{A}_1 = \begin{pmatrix} 1 & \sin(\omega) & \cos(\omega)\\ 1 & \sin(4\omega) & \cos(4\omega)\\ 1 & \sin(8\omega) & \cos(8\omega)\\ 1 & \sin(12\omega) & \cos(12\omega)\\ 1 & \sin(14\omega) & \cos(14\omega)\\ 1 & \sin(16\omega) & \cos(16\omega)\\ 1 & \sin(18\omega) & \cos(18\omega)\\ 1 & \sin(20\omega) & \cos(20\omega)\\ 1 & \sin(22\omega) & \cos(22\omega)\\ 1 & \sin(24\omega) & \cos(24\omega) \end{pmatrix}, \quad \boldsymbol{A}_2 = \begin{pmatrix} \sin(2\omega)\\ \sin(4*2\omega)\\ \sin(8*2\omega)\\ \sin(12*2\omega)\\ \sin(14*2\omega)\\ \sin(16*2\omega)\\ \sin(18*2\omega)\\ \sin(20*2\omega)\\ \sin(22*2\omega)\\ \sin(24*2\omega) \end{pmatrix}, \quad \boldsymbol{A}_3 = \begin{pmatrix} \cos(2\omega)\\ \cos(4*2\omega)\\ \cos(8*2\omega)\\ \cos(12*2\omega)\\ \cos(14*2\omega)\\ \cos(16*2\omega)\\ \cos(18*2\omega)\\ \cos(20*2\omega)\\ \cos(22*2\omega)\\ \cos(24*2\omega) \end{pmatrix},$$

$$\boldsymbol{C}_1 = (\boldsymbol{1}_{10}' \otimes \begin{pmatrix}1\\0\\0\end{pmatrix} : \boldsymbol{1}_{15}' \otimes \begin{pmatrix}0\\1\\0\end{pmatrix} : \boldsymbol{1}_{20}' \otimes \begin{pmatrix}0\\0\\1\end{pmatrix}),$$

$$\boldsymbol{C}_2 = (\boldsymbol{1}_{10}' \otimes \begin{pmatrix}1\\0\end{pmatrix} : \boldsymbol{1}_{15}' \otimes \begin{pmatrix}0\\1\end{pmatrix} : \boldsymbol{1}_{20}' \otimes \begin{pmatrix}0\\0\end{pmatrix}), \quad \boldsymbol{C}_3 = (\boldsymbol{1}_{10}' : \boldsymbol{1}_{35}' \otimes 0).$$

Here $\mathcal{C}(\boldsymbol{C}_3') \subseteq \mathcal{C}(\boldsymbol{C}_2') \subseteq \mathcal{C}(\boldsymbol{C}_1')$ is satisfied and in order to generate data, the remaining task is to specify the parameters:

$$\boldsymbol{B}_1 = \begin{pmatrix} 0.01 & 0.14 & 0.20 \\ 0.21 & -0.01 & -0.004 \\ 0.02 & 0.03 & -0.01 \end{pmatrix}, \quad \boldsymbol{B}_2 = \begin{pmatrix} -0.04 & -0.06 \end{pmatrix}, \quad \boldsymbol{B}_3 = (0.10),$$

$$10^2\boldsymbol{\Sigma} = \begin{pmatrix} 0.25 & -0.10 & 0.10 & -0.10 & 0.10 & 0.20 & 0.05 & 0.00 & -0.05 & 0.05 \\ -0.10 & 0.29 & -0.14 & 0.09 & -0.04 & -0.13 & -0.07 & 0.05 & 0.07 & -0.02 \\ 0.10 & -0.14 & 0.33 & -0.01 & 0.04 & 0.15 & -0.01 & 0.03 & 0.11 & 0.12 \\ -0.10 & 0.09 & -0.01 & 0.31 & 0.01 & -0.13 & -0.09 & -0.03 & 0.11 & 0.05 \\ 0.10 & -0.04 & 0.04 & 0.01 & 0.21 & 0.03 & 0.01 & 0.03 & -0.05 & 0.03 \\ 0.20 & -0.13 & 0.15 & -0.13 & 0.03 & 0.45 & 0.10 & 0.05 & 0.03 & 0.05 \\ 0.05 & -0.07 & -0.01 & -0.09 & 0.01 & 0.10 & 0.30 & 0.00 & -0.15 & 0.13 \\ 0.00 & 0.05 & 0.03 & -0.03 & 0.03 & 0.05 & 0.00 & 0.21 & 0.07 & -0.11 \\ -0.05 & 0.07 & 0.11 & 0.11 & -0.05 & 0.03 & -0.15 & 0.07 & 0.28 & -0.06 \\ 0.05 & -0.02 & 0.12 & 0.05 & 0.03 & 0.05 & 0.13 & -0.11 & -0.06 & 0.34 \end{pmatrix}.$$

The choice of parameters is directed by the values presented in Fig. 1.3. In this figure two groups of individuals follow a day-and-night cycle, whereas in the present example a third group of individuals has been added which does not show any nocturnal peak level (see Fig. 1.3). Later, in Sect. 6.6, the data will be contaminated and the effect of this contamination on various residuals will be studied. □

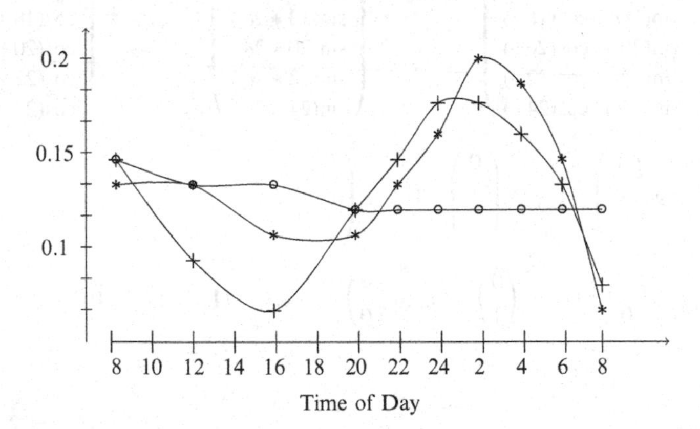

Fig. 1.3 Based on the serum melatonin data presented in Example 1.6 a new data set with three groups of individuals has been generated. Group 1, Group 2 and Group 3 are indicated by asterisk symbol, plus symbol and open circle, respectively, and follow the model in Example 1.9

Example 1.10 The model in Example 1.8 is now reconsidered. This example indicates how the $EBRM_B^3$ and $EBRM_W^3$ are related. However, in general the relation between the $EBRM_B^3$ and $EBRM_W^3$ is not so clear. The following model is equivalent to the model in Example 1.8:

$$\boldsymbol{X} = \boldsymbol{A}_1\boldsymbol{\Theta}_1\boldsymbol{C}_1 + \boldsymbol{A}_2\boldsymbol{\Theta}_2\boldsymbol{C}_2 + \boldsymbol{A}_3\boldsymbol{\Theta}_3\boldsymbol{C}_3 + \boldsymbol{E},$$

where

$$\boldsymbol{C}_1 = \big(1\,1\ldots1\,0\,0\ldots0\,0\,0\ldots0\big),$$
$$\boldsymbol{C}_2 = \big(0\,0\ldots0\,1\,1\ldots1\,0\,0\ldots0\big),$$
$$\boldsymbol{C}_3 = \big(0\,0\ldots0\,0\,0\ldots0\,1\,1\ldots1\big),$$

$$\boldsymbol{A}_1 = \begin{pmatrix} 1 & t_1 & \ldots & t_1^{q-1} \\ 1 & t_2 & \ldots & t_2^{q-1} \\ \vdots & \vdots & \ddots & \vdots \\ 1 & t_p & \ldots & t_p^{q-1} \end{pmatrix}, \qquad \boldsymbol{\Theta}_1 = (\boldsymbol{\beta}_1', \beta_3, \beta_5)',$$

$$\boldsymbol{A}_2 = \begin{pmatrix} 1 & t_1 & \ldots & t_1^{q-2} \\ 1 & t_2 & \ldots & t_2^{q-2} \\ \vdots & \vdots & \ddots & \vdots \\ 1 & t_p & \ldots & t_p^{q-2} \end{pmatrix}, \qquad \boldsymbol{\Theta}_2 = (\boldsymbol{\beta}_2', \beta_4)',$$

$$\boldsymbol{A}_3 = \begin{pmatrix} 1 & t_1 & \ldots & t_1^{q-3} \\ 1 & t_2 & \ldots & t_2^{q-3} \\ \vdots & \vdots & \ddots & \vdots \\ 1 & t_p & \ldots & t_p^{q-3} \end{pmatrix}, \qquad \boldsymbol{\Theta}_3 = \boldsymbol{\beta}_3.$$

The interesting point is that now $\mathcal{C}(\boldsymbol{A}_3) \subseteq \mathcal{C}(\boldsymbol{A}_2) \subseteq \mathcal{C}(\boldsymbol{A}_1)$ holds instead of $\mathcal{C}(\boldsymbol{C}_3') \subseteq \mathcal{C}(\boldsymbol{C}_2') \subseteq \mathcal{C}(\boldsymbol{C}_1')$. Moreover, when considering the $EBRM_B^3$, $\{\boldsymbol{B}_i\}$, $i = 1, 2, 3$, are the objects of interest, whereas in the $EBRM_W^3$ the parameters $\{\boldsymbol{\Theta}_i\}$, $i = 1, 2, 3$, are of interest. For example, if the estimability conditions are considered, the estimability of $\boldsymbol{B}_1$ does not necessarily imply the estimability of $\boldsymbol{\Theta}_1$. Of course, if $\{\boldsymbol{B}_i\}$ is estimable, then so too are $\{\boldsymbol{\Theta}_i\}$, $i = 1, 2, 3$, but usually we are not interested in estimating all the parameters in $\{\boldsymbol{B}_i\}$, $i = 1, 2, 3$, uniquely and then it is not so easy to find out the estimability conditions for $\boldsymbol{\Theta}_i$. Moreover, deriving $D[\widehat{\boldsymbol{\Theta}}_i]$ from $D[\widehat{\boldsymbol{B}}_i]$ without knowledge about the covariance $C[\widehat{\boldsymbol{B}}_i, \widehat{\boldsymbol{B}}_j]$, $i \neq j$, is impossible (see Appendix A, Sect. A.10 for definitions of these moments). □

The next example involves a relatively complicated between-individuals design, together with an easily interpretable within-individuals structure.

Example 1.11 $EBRM_W^3$: This example presents a so-called interference model, see Filipiak and von Rosen (2012) and Filipiak and Markiewicz (2017), among other presentations. Consider an agricultural experiment and suppose that one wants to compare t different varieties of spring barley, for example. There is likely to be an interaction between the environment (the type of soil, rainfall, drainage, etc.) and the variety of grain which will affect the yield. Therefore, b blocks are chosen where the environment is fairly consistent throughout the blocks.

Let n experimental units (plots) be divided into the b blocks each of size k. Let the t treatments be applied to the units so that each unit receives one treatment. The treatment which is applied to unit j in block i is determined by the design d. Within the blocks the effect of the treatments applied to each unit can be quantified via a random variable $\boldsymbol{x}$.

Assume that the response of a given plot may be affected by treatments of neighbouring plots, as well as by the treatment applied to that plot. Moreover, consider experiments with a one-dimensional arrangement of plots in each block, and in which the treatments have different left and right neighbour interference effects.

The linear model associated with the design d can be written as follows:

$$\boldsymbol{x}' = \boldsymbol{\beta}_1 \boldsymbol{C}_{1,d} + \boldsymbol{\beta}_2 \boldsymbol{C}_{2,d} + \boldsymbol{\beta}_3 \boldsymbol{C}_3 + \boldsymbol{e}', \tag{1.12}$$

where $\boldsymbol{\beta}_i$, $i = 1, 2, 3$, are the unknown vectors of treatment effects, neighbour effects and block effects, respectively, and $\boldsymbol{e}$ is the vector of random errors. The matrix $\boldsymbol{C}_{1,d} \in \mathbb{R}^{v \times n}$ depends on the design and it is a matrix with binary entries which satisfies $\boldsymbol{C}'_{1,d}\mathbf{1_v} = \mathbf{1_n}$. The matrix $\boldsymbol{C}'_{2,d} = ((\boldsymbol{I}_b \otimes \boldsymbol{H})\boldsymbol{C}'_{1,d} : (\boldsymbol{I}_b \otimes \boldsymbol{H}')\boldsymbol{C}'_{1,d})$ is a known matrix of neighbour effects, where

$$\boldsymbol{H}' = \begin{pmatrix} \mathbf{0}'_{k-1} & 1 \\ \mathbf{I}_{k-1} & \mathbf{0}_{k-1} \end{pmatrix} \quad \text{or} \quad \mathbf{H}' = \begin{pmatrix} \mathbf{0}'_{k-1} & 0 \\ \mathbf{I}_{k-1} & \mathbf{0}_{k-1} \end{pmatrix}$$

for a circular design (Druilhet, 1999) and for a design without border plots (Kunert and Martin, 2000), respectively ($\mathbf{0}_{k-1}$ is a $k-1$ dimensional vector of zeros). The matrix $\boldsymbol{C}_3 = \boldsymbol{I}_b \otimes \mathbf{1}'_k$ is the design matrix of block effects. In the literature such a model as the one presented above is called an interference model with neighbour effects.

Suppose that for each treatment, we are measuring a response which consists of p characteristics. Then the following extension of the interference model (1.12) appears:

$$X = A_1B_1C_{1,d} + A_2B_2C_{2,d} + A_3B_3C_3 + E,$$

where $X \in \mathbb{R}^{p\times n}$ is the matrix of observations, B_i, $i = 1, 2, 3$, are the unknown matrices of treatment, neighbour and block effects, respectively, and A_i, $i = 1, 2, 3$, are within-individuals design matrices, which now will be specified. It is assumed that in the experiment there is no left- and right-neighbour effect and no block effect for the last characteristic, and for the second last characteristic there is no block effect. Then $A_1 = I_p$, $A_2 = (I_{p-1}, 0_{p-1})'$ and $A_3 = (I_{p-2}, 0_{p-2}, 0_{p-2})'$, which obviously satisfy $\mathcal{C}(A_3) \subseteq \mathcal{C}(A_2) \subseteq \mathcal{C}(A_1)$. Finally it is noted that $E \sim N_{p,n}(0, \Sigma, I)$, where $\Sigma > 0$ is an unstructured dispersion matrix. □

Problems

1 Generate data according to $X \sim N_{5,20}(ABC, \Sigma, I_{20})$, where

$$A = \begin{pmatrix} 1 & 2 & 4 \\ 1 & 3 & 9 \\ 1 & 4 & 16 \\ 1 & 5 & 25 \\ 1 & 6 & 36 \end{pmatrix}, \quad \Sigma = \begin{pmatrix} 3.0 & 1.0 & 0.5 & 0.5 & 1.0 \\ 1.0 & 4.0 & 1.5 & 1.5 & 1.0 \\ 0.5 & 1.5 & 2.0 & 1.0 & 0.5 \\ 0.5 & 1.5 & 1.0 & 2.0 & 0.5 \\ 1.0 & 1.0 & 0.5 & 0.5 & 2.0 \end{pmatrix}, \quad B = \begin{pmatrix} 1 & 0.5 \\ 3 & 4 \end{pmatrix}$$

$$C = \begin{pmatrix} 1 & 1 & 1 & 1 & 1 & 1 & 1 & 1 & 1 & 1 & 0 & 0 & 0 & 0 & 0 & 0 & 0 & 0 & 0 & 0 \\ 0 & 0 & 0 & 0 & 0 & 0 & 0 & 0 & 0 & 0 & 1 & 1 & 1 & 1 & 1 & 1 & 1 & 1 & 1 & 1 \end{pmatrix}.$$

Present informative plot(s) of the data.

2 Let $x_i \sim N_5(\mu, \Sigma)$, $i = 1, \ldots, n$, be independently distributed, where

$$\mu = \begin{pmatrix} 1 \\ 2 \\ 4 \\ 5 \\ 3 \end{pmatrix}, \quad \Sigma = \begin{pmatrix} 4.0 & 2.0 & 1.5 & 2.5 & 1.0 \\ 2.0 & 5.0 & 0.5 & 2.5 & 2.0 \\ 1.5 & 0.5 & 2.0 & 1.0 & 0.5 \\ 2.5 & 2.5 & 2.0 & 2.0 & 1.5 \\ 1.0 & 2.0 & 0.5 & 1.5 & 3.0 \end{pmatrix}.$$

Put

$$\widehat{\mu} = \frac{1}{n}\sum_{l=n}^{n} x_i.$$

(i) Formulate the weak law of large numbers, i.e. $\widehat{\mu}$ converges in probability to μ, and indicate through simulations that the error is of order n^{-1}. (ii) Formulate the multivariate central limit theorem, i.e. $\widehat{\mu}$ converges in distribution to the multivariate normal distribution, and indicate through simulations that the error is of order $n^{-1/2}$.

3 (i) Formulate a three-way ANOVA model with two-way interactions. (ii) Formulate a multiple regression model with three independent variables and an intercept. (iii) Present the proposed models in (i) and (ii) using matrix notation. (iv) Formulate, using matrix notation, an analysis of covariance model.

4 Let

$$A = \begin{pmatrix} 1 & 8 \\ 1 & 12 \\ 1 & 14 \\ 1 & 16 \end{pmatrix}.$$

Find an orthogonal matrix $\boldsymbol{\Gamma}$ and a non-singular matrix $\boldsymbol{H}$ such that $\boldsymbol{A}' = \boldsymbol{H}(\boldsymbol{I}_2 : \boldsymbol{0})\boldsymbol{\Gamma}$. (*Hint: Utilize some linear algebra book.*)

5 Let $\boldsymbol{P}_{A,V} = \boldsymbol{A}(\boldsymbol{A}'\boldsymbol{V}^{-1}\boldsymbol{A})^{-}\boldsymbol{A}'\boldsymbol{V}^{-1}$, where $\boldsymbol{V}$ is positive definite. Show (i) $\mathrm{tr}\{\boldsymbol{P}_{A,V}\} = r(\boldsymbol{A})$; (ii) $\boldsymbol{P}_{A,V}\boldsymbol{P}_{A,V} = \boldsymbol{P}_{A,V}$; (iii) $\mathcal{C}(\boldsymbol{P}_{A,V}) = \mathcal{C}(\boldsymbol{A})$; and (iv) $\mathcal{N}(\boldsymbol{I} - \boldsymbol{P}_{A,V}) = \mathcal{C}(\boldsymbol{A})$. (For an explanation of the notation, see Appendix A, Sect. A.7 and Appendix A, Sect. A.8.)

6 Let $\boldsymbol{A}$ be non-singular. Show that the inverse matrix $\boldsymbol{A}^{-1}$ is unique.

7 Show that if a matrix $\boldsymbol{\Gamma}$ of size $p \times p$ satisfies $\boldsymbol{\Gamma}\boldsymbol{\Gamma}' = \boldsymbol{I}_p$, then $\boldsymbol{\Gamma}'\boldsymbol{\Gamma} = \boldsymbol{I}_p$.

8 Show that the commutation matrix (for a definition of the matrix see Appendix A, Sect. A.5) is an orthogonal matrix.

9 Show that the square matrices $\boldsymbol{A}$ and $\boldsymbol{A}'$ have the same eigenvalues.

10 Show that if all the eigenvalues of the square matrix $\boldsymbol{A}$ are real and k of them are non-zero, then $(\mathrm{tr}\{\boldsymbol{A}\})^2 \leq k\,\mathrm{tr}\{\boldsymbol{A}^2\}$.

Literature

The following literature review reflects the historical development of some part of statistical science and includes background information on linear and bilinear models. No details are provided, meaning, for example, that the techniques and tools used by the various authors are omitted. Instead it is recommended that one should study the original articles. Moreover, it should be noted that it is impossible, in few pages, to present a complete survey of literature published on the topics under consideration.

Nowadays statistical science is mainly based on probability theory. One has merged stochastics with statistics but this has not always been the case. Today statisticians use probabilities to describe uncertainty, and probability and probability distributions are used for the following purposes: (i) to build models, (ii) to create random experiments (sampling), and (iii) to support conclusions. One challenge has been to handle "continuous" data, and this is a problem which statisticians are still faced with today. Fundamental theory was established at the beginning of the twentieth century, including Kolmogorov's (1933) famous axiomatic probability proposal. The philosophy behind Kolmogorov's work and alternative proposals, as well as an interesting and beneficial historical perspective, has been presented by Schafer and Vovk (2006). It is interesting to look into early works on probability theory, for example, von Bortkiewicz (1917), where also references to earlier works can be found.

An embryo of multivariate statistics was introduced by Galton (1886, 1888, 1889), who, among other things, exploited bivariate problems (see Anderson, 1996). The normal distribution has always played a fundamental role when it comes to analysing continuous data. Two very well-known results/notion, which are connected to the normal distribution and which appeared more than a hundred years ago, are the t-test (Student, 1908) and Pearson's product correlation coefficient (Pearson, 1896). Concerning correlation, it was, however, Galton (1886, 1888) who came up with the fundamental ideas, including the concept of conditional expectation; see Bulmer (2003) and Stigler (2012), for interesting reading about Galton. Pearson, besides referring to Galton, also refers to Bravais (1846), who used the correlation coefficient (see Monhor, 2012). Cowles (2001) points out that Galton's half-cousin Charles Darwin used the term correlated variation in his renowned book "The Origin of Species".

Many references concerning the bivariate normal distribution can be found in Kotz et al. (2000). Edgeworth (1892) presented a three-dimensional normal distribution which was generalized by Pearson (1896) to a p-dimensional version. Fisher (1915) derived the distribution of the sample Pearson correlation coefficient. Hence, we can conclude that around 1900 it became possible to analyse continuous multi-response data in a systematic way. To understand how important and impressive the development of statistics was during the above-mentioned years, we refer to historically oriented books and articles, for example see Stigler (1986, 2012) and Cowles (2001).

Fisher's result concerning the correlation coefficient was generalized by Wishart (1928), who derived the distribution of a quadratic form of a p-variate normally distributed variable, i.e. the joint distribution of sample variances and sample covariances. Wishart's result has been very fundamental to multivariate statistics; see Aitken (1949) for additional references.

Matrices were not used in statistics during the period stretching from 1880s to 1920s. However, determinants were frequently applied, and for example, the inverse dispersion matrix in the multivariate normal density was expressed with the help of the determinant and minors. Today multivariate analysis is mostly presented via matrices, but sometimes more abstract/geometric presentations are available;

see, for example, Drygas (1970), Stone (1977, 1987), Herr (1980), Eaton (1983) and Wichura (2006). Matrices can play different roles, and can, for example, be used as a collection of elements or as representations of linear transformations. It is advantageous to use both interpretations simultaneously, but this will not be promoted in the present book. It should be noted that the concept of matrices has existed for more than 150 years, but matrices and statistics established contact with each other much later in the history of statistics. Searle (2000, 2005) (see also David, 2006) states that it was around 1930 that matrices started to be used. Early work using matrices was performed by Bartlett (1934b), Cochran (1934) and Aitken (1935). Algebra has also entered multivariate analysis, which was highlighted by Perlman (1987), for example. Now the use of algebra can be found in many branches of multivariate analysis and one area is the derivation of moments and cumulants (e.g. see Letac and Massam, 2008; Withers and Nadarajah, 2012).

In the following, a very brief overview is presented of the literature dealing with the "chain": linear models—multivariate linear models—bilinear models—extended bilinear models. Least squares (different versions) and their applications (data analysis) have a very long history in which many famous scientists have been involved, such as Laplace, Legendre and Gauss (e.g. see Seal, 1967; Stigler, 1986; Aldrich, 1999; Farebrother, 1999). The development of least squares theory has been driven forward through applications. However, according to Seal (1967), based on sums of squares the underlying linear models which were used were analysed intuitively. It was Yates (1933) who first connected linear models to least squares (see also Irwin, 1934; Aitken, 1936; Kolodziejczyk, 1935). However, it has been clearly demonstrated by Hald (1981, 2002) that within the actuarial sciences, the Danish statisticians Gram (1879) and Thiele (1889) worked with linear models and least squares. There are also other interesting works written by these authors (see Hald, 1981). Although regression analysis and analysis of variance models have been applied for more than 100 years, it was not until the 1950s that these subject areas were put under the same umbrella, for example, in a paper by Tocher (1952) and in the impressive book by Kempthorne (1952).

As noted above, Galton, Thiele, Edgeworth, Pearson, Fisher and indeed several others, at the beginning of the twentieth century, dealt with the concept of multi-response. Thereafter followed an impressive period, 1930–1940, when multivariate analysis was really blossoming with many new published ideas, covering topics such as generalized distance: (Mahalanobis (1930, 1936) who was heavily influenced by Pearson's work, see Nayak (2009)); generalized variance (Wilks, 1932), including the test statistic Wilks' Λ (a term introduced by Rao (1948), in an excellent survey of multivariate testing); principal components analysis (Pearson, 1901; Hotelling, 1933); canonical correlation analysis (Hotelling, 1936); discriminant analysis (Bose, 1936; Fisher, 1936, 1938) (according to Kendall (1957), Karl Pearson around 1920 introduced the idea of discriminating between multivariate populations); precise derivations of distributions of various statistics (Wishart, 1928; Hotelling, 1931; Bartlett, 1934a; Cochran, 1934; Bose, 1936; Bose and Roy, 1938) (in these works references are often made to earlier works of Fisher); distribution of eigenvalues of, for example, certain functions of Wishart matrices (Fisher, 1939;

Girshick, 1939; Hsu, 1939; Roy, 1939) (see also Anderson (2007), about the connections between these publications); multivariate testing (Wilks, 1932; Bartlett, 1934b, 1939). A general probabilistically oriented review of multivariate analysis in its early years was presented by Madow (1938). There are several other interesting articles which were published during this period and many of the above references cross-refer to each other (see e.g. Bartlett, 1974; Anderson, 1996, for some details). One should also note that many of the above-mentioned fundamental ideas were backed up by geometrical arguments; i.e. intuition and mathematics went hand in hand.

During the next decade (the 1940s) structured dispersion matrices started to be studied. Among others, Wilks (1946) (with his study of the intraclass structure, also termed the uniform structure) and Votaw (1948) (with his study of compound symmetry, block symmetry) contributed to the development of the treatment of patterned dispersion matrices. Nowadays many dispersion structures are treated, although there is no general reference available. Time series structures, spatial-temporal structures, structures fulfilling some invariance conditions, variance components structures and several other structures are treated by various authors. However, if one is interested in obtaining explicit estimators, structures satisfying a Jordan algebra condition (a quadratic subspace condition, Seely, 1971) are the natural structures to consider (e.g. see Jensen, 1988).

It took rather a long time before the first books on multivariate analysis appeared, i.e. the seminal works of Roy (1957), Kendall (1957) and Anderson (1958). It is interesting to note that Anderson's book has been published in a third edition, Anderson (2003), and is still in use. With the development of computational facilities, the subject has also changed. Schervish (1987) made a number of interesting reflections about multivariate analysis when comparing the second edition of the book by Anderson (1958), i.e. Anderson (1984), with a book by Dillon and Goldstein (1984). Schervish's article, together with the discussion by Anderson, Gnanadesikan and Kettenring, Goldstein, Perlman, Press and Sen, makes very interesting reading. Now, more than 25 years since the discussion took place, we can study how multivariate analysis has developed since then. Several new methods have appeared, new classes of distributions (e.g. elliptical distributions) are used and Bayesian analysts have acquired tools for obtaining posterior distributions. Right now multivariate analysis is slowly moving towards the analysis of large-dimensional observations (e.g. see Fujikoshi et al., 2013; Imori and von Rosen, 2015).

A number of books which treat classical multivariate analysis have been produced over the years, for example, Dempster (1969), Srivastava and Khatri (1979), Mardia et al. (1979), Muirhead (1982), Takeuchi et al. (1982), Eaton (1983), Srivastava and Carter (1983), Seber (1984), Siotani et al. (1985), Bilodeau and Brenner (1999), Morrison (2005) and Rencher and Christensen (2012). All these works include a large number of references to works within classical multivariate analysis. However, it should be emphasized that this list of interesting books in this field could be extended considerably. The above selection is just a personal choice indicating the broad spectrum of multivariate analysis. Fujikoshi et al. (2010)

considered many classical multivariate analysis approaches through expansions of distributions and, via the expansions, also considered high-dimensional problems. Furthermore, over the years a number of specialized books have been published, such as books on principal components analysis (Jolliffe, 2002), discriminant analysis (McLachlan, 1992), correspondence analysis (Greenacre, 1984), cluster analysis (Everitt et al., 2011), independent component analysis (Hyvärinen et al., 2001), (which is related to projection pursuit), confirmatory and explorative factor analysis, latent structural equations (Bartholomew et al., 2011) and graphical models (Whittaker, 1990; Lauritzen, 1996; Cox and Wermuth, 1996; Andersson and Perlman, 1998). Part of the theory around graphical models has many connections with the subject matter of this book, although the links are usually not mentioned. Moreover, distribution theory has been developed to fit the statistical problems connected to multivariate analysis.

Above, a selection of the relatively rich body of literature concerning multivariate analysis has been presented. A few of the references provided mention the BRM, either under the heading of the growth curve model or GMANOVA. The history of the analysis of growth curves through a repeated measurements analysis can be traced back to works such as those by Wishart (1938) and Box (1950), which are two well-known contributions. Both papers are of interest from a historical perspective, with Box, for example, taking care of the dependency within repeated measurements via split-plot analysis, as well as by assuming unstructured dispersion matrices. Rao (1958) is another early contribution and in the above-mentioned book by Roy (1957), bilinear hypothesis testing is presented; this topic is also dealt with in a work by Anderson (1951) and in an abstract by Olkin and Shrikhande (1954). The article by Potthoff and Roy (1964) is often considered to be the first paper where the growth curve model was treated, but a similar model had already been discussed by Rao (1958), as well as by other authors (e.g. see the reference list of Gleser and Olkin, 1970). Moreover, an article by Burnaby (1966) which is related to the article by Potthoff and Roy (1964) dealt with the discrimination of growth curves (see also Rao, 1966a) and included more precise mathematical results than Potthoff and Roy (1964). Soon after the article by Potthoff and Roy (1964), a number of important contributions appeared, in particular, Rao (1965, 1966b, 1967), Khatri (1966), Grizzle and Allen (1969) and Gleser and Olkin (1970) (the last of these aforementioned papers was written much earlier than its publication date). Reviews of the growth curve model have been written by Woolson and Leeper (1980), Seber (1984, Chapter 9.7), von Rosen (1991), Kanda (1994) and Srivastava and von Rosen (1999). The first book dedicated to the growth curve model was written by Kariya (1985), who focused on testing hypothesis. Kariya and Sinha (1989) discussed the model and provided many references, in particular it was noted that the model belongs to the curved exponential family. Kshirsagar and Smith (1995) wrote a book on the growth curve model which to some extent summarizes the earlier works on the model. Pan and Fang (2002) considered model validation of the BRM, in particular the recognition of influential observations. Timm (1997), in an interesting review, considered extensions of the BRM, in particular the $EBRM_{\bullet}^{m}$.

Extended growth curve models have been presented in papers by Gleser and Olkin (1970), Verbyla and Venables (1988), von Rosen (1989), Timm (1997), Fujikoshi et al. (1999) and others. In particular, Srivastava and Khatri (1979, Problem 6.9, p. 196) indicated one way to estimate the parameters. It is interesting to note that in order to estimate parameters in a MANOVA model under bilinear restrictions, an $EBRM_{\bullet}^{m}$ is useful. However, when testing bilinear hypotheses this can be performed without any knowledge of the $EBRM_{\bullet}^{m}$. Perhaps this is one reason why the $EBRM_{\bullet}^{m}$ has not been discussed so much. However, to test a hypothesis without estimating the appropriate parameters does not usually constitute a complete analysis. Moreover, in relation to the $EBRM_{\bullet}^{m}$, lattice models, considered by Andersson and Perlman (1993) and the approach of Andersson et al. (1993), among others, are very interesting.

The term bilinear has previously been used in the context of statistical model building by Gabriel (1998), for example, (see also Drton and Richardson, 2004; Hoff, 2015), although the term has been used more often in the chemometrics literature (e.g. see Linder and Sundberg, 2002). Moreover, a current topic of discussion is the so-called bilinear least squares approach (see Valderrama and Poppi, 2008).

Models partly overlapping the above-mentioned classes are mixed linear models and variance components models. The latter class of models usually assumes an unstructured mean and thus does not belong to the same class as the BRM and its extensions. The book by Rao and Kleffe (1988) is one of several interesting works dealing with the estimation of variance components. Concerning mixed linear models (i.e. linear models with fixed and random effects), this class has an extensive scope and comprises all the above-mentioned models. However, the treatment of mixed linear models, except in a few special cases, is completely based on asymptotics, and this approach is inconsistent with the philosophy of the book, where a great deal of energy is devoted to obtaining explicit finite sample results. One reference with a focus on mixed linear models and applications is Verbeke and Molenberghs (2000).

Finally, a few comments follow on the growth curve model, i.e. the BRM. Potthoff and Roy (1964) presented the model as a model for modelling growth curves, but this is slightly misleading. The model calls for balanced data, which means that each "individual", which is supposed to be the independent unit, has to be observed at the same points in time and the same number of times. However, usually growth curves consist of the so-called unbalanced data and a better approach for studying growth curves (estimating parameters, testing hypotheses, predicting new observations) than using the growth curve model is to consider random coefficient regression models (see Rao, 1965). Random coefficient regression models use the idea of analysing individual growth curves and this approach has natural generalizations, for example, for the analysis of non-linear growth. Moreover, there are interesting Bayesian approaches to the analysis of growth curves (e.g. see Fearn, 1975; Geisser, 1980). Nowadays the term "latent growth curves" is in use, but these models differ significantly from the BRM (see Geiser et al., 2013).

References

Aitken, A. C. (1935). Note on selection from a multivariate normal population. *Proceedings of the Edinburgh Mathematical Society, Series 2, 4*, 106–110.

Aitken, A. C. (1936). On least squares and linear combinations of observations. *Proceedings of the Royal Society of Edinburgh, Section A, 55*, 42–48.

Aitken, A. C. (1949). On the Wishart distribution in Statistics. *Biometrika, 36*, 59–62.

Aldrich, J. (1999). Determinacy in the linear model: Gauss to Bose and Koopmans. *International Statistical Review, 67*, 211–219.

Anderson, T. W. (1951). Estimating linear restrictions on regression coefficients for multivariate normal distributions. *Annals of Mathematical Statistics, 22*, 327–351.

Anderson, T. W. (1958). *An introduction to multivariate statistical analysis*. New York/London: Wiley/Chapman & Hall.

Anderson, T. W. (1984). *An introduction to multivariate statistical analysis* (2nd ed.). New York: Wiley.

Anderson, T. W. (1996). R.A. Fisher and multivariate analysis. *Statistical Science, 11*, 20–34.

Anderson, T. W. (2003). *An introduction to multivariate statistical analysis. Wiley series in probability and statistics* (3rd ed.). Hoboken: Wiley-Interscience.

Anderson, T. W. (2007). Multiple discoveries: Distribution of roots of determinantal equations. *The Journal of Statistical Planning and Inference, 137*, 3240–3248.

Andersson, S. A., Marden, J. I., & Perlman, M. D. (1993). Totally ordered multivariate linear models. *Sankhyā, Series A, 55*, 370–394.

Andersson, S. A., & Perlman, M. D. (1993). Lattice models for conditional independence in a multivariate normal distribution. *The Annals of Statistics, 21*, 1318–1358.

Andersson, S. A., & Perlman, M. D. (1998). Normal linear regression models with recursive graphical Markov structure. *Journal of Multivariate Analysis, 66*, 133–187.

Bartholomew, D., Knott, M., & Moustaki, I. (2011). *Latent variable models and factor analysis. A unified approach. Wiley series in probability and statistics* (3rd ed.). Chichester: Wiley.

Bartlett, M. S. (1934a). On the theory of statistical regression. *Proceedings of the Royal Society of Edinburgh, 53*, 260–283.

Bartlett, M. S. (1934b). The vector representation of a sample. *Mathematical Proceedings of the Cambridge Philosophical Society, 30*, 327–340.

Bartlett, M. S. (1939). A note on tests of significance in multivariate analysis. *Mathematical Proceedings of the Cambridge Philosophical Society, 35*, 180–185.

Bartlett, M. S. (1974). Historical remarks and recollections on multivariate analysis. *Sankhyā, Series B, 36*, 107–114.

Berger, J. O., & Molina, G. (2004). Some recent developments in Bayesian variable selection. In *Bayesian Inference and Maximum Entropy Methods in Science and Engineering. AIP Conference Proceedings* (Vol. 735, pp. 417–428). Melville: American Institute of Physics.

Bilodeau, M., & Brenner, D. (1999). *Theory of multivariate statistics. Springer texts in statistics.* New York: Springer.

Bose, R. C. (1936). On the exact distribution of D^2-statistic. *Sankhyā, 2*, 143–154.

Bose, R. C., & Roy, S. N. (1938). The distribution of the studentized D^2-statistic. *Sankhyā, 4*, 19–38.

Box, G. E. P. (1950). Problems in the analysis of growth and wear curves. *Biometrics, 6*, 362–389.

Bravais, A. (1846). Analyse mathématique sur les probabilités des erreurs de situation d'un point. *Mémoires de l'Institute de France, IX*, 255–332 (in French).

Bulmer, M. (2003). *Francis Galton: Pioneer of heredity and biometry*. Baltimore: Johns Hopkins University Press.

Burnaby, T. P. (1966). Growth invariant discriminant functions and generalized distances. *Biometrics, 22*, 96–110.

Cochran, W. G. (1934). The distribution of quadratic forms in a normal system, with applications to the analysis of covariance. *Mathematical Proceedings of the Cambridge Philosophical Society, 30*, 178–191.

Cowles, M. (2001). *Statistics in psychology: An historical perspective* (2nd ed.). Mahwah: Lawrence Erlbaum Associates.

Cox, D. R. (2006). *Principles of statistical inference*. Cambridge: Cambridge University Press.

Cox, D. R., & Wermuth, N. (1996). *Multivariate dependencies. Models, analysis and interpretation. Monographs on statistics and applied probability* (Vol. 67). London: Chapman & Hall.

David, H. A. (2006). The introduction of matrix algebra into statistics. *The American Statistician, 60*, 162.

Davison, A. C. (2003). *Statistical models. Cambridge series in statistical and probabilistic mathematics* (Vol. 11). Cambridge: Cambridge University Press.

Dempster, A. P. (1969). *Elements of continuous multivariate analysis*. New York: Addison-Wesley.

Dillon, W. R., & Goldstein, M. (1984). *Multivariate analysis: Methods and applications*. New York: Wiley.

Drton, M., & Richardson, T. S. (2004). Multimodality of the likelihood in the bivariate seemingly unrelated regressions model. *Biometrika, 91*, 383–392.

Druilhet, P. (1999). Optimality of neighbour balanced designs. *The Journal of Statistical Planning and Inference, 81*, 141–152.

Drygas, H. (1970). *The coordinate-free approach to Gauss-Markov estimation. Lecture notes in operations research and mathematical systems* (Vol. 40). New York: Springer.

Eaton, M. L. (1983). *Multivariate statistics. A vector space approach*. New York: Wiley.

Edgeworth, F. Y. (1892). Correlated averages. *Philosophical Magazine (5th Series), 34*, 190–204.

Evans, M. J., Fraser, D. A. S., & Monette, G. (1986). On principles and arguments to likelihood. With discussion and a rejoinder by the authors. *The Canadian Journal of Statistics, 14*, 181–199.

Everitt, B. S., Landau, S., Leese, M., & Stahl, D. (2011). *Cluster analysis. Wiley series in probability and statistics* (5th ed.). Chichester: Wiley.

Farebrother, R. W. (1999). *Fitting linear relationships: A history of the calculus of observations 1750–1900*. New York: Springer.

Fearn, T. (1975). A Bayesian approach to growth curves. *Biometrika, 62*, 89–100.

Filipiak, K., & Markiewicz, A. (2017). Universally optimal designs under interference models with and without block effects. *Communications in Statistics: Theory and Methods, 46*, 1127–1143.

Filipiak, K., & von Rosen, D. (2012). On MLEs in an extended multivariate linear growth curve model. *Metrika, 75*, 1069–1092.

Fisher, R. A. (1915). Frequency distribution of the values of the correlation coefficient in samples from an indefinitely large population. *Biometrika, 10*, 507–521.

Fisher, R. A. (1936). The use of multiple measurements in taxonomic problems. *Annals of Eugenics, 7*, 179–188.

Fisher, R. A. (1938). The statistical utilization of multiple measurements. *Annals of Eugenics, 8*, 376–386.

Fisher, R. A. (1939). The sampling distribution of some statistics obtained from non-linear equations. *Annals of Eugenics, 9*, 238–249.

Fujikoshi, Y., Enomoto, R., & Sakurai, T. (2013). High-dimensional AIC in the growth curve model. *Journal of Multivariate Analysis, 122*, 239–250.

Fujikoshi, Y., Kanda, T., & Ohtaki, M. (1999). Growth curve model with hierarchical within-individuals design matrices. *Annals of the Institute of Statistical Mathematics, 51*, 707–721.

Fujikoshi, Y, Ulyanov, V. V., & Shimizu, R. (2010). *Multivariate statistics. High-dimensional and large-sample approximations. Wiley series in probability and statistics*. Hoboken: Wiley.

Gabriel, K. R. (1998). Generalised bilinear regression. *Biometrika, 85*, 689–700.

Galton, F. (1886). Regression towards mediocrity in hereditary stature. *Journal of the Anthropological Institute of Great Britain and Ireland, 15*, 246–263.

Galton, F. (1888). Co-relations and their measurement, chiefly from anthropometric data. *Proceedings of the Royal Society of London, 45*, 135–145.

Galton, F. (1889). *Natural inheritance*. London: Macmillan.

Geiser, C., Keller, B. T., & Lockhart, G. (2013). First- versus second-order latent growth curve models: Some insights from latent state-trait theory. *Structural Equation Modeling, 20*, 479–503.

Geisser, S. (1980). Growth curve analysis. In P. R. Krishnaiah (Ed.), *Handbook of statistics* (Vol. 1, pp. 89–115). New York: North-Holland.

Geisser, S. (2006). *Modes of parametric statistical inference*. With the assistance of Wesley Johnson. With a foreword by Anne Flaxman Geisser. *Wiley series in probability and statistics*. Hoboken: Wiley-Interscience.

Girshick, M. A. (1939). On the sampling theory of roots of determinantal equations. *Annals of Mathematical Statistics, 10*, 203–224.

Gleser, L. J., & Olkin, I. (1970). Linear models in multivariate analysis. In *Essays in probability and statistics* (pp. 267–292). Chapel Hill: University of North Carolina Press.

Gram, J. P. (1879). *Om ræckkeudviklinger, bestemte ved hjælp af de mindste kvadraters methode*. Dissertation, Høst og Søn, København (in Danish).

Greenacre, M. J. (1984). *Theory and applications of correspondence analysis*. London: Academic.

Grizzle, J. E., & Allen, D. M. (1969). Analysis of growth and dose response curves. *Biometrics, 25*, 357–381.

Hald, A. (1981). T.N. Thiele's contributions to statistics. *International Statistical Review, 49*, 1–20.

Hald, A. (2002). On the history of series expansions of frequency functions and sampling distributions, 1873–1944. *Matematisk-fysiske meddelelser, 49*. ISSN: 00233323.

Herr, D. G. (1980). On the history of the use of geometry in the general linear model. *The American Statistician, 34*, 43–47.

Hoff, P. (2015). Multilinear tensor regression for longitudinal relational data. *Annals of Applied Statistics, 9*, 1169–1193.

Hotelling, H. (1931). The generalization of Student's ratio. *Annals of Mathematical Statistics, 2*, 170–198.

Hotelling, H. (1933). Analysis of a complex of statistical variables into principal components. *The Journal of Educational Psychology, 24*, 417–441, 498–520.

Hotelling, H. (1936). Relations between two sets of variates. *Biometrika, 28*, 321–377.

Hsu, P. L. (1939). On the distribution of roots of certain determinantal equations. *Annals of Eugenics, 9*, 250–258.

Hyvärinen, A., Karhunen, J., & Oja, E. (2001). *Independent component analysis*. New York: Wiley.

Imori, S., & von Rosen, D. (2015). Covariance components selection in high-dimensional growth curve model with random coefficients. *Journal of Multivariate Analysis, 136*, 86–94.

Irwin, J. O. (1934). On the independence of the constituent items in the analysis of variance. *Journal of the Royal Statistical Society Supplements, 1*, 236–251.

Jensen, S. T. (1988). Covariance hypotheses which are linear in both the covariance and the inverse covariance. *The Annals of Statistics, 16*, 302–322.

Jolliffe, I. T. (2002). *Principal component analysis* (2nd ed.). New York: Springer.

Kanda, T. (1994). Growth curve model with covariance structures. *Hiroshima Mathematical Journal, 24*, 135–176.

Kariya, T. (1985). *Testing in the multivariate general linear model*. New York: Kinokuniya.

Kariya, T., & Kurata, H. (2004). *Generalized least squares*. Chichester: Wiley.

Kariya, T., & Sinha, B. K. (1989). *Robustness of statistical tests. Statistical modeling and decision science*. Boston: Academic.

Kempthorne, O. (1952). *The design and analysis of experiments*. New York/London: Wiley/Chapman & Hall.

Kendall, M. G. (1957). *A course in multivariate analysis. Griffin's statistical monographs & courses* (Vol. 2). New York: Hafner Publishing Company.

Khatri, C. G. (1966). A note on a MANOVA model applied to problems in growth curves. *Annals of the Institute of Statistical Mathematics, 18*, 75–86.

Kolmogorov, A. N. (1933). *Grundbegriffe der Wahrscheinlichkeitsrechnung*. Berlin: Springer (in German).

Kolodziejczyk, S. (1935). On an important class of statistical hypotheses. *Biometrika, 27*, 161–190.
Kotz, S., Balakrishnan, N., & Johnson, N. L. (2000). *Continuous multivariate distributions, 1. Models and applications. Wiley series in probability and statistics: Applied probability and statistics* (2nd ed.). New York: Wiley.
Kshirsagar, A. M., & Smith, W. B. (1995). *Growth curves*. New York: Marcel Dekker.
Kunert, J., & Martin, R. J. (2000). On the determination of optimal designs for an interference model. *The Annals of Statistics, 28*, 1728–1742.
Lauritzen, S. L. (1996). *Graphical models. Oxford statistical science series* (Vol. 17). New York/Oxford: The Clarendon Press/Oxford University Press.
Letac, G., & Massam, H. (2008). The noncentral Wishart as an exponential family, and its moments. *Journal of Multivariate Analysis, 99*, 1393–1417.
Linder, M., & Sundberg, R. (2002). Precision of prediction in second-order calibration, with focus on bilinear regression methods. *Journal of Chemometrics, 16*, 12–27.
Madow, W. G. (1938). Contributions to the theory of multivariate statistical analysis. *Transactions of the American Mathematical Society, 44*, 454–490.
Mahalanobis, P. C. (1930). On tests and measures of group divergence. Part I. Theoretical formulae. *Journal of the Asiatic Society of Bengal, 26*, 541–588.
Mahalanobis, P. C. (1936). On the generalised distance in statistics. *Proceedings of National Institute of Sciences (India), 2*, 49–55.
Mardia, K. V., Kent, J. T., & Bibby, J. M. (1979). *Multivariate analysis. Probability and mathematical statistics: A series of monographs and textbooks*. New York: Academic.
Mayo, D. G., & Cox, D. R. (2006). Frequentist statistics as a theory of inductive inference. In *2nd Lehmann Symposium—Optimality. IMS Lecture Notes—Monograph Series* (Vol. 49, pp. 77–97). Beachwood: Institute of Mathematical Statistics.
McLachlan, G. J. (1992). *Discriminant analysis and statistical pattern recognition. Wiley series in probability and mathematical statistics: Applied probability and statistics*. New York: Wiley.
Monhor, D. (2012). A very short note on the origins of correlated bivariate normal distribution with particular relevance to earth sciences. *Acta Geodaetica et Geophysica Hungarica, 47*, 117–122.
Morrison, D. F. (2005). *Multivariate statistical methods. McGraw-Hill series in probability and statistics* (4th ed.). Belmont: Thomson/Brooks/Cole.
Muirhead, R. J. (1982). *Aspects of multivariate statistical theory*. New York: Wiley.
Nayak, T. P. (2009). Impact of Karl Pearson's work on statistical developments in India. *International Statistical Review, 77*, 72–80.
Olkin, I., & Shrikhande, S. S. (1954). On a modified T^2 problem. *Annals of Mathematical Statistics, 25*, 808 (abstract).
Pan, J.-X., & Fang, K. T. (2002). *Growth curve models and statistical diagnostics*. New York: Springer.
Pearson, K. (1896). Mathematical contributions to the theory of evolution. III. Regression, heredity and panmixia. *Philosophical Transactions of the Royal Society A, 187*, 253–318.
Pearson, K. (1901). On lines and planes of closest fit to systems of points in space. *Philosophical Magazine (6th series), 2*, 559–572.
Perlman, M. D. (1987). Group symmetry covariance models. (Discussion of "A Review of Multivariate Analysis" by Mark Schervish.) *Statistical Science, 2*, 421–425.
Potthoff, R. F., & Roy, S. N. (1964). A generalized multivariate analysis of variance model useful especially for growth curve problems. *Biometrika, 51*, 313–326.
Rao, C. R. (1948). Tests of significance in multivariate analysis. *Biometrika, 35*, 58–79.
Rao, C. R. (1958). Some statistical methods for comparison of growth curves. *Biometrics, 14*, 1–17.
Rao, C. R. (1965). The theory of least squares when the parameters are stochastic and its application to the analysis of growth curves. *Biometrika, 52*, 447–458.
Rao, C. R. (1966a). Discriminant function between composite hypotheses and related problems. *Biometrika, 53*, 339–345.
Rao, C. R. (1966b). Covariance adjustment and related problems in multivariate analysis. In P. R. Krishnaiah (Ed.), *Multivariate analysis*, (pp. 87–103). New York: Academic.

Rao, C. R. (1967). Least squares theory using an estimated dispersion matrix and its application to measurement of signals. In *Proceedings of the Fifth Berkeley Symposium on Mathematical Statistics and Probability, Volume 1: Statistics, Berkeley, 1965/1966* (pp. 355–372). Berkeley: University of California Press.

Rao, C. R., & Kleffe, J. (1988). *Estimation of variance components and applications. North-Holland series in statistics and probability* (Vol. 3), Amsterdam: North-Holland.

Rencher, A. C., & Christensen, W. F. (2012). *Methods of multivariate analysis. Wiley series in probability and statistics* (3rd ed.). Hoboken: Wiley.

Roy, S. N. (1939). p-Statistics or some generalisations in analysis of variance appropriate to multivariate problems. *Sankhyā, 4*, 381–396.

Roy, S. N. (1957) *Some aspects of multivariate analysis*. New York/Calcutta: Wiley/Indian Statistical Institute.

Schafer, G., & Vovk, V. (2006). The sources of Kolmogorov's Grundbegriffe. *Statistical Science, 21*, 70–98.

Schervish, M. J. (1987). A review of multivariate analysis. With discussion and a reply by the author. *Statistical Science, 2*, 396–433.

Seal, H. L. (1967). Studies in the history of probability and statistics. XV: The historical development of the Gauss linear model. *Biometrika, 54*, 1–24.

Searle, S. R. (2000). The infusion of matrices into statistics. *IMAGE, 24*, 25–32.

Searle, S. R. (2005). Recollections from a 50-year random walk midst matrices, statistics and computing. In P. S. P. Cowpertwait (Ed.), *Proceedings of the 14th workshop on matrices and statistics. Research letters in the information and mathematical sciences* (Vol. 8, pp. 45–52). Palmerston North: Massey University.

Seber, G. A. F. (1984). *Multivariate observations. Wiley series in probability and mathematical statistics: Probability and mathematical statistics*. New York: Wiley.

Seely, J. (1971). Quadratic subspaces and completeness. *Annals of Mathematical Statistics, 42*, 710–721.

Shao, J. (2003). *Mathematical statistics. Springer texts in statistics* (2nd ed.). New York: Springer.

Siotani, M., Hayakawa, T., & Fujikoshi, Y. (1985). *Modern multivariate statistical analysis: A graduate course and handbook. American sciences press series in mathematical and management sciences* (Vol. 9). Columbus: American Sciences Press.

Srivastava, M. S., & Carter, E. M. (1983). *An introduction to applied multivariate statistics*. New York: North-Holland.

Srivastava, M. S., & Khatri, C. G. (1979). *An introduction to multivariate statistics*. New York: North-Holland.

Srivastava, M. S., & von Rosen, D. (1999). Growth curve models. In *Multivariate analysis, design of experiments, and survey sampling. Statistics: A series of textbooks and monographs* (Vol. 159, pp. 547–578). New York: Dekker.

Stigler, S. M. (1986). *The history of statistics: The quantification of uncertainty before 1900*. Cambridge: Harvard University Press.

Stigler, S. M. (2012). Karl Pearson and the rule of three. *Biometrika, 99*, 1–14.

Stone, M. (1977). A unified approach to coordinate-free multivariate analysis. *Annals of the Institute of Statistical Mathematics, 29*, 43–57.

Stone, M. (1987). *Coordinate-free multivariable statistics. An illustrated geometric progression from Halmos to Gauss and Bayes. Oxford statistical science series* (Vol. 2). New York: The Clarendon Press/Oxford University Press.

Student. (1908). The probable error of a mean. *Biometrika, 6*, 1–25.

Takeuchi, K., Yanai, H., & Mukherjee, B. N. (1982). *The foundations of multivariate analysis. A unified approach by means of projection onto linear subspaces*. New York: A Halsted Press Book/Wiley.

Thiele, T. N. (1889). *Forelæsninger over almindelig iagttagelseslære: Sandsynlighedsregning og mindste kvadraters methode* (in Danish). København: Reitzel.

Timm, N. H. (1997). The CGMANOVA model. *Communications in Statistics: Theory and Methods, 26*, 1083–1098.

Tocher, K. D. (1952). On the concurrence of a set of regression lines. *Biometrika, 39*, 109–117.
Valderrama, P., & Poppi, R. J. (2008). Bilinear least squares (BLLS) and molecular fluorescence in the quantification of the propranolol enantiomers. *Analytica Chimica Acta, 623*, 38–45.
Verbeke, G., & Molenberghs, G. (2000). *Linear mixed models for longitudinal data. Springer series in statistics*. New York: Springer.
Verbyla, A. P., & Venables, W. N. (1988). An extension of the growth curve model. *Biometrika, 75*, 129–138.
von Bortkiewicz, Dr. L. (1917). *Die Iterationen. Ein Beitrag zur Wahrscheinlichkeitstheorie*. Berlin: Julius Springer (in German).
von Rosen, D. (1989). Maximum likelihood estimators in multivariate linear normal models. *Journal of Multivariate Analysis, 31*, 187–200.
von Rosen, D. (1991). The growth curve model: A review. *Communications in Statistics: Theory and Methods, 20*, 2791–2822.
Votaw, D. F. (1948). Testing compound symmetry in a normal multivariate distribution. *Annals of Mathematical Statistics, 19*, 447–473.
Whittaker, J. (1990). *Graphical models in applied multivariate statistics. Wiley series in probability and mathematical statistics: Probability and mathematical statistics*. Chichester: Wiley.
Wichura, M. J. (2006). *The coordinate-free approach to linear models. Cambridge series in statistical and probabilistic mathematics*. Cambridge: Cambridge University Press.
Wilks, S. S. (1932). Certain generalizations in the analysis of variance. *Biometrika, 24*, 471–494.
Wilks, S. S. (1946). Sample criteria for testing equality of means, equality of variances, and equality of covariances in a normal multivariate distribution. *Annals of Mathematical Statistics, 17*, 257–281.
Wishart, J. (1928). The generalised product moment distribution in samples from a normal multivariate population. *Biometrika, 20 A*, 32–52.
Wishart, J. (1938). Growth-rate determinations in nutrition studies with the bacon pig, and their analysis. *Biometrika, 30*, 16–28.
Withers, C. S., & Nadarajah, S. (2012). Moments and cumulants for the complex Wishart. *Journal of Multivariate Analysis, 112*, 242–247.
Woolson, R. F., & Leeper, J. D. (1980). Growth curve analysis of complete and incomplete longitudinal data. *Communications in Statistics: Theory and Methods, 9*, 1491–1513.
Yates, F. (1933). The analysis of replicated experiments when the field results are incomplete. *Empire Journal of Experimental Agriculture, 1*, 129–142.

Chapter 2
The Basic Ideas of Obtaining MLEs: A Known Dispersion

2.1 Introduction

Multivariate linear models, as well as the bilinear regression models, are extensions of univariate linear models. Therefore, possessing a good knowledge of linear models theory helps one understand the BRM and $EBRM_{\bullet}^{m}$. If the dispersion matrix in the BRM or $EBRM_{\bullet}^{m}$ is supposed to be known, these models belong to the class of univariate linear models (the Gauss-Markov model, after a vectorization). It is well known that for this class of models a decomposition of subspaces is essential. This decomposition is important for the mathematical treatment, as well as for the understanding of the analysis based on these models. In this chapter, first the singular Gauss-Markov model is treated, and thereafter the models which are the main subject of this book are discussed in some detail. Note that the singular Gauss-Markov model is the most general linear model when only a single variance component (error variance) is present.

2.2 Linear Models with a Focus on the Singular Gauss-Markov Model

The inference method adopted in this book is mainly based on the likelihood function. The purpose of this section is to introduce vector space decompositions and show their roles when estimating parameters. In Appendix B, Theorems B.3 and B.11, a few important results about the linear space $\mathcal{C}(\bullet)$, its orthogonal complement $\mathcal{C}(\bullet)^{\perp}$ and projections $\boldsymbol{P}_A = \boldsymbol{A}(\boldsymbol{A}'\boldsymbol{A})^{-}\boldsymbol{A}'$ are presented. Once again the univariate linear model

$$\boldsymbol{x}' = \boldsymbol{\beta}'\boldsymbol{C} + \boldsymbol{e}', \quad \boldsymbol{e} \sim N_n(\boldsymbol{0}, \sigma^2\boldsymbol{I}). \tag{2.1}$$

D. von Rosen, *Bilinear Regression Analysis*, Lecture Notes in Statistics 220,
https://doi.org/10.1007/978-3-319-78784-8_2

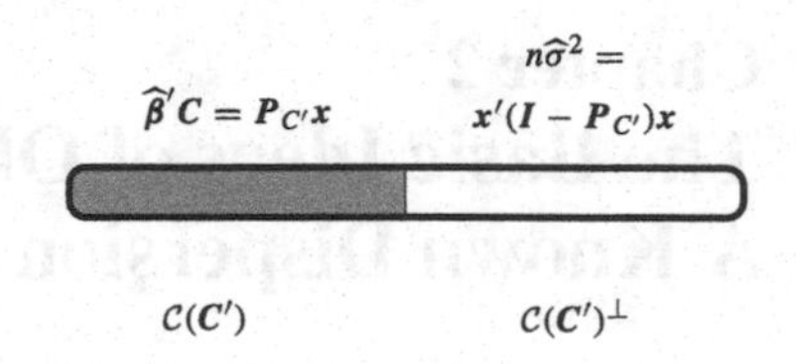

Fig. 2.1 Consider the model given in (2.1). Decomposition of the whole space according to the design matrix C' is presented

will be studied. In Example 1.1 it was noted that $\widehat{\mu}' = \widehat{\beta}'C$ and the maximum likelihood estimator of σ^2 equalled $n\widehat{\sigma}^2 = r'r$, where the "mean" $\widehat{\mu} = P_{C'}x$ and "residuals" $r = (I - P_{C'})x$. Hence, the estimators and residuals are obtained by projecting x on the column space $\mathcal{C}(C')$ and on its orthogonal complement $\mathcal{C}(C')^{\perp}$, respectively. The estimates are obtained by replacing x by x_o in the expressions given above. Moreover, under normality, $\widehat{\mu}$ and r are independently distributed and constitute the building blocks of the complete and sufficient statistics. Thus, $\widehat{\mu}$ and r are very fundamental quantities for carrying out inference according to the statistical paradigm, i.e. parameter estimation and model evaluation. Indeed, this is the basic philosophy adopted throughout this book, even if the models presented later become much more complicated. Consequently, the following space decomposition is of interest:

$$\mathcal{R}^n = \mathcal{C}(C') \boxplus \mathcal{C}(C')^{\perp},$$

where $\boxplus$ denotes the orthogonal sum (see Appendix A, Sect. A.8), which is illustrated in Fig. 2.1.

Suppose now that in the model $x' = \beta'C + e'$, the restrictions

$$\beta'G = 0$$

hold. The restrictions mean that there is some prior information about β or some hypothesis has been postulated about the parameters in β. Then it follows from Sect. 1.3 that

$$\widehat{\beta}'C = x'C'G^o(G^{o\prime}CC'G^o)^-G^{o\prime}C = x'P_{C'G^o}.$$

An important property is that if $\mathcal{C}(G) \subseteq \mathcal{C}(C)$, then $\widehat{\beta}'G = 0$ because

$$\widehat{\beta}'G = \widehat{\beta}'CC'(CC')^-G = 0.$$

Moreover, $\widehat{\sigma}^2$ is proportional to the squared residuals $r = (I - P_{C'G^o})x$, where

$$r'r = x'(I - P_{C'G^o})x = x'(P_{C'(CC'G^o)^o} + I - P_{C'})x,$$

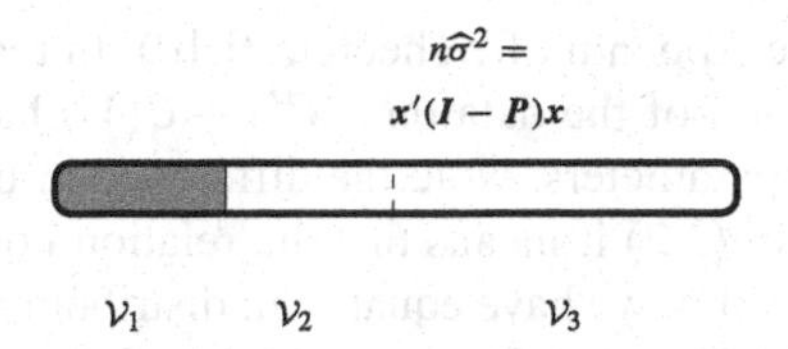

Fig. 2.2 Consider the model given in (2.1). Decomposition of the whole space according to the design and the restriction $\boldsymbol{\beta}'\boldsymbol{G} = \boldsymbol{0}$; $\mathcal{V}_1 = \mathcal{C}(\boldsymbol{C}'\boldsymbol{G}^o)$, $\mathcal{V}_2 = \mathcal{C}(\boldsymbol{C}'\boldsymbol{G}^o)^\perp \cap \mathcal{C}(\boldsymbol{C}')$, $\mathcal{V}_3 = \mathcal{C}(\boldsymbol{C}')^\perp$ and $\boldsymbol{P} = \boldsymbol{P}_{\boldsymbol{C}'\boldsymbol{G}^o}$

since $\mathcal{C}(\boldsymbol{C}'(\boldsymbol{C}\boldsymbol{C}'\boldsymbol{G}^o)^o) = \mathcal{C}(\boldsymbol{C}'\boldsymbol{G}^o)^\perp \cap \mathcal{C}(\boldsymbol{C}')$ (see Appendix B, Theorem B.3 (vi)). The estimators are obtained by projections of $\boldsymbol{x}$ using the space decomposition

$$\mathcal{R}^n = \mathcal{C}(\boldsymbol{C}'\boldsymbol{G}^o) \boxplus \mathcal{C}(\boldsymbol{C}'\boldsymbol{G}^o)^\perp \cap \mathcal{C}(\boldsymbol{C}') \boxplus \mathcal{C}(\boldsymbol{C}')^\perp,$$

which is illustrated in Fig. 2.2.

Note that we have decomposed the whole space into three orthogonal subspaces. It is easy to imagine that one can continue decomposing until spaces of dimension 1 occur. This can always be performed, but the procedure is only meaningful if the subspaces can be interpreted. Usually applications induce restrictions on $\mathcal{C}(\boldsymbol{C}')$ and then, if a decomposition into orthogonal subspaces can be achieved, an easily interpretable model is obtained. Unfortunately, the majority of linear models which are to be analysed do not share this property, for example regression models and many analysis of variance models which are unbalanced, i.e. models suitable to handle a different number of observations in the "cells", such as models for k-way tables. A lack of orthogonality does not mean that one is unable to use the model, but it indicates that many competitive models can exist. Choosing between models is challenging and is at least partly a matter of taste.

Now the Gauss-Markov model presented in Sect. 1.3 and Example 1.2, i.e.

$$\boldsymbol{x}' = \boldsymbol{\beta}'\boldsymbol{C} + \boldsymbol{\epsilon}', \quad \boldsymbol{\epsilon} \sim N_n(\boldsymbol{0}, \sigma^2\boldsymbol{V}), \quad \boldsymbol{V} \text{ p.s.d.},$$

will be studied in some detail, because it provides a deeper understanding of how to relate subspace decompositions to statistical inference. An unknown variance parameter, σ^2, is now also included. Let $\boldsymbol{V} = \boldsymbol{H}\boldsymbol{H}'$, where $\boldsymbol{H}$: $n \times r$, $r = r(\boldsymbol{V})$ and put $\boldsymbol{G} = (\boldsymbol{H}'\boldsymbol{H})^{-1}\boldsymbol{H}'$. Post-multiplying $\boldsymbol{x}'$ by $(\boldsymbol{G}' : \boldsymbol{H}^o)$ is a one-to-one transformation, i.e. there is no loss of information, and

$$\boldsymbol{x}_o'\boldsymbol{H}^o = \boldsymbol{\beta}'\boldsymbol{C}\boldsymbol{H}^o, \tag{2.2}$$

$$\boldsymbol{x}'\boldsymbol{G}' = \boldsymbol{\beta}'\boldsymbol{C}\boldsymbol{G}' + \widetilde{\boldsymbol{\epsilon}}', \quad \widetilde{\boldsymbol{\epsilon}} \sim N_r(\boldsymbol{0}, \sigma^2\boldsymbol{I}) \tag{2.3}$$

is obtained. In comparison with Sect. 1.3 the approach is slightly different. The presentation has been altered because now a very natural variance estimator is obtained immediately. If (2.2) is to have a solution, it has to be assumed that

$\boldsymbol{x}_o \in \mathcal{C}(\boldsymbol{C}') + \mathcal{C}(\boldsymbol{V})$ (see Appendix B, Theorem B.10). In reality this may not hold and, therefore, a projection of the data on $\mathcal{C}(\boldsymbol{C}') + \mathcal{C}(\boldsymbol{V})$ has to take place before starting to estimate the parameters. Note the difference in using the equality sign "=" in (2.2) and (2.3). In (2.2) it means that the relation holds with probability 1, whereas in (2.3) it means that we have equality in distribution.

Hence, according to (2.2) and (2.3), the original model with a singular dispersion matrix has been transformed into a model where a normal density is involved, but where there are now also some restrictions on the mean induced by the data. Note that in (2.2) the random variable $\boldsymbol{x}$ has been replaced by the observation vector $\boldsymbol{x}_o$. Since the restrictions depend on the data one may question if this is a statistical model and there are definitely problems with the interpretation of the estimate. Solving (2.2) implies that $\boldsymbol{\beta}$ can be written as follows (see Appendix B, Theorem B.10):

$$\boldsymbol{\beta}' = \boldsymbol{x}_o'\boldsymbol{H}^o(\boldsymbol{C}\boldsymbol{H}^o)^- + \boldsymbol{\theta}(\boldsymbol{C}\boldsymbol{H}^o)^{o'}, \tag{2.4}$$

where $\boldsymbol{\theta}$ is a new arbitrary parameter vector. Inserting the solution in (2.3) yields the following linear model:

$$\boldsymbol{x}'\boldsymbol{G}' = \boldsymbol{x}_o'\boldsymbol{H}^o(\boldsymbol{C}\boldsymbol{H}^o)^-\boldsymbol{C}\boldsymbol{G}' + \boldsymbol{\theta}(\boldsymbol{C}\boldsymbol{H}^o)^{o'}\boldsymbol{C}\boldsymbol{G}' + \widetilde{\boldsymbol{\epsilon}}'. \tag{2.5}$$

Now standard methods for obtaining MLEs can be applied. Put $\boldsymbol{F} = (\boldsymbol{C}\boldsymbol{H}^o)^{o'}\boldsymbol{C}\boldsymbol{G}'$. Then the MLE of $\boldsymbol{\theta}$ is given by

$$\widehat{\boldsymbol{\theta}}_o = \boldsymbol{x}_o'(\boldsymbol{I} - \boldsymbol{H}^o(\boldsymbol{C}\boldsymbol{H}^o)^-\boldsymbol{C})\boldsymbol{G}'\boldsymbol{F}'(\boldsymbol{F}\boldsymbol{F}')^- + \boldsymbol{z}'\boldsymbol{F}^{o'},$$

where $\boldsymbol{z}$ is arbitrary. Since $\boldsymbol{G}'\boldsymbol{G} = \boldsymbol{H}(\boldsymbol{H}'\boldsymbol{V}\boldsymbol{H})^{-1}\boldsymbol{H}'$, this expression is the same as the one presented in (1.6). It follows that

$$\begin{aligned}\mathcal{C}(\boldsymbol{F}) &= \mathcal{C}((\boldsymbol{C}\boldsymbol{H}^o)^{o'}\boldsymbol{C}\boldsymbol{G}') = \mathcal{C}((\boldsymbol{C}\boldsymbol{H}^o)^{o'}\boldsymbol{C}\boldsymbol{H}(\boldsymbol{H}'\boldsymbol{H})^{-1}\boldsymbol{H}') \\ &= \mathcal{C}((\boldsymbol{C}\boldsymbol{H}^o)^{o'}\boldsymbol{C}(\boldsymbol{I} - \boldsymbol{H}^o(\boldsymbol{H}^{o'}\boldsymbol{H}^o)^-\boldsymbol{H}^{o'})) = \mathcal{C}((\boldsymbol{C}\boldsymbol{H}^o)^{o'}\boldsymbol{C})\end{aligned}$$

and, since $\boldsymbol{F}^{o'}(\boldsymbol{C}\boldsymbol{H}^o)^{o'}\boldsymbol{C} = \boldsymbol{0}$,

$$\widehat{\boldsymbol{\beta}}_o'\boldsymbol{C} = \boldsymbol{x}_o'\boldsymbol{H}^o(\boldsymbol{C}\boldsymbol{H}^o)^-\boldsymbol{C} + \boldsymbol{x}_o'(\boldsymbol{I} - \boldsymbol{H}^o(\boldsymbol{C}\boldsymbol{H}^o)^-\boldsymbol{C})\boldsymbol{G}'\boldsymbol{F}'(\boldsymbol{F}\boldsymbol{F}')^-(\boldsymbol{C}\boldsymbol{H}^o)^{o'}\boldsymbol{C}. \tag{2.6}$$

Moreover, it is important to note that this expression does not depend on any specific choice of $\boldsymbol{H}^o$. The estimator can be rewritten as

$$\widehat{\boldsymbol{\beta}}'\boldsymbol{C} = \boldsymbol{x}'\boldsymbol{H}^o(\boldsymbol{C}\boldsymbol{H}^o)^-\boldsymbol{C}(\boldsymbol{I} - \boldsymbol{G}'\boldsymbol{F}'(\boldsymbol{F}\boldsymbol{F}')^-(\boldsymbol{C}\boldsymbol{H}^o)^{o'}\boldsymbol{C}) + \boldsymbol{x}'\boldsymbol{G}'\boldsymbol{F}'(\boldsymbol{F}\boldsymbol{F}')^-(\boldsymbol{C}\boldsymbol{H}^o)^{o'}\boldsymbol{C}, \tag{2.7}$$

which thus is split into a deterministic and a stochastic part, since $\mathbf{x}'\mathbf{H}^o$ is constant with probability 1. However, note that the deterministic part is data-dependent. If we consider the estimates, there is no conceptual difference between the deterministic and the stochastic parts. On the other hand, if we want to evaluate the model, as the statistical paradigm requires, there are problems concerning how to evaluate the deterministic part, since distribution theory will not help us, for example, to identify what an extreme observation is. An alternative way of expressing $\widehat{\boldsymbol{\beta}'\mathbf{C}}$ is given by

$$\widehat{\boldsymbol{\beta}'\mathbf{C}} = \mathbf{x}'(\mathbf{I} - (\mathbf{C}')^o((\mathbf{C}')^{o'}\mathbf{V}(\mathbf{C}')^o)^-(\mathbf{C}')^{o'}\mathbf{V}). \tag{2.8}$$

This expression is presented because there are good and simple geometrical interpretations which can take place, which we will return to later. The relation is obtained in the following way. Start from (2.6) and then (letting $\mathbf{P}_H = \mathbf{H}(\mathbf{H}'\mathbf{H})^{-1}\mathbf{H}'$)

$$\mathbf{G}'\mathbf{F}'(\mathbf{F}\mathbf{F}')^-(\mathbf{C}\mathbf{H}^o)^{o'}\mathbf{C} = \mathbf{P}_H(\mathbf{I} - (\mathbf{C}')^o((\mathbf{C}')^{o'}\mathbf{H}\mathbf{H}'(\mathbf{C}')^o)^-(\mathbf{C}')^{o'}\mathbf{H}\mathbf{H}'),$$

because $\mathcal{C}(\mathbf{C}'(\mathbf{C}\mathbf{H}^o)^o) = \mathcal{C}(\mathbf{H}(\mathbf{H}'(\mathbf{C}')^o)^o)$ (see Appendix B, Theorem B.3 (v)), and thereafter, applying the special case in Appendix B, Theorem B.13,

$$\mathbf{x}_o'\mathbf{H}^o(\mathbf{C}\mathbf{H}^o)^-\mathbf{C}\mathbf{P}_H = \mathbf{x}_o'\mathbf{H}^o(\mathbf{C}\mathbf{H}^o)^-\mathbf{C} - \mathbf{x}_o'\mathbf{P}_{H^o},$$

where (2.2) has been utilized, and

$$\mathbf{x}_o'\mathbf{H}^o(\mathbf{C}\mathbf{H}^o)^-\mathbf{C}\mathbf{P}_H(\mathbf{C}')^o = -\mathbf{x}_o'\mathbf{H}^o\mathbf{P}_H(\mathbf{C}')^o.$$

All these relations establish the proposed estimator in (2.8).

Since the estimator $\widehat{\boldsymbol{\beta}'\mathbf{C}}$ is linear in $\mathbf{x}$, it is normally distributed. Using (2.7), the mean can be derived and it can be shown that the estimator is unbiased, i.e.

$$E[\widehat{\boldsymbol{\beta}'\mathbf{C}}] = \boldsymbol{\beta}'\mathbf{C}.$$

Concerning the dispersion, since the deterministic part of the estimator does not have to be considered,

$$D[\widehat{\boldsymbol{\beta}'\mathbf{C}}] = D[\mathbf{C}'\widehat{\boldsymbol{\beta}}] = \sigma^2\mathbf{C}'(\mathbf{C}\mathbf{H}^o)^o(\mathbf{F}\mathbf{F}')^-(\mathbf{C}\mathbf{H}^o)^{o'}\mathbf{C},$$

which does not depend on the choice of $(\mathbf{F}\mathbf{F}')^-$; i.e. it is unique. Moreover, the unbiased, quadratic, minimum variance estimator is given by

$$(r - r(\mathbf{F}))\widehat{\sigma}^2 = \mathbf{x}'\mathbf{R}(\mathbf{I} - \mathbf{F}'(\mathbf{F}\mathbf{F}')^-\mathbf{F})\mathbf{R}'\mathbf{x}, \tag{2.9}$$

where

$$\mathbf{R} = (\mathbf{I} - \mathbf{H}^o(\mathbf{C}\mathbf{H}^o)^-\mathbf{C})\mathbf{G}'.$$

To show that the expression in (2.9) is unbiased, it is noted that $E[\boldsymbol{x}'\boldsymbol{R}(\boldsymbol{F}')^o] = \boldsymbol{0}$ and $\operatorname{tr}\{\boldsymbol{R}(\boldsymbol{I} - \boldsymbol{F}'(\boldsymbol{F}\boldsymbol{F}')^-\boldsymbol{F})\boldsymbol{R}'\boldsymbol{V}\} = \operatorname{tr}\{\boldsymbol{I} - \boldsymbol{F}'(\boldsymbol{F}\boldsymbol{F}')^-\boldsymbol{F}\}$, since $\boldsymbol{H}'\boldsymbol{G}' = \boldsymbol{I}_r$. It can also be observed that

$$\begin{aligned}\boldsymbol{G}'(\boldsymbol{I} - \boldsymbol{F}'(\boldsymbol{F}\boldsymbol{F}')^-\boldsymbol{F})\boldsymbol{G} &= \boldsymbol{G}'(\boldsymbol{F}')^o((\boldsymbol{F}')^{o'}(\boldsymbol{F}')^o)^-(\boldsymbol{F}')^{o'}\boldsymbol{G}\\ &= \boldsymbol{H}(\boldsymbol{H}'\boldsymbol{H})^{-1}\boldsymbol{H}'(\boldsymbol{C}')^o((\boldsymbol{C}')^{o'}\boldsymbol{V}(\boldsymbol{C}')^o)^-(\boldsymbol{C}')^{o'}\boldsymbol{H}(\boldsymbol{H}'\boldsymbol{H})^{-1}\boldsymbol{H}'\end{aligned}$$

and

$$\begin{aligned}&\boldsymbol{x}'(\boldsymbol{I} - \boldsymbol{H}^o(\boldsymbol{C}\boldsymbol{H}^o)^-\boldsymbol{C})\boldsymbol{H}(\boldsymbol{H}'\boldsymbol{H})^{-1}\boldsymbol{H}'(\boldsymbol{C}')^o\\ &\quad= \boldsymbol{x}'(\boldsymbol{I} - \boldsymbol{H}^o(\boldsymbol{C}\boldsymbol{H}^o)^-\boldsymbol{C})(\boldsymbol{I} - \boldsymbol{H}^o(\boldsymbol{H}^{o'}\boldsymbol{H}^o)^-\boldsymbol{H}^{o'})(\boldsymbol{C}')^o = \boldsymbol{x}'(\boldsymbol{C}')^o,\end{aligned}$$

since $\boldsymbol{x} \in \mathcal{C}(\boldsymbol{C}' : \boldsymbol{V})$. Note that $\boldsymbol{x} \in \mathcal{C}(\boldsymbol{C}' : \boldsymbol{V})$ is always true, but data $\boldsymbol{x}_o$ may not share this property. The relations given above imply that (2.9) can be written as follows:

$$(r - r(\boldsymbol{F}))\widehat{\sigma}^2 = \boldsymbol{x}'(\boldsymbol{C}')^o((\boldsymbol{C}')^{o'}\boldsymbol{V}(\boldsymbol{C}')^o)^-(\boldsymbol{C}')^{o'}\boldsymbol{x}, \tag{2.10}$$

where it is important to note that $r - r(\boldsymbol{F})$ is identical to the dimension of $(\mathcal{C}(\boldsymbol{C}') \cap \mathcal{C}(\boldsymbol{V}))^\perp$, which also means that if $\boldsymbol{V}$ is positive definite, $r(\boldsymbol{F}) = r(\boldsymbol{C})$.

Now we study which spaces are involved when $\boldsymbol{\beta}'\boldsymbol{C}$ is estimated and will later study how linear spaces are connected to the estimation of σ^2. Let $\boldsymbol{P}$ be an orthogonal projector on $\mathcal{C}(\boldsymbol{C}' : \boldsymbol{V})$, i.e. by assumption $\boldsymbol{P}\boldsymbol{x} = \boldsymbol{x}$. Then,

$$\boldsymbol{C}'\widehat{\boldsymbol{\beta}} = \boldsymbol{P}_1\boldsymbol{x} + \boldsymbol{P}_2\boldsymbol{x},$$

where

$$\begin{aligned}\boldsymbol{P}_1 &= \boldsymbol{C}'(\boldsymbol{H}^{o'}\boldsymbol{C}')^-\boldsymbol{H}^{o'}\boldsymbol{P},\\ \boldsymbol{P}_2 &= \boldsymbol{C}'(\boldsymbol{C}\boldsymbol{H}^o)^o(\boldsymbol{F}\boldsymbol{F}')^-\boldsymbol{F}\boldsymbol{G}(\boldsymbol{I} - \boldsymbol{C}'(\boldsymbol{H}^{o'}\boldsymbol{C}')^-\boldsymbol{H}^{o'})\boldsymbol{P}.\end{aligned}$$

One can show that $\boldsymbol{P}_1\boldsymbol{P}_2 = \boldsymbol{P}_2\boldsymbol{P}_1 = \boldsymbol{0}$ and

$$\mathcal{C}(\boldsymbol{C}') = \mathcal{C}(\boldsymbol{P}_1) \oplus \mathcal{C}(\boldsymbol{P}_2) = \mathcal{C}(\boldsymbol{C}'(\boldsymbol{H}^{o'}\boldsymbol{C}')^-\boldsymbol{H}^{o'}\boldsymbol{C}') \oplus \mathcal{C}(\boldsymbol{C}') \cap \mathcal{C}(\boldsymbol{H}).$$

It is interesting to note that by choosing $(\boldsymbol{H}^{o'}\boldsymbol{C}')^-$ we obtain different types of decompositions. Consider a general expression (not the most general), which is obtained by solving the linear equation system defining any g-inverse ($\boldsymbol{Q}\boldsymbol{Q}^-\boldsymbol{Q} = \boldsymbol{Q}$),

$$(\boldsymbol{H}^{o'}\boldsymbol{C}')^- = (\boldsymbol{H}^{o'}\boldsymbol{C}')^+ + (\boldsymbol{C}\boldsymbol{H}^o)^o\boldsymbol{Z},$$

where "+" indicates the use of the unique Moore-Penrose inverse (see Appendix A, Sect. A.6) and $\boldsymbol{Z}$ is an arbitrary matrix. If $\boldsymbol{Z} = \boldsymbol{0}$, then

$$\mathcal{C}(\boldsymbol{C}'(\boldsymbol{H}^{o'}\boldsymbol{C}')^{-}\boldsymbol{H}^{o'}\boldsymbol{C}') = \mathcal{C}(\boldsymbol{C}'(\boldsymbol{H}^{o'}\boldsymbol{C}')^{+}\boldsymbol{H}^{o'}\boldsymbol{C}') = \mathcal{C}(\boldsymbol{C}'\boldsymbol{C}\boldsymbol{H}^{o}),$$

but if

$$\boldsymbol{Z} = -((\boldsymbol{C}\boldsymbol{H}^{o})^{o'}\boldsymbol{C}\boldsymbol{C}'(\boldsymbol{C}\boldsymbol{H}^{o})^{o})^{-}(\boldsymbol{C}\boldsymbol{H}^{o})^{o'}\boldsymbol{C}\boldsymbol{C}'(\boldsymbol{H}^{o'}\boldsymbol{C}')^{+},$$

$$\begin{aligned}
&\mathcal{C}(\boldsymbol{C}'(\boldsymbol{H}^{o'}\boldsymbol{C}')^{-}\boldsymbol{H}^{o'}\boldsymbol{C}')\\
&\quad = \mathcal{C}((\boldsymbol{I} - \boldsymbol{C}'(\boldsymbol{C}\boldsymbol{H}^{o})^{o}((\boldsymbol{C}\boldsymbol{H}^{o})^{o'}\boldsymbol{C}\boldsymbol{C}'(\boldsymbol{C}\boldsymbol{H}^{o})^{o})^{-}(\boldsymbol{C}\boldsymbol{H}^{o})^{o'}\boldsymbol{C})\boldsymbol{C}'(\boldsymbol{H}^{o'}\boldsymbol{C}')^{+}\boldsymbol{H}^{o'}\boldsymbol{C}')\\
&\quad = (\mathcal{C}(\boldsymbol{C}') \cap \mathcal{C}(\boldsymbol{H}))^{\perp} \cap (\mathcal{C}(\boldsymbol{C}') \cap \mathcal{C}(\boldsymbol{H}) + \mathcal{C}(\boldsymbol{C}'(\boldsymbol{H}^{o'}\boldsymbol{C}')^{+}\boldsymbol{H}^{o'}\boldsymbol{C}'))\\
&\quad = (\mathcal{C}(\boldsymbol{C}') \cap \mathcal{C}(\boldsymbol{H}))^{\perp} \cap \mathcal{C}(\boldsymbol{C}'),
\end{aligned}$$

since

$$\begin{aligned}
\mathcal{C}(\boldsymbol{C}') \cap \mathcal{C}(\boldsymbol{H}) + \mathcal{C}(\boldsymbol{C}'(\boldsymbol{H}^{o'}\boldsymbol{C}')^{+}\boldsymbol{H}^{o'}\boldsymbol{C}') &= \mathcal{C}(\boldsymbol{C}') \cap \mathcal{C}(\boldsymbol{H}) + \mathcal{C}(\boldsymbol{C}'\boldsymbol{C}\boldsymbol{H}^{o})\\
&= \mathcal{C}(\boldsymbol{C}'(\boldsymbol{C}\boldsymbol{H}^{o})^{o}) + \mathcal{C}(\boldsymbol{C}'\boldsymbol{C}\boldsymbol{H}^{o}) = \mathcal{C}(\boldsymbol{C}').
\end{aligned}$$

One can sum up by stating that the following general decomposition holds:

$$\mathcal{R}^{n} = \{\mathcal{C}(\boldsymbol{C}'(\boldsymbol{H}^{o'}\boldsymbol{C}')^{-}\boldsymbol{H}^{o'}\boldsymbol{C}') \oplus \mathcal{C}(\boldsymbol{C}') \cap \mathcal{C}(\boldsymbol{V})\} \oplus \mathcal{C}(\boldsymbol{V}(\boldsymbol{C}')^{o}) \boxplus (\mathcal{C}(\boldsymbol{C}') + \mathcal{C}(\boldsymbol{V}))^{\perp},$$

since $\mathcal{C}(\boldsymbol{C}') + \mathcal{C}(\boldsymbol{V}) = \mathcal{C}(\boldsymbol{C}') \oplus \mathcal{C}(\boldsymbol{V}(\boldsymbol{C}')^{o})$, and this is illustrated in Fig. 2.3. For the two special cases considered above,

$$\mathcal{R}^{n} = \{\mathcal{C}(\boldsymbol{C}'\boldsymbol{C}\boldsymbol{V}^{o}) \oplus \mathcal{C}(\boldsymbol{C}') \cap \mathcal{C}(\boldsymbol{V})\} \oplus \mathcal{C}(\boldsymbol{V}(\boldsymbol{C}')^{o}) \boxplus (\mathcal{C}(\boldsymbol{C}') + \mathcal{C}(\boldsymbol{V}))^{\perp},$$

if $\boldsymbol{Z} = \boldsymbol{0}$, and the second choice of $\boldsymbol{Z}$ leads to

$$\mathcal{R}^{n} = \{\mathcal{C}(\boldsymbol{C}') \cap (\mathcal{C}(\boldsymbol{C}') \cap \mathcal{C}(\boldsymbol{V}))^{\perp} \boxplus \mathcal{C}(\boldsymbol{C}') \cap \mathcal{C}(\boldsymbol{V})\} \oplus \mathcal{C}(\boldsymbol{V}(\boldsymbol{C}')^{o}) \boxplus (\mathcal{C}(\boldsymbol{C}') + \mathcal{C}(\boldsymbol{V}))^{\perp}.$$

Other types of decompositions of $\mathcal{R}^{n}$ which are expressed as subspace functions of $\mathcal{C}(\boldsymbol{C}')$ and $\mathcal{C}(\boldsymbol{V})$ exist, for example

$$\begin{aligned}
\mathcal{R}^{n} = ((\mathcal{C}(\boldsymbol{C}') + \mathcal{C}(\boldsymbol{V})) \cap \mathcal{C}(\boldsymbol{C}')^{\perp} \oplus ((\mathcal{C}(\boldsymbol{C}') + \mathcal{C}(\boldsymbol{V})) \cap \mathcal{C}(\boldsymbol{V})^{\perp}) \boxplus \mathcal{C}(\boldsymbol{C}') \cap \mathcal{C}(\boldsymbol{V})\\
\boxplus(\mathcal{C}(\boldsymbol{C}') + \mathcal{C}(\boldsymbol{V}))^{\perp}
\end{aligned}$$

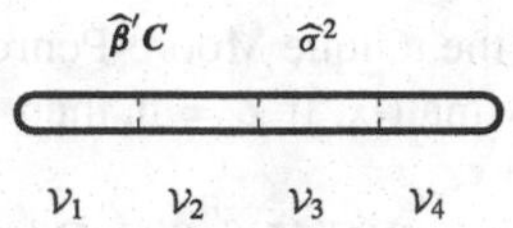

Fig. 2.3 Decomposition of the whole space in the strongly singular Gauss-Markov model; $\mathcal{V}_1 = \mathcal{C}(\boldsymbol{C}'(\boldsymbol{H}^{o'}\boldsymbol{C}')^-\boldsymbol{H}^{o'}\boldsymbol{C})$, $\mathcal{V}_2 = \mathcal{C}(\boldsymbol{C}') \cap \mathcal{C}(\boldsymbol{V})$, $\mathcal{V}_3 = \mathcal{C}(\boldsymbol{V}(\boldsymbol{C}')^o)$ and $\mathcal{V}_4 = (\mathcal{C}(\boldsymbol{C}') + \mathcal{C}(\boldsymbol{V}))^\perp$

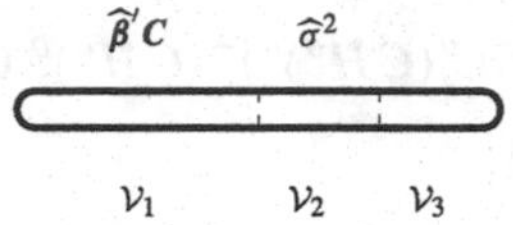

Fig. 2.4 Decomposition of the whole space in the weakly singular Gauss-Markov model; $\mathcal{V}_1 = \mathcal{C}(\boldsymbol{C}')$, $\mathcal{V}_2 = \mathcal{C}(\boldsymbol{V}(\boldsymbol{C}')^o)$ and $\mathcal{V}_3 = \mathcal{C}(\boldsymbol{V})^\perp$

and

$$\mathcal{R}^n = (\mathcal{C}(\boldsymbol{C}') + \mathcal{C}(\boldsymbol{V})) \cap \mathcal{C}(\boldsymbol{C}')^\perp \boxplus (\mathcal{C}(\boldsymbol{C}') + \mathcal{C}(\boldsymbol{V}))^\perp \cap \mathcal{C}(\boldsymbol{C}') \boxplus \mathcal{C}(\boldsymbol{C}') \cap \mathcal{C}(\boldsymbol{V}) \boxplus (\mathcal{C}(\boldsymbol{C}') + \mathcal{C}(\boldsymbol{V}))^\perp,$$

but they will not be considered. More importantly, one conclusion from the above discussion is that one should be very careful when estimating the mean parameters if this involves $\mathcal{C}(\boldsymbol{C}'(\boldsymbol{H}^{o'}\boldsymbol{C}')^-\boldsymbol{H}^{o'}\boldsymbol{C})$. In the literature the above general situation is called strongly singular (see also Fig. 2.3). If $\mathcal{C}(\boldsymbol{C}') \subseteq \mathcal{C}(\boldsymbol{V})$, one refers to the model as a weakly singular Gauss-Markov model (see Nordström, 1985). In this case

$$\mathcal{R}^n = \{\mathcal{C}(\boldsymbol{C}') \oplus \mathcal{C}(\boldsymbol{V}(\boldsymbol{C}')^o)\} \boxplus \mathcal{C}(\boldsymbol{V})^\perp,$$

which is illustrated in Fig. 2.4.

Moreover, some light is now shed on the decomposition

$$\mathcal{C}(\boldsymbol{C}') + \mathcal{C}(\boldsymbol{V}) = \mathcal{C}(\boldsymbol{C}') \oplus \mathcal{C}(\boldsymbol{V}(\boldsymbol{C}')^o). \tag{2.11}$$

Although it may look mysterious, this is a natural expression and in full agreement with the results for the model in (2.1). For the Gauss-Markov model, a subspace decomposition has been presented with a standard inner product. However, the "natural" inner product is based on $\boldsymbol{V}$; i.e. for any pair of vectors $\boldsymbol{u}, \boldsymbol{v}$ the inner product is defined as $(\boldsymbol{u}, \boldsymbol{v}) = \boldsymbol{u}'\boldsymbol{V}^{-1}\boldsymbol{v}$, if $\boldsymbol{V}^{-1}$ exists. If $\boldsymbol{V}$ is singular and the vectors $\boldsymbol{u}, \boldsymbol{v}$ belong to $\mathcal{C}(\boldsymbol{V})$, one can use $(\boldsymbol{u}, \boldsymbol{v}) = \boldsymbol{u}'\boldsymbol{V}^-\boldsymbol{v}$. If either of the vectors $\boldsymbol{u}, \boldsymbol{v}$ does not belong to $\mathcal{C}(\boldsymbol{V})$, the inner product does not make sense. Let us return to (2.11). If $\boldsymbol{V}$ is non-singular, (2.11) can be written

$$\mathcal{R}^n = \mathcal{C}_V(\boldsymbol{C}') \boxplus \mathcal{C}_V(\boldsymbol{V}(\boldsymbol{C}')^o).$$

If V is singular and $\mathcal{C}(C') \subseteq \mathcal{C}(V)$,

$$\mathcal{C}_V(V) = \mathcal{C}_V(C') \boxplus \mathcal{C}_V(V(C')^o).$$

Thus we have an informative orthogonal decomposition,

$$\mathcal{R}^n = \mathcal{C}_V(C') \boxplus \mathcal{C}_V(V(C')^o) \boxplus \mathcal{C}_V(V)^{\perp}.$$

Estimators are obtained by projecting random variables corresponding to data on these spaces, with the additional assumption that $x \in \mathcal{C}(V)$. If (2.8) is rewritten as

$$\widehat{\beta}'C = x'(I - V^- V(C')^o((C')^{o'} VV^- V(C')^o)^-(C')^{o'} V), \qquad (2.12)$$

the orthogonal projection of x on $\mathcal{C}_V(V(C')^o)^{\perp}$ is uncovered. Moreover, (2.10) can be written as follows:

$$(r - r(F))\widehat{\sigma}^2 = r'V^- r,$$

which means that we have multiplied the residual r by itself, using the inner product, with the residual being equal to

$$r = V(C')^o((C')^{o'} VV^- V(C')^o)^-(C')^{o'} VV^- x.$$

Thus, similar to the linear model with a non-singular dispersion matrix, the estimators for the weakly singular Gauss-Markov model are also obtained with the help of projections.

Turning to the strongly singular Gauss-Markov model, it follows immediately from (2.10) and (2.12) that V^- cannot be used as an inner product if one wants to apply a geometrical approach based on projections. Hence, the question is what inner product should be used. It follows from (2.12) that an inner product based on a matrix W has to satisfy

$$(C')^{o'} W = (C')^{o'} V, \quad \text{for any} (C')^{o'}$$
$$(C')^{o'} WW^- x = (C')^{o'} x, \qquad x \in \mathcal{C}(C') + \mathcal{C}(V).$$

We will not discuss these equations in detail, but note that one choice of solution is $W = C'C + V$. Hence, $C'C + V$ is used to define the inner product instead of V. However, $W = C'MC + V$, where M is any p.d. matrix, could also have been used as a solution. Moreover, instead of (2.12),

$$\widehat{\beta}'C = x'(I - (C'C + V)^- V(C')^o((C')^{o'} V(C'C + V)^- V(C')^o)^-(C')^{o'} V)$$

and instead of (2.10)

$$(r - r(\boldsymbol{F}))\widehat{\sigma}^2 = \boldsymbol{r}'(\boldsymbol{C}'\boldsymbol{C} + \boldsymbol{V})^{-}\boldsymbol{r},$$

where

$$\boldsymbol{r} = \boldsymbol{V}(\boldsymbol{C}')^{o}((\boldsymbol{C}')^{o'}\boldsymbol{V}(\boldsymbol{C}'\boldsymbol{C} + \boldsymbol{V})^{-}\boldsymbol{V}(\boldsymbol{C}')^{o})^{-}(\boldsymbol{C}')^{o'}\boldsymbol{V}(\boldsymbol{C}'\boldsymbol{C} + \boldsymbol{V})^{-}\boldsymbol{x}.$$

Therefore, we have the following spaces which can serve as a basis for the statistical inference and evaluations:

$$\mathcal{R}^n = \mathcal{C}_W(\boldsymbol{C}') \boxplus \mathcal{C}_W(\boldsymbol{V}(\boldsymbol{C}')^{o}) \boxplus \mathcal{C}_W(\boldsymbol{C}' : \boldsymbol{V})^{\perp},$$

where $\boldsymbol{W} = \boldsymbol{C}'\boldsymbol{C} + \boldsymbol{V}$, and when calculating the inner product, the Moore-Penrose inverse is used, i.e. $(\boldsymbol{u}, \boldsymbol{v}) = \boldsymbol{u}'\boldsymbol{W}^{+}\boldsymbol{v}$, for $\boldsymbol{u}$ and $\boldsymbol{v}$ in $\mathcal{C}(\boldsymbol{W})$. Among other things, this implies that $\mathcal{C}_W(\boldsymbol{C}' : \boldsymbol{V})^{\perp}$ is orthogonal to the other spaces and does not bear any information. Hence, we have obtained a general basic decomposition for analysing the strongly singular Gauss-Markov model. From the space decomposition we cannot identify what role the deterministic part of the model plays. On the other hand, if we choose the g-inverse $(\boldsymbol{H}^{o'}\boldsymbol{C}')^{-}$ to be the Moore-Penrose inverse, then one can show that

$$\begin{aligned}
\mathcal{R}^n &= \mathcal{C}_W(\boldsymbol{C}'(\boldsymbol{H}^{o'}\boldsymbol{C}')^{+}\boldsymbol{H}^{o'}\boldsymbol{C}') \\
&\quad \boxplus \mathcal{C}_W(\boldsymbol{C}') \cap \mathcal{C}_W(\boldsymbol{V}) \boxplus \mathcal{C}_W(\boldsymbol{V}(\boldsymbol{C}')^{o}) \boxplus (\mathcal{C}_W(\boldsymbol{C}') + \mathcal{C}_W(\boldsymbol{V}))^{\perp} \\
&= \mathcal{C}_W(\boldsymbol{C}'\boldsymbol{C}\boldsymbol{V}^{o}) \boxplus \mathcal{C}_W(\boldsymbol{C}') \cap \mathcal{C}_W(\boldsymbol{V}) \boxplus \mathcal{C}_W(\boldsymbol{V}(\boldsymbol{C}')^{o}) \boxplus (\mathcal{C}_W(\boldsymbol{C}') + \mathcal{C}_W(\boldsymbol{V}))^{\perp}.
\end{aligned}$$

By projecting observations on these spaces, estimators of parameters can be derived, non-random parts can be identified and residuals can be derived, in order to validate the model and estimate the variance parameter.

Finally, restrictions on the mean parameter space,

$$\boldsymbol{\beta}'\boldsymbol{K} = \boldsymbol{0},$$

are briefly considered. These restrictions are used, for example, when hypotheses are tested. In this case

$$\boldsymbol{\beta}' = \boldsymbol{\gamma}\boldsymbol{K}^{o'},$$

where $\boldsymbol{\gamma}$ is a new parameter and, instead of (2.2) and (2.3), the following equations hold:

$$\begin{aligned}
\boldsymbol{x}_o'\boldsymbol{H}^{o} &= \boldsymbol{\beta}'\boldsymbol{K}^{o'}\boldsymbol{C}\boldsymbol{H}^{o}, \\
\boldsymbol{x}'\boldsymbol{G}' &= \boldsymbol{\beta}'\boldsymbol{K}^{o'}\boldsymbol{C}\boldsymbol{G}' + \widetilde{\boldsymbol{\epsilon}}, \quad \widetilde{\boldsymbol{\epsilon}} \sim N_r(\boldsymbol{0}, \sigma^2\boldsymbol{I}).
\end{aligned}$$

Note that $x \in \mathcal{C}(C'K^o) + \mathcal{C}(V)$. Thus, the above approach can be copied and the following estimators are obtained:

$$
\begin{aligned}
\widehat{\beta}'C &= x'(I - (C'K^oK^{o'}C + V)^- V(C'K^o)^o \\
&\quad \times ((C'K^o)^{o'} V(C'K^oK^{o'}C + V)^- V(C'K^o)^o)^- (C'K^o)^{o'} V), \\
(r - r(F))\widehat{\sigma}^2 &= r'(C'K^oK^{o'}C + V)^- r, \\
r &= V(C'K^o)^o \\
&\quad \times ((C'K^o)^{o'} V(C'K^oK^{o'}C + V)^- V(C'K^o)^o)^- (C'K^o)^{o'} V(C'K^oK^{o'}C + V)^- x,
\end{aligned}
$$

as well as the orthogonal subspace decomposition

$$
\begin{aligned}
\mathcal{R}^n &= \mathcal{C}_{W_0}(C'K^oK^{o'}CV^o) \boxplus \mathcal{C}_{W_0}(C'K^o) \cap \mathcal{C}_{W_0}(V) \\
&\quad \boxplus \mathcal{C}_{W_0}(V(C'K^o)^o) \boxplus (\mathcal{C}_{W_0}(C'K^o) + \mathcal{C}_{W_0}(V))^\perp, \qquad W_0 = C'K^oK^{o'}C + V.
\end{aligned}
$$

These relations are natural, but it would have been interesting to have been able to decompose $\mathcal{C}_{W_0}(C') \cap \mathcal{C}_{W_0}(V)$ into two orthogonal subspaces $\mathcal{C}_{W_0}(C'K^o) \cap \mathcal{C}_{W_0}(V) \boxplus \mathcal{C}_{W_0}(C'K^o)^\perp \cap \mathcal{C}_{W_0}(C') \cap \mathcal{C}_{W_0}(V)$. This would have meant that $\mathcal{C}_{W_0}(C'K^o)$ would have had to commute with $\mathcal{C}_{W_0}(C') \cap \mathcal{C}_{W_0}(V)$ (for a definition of commutativity see Kollo and von Rosen (2005, p. 31)), which, for example, takes place if $\mathcal{C}_{W_0}(K^o) \subseteq \mathcal{C}_{W_0}((CV^o)^o)$, because in this case $\mathcal{C}_{W_0}(C'K^o)$ is a subspace to $\mathcal{C}_{W_0}(C') \cap \mathcal{C}_{W_0}(V)$ (see Appendix B, Theorem B.3).

2.3 Multivariate Linear Models

In this short section, an MLE for $\boldsymbol{\Sigma}$ is additionally given, for comparisons with the estimator of the variance in univariate linear models (see Fig. 2.5). The purpose of this section is to link univariate linear models with multivariate linear models, which will later be linked to the BRM. The multivariate linear model was presented in Sect. 1.4 and its MLEs were given by

$$
\begin{aligned}
\widehat{B}_o C &= X_o P_{C'}, \\
n\widehat{\boldsymbol{\Sigma}}_o &= r_o r_o', \qquad r_o' = (I - P_{C'})X_o'.
\end{aligned} \tag{2.13}
$$

In comparison with univariate linear models, the only difference when estimating parameters is that instead of x': $1 \times n$, we have X: $p \times n$. Thus, in some sense, from a mathematical point of view, the treatment of the univariate and multivariate models concerning estimation is the same. Indeed it would be mathematically more correct to say "linear multivariate model" instead of "multivariate linear model". However, if one considers properties of the estimators, then differences appear. This is mainly

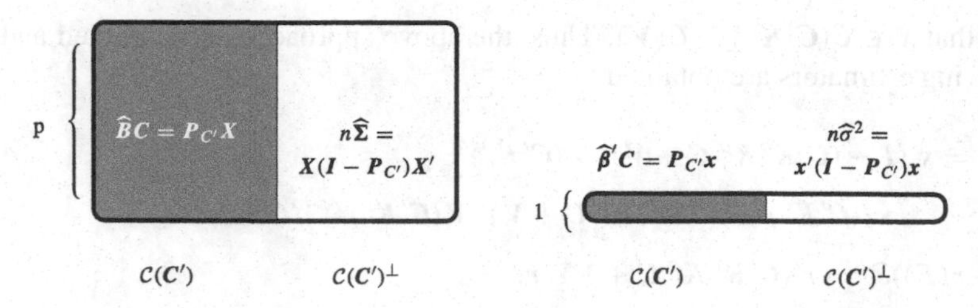

Fig. 2.5 Decomposition of the whole space according to the transpose of the design matrix C, which is valid for both the multivariate and univariate linear models. The difference in size of the figures indicates an observation space which is p-dimensional versus a space which is one-dimensional

due to the difference between the Wishart distribution and the χ^2 distribution (see Appendix A, Sect. A.9, for definitions of the distributions). Moreover, from a practical point of view, since in the multivariate case one is dealing with several variables simultaneously, the data analysis also becomes more complicated. For example, dependencies among the variables have to be taken into account, which of course is not necessary in the univariate case. Obviously there are more questions which are to be considered in the multivariate model. The differences between the univariate linear and multivariate linear models are illustrated in Fig. 2.5.

It is worth noting that any multivariate linear model via a vectorization can be written as a univariate linear model. Consider the multivariate linear model

$$X = BC + E, \qquad E \sim N_{p,n}(\mathbf{0}, \Sigma, I), \quad \Sigma > 0, \tag{2.14}$$

which can also be written as follows:

$$\text{vec}X = (C' \otimes I)\text{vec}B + e, \qquad e \sim N_{pn}(\mathbf{0}, I \otimes \Sigma), \quad \Sigma > 0. \tag{2.15}$$

However, stating that any one of the representations given above has some general advantages does not make sense from a statistical point of view. Finally, it is noted that a general inference strategy in multivariate analysis is to take an arbitrary linear combination of X, let us say $l'X$, leading to a univariate model, and then to try to choose in some sense the best l (e.g. see Rao, 1973, Chapter 8).

2.4 *BRM* with a Known Dispersion Matrix

It should be stressed that the multivariate model illustrated in Fig. 2.5 is a special case of the model given in (1.9), which will serve as a basic model for the presentation of the subject matter of this book. Before starting the technical presentation, a formal definition of the *BRM* is provided.

Definition 2.1 (*BRM*) Let $\boldsymbol{X}$: $p \times n$, $\boldsymbol{A} : p \times q, q \leq p$, $\boldsymbol{B}$: $q \times k$, $\boldsymbol{C}$: $k \times n$, $r(\boldsymbol{C}) + p \leq n$ and $\boldsymbol{\Sigma}$: $p \times p$ be p.d. Then

$$\boldsymbol{X} = \boldsymbol{ABC} + \boldsymbol{E} \tag{2.16}$$

defines the *BRM*, where $\boldsymbol{E} \sim N_{p,n}(\boldsymbol{0}, \boldsymbol{\Sigma}, \boldsymbol{I})$, $\boldsymbol{A}$ and $\boldsymbol{C}$ are known matrices, and $\boldsymbol{B}$ and $\boldsymbol{\Sigma}$ are unknown parameter matrices.

The condition $r(\boldsymbol{C}) + p \leq n$ is an estimability condition when $\boldsymbol{\Sigma}$ is unknown. However, for ease of presentation in this section, it is assumed that the dispersion matrix $\boldsymbol{\Sigma}$ is known. The idea is to give a general overview and leave many details for the subsequent sections.

For the likelihood, $L(\boldsymbol{B})$, we have

$$L(\boldsymbol{B}) \propto |\boldsymbol{\Sigma}|^{-n/2} e^{-1/2\mathrm{tr}\{\boldsymbol{\Sigma}^{-1}(\boldsymbol{X}_o - \boldsymbol{ABC})(\boldsymbol{X}_o - \boldsymbol{ABC})'\}}.$$

From (2.16) it is seen that there exists a design matrix $\boldsymbol{A}$ which describes the expectation of the rows of $\boldsymbol{X}$ (a within-individuals design matrix), as well as a design matrix $\boldsymbol{C}$ which describes the mean of the columns of $\boldsymbol{X}$ (a between-individuals design matrix). It is known that if one pre- and post-multiplies a matrix, a bilinear transformation is performed. Thus, in a comparison of (1.7) and (2.16), instead of a linear model in (1.7), there is a bilinear one in (2.16). The previous techniques used when R^n was decomposed into $\mathcal{C}(\boldsymbol{C}') \boxplus \mathcal{C}(\boldsymbol{C}')^{\perp}$ are adopted; i.e. due to bilinearity the tensor product $R^p \otimes R^n$ is decomposed as

$$(\mathcal{C}(\boldsymbol{A}) \otimes \mathcal{C}(\boldsymbol{C}')) \boxplus (\mathcal{C}(\boldsymbol{A}) \otimes \mathcal{C}(\boldsymbol{C}')^{\perp}) \boxplus (\mathcal{C}(\boldsymbol{A})^{\perp} \otimes \mathcal{C}(\boldsymbol{C}')) \boxplus (\mathcal{C}(\boldsymbol{A})^{\perp} \otimes \mathcal{C}(\boldsymbol{C}')^{\perp}).$$

Let the projections $\boldsymbol{P}_{A,\Sigma} = \boldsymbol{A}(\boldsymbol{A}'\boldsymbol{\Sigma}^{-1}\boldsymbol{A})^{-}\boldsymbol{A}'\boldsymbol{\Sigma}^{-1}$ and $\boldsymbol{P}_{C'}$ be as before (see Appendix A, Sect. A.7). It appears that the likelihood can be decomposed as follows (omitting the proportionality constant $(2\pi)^{-np/2}$):

$$\begin{aligned} L(\boldsymbol{B}) \propto\, & |\boldsymbol{\Sigma}|^{-n/2}\exp\{-1/2\mathrm{tr}\{\boldsymbol{\Sigma}^{-1}\boldsymbol{P}_{A,\Sigma}(\boldsymbol{X}_o - \boldsymbol{ABC})(\boldsymbol{X}_o - \boldsymbol{ABC})'\boldsymbol{P}'_{A,\Sigma}\}\} \\ & \times\exp\{-1/2\mathrm{tr}\{\boldsymbol{\Sigma}^{-1}(\boldsymbol{I} - \boldsymbol{P}_{A,\Sigma})(\boldsymbol{X}_o - \boldsymbol{ABC})(\boldsymbol{X}_o - \boldsymbol{ABC})'(\boldsymbol{I} - \boldsymbol{P}'_{A,\Sigma})\}\}, \end{aligned}$$

since $(\boldsymbol{I} - \boldsymbol{P}'_{A,\Sigma})\boldsymbol{\Sigma}^{-1}\boldsymbol{P}_{A,\Sigma} = \boldsymbol{0}$. Thus, a decomposition of $\mathcal{R}^p$ into two orthogonal subspaces has been utilized. Continuing as in the linear case, i.e. using $\boldsymbol{P}_{C'}$ and $\boldsymbol{I} - \boldsymbol{P}_{C'}$, the following expression for the likelihood is obtained:

$$\begin{aligned} L(\boldsymbol{B}) \propto\, & |\boldsymbol{\Sigma}|^{-n/2}\exp\{-1/2\mathrm{tr}\{\boldsymbol{\Sigma}^{-1}\boldsymbol{P}_{A,\Sigma}(\boldsymbol{X}_o - \boldsymbol{ABC})\boldsymbol{P}_{C'}(\boldsymbol{X}_o - \boldsymbol{ABC})'\boldsymbol{P}'_{A,\Sigma}\}\} \\ & \times\exp\{-1/2\mathrm{tr}\{\boldsymbol{\Sigma}^{-1}\boldsymbol{P}_{A,\Sigma}(\boldsymbol{X}_o - \boldsymbol{ABC})(\boldsymbol{I} - \boldsymbol{P}_{C'})(\boldsymbol{X}_o - \boldsymbol{ABC})'\boldsymbol{P}'_{A,\Sigma}\}\} \\ & \times\exp\{-1/2\mathrm{tr}\{\boldsymbol{\Sigma}^{-1}(\boldsymbol{I} - \boldsymbol{P}_{A,\Sigma})(\boldsymbol{X}_o - \boldsymbol{ABC})\boldsymbol{P}_{C'}(\boldsymbol{X}_o - \boldsymbol{ABC})'(\boldsymbol{I} - \boldsymbol{P}'_{A,\Sigma})\}\} \\ & \times\exp\{-1/2\mathrm{tr}\{\boldsymbol{\Sigma}^{-1}(\boldsymbol{I} - \boldsymbol{P}_{A,\Sigma})(\boldsymbol{X}_o - \boldsymbol{ABC})(\boldsymbol{I} - \boldsymbol{P}_{C'})(\boldsymbol{X}_o - \boldsymbol{ABC})'(\boldsymbol{I} - \boldsymbol{P}'_{A,\Sigma})\}\}; \end{aligned}$$

i.e. the likelihood consists of four factors. Utilizing $(\boldsymbol{I} - \boldsymbol{P}_{A,\Sigma})\boldsymbol{A} = \boldsymbol{0}$ and $(\boldsymbol{I} - \boldsymbol{P}_{C'})\boldsymbol{C}' = \boldsymbol{0}$, this expression reduces to

$$
\begin{aligned}
L(\boldsymbol{B}) \propto |\boldsymbol{\Sigma}|^{-n/2}&\exp\{-1/2\mathrm{tr}\{\boldsymbol{\Sigma}^{-1}\boldsymbol{P}_{A,\Sigma}(\boldsymbol{X}_o - \boldsymbol{ABC})\boldsymbol{P}_{C'}(\boldsymbol{X}_o - \boldsymbol{ABC})'\boldsymbol{P}'_{A,\Sigma}\}\}\\
&\times\exp\{-1/2\mathrm{tr}\{\boldsymbol{\Sigma}^{-1}\boldsymbol{P}_{A,\Sigma}\boldsymbol{X}_o(\boldsymbol{I} - \boldsymbol{P}_{C'})\boldsymbol{X}'_o\boldsymbol{P}'_{A,\Sigma}\}\}\\
&\times\exp\{-1/2\mathrm{tr}\{\boldsymbol{\Sigma}^{-1}(\boldsymbol{I} - \boldsymbol{P}_{A,\Sigma})\boldsymbol{X}_o\boldsymbol{P}_{C'}\boldsymbol{X}'_o(\boldsymbol{I} - \boldsymbol{P}'_{A,\Sigma})\}\}\\
&\times\exp\{-1/2\mathrm{tr}\{\boldsymbol{\Sigma}^{-1}(\boldsymbol{I} - \boldsymbol{P}_{A,\Sigma})\boldsymbol{X}_o(\boldsymbol{I} - \boldsymbol{P}_{C'})\boldsymbol{X}'_o(\boldsymbol{I} - \boldsymbol{P}'_{A,\Sigma})\}\},
\end{aligned}
\tag{2.17}
$$

and only the first term involves the unknown parameter. Since $\boldsymbol{\Sigma}$ is supposed to be known, the maximum of the likelihood occurs when

$$
\begin{aligned}
\boldsymbol{A}\widehat{\boldsymbol{B}}_o\boldsymbol{C} &= \boldsymbol{P}_{A,\Sigma}\boldsymbol{X}_o\boldsymbol{P}_{C'}\\
&= \boldsymbol{A}(\boldsymbol{A}'\boldsymbol{\Sigma}^{-1}\boldsymbol{A})^{-}\boldsymbol{A}'\boldsymbol{\Sigma}^{-1}\boldsymbol{X}_o\boldsymbol{C}'(\boldsymbol{C}\boldsymbol{C}')^{-}\boldsymbol{C},
\end{aligned}
\tag{2.18}
$$

because in (2.17) one term smaller than one cancels. If a vectorized form of the model had been used, i.e.

$$
\mathrm{vec}\boldsymbol{X} = (\boldsymbol{C}' \otimes \boldsymbol{A})\mathrm{vec}\boldsymbol{B} + e, \quad e \sim N_{pn}(\boldsymbol{0}, \boldsymbol{I} \otimes \boldsymbol{\Sigma}),
$$

we would have obtained, applying standard linear models theory, the estimator given in Sect. 2.2, which is a BLUE (best linear unbiased estimator). In the next section the "real" case when $\boldsymbol{\Sigma}$ is unknown will be considered. The decomposition of $\mathcal{R}^p \otimes \mathcal{R}^n$ when estimating the parameters is illustrated in Fig. 2.6.

Note that $\mathcal{C}_\Sigma(\boldsymbol{A})$ means that the inner product is defined through $\boldsymbol{\Sigma}^{-1}$; i.e. take any two vectors $\boldsymbol{x}$ and $\boldsymbol{y}$ from $\mathcal{C}_\Sigma(\boldsymbol{A})$ and then the inner product is defined by the operation $\boldsymbol{x}'\boldsymbol{\Sigma}^{-1}\boldsymbol{y}$. When $\boldsymbol{A}\widehat{\boldsymbol{B}}\boldsymbol{C}$ is estimated, $\boldsymbol{X}$ is projected on the tensor space $\mathcal{C}_\Sigma(\boldsymbol{A}) \otimes \mathcal{C}(\boldsymbol{C}')$. If $\mathcal{C}_\Sigma(\boldsymbol{A})$ is the whole space, $\boldsymbol{P}_A = \boldsymbol{I}$, which for example takes

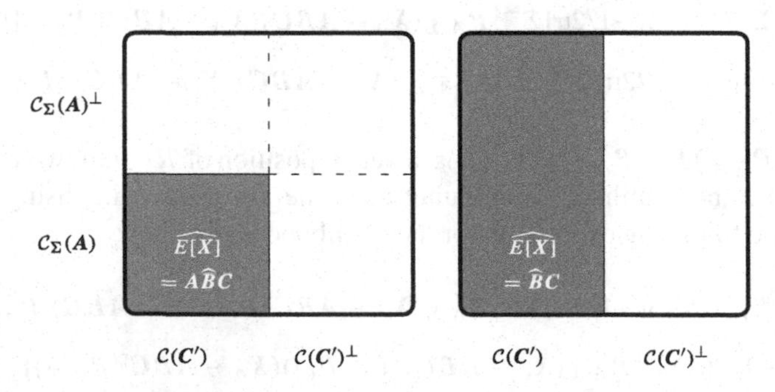

Fig. 2.6 Decomposition of the whole space according to the within-individuals and between-individuals designs, illustrating the mean and residual spaces in the BRM, and a comparison with the multivariate linear model (MANOVA)

place when $\boldsymbol{A}$: $p \times p$ is non-singular. Moreover, in Fig. 2.6, $\mathcal{C}_\Sigma(\boldsymbol{A})^\perp$ stands for the space where any element, let us say $\boldsymbol{u}$, satisfies $\boldsymbol{u}'\boldsymbol{\Sigma}^{-1}\boldsymbol{A} = \boldsymbol{0}$.

2.5 $EBRM_B^m$ with a Known Dispersion Matrix

In Sect. 1.5 two extensions of the BRM were presented, i.e. the $EBRM_B^m$ and $EBRM_W^m$, together with examples of the application of these models. In this section the reader is introduced to the mathematics concerning the $EBRM_B^m$, with $m = 3$, which will also be used later when studying the model without a known dispersion matrix. Now (2.16) is formally generalized and the $EBRM_B^m$ is specified in detail.

Definition 2.2 ($EBRM_B^m$) Let $\boldsymbol{X}$: $p \times n$, $\boldsymbol{A}_i : p \times q_i$, $q_i \leq p$, $\boldsymbol{B}_i$: $q_i \times k_i$, $\boldsymbol{C}_i$: $k_i \times n$, $i = 1, 2, \ldots, m$, $r(\boldsymbol{C}_1) + p \leq n$, $\mathcal{C}(\boldsymbol{C}_i') \subseteq \mathcal{C}(\boldsymbol{C}_{i-1}')$, $i = 2, 3, \ldots, m$, and $\boldsymbol{\Sigma}$: $p \times p$ be p.d. Then

$$\boldsymbol{X} = \sum_{i=1}^{m} \boldsymbol{A}_i\boldsymbol{B}_i\boldsymbol{C}_i + \boldsymbol{E} \tag{2.19}$$

defines the $EBRM_B^m$, where $\boldsymbol{E} \sim N_{p,n}(\boldsymbol{0}, \boldsymbol{\Sigma}, \boldsymbol{I})$, $\{\boldsymbol{A}_i\}$ and $\{\boldsymbol{C}_i\}$ are known matrices, and $\{\boldsymbol{B}_i\}$ and $\boldsymbol{\Sigma}$ are unknown parameter matrices.

In the present book it is usually assumed that $m = 2, 3$, and in this section $\boldsymbol{\Sigma}$ is supposed to be known. In that case, $r(\boldsymbol{C}_1) + p \leq n$, $\mathcal{C}(\boldsymbol{C}_i') \subseteq \mathcal{C}(\boldsymbol{C}_{i-1}')$, $i = 2, 3, \ldots, m$ are not needed when estimating $\boldsymbol{B}_i$. However, since the results from this chapter will be utilized in the next chapter, it is assumed that $\mathcal{C}(\boldsymbol{C}_i') \subseteq \mathcal{C}(\boldsymbol{C}_{i-1}')$, $i = 2, 3, \ldots, m$, holds. Thus, the following model will be handled:

$$\boldsymbol{X} = \boldsymbol{A}_1\boldsymbol{B}_1\boldsymbol{C}_1 + \boldsymbol{A}_2\boldsymbol{B}_2\boldsymbol{C}_2 + \boldsymbol{A}_3\boldsymbol{B}_3\boldsymbol{C}_3 + \boldsymbol{E}, \quad \boldsymbol{E} \sim N_{p,n}(\boldsymbol{0}, \boldsymbol{\Sigma}, \boldsymbol{I}), \tag{2.20}$$

where $\mathcal{C}(\boldsymbol{C}_3') \subseteq \mathcal{C}(\boldsymbol{C}_2') \subseteq \mathcal{C}(\boldsymbol{C}_1')$, $\boldsymbol{A}_i$: $p \times q_i$, the parameter $\boldsymbol{B}_i : p \times q_i$, is unknown, $\boldsymbol{C}_i : k_i \times n$ and the dispersion matrix $\boldsymbol{\Sigma}$ is supposed to be known. It has already been noted in Sect. 1.5 that without the subspace condition on $\mathcal{C}(\boldsymbol{C}_i)$, we would have the general "sum of profiles model" (a multivariate seemingly unrelated regression (SUR) model). Later (2.20) is studied when $\mathcal{C}(\boldsymbol{A}_3) \subseteq \mathcal{C}(\boldsymbol{A}_2) \subseteq \mathcal{C}(\boldsymbol{A}_1)$ replaces $\mathcal{C}(\boldsymbol{C}_3') \subseteq \mathcal{C}(\boldsymbol{C}_2') \subseteq \mathcal{C}(\boldsymbol{C}_1')$, i.e. we have an $EBRM_W^3$. Since the model under the assumption $\mathcal{C}(\boldsymbol{A}_3) \subseteq \mathcal{C}(\boldsymbol{A}_2) \subseteq \mathcal{C}(\boldsymbol{A}_1)$ through a reparametrization can be converted to (2.20) and vice versa, i.e. $EBRM_B^3 \rightleftarrows EBRM_W^3$, the models are in some sense equivalent. However, because of non-linearity in estimators of mean parameters, this does not imply that all the results for the models can easily be transferred from one model to the other.

From now on, under the nested subspace condition $\mathcal{C}(\boldsymbol{C}_3') \subseteq \mathcal{C}(\boldsymbol{C}_2') \subseteq \mathcal{C}(\boldsymbol{C}_1')$, MLEs will be derived when $\boldsymbol{\Sigma} > 0$ is known. The likelihood is proportional to

$$|\boldsymbol{\Sigma}|^{-n/2}\exp\{-1/2\mathrm{tr}\{\boldsymbol{\Sigma}^{-1}(\boldsymbol{X}_o - E[\boldsymbol{X}])()'\}\}, \tag{2.21}$$

where $E[\boldsymbol{X}] = \boldsymbol{A}_1\boldsymbol{B}_1\boldsymbol{C}_1 + \boldsymbol{A}_2\boldsymbol{B}_2\boldsymbol{C}_2 + \boldsymbol{A}_3\boldsymbol{B}_3\boldsymbol{C}_3$. A chain consisting of three links of relatively straightforward calculations involving the trace function will start. The calculations will involve the following three basic quantities:

$$\boldsymbol{S}_1 = \boldsymbol{X}_o(\boldsymbol{I} - \boldsymbol{P}_{C_1'})\boldsymbol{X}_o', \tag{2.22}$$

$$\boldsymbol{P}_{A_1^o,\Sigma^{-1}} = \boldsymbol{A}_1^o(\boldsymbol{A}_1^{o\prime}\boldsymbol{\Sigma}\boldsymbol{A}_1^o)^-\boldsymbol{A}_1^{o\prime}\boldsymbol{\Sigma}, \tag{2.23}$$

$$\boldsymbol{P}_{A_1,\Sigma} = \boldsymbol{A}_1(\boldsymbol{A}_1'\boldsymbol{\Sigma}^{-1}\boldsymbol{A}_1)^-\boldsymbol{A}_1'\boldsymbol{\Sigma}^{-1}. \tag{2.24}$$

For notational convenience $\boldsymbol{Q}_1 = \boldsymbol{P}_{A_1^o,\Sigma^{-1}}$ and $\boldsymbol{P}_1 = \boldsymbol{P}_{A_1,\Sigma}$ will be used. Note that $\boldsymbol{S}_1$ is positive definite with probability 1 and both $\boldsymbol{Q}_1$ and $\boldsymbol{P}_1$ are projectors which are related, i.e. $\boldsymbol{P}_1 = \boldsymbol{I} - \boldsymbol{Q}_1'$ (see Appendix B, Theorem B.11 (v)). Thus,

$$\mathrm{tr}\{\boldsymbol{\Sigma}^{-1}(\boldsymbol{X}_o - E[\boldsymbol{X}])()'\} = \mathrm{tr}\{\boldsymbol{\Sigma}^{-1}\boldsymbol{S}_1\} + \mathrm{tr}\{\boldsymbol{\Sigma}^{-1}(\boldsymbol{X}_o\boldsymbol{P}_{C_1'} - E[\boldsymbol{X}])()'\}$$

(because $\mathcal{C}(\boldsymbol{C}_3') \subseteq \mathcal{C}(\boldsymbol{C}_2') \subseteq \mathcal{C}(\boldsymbol{C}_1')$)

$$= \mathrm{tr}\{\boldsymbol{\Sigma}^{-1}\boldsymbol{S}_1\} + \mathrm{tr}\{(\boldsymbol{X}_o\boldsymbol{P}_{C_1'} - E[\boldsymbol{X}])'\boldsymbol{\Sigma}^{-1}(\boldsymbol{X}_o\boldsymbol{P}_{C_1'} - E[\boldsymbol{X}])\}$$

(because $\mathrm{tr}(\boldsymbol{U}\boldsymbol{V}) = \mathrm{tr}(\boldsymbol{V}\boldsymbol{U})$)

$$= \mathrm{tr}\{\boldsymbol{\Sigma}^{-1}\boldsymbol{S}_1\} + \mathrm{tr}\{(\boldsymbol{X}_o\boldsymbol{P}_{C_1'} - E[\boldsymbol{X}])'\boldsymbol{\Sigma}^{-1}\boldsymbol{P}_1(\boldsymbol{X}_o\boldsymbol{P}_{C_1'} - E[\boldsymbol{X}])\}$$
$$+\mathrm{tr}\{(\boldsymbol{X}_o\boldsymbol{P}_{C_1'} - E[\boldsymbol{X}])'\boldsymbol{Q}_1\boldsymbol{\Sigma}^{-1}(\boldsymbol{X}_o\boldsymbol{P}_{C_1'} - E[\boldsymbol{X}])\}$$

(because $\boldsymbol{Q}_1\boldsymbol{\Sigma}^{-1} + \boldsymbol{\Sigma}^{-1}\boldsymbol{P}_1 = \boldsymbol{\Sigma}^{-1}$) (see Appendix B, Theorem B.11 (v))

$$\geq \mathrm{tr}\{\boldsymbol{\Sigma}^{-1}\boldsymbol{S}_1\} + \mathrm{tr}\{(\boldsymbol{X}_o\boldsymbol{P}_{C_1'} - E[\boldsymbol{X}])'\boldsymbol{Q}_1\boldsymbol{\Sigma}^{-1}\boldsymbol{Q}_1'(\boldsymbol{X}_o\boldsymbol{P}_{C_1'} - E[\boldsymbol{X}])\}$$

(because $\boldsymbol{Q}_1\boldsymbol{\Sigma}^{-1} = \boldsymbol{Q}_1\boldsymbol{\Sigma}^{-1}\boldsymbol{Q}_1'$)

$$= \mathrm{tr}\{\boldsymbol{\Sigma}^{-1}\boldsymbol{S}_1\} + \mathrm{tr}\{\boldsymbol{\Sigma}^{-1}(\boldsymbol{Q}_1'\boldsymbol{X}_o\boldsymbol{P}_{C_1'} - E[\boldsymbol{Q}_1'\boldsymbol{X}])()'\} \tag{2.25}$$

(because $\mathrm{tr}(\boldsymbol{U}\boldsymbol{V}) = \mathrm{tr}(\boldsymbol{V}\boldsymbol{U})$).

Note that $E[\boldsymbol{Q}_1'\boldsymbol{X}] = \boldsymbol{Q}_1'\boldsymbol{A}_2\boldsymbol{B}_2\boldsymbol{C}_2 + \boldsymbol{Q}_1'\boldsymbol{A}_3\boldsymbol{B}_3\boldsymbol{C}_3$; i.e. the parameter $\boldsymbol{B}_1$ has been excluded (filtered) and thereby the number of parameters has been reduced. Equality holds in (2.25) if and only if

$$\boldsymbol{A}_1'\boldsymbol{\Sigma}^{-1}(\boldsymbol{X}_o\boldsymbol{P}_{C_1'} - \boldsymbol{A}_1\boldsymbol{B}_1\boldsymbol{C}_1 - \boldsymbol{A}_2\boldsymbol{B}_2\boldsymbol{C}_2 - \boldsymbol{A}_3\boldsymbol{B}_3\boldsymbol{C}_3) = \boldsymbol{0}, \tag{2.26}$$

and this expression will later be used in order to determine $\widehat{B}_1$. When continuing, the calculations which started with (2.22) will be repeated, but now using matrices which have been projected on $\mathcal{C}(A_1)^{\perp}$. Put

$$S_2 = S_1 + Q_1'X_oP_{C_1'}(I - P_{C_2'})P_{C_1'}X_o'Q_1, \tag{2.27}$$

$$Q_2 = P_{(Q_1'A_2)^o,\Sigma^{-1}} = (Q_1'A_2)^o((Q_1'A_2)^{o'}\Sigma(Q_1'A_2)^o)^-(Q_1'A_2)^{o'}\Sigma, \tag{2.28}$$

$$P_2 = P_{Q_1'A_2,\Sigma} = Q_1'A_2(A_2'Q_1\Sigma^{-1}Q_1'A_2)^-A_2'Q_1\Sigma^{-1} \tag{2.29}$$

and then continuing from (2.25), as well as repeating the arguments used in (2.25), yields

$$\begin{aligned}
&\mathrm{tr}\{\Sigma^{-1}S_2\} + \mathrm{tr}\{(Q_1'X_oP_{C_2'} - E[Q_1'X])'\Sigma^{-1}(Q_1'X_oP_{C_2'} - E[Q_1'X])\}\\
&= \mathrm{tr}\{\Sigma^{-1}S_2\} + \mathrm{tr}\{(Q_1'X_oP_{C_2'} - E[Q_1'X])'\Sigma^{-1}P_2(Q_1'X_oP_{C_2'} - E[Q_1'X])\}\\
&\quad +\mathrm{tr}\{(Q_1'X_oP_{C_2'} - E[Q_1'X])'Q_2\Sigma^{-1}(Q_1'X_oP_{C_2'} - E[Q_1'X])\}\\
&\geq \mathrm{tr}\{\Sigma^{-1}S_2\} + \mathrm{tr}\{(Q_1'X_oP_{C_2'} - E[Q_1'X])'Q_2\Sigma^{-1}Q_2(Q_1'X_oP_{C_2'} - E[Q_1'X])\}\\
&= \mathrm{tr}\{\Sigma^{-1}S_2\} + \mathrm{tr}\{\Sigma^{-1}(Q_2'Q_1'X_oP_{C_2'} - E[Q_2'Q_1'X])()'\}.
\end{aligned} \tag{2.30}$$

Equality holds in (2.30) if and only if

$$A_2'Q_1\Sigma^{-1}(Q_1'X_oP_{C_2'} - Q_1'A_2B_2C_2 - Q_1'A_3B_3C_3) = 0. \tag{2.31}$$

Moreover, since in (2.30) $E[Q_2'Q_1'X] = Q_2'Q_1'A_3B_3C_3$, we have in two steps reduced the $EBRM_B^3$ to a BRM. Let

$$S_3 = S_2 + Q_2'Q_1'X_oP_{C_2'}(I - P_{C_3'})P_{C_2'}X_o'Q_1Q_2, \tag{2.32}$$

$$Q_3 = P_{(Q_2'Q_1'A_3)^o,\Sigma^{-1}} = (Q_2'Q_1'A_3)^o((Q_2'Q_1'A_3)^{o'}\Sigma(Q_2'Q_1'A_3)^o)^-(Q_2'Q_1'A_3)^{o'}\Sigma, \tag{2.33}$$

$$P_3 = P_{Q_2'Q_1'A_3,\Sigma} = Q_2'Q_1'A_3(A_3'Q_1Q_2\Sigma^{-1}Q_2'Q_1'A_3)^-A_3'Q_1Q_2\Sigma^{-1} \tag{2.34}$$

and then advancing from (2.30) yields

$$\begin{aligned}
&\mathrm{tr}\{\Sigma^{-1}S_3\} + \mathrm{tr}\{(Q_2'Q_1'X_oP_{C_3'} - E[Q_2'Q_1'X])'\Sigma^{-1}(Q_2'Q_1'X_oP_{C_3'} - E[Q_2'Q_1'X])\}\\
&= \mathrm{tr}\{\Sigma^{-1}S_3\}\\
&\quad +\mathrm{tr}\{(Q_2'Q_1'X_oP_{C_3'} - E[Q_2'Q_1'X])'\Sigma^{-1}P_3(Q_2'Q_1'X_oP_{C_3'} - E[Q_2'Q_1'X])\}\\
&\quad +\mathrm{tr}\{(Q_2'Q_1'X_oP_{C_3'} - E[Q_2'Q_1'X])'Q_3\Sigma^{-1}(Q_2'Q_1'X_oP_{C_3'} - E[Q_2'Q_1'X])\}
\end{aligned}$$

$$
\begin{aligned}
&\geq \mathrm{tr}\{\boldsymbol{\Sigma}^{-1}\boldsymbol{S}_3\} + \mathrm{tr}\{(\boldsymbol{Q}_2'\boldsymbol{Q}_1'\boldsymbol{X}_o\boldsymbol{P}_{C_1'})'\boldsymbol{Q}_3\boldsymbol{\Sigma}^{-1}\boldsymbol{Q}_3'(\boldsymbol{Q}_2'\boldsymbol{Q}_1'\boldsymbol{X}_o\boldsymbol{P}_{C_1'})\}\\
&= \mathrm{tr}\{\boldsymbol{\Sigma}^{-1}\boldsymbol{S}_3\} + \mathrm{tr}\{\boldsymbol{\Sigma}^{-1}\boldsymbol{Q}_3'\boldsymbol{Q}_2'\boldsymbol{Q}_1'\boldsymbol{X}_o\boldsymbol{P}_{C_3'}\boldsymbol{X}_o'\boldsymbol{Q}_1\boldsymbol{Q}_2\boldsymbol{Q}_3\} \qquad (2.35)
\end{aligned}
$$

with equality if and only if

$$
\boldsymbol{A}_3'\boldsymbol{Q}_1\boldsymbol{Q}_2\boldsymbol{\Sigma}^{-1}(\boldsymbol{Q}_2'\boldsymbol{Q}_1'\boldsymbol{X}_o\boldsymbol{P}_{C_3'} - \boldsymbol{Q}_2'\boldsymbol{Q}_1'\boldsymbol{A}_3\boldsymbol{B}_3\boldsymbol{C}_3) = \mathbf{0}. \qquad (2.36)
$$

It follows that the last line in (2.35) is independent of the parameters $\boldsymbol{B}_i, i = 1, 2, 3$, and if we can find estimators of $\boldsymbol{B}_i$ so that the lower bound is obtained, we have found the MLEs.

From the above-presented chain of calculations, it follows from (2.26), (2.31) and (2.36) that three linear equations in three unknown parameters appear which then have to be solved. This means that if we can find solutions to these equations, the lower bound given in (2.35) can be attained. Thus we have to verify the existence of a solution. From (2.36) it follows that

$$
\mathcal{C}(\boldsymbol{A}_3'\boldsymbol{Q}_1\boldsymbol{Q}_2\boldsymbol{\Sigma}^{-1}\boldsymbol{Q}_2'\boldsymbol{Q}_1'\boldsymbol{X}_o\boldsymbol{P}_{C_3'}) \subseteq \mathcal{C}(\boldsymbol{A}_3'\boldsymbol{Q}_1\boldsymbol{Q}_2\boldsymbol{\Sigma}^{-1}\boldsymbol{Q}_2'\boldsymbol{Q}_1'\boldsymbol{A}_3) = \mathcal{C}(\boldsymbol{A}_3'\boldsymbol{Q}_1\boldsymbol{Q}_2)
$$

and thus there always exists a $\widehat{\boldsymbol{B}}_3$ (see Appendix B, Theorem B.10 (ii)). Moreover, for (2.31) there is a solution with respect to $\boldsymbol{B}_2$ if and only if

$$
\mathcal{C}(\boldsymbol{A}_2'\boldsymbol{Q}_1\boldsymbol{\Sigma}^{-1}\boldsymbol{Q}_1'(\boldsymbol{X}_o\boldsymbol{P}_{C_2'} - \boldsymbol{A}_3\boldsymbol{B}_3\boldsymbol{C}_3)) \subseteq \mathcal{C}(\boldsymbol{A}_2'\boldsymbol{Q}_1)
$$

holds, which is always true, and finally (2.26) implies that a solution with respect to $\boldsymbol{B}_3$ exists if and only if

$$
\mathcal{C}(\boldsymbol{A}_1\boldsymbol{\Sigma}^{-1}(\boldsymbol{X}_o\boldsymbol{P}_{C_1'} - \boldsymbol{A}_2\boldsymbol{B}_2\boldsymbol{C}_2 - \boldsymbol{A}_3\boldsymbol{B}_3\boldsymbol{C}_3)) \subseteq \mathcal{C}(\boldsymbol{A}_1),
$$

which also is trivially true. Thus there exists at least one solution. To estimate $\boldsymbol{B}_i$, $i = 1, 2, 3$, uniquely, we need conditions on $\mathcal{C}(\boldsymbol{A}_i)$, $i = 1, 2, 3$, which will be considered in Chap. 4. However, the general mean $E[\boldsymbol{X}]$ can always be uniquely estimated:

$$
\begin{aligned}
\widehat{E[\boldsymbol{X}]} &= \boldsymbol{A}_1\widehat{\boldsymbol{B}}_{10}\boldsymbol{C}_1 + \boldsymbol{A}_2\widehat{\boldsymbol{B}}_{20}\boldsymbol{C}_2 + \boldsymbol{A}_3\widehat{\boldsymbol{B}}_{30}\boldsymbol{C}_3\\
&= \boldsymbol{P}_1\boldsymbol{X}_o\boldsymbol{P}_{C_1'} + (\boldsymbol{I} - \boldsymbol{P}_1)(\boldsymbol{A}_2\widehat{\boldsymbol{B}}_{20}\boldsymbol{C}_2 + \boldsymbol{A}_3\widehat{\boldsymbol{B}}_{30}\boldsymbol{C}_3)\\
&= \boldsymbol{P}_1\boldsymbol{X}_o\boldsymbol{P}_{C_1'} + \boldsymbol{Q}_1'(\boldsymbol{A}_2\widehat{\boldsymbol{B}}_{20}\boldsymbol{C}_2 + \boldsymbol{A}_3\widehat{\boldsymbol{B}}_{30}\boldsymbol{C}_3)\\
&= \boldsymbol{P}_1\boldsymbol{X}_o\boldsymbol{P}_{C_1'} + \boldsymbol{P}_2\boldsymbol{Q}_1'\boldsymbol{X}_o\boldsymbol{P}_{C_2'} + \boldsymbol{Q}_2'\boldsymbol{Q}_1'\boldsymbol{A}_3\widehat{\boldsymbol{B}}_{30}\boldsymbol{C}_3\\
&= \boldsymbol{P}_1\boldsymbol{X}_o\boldsymbol{P}_{C_1'} + \boldsymbol{P}_2\boldsymbol{Q}_1'\boldsymbol{X}_o\boldsymbol{P}_{C_2'} + \boldsymbol{P}_3\boldsymbol{Q}_2'\boldsymbol{Q}_1'\boldsymbol{X}_o\boldsymbol{P}_{C_3'}. \qquad (2.37)
\end{aligned}
$$

In order to understand $\widehat{E[\boldsymbol{X}]}$, as well as the calculations leading to the final expression, it is of interest to note that calculations constitute projections of observations. Therefore, it is informative to know which spaces the observations are projected onto. Moreover, since $\boldsymbol{\Sigma}$ is known, standard linear models theory (see Sect. 2.2) implies that $\widehat{E[\boldsymbol{X}]}$ should be expressed through a projector. Therefore, the projectors $\boldsymbol{P}_1$, $\boldsymbol{P}_2$ and $\boldsymbol{P}_3$ will be exploited. To establish that $\boldsymbol{P}_1$, $\boldsymbol{P}_2$ and $\boldsymbol{P}_3$ are projectors, straightforward calculations show that each of the three matrices is idempotent. From (2.23) it follows that

$$\mathcal{C}(\boldsymbol{P}_1) = \mathcal{C}(\boldsymbol{A}_1),$$

and using (2.29) and the projection theorem (Appendix B, Theorem B.11 (iv)) yields

$$\mathcal{C}(\boldsymbol{P}_2) = \mathcal{C}(\boldsymbol{Q}_1'\boldsymbol{A}_2) = \mathcal{C}(\boldsymbol{\Sigma}\boldsymbol{A}_1^o) \cap (\mathcal{C}(\boldsymbol{A}_1) + \mathcal{C}(\boldsymbol{A}_2)) = \mathcal{C}_\Sigma(\boldsymbol{A}_1)^\perp \cap (\mathcal{C}_\Sigma(\boldsymbol{A}_1 : \boldsymbol{A}_2)). \quad (2.38)$$

Moreover, (2.34) implies

$$\mathcal{C}(\boldsymbol{P}_3) = \mathcal{C}(\boldsymbol{Q}_2'\boldsymbol{Q}_1'\boldsymbol{A}_3) = \mathcal{C}(\boldsymbol{\Sigma}(\boldsymbol{Q}_1'\boldsymbol{A}_2)^o) \cap (\mathcal{C}(\boldsymbol{Q}_1'\boldsymbol{A}_2) + \mathcal{C}(\boldsymbol{Q}_1'\boldsymbol{A}_3))$$

(because of the projection theorem, i.e. Appendix B, Theorem B.11 (iv))

$$= \mathcal{C}(\boldsymbol{\Sigma}(\boldsymbol{Q}_1'\boldsymbol{A}_2)^o) \cap \mathcal{C}(\boldsymbol{Q}_1') \cap (\mathcal{C}(\boldsymbol{A}_1 : \boldsymbol{A}_2 : \boldsymbol{A}_3)$$

(because of the projection theorem, i.e. Appendix B, Theorem B.11 (iv), and (2.38))

$$= (\mathcal{C}(\boldsymbol{A}_1) + \mathcal{C}(\boldsymbol{\Sigma}(\boldsymbol{A}_1 : \boldsymbol{A}_2)^o)) \cap \mathcal{C}(\boldsymbol{\Sigma}\boldsymbol{A}_1^o) \cap (\mathcal{C}(\boldsymbol{A}_1 : \boldsymbol{A}_2 : \boldsymbol{A}_3)$$
$$= (\mathcal{C}(\boldsymbol{A}_1) \cap \mathcal{C}(\boldsymbol{\Sigma}\boldsymbol{A}_1^o) + \mathcal{C}(\boldsymbol{\Sigma}(\boldsymbol{A}_1 : \boldsymbol{A}_2)^o)) \cap \mathcal{C}(\boldsymbol{A}_1 : \boldsymbol{A}_2 : \boldsymbol{A}_3)$$

(through application of the modular identity, see Appendix B, Theorem B.3 (iv))

$$= \mathcal{C}(\boldsymbol{\Sigma}(\boldsymbol{A}_1 : \boldsymbol{A}_2)^o) \cap \mathcal{C}(\boldsymbol{A}_1 : \boldsymbol{A}_2 : \boldsymbol{A}_3)$$

(because $\mathcal{C}(\boldsymbol{A}_1) \cap \mathcal{C}(\boldsymbol{\Sigma}\boldsymbol{A}_1^o) = \{\boldsymbol{0}\}$)

$$= \mathcal{C}_\Sigma(\boldsymbol{A}_1 : \boldsymbol{A}_2)^\perp \cap \mathcal{C}_\Sigma(\boldsymbol{A}_1 : \boldsymbol{A}_2 : \boldsymbol{A}_3).$$

Note that these relations imply that $\boldsymbol{P}_2\boldsymbol{Q}_1' = \boldsymbol{P}_2$ and $\boldsymbol{P}_3\boldsymbol{Q}_2'\boldsymbol{Q}_1' = \boldsymbol{P}_3$, which means that instead of (2.37),

$$\widehat{E[\boldsymbol{X}]} = \boldsymbol{P}_1\boldsymbol{X}_o\boldsymbol{P}_{C_1'} + \boldsymbol{P}_2\boldsymbol{X}_o\boldsymbol{P}_{C_2'} + \boldsymbol{P}_3\boldsymbol{X}_o\boldsymbol{P}_{C_3'}. \quad (2.39)$$

Furthermore, when the inner product is defined via $\boldsymbol{\Sigma}$, the projectors $\boldsymbol{P}_1$, $\boldsymbol{P}_2$ and $\boldsymbol{P}_3$ project onto orthogonal subspaces. Thus, there is enough information to generalize Figs. 2.3 and 2.6 so that the $EBRM_B^3$ can also be described graphically, for example as in Fig. 2.7.

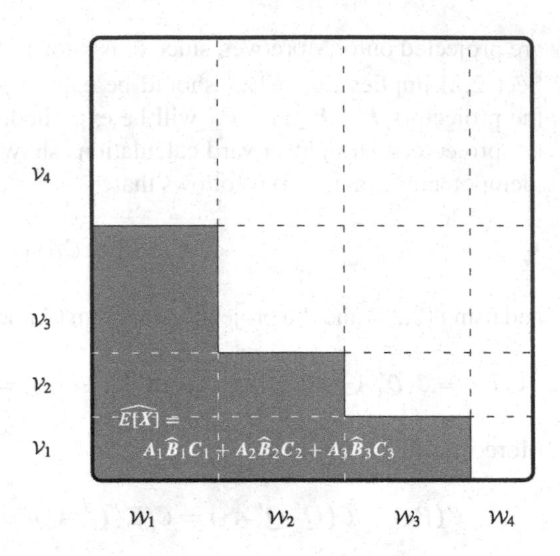

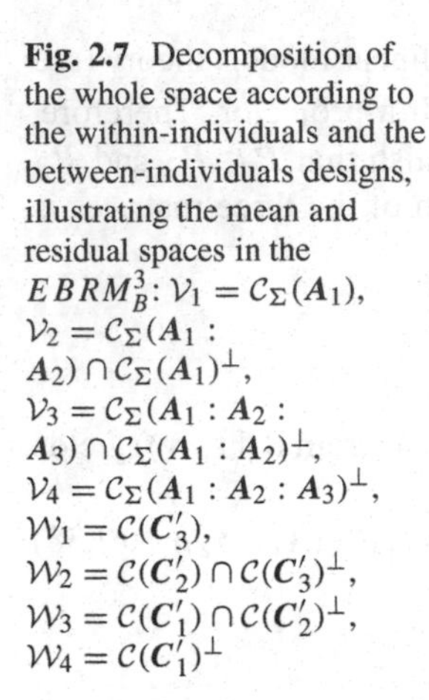
Fig. 2.7 Decomposition of the whole space according to the within-individuals and the between-individuals designs, illustrating the mean and residual spaces in the $EBRM_B^3$: $\mathcal{V}_1 = \mathcal{C}_\Sigma(\boldsymbol{A}_1)$, $\mathcal{V}_2 = \mathcal{C}_\Sigma(\boldsymbol{A}_1 : \boldsymbol{A}_2) \cap \mathcal{C}_\Sigma(\boldsymbol{A}_1)^\perp$, $\mathcal{V}_3 = \mathcal{C}_\Sigma(\boldsymbol{A}_1 : \boldsymbol{A}_2 : \boldsymbol{A}_3) \cap \mathcal{C}_\Sigma(\boldsymbol{A}_1 : \boldsymbol{A}_2)^\perp$, $\mathcal{V}_4 = \mathcal{C}_\Sigma(\boldsymbol{A}_1 : \boldsymbol{A}_2 : \boldsymbol{A}_3)^\perp$, $\mathcal{W}_1 = \mathcal{C}(\boldsymbol{C}_3')$, $\mathcal{W}_2 = \mathcal{C}(\boldsymbol{C}_2') \cap \mathcal{C}(\boldsymbol{C}_3')^\perp$, $\mathcal{W}_3 = \mathcal{C}(\boldsymbol{C}_1') \cap \mathcal{C}(\boldsymbol{C}_2')^\perp$, $\mathcal{W}_4 = \mathcal{C}(\boldsymbol{C}_1')^\perp$

Note that in Fig. 2.7 the so-called stairs structure is indicated, which is a distinctive feature of the $EBRM_\bullet^\bullet$.

The estimation procedure for obtaining $\widehat{E[\boldsymbol{X}]}$ will now be graphically illustrated. The fact is that if one understands the link between Fig. 2.7 and the derivation of the maximum likelihood estimators, more general models can be treated and, for example, expressions for the $EBRM_B^m$ can be derived. Moreover, similar figures will be used when working with the $EBRM_W^3$. First it is noted that $\mathrm{vec}(E[\boldsymbol{X}])$ belongs to the mean space

$$(\mathcal{V}_1 \otimes (\mathcal{W}_1 \boxplus \mathcal{W}_1 \boxplus \mathcal{W}_1)) \boxplus (\mathcal{V}_2 \otimes (\mathcal{W}_1 \boxplus \mathcal{W}_1)) \boxplus (\mathcal{V}_3 \otimes \mathcal{W}_1);$$

the notation used here, including the definition of the subspaces, and the reasons for using the expressions employed follow from Fig. 2.7.

The estimation of the parameters follows a three-step procedure with a final updating of expressions. The process is illustrated in Figs. 2.8 and 2.9. Let $\mathcal{V}_i$ be as in Fig. 2.7. In the first step of the estimation procedure the tensor space $\mathcal{C}(\boldsymbol{C}_1') \otimes \mathcal{C}_\Sigma(\boldsymbol{I})$ is decomposed into two parts and the observation vector is projected on $\mathcal{C}(\boldsymbol{C}_1') \otimes \mathcal{V}_1$ and $\mathcal{C}(\boldsymbol{C}_1') \otimes (\mathcal{V}_2 \boxplus \mathcal{V}_3 \boxplus \mathcal{V}_4)$, via the projections $(\boldsymbol{P}_{C_1'} \otimes \boldsymbol{P}_1)\boldsymbol{x}_o$ and $(\boldsymbol{P}_{C_1'} \otimes \boldsymbol{Q}_1')\boldsymbol{x}_o$, where $\boldsymbol{P}_1$ and $\boldsymbol{Q}_1$ are defined by (2.24) and (2.23), and $\boldsymbol{x}_o = \mathrm{vec}\boldsymbol{X}_o$ (see Fig. 2.8). The projection $(\boldsymbol{P}_{C_1'} \otimes \boldsymbol{P}_1)\boldsymbol{x}_o$ is used for estimating $\boldsymbol{B}_1$ and one can, according to (2.26), express $\widehat{\boldsymbol{B}}_{1o}$ as a function of $\boldsymbol{B}_2$ and $\boldsymbol{B}_3$. Moreover, the second projection does not include $\boldsymbol{B}_1$, which is essential. Relative to $\boldsymbol{B}_1$ the second projection generates a residual space which is part of the total residual space (see Figs. 2.8 and 2.9). This space will be utilized when estimating $\boldsymbol{B}_2$ and $\boldsymbol{B}_3$. In Fig. 2.8, $\mathcal{P}_1$ symbolizes the projection.

In the second step the ideas from the first step are repeated and $\mathcal{C}(\boldsymbol{C}_2') \otimes (\mathcal{V}_2 \boxplus \mathcal{V}_3 \boxplus \mathcal{V}_4)$ is decomposed into two parts, $\mathcal{C}(\boldsymbol{C}_2') \otimes \mathcal{V}_2$ and $\mathcal{C}(\boldsymbol{C}_2') \otimes (\mathcal{V}_3 \boxplus \mathcal{V}_4)$. Therefore, $(\boldsymbol{P}_{C_2'} \otimes \boldsymbol{P}_2)(\boldsymbol{P}_{C_1'} \otimes \boldsymbol{Q}_1')\boldsymbol{x}_o$ and $(\boldsymbol{P}_{C_2'} \otimes \boldsymbol{Q}_2')(\boldsymbol{P}_{C_1'} \otimes \boldsymbol{Q}_1')\boldsymbol{x}_o$ will be utilized. However,

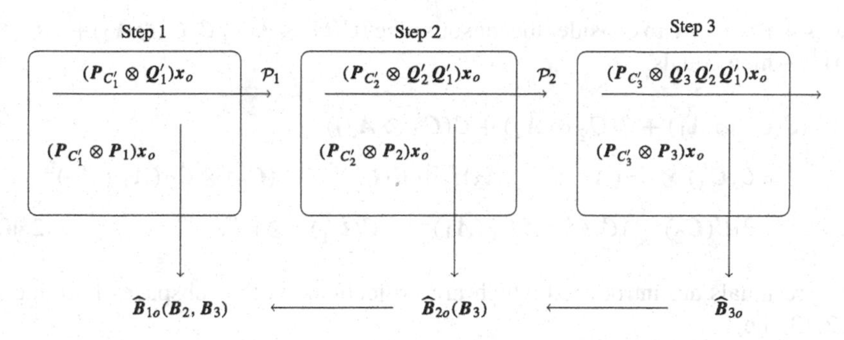

Backwards determination yields

$$\widehat{E[X]} = \sum_{i=1}^{3} A_i \widehat{B}_i C_i = P_1 X_o P_{C_1'} + P_2 X_o P_{C_2'} + P_3 X_o P_{C_3'}.$$

Fig. 2.8 Illustration of the various steps in the maximum likelihood estimation procedure. For details, the reader is referred to the text

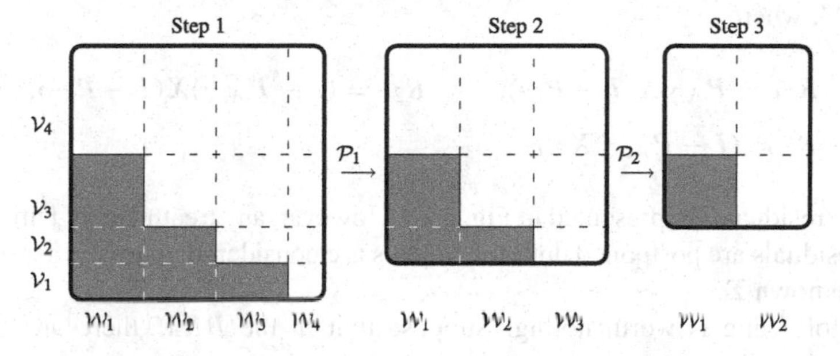

Fig. 2.9 Illustration of the steps when obtaining maximum likelihood estimators. For the notation see Fig. 2.7 and the text

$(P_{C_2'} \otimes P_2)(P_{C_1'} \otimes Q_1') = P_{C_2'} \otimes P_2$ and $(P_{C_2'} \otimes Q_2')(P_{C_1'} \otimes Q_1') = P_{C_2'} \otimes Q_2'Q_1'$. According to (2.31) and $P_{C_2'} \otimes P_2$, $\widehat{B}_{2o}$ can be expressed as a function of B_3. Moreover, the projection on the new residual space is in Fig. 2.8 indicated by $\mathcal{P}_2$.

In the third step $\mathcal{C}(C_3') \otimes (\mathcal{V}_2 \boxplus \mathcal{V}_3 \boxplus \mathcal{V}_4)$ is also decomposed into two parts and the part which is obtained from the projection $(P_{C_3'} \otimes P_3)x_o$ is used to estimate B_3. The explicit expression for $\widehat{B}_{3o}$ is obtained from (2.36). Since there are no more unknown parameters involved in $\widehat{B}_{3o}$, all the estimators can be found via a final backwards updating; i.e. $\widehat{B}_{3o}$ is used in (2.31) in order to find $\widehat{B}_{2o}$ and then $\widehat{B}_{3o}$ and $\widehat{B}_{2o}$ are used in (2.26).

So far we have only considered how to estimate the parameters of the model. The statistical paradigm, however, demands that methods for validating the $EBRM_B^m$ should be developed. Many natural methods are based on the exploration of residual spaces; i.e. we have to consider the tensor space $(\mathcal{C}(\boldsymbol{C}_1'\otimes\boldsymbol{A}_1)+\mathcal{C}(\boldsymbol{C}_2'\otimes\boldsymbol{A}_2)+\mathcal{C}(\boldsymbol{C}_3'\otimes\boldsymbol{A}_3))^\perp$, which equals

$$\begin{aligned}
&(\mathcal{C}(\boldsymbol{C}_1'\otimes\boldsymbol{A}_1)+\mathcal{C}(\boldsymbol{C}_2'\otimes\boldsymbol{A}_2)+\mathcal{C}(\boldsymbol{C}_3'\otimes\boldsymbol{A}_3))^\perp\\
&=\mathcal{C}(\boldsymbol{C}_3')\otimes\mathcal{C}_\Sigma(\boldsymbol{A}_1:\boldsymbol{A}_2:\boldsymbol{A}_3)^\perp\boxplus\mathcal{C}(\boldsymbol{C}_3')^\perp\cap\mathcal{C}(\boldsymbol{C}_2')\otimes\mathcal{C}_\Sigma(\boldsymbol{A}_1:\boldsymbol{A}_2)^\perp\\
&\boxplus\mathcal{C}(\boldsymbol{C}_2')^\perp\cap\mathcal{C}(\boldsymbol{C}_1')\otimes\mathcal{C}_\Sigma(\boldsymbol{A}_1)^\perp\boxplus\mathcal{C}(\boldsymbol{C}_1')^\perp\otimes\mathbb{R}^p.
\end{aligned}\tag{2.40}$$

Thus, residuals are introduced which are projections on the subspaces introduced in (2.40), i.e.

$$\boldsymbol{R}_1=\boldsymbol{X}(\boldsymbol{I}-\boldsymbol{P}_{C_1'}),\qquad \boldsymbol{R}_2=\boldsymbol{Q}_1'\boldsymbol{X}\boldsymbol{P}_{C_1'},$$
$$\boldsymbol{R}_3=\boldsymbol{Q}_2'\boldsymbol{Q}_1'\boldsymbol{X}\boldsymbol{P}_{C_2'},\qquad \boldsymbol{R}_4=\boldsymbol{Q}_3'\boldsymbol{Q}_2'\boldsymbol{Q}_1'\boldsymbol{X}\boldsymbol{P}_{C_3'}.$$

Indeed, a finer division of the subspaces can be performed and this is illustrated via the BRM, where

$$\boldsymbol{R}_{11}=\boldsymbol{P}_{A,\Sigma}\boldsymbol{X}(\boldsymbol{I}-\boldsymbol{P}_{C'}),\qquad \boldsymbol{R}_{21}=(\boldsymbol{I}-\boldsymbol{P}_{A,\Sigma})\boldsymbol{X}(\boldsymbol{I}-\boldsymbol{P}_{C'}),\tag{2.41}$$
$$\boldsymbol{R}_2=(\boldsymbol{I}-\boldsymbol{P}_{A,\Sigma})\boldsymbol{X}\boldsymbol{P}_{C'}.\tag{2.42}$$

All these residuals are presented in Fig. 2.10. However, any treatment and utilization of the residuals are postponed until the models are considered under the assumption of an unknown $\boldsymbol{\Sigma}$.

The following is worth noting. Suppose that in the BRM there are bilinear restrictions on the mean parameters, i.e.

$$E[\boldsymbol{X}]=\boldsymbol{ABC},\qquad \boldsymbol{FBG}=\boldsymbol{0},$$

where $\boldsymbol{F}$ and $\boldsymbol{G}$ are known matrices. Because $\boldsymbol{FBG}=\boldsymbol{0}$ forms a linear system of equations, the restriction $\boldsymbol{FBG}=\boldsymbol{0}$ can be reformulated as follows (see Appendix B, Theorem B.10 (i)):

$$\boldsymbol{B}=(\boldsymbol{F}')^o\boldsymbol{\Theta}_1+\boldsymbol{F}'\boldsymbol{\Theta}_2\boldsymbol{G}^{o'},$$

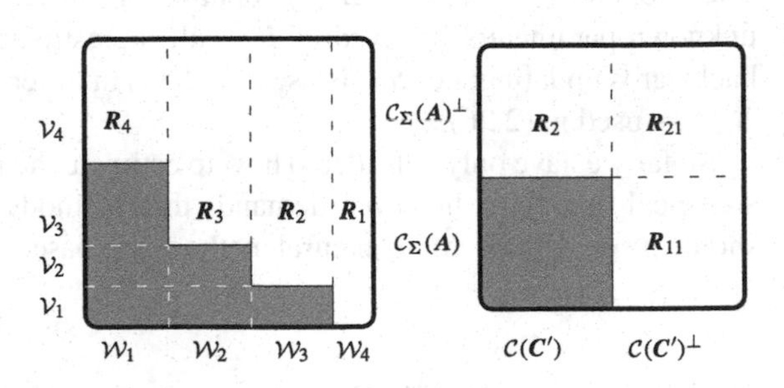

Fig. 2.10 Illustration of four residual spaces in the $EBRM_B^3$ and the three residual spaces in the BRM. For the notation see Fig. 2.7

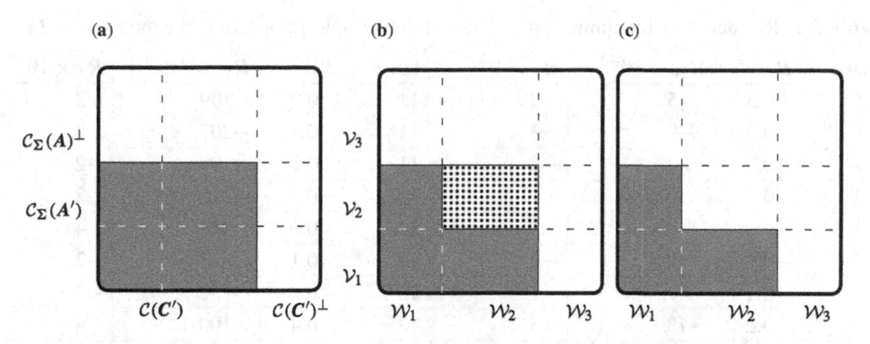

Fig. 2.11 In **(a)**, a BRM without restrictions is shown, in **(b)**, the area where $\boldsymbol{FBG} = \boldsymbol{0}$ may have an effect is illustrated and in **(c)**, $\boldsymbol{FBG} = \boldsymbol{0}$ holds, leading to a stairs structure, i.e. an $EBRM_B^2$. Furthermore, $\mathcal{V}_1 = \mathcal{C}_\Sigma(\boldsymbol{A}(\boldsymbol{F}')^o)$, $\mathcal{V}_2 = \mathcal{C}_\Sigma(\boldsymbol{A}) \cap \mathcal{C}_\Sigma(\boldsymbol{A}(\boldsymbol{F}')^o)^\perp$, $\mathcal{V}_3 = \mathcal{C}_\Sigma(\boldsymbol{A})^\perp$, $\mathcal{W}_1 = \mathcal{C}(\boldsymbol{C}'\boldsymbol{G}^o)$, $\mathcal{W}_2 = \mathcal{C}(\boldsymbol{C}') \cap \mathcal{C}(\boldsymbol{C}'\boldsymbol{G}^o)^\perp$ and $\mathcal{W}_3 = \mathcal{C}(\boldsymbol{C}')^\perp$

where $\boldsymbol{\Theta}_1$ and $\boldsymbol{\Theta}_2$ are new parameters. Thus the BRM with bilinear restrictions turns into an $EBRM_B^2$. This is illustrated in Fig. 2.11. Later in Chaps. 3 and 7 a complete theory is presented concerning how to estimate parameters and test hypotheses when bilinear restrictions exist.

This section is ended by briefly considering residuals for the liming data presented in Example 1.5.

Example 2.1 In Example 1.5, liming data for 20 Swedish lakes were presented. A BRM with $\boldsymbol{\Sigma} = \boldsymbol{I}_3$ and $\boldsymbol{A}$, given in Example 1.5, was applied and led to

$$\widehat{\boldsymbol{B}}_o = \begin{pmatrix} 7.09 & 7.03 \\ -0.03 & -0.04 \end{pmatrix}. \tag{2.43}$$

The residuals $\boldsymbol{R}_{11}$, $\boldsymbol{R}_{21}$ and $\boldsymbol{R}_2$ in Fig. 2.10 were calculated according to (2.41) and (2.42), and are presented in Table 2.1. Now the problem is to interpret the residuals and decide if there are any extreme residuals. This can be accomplished in many ways. It is, however, crucial that we derive the distributions for the residuals (e.g. for the largest or the smallest residual). A detailed handling of the residuals will be provided in Chap. 6. Moreover, it should be noted that if, for example, the value for Lake 1, depth 0.5 m is changed from 6.72 to 10, this will affect the residuals in Region 1, whereas the residuals in Region 2 will be unaffected. The residual for Lake 1, depth 0.5 m changes from −0.3 to 2.1. Other changes also appear, but are not very pronounced. If the values for Lake 1, depth 5 and 10 m are also altered, supposed to equal 10, the three residuals $\boldsymbol{R}_{11}$ for Lake 1 equal 2.6, 2.7 and 2.8, respectively, are much larger than the other residuals. Thus, it has been demonstrated that outstanding observations can be identified via the residuals. □

Table 2.1 Residuals for the liming data presented in Example 1.5 where in the model $\boldsymbol{\Sigma} = \boldsymbol{I}_3$

Lake	$\boldsymbol{R}_{11}$	$\boldsymbol{R}_{21} \times 10^{-3}$	$\boldsymbol{R}_2 \times 10^{-2}$	Lake	$\boldsymbol{R}_{11}$	$\boldsymbol{R}_{21} \times 10^{-3}$	$\boldsymbol{R}_2 \times 10^{-2}$
1	−0.3	5	−2	11	0.2	109	−2
1	−0.3	−9	3	11	0.1	−207	4
1	−0.3	4	−2	11	0.1	98	−2
2	−0.3	0.9	−2	12	−0.1	−15	−2
2	−0.2	−2	3	12	0.0	28	4
2	−0.0	0.8	−2	12	0.1	−13	−2
3	0.1	7	−2	13	0.3	−52	−2
3	0.2	−13	3	13	0.4	100	4
3	0.3	6	−2	13	0.6	−47	−2
4	0.1	−8	−2	14	−0.1	41	−2
4	0.2	15	3	14	−0.2	77	4
4	0.3	−7	−2	14	−0.4	−37	−2
5	−0.1	36	−2	15	−0.3	4	−2
5	−0.2	−70	3	15	−0.4	−7	4
5	−0.3	32	−2	15	−0.4	3	−2
6	0.2	20	−2	16	−0.1	7	−2
6	0.1	−37	3	16	−0.2	−14	4
6	0.0	18	−2	16	−0.4	6	−2
7	−0.2	−7	−2	17	−0.0	15	−2
7	−0.2	12	3	17	−0.2	−28	4
7	−0.3	−6	−2	17	0.4	13	2
8	0.1	−51	−2	18	−0.1	−56	−2
8	0.1	97	3	18	0.1	105	4
8	0.1	−46	−2	18	0.2	−50	−2
9	0.2	5	−2	19	0.0	22	−2
9	0.1	−9	3	19	0.1	−42	4
9	−0.0	4	−2	19	0.2	20	−2
10	0.2	7	−2	20	0.2	7	−2
10	0.2	12	3	20	0.3	−14	4
10	0.3	−6	−2	20	0.5	6	−2

2.6 $EBRM_W^m$ with a Known Dispersion Matrix

Here the estimators for the $EBRM_W^3$ when $\boldsymbol{\Sigma}$ is known are derived and compared with the estimators for the $EBRM_B^3$, which were obtained in the previous section. For completeness, the definition of the model under consideration is given below.

Definition 2.3 ($EBRM_W^m$) Let $\boldsymbol{X}: p\times n$, $\boldsymbol{A}_i : p\times q_i, q_i \leq p$, $\boldsymbol{B}_i: q_i\times k_i$, $\boldsymbol{C}_i: k_i\times n$, $i = 1, 2, \ldots, m$, $r(\boldsymbol{C}_1' : \boldsymbol{C}_2' : \boldsymbol{C}_3') + p \leq n$, $\mathcal{C}(\boldsymbol{A}_i) \subseteq \mathcal{C}(\boldsymbol{A}_{i-1})$, $i = 2, 3, \ldots, m$, and

Σ: $p \times p$ be p.d. Then

$$X = \sum_{i=1}^{m} A_i B_i C_i + E \tag{2.44}$$

defines the $EBRM_W^m$, where $E \sim N_{p,n}(\mathbf{0}, \Sigma, I)$, $\{A_i\}$ and $\{C_i\}$ are known matrices, and $\{B_i\}$ and Σ are unknown parameter matrices.

When estimating the parameters of the $EBRM_B^3$, a chain of straightforwardly performed calculations was presented. Now, in order to estimate the parameters in the $EBRM_W^3$, a between-individuals subspace decomposition is utilized and it is noted that (use Appendix B, Theorem B.3 (iii))

$$\mathcal{R}^n = \mathcal{C}(C_1') \boxplus \mathcal{C}(C_1')^{\perp} \cap \mathcal{C}(C_1' : C_2') \boxplus \mathcal{C}(C_1' : C_2')^{\perp} \cap \mathcal{C}(C_1' : C_2' : C_3') \boxplus \mathcal{C}(C_1' : C_2' : C_3')^{\perp}.$$

Let P_i, $i = 1, 2, 3, 4$, be orthogonal projections on these spaces, i.e.

$$P_1 = P_{C_1'}, \quad P_2 = P_{Q_1 C_2'}, \quad P_3 = P_{Q_2 Q_1 C_3'}, \quad P_4 = P_{(C_1':C_2':C_3')^o}, \tag{2.45}$$

where

$$Q_1 = P_{(C_1')^o}, \quad Q_2 = P_{(C_1':C_2')^o}.$$

The likelihood up to proportionality is stated in (2.21) and from there it follows that one should consider

$$\mathrm{tr}\{\Sigma^{-1}(X_o - E[X])(X_o - E[X])'\} = \sum_{i=1}^{4} \mathrm{tr}\{\Sigma^{-1}(X_o - E[X])P_i(X_o - E[X])'\},$$

where one has utilized the fact that $P_1 + P_2 + P_3 + P_4 = I$, since $\sum_{i=1}^4 P_i$ is a projector on the whole space. Because of the stairs structure, the within-individuals space, i.e. $\mathcal{R}^p$, is split. Hence,

$$\mathrm{tr}\{\Sigma^{-1}(X_o - E[X])(X_o - E[X])'\} = \mathrm{tr}\{\Sigma^{-1}(X_o - E[X])P_4(X_o - E[X])'\} \tag{2.46}$$

$$+ \sum_{i=1}^{3} \mathrm{tr}\{\Sigma^{-1} P_{A_i,\Sigma}(X_o - E[X])P_i(X_o - E[X])' P'_{A_i,\Sigma}\} \tag{2.47}$$

$$+ \sum_{i=1}^{3} \mathrm{tr}\{\Sigma^{-1} P'_{A_i^o,\Sigma^{-1}}(X_o - E[X])P_i(X_o - E[X])' P_{A_i^o,\Sigma^{-1}}\}. \tag{2.48}$$

Note that the right side of (2.46) and (2.48) are free of $\boldsymbol{B}_1$, $\boldsymbol{B}_2$ and $\boldsymbol{B}_3$, and thus MLEs are obtained if estimators can be found so that (2.47) equals 0; i.e. in this case there is an upper bound of the likelihood which is attainable and which is free of parameters. The condition that (2.47) should equal 0 is equivalent to the following system of linear equations:

$$\boldsymbol{A}_1'\boldsymbol{\Sigma}^{-1}(\boldsymbol{X}_o - \boldsymbol{A}_1\boldsymbol{B}_1\boldsymbol{C}_1 - \boldsymbol{A}_2\boldsymbol{B}_2\boldsymbol{C}_2 - \boldsymbol{A}_3\boldsymbol{B}_3\boldsymbol{C}_3)\boldsymbol{P}_1 = \boldsymbol{0}, \tag{2.49}$$

$$\boldsymbol{A}_2'\boldsymbol{\Sigma}^{-1}(\boldsymbol{X}_o - \boldsymbol{A}_2\boldsymbol{B}_2\boldsymbol{C}_2 - \boldsymbol{A}_3\boldsymbol{B}_3\boldsymbol{C}_3)\boldsymbol{P}_2 = \boldsymbol{0}, \tag{2.50}$$

$$\boldsymbol{A}_3'\boldsymbol{\Sigma}^{-1}(\boldsymbol{X}_o - \boldsymbol{A}_3\boldsymbol{B}_3\boldsymbol{C}_3)\boldsymbol{P}_3 = \boldsymbol{0}. \tag{2.51}$$

In order to find the estimates $\widehat{\boldsymbol{B}}_{io}$, $i = 1, 2, 3$, (2.49)–(2.51) have to be solved. It can be shown that these linear equations are consistent, but, as for the $EBRM_B^3$ it is meaningless to consider the parameters separately without additional assumptions. Thus, once again the focus will be on $\widehat{E[\boldsymbol{X}]}$, i.e.

$$\widehat{E[\boldsymbol{X}]} = \boldsymbol{P}_{A_1,\Sigma}\boldsymbol{X}_o\boldsymbol{P}_{C_1'} + \boldsymbol{P}_{A_2,\Sigma}\boldsymbol{X}_o\boldsymbol{P}_{Q_1C_2'} + \boldsymbol{P}_{A_3,\Sigma}\boldsymbol{X}_o\boldsymbol{P}_{Q_2Q_1C_3'}, \tag{2.52}$$

which through the following calculations will be shown to hold. Solving (2.49)–(2.51) yields

$$\begin{aligned}
\widehat{E[\boldsymbol{X}]} &= \boldsymbol{A}_1\widehat{\boldsymbol{B}}_1\boldsymbol{C}_1 + \boldsymbol{A}_2\widehat{\boldsymbol{B}}_2\boldsymbol{C}_2 + \boldsymbol{A}_3\widehat{\boldsymbol{B}}_3\boldsymbol{C}_3 \\
&= \boldsymbol{P}_{A_1,\Sigma}\boldsymbol{X}_o\boldsymbol{P}_1 + \boldsymbol{A}_2\widehat{\boldsymbol{B}}_2\boldsymbol{C}_2(\boldsymbol{I} - \boldsymbol{P}_1) + \boldsymbol{A}_3\widehat{\boldsymbol{B}}_3\boldsymbol{C}_3(\boldsymbol{I} - \boldsymbol{P}_1) \\
&= \boldsymbol{P}_{A_1,\Sigma}\boldsymbol{X}_o\boldsymbol{P}_1 + \boldsymbol{P}_{A_2,\Sigma}\boldsymbol{X}_o\boldsymbol{P}_2(\boldsymbol{I} - \boldsymbol{P}_1) + \boldsymbol{A}_3\widehat{\boldsymbol{B}}_3\boldsymbol{C}_3(\boldsymbol{I} - \boldsymbol{P}_2)(\boldsymbol{I} - \boldsymbol{P}_1) \\
&= \boldsymbol{P}_{A_1,\Sigma}\boldsymbol{X}_o\boldsymbol{P}_1 + \boldsymbol{P}_{A_2,\Sigma}\boldsymbol{X}_o\boldsymbol{P}_2(\boldsymbol{I} - \boldsymbol{P}_1) + \boldsymbol{P}_{A_3,\Sigma}\boldsymbol{X}_o\boldsymbol{P}_3(\boldsymbol{I} - \boldsymbol{P}_2)(\boldsymbol{I} - \boldsymbol{P}_1),
\end{aligned}$$

which is identical to (2.52) since $\boldsymbol{P}_2(\boldsymbol{I}-\boldsymbol{P}_1) = \boldsymbol{P}_2$ and $\boldsymbol{P}_3(\boldsymbol{I}-\boldsymbol{P}_2)(\boldsymbol{I}-\boldsymbol{P}_1) = \boldsymbol{P}_3$.

While Fig. 2.7 shows a decomposition of the tensor space for the $EBRM_B^3$, Fig. 2.12 provides the corresponding information for the $EBRM_W^3$.

Moreover, while Fig. 2.10 illustrates the four residual spaces in the $EBRM_B^3$, Fig. 2.13 presents the four residual spaces in the $EBRM_W^3$. In Fig. 2.13 the natural residuals are given by

$$\begin{aligned}
\boldsymbol{R}_1 &= \boldsymbol{X}(\boldsymbol{I} - \boldsymbol{P}_4), & \boldsymbol{R}_2 &= (\boldsymbol{I} - \boldsymbol{P}_{A_3,\Sigma})\boldsymbol{X}(\boldsymbol{I} - \boldsymbol{P}_3), \\
\boldsymbol{R}_3 &= (\boldsymbol{I} - \boldsymbol{P}_{A_2,\Sigma})\boldsymbol{X}(\boldsymbol{I} - \boldsymbol{P}_2), & \boldsymbol{R}_4 &= (\boldsymbol{I} - \boldsymbol{P}_{A_1,\Sigma})\boldsymbol{X}(\boldsymbol{I} - \boldsymbol{P}_1);
\end{aligned} \tag{2.53}$$

$\boldsymbol{P}_i$, $i = 1, 2, 3, 4$, are defined in (2.45).

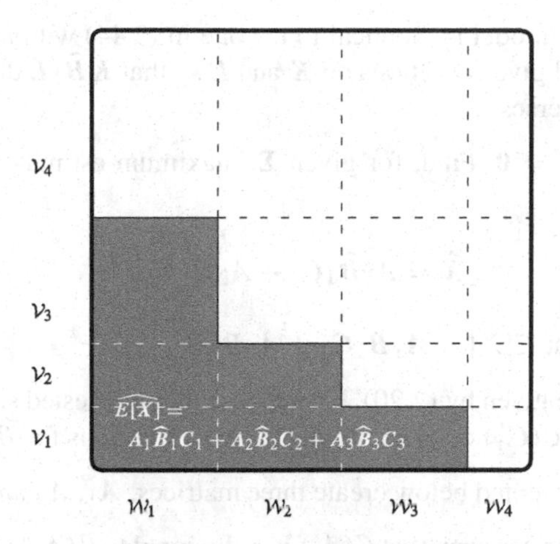

Fig. 2.12 Decomposition of the whole space according to the within-individuals and the between-individuals designs, illustrating the mean and residual spaces in the $EBRM_W^3$: $\mathcal{V}_1 = \mathcal{C}_\Sigma(A_3)$, $\mathcal{V}_2 = \mathcal{C}_\Sigma(A_2) \cap \mathcal{C}_\Sigma(A_3)^\perp$, $\mathcal{V}_3 = \mathcal{C}_\Sigma(A_1) \cap \mathcal{C}_\Sigma(A_2)^\perp$, $\mathcal{V}_4 = \mathcal{C}_\Sigma(A_1)^\perp$, $\mathcal{W}_1 = \mathcal{C}(C_1')$, $\mathcal{W}_2 = \mathcal{C}(C_1' : C_2') \cap \mathcal{C}(C_1')^\perp$, $\mathcal{W}_3 = \mathcal{C}(C_1' : C_2' : C_3') \cap \mathcal{C}(C_1' : C_2')^\perp$, $\mathcal{W}_4 = \mathcal{C}(C_1' : C_2' : C_3')^\perp$. The estimator $\widehat{E[X]}$ is presented in (2.52)

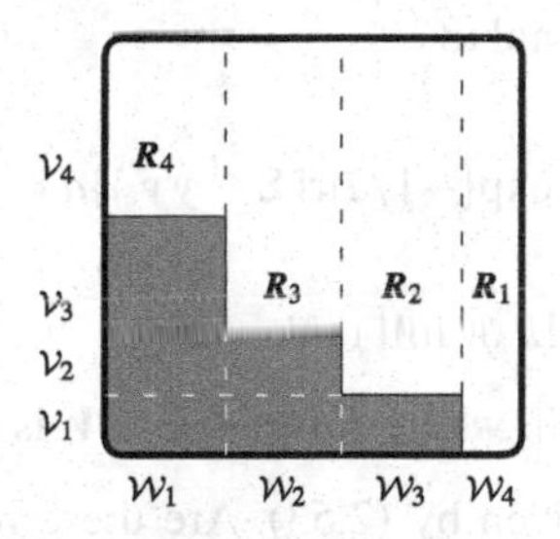

Fig. 2.13 Illustration of the four residual spaces in the $EBRM_W^3$. For the notation see Fig. 2.12

Problems

1 Give examples, i.e. specify appropriate matrices, of a weakly singular and a strongly singular Gauss-Markov model.

2 Let

$$x' = \beta' C + \epsilon, \qquad \epsilon \sim N_n(0, \sigma^2 V), \qquad V \ p.s.d.$$

and suppose that $\beta' L = 0$, for some known matrix L. Estimate the parameters β and σ^2.

3 Suppose that the model is identical to the one in (2.44) with $m = 2$ and known $\boldsymbol{\Sigma}$. Estimate $\boldsymbol{B}_1$ and give conditions on $\boldsymbol{K}$ and $\boldsymbol{L}$ so that $\boldsymbol{K}\widehat{\boldsymbol{B}}_1\boldsymbol{L}$ does not depend on any choice of g-inverses.

4 In (2.20) let $\boldsymbol{A}_3 = \boldsymbol{0}$. Find, for given $\boldsymbol{\Sigma}$, maximum estimators of $\boldsymbol{B}_1$, $\boldsymbol{B}_2$ and determine

$$\widehat{\boldsymbol{X}} = \boldsymbol{A}_1\widehat{\boldsymbol{B}}_1\boldsymbol{C}_1 + \boldsymbol{A}_2\widehat{\boldsymbol{B}}_2\boldsymbol{C}_2.$$

Moreover, show that $E[\widehat{\boldsymbol{X}}] = \boldsymbol{A}_1\boldsymbol{B}_1\boldsymbol{C}_1 + \boldsymbol{A}_2\boldsymbol{B}_2\boldsymbol{C}_2$.

5 Let the model be given by (2.20), but suppose that the nested subspace condition $\mathcal{C}(\boldsymbol{C}_3') \subseteq \mathcal{C}(\boldsymbol{C}_2') \subseteq \mathcal{C}(\boldsymbol{C}_1')$ does not hold. Derive expressions for $\widehat{\boldsymbol{B}}_i$, $i = 1, 2, 3$.

6 For each task presented below create three matrices: $\boldsymbol{A}_1$, $\boldsymbol{A}_2$ and $\boldsymbol{A}_3$.

(i) Create the matrices such that $\mathcal{C}(\boldsymbol{A}_i)$ is orthogonal to $\mathcal{C}(\boldsymbol{A}_j)$, $i \neq j$.
(ii) Create the matrices such that $\mathcal{C}(\boldsymbol{A}_i)$ is disjoint with $\mathcal{C}(\boldsymbol{A}_j)$, $i \neq j$, but not orthogonal.
(iii) Create matrices such that $\mathcal{C}(\boldsymbol{A}_1) \cap \mathcal{C}(\boldsymbol{A}_2) = \{\boldsymbol{0}\}$, $\mathcal{C}(\boldsymbol{A}_1) \cap \mathcal{C}(\boldsymbol{A}_3) = \{\boldsymbol{0}\}$, but $\mathcal{C}(\boldsymbol{A}_1) \cap \mathcal{C}(\boldsymbol{A}_2 : \boldsymbol{A}_3) \neq \{\boldsymbol{0}\}$.

7 Show that $|\boldsymbol{\Sigma}|$ is proportional to

$$\int \exp\{-1/2\mathrm{tr}\{\boldsymbol{\Sigma}^{-1}\boldsymbol{y}\boldsymbol{y}'\}\}d\boldsymbol{y},$$

where $\boldsymbol{\Sigma}$ is a dispersion matrix of full rank.

8 Show that $|\boldsymbol{S} + \boldsymbol{V}\boldsymbol{V}'| \geq |\boldsymbol{S}|$, where $\boldsymbol{S}$ is p.d. and $\boldsymbol{V}$ is any matrix of a proper size.

9 Let $\boldsymbol{R}_i$, $i = 1, 2, 3$, be given by (2.53). Are these residuals mutually independently distributed? Why/why not?

10 Solve (2.49)–(2.51).

Literature

In this chapter the dispersion matrix was supposed to be known, and therefore we have the obvious connections between the BRM, the $EBRM_{\bullet}^{m}$ and univariate linear models, generally speaking the Gauss-Markov model. Therefore, it is appropriate here to provide some background references on univariate linear models. Before commencing, from a practical point of view it is worth noting that analysis of variance, regression analysis and covariance analysis can all be treated in the same fashion within linear models theory. However, for each of these topics, of course, special problems and ideas have been dealt with and exploited, for example balancedness, multiple testing problems, variable selection and a huge range of methods for performing model validation, including the topic of influential observations (see Chap. 8 for references). A general ultimate goal has been to develop corresponding results for the BRM and its extensions, but this has only been partly fulfilled.

In his classical book entitled "The Design and Analysis of Experiments", Kempthorne (1952) presented, among other things, general linear univariate models with the help of matrices (see also Hinkelmann and Kempthorne, 2005, 2008). The main topic of Kempthorne's book was analysis of variance methods, which were treated in great detail, and even today this book is still highly useful. It constitutes a basis for a solid handling of models connected to least squares. The development of methods for handling models via least squares was to a large extent complete in the 1960s. Some other well-known books on linear models and their theory have been presented by Scheffé (1959), Graybill (1961, 1976), Seber (1966), Searle (1971, 1987) and Rao (1973). In contrast to Kempthorne's work, the authors who came after him (in particular Rao) started to use generalized inverses (g-inverses) instead of performing reparametrizations, in order to handle the rank deficiencies of the design matrix in the general linear model. In the 1960s a large amount of research activities on g-inverses started, although the concept is much older. Today many books are available which specialize in g-inverses, for example, the classical work by Rao and Mitra (1971) or the newer book by Ben-Israel and Greville (2003), which among other things includes many references connected to g-inverses (note that the first edition of the book by Ben-Israel and Greville appeared in the 1970s). In parallel with all the above-mentioned publications, interesting work on linear models (slightly more abstract in nature and based on linear spaces and a coordinate-free approach) was performed by Kruskal (1961), Drygas (1970), Eaton (1970) (see Eaton, 2007, for some notes on Kruskal's work), Stone (1977, 1987) and Wong (1993), among others. Among the more recently published works on linear models is the book by Sengupta and Jammalamadaka (2003), who present the topic in a clear and interesting way.

After the basic theory on linear models had been established the academic challenge was then to develop methods for handling a general linear model with a known singular dispersion matrix. Under the assumption of a singular dispersion matrix, there exist random variables which equal a constant with probability 1, which is indeed quite special. This leads to some philosophical concerns (see Baksalary et al., 1992). With regard to non-singular dispersion Aitken (1936) had already presented work on estimation and least squares, i.e. had derived the best linear unbiased estimator of the mean parameter. There exists a huge volume of literature on the singular Gauss-Markov model, for example Zyskind and Martin (1969), Rao (1973, Chapter 4i), Alalouf (1978), Baksalary and Kala (1979, 1981), Nordström (1985), Tian et al. (2008) and Baksalary and Trenkler (2011). In particular we refer to Nordström, because he divided the singular Gauss-Markov model into two cases, i.e. the weakly singular and the strongly singular Gauss-Markov model, and to Baksalary & Trenkler for a number of recent references.

Concerning the BRM, it is of interest to discuss weighted versus unweighted estimators of the mean parameters. This topic has a long history within the Gauss-Markov model framework (see Puntanen et al., 2011, Chapter 10; Haslett et al., 2014). For a complete set of references on the topic up to 1989, one should consult Puntanen and Styan (1989).

It should be noted that there are articles which treat in detail the $EBRM_{\bullet}^{m}$ (and the BRM) with almost-known dispersion matrices (proportional to an unknown constant), i.e. a Gauss-Markov model where the overall design matrix is a sum of Kronecker products of matrices and thus the corresponding linear space is a tensor product. Examples of such articles are those written by Tian and Takane (2007, 2009), Beganu (2009), Song (2011) and Song and Wang (2014), who considered best linear unbiased estimators (see also Zhang and Zhu, 2000; Xu and Wang, 2011). Also relevant for this book are the results and ideas of Hu (2010), who proposed, by first assuming a known dispersion matrix, a two-stage estimator of the mean parameters. Admissibility of linear estimators for the BRM with known correlation, under some specific restrictions, was obtained by Zhang and Gui (2008) and Zhang et al. (2009, 2011).

References

Aitken, A. C. (1936). On least squares and linear combinations of observations. *Proceedings of the Royal Society of Edinburgh, Section A, 55*, 42–48.

Alalouf, I. S. (1978). An explicit treatment of the general linear model with singular covariance matrix. *Sankhyā, Series B, 40*, 65–73.

Baksalary, J. K., & Kala, R. (1979). Best linear unbiased estimation in the restricted general linear model. *Mathematische Operationsforschung und Statistik, Series Statistics, 10*, 27–35.

Baksalary, J. K., & Kala, R. (1981). Linear transformations preserving best linear unbiased estimators in a general Gauss-Markoff model. *Annals of Statistics, 9*, 913–916.

Baksalary, J. K., Rao, C. R., & Markiewicz, A. (1992). A study of the influence of the "natural restrictions" on estimation problems in the singular Gauss-Markov model. *The Journal of Statistical Planning and Inference, 31*, 335–351.

Baksalary, O. M., & Trenkler, G. (2011). Between OLSE and BLUE. *Australian and New Zealand Journal of Statistics, 53*, 289–303.

Beganu, G. (2009). Some properties of the best linear unbiased estimators in multivariate growth curve models. *RACSAM - Revista de la Real Academia de Ciencias Exactas, Fisicas y Naturales. Serie A. Matematicas, 103*, 161–166.

Ben-Israel, A., & Greville, T. N. E. (2003). *Generalized inverses. Theory and applications. CMS books in mathematics/Ouvrages de Mathématiques de la SMC* (Vol. 15, 2nd ed.). New York: Springer.

Drygas, H. (1970). *The coordinate-free approach to Gauss-Markov estimation. Lecture notes in operations research and mathematical systems* (Vol. 40). New York: Springer.

Eaton, M. L. (1970). Gauss-Markov estimation for multivariate linear models: A coordinate free approach. *Annals of Mathematical Statistics, 41*, 528–538.

Eaton, M. L. (2007). William H. Kruskal and the development of coordinate-free methods. *Statistical Science, 22*, 264–265.

Graybill, F. A. (1961). *An introduction to linear statistical models. McGraw-Hill series in probability and statistics* (Vol. I). New York: McGraw-Hill.

Graybill, F. A. (1976). *Theory and application of the linear model*. North Scituate: Duxbury Press.
Haslett, S. J., Isotalo, J., Liu, Y., & Puntanen, S. (2014). Equalities between OLSE, BLUE and BLUP in the linear model. *Statistical Papers, 55*, 543–561.
Hinkelmann, K., & Kempthorne, O. (2005). *Design and analysis of experiments. Vol. 2. Advanced experimental design. Wiley series in probability and statistics*. Hoboken: Wiley.
Hinkelmann, K., & Kempthorne, O. (2008). *Design and analysis of experiments. Vol. 1. Introduction to experimental design. Wiley series in probability and statistics* (2nd ed.). Hoboken: Wiley.
Hu, J. (2010). Properties of the explicit estimators in the extended growth curve model. *Statistics: A Journal of Theoretical and Applied Statistics, 44*, 477–492.
Kempthorne, O. (1952). *The design and analysis of experiments*. New York/London: Wiley/Chapman & Hall.
Kollo, T., & von Rosen, D. (2005). *Advanced multivariate statistics with matrices. Mathematics and its applications* (Vol. 579). Dordrecht: Springer.
Kruskal, W. (1961). The coordinate-free approach to Gauss-Markov estimation, and its application to missing and extra observations. In *Proceedings of the Fourth Berkeley Symposium on Mathematical Statistics and Probability* (Vol. I, pp. 435–451). Berkeley: University of California Press.
Nordström, K. (1985). On a decomposition of the singular Gauss-Markov model. In: *Linear statistical inference (Poznan, 1984). Lecture notes in statistics* (Vol. 35, pp. 231–245). Berlin: Springer.
Puntanen, S., & Styan, G. P. H. (1989). The equality of the ordinary least squares estimator and the best linear unbiased estimator. With comments by Oscar Kempthorne and Shayle R. Searle and a reply by the authors. *The American Statistician, 43*, 153–164.
Puntanen, S., Styan, G. P. H., & Isotalo, J. (2011). *Matrix tricks for linear statistical models. Our personal top twenty*. Heidelberg: Springer.
Rao, C. R. (1973). *Linear statistical inference and its applications. Wiley series in probability and mathematical statistics* (2nd ed.). New York: Wiley.
Rao, C. R., & Mitra, S. K. (1971). *Generalized inverse of matrices and its applications*. New York: Wiley.
Scheffé, H. (1959). *The analysis of variance*. New York/London: Wiley/Chapman & Hall.
Searle, S. R. (1971). *Linear models*. New York: Wiley.
Searle, S. R. (1987). *Linear models for unbalanced data. Wiley series in probability and mathematical statistics: Applied probability and statistics*. New York: Wiley.
Seber, G. A. F. (1966). *The linear hypothesis: A general theory. Griffin's statistical monographs & courses* (Vol. 19). London: Charles Griffin.
Sengupta, D., & Jammalamadaka, S. R. (2003). *Linear models. An integrated approach. Series on multivariate analysis*. (Vol. 6). River Edge: World Scientific.
Song, G. J. (2011). On the best linear unbiased estimator and the linear sufficiency of a general growth curve model. *The Journal of Statistical Planning and Inference, 141*, 2700–2710.
Song, G. J., & Wang, Q. W. (2014). On the weighted least-squares, the ordinary least-squares and the best linear unbiased estimators under a restricted growth curve model. *Statistical Papers, 55*, 375–392.
Stone, M. (1977). A unified approach to coordinate-free multivariate analysis. *Annals of the Institute of Statistical Mathematics, 29*, 43–57.
Stone, M. (1987). *Coordinate-free multivariable statistics. An illustrated geometric progression from Halmos to Gauss and Bayes. Oxford statistical science series* (Vol. 2). New York: The Clarendon Press/Oxford University Press.
Tian, Y., Beisiegel, M., Dagenais, E., & Haines, C. (2008). On the natural restrictions in the singular Gauss-Markov model. *Statistical Papers, 49*, 553–564.
Tian, Y., & Takane, Y. (2007). Some algebraic and statistical properties of WLSEs under a general growth curve model. *Electronic Journal of Linear Algebra, 16*, 187–203.

Tian, Y., & Takane, Y. (2009). On consistency, natural restrictions and estimability under classical and extended growth curve models. *The Journal of Statistical Planning and Inference, 139*, 2445–2458.

Wong, C. S. (1993). Linear models in a general parametric form. *Sankhyā, Series A, 55*, 130–149.

Xu, L.-W., & Wang, S.-G. (2011). Linear sufficiency in a general growth curve model. *Linear Algebra and Its Applications, 434*, 593–604.

Zhang, B. X., & Zhu, X. H. (2000). Gauss-Markov and weighted least-squares estimation under a general growth curve model. *Linear Algebra and Its Applications, 321*, 387–398.

Zhang, S., Fang, Z., Qin, H., & Han, L. (2011). Characterization of admissible linear estimators in the growth curve model with respect to inequality constraints. *Journal of the Korean Statistical Society, 40*, 173–179.

Zhang, S., & Gui, W. (2008). Admissibility of linear estimators in a growth curve model subject to an incomplete ellipsoidal restriction. *Acta Mathematica Scientia. Series B. English Edition, 28*, 194–200.

Zhang, S., Gui, W., & Liu, G. (2009). Characterization of admissible linear estimators in the general growth curve model with respect to an incomplete ellipsoidal restriction. *Linear Algebra and Its Applications, 431*, 120–131.

Zyskind, G., & Martin, F. B. (1969). On best linear estimation and general Gauss-Markov theorem in linear models with arbitrary nonnegative covariance structure. *SIAM Journal on Applied Mathematics, 17*, 1190–1202.

Chapter 3
The Basic Ideas of Obtaining MLEs: Unknown Dispersion

3.1 Introduction

In this chapter, the maximum likelihood estimators of all the parameters in the BRM, $EBRM_W^3$ and $EBRM_B^3$ are derived when the dispersion is supposed to be unknown; i.e. when following the statistical paradigm, it is supposed that the experiment has been designed and accomplished, and now it is time to estimate the parameters of the model. Only the estimators are obtained, while statistical properties such as their distributions are left to subsequent chapters. The subject matter of this chapter is essential for the book and it is worthwhile devoting some time to reflection on the derivations and results.

3.2 BRM and Its MLEs

Let

$$X = ABC + E, \quad E \sim N_{p,n}(\mathbf{0}, \boldsymbol{\Sigma}, \boldsymbol{I}), \quad \boldsymbol{\Sigma} > 0, \tag{3.1}$$

where all matrices are specified in Definition 2.1. From general maximum likelihood theory we know that estimators are consistent. This means that the MLE of $\boldsymbol{\Sigma}$, should converge to $\boldsymbol{\Sigma}$ and, therefore, intuitively, the estimators of $\boldsymbol{B}$ with a known or estimated $\boldsymbol{\Sigma}$ should be of a similar form. Let us restate the appropriate part of Fig. 2.6 as Fig. 3.1 which will serve as a basis for understanding how subspaces are connected to the MLEs.

D. von Rosen, *Bilinear Regression Analysis*, Lecture Notes in Statistics 220,
https://doi.org/10.1007/978-3-319-78784-8_3

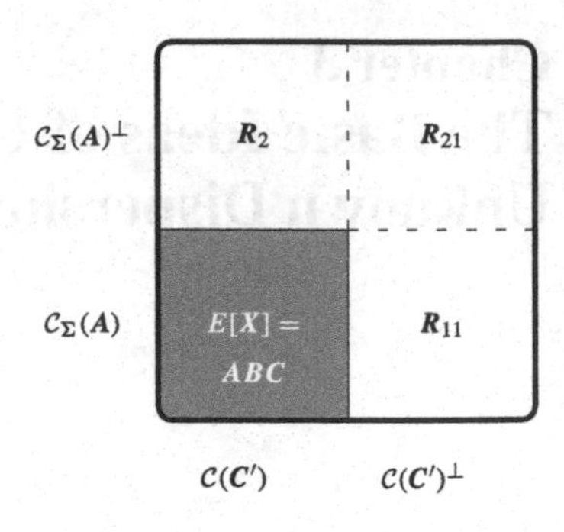

Fig. 3.1 Consider the model given in (3.1). Decomposition of the whole space according to the within-individuals and between-individuals designs, illustrating the mean and residuals in the BRM, is presented

First a strict mathematical treatment of the model is presented and thereafter the mathematics is illustrated graphically in Fig. 3.2. It follows from (3.1) that the likelihood, $L(\boldsymbol{B}, \boldsymbol{\Sigma})$, is given by

$$L(\boldsymbol{B}, \boldsymbol{\Sigma}) = (2\pi)^{-np/2}|\boldsymbol{\Sigma}|^{-n/2}e^{-1/2\mathrm{tr}\{\boldsymbol{\Sigma}^{-1}(\boldsymbol{X}_o-\boldsymbol{ABC})(\boldsymbol{X}_o-\boldsymbol{ABC})'\}}.$$

Using the results from Sect. 2.4 when $\boldsymbol{\Sigma}$ was known, the likelihood, $L(\boldsymbol{B}, \boldsymbol{\Sigma})$, in agreement with Fig. 3.1, can be decomposed as

$$\begin{aligned} L(\boldsymbol{B}, \boldsymbol{\Sigma}) &= (2\pi)^{-np/2}|\boldsymbol{\Sigma}|^{-n/2} \\ &\times \exp\{-1/2\mathrm{tr}\{\boldsymbol{\Sigma}^{-1}\boldsymbol{P}_{A,\Sigma}(\boldsymbol{X}_o - \boldsymbol{ABC})\boldsymbol{P}_{C'}(\boldsymbol{X}_o - \boldsymbol{ABC})'\boldsymbol{P}'_{A,\Sigma}\}\} \\ &\times \exp\{-1/2\mathrm{tr}\{\boldsymbol{\Sigma}^{-1}\boldsymbol{X}_o(\boldsymbol{I} - \boldsymbol{P}_{C'})\boldsymbol{X}'_o\}\} \\ &\times \exp\{-1/2\mathrm{tr}\{\boldsymbol{\Sigma}^{-1}(\boldsymbol{I} - \boldsymbol{P}_{A,\Sigma})\boldsymbol{X}_o\boldsymbol{P}_{C'}\boldsymbol{X}'_o(\boldsymbol{I} - \boldsymbol{P}_{A,\Sigma})'\}\}. \end{aligned}$$

This expression is smaller than or equal to the profile likelihood

$$\begin{aligned} &(2\pi)^{-np/2}|\boldsymbol{\Sigma}|^{-n/2} \\ &\times \exp\{-1/2\mathrm{tr}\{\boldsymbol{\Sigma}^{-1}(\boldsymbol{X}_o(\boldsymbol{I} - \boldsymbol{P}_{C'})\boldsymbol{X}'_o + (\boldsymbol{I} - \boldsymbol{P}_{A,\Sigma})\boldsymbol{X}_o\boldsymbol{P}_{C'}\boldsymbol{X}'_o(\boldsymbol{I} - \boldsymbol{P}_{A,\Sigma})')\}\} \end{aligned} \tag{3.2}$$

with equality if and only if

$$\begin{aligned} \boldsymbol{ABC} &= \boldsymbol{P}_{A,\Sigma}\boldsymbol{X}_o\boldsymbol{P}_{C'} \\ &= \boldsymbol{A}(\boldsymbol{A}'\boldsymbol{\Sigma}^{-1}\boldsymbol{A})^{-}\boldsymbol{A}'\boldsymbol{\Sigma}^{-1}\boldsymbol{X}_o\boldsymbol{C}'(\boldsymbol{CC}')^{-}\boldsymbol{C}. \end{aligned} \tag{3.3}$$

In Fig. 3.1 this implies that the part of the likelihood which is connected to the mean ($E[\boldsymbol{X}] = \boldsymbol{ABC}$) has been eliminated. Moreover, from Appendix B, Theorem B.9 (iv) it follows that (3.2) is smaller than or equal to

$$(2\pi)^{-np/2}|(\boldsymbol{S}_o+(\boldsymbol{I}-\boldsymbol{P}_{A,\Sigma})\boldsymbol{X}_o\boldsymbol{P}_{C'}\boldsymbol{X}'_o(\boldsymbol{I}-\boldsymbol{P}_{A,\Sigma})')/n|^{-n/2}\exp\{-np/2\}, \tag{3.4}$$

where $S_o = X_o(I - P_{C'})X_o'$, which is obtained if

$$n\Sigma = S_o + (I - P_{A,\Sigma})X_o P_{C'} X_o'(I - P_{A,\Sigma})' \tag{3.5}$$

is inserted in (3.2). Since the right-hand side of (3.5) equals $(X_o - ABC)()'$, there is no problem applying Theorem B.9 (iv) in Appendix B. It is less clear if this theorem can be applied for optimization purposes, if instead of B, we have a function in Σ; i.e. $B(\Sigma)$, which sometimes appears.

Using (2.41) and (2.42), it follows from (3.5) that $n\Sigma = R_{11}R_{11}' + R_{21}R_{21}' + R_2R_2'$, among other things showing the whole tensor space $\mathcal{R}^n \otimes \mathcal{R}^p$ to be included in the estimation process. Both Eqs. (3.3) and (3.5) are complicated functions in Σ, but fortunately the only requirement for finding explicit MLEs are a few straightforward calculations. Pre-multiplying (3.5) by $A'\Sigma^{-1}$ yields

$$nA' = A'\Sigma^{-1}S_o,$$

and thus under the assumption that S_o^{-1} exists

$$\widehat{A'\Sigma^{-1}} = nA'S_o^{-1}. \tag{3.6}$$

This means that $A'\Sigma^{-1}$ has been estimated, which is exactly what is needed in (3.3) and (3.5) because $P_{A,\Sigma}$ is used, and now it is known that $P_{A,\Sigma} = P_{A,S_o}$. It follows that the upper bound in (3.4) does not depend on any unknown parameter and is obtained by inserting the estimates given in (3.3) and (3.5), in the likelihood, which thus yields MLEs. Moreover, $\widehat{A'\Sigma^{-1}} = A'\widehat{\Sigma}^{-1}$. We may summarize our finding as follows. Out of all the relations, the relation shown in (3.6) is the most important one because it implies:

1. the finding of an upper bound of the likelihood function;
2. the finding of MLEs;
3. establishment of the relation $P_{A,\widehat{\Sigma}} = P_{A,S}$.

In particular, implication (3) tells us that there is no great difference between obtaining MLEs when Σ is known and obtaining them when Σ is unknown, since all the estimators, including the estimators of the residuals R_{11}, R_{21} and R_2 are similar, i.e. the projection operators used in the estimation process project on the same spaces.

In the next theorem the above results are summarized and the MLEs of B and Σ are explicitly presented.

Theorem 3.1 *For the BRM given in Definition 2.1 and with $S = X(I - P_{C'})X'$ supposed to be p.d., with $n - r(C) \geq p$, the MLEs are given by*

$$A\widehat{B}C = A(A'S^{-1}A)^{-}A'S^{-1}XC'(CC')^{-}C,$$
$$n\widehat{\Sigma} = S + (I - A(A'S^{-1}A)^{-}A'S^{-1})XC'(CC')^{-}CX'(I - S^{-1}A(A'S^{-1}A)^{-}A').$$

The assumption that $\boldsymbol{S}$ is p.d. holds with probability 1, if $n - r(\boldsymbol{C}) \geq p$. Moreover, $\widehat{\boldsymbol{\Sigma}}$ is always unique, i.e. does not depend on any choice of g-inverse.

Corollary 3.1 *Let $\widehat{\boldsymbol{B}}$ satisfy the relation $\boldsymbol{A}\widehat{\boldsymbol{B}}\boldsymbol{C}$ given in Theorem 3.1. Then*

$$\widehat{\boldsymbol{B}} = (\boldsymbol{A}'\boldsymbol{S}^{-1}\boldsymbol{A})^{-}\boldsymbol{A}'\boldsymbol{S}^{-1}\boldsymbol{X}\boldsymbol{C}'(\boldsymbol{C}\boldsymbol{C}')^{-} + (\boldsymbol{A}')^{o}\boldsymbol{Z}_1 + \boldsymbol{A}'\boldsymbol{Z}_2\boldsymbol{C}^{o\prime},$$

where $\boldsymbol{Z}_1$ and $\boldsymbol{Z}_2$ are arbitrary matrices.

If the estimability conditions $\mathcal{C}(\boldsymbol{K}') \subseteq \mathcal{C}(\boldsymbol{A}')$ and $\mathcal{C}(\boldsymbol{L}) \subseteq \mathcal{C}(\boldsymbol{C})$ are fulfilled, then

$$\boldsymbol{K}\widehat{\boldsymbol{B}}\boldsymbol{L} = \boldsymbol{K}(\boldsymbol{A}'\boldsymbol{S}^{-1}\boldsymbol{A})^{-}\boldsymbol{A}'\boldsymbol{S}^{-1}\boldsymbol{X}\boldsymbol{C}'(\boldsymbol{C}\boldsymbol{C}')^{-}\boldsymbol{L},$$

which is independent of any choice of g-inverse, i.e. is unique.

If $\rho(\boldsymbol{A}) = q$ and $\rho(\boldsymbol{C}) = k$, then

$$\widehat{\boldsymbol{B}} = (\boldsymbol{A}'\boldsymbol{S}^{-1}\boldsymbol{A})^{-1}\boldsymbol{A}'\boldsymbol{S}^{-1}\boldsymbol{X}\boldsymbol{C}'(\boldsymbol{C}\boldsymbol{C}')^{-1}.$$

It is questionable whether $\widehat{\boldsymbol{B}}$ under non-estimability should be called an estimator, because $\boldsymbol{Z}_1$ and $\boldsymbol{Z}_2$ are both unknown and unrestricted. For this reason $\widehat{\boldsymbol{B}}$, in this case, is definitely not a very useful quantity.

Corollary 3.2 *If $\boldsymbol{A} = \boldsymbol{I}$, then*

$$\widehat{\boldsymbol{B}}\boldsymbol{C} = \boldsymbol{X}\boldsymbol{C}'(\boldsymbol{C}\boldsymbol{C}')^{-}\boldsymbol{C},$$
$$n\widehat{\boldsymbol{\Sigma}} = \boldsymbol{S}.$$

In Corollary 3.2 the MLEs for the classical multivariate analysis of variance model (MANOVA) are presented. The estimators should be compared to those given in Theorem 3.1. It is clearly seen that a member of the exponential family is easier to deal with than with a member from the curved exponential family. Among others, for the BRM the mean estimator is non-linear. This implies that many statistical properties are more difficult to verify for the BRM than for the MANOVA model. The mathematics behind the above presented estimation approach is illustrated in Fig. 3.2. Note that we can consider the approach to consist of two steps.

For completeness and to illustrate how the decomposition of subspaces and projections leads to three different residuals (see Figs. 3.1 and 3.2), the next relations are presented:

$$\widehat{\boldsymbol{R}}_{11} = \boldsymbol{P}_{A,S}\boldsymbol{X}(\boldsymbol{I} - \boldsymbol{P}_{C'}); \tag{3.7}$$

$$\widehat{\boldsymbol{R}}_{21} = (\boldsymbol{I} - \boldsymbol{P}_{A,S})\boldsymbol{X}(\boldsymbol{I} - \boldsymbol{P}_{C'}); \tag{3.8}$$

$$\widehat{\boldsymbol{R}}_{2} = (\boldsymbol{I} - \boldsymbol{P}_{A,S})\boldsymbol{X}\boldsymbol{P}_{C'}. \tag{3.9}$$

All these relations bear information about the BRM. Later, in Chap. 6, the above residuals will be studied in detail.

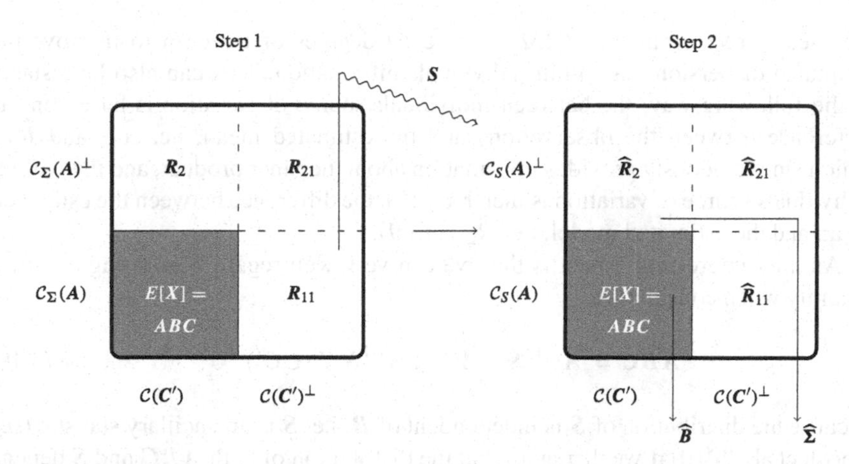

Fig. 3.2 Step 1 is used to find information about the inner product, which is then estimated using $S = X(I - P_{C'})X' = R_{11}R_{11}' + R_{21}R_{21}'$. In Step 2 the MLEs are constructed via projections on appropriate subspaces

The MLEs given in Theorem 3.1 provide interesting information and also force us to examine more deeply the estimation process of the parameters of the BRM. It appears that $\boldsymbol{\Sigma}$ plays two roles. One role is to reflect the uncertainty in the data and another role is to determine the inner product when the mean estimator $A\widehat{B}C$ is to be derived. Mathematically this means that when quantifying uncertainty, we are operating with an outer product of vectors, i.e. $I \otimes \boldsymbol{\Sigma} = E[\text{vec}(X - ABC)\text{vec}'(X - ABC)]$, whereas when considering the estimators of the mean parameters $\boldsymbol{\Sigma}$ is used in the definition of an inner product. On the other hand, we do not have to distinguish between these two roles of $\boldsymbol{\Sigma}$, because the use of $\boldsymbol{\Sigma}$ when defining the inner product is taken care of through the relation $A'\widehat{\boldsymbol{\Sigma}}^{-1} = nA'S^{-1}$, implying that automatically only the variation connected to $\mathcal{C}(C')^\perp$, i.e. $S = \widehat{R}_{11}\widehat{R}_{11}' + \widehat{R}_{12}\widehat{R}_{12}'$, will be involved, omitting $\widehat{R}_2\widehat{R}_2'$ (see (3.7)–(3.9)). However, it is conceptually beneficial to regard $\boldsymbol{\Sigma}$ as having two roles.

The residuals $\widehat{R}_{11}$, $\widehat{R}_{21}$ and $\widehat{R}_2$ all carry information about $\boldsymbol{\Sigma}$, and it was shown in the proof of Theorem 3.1 that the sum of the squared residuals will form the MLE of $\boldsymbol{\Sigma}$. However, it is really worthwhile to complicate the picture somewhat and not just think of $\boldsymbol{\Sigma}$ as an object summarizing the variation, because if $\boldsymbol{\Sigma}$ is structured, e.g. banded, we can use some basic principles for estimating $\boldsymbol{\Sigma}$ in a straightforward manner. For example, we can use projections on subspaces and then adjust the estimator so that it becomes banded.

Moreover, as noted above, the parameter $\boldsymbol{\Sigma}$ represents the dispersion (variances/covariances) within individuals. Usually, in order to estimate the dispersion, independent observations are needed. However, for the BRM it appears that once there are enough independent observations, one can also utilize within-individuals information, i.e. $\widehat{R}_2$, to estimate $\boldsymbol{\Sigma}$. The idea is that based on the independent observations, one can estimate the inner product defining the dependency within individuals ($\boldsymbol{\Sigma}$ in $\mathcal{C}_\Sigma(A)$), via $\widehat{R}_{11}$ in (3.7) and $\widehat{R}_{21}$ in (3.8), and then due to the mean structure in the BRM, there exist degrees of freedom to improve the estimated dispersion via within-individuals information. This can also be restated in the following way: the between-individuals source of variation is based on the difference between the observations and the estimated mean, i.e. $\widehat{\boldsymbol{R}}_{11}$ and $\widehat{\boldsymbol{R}}_{21}$, which simultaneously provides information about the inner product, and the within-individuals source of variation is then based on the difference between the estimated mean and the estimated model, i.e. $\widehat{\boldsymbol{R}}_2$ in (3.9).

Another interesting aspect is that we can very well regard $\boldsymbol{S}$ as being a known quantity when considering

$$\boldsymbol{A}\widehat{\boldsymbol{B}}\boldsymbol{C} = \boldsymbol{A}(\boldsymbol{A}'\boldsymbol{S}^{-1}\boldsymbol{A})^{-}\boldsymbol{A}'\boldsymbol{S}^{-1}\boldsymbol{X}\boldsymbol{C}'(\boldsymbol{C}\boldsymbol{C}')^{-}\boldsymbol{C}, \tag{3.10}$$

because the distribution of $\boldsymbol{S}$ is independent of $\boldsymbol{B}$, i.e. $\boldsymbol{S}$ is an ancillary statistic (see Ghosh et al., 2010) if we disregard that the distribution of both $\boldsymbol{A}\widehat{\boldsymbol{B}}\boldsymbol{C}$ and $\boldsymbol{S}$ depend on $\boldsymbol{\Sigma}$. The projection $\boldsymbol{A}(\boldsymbol{A}'\boldsymbol{S}^{-1}\boldsymbol{A})^{-}\boldsymbol{A}'\boldsymbol{S}^{-1}$ which is a function of $\boldsymbol{S}$ can be used to improve the unbiased estimator $\boldsymbol{X}\boldsymbol{C}'(\boldsymbol{C}\boldsymbol{C}')^{-}\boldsymbol{C}$ through the possibility to improve its dispersion. However, there do not exist any results which indicate that this way of performing inference, in general, will improve non-conditional inference. Moreover, note that the variation introduced by $\boldsymbol{S}$ in (3.10) is in some way artificial. If an experiment which is analysed by the BRM is intended to be repeated, the new estimate will differ from (3.10) (with inserted data), which will be partly due to the fact that $\boldsymbol{S}$ is not constant, and if conditioning with respect to $\boldsymbol{S}$, this has to be taken into account. However, if only a single study is performed, one can very well condition with respect to $\boldsymbol{S}$, which simplifies inference significantly.

Above, in (3.10), a weighted estimator was presented. Alternatively, an unweighted estimator,

$$\boldsymbol{A}\widetilde{\boldsymbol{B}}\boldsymbol{C} = \boldsymbol{A}(\boldsymbol{A}'\boldsymbol{A})^{-}\boldsymbol{A}'\boldsymbol{X}\boldsymbol{C}'(\boldsymbol{C}\boldsymbol{C}')^{-}\boldsymbol{C}, \tag{3.11}$$

can also be used. The difference between (3.10) and (3.11) equals (see Appendix B, Theorem B.13)

$$\boldsymbol{A}\widehat{\boldsymbol{B}}\boldsymbol{C} = \boldsymbol{A}\widetilde{\boldsymbol{B}}\boldsymbol{C} - \boldsymbol{A}(\boldsymbol{A}'\boldsymbol{A})^{-}\boldsymbol{A}'\boldsymbol{S}\boldsymbol{A}^{o}(\boldsymbol{A}^{o'}\boldsymbol{S}\boldsymbol{A}^{o})^{-}\boldsymbol{A}^{o'}\boldsymbol{X}\boldsymbol{C}'(\boldsymbol{C}\boldsymbol{C}')^{-}\boldsymbol{C}. \tag{3.12}$$

However, since the two terms on the right-hand side of (3.12) are not independently distributed it is not obvious how (3.12) should be interpreted.

Example 3.1 Consider the Potthoff and Roy data presented in Table 1.2. In a preliminary analysis of the data, the results for two different model versions and two types of estimates are now shown. The model equals $\boldsymbol{X} \sim N_{p,n}(\boldsymbol{A}_{\bullet}\boldsymbol{B}_{\bullet}\boldsymbol{C}, \boldsymbol{\Sigma}_{\bullet}, \boldsymbol{I})$, where $\boldsymbol{A}_{\bullet}$ indicates that different choices of the within-individuals design matrix will be used and $\boldsymbol{B}_{\bullet}, \boldsymbol{\Sigma}_{\bullet}$ means that different estimates will be obtained in the different model versions applied below. In the formulas, $\boldsymbol{S}_o = \boldsymbol{X}_o(\boldsymbol{I}_{27} - \boldsymbol{P}_{C'})\boldsymbol{X}'_o$.

Model Ia
The MLEs for a model where the linear growth is defined through

$$A_1 = \begin{pmatrix} 1 & 8 \\ 1 & 10 \\ 1 & 12 \\ 1 & 14 \end{pmatrix}$$

are derived:

$$\widehat{B}_{1o} = (A_1' S_o^{-1} A_1)^{-1} A_1' S_o^{-1} X_o C'(CC')^{-1} = \begin{pmatrix} 17.4 & 15.8 \\ 0.48 & 0.83 \end{pmatrix},$$

$$\widehat{\Sigma}_{1o} = \begin{pmatrix} 5.1 & 2.4 & 3.6 & 2.5 \\ & 3.9 & 2.7 & 3.1 \\ & & 6.0 & 3.8 \\ & & & 4.6 \end{pmatrix}.$$

The first column in $\widehat{B}_{1o}$ refers to the girls and the second to the boys. Since there does not seem to be any structure in $\widehat{\Sigma}_{1o}$, the assumption about an unstructured dispersion matrix is reasonable.

Model Ib
This model is the same as Model Ia, but now an unweighted estimate of the mean parameters is derived, and $n\widehat{\Sigma}_{2o} = (X_o - A_1\widehat{B}_{2o}C)()'$:

$$\widehat{B}_{2o} = (A_1' A_1)^{-1} A_1' X_o C'(CC')^{-1} = \begin{pmatrix} 17.4 & 16.3 \\ 0.48 & 0.78 \end{pmatrix},$$

$$\widehat{\Sigma}_{2o} = \begin{pmatrix} 5.1 & 2.5 & 3.6 & 2.5 \\ & 4.0 & 2.7 & 3.0 \\ & & 6.0 & 3.8 \\ & & & 4.6 \end{pmatrix}.$$

In comparison with Model Ia there does not seem to be any big numerical differences. However, the distributions for the estimators in Model Ib are much easier to work out than those in Model Ia.

Model IIa
The MLEs for a model with quadratic growth are now presented, i.e.

$$A_2 = \begin{pmatrix} 1 & 8 & 64 \\ 1 & 10 & 100 \\ 1 & 12 & 144 \\ 1 & 14 & 196 \end{pmatrix},$$

$$\widehat{\boldsymbol{B}}_{3o} = (\boldsymbol{A}_2'\boldsymbol{S}_o^{-1}\boldsymbol{A}_2)^{-1}\boldsymbol{A}_2'\boldsymbol{S}_o^{-1}\boldsymbol{X}_o\boldsymbol{C}'(\boldsymbol{C}\boldsymbol{C}')^{-1} = \begin{pmatrix} 17.1 & 22.0 \\ 0.54 & -0.31 \\ -0.003 & 0.050 \end{pmatrix},$$

$$\widehat{\boldsymbol{\Sigma}}_{3o} = \begin{pmatrix} 5.0 & 2.5 & 3.6 & 2.5 \\ & 3.9 & 2.7 & 3.1 \\ & & 6.0 & 3.8 \\ & & & 4.6 \end{pmatrix}.$$

In comparison with Models Ia, b, the intercept for the boys has increased, whereas for the girls not much has been altered. Thus, the data indicate that the growth patterns for the girls and the boys differ and the use of a BRM may be questionable.

Model IIb

This model is the same as Model IIa, but now an unweighted estimate of the mean parameters is derived, and $n\widehat{\boldsymbol{\Sigma}}_{4o} = (\boldsymbol{X} - \boldsymbol{A}_2\widehat{\boldsymbol{B}}_{4o}\boldsymbol{C})()'$:

$$\widehat{\boldsymbol{B}}_{4o} = (\boldsymbol{A}_2'\boldsymbol{A}_2)^{-1}\boldsymbol{A}_2'\boldsymbol{X}_o\boldsymbol{C}'(\boldsymbol{C}\boldsymbol{C}')^{-1} = \begin{pmatrix} 17.0 & 22.2 \\ 0.54 & -0.31 \\ -0.003 & 0.050 \end{pmatrix},$$

$$\widehat{\boldsymbol{\Sigma}}_{4o} = \begin{pmatrix} 5.0 & 2.5 & 3.6 & 2.5 \\ & 3.9 & 2.7 & 3.1 \\ & & 6.0 & 3.8 \\ & & & 4.6 \end{pmatrix}.$$

The estimators in Model IIb are almost identical to those in Model IIa.

Figure 3.3 illustrates the data. The most striking revelation in Fig. 3.3 is that there are some indications that the boys may follow a quadratic growth. This

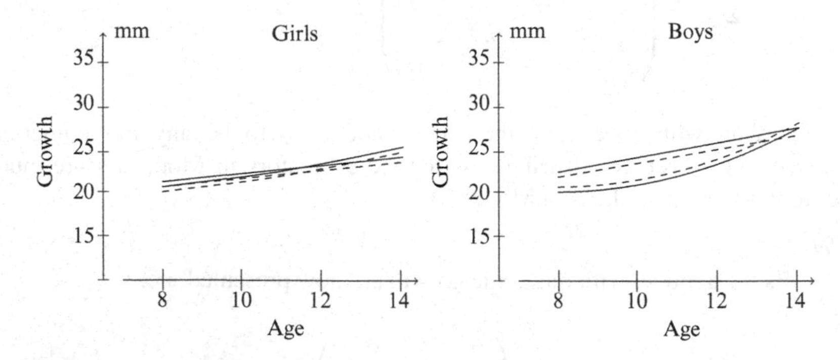

Fig. 3.3 The growth in the Potthoff and Roy (1964) data set (see Table 1.2) is illustrated for boys and girls, separately. In each figure the four models presented in Example 3.1 are given. The dashed lines indicate the unweighted estimators

will be investigated in subsequent sections. Moreover, the differences between the MLEs and the unweighted estimates are minor. Thus, considering the BRM for data analysis, one has to consider seriously if it is advantageous to use MLEs, since the distribution for these estimators is much more complicated than the distribution for the unweighted estimators, for example. □

3.3 $EBRM_B^3$ and Its MLEs

Let

$$X = A_1B_1C_1 + A_2B_2C_2 + A_3B_3C_3 + E, \quad E \sim N_{p,n}(\mathbf{0}, \Sigma, I), \quad \Sigma > 0,$$
$$\mathcal{C}(C_3') \subseteq \mathcal{C}(C_2') \subseteq \mathcal{C}(C_1'),$$

where all sizes of matrices are given in Definition 2.2. Following the structure of the previous section, first the derivation of the MLEs is performed in a rigorous way, culminating in Theorem 3.2, and thereafter the mathematics is illustrated in Fig. 3.4. Note that a major part of the derivation for obtaining MLEs has already been carried out in Sect. 2.5. The likelihood, $L(B_1, B_2, B_3, \Sigma)$, equals

$$L(B_1, B_2, B_3, \Sigma) = (2\pi)^{-np/2}|\Sigma|^{-n/2}e^{-1/2\mathrm{tr}\{\Sigma^{-1}(X_o-A_1B_1C_1-A_2B_2C_2-A_3B_3C_3)()'\}}.$$

Let, as in Sect. 2.5,

$$P_1 = I - Q_1' = P_{A_1,\Sigma}, \quad P_2 = I - Q_2' = P_{Q_1'A_2,\Sigma}, \quad P_3 = I - Q_3' = P_{Q_2'Q_1'A_3,\Sigma}, \tag{3.13}$$

$$S_1 = X_o(I - P_{C_1'})X_o', \text{ or } X(I - P_{C_1'})X', \tag{3.14}$$

$$S_2 = S_1 + Q_1'X_o(P_{C_1'} - P_{C_2'})X_o'Q_1, \text{ or } S_1 + Q_1'X(P_{C_1'} - P_{C_2'})X'Q_1, \tag{3.15}$$

$$S_3 = S_2 + Q_2'Q_1'X_o(P_{C_2'} - P_{C_3'})X_o'Q_1Q_2, \text{ or } S_2 + Q_2'Q_1'X(P_{C_2'} - P_{C_3'})X'Q_1Q_2. \tag{3.16}$$

Adopting the results from Sect. 2.5 when Σ is known, it is seen that the likelihood can be factored in the following way:

$$\begin{aligned}
L(B_1, B_2, B_3, \Sigma) &= (2\pi)^{-np/2}|\Sigma|^{-n/2} \\
&\quad \times \exp\{-1/2\mathrm{tr}\{\Sigma^{-1}S_1\}\}\exp\{-1/2\mathrm{tr}\{(X_oP_{C_1'} - E[X])'\Sigma^{-1}P_1()\}\} \\
&\quad \times \exp\{-1/2\mathrm{tr}\{\Sigma^{-1}(Q_1'X_oP_{C_1'} - E[Q_1'X])()'\}\} \\
&= (2\pi)^{-np/2}|\Sigma|^{-n/2} \\
&\quad \times \exp\{-1/2\mathrm{tr}\{\Sigma^{-1}S_2\}\}\exp\{-1/2\mathrm{tr}\{(X_oP_{C_1'} - E[X])'\Sigma^{-1}P_1()\}\}
\end{aligned}$$

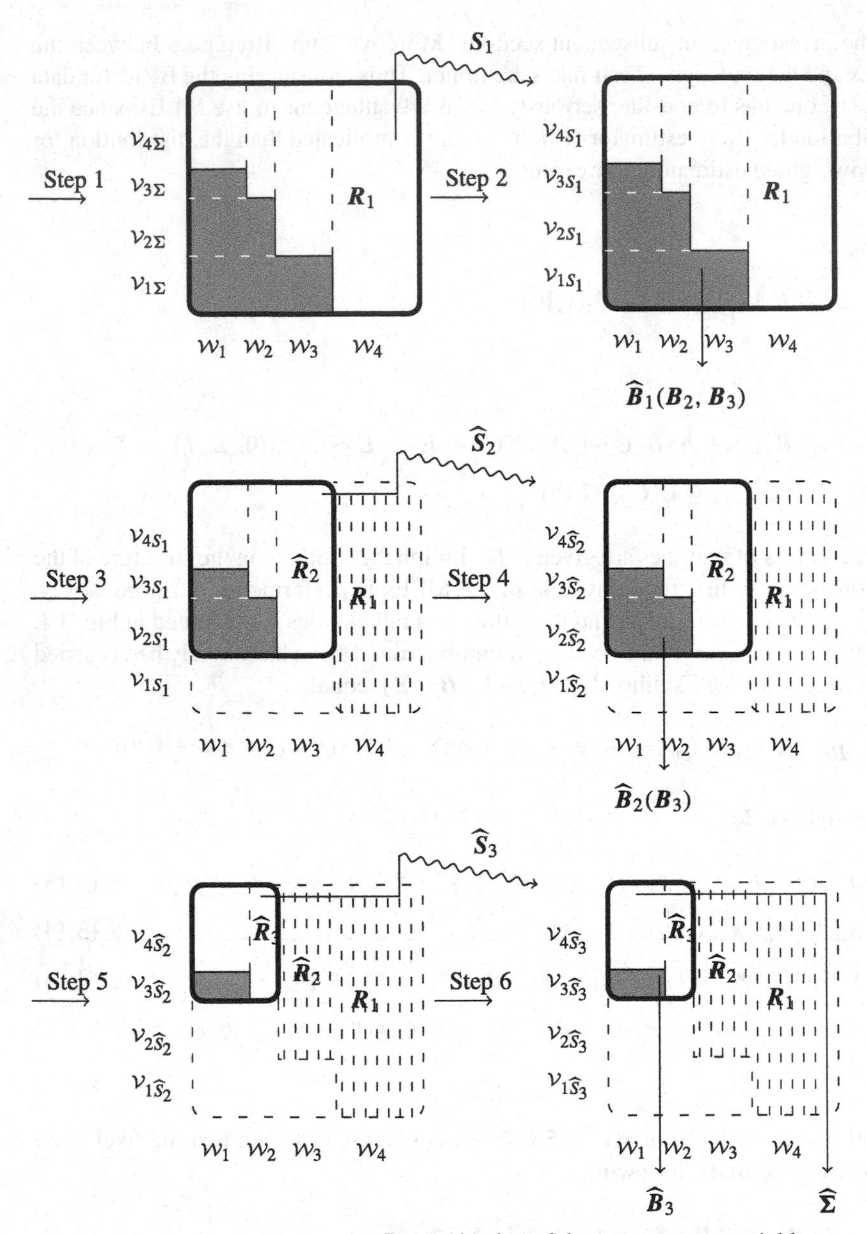

$$\widehat{E[X]} = \sum_{i=1}^{3} A_i\widehat{B}_iC_i = P_{A_1,S_1}XP_{C_1'} + P_{\widehat{Q}_1'A_2,\widehat{S}_2}XP_{C_2'} + P_{\widehat{Q}_2'\widehat{Q}_1'A_3,\widehat{S}_3}XP_{C_3'}.$$

Fig. 3.4 Estimation flow for the $EBRM_B^3$. For a detailed explanation of the various steps and notation see Sect. 3.3. $\mathcal{W}_1 = \mathcal{C}(C_3')$, $\mathcal{W}_2 = \mathcal{C}(C_2') \cap \mathcal{C}(C_3')^{\perp}$, $\mathcal{W}_3 = \mathcal{C}(C_1') \cap \mathcal{C}(C_2')^{\perp}$, $\mathcal{W}_4 = \mathcal{C}(C_1')^{\perp}$; $\mathcal{V}_{1\bullet} = \mathcal{C}_\bullet(A_1)$, $\mathcal{V}_{2\bullet} = \mathcal{C}_\bullet(A_1)^{\perp} \cap \mathcal{C}_\bullet(A_1 : A_2)$, $\mathcal{V}_{3\bullet} = \mathcal{C}_\bullet(A_1 : A_2)^{\perp} \cap \mathcal{C}_\bullet(A_1 : A_2 : A_3)$, $\mathcal{V}_{4\bullet} = \mathcal{C}_\bullet(A_1 : A_2 : A_3)^{\perp}$, where $\bullet$ represents Σ, S_1, $\widehat{S}_2$ or $\widehat{S}_3$. In the expressions $\perp$ is interpreted as denoting the orthogonal complement relative to the inner product

$$
\begin{aligned}
&\times\exp\{-1/2\mathrm{tr}\{(\boldsymbol{Q}_1'\boldsymbol{X}_o\boldsymbol{P}_{\boldsymbol{C}_2'} - E[\boldsymbol{Q}_1'\boldsymbol{X}])'\boldsymbol{\Sigma}^{-1}\boldsymbol{P}_2()\}\}\\
&\times\exp\{-1/2\mathrm{tr}\{\boldsymbol{\Sigma}^{-1}(\boldsymbol{Q}_2'\boldsymbol{Q}_1'\boldsymbol{X}_o\boldsymbol{P}_{\boldsymbol{C}_2'} - E[\boldsymbol{Q}_2'\boldsymbol{Q}_1'\boldsymbol{X}])()'\}\}\\
&= (2\pi)^{-np/2}|\boldsymbol{\Sigma}|^{-n/2}\\
&\times\exp\{-1/2\mathrm{tr}\{\boldsymbol{\Sigma}^{-1}\boldsymbol{S}_3\}\}\exp\{-1/2\mathrm{tr}\{(\boldsymbol{X}_o\boldsymbol{P}_{\boldsymbol{C}_1'} - E[\boldsymbol{X}])'\boldsymbol{\Sigma}^{-1}\boldsymbol{P}_1()\}\}\\
&\times\exp\{-1/2\mathrm{tr}\{(\boldsymbol{Q}_1'\boldsymbol{X}_o\boldsymbol{P}_{\boldsymbol{C}_2'} - E[\boldsymbol{Q}_1'\boldsymbol{X}])'\boldsymbol{\Sigma}^{-1}\boldsymbol{P}_2()\}\}\\
&\times\exp\{-1/2\mathrm{tr}\{(\boldsymbol{Q}_2'\boldsymbol{Q}_1'\boldsymbol{X}_o\boldsymbol{P}_{\boldsymbol{C}_3'} - E[\boldsymbol{Q}_2'\boldsymbol{Q}_1'\boldsymbol{X}_o])'\boldsymbol{\Sigma}^{-1}\boldsymbol{P}_3()\}\}\\
&\times\exp\{-1/2\mathrm{tr}\{\boldsymbol{\Sigma}^{-1}\boldsymbol{Q}_3'\boldsymbol{Q}_2'\boldsymbol{Q}_1'\boldsymbol{X}_o\boldsymbol{P}_{\boldsymbol{C}_3'}\boldsymbol{X}_o'\boldsymbol{Q}_1\boldsymbol{Q}_2\boldsymbol{Q}_3\}\}.
\end{aligned}
$$

This expression is smaller than or equal to

$$
(2\pi)^{-np/2}|\boldsymbol{\Sigma}|^{-n/2}\exp\{-1/2\mathrm{tr}\{\boldsymbol{\Sigma}^{-1}\boldsymbol{S}_3 + \boldsymbol{\Sigma}^{-1}\boldsymbol{Q}_3'\boldsymbol{Q}_2'\boldsymbol{Q}_1'\boldsymbol{X}_o\boldsymbol{P}_{\boldsymbol{C}_3'}\boldsymbol{X}_o'\boldsymbol{Q}_1\boldsymbol{Q}_2\boldsymbol{Q}_3\}\} \quad (3.17)
$$

with equality if and only if (see (2.26), (2.31) and (2.36))

$$
\boldsymbol{A}_1'\boldsymbol{\Sigma}^{-1}(\boldsymbol{X}_o\boldsymbol{P}_{\boldsymbol{C}_1'} - \boldsymbol{A}_1\boldsymbol{B}_1\boldsymbol{C}_1 - \boldsymbol{A}_2\boldsymbol{B}_2\boldsymbol{C}_2 - \boldsymbol{A}_3\boldsymbol{B}_3\boldsymbol{C}_3) = \boldsymbol{0}, \quad (3.18)
$$

$$
\boldsymbol{A}_2'\boldsymbol{Q}_1\boldsymbol{\Sigma}^{-1}(\boldsymbol{Q}_1'\boldsymbol{X}_o\boldsymbol{P}_{\boldsymbol{C}_2'} - \boldsymbol{Q}_1'\boldsymbol{A}_2\boldsymbol{B}_2\boldsymbol{C}_2 - \boldsymbol{Q}_1'\boldsymbol{A}_3\boldsymbol{B}_3\boldsymbol{C}_3) = \boldsymbol{0}, \quad (3.19)
$$

$$
\boldsymbol{A}_3'\boldsymbol{Q}_1\boldsymbol{Q}_2\boldsymbol{\Sigma}^{-1}(\boldsymbol{Q}_2'\boldsymbol{Q}_1'\boldsymbol{X}_o\boldsymbol{P}_{\boldsymbol{C}_3'} - \boldsymbol{Q}_2'\boldsymbol{Q}_1'\boldsymbol{A}_3\boldsymbol{B}_3\boldsymbol{C}_3) = \boldsymbol{0}. \quad (3.20)
$$

Moreover, using (3.18)–(3.20) and the equality

$$
\boldsymbol{S}_3 + \boldsymbol{Q}_3'\boldsymbol{Q}_2'\boldsymbol{Q}_1'\boldsymbol{X}_o\boldsymbol{P}_{\boldsymbol{C}_3'}\boldsymbol{X}_o'\boldsymbol{Q}_1\boldsymbol{Q}_2\boldsymbol{Q}_3 = (\boldsymbol{X}_o - \sum_{i=1}^{3}\boldsymbol{A}_i\boldsymbol{B}_i\boldsymbol{C}_i)()',
$$

which is independent of $\boldsymbol{\Sigma}$, it is established that the likelihood $L(\boldsymbol{B}_1, \boldsymbol{B}_2, \boldsymbol{B}_3, \boldsymbol{\Sigma})$ is smaller than or equal to (see Appendix B, Theorem B.9 (iv))

$$
(2n\pi)^{-np/2}|\boldsymbol{S}_3 + \boldsymbol{Q}_3'\boldsymbol{Q}_2'\boldsymbol{Q}_1'\boldsymbol{X}_o\boldsymbol{P}_{\boldsymbol{C}_3'}\boldsymbol{X}_o'\boldsymbol{Q}_1\boldsymbol{Q}_2\boldsymbol{Q}_3|^{-n/2}\exp\{-np/2\} \quad (3.21)
$$

and (3.21) is obtained if and only if

$$
n\boldsymbol{\Sigma} = \boldsymbol{S}_3 + \boldsymbol{Q}_3'\boldsymbol{Q}_2'\boldsymbol{Q}_1'\boldsymbol{X}_o\boldsymbol{P}_{\boldsymbol{C}_3'}\boldsymbol{X}_o'\boldsymbol{Q}_1\boldsymbol{Q}_2\boldsymbol{Q}_3, \quad (3.22)
$$

which is an equation in $\boldsymbol{\Sigma}$ since $\boldsymbol{Q}_i$, $i = 1, 2, 3$, are functions of $\boldsymbol{\Sigma}$. Thus, if we are able to solve (3.18)–(3.20) and (3.22), the MLEs will be found, because then it has been shown that these equations determine (3.21), i.e. (3.21) will be independent of any unknown parameter which becomes the upper bound of the likelihood.

From now on, for notational convenience, only estimators are considered. Note that (see Appendix B, Theorem B.11 (iv))

$$\begin{aligned}\mathcal{C}(\boldsymbol{Q}_1') &= \mathcal{C}_{\Sigma}(\boldsymbol{A}_1)^{\perp} = \mathcal{C}(\boldsymbol{\Sigma}^{-1}\boldsymbol{A}_1)^{\perp},\\ \mathcal{C}(\boldsymbol{Q}_2'\boldsymbol{Q}_1') &= \mathcal{C}(\boldsymbol{\Sigma}^{-1}\boldsymbol{Q}_1'\boldsymbol{A}_2)^{\perp} \cap \mathcal{C}(\boldsymbol{Q}_1') = \mathcal{C}(\boldsymbol{\Sigma}^{-1}\boldsymbol{Q}_1'\boldsymbol{A}_2)^{\perp} \cap \mathcal{C}(\boldsymbol{\Sigma}^{-1}\boldsymbol{A}_1)^{\perp},\\ \mathcal{C}(\boldsymbol{Q}_3'\boldsymbol{Q}_2'\boldsymbol{Q}_1') &= \mathcal{C}(\boldsymbol{\Sigma}^{-1}\boldsymbol{Q}_2'\boldsymbol{Q}_1'\boldsymbol{A}_3)^{\perp} \cap \mathcal{C}(\boldsymbol{\Sigma}^{-1}\boldsymbol{Q}_1'\boldsymbol{A}_2)^{\perp} \cap \mathcal{C}(\boldsymbol{\Sigma}^{-1}\boldsymbol{A}_1)^{\perp}.\end{aligned}$$

Hence, pre-multiplying (3.22) by $\boldsymbol{A}_1'\boldsymbol{\Sigma}^{-1}$, $\boldsymbol{A}_2'\boldsymbol{Q}_1'\boldsymbol{\Sigma}^{-1}$ and $\boldsymbol{A}_3'\boldsymbol{Q}_2'\boldsymbol{Q}_1'\boldsymbol{\Sigma}^{-1}$ yields the important relations

$$\boldsymbol{A}_1'\boldsymbol{\Sigma}^{-1} = n\boldsymbol{A}_1'\boldsymbol{S}_1^{-1}, \tag{3.23}$$

$$\boldsymbol{A}_2'\boldsymbol{Q}_1\boldsymbol{\Sigma}^{-1} = n\boldsymbol{A}_2'\boldsymbol{Q}_1\boldsymbol{S}_2^{-1}, \tag{3.24}$$

$$\boldsymbol{A}_3'\boldsymbol{Q}_2\boldsymbol{Q}_1\boldsymbol{\Sigma}^{-1} = n\boldsymbol{A}_3'\boldsymbol{Q}_2\boldsymbol{Q}_1\boldsymbol{S}_3^{-1}. \tag{3.25}$$

Equation (3.23) implies that $\boldsymbol{\Sigma}$ in $\boldsymbol{Q}_1$ can be replaced by $\boldsymbol{S}_1$ and then $\boldsymbol{Q}_1$ will be denoted $\widehat{\boldsymbol{Q}}_1$. Let $\widehat{\boldsymbol{S}}_2$ be $\boldsymbol{S}_2$, with $\boldsymbol{Q}_1$ having been replaced by $\widehat{\boldsymbol{Q}}_1$. Moreover, (3.24) implies that $\boldsymbol{\Sigma}$ in $\boldsymbol{Q}_2$ can be replaced by $\widehat{\boldsymbol{S}}_2$ which will then be denoted by $\widehat{\boldsymbol{Q}}_2$ with the additional supposition that $\boldsymbol{Q}_1$ has been replaced by $\widehat{\boldsymbol{Q}}_1$. Let $\widehat{\boldsymbol{S}}_3$ be $\boldsymbol{S}_3$ with $\boldsymbol{S}_2$, $\boldsymbol{Q}_2$ and $\boldsymbol{Q}_1$ having been replaced by $\widehat{\boldsymbol{S}}_2$, $\widehat{\boldsymbol{Q}}_2$ and $\widehat{\boldsymbol{Q}}_1$, respectively. The facts and notations given above yield that instead of (3.18)–(3.20), a consistent linear equation system in $\boldsymbol{B}_1$, $\boldsymbol{B}_2$ and $\boldsymbol{B}_3$ has emerged which equals

$$\begin{aligned}&\boldsymbol{A}_1'\boldsymbol{S}_1^{-1}(\boldsymbol{X}\boldsymbol{P}_{\boldsymbol{C}_1'} - \boldsymbol{A}_1\boldsymbol{B}_1\boldsymbol{C}_1 - \boldsymbol{A}_2\boldsymbol{B}_2\boldsymbol{C}_2 - \boldsymbol{A}_3\boldsymbol{B}_3\boldsymbol{C}_3) = \boldsymbol{0},\\ &\boldsymbol{A}_2'\widehat{\boldsymbol{Q}}_1\widehat{\boldsymbol{S}}_2^{-1}(\widehat{\boldsymbol{Q}}_1'\boldsymbol{X}\boldsymbol{P}_{\boldsymbol{C}_2'} - \widehat{\boldsymbol{Q}}_1'\boldsymbol{A}_2\boldsymbol{B}_2\boldsymbol{C}_2 - \widehat{\boldsymbol{Q}}_1'\boldsymbol{A}_3\boldsymbol{B}_3\boldsymbol{C}_3) = \boldsymbol{0},\\ &\boldsymbol{A}_3'\widehat{\boldsymbol{Q}}_1\widehat{\boldsymbol{Q}}_2\widehat{\boldsymbol{S}}_3^{-1}(\widehat{\boldsymbol{Q}}_2'\widehat{\boldsymbol{Q}}_1'\boldsymbol{X}\boldsymbol{P}_{\boldsymbol{C}_3'} - \widehat{\boldsymbol{Q}}_2'\widehat{\boldsymbol{Q}}_1'\boldsymbol{A}_3\boldsymbol{B}_3\boldsymbol{C}_3) = \boldsymbol{0}.\end{aligned}$$

These equations compose a nested structure; i.e. in the first equation $\boldsymbol{B}_1$, $\boldsymbol{B}_2$ and $\boldsymbol{B}_3$ are included, in the second equation $\boldsymbol{B}_2$ and $\boldsymbol{B}_3$ are included and in the last equation only $\boldsymbol{B}_3$ is included. Thus, we can solve for $\boldsymbol{B}_3$, insert the solution in the other equations, and then solve for $\boldsymbol{B}_2$, etc. The solution is presented in the next theorem:

Theorem 3.2 *For the $EBRM_B^3$ given in Definition 2.2 and with $\boldsymbol{S}_1 = \boldsymbol{X}(\boldsymbol{I} - \boldsymbol{P}_{\boldsymbol{C}_1'})\boldsymbol{X}'$ supposed to be p.d., with $n - r(\boldsymbol{C}_1') \geq p$, the MLEs are given by*

$$\begin{aligned}\widehat{\boldsymbol{B}}_1 &= (\boldsymbol{A}_1'\boldsymbol{S}_1^{-1}\boldsymbol{A}_1)^{-}\boldsymbol{A}_1'\boldsymbol{S}_1^{-1}(\boldsymbol{X} - \boldsymbol{A}_2\widehat{\boldsymbol{B}}_2\boldsymbol{C}_2 - \boldsymbol{A}_3\widehat{\boldsymbol{B}}_3\boldsymbol{C}_3)\boldsymbol{C}_1'(\boldsymbol{C}_1\boldsymbol{C}_1')^{-}\\ &\quad+(\boldsymbol{A}_1')^{o}\boldsymbol{Z}_{11} + \boldsymbol{A}_1'\boldsymbol{Z}_{12}\boldsymbol{C}_1^{o'},\\ \widehat{\boldsymbol{B}}_2 &= (\boldsymbol{A}_2'\widehat{\boldsymbol{Q}}_1\widehat{\boldsymbol{S}}_2^{-1}\widehat{\boldsymbol{Q}}_1'\boldsymbol{A}_2)^{-}\boldsymbol{A}_2'\widehat{\boldsymbol{Q}}_1\widehat{\boldsymbol{S}}_2^{-1}\widehat{\boldsymbol{Q}}_1'(\boldsymbol{X} - \boldsymbol{A}_3\widehat{\boldsymbol{B}}_3\boldsymbol{C}_3)\boldsymbol{C}_2'(\boldsymbol{C}_2\boldsymbol{C}_2')^{-}\end{aligned}$$

$$
\begin{aligned}
&+(A_2'\widehat{Q}_1)^o Z_{21} + A_2'\widehat{Q}_1 Z_{2,2} C_2^{o'},\\
\widehat{B}_3 &= (A_3'\widehat{Q}_1\widehat{Q}_2\widehat{S}_3^{-1}\widehat{Q}_2'\widehat{Q}_1'A_3)^- A_3'\widehat{Q}_1\widehat{Q}_2\widehat{S}_3^{-1}\widehat{Q}_2'\widehat{Q}_1'XC_3'(C_3C_3')^-\\
&+(A_3'\widehat{Q}_1\widehat{Q}_2)^o Z_{31} + A_3'\widehat{Q}_1\widehat{Q}_2 Z_{32} C_3^{o'},\\
n\widehat{\Sigma} &= (X - A_1\widehat{B}_1C_1 - A_2\widehat{B}_2C_2 - A_3\widehat{B}_3C_3)()'\\
&= \widehat{S}_3 + \widehat{Q}_3'\widehat{Q}_2'\widehat{Q}_1'XP_{C_3'}X'\widehat{Q}_1\widehat{Q}_2\widehat{Q}_3,
\end{aligned}
$$

where Z_{ij}, $i = 1, 2, 3$, $j = 1, 2$, are arbitrary matrices, $\widehat{Q}_1 = I - P'_{A_1,S_1}$, $\widehat{Q}_2 = I - P'_{\widehat{Q}_1'A_2,\widehat{S}_2}$, $\widehat{Q}_3 = I - P'_{\widehat{Q}_2'\widehat{Q}_1'A_3,\widehat{S}_3}$, and $\widehat{S}_2$ and $\widehat{S}_3$ are estimators of S_2 and S_3, with Q_i having been replaced by $\widehat{Q}_i$, $i = 2, 3$; S_2 and S_3 are defined in (3.15) and (3.16), respectively. The assumption that S_1 is p.d. holds with probability 1, since $n \geq p + r(C_1)$ is assumed to hold.

From this theorem it follows that the upper bound of the likelihood is obtained when one inserts the estimators presented in the theorem in the likelihood; i.e. the upper bound equals

$$
(2n\pi)^{-np/2}|\widehat{S}_3 + \widehat{Q}_3'\widehat{Q}_2'\widehat{Q}_1'XP_{C_3'}X'\widehat{Q}_1\widehat{Q}_2\widehat{Q}_3|^{-n/2}\exp\{-np/2\}.
$$

Corollary 3.3

$$
\begin{aligned}
\widehat{E[X]} &= A_1\widehat{B}_1C_1 + A_2\widehat{B}_2C_2 + A_3\widehat{B}_3C_3\\
&= P_{A_1,S_1}XP_{C_1'} + P_{\widehat{Q}_1'A_2,\widehat{S}_2}XP_{C_2'} + P_{\widehat{Q}_2'\widehat{Q}_1'A_3,\widehat{S}_3}XP_{C_3'}.
\end{aligned}
$$

Now the estimation process will be described in more heuristic terms, similar to the discussion connected to Figs. 2.9 and 2.10. This is important, because one needs to develop one's intuition in order to generalize the above-presented treatment in a meaningful way.

In Sect. 2.5, where Σ was supposed to be known, we established how the estimation was performed via projections. It appeared that Σ was involved only as a matrix defining the inner product. Thus, the estimation strategy will be, as with the BRM with an unknown dispersion matrix, to estimate the inner product first and then project observations on suitable spaces, i.e. the same spaces as when Σ is known.

In Fig. 3.4 a particular estimation scheme for the $EBRM_B^3$ is presented. It switches between estimating the inner product in certain regression spaces and then projecting observations on appropriate spaces in order to obtain estimators of the parameters of the mean, or to be more precise, to obtain estimators of estimable linear combinations of B_i, $i = 1, 2, 3$. The estimation scheme appears when solving the likelihood equations

$$A_i'\boldsymbol{\Sigma}^{-1}(\boldsymbol{X}-E[\boldsymbol{X}])\boldsymbol{C}_i'=\boldsymbol{0}, \quad i=1,2,3, \quad n\boldsymbol{\Sigma}=(\boldsymbol{X}-E[\boldsymbol{X}])()',$$

starting with $\boldsymbol{A}_1'\boldsymbol{\Sigma}^{-1}(\boldsymbol{X}-E[\boldsymbol{X}])\boldsymbol{C}_1'=\boldsymbol{0}$.

From the estimation of the parameters in the BRM it follows that in Step 1 the natural starting point is to construct $\boldsymbol{S}_1=\boldsymbol{R}_1\boldsymbol{R}_1'$, where $\boldsymbol{R}_1=\boldsymbol{X}(\boldsymbol{I}-\boldsymbol{P}_{C_1'})$ which then in Step 2 will replace $\boldsymbol{\Sigma}$ in $\mathcal{V}_{i\Sigma}$, i.e. the space $\mathcal{V}_i$ with the inner product defined by $\boldsymbol{\Sigma}$, $i=1,2,3,4$ (see Fig. 3.4 for a definition of $\mathcal{V}_i$). Note that we do not have to involve n such that instead $\boldsymbol{\Sigma}$ the matrix $n^{-1}\boldsymbol{S}_1$ (it is a consistent estimator) is used because in the projector the scalar n is not included. Thereafter in Step 2, two projections are performed. One projection gives an estimator of linear combinations of $\boldsymbol{B}_1$ as a function of $\boldsymbol{B}_2$ and $\boldsymbol{B}_3$, while the other projection projects observations on the tensor space $\mathcal{C}(\boldsymbol{C}_1')\otimes\mathcal{C}_{S_1}(\widehat{\boldsymbol{Q}}_1'(A_2,A_3,A_4))$ for further manipulations. Remember that $\widehat{\boldsymbol{Q}}_1'$ is a projector.

In Step 3 the information in $\boldsymbol{R}_1$ is directly used via $\boldsymbol{S}_1$ in the calculations of $\widehat{\boldsymbol{S}}_2$ given by

$$\widehat{\boldsymbol{S}}_2=\boldsymbol{S}_1+\widehat{\boldsymbol{R}}_2\widehat{\boldsymbol{R}}_2',$$

where $\widehat{\boldsymbol{R}}_2=\widehat{\boldsymbol{Q}}_1'\boldsymbol{X}(\boldsymbol{P}_{C_1'}-\boldsymbol{P}_{C_2'})$. It is interesting to observe that after the application of Step 2, we have an $EBRM_B^2$ model, which can also be seen in the illustration in Fig. 3.4 in Step 3. Moreover, in this figure it is indicated that the spaces connected with the estimation of $\boldsymbol{B}_1$, as well as $\mathcal{R}^p\otimes\mathcal{C}(\boldsymbol{C}_1')^{\perp}$, where $\mathcal{R}^p=\sum_{i=1}^4\mathcal{V}_i=\mathcal{C}_\Sigma(\boldsymbol{I})$, will not be used anymore.

Now, going from Step 3 to Step 4 is identical to going from Step 1 to Step 2. Instead of the sum of squares matrix $\boldsymbol{S}_1$, the matrix $\widehat{\boldsymbol{S}}_2$ appears as an inner product estimator. Two projections are carried out, one via $\boldsymbol{P}_{C_2'}\otimes\widehat{\boldsymbol{Q}}_2'\widehat{\boldsymbol{Q}}_1'$ and one which is used to estimate linear combinations of the mean parameter $\boldsymbol{B}_2$ as a function of $\boldsymbol{B}_3$, which is indicated by $\widehat{\boldsymbol{B}}_2(\boldsymbol{B}_3)$ in Fig. 3.4.

In Step 5 in Fig. 3.4 it can be seen that the BRM structure has been obtained and we can continue as before, i.e. the inner product is updated with the help of $\widehat{\boldsymbol{S}}_3=\widehat{\boldsymbol{S}}_2+\widehat{\boldsymbol{R}}_3\widehat{\boldsymbol{R}}_3'$, where $\widehat{\boldsymbol{R}}_3$ is obtained from $\boldsymbol{R}_3$, with $\boldsymbol{S}_2$, $\boldsymbol{Q}_2$ and $\boldsymbol{Q}_1$ having been replaced by $\widehat{\boldsymbol{S}}_2$, $\widehat{\boldsymbol{Q}}_2$ and $\widehat{\boldsymbol{Q}}_1$, respectively. Thereafter, in Step 6, projections on the mean space and its orthogonal complement are carried out. Thus, $\boldsymbol{B}_3$ can be estimated and by backwards updating $\widehat{\boldsymbol{B}}_2$, $\widehat{\boldsymbol{B}}_1$ and $\widehat{E[\boldsymbol{X}]}$ are obtained. Moreover, since this is the last step, $\boldsymbol{\Sigma}$ is estimated via $\boldsymbol{S}_3$ and a projection on $\mathcal{C}(\boldsymbol{C}_3')\otimes\mathcal{C}(\widehat{\boldsymbol{Q}}_3'\widehat{\boldsymbol{Q}}_2'\widehat{\boldsymbol{Q}}_1')$, i.e. $n\widehat{\boldsymbol{\Sigma}}=\widehat{\boldsymbol{S}}_3+\widehat{\boldsymbol{Q}}_3'\widehat{\boldsymbol{Q}}_2'\widehat{\boldsymbol{Q}}_1'\boldsymbol{X}\boldsymbol{P}_{C_3'}\boldsymbol{X}'\widehat{\boldsymbol{Q}}_1\widehat{\boldsymbol{Q}}_2\widehat{\boldsymbol{Q}}_3$. However, note that any of properly scaled $\boldsymbol{S}_1$ and $\widehat{\boldsymbol{S}}_i$, $i=2,3$, can be used as an estimator of $\boldsymbol{\Sigma}$ and serve as alternative estimators to the MLE.

3.4 $EBRM_W^3$ and Its MLEs

Now

$$X = A_1B_1C_1 + A_2B_2C_2 + A_3B_3C_3 + E, \quad E \sim N_{p,n}(\mathbf{0}, \Sigma, I), \quad \Sigma > 0,$$
$$\mathcal{C}(A_3) \subseteq \mathcal{C}(A_2) \subseteq \mathcal{C}(A_1),$$

is studied where all the sizes of the matrices are presented in Definition 2.3. Once again the mathematical derivation of the estimators is given first, and then the approach is illustrated. It is interesting to compare the results for the $EBRM_W^3$ with those for the $EBRM_B^3$.

At the beginning of the mathematical derivation, we completely rely on Sect. 2.6, where MLEs were obtained for a known Σ. The likelihood, $L(B_1, B_2, B_3, \Sigma)$, equals

$$L(B_1, B_2, B_3, \Sigma) = (2\pi)^{-np/2}|\Sigma|^{-n/2}e^{-1/2\mathrm{tr}\{\Sigma^{-1}(X_o - A_1B_1C_1 - A_2B_2C_2 - A_3B_3C_3)()'\}}. \tag{3.26}$$

Let, as previously in Sect. 2.6,

$$P_1 = P_{C_1'}, \quad P_2 = P_{Q_1C_2'}, \quad P_3 = P_{Q_2C_3'}, \quad P_4 = P_{(C_1':C_2':C_3')^o}, \tag{3.27}$$

where

$$Q_1 = P_{(C_1')^o}, \quad Q_2 = P_{(C_1':C_2')^o}. \tag{3.28}$$

Thus, the likelihood can be written as follows:

$$L(B_1, B_2, B_3, \Sigma)$$
$$= (2\pi)^{-np/2}|\Sigma|^{-n/2}\exp\{-1/2\sum_{i=1}^{4}\mathrm{tr}\{\Sigma^{-1}(X_o - E[X])P_i()'\}\}. \tag{3.29}$$

From Sect. 2.6 it follows that an upper bound of the likelihood is achieved if a solution can be found to the system of equations consisting of (2.49)–(2.51), i.e. the nested system

$$A_1'\Sigma^{-1}(X_o - A_1B_1C_1 - A_2B_2C_2 - A_3B_3C_3)P_1 = \mathbf{0}, \tag{3.30}$$
$$A_2'\Sigma^{-1}(X_o - A_2B_2C_2 - A_3B_3C_3)P_2 = \mathbf{0}, \tag{3.31}$$
$$A_3'\Sigma^{-1}(X_o - A_3B_3C_3)P_3 = \mathbf{0}. \tag{3.32}$$

Based on (2.46), (2.48), (3.26) and (3.29), it follows that $\boldsymbol{\Sigma}$ has to satisfy (see Appendix B, Theorem B.9 (iv))

$$n\boldsymbol{\Sigma} = (\boldsymbol{X}_o - E[\boldsymbol{X}])()' = \boldsymbol{X}_o\boldsymbol{P}_4\boldsymbol{X}_o' + \sum_{i=1}^{3} \boldsymbol{P}'_{A_i^o,\Sigma^{-1}}\boldsymbol{X}_o\boldsymbol{P}_i\boldsymbol{X}_o'\boldsymbol{P}_{A_i^o,\Sigma^{-1}}. \quad (3.33)$$

In order to find estimators for $\boldsymbol{B}_i$ which are independent of $\boldsymbol{\Sigma}$, explicit expressions for $\boldsymbol{A}_i'\boldsymbol{\Sigma}^{-1}$, $i = 1, 2, 3$, are required. However, it is straightforward to obtain such expressions from (3.33), since pre-multiplying (3.33) by $\boldsymbol{A}_i'\boldsymbol{\Sigma}^{-1}$, i=1,2,3, leads to the following important relations:

$$n\boldsymbol{A}_3'\boldsymbol{S}_{1o}^{-1} = \boldsymbol{A}_3'\boldsymbol{\Sigma}^{-1}, \quad n\boldsymbol{A}_2'\widehat{\boldsymbol{S}}_{2o}^{-1} = \boldsymbol{A}_2'\boldsymbol{\Sigma}^{-1}, \quad n\boldsymbol{A}_1'\widehat{\boldsymbol{S}}_{3o}^{-1} = \boldsymbol{A}_1'\boldsymbol{\Sigma}^{-1}, \quad (3.34)$$

where

$$\boldsymbol{S}_{1o} = \boldsymbol{X}_o\boldsymbol{P}_4\boldsymbol{X}_o', \quad \widehat{\boldsymbol{S}}_{2o} = \boldsymbol{S}_{1o} + \boldsymbol{P}'_{A_3^o,S_{1o}^{-1}}\boldsymbol{X}_o\boldsymbol{P}_3\boldsymbol{X}_o'\boldsymbol{P}_{A_3^o,S_{1o}^{-1}}, \quad (3.35)$$

$$\widehat{\boldsymbol{S}}_{3o} = \widehat{\boldsymbol{S}}_{2o} + \boldsymbol{P}'_{A_2^o,\widehat{S}_{2o}^{-1}}\boldsymbol{X}_o\boldsymbol{P}_2\boldsymbol{X}_o'\boldsymbol{P}_{A_2^o,\widehat{S}_{2o}^{-1}}. \quad (3.36)$$

As before, the $\widehat{\ }$ on $\boldsymbol{S}_{2o}$ and $\boldsymbol{S}_{3o}$ indicates that an inner product has been estimated. It follows that, instead of (3.30)–(3.32), a system of consistent linear equations in $\boldsymbol{B}_i$, $i = 1, 2, 3$, has been obtained, which equals

$$\boldsymbol{A}_1'\widehat{\boldsymbol{S}}_{3o}^{-1}(\boldsymbol{X}_o - \boldsymbol{A}_1\boldsymbol{B}_1\boldsymbol{C}_1 - \boldsymbol{A}_2\boldsymbol{B}_2\boldsymbol{C}_2 - \boldsymbol{A}_3\boldsymbol{B}_3\boldsymbol{C}_3)\boldsymbol{P}_1 = \boldsymbol{0}, \quad (3.37)$$

$$\boldsymbol{A}_2'\widehat{\boldsymbol{S}}_{2o}^{-1}(\boldsymbol{X}_o - \boldsymbol{A}_2\boldsymbol{B}_2\boldsymbol{C}_2 - \boldsymbol{A}_3\boldsymbol{B}_3\boldsymbol{C}_3)\boldsymbol{P}_2 = \boldsymbol{0}, \quad (3.38)$$

$$\boldsymbol{A}_3'\boldsymbol{S}_{1o}^{-1}(\boldsymbol{X}_o - \boldsymbol{A}_3\boldsymbol{B}_3\boldsymbol{C}_3)\boldsymbol{P}_3 = \boldsymbol{0}. \quad (3.39)$$

Hence, from these hierarchically structured equations $\widehat{\boldsymbol{B}}_i$, $i = 1, 2, 3$, are derived. Moreover, $\widehat{\boldsymbol{\Sigma}}$ is obtained via (3.33). The results are summarized in the next theorem, but we alter the presentation by using random variables instead of observations.

Theorem 3.3 *For the $EBRM_W^3$ presented in Definition 2.3 let $\boldsymbol{S}_1$ and $\widehat{\boldsymbol{S}}_i$ $i = 2, 3$, be defined through (3.35) and (3.36), respectively; $\boldsymbol{Q}_i$, $i = 1, 2$, is defined in (3.28) and $\boldsymbol{P}_i$, $i = 1, 2, 3, 4$, in (3.27). Moreover, $\boldsymbol{S}_1 = \boldsymbol{X}\boldsymbol{P}_4\boldsymbol{X}'$ is supposed to be p.d., which holds with probability 1 if $n - r(\boldsymbol{C}_1' : \boldsymbol{C}_2' : \boldsymbol{C}_3') \geq p$. Then the MLEs are given by*

$$\widehat{\boldsymbol{B}}_1 = (\boldsymbol{A}_1'\widehat{\boldsymbol{S}}_3^{-1}\boldsymbol{A}_1)^-\boldsymbol{A}_1'\widehat{\boldsymbol{S}}_3^{-1}(\boldsymbol{X} - \boldsymbol{A}_2\widehat{\boldsymbol{B}}_2\boldsymbol{C}_2 - \boldsymbol{A}_3\widehat{\boldsymbol{B}}_3\boldsymbol{C}_3)\boldsymbol{C}_1'(\boldsymbol{C}_1\boldsymbol{C}_1')^-$$
$$+(\boldsymbol{A}_1')^o\boldsymbol{Z}_{11} + \boldsymbol{A}_1'\boldsymbol{Z}_{12}\boldsymbol{C}_1^{o'},$$
$$\widehat{\boldsymbol{B}}_2 = (\boldsymbol{A}_2'\widehat{\boldsymbol{S}}_2^{-1}\boldsymbol{A}_2)^-\boldsymbol{A}_2'\widehat{\boldsymbol{S}}_2^{-1}(\boldsymbol{X} - \boldsymbol{A}_3\widehat{\boldsymbol{B}}_3\boldsymbol{C}_3)\boldsymbol{Q}_1\boldsymbol{C}_2'(\boldsymbol{C}_2\boldsymbol{Q}_1\boldsymbol{C}_2')^-$$

$$
\begin{aligned}
&\quad +(A_2')^o Z_{21} + A_2' Z_{2,2}(C_2 Q_1)^{o'},\\
\widehat{B}_3 &= (A_3' S_1^{-1} A_3)^- A_3' S_1^{-1} X Q_2 C_3' (C_3 Q_2 C_3')^-\\
&\quad +(A_3')^o Z_{31} + A_3' Z_{32}(C_3 Q_2)^{o'},\\
n\widehat{\Sigma} &= (X - A_1\widehat{B}_1 C_1 - A_2\widehat{B}_2 C_2 - A_3\widehat{B}_3 C_3)()'\\
&= \widehat{S}_3 + P'_{A_1^o, \widehat{S}_3^{-1}} X P_{C_1'} X' P_{A_1^o, \widehat{S}_3^{-1}},
\end{aligned}
$$

where Z_{ij}, $i = 1, 2, 3$, $j = 1, 2$, are arbitrary matrices.

Corollary 3.4 *Let $\widehat{B}_i$ be given in Theorem 3.3. Then*

$$
\begin{aligned}
\widehat{E[X]} &= A_1\widehat{B}_1 C_1 + A_2\widehat{B}_2 C_2 + A_3\widehat{B}_3 C_3\\
&= P_{A_1, \widehat{S}_3} X P_{C_1'} + P_{A_2, \widehat{S}_2} X P_{Q_1 C_2'} + P_{A_3, S_1} X P_{Q_2 C_3'}.
\end{aligned}
$$

Corollary 3.5 *Let $\widehat{B}_i$ be given in Theorem 3.3, and suppose that $\mathcal{C}(C_1')$ is orthogonal to $\mathcal{C}(C_2' : C_3')$ and $\mathcal{C}(C_2')$ is orthogonal to $\mathcal{C}(C_1' : C_3')$. Then, the MLEs are given by*

$$
\begin{aligned}
\widehat{B}_1 &= (A_1'\widehat{S}_3^{-1} A_1)^- A_1'\widehat{S}_3^{-1} X C_1'(C_1 C_1')^- + (A_1')^o Z_{11} + A_1' Z_{12} C_1^{o'},\\
\widehat{B}_2 &= (A_2'\widehat{S}_2^{-1} A_2)^- A_2'\widehat{S}_2^{-1} X C_2'(C_2 C_2')^- + (A_2')^o Z_{21} + A_2' Z_{2,2} C_2^{o'},\\
\widehat{B}_3 &= (A_3' S_1^{-1} A_3)^- A_3' S_1^{-1} X C_3'(C_3 C_3')^- + (A_3')^o Z_{31} + A_3' Z_{32} C_3^{o'},\\
n\widehat{\Sigma} &= (X - A_1\widehat{B}_1 C_1 - A_2\widehat{B}_2 C_2 - A_3\widehat{B}_3 C_3)()'\\
&= \widehat{S}_3 + P'_{A_1^o, \widehat{S}_3^{-1}} X P_{C_1'} X' P_{A_1^o, \widehat{S}_3^{-1}},
\end{aligned}
$$

where

$$
S_1 = X(I - P_{C_1':C_2':C_3'})X', \quad \widehat{S}_2 = S_1 + P'_{A_3^o, S_1^{-1}} X P_{Q_2 C_3'} X' P_{A_3^o, S_1^{-1}},
$$

$$
\widehat{S}_3 = \widehat{S}_2 + P'_{A_2^o, \widehat{S}_2^{-1}} X P_{Q_1 C_2'} X' P_{A_2^o, \widehat{S}_2^{-1}}.
$$

There is one interesting aspect of Corollary 3.5. In the $EBRM_B^3$, because of the unknown dispersion Σ, it is not possible to interpret any orthogonal relations among A_i, immediately. However, for the $EBRM_W^3$ it makes sense to include orthogonality restrictions for C_i', $i = 1, 2, 3$, which, as seen in Corollary 3.5, then also simplifies the expressions of the estimators. In fact, in many applications one can reformulate an $EBRM_B^3$ and transform it into an $EBRM_W^3$ with an orthogonal between-individuals structure and interpretable parameters, for example when studying growth curves in different treatment groups.

Similar to the description of the estimation of the parameters in the $EBRM_B^3$, which was presented in Fig. 3.4, an estimation algorithm for the $EBRM_W^3$ is now described. Moreover, $\boldsymbol{P}_{A_i,\Sigma}$, $i = 1, 2, 3$, are determined by (3.34), i.e. $\widehat{\boldsymbol{P}}_{A_1,\Sigma} = \boldsymbol{P}_{A_3,S_1}$, $\widehat{\boldsymbol{P}}_{A_2,\Sigma} = \boldsymbol{P}_{A_2,\widehat{S}_2}$ and $\widehat{\boldsymbol{P}}_{A_1,\Sigma} = \boldsymbol{P}_{A_1,\widehat{S}_3}$. The estimation scheme in Fig. 3.5 follows in principle (3.30)–(3.32), starting with (3.32), then using (3.31) and, finally, considering (3.30).

We can summarize the estimation in six steps. In Step 1 a sums of squares matrix $\boldsymbol{S}_1 = \boldsymbol{R}_1\boldsymbol{R}_1'$, where $\boldsymbol{R}_1 = \boldsymbol{X}(\boldsymbol{I} - \boldsymbol{P}_{C_1':C_2':C_3'})$, is constructed which is used to replace $\boldsymbol{\Sigma}$ in Step 2. Moreover, in Step 2, $\boldsymbol{B}_3$ is estimated. In Step 3 the inner product estimator is updated with the help of $\widehat{\boldsymbol{R}}_2 = \boldsymbol{P}_{A_3^o,S_1^{-1}}\boldsymbol{X}\boldsymbol{P}_{Q_2C_3'}$. It is also indicated in Fig. 3.5 that $\boldsymbol{R}_1$ is not needed anymore in the estimation process. Proceeding to Step 4, $\widehat{\boldsymbol{B}}_2$ is obtained as a function of $\widehat{\boldsymbol{B}}_3$. The arguments from Step 3 and Step 4 are then repeated in Step 5 and Step 6, and Step 6 produces $\widehat{\boldsymbol{B}}_1$ as a function of $\widehat{\boldsymbol{B}}_2$ and $\widehat{\boldsymbol{B}}_3$, as well as $\widehat{\boldsymbol{\Sigma}}$, where $\widehat{\boldsymbol{R}}_4 = \boldsymbol{P}_{A_1^o,\widehat{S}_3^{-1}}\boldsymbol{X}\boldsymbol{P}_{C_1'}$ and $\widehat{\boldsymbol{R}}_3 = \boldsymbol{P}_{A_2^o,\widehat{S}_2^{-1}}\boldsymbol{X}\boldsymbol{P}_{Q_1C_2'}$ are used.

A comparison of Figs. 3.4 and 3.5 uncovers both similarities and some principal differences. If one examines the spaces which are involved, for the $EBRM_B^3$ there are two decompositions,

$$\mathcal{C}(\boldsymbol{C}_3') \boxplus \mathcal{C}(\boldsymbol{C}_2') \cap \mathcal{C}(\boldsymbol{C}_3')^\perp \boxplus \mathcal{C}(\boldsymbol{C}_1') \cap \mathcal{C}(\boldsymbol{C}_2')^\perp \boxplus \mathcal{C}(\boldsymbol{C}_1')^\perp,$$

$$\mathcal{C}(\boldsymbol{A}_1) \boxplus \mathcal{C}(\boldsymbol{A}_1)^\perp \cap \mathcal{C}(\boldsymbol{A}_1 : \boldsymbol{A}_2) \boxplus \mathcal{C}(\boldsymbol{A}_1 : \boldsymbol{A}_2)^\perp \cap \mathcal{C}(\boldsymbol{A}_1 : \boldsymbol{A}_2 : \boldsymbol{A}_3)$$
$$\boxplus \mathcal{C}(\boldsymbol{A}_1 : \boldsymbol{A}_2 : \boldsymbol{A}_3)^\perp,$$

which build up the tensor space, illustrated in Fig. 3.4, whereas for the $EBRM_W^3$ in Fig. 3.5 the corresponding spaces are

$$\mathcal{C}(\boldsymbol{C}_1') \boxplus \mathcal{C}(\boldsymbol{C}_1 : \boldsymbol{C}_2') \cap \mathcal{C}(\boldsymbol{C}_1')^\perp \boxplus \mathcal{C}(\boldsymbol{C}_1' : \boldsymbol{C}_2' : \boldsymbol{C}_3') \cap \mathcal{C}(\boldsymbol{C}_1' : \boldsymbol{C}_2')^\perp$$
$$\boxplus \mathcal{C}(\boldsymbol{C}_1' : \boldsymbol{C}_2' : \boldsymbol{C}_3')^\perp,$$

$$\mathcal{C}(\boldsymbol{A}_3) \boxplus \mathcal{C}(\boldsymbol{A}_3)^\perp \cap \mathcal{C}(\boldsymbol{A}_2) \boxplus \mathcal{C}(\boldsymbol{A}_2)^\perp \cap \mathcal{C}(\boldsymbol{A}_1) \boxplus \mathcal{C}(\boldsymbol{A}_1)^\perp.$$

For the $EBRM_B^3$ the condition $\mathcal{C}(\boldsymbol{C}_3') \subseteq \mathcal{C}(\boldsymbol{C}_2') \subseteq \mathcal{C}(\boldsymbol{C}_1')$ means that the spaces are nested within $\mathcal{C}(\boldsymbol{C}_1')$, whereas for the $EBRM_W^3$ there are three arbitrary spaces, $\mathcal{C}(\boldsymbol{C}_3')$, $\mathcal{C}(\boldsymbol{C}_2')$ and $\mathcal{C}(\boldsymbol{C}_1')$, which are comparable but do not have to be nested in any way. The nestedness applies to $\mathcal{C}(\boldsymbol{A}_i)$, $i = 1, 2, 3$, when working with the $EBRM_W^3$. However, what the two models have common is the fact that the estimation in both of them starts with $\mathcal{W}_4$ from where $\boldsymbol{\Sigma}$ is estimated when $\boldsymbol{\Sigma}$ is used to define the inner product. Thereafter, one transmits the information, via $\widehat{\boldsymbol{S}}_2$, to $\mathcal{W}_3$, updates the estimation of the inner product, transmits the information, via $\widehat{\boldsymbol{S}}_3$, to $\mathcal{W}_2$, obtains a new estimator of the inner product, and finally transmits the information to $\mathcal{W}_1$, after which $\boldsymbol{\Sigma}$ is estimated as a dispersion matrix. However, the procedures for finding the estimators of the mean parameters in $EBRM_B^3$ and $EBRM_W^3$ are different.

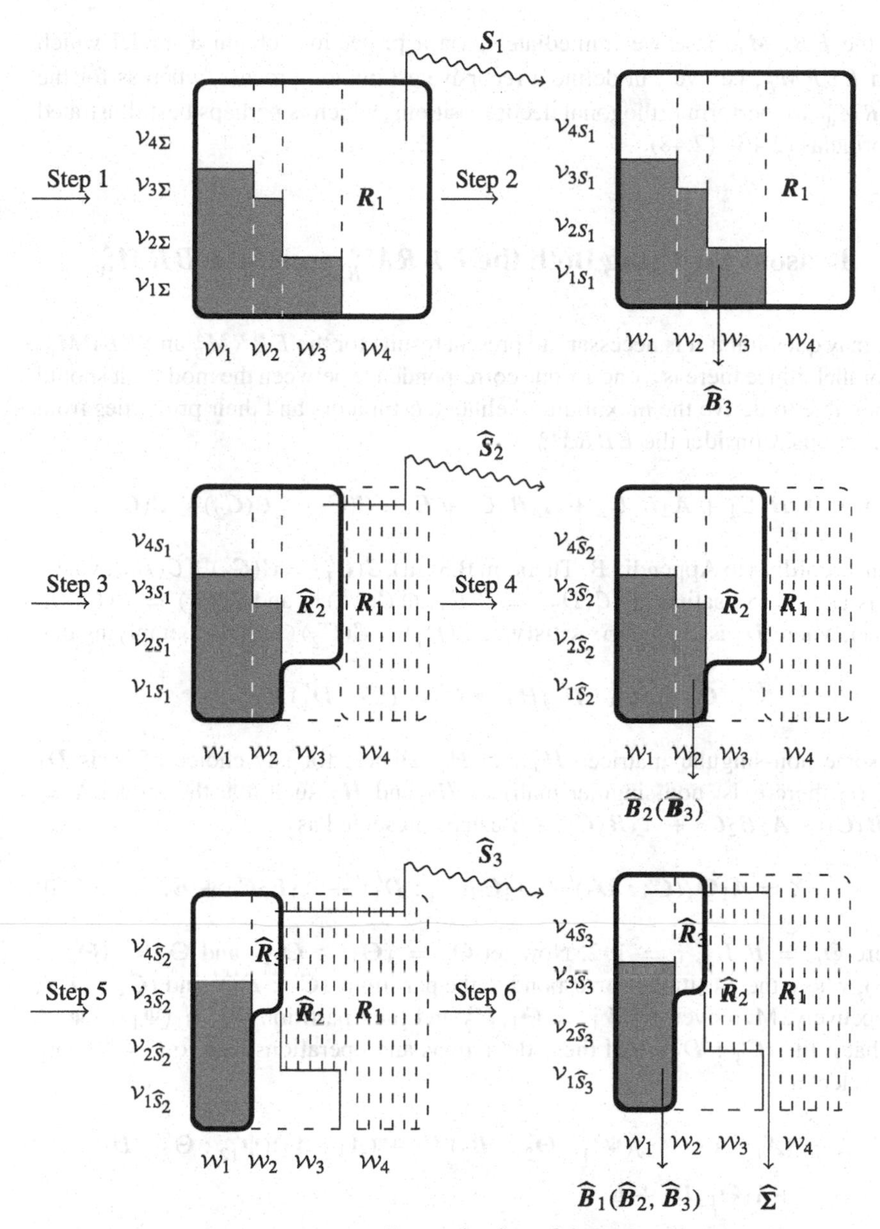

Fig. 3.5 Estimation flow for the $EBRM_W^3$. For a detailed explanation of the various steps and notation see Sect. 3.4. $\mathcal{W}_1 = \mathcal{C}(C_1')$, $\mathcal{W}_2 = \mathcal{C}(C_1' : C_2') \cap \mathcal{C}(C_1')^{\perp}$, $\mathcal{W}_3 = \mathcal{C}(C_1' : C_2' : C_3') \cap \mathcal{C}(C_1' : C_2')^{\perp}$, $\mathcal{W}_4 = \mathcal{C}(C_1' : C_2' : C_3')^{\perp}$; $\mathcal{V}_{1\bullet} = \mathcal{C}_{\bullet}(A_3)$, $\mathcal{V}_{2\bullet} = \mathcal{C}_{\bullet}(A_3)^{\perp} \cap \mathcal{C}_{\bullet}(A_2)$, $\mathcal{V}_{3\bullet} = \mathcal{C}_{\bullet}(A_2)^{\perp} \cap \mathcal{C}_{\bullet}(A_1)$, $\mathcal{V}_{4\bullet} = \mathcal{C}_{\bullet}(A_1)^{\perp}$, where $\bullet$ represents Σ, S_1, $\widehat{S}_2$ or $\widehat{S}_3$

For the $EBRM_B^3$ case we immediately, via a projection, obtain a model which is an $EBRM_B^2$, i.e. we can define a recursive estimation process, whereas for the $EBRM_W^3$ we perform orthogonal decompositions, which is perhaps best illustrated in formulas (2.46)–(2.48).

3.5 Reasons for Using Both the $EBRM_B^3$ and the $EBRM_W^3$

One may question if it is necessary to present results for the $EBRM_B^3$ and $EBRM_W^3$ in parallel. Since there is a one-to-one correspondence between the models, it should be possible to derive the maximum likelihood estimators and their properties from both set-ups. Consider the $EBRM_B^3$

$$X = A_1B_1C_1 + A_2B_2C_2 + A_3B_3C_3 + E, \quad \mathcal{C}(C_3') \subseteq \mathcal{C}(C_2') \subseteq \mathcal{C}(C_1').$$

Then, according to Appendix B, Theorem B.3 (iii), $\mathcal{C}(C_1') = \mathcal{C}(C_2') \boxplus \mathcal{C}(D_2')$, where D_2 is any matrix satisfying $\mathcal{C}(D_2') = \mathcal{C}(C_1') \cap \mathcal{C}(C_2')^{\perp}$, and $\mathcal{C}(C_2') = \mathcal{C}(C_3') \boxplus \mathcal{C}(D_1')$, where D_1 is any matrix satisfying $\mathcal{C}(D_1') = \mathcal{C}(C_2') \cap \mathcal{C}(C_3')^{\perp}$, implying that

$$C_1' = (C_2' : D_2')H_1, \quad C_2' = (C_3' : D_1')H_2$$

for some non-singular matrices H_1 and H_2. Hence, for any choice of basis D_1 and D_2 there exist non-singular matrices H_1 and H_2 such that the model $X = A_1B_1C_1 + A_2B_2C_2 + A_3B_3C_3 + E$ can be presented as

$$X = A_1\Theta_1(C_2' : D_2')' + A_2\Theta_2(C_3' : D_1')' + A_3B_3C_3 + E, \tag{3.40}$$

where $\Theta_i = B_iH_i'$, $i = 1, 2$. Now let $\Theta_1 = (\Theta_{11} : \Theta_{12})$ and $\Theta_2 = (\Theta_{21} : \Theta_{22})$, where the partitions correspond to the partitions $(C_2' : D_2')'$ and $(C_3' : D_1')'$, respectively. Moreover, let $\Psi_1 = \Theta_{11}H_2'$ and then partition $\Psi_1 = (\Psi_{11} : \Psi_{12})$ so that it fits $(C_3' : D_1')'$. All these definitions and operations lead to (3.40) being equivalent to

$$\begin{aligned} X = &(A_1 : A_2 : A_3)(\Psi_{11}' : \Theta_{21}' : B_3')'C_3 + (A_1 : A_2)(\Psi_{12}' : \Theta_{22}')'D_1 \\ &+ A_1\Theta_{12}D_2 + E, \end{aligned}$$

which is an $EBRM_W^3$. Hence, it has been shown how, by a reparametrization, any $EBRM_B^3$ can be formulated as an $EBRM_W^3$. The opposite is, of course, also true, i.e. any $EBRM_W^3$ can be formulated as an $EBRM_B^3$. In principle one might believe that it would be sufficient to, for example, only consider the $EBRM_B^3$. However, there are some problems with this approach. Firstly there are several reparametrizations and several partitions involved, which means that individual parameter estimates may be difficult to interpret, and secondly all MLEs are non-linear estimators and, therefore, it is not so easy to work out how to transmit properties, for example knowledge about moments of the MLEs, from one model to another, i.e. from the $EBRM_B^3$ to the $EBRM_W^3$ or vice versa. Thus, to achieve greater ease of application and clarity, one should work with the two different types of models separately.

Problems

1 For the BRM, calculate the residuals $\widehat{\boldsymbol{R}}_{11}$, $\widehat{\boldsymbol{R}}_{21}$ and $\widehat{\boldsymbol{R}}_2$ in (3.7), (3.8) and (3.9), respectively, and compare with the data in Table 2.1. What conclusions can be drawn?

2 (*GMANOVA* + *MANOVA*) Let

$$\boldsymbol{X} = \boldsymbol{A}\boldsymbol{B}_1\boldsymbol{C}_1 + \boldsymbol{B}_2\boldsymbol{C}_2 + \boldsymbol{E},$$

where the observation matrix $\boldsymbol{X}$: $p \times n$, the unknown mean parameter matrices $\boldsymbol{B}_1$: $q \times k_1$ and $\boldsymbol{B}_2$: $p \times k_2$, the three known design matrices $\boldsymbol{A}$: $p \times q$, $\boldsymbol{C}_1$: $k_1 \times n$ and $\boldsymbol{C}_2$: $k_2 \times n$, and the error matrix $\boldsymbol{E}$ form the model. Moreover, let $\boldsymbol{E}$ be normally distributed with independent columns, with mean $\boldsymbol{0}$, and an unknown positive definite dispersion matrix $\boldsymbol{\Sigma}$ for the elements within each column of $\boldsymbol{E}$. Find maximum likelihood estimates of the parameters. Can the model be used when there is a MANOVA model with some specific background information? Can the model be used when there is a GMANOVA model (BRM) with some specific background information?

3 Let

$$\boldsymbol{X} = \boldsymbol{A}\boldsymbol{B}_1\boldsymbol{C}_1 + \boldsymbol{A}_2\boldsymbol{B}_2\boldsymbol{C}_2 + \boldsymbol{E}, \quad \mathcal{C}(\boldsymbol{C}_2') \subseteq \mathcal{C}(\boldsymbol{C}_1'),$$

where the observation matrix $\boldsymbol{X}$: $p \times n$, the unknown mean parameter matrices $\boldsymbol{B}_1$: $q_1 \times k_1$ and $\boldsymbol{B}_2$: $q_2 \times k_2$, the four known design matrices $\boldsymbol{A}_1$: $p \times q_1$, $\boldsymbol{A}_2$: $p \times q_2$, $\boldsymbol{C}_1$: $k_1 \times n$ and $\boldsymbol{C}_2$: $k_2 \times n$, and the error matrix $\boldsymbol{E} \sim N_{p,n}(\boldsymbol{0}, \boldsymbol{\Sigma}, \boldsymbol{I})$, where $\boldsymbol{\Sigma} > 0$, form the model. Find maximum likelihood estimates of the parameters.

4 In Problems 2 and 3 suppose that $\boldsymbol{\Sigma} = \boldsymbol{I}$ and estimate the parameters in both models. Moreover, generate $\boldsymbol{X}_o$ according to the models in Problems 2 and 3 (choose matrices $\boldsymbol{A}_i$, $\boldsymbol{B}_i$, $\boldsymbol{C}_i$ and $\boldsymbol{\Sigma}$). Compare the unweighted estimates (assuming $\boldsymbol{\Sigma} = \boldsymbol{I}$) with the MLEs, assuming $\boldsymbol{\Sigma}$ to be an unknown parameter.

5 In Problem 3 replace $\mathcal{C}(\boldsymbol{C}_2') \subseteq \mathcal{C}(\boldsymbol{C}_1')$ by $\mathcal{C}(\boldsymbol{A}_2) \subseteq \mathcal{C}(\boldsymbol{A}_1)$ and derive the parameter estimators.

6 Let $\boldsymbol{W} \sim W_p(\boldsymbol{\Sigma}, n)$, $\boldsymbol{\Sigma}$ is p.d., and let $\boldsymbol{A}$ be of size $p \times q$.

(i) Show that $\boldsymbol{A}(\boldsymbol{A}'\boldsymbol{W}^{-1}\boldsymbol{A})^{-}\boldsymbol{A}'$ and $\boldsymbol{W} - \boldsymbol{A}(\boldsymbol{A}'\boldsymbol{W}^{-1}\boldsymbol{A})^{-}\boldsymbol{A}'$ are independently distributed. (Hint: note that the g-inverse can be replaced by the inverse and a matrix $\underline{\boldsymbol{A}}$ of full rank. Thereafter factorize $\underline{\boldsymbol{A}}$.)
(ii) Show that $\boldsymbol{A}(\boldsymbol{A}'\boldsymbol{W}^{-1}\boldsymbol{A})^{-}\boldsymbol{A}'$ and $\boldsymbol{I} - \boldsymbol{P}_{A,W}$ are independently distributed.

7 Let $\boldsymbol{W} \sim W_p(\boldsymbol{\Sigma}, n)$. Show that with probability 1, $\mathcal{C}(\boldsymbol{W}) \subseteq \mathcal{C}(\boldsymbol{\Sigma})$ and if $n \geq r(\boldsymbol{\Sigma})$, $\mathcal{C}(\boldsymbol{W}) = \mathcal{C}(\boldsymbol{\Sigma})$.

8 Consider Example 1.9 and generate data according to the proposed model. Estimate the parameters of the model.

9 Analyse the data presented in Example 1.5. Discuss the model fit via appropriately chosen residuals.

10 In the $EBRM_W^3$ suppose that the condition $\mathcal{C}(\boldsymbol{A}_3) \subseteq \mathcal{C}(\boldsymbol{A}_2) \subseteq \mathcal{C}(\boldsymbol{A}_1)$ does not hold. Try to understand why in this case it is so difficult to obtain explicit maximum likelihood estimators.

Literature

Potthoff and Roy (1964) formulated the BRM but did not derive MLEs. They provided the structure which "natural" estimators should satisfy and, undoubtedly, stimulated many other authors. Explicit maximum likelihood estimators were obtained by Khatri (1966), who derived the results using precise matrix manipulations. A completely different approach was taken by Rao (1965, 1966), who applied a variable selection approach together with multivariate covariance analysis (see also Baksalary et al., 1978; Kenward, 1985; Verbyla, 1986; Fujikoshi and Rao, 1991; Mikulich et al., 1999; Soler and Singer, 2000; Vasdekis, 2008). Rao's estimator appears to comprise Khatri's and Rao showed that the approach taken by Potthoff and Roy did not take care of all the information in the data. Grizzle and Allen (1969) provided a number of insightful comments on the approaches taken by Rao and Khatri. A "canonical reduction" of the BRM through singular value decompositions of the known within-individuals and between-individuals design matrices, leading to a canonical formulation of the BRM, was performed by Gleser and Olkin (1970). Estimators of the model were obtained with the help of a fundamental inequality applied to the likelihood function. Anderson and Olkin (1985) presented a general overview of techniques of finding MLEs in the BRM, as well as for finding them when there are some restrictions on the mean parameters. The elegant work by Gleser and Olkin (1970) inspired many others, including Kariya (1978, 1985), Banken (1984a,b), Fujikoshi and Satoh (1996) and Kariya and Sinha (1989). Kariya, as well as Banken, applied group symmetry arguments when working with the BRM. A monograph by Srivastava and Khatri (1979) was the first book where inequalities were used to derive the MLEs in the BRM. In contrast to

Gleser and Olkin, Srivastava and Khatri used the original matrices in the derivation of the MLEs (see also Gleser and Olkin, 1972). Another approach is to solve the likelihood equations. Elswick (1985), Chinchilli and Elswick (1985) and von Rosen (1985, 1989), among others, all showed how to solve the likelihood equations. These equations look complicated and are clearly non-linear, and therefore, from a mathematical point of view, it is somewhat surprising that explicit solutions exist and that, in fact, all the solutions can be explicitly presented.

The estimation of parameters in the BRM with a bilinear restriction such as $\boldsymbol{FBG} = \mathbf{0}$ was considered by Tubbs et al. (1975), where $\boldsymbol{F}$ and $\boldsymbol{G}$ are known matrices. Kabe (1981) discussed more general restrictions. The estimators proposed by these authors are not MLEs (see also Lewis and van Knippenberg, 1984). Gleser and Olkin (1970) and Fujikoshi et al. (1999) put restrictions on the mean parameters in the canonical formulation of the model, which was fully exploited by Banken (1984b). Srivastava and Khatri (1979, Problem 6.9, p. 196) indicated how to obtain MLEs under bilinear restrictions (Srivastava, 2002, gave some more details). von Rosen (1989) considered $\boldsymbol{F}_i\boldsymbol{B}\boldsymbol{G}_i = \mathbf{0}, i = 1, 2, \ldots, s$, where $\boldsymbol{F}_i$ and $\boldsymbol{G}_i$ are known, and $\mathcal{C}(\boldsymbol{G}_s) \subseteq \mathcal{C}(\boldsymbol{G}_{s-1}) \subseteq \cdots \subseteq \mathcal{C}(\boldsymbol{G}_1)$, and showed how MLEs can be obtained.

Estimating parameters in the BRM under bilinear restrictions on the mean parameters is equivalent to estimating the parameters in the $EBRM_\bullet^m$, although, in order to have nested subspace relations, sometimes additional restrictions have to be put on the design matrices or the matrices defining the restrictions (see von Rosen, 1989; Kollo and von Rosen, 2005, Chapter 4). Verbyla and Venables (1988), in an interesting article, presented an extended growth curve model ($EBRM_\bullet^m$), which was termed "the sum of profiles model", and the authors came up with several important observations, for instance that the $EBRM_\bullet^m$ without a nested subspace condition is a multivariate seemingly unrelated regression (SUR) model. The estimation algorithm proposed by Verbyla and Venables, designed to estimate the parameters of the SUR model, will stop in one iteration if either a within-individuals or a between-individuals nested subspace condition holds (see also Stanek and Koch, 1985; Kabe, 1992, Timm, 1997; Drton et al., 2006). von Rosen (1989) presented explicit MLEs for the $EBRM_B^m$, where estimators were recursively presented. Takane and Zhou (2012) discussed the MLEs provided by Verbyla and Venables' estimation algorithm and von Rosen's solution.

Moreover, Verbyla and Venables (1988) also studied a special $EBRM_W^2$ which is a combination of a GMANOVA and a MANOVA model (GMANOVA+MANOVA), i.e. $E[\boldsymbol{X}] = \boldsymbol{A}\boldsymbol{B}_1\boldsymbol{C}_1 + \boldsymbol{B}_2\boldsymbol{C}_2$, where $\boldsymbol{B}_i, i = 1, 2$, are the unknown parameters. This model had also been studied by von Rosen (1985), Elswick (1985) and Chinchilli and Elswick (1985). All these authors presented MLEs. Note that this model is a special case of the $EBRM_W^2$. Klein and Žežula (2015) studied an $EBRM_W^m$ with mutually orthogonal between-individuals design matrices (see also Hu et al., 2011).

As noted above, Gleser and Olkin (1970) presented a canonical version of the $EBRM_\bullet^2$, showed how to reduce the original model to be of a canonical form (see also Fujikoshi and Satoh, 1996) and derived the MLEs. This approach was later generalized, to cover a general $EBRM_\bullet^m$, by Banken (1984b), who also presented MLEs. Furthermore, Fujikoshi et al. (1999) presented estimators and discussed variable selection in the $EBRM_W^2$ (see also Srivastava, 2002; Filipiak and von Rosen, 2012).

An interesting generalization of Gleser and Olkin's (1970) approach was presented in an article by Andersson et al. (1993), where the concept of totally ordered subspaces was introduced in the context of estimating mean parameters and an unstructured dispersion matrix. Explicit MLEs were obtained. Note that a chain of nested subspaces implies that the spaces are totally ordered subspaces. In general the presentation by Andersson et al. (1993) is more mathematical than other presentations. Moreover, this work was extended in Andersson and Perlman (1993), where other references can also be found.

Wong and Cheng (2001) also used a mathematical language when considering the BRM, but instead of a positive definite dispersion matrix, they treated a singular dispersion matrix (see also Wong et al., 1995). The BRM with a singular dispersion matrix was also discussed by Srivastava and von Rosen (2002).

Above we have mostly been considering MLEs which also constitute the main theme of this chapter. However, alternative estimating approaches have been used over the years. Probably the most frequently applied estimation alternatives are Bayesian oriented approaches or different versions of a two-step approach.

Geisser (1980) presented a Bayesian review of the BRM. Among other things, it was noted that the posterior mean estimator of the mean parameters is identical to the corresponding MLE. Furthermore, Geisser presented a number of results concerning prediction (see also Geisser, 1970; Lee and Geisser, 1972, 1975; Fearn, 1975; He and Xu, 2014).

A two-step approach usually means that first an estimator is constructed when the dispersion matrix is known and thereafter, in a second step the dispersion matrix is replaced by an estimator. For examples, see Rao (1967), Fearn (1977), Kariya and Kurata (2004, Chapter 9), Hu and Yan (2008), Hu et al. (2012a,b) and Liu et al. (2015).

Other types of estimators for the BRM have also been suggested. For example, Fang et al. (2006) introduced an approach termed restricted expected multivariate least squares. Tan (1991), in an interesting article, showed how to improve the MLE of the mean parameter in the BRM via different types of loss functions. Other authors who have used loss functions to improve MLEs are Kariya (1989), Kubokawa et al. (1992), Kariya et al. (1996, 1999). Moreover, for the $EBRM_B^m$ minimum risk estimators were considered by Wu (1998, 2000), and Wu et al. (2006) applied a MINQUE-related approach and estimated both the mean parameters and the dispersion matrix simultaneously. Kubokawa and Srivastava (2001) studied robustness of mean estimators in the BRM. Kanda et al. (2002) considered simultaneous confidence regions for $EBRM_W^k$ using a canonical formulation of the model.

In the above-presented literature review, two large areas have not been covered. One of them is the estimation of parameters in the BRM and $EBRM_\bullet^m$ when there exist data which are missing at random. The other uncovered area is the estimation of parameters when the models include structured dispersion matrices.

References

Anderson, T. W., & Olkin, I. (1985). Maximum-likelihood estimation of the parameters of a multivariate normal distribution. *Linear Algebra and Its Applications, 70*, 147–171.

Andersson, S. A., Marden, J. I., & Perlman, M. D. (1993). Totally ordered multivariate linear models. *Sankhyā, Series A, 55*, 370–394.

Andersson, S. A., & Perlman, M. D. (1993). Lattice models for conditional independence in a multivariate normal distribution. *The Annals of Statistics, 21*, 1318–1358.

Baksalary, J. K., Corsten, L. C. A., & Kala, R. (1978). Reconciliation of two different views on estimation of growth curve parameters. *Biometrika, 65*, 662–665.

Banken, L. (1984a). *On the reduction of the general MANOVA model*. Technical report. University of Trier, Trier.

Banken, L. (1984b). *Eine Verallgemeinerung des GMANOVA-Modells*. Dissertation, University of Trier, Trier.

Chinchilli, V. M., & Elswick, R. K. (1985). A mixture of the MANOVA and GMANOVA models. *Communications in Statistics A—Theory Methods, 14*, 3075–3089.

Drton, M., Andersson, S. A., & Perlman, M. D. (2006). Conditional independence models for seemingly unrelated regressions with incomplete data. *Journal of Multivariate Analysis, 97*, 385–411.

Elswick, R. K. (1985). *The Missing Data Problem as Applied to the Extended Version of the GMANOVA Model*. Dissertation, Virginia Commonwealth University, Richmond.

Fang, K.-T., Wang, S.-G., & von Rosen, D. (2006). Restricted expected multivariate least squares. *Journal of Multivariate Analysis, 97*, 619–632.

Fearn, T. (1975). A Bayesian approach to growth curves. *Biometrika, 62*, 89–100.

Fearn, T. (1977). A two-stage model for growth curves which leads to Rao's covariance adjusted estimators. *Biometrika, 64*, 141–143.

Filipiak, K., & von Rosen, D. (2012). On MLEs in an extended multivariate linear growth curve model. *Metrika, 75*, 1069–1092.

Fujikoshi, Y., Kanda, T., & Ohtaki, M. (1999). Growth curve model with hierarchical within-individuals design matrices. *Annals of the Institute of Statistical Mathematics, 51*, 707–721.

Fujikoshi, Y., & Rao, C. R. (1991). Selection of covariables in the growth curve model. *Biometrika, 78*, 779–785.

Fujikoshi, Y., & Satoh, K. (1996). Estimation and model selection in an extended growth curve model. *Hiroshima Mathematical Journal, 26*, 635–647.

Geisser, S. (1970). Bayesian analysis of growth curves. *Sankhyā, Series A, 32*, 53–64.

Geisser, S. (1980). Growth curve analysis. In P. R. Krishnaiah (Ed.), *Handbook of statistics* (Vol. 1, pp. 89–115). New York: North-Holland.

Ghosh, M., Reid, N., & Fraser, D. A. S. (2010). Ancillary statistics: A review. *Statistica Sinica, 20*, 1309–1332.

Gleser, L. J., & Olkin, I. (1970). Linear models in multivariate analysis. In *Essays in probability and statistics* (pp. 267–292). Chapel Hill: University of North Carolina Press.

Gleser, L. J., & Olkin, I. (1972). Estimation for a regression model with an unknown covariance matrix. In *Proceedings of the Sixth Berkeley Symposium on Mathematical Statistics and Probability (University of California, Berkeley, 1970/1971), I: Theory of Statistics* (pp. 541–568). Berkeley: University of California Press.

Grizzle, J. E, & Allen, D. M. (1969). Analysis of growth and dose response curves. *Biometrics, 25*, 357–381.

He, D., & Xu, K. (2014). Reference priors for the growth curve model with general covariance structures. *Chinese Journal of Applied Probability and Statistics, 30*, 57–71.

Hu, J., Liu, F., & Ahmed, S. E. (2012a). Estimation of parameters in the growth curve model via an outer product least squares approach for covariance. *Journal of Multivariate Analysis, 108*, 53–66.

Hu, J., Liu, F., & You, J. (2012b). Estimation of parameters in a generalized GMANOVA model based on an outer product analogy and least squares. *Journal of Statistical Planning and Inference, 142*, 2017–2031.
Hu, J., & Yan, G. (2008). Asymptotic normality and consistency of a two-stage generalized least squares estimator in the growth curve model. *Bernoulli, 14*, 623–636.
Hu, J., Yan, G., & You, J. (2011). Estimation for an additive growth curve model with orthogonal design matrices. *Bernoulli, 17*, 1400–1419.
Kabe, D. G. (1981). MANOVA double linear hypothesis with double linear restrictions. *Communications in Statistics A—Theory Methods, 10*, 2545–2550.
Kabe, D. G. (1992). Equivalence of GMANOVA and SUR models. *Industrial Mathematics, 41*, 53–60.
Kanda, T., Ohtaki. M., & Fujikoshi, Y. (2002). Simultaneous confidence regions in an extended growth curve model with k hierarchical within-individuals design matrices. *Communications in Statistics—Theory and Methods, 31*, 1605–1616.
Kariya, T. (1978). The general MANOVA problem. *The Annals of Statistics, 6*, 200–214.
Kariya, T. (1985). *Testing in the multivariate general linear model*. Tokyo: Kinokuniya.
Kariya, T. (1989). Equivariant estimation in a model with an ancillary statistic. *The Annals of Statistics, 17*, 920–928.
Kariya, T., Konno, Y., & Strawderman, W. E. (1996). Double shrinkage estimators in the GMANOVA model. *Journal of Multivariate Analysis, 56*, 245–258.
Kariya, T., Konno, Y., & Strawderman, W. E. (1999). Construction of shrinkage estimators for the regression coefficient matrix in the GMANOVA model. Statistical inference and data analysis (Tokyo, 1997). *Communications in Statistics—Theory and Methods, 28*, 597–611.
Kariya, T., & Kurata, H. (2004). *Generalized least squares. Wiley series in probability and statistics*. Chichester: Wiley.
Kariya, T., & Sinha, B. K. (1989). *Robustness of statistical tests. Statistical modeling and decision science*. Boston: Academic.
Kenward, M. G. (1985). The use of fitted higher-order polynomial coefficients as covariates in the analysis of growth curves. *Biometrics, 41*, 19–28.
Khatri, C. G. (1966). A note on a MANOVA model applied to problems in growth curves. *Annals of the Institute of Statistical Mathematics, 18*, 75–86.
Klein, D., & Žežula, I. (2015). Maximum likelihood estimators for extended growth curve model with orthogonal between-individual design matrices. *Statistical Methodology, 23*, 59–72.
Kollo, T., & von Rosen, D. (2005). *Advanced multivariate statistics with matrices: Vol. 579. Mathematics and its applications*. Dordrecht: Springer.
Kubokawa, T., Saleh, A. K. Md. E., & Morita, K. (1992). Improving on MLE of coefficient matrix in a growth curve model. *Journal of Statistical Planning and Inference, 31*, 169–177.
Kubokawa, T., & Srivastava, M. S. (2001). Robust improvement in estimation of a mean matrix in an elliptically contoured distribution. *Journal of Multivariate Analysis, 76*, 138–152.
Lee, J. C., & Geisser, S. (1972). Growth curve prediction. *Sankhyā, Series A, 34*, 393–412.
Lee, J. C., & Geisser, S. (1975). Applications of growth curve prediction. *Sankhyā, Series A, 37*, 239–256.
Lewis, C., & van Knippenberg, C. (1984). Estimation and model comparisons for repeated measures data. *Psychological Bulletin, 96*, 182–194.
Liu, F., Hu, J., & Chu, G. (2015). Estimation of parameters in the extended growth curve model via outer product least squares for covariance. *Linear Algebra and Its Applications, 473*, 236–260.
Mikulich, S. K., Zerbe, G. O., Jones, R. H., & Crowley, T. J. (1999). Relating the classical covariance adjustment techniques of multivariate growth curve models to modern univariate mixed effects models. *Biometrics, 55*, 957–964.
Potthoff, R. F., & Roy, S. N. (1964). A generalized multivariate analysis of variance model useful especially for growth curve problems. *Biometrika, 51*, 313–326.
Rao, C. R. (1965). The theory of least squares when the parameters are stochastic and its application to the analysis of growth curves. *Biometrika, 52*, 447–458.

Rao, C. R. (1966). Covariance adjustment and related problems in multivariate analysis. In P. R. Krishnaiah (Ed.), *Multivariate analysis* (pp. 87–103). New York: Academic.

Rao, C. R. (1967). Least squares theory using an estimated dispersion matrix and its application to measurement of signals. In *Proceedings of the Fifth Berkeley Symposium on Mathematical Statistics and Probability (Berkeley, CA, 1965/66), I: Statistics* (pp. 355–372). Berkeley: University of California Press.

Soler, J. M. P., & Singer, J. M. (2000). Optimal covariance adjustment in growth curve models. *Computational Statistics and Data Analysis, 33*, 101–110.

Srivastava, M. S. (2002). Nested growth curve models. Selected articles from San Antonio Conference in honour of C. Radhakrishna Rao (San Antonio, TX, 2000). *Sankhyā, Series A, 64*, 379–408.

Srivastava, M. S., & Khatri, C. G. (1979). *An introduction to multivariate statistics*. New York: North-Holland.

Srivastava, M. S., & von Rosen, D. (2002). Regression models with unknown singular covariance matrix. *Linear Algebra and Its Applications, 354*, 255–273.

Stanek, E. J. III, & Koch, G. G. (1985). The equivalence of parameter estimates from growth curve models and seemingly unrelated regression models. *The American Statistician, 39*, 149–152.

Takane, Y., & Zhou, L. (2012). On two expressions of the MLE for a special case of the extended growth curve models. *Linear Algebra and Its Applications, 436*, 2567–2577.

Tan, M. (1991). Improved estimators for the GMANOVA problem with application to Monte Carlo simulation. *Journal of Multivariate Analysis, 38*, 262–274.

Timm, N. H. (1997). The CGMANOVA model. *Communications in Statistics—Theory and Methods, 26*, 1083–1098.

Tubbs, J. D., Lewis, T. O., & Duran, B. S. (1975). A note on the analysis of the MANOVA model and its application to growth curves. *Communications in Statistics, 4*, 643–653.

Vasdekis, V. G. S. (2008). A comparison of REML and covariance adjustment method in the estimation of growth curve models. *Communications in Statistics—Theory and Methods, 37*, 3287–3297.

Verbyla, A. P. (1986). Conditioning in the growth curve model. *Biometrika, 73*, 475–483.

Verbyla, A. P., & Venables, W. N. (1988). An extension of the growth curve model. *Biometrika, 75*, 129–138.

von Rosen, D. (1985). *Multivariate Linear Normal Models with Special References to the Growth Curve Model*. Dissertation, Stockholm University.

von Rosen, D. (1989). Maximum likelihood estimators in multivariate linear normal models. *Journal of Multivariate Analysis, 31*, 187–200.

Wong, C. S., & Cheng, H. (2001). Estimation in a growth curve model with singular covariance. *Journal of Statistical Planning and Inference, 97*, 323–342.

Wong, C. S., Masaro, J., & Deng, W. C. (1995). Estimating covariance in a growth curve model. *Linear Algebra and Its Applications, 214*, 103–118.

Wu, Q.-G. (1998). Existence conditions of the uniformly minimum risk unbiased estimators in extended growth curve models. *Journal of Statistical Planning and Inference, 69*, 101–114.

Wu, Q.-G. (2000). Some results on parameter estimation in extended growth curve models. *Journal of Statistical Planning and Inference, 88*, 285–300.

Wu, X., Zou, G., & Chen, J. (2006). Unbiased invariant minimum norm estimation in generalized growth curve model. *Journal of Multivariate Analysis, 97*, 1718–1741.

Chapter 4
Basic Properties of Estimators

4.1 Introduction

Since statistical models usually consist of unknown parameters, these parameters have to be estimated in order to make the models interpretable. A general strategy (plugging-in strategy) is to replace the original unknown parameters with estimated quantities, i.e. to create an estimated model and then hope that this procedure will provide useful information. In order to draw firm statistical conclusions, one needs to know the distribution of the estimated model, the estimated parameters or in general the distribution of any statistic of interest. One consequence of the estimation procedure is that the produced estimators of the parameters in a model are usually dependent (correlated), which obviously cannot be the case in the original model where there is no distribution put on the parameters. This deviance from the original model may be essential for the interpretation of the output from any analysis based on the model.

Unfortunately, exact distributions may be difficult to derive. Therefore one has mostly to rely on approximations. There are many ways of performing approximations. One is to approximate the original model with a model where the necessary distributions can be obtained. For example, a non-linear model can be approximated by a linear model, and if one additionally supposes an error which is normally distributed, the basic distributions are available for applying the model to real data. Sometimes this is a good idea, but sometimes the original model has a specific meaning, including an understanding of the parameters, whereas its linearization is more difficult to interpret.

Another type of approximation is implemented when a multivariate set-up, with an unknown dispersion matrix, is approximated with a number of independent univariate models, for example, when a p-dimensional multivariate linear model is approximated by p independent univariate linear models.

A third type of approximation is to consider the approximation from an asymptotic perspective, i.e. to suppose that many independent observations, let us say n,

D. von Rosen, *Bilinear Regression Analysis*, Lecture Notes in Statistics 220,
https://doi.org/10.1007/978-3-319-78784-8_4

are available. The mathematics usually requires that $n \to \infty$, but, of course, we always have a finite number of independent observations. One rarely knows how many observations are needed in order to trust results based on $n \to \infty$.

In statistics and, in particular, multivariate analysis, functions of the inverse dispersion matrix, $\boldsymbol{\Sigma}^{-1}$: $p \times p$, are often used. However, there may be a problem estimating the inverse, e.g. due to multicollinearity in "specific functions of data" or there may simply be too few independent observations. In this case one can use the Cayley-Hamilton theorem (see Rao, 1973, pp. 44–45), which implies

$$\boldsymbol{\Sigma}^{-1} = \sum_{i=0}^{p-1} c_i \boldsymbol{\Sigma}^i, \qquad c_i \text{ are functions of } \boldsymbol{\Sigma}, \quad \boldsymbol{\Sigma}^0 = \boldsymbol{I}_p,$$

with the following approximation (pretending that c_i are unknown constants):

$$\boldsymbol{\Sigma}^{-1} \approx \sum_{i=0}^{a-1} c_i \boldsymbol{\Sigma}^i, \qquad \text{for some } a < p.$$

This type of approximation can motivate the use of partial least squares (PLS) (see Li et al., 2015). There exist several other types of approximations of $\boldsymbol{\Sigma}^{-1}$, among others the Moore-Penrose inverse $\boldsymbol{\Sigma}^{+}$ (see Appendix A, Sect. A.6) or the regularized dispersion matrix $(\boldsymbol{\Sigma} + \lambda \boldsymbol{I})^{-1}$ with some particularly chosen λ.

When approximating distributions it is fairly straightforward to base the approximations on moments, if they can be explicitly derived or approximated in a reasonable way. For distributions with compact support, moments contain the necessary information for determining the distribution. However, if the support is not compact moments can still be used in the approximations. Deciding the order of moments to be used in the approximations is similar to the problem of deciding which polynomial degree should be used when approximating a non-linear function, e.g. via a Taylor series expansion. In this book we use the so-called Edgeworth-type expansions, which in principle involve the approximation of one density based on another density via knowledge about moments from both the original distribution and the approximating distribution.

In Chap. 3, MLEs were presented for the BRM, as well as for the $EBRM_B^3$ and $EBRM_W^3$. Unfortunately all the estimators are non-linear functions of the random variables of the model. Therefore, no expressions for exact distributions are available which can be of practical use. Since the estimators are MLEs, it is known that they are consistent and asymptotically normally distributed, but usually in applications the difference between the number of unknown parameters and the number of independent observations is relatively small and utilizing asymptotic theory is questionable.

Approximations of distributions via simulations can be useful when there are a few parameters of interest. However, with a larger number of parameters, it can become too complicated to perform such approximations via simulations. For example, there may be a large number of nuisance parameters, e.g. $\boldsymbol{\Sigma}$ in the BRM when $\boldsymbol{B}$ is of primary interest. In principle the size of $\boldsymbol{\Sigma}$ may approach infinity and then there is the problem of how to estimate $\boldsymbol{B}$.

Finally, it is noted that for the BRM, as well as the $EBRM_B^m$ and $EBRM_W^m$, which all belong to the curved exponential family, there are no optimal properties available, such as minimum variance estimators or most powerful tests. Therefore, there are many more possibilities for choosing strategies and methods when applying bilinear regression models than when dealing with models belonging to the exponential family. In this book, we mainly use maximum likelihood theory, which makes it possible to obtain optimal asymptotic properties, which unfortunately are rarely of use when analysing medium-sized data sets. When testing hypotheses, the likelihood ratio test is based on maximum likelihood estimators which replace the unknown parameters of the likelihood. This, however, does not mean that maximum likelihood estimators have to be used when interpreting models and their parameters. One can very well use other classes of estimators for the interpretation of parameters and models, and use maximum likelihood estimators solely for constructing likelihood ratio tests, where the estimators are used so that correct levels and high powers are obtained. Hence, it can be concluded that maximum likelihood estimators are of the utmost interest, but there can be many reasons for using other estimators when evaluating statistical models.

4.2 Asymptotic Properties of Estimators of Parameters in the BRM

The statistics presented in the following are all functions of the number of independent observations, n. Thus, when writing $n \to \infty$, we imagine a sequence of statistics under consideration which can be exploited in many ways. In the following we only elucidate whether a sequence converges and not how fast it converges. There exists a huge body of mathematical literature which studies sequences, in particular the convergence of sequences, and in this book we follow statistical tradition in our use of convergence in probability and in distribution (see Appendix A, Sect. A.11 for definitions).

The next lemma is fundamental for the following presentation of asymptotic results for the BRM (see also Appendix B, Theorem B.18).

Lemma 4.1 *Let $\boldsymbol{S} = \boldsymbol{X}(\boldsymbol{I} - \boldsymbol{P}_{\boldsymbol{C}'})\boldsymbol{X}'$, where $\boldsymbol{X}$ follows the BRM presented in Definition 2.1. Then, if $n \to \infty$, and $r(\boldsymbol{C}) \leq k$ is independent of n,*

(i) $n^{-1}\boldsymbol{S} \xrightarrow{P} \boldsymbol{\Sigma}$;

(ii) $\frac{1}{\sqrt{n}}\mathrm{vec}(\boldsymbol{S} - \boldsymbol{\Sigma}) \xrightarrow{D} N_{p^2}(\boldsymbol{0}, \boldsymbol{\Pi}), \qquad \boldsymbol{\Pi} = (\boldsymbol{I}_{p^2} + \boldsymbol{K}_{p,p})(\boldsymbol{\Sigma} \otimes \boldsymbol{\Sigma})$,

where $\boldsymbol{K}_{p,p}$ is the commutation matrix. See Appendix A, Sects. A.5 and A.6 for definitions of $\boldsymbol{K}_{p,p}$ and $\mathrm{vec}(\bullet)$, respectively.

Proof Since $S = \sum_{i=1}^{n-r(C)} y_i y_i'$, for some $y_i \sim N_p(\mathbf{0}, \Sigma)$, where y_i and y_j, $i \neq j$, are independent, statement (i) follows from the law of large numbers and statement (ii) from the central limit theorem (see Appendix B, Theorem B.18 (ii) and (v)) and that $D[S] = (n - r(C))(I_{p^2} + K_{p,p})(\Sigma \otimes \Sigma)$. □

Suppose that there are two matrices K and L, such that the following estimation conditions hold: $\mathcal{C}(K') \subseteq \mathcal{C}(A')$, and $\mathcal{C}(L) \subseteq \mathcal{C}(C_v) \subseteq \mathcal{C}(C)$ for some fixed number v, where C_v is a matrix which consists of the first v columns in C. The reason for the latter assumption is that when $n \to \infty$, the number of columns in C increases and without this assumption it would not make sense to consider $K\widehat{B}L$, where $\widehat{B}$ is the MLE of the mean parameter of the BRM.

The estimability conditions given above and Theorem 3.1 together provide

$$K\widehat{B}L = K(A'S^{-1}A)^- A'S^{-1}XC'(CC')^- L. \tag{4.1}$$

Among other things, it is noted that this expression does not depend on the choice of g-inverse (see Appendix B, Theorem B.7 (ii)), and $K\widehat{B}L$ is built up with the help of two independent quantities (jointly sufficient statistics), $S \sim W_p(\Sigma, n-k)$, and $XC'(CC')^- L \sim N_{p,k}(ABL, \Sigma, L(C'C)^- L')$. From Lemma 4.1 (i), since for any continuous function $h(\bullet)$, $h(\frac{1}{n}S) \to h(\Sigma)$, in probability, it follows that

$$\begin{aligned} K(A'S^{-1}A)^- A'S^{-1} &= K(A'(n^{-1}S)^{-1}A)^- A'(n^{-1}S)^{-1} \\ &\xrightarrow{P} K(A'\Sigma^{-1}A)^- A'\Sigma^{-1}, \qquad n \to \infty. \end{aligned} \tag{4.2}$$

Let

$$KB_\Sigma L = K(A'\Sigma^{-1}A)^- A'\Sigma^{-1}XC'(CC')^- L$$

and it will be demonstrated that the tr-distance, $|| \bullet ||$ (see Appendix A, Sect. A.6), converges to zero, i.e.

$$||K\widehat{B}L - KB_\Sigma L|| = \mathrm{tr}\{(K\widehat{B}L - KB_\Sigma L)(K\widehat{B}L - KB_\Sigma L)'\} \xrightarrow{P} 0, \quad n \to \infty. \tag{4.3}$$

This means that under the tr-distance $K\widehat{B}L$ is asymptotically equivalent to $KB_\Sigma L$. Note that (see Appendix B, Theorem B.9 (iii)) $||AQB - APB|| > ||CQD - CPD||$ for all P and Q if and only if $BB' \otimes A'A - DD' \otimes C'C$ is p.d., where it is supposed that the matrices are of proper sizes.

Now let ϵ be any small quantity and

$$P(||K\widehat{B}L - KB_\Sigma L|| > \epsilon) = P(||D(S, \Sigma)XC'(CC')^- L|| > \epsilon), \tag{4.4}$$

where

$$D(S, \Sigma) = K((A'S^{-1}A)^{-}A'S^{-1} - (A'\Sigma^{-1}A)^{-}A'\Sigma^{-1}). \tag{4.5}$$

Note that from (4.2) it follows that $D(S, \Sigma) \xrightarrow{P} 0$. Let M be any arbitrary non-stochastic matrix and $Y = X - ABC$. Then, (4.4) equals

$$\begin{aligned}
&P(\|K\widehat{B}L - KB_{\Sigma}L\| > \epsilon)\\
&= P(\|D(S, \Sigma)YC'(CC')^{-}L\| > \epsilon,\ MM' - YC'(CC')^{-}LL'(CC')^{-}CY' \text{ is p.d.})\\
&\quad + P(\|D(S, \Sigma)YC'(CC')^{-}L\| > \epsilon,\ MM' - YC'(CC')^{-}LL'(CC')^{-}CY' \text{ is not p.d.})\\
&\leq P(\|D(S, \Sigma)M\| > \epsilon) + P(MM' - YC'(CC')^{-}LL'(CC')^{-}CY' \text{ is not p.d.}). \qquad (4.6)
\end{aligned}$$

The first term in (4.6) converges to zero and the second one is discussed now. Since the number of columns in C is increasing when $n \to \infty$, one most proceed with a certain degree of caution. Note that, based on Markov's inequality (see Appendix B, Theorem B.9 (i)),

$$\begin{aligned}
&P(MM' - YC'(CC')^{-}LL'(CC')^{-}CY' \text{ is not p.d.})\\
&\quad = P(\alpha'YC'(CC')^{-}LL'(CC')^{-}CY'\alpha \geq \alpha'MM'\alpha, \text{ for some } \alpha)\\
&\quad \leq \frac{\mathrm{tr}\{L'(CC')^{-}L\}\alpha'\Sigma\alpha}{\alpha'MM'\alpha} \leq \frac{\mathrm{tr}\{L'(C_vC_v')^{-}L\}\alpha'\Sigma\alpha}{\alpha'MM'\alpha},
\end{aligned}$$

and the right-hand side does not depend on n. Thus, by choosing M appropriately, the probability given above can be made smaller than any pre-requested quantity. Hence, from (4.6) it follows that $K\widehat{B}L$ is asymptotically equivalent to $KB_{\Sigma}L$. Moreover, since $KB_{\Sigma}L$ converges to KBL the next theorem has been established.

Theorem 4.1 *Let $K\widehat{B}L$ be given by (4.1), where K: $r \times q$ and L: $k \times s$. Then, if $n \to \infty$,*

(i) $\sqrt{n}(K\widehat{B}L - KBL) \xrightarrow{D} N_{r,s}(0, K(A'\Sigma^{-1}A)^{-}K', L'(CC')^{-}L)$;
(ii) $K\widehat{B}L \xrightarrow{P} KBL$.

Concerning asymptotic results for $\widehat{\Sigma}$, the following expression, obtained from Theorem 3.1, is now considered in some detail:

$$n\widehat{\Sigma} = S + (I - A(A'S^{-1}A)^{-}A'S^{-1})XP_{C'}X'(I - S^{-1}A(A'S^{-1}A)^{-}A'). \tag{4.7}$$

It can be shown that this expression is asymptotically equivalent to

$$n\Sigma_{\Sigma} = S + (I - A(A'\Sigma^{-1}A)^{-}A'\Sigma^{-1})XP_{C'}X'(I - \Sigma^{-1}A(A'\Sigma^{-1}A)^{-}A'),$$

since

$$(\boldsymbol{I} - \boldsymbol{A}(\boldsymbol{A}'\boldsymbol{S}^{-1}\boldsymbol{A})^{-}\boldsymbol{A}'\boldsymbol{S}^{-1})\boldsymbol{X}\boldsymbol{P}_{C'}$$

and

$$(\boldsymbol{I} - \boldsymbol{A}(\boldsymbol{A}'\boldsymbol{\Sigma}^{-1}\boldsymbol{A})^{-}\boldsymbol{A}'\boldsymbol{\Sigma}^{-1})\boldsymbol{X}\boldsymbol{P}_{C'}$$

are asymptotically equivalent, which follows from (4.3); i.e. when the asymptotic equivalence of $\boldsymbol{K}\widehat{\boldsymbol{B}}\boldsymbol{L}$ and $\boldsymbol{K}\boldsymbol{B}_{\Sigma}\boldsymbol{L}$ is proven. The distribution of $n\boldsymbol{\Sigma}_{\Sigma}$ equals the sum of two independent Wishart-distributed variables, and the Wishart distribution is a much simpler distribution to deal with than the distribution for $n\widehat{\boldsymbol{\Sigma}}$.

The matrix $\boldsymbol{X}$ in (4.7) can be replaced by $\boldsymbol{Y} = \boldsymbol{X} - \boldsymbol{A}\boldsymbol{B}\boldsymbol{C}$. Moreover, $\boldsymbol{Y}\boldsymbol{P}_{C'}\boldsymbol{Y}'$ is independent of n, if $r(\boldsymbol{C}) = k$, which is supposed to hold. Therefore, $\frac{1}{\sqrt{n}}\boldsymbol{Y}\boldsymbol{P}_{C'}\boldsymbol{Y}' \xrightarrow{P} \boldsymbol{0}$. Thus, applying Lemma 4.1 and Appendix B, Theorem B.17 (iii), the next theorem is established.

Theorem 4.2 *Let $\widehat{\boldsymbol{\Sigma}}$ be given in Theorem 3.1. Then, if $n \to \infty$,*

(i) $\sqrt{n}\mathrm{vec}(\widehat{\boldsymbol{\Sigma}} - \boldsymbol{\Sigma}) \xrightarrow{D} N_{p^2}(\boldsymbol{0}, \boldsymbol{\Pi}), \quad \boldsymbol{\Pi} = (\boldsymbol{I}_{p^2} + \boldsymbol{K}_{p,p})(\boldsymbol{\Sigma} \otimes \boldsymbol{\Sigma})$;

(ii) $\widehat{\boldsymbol{\Sigma}} \xrightarrow{P} \boldsymbol{\Sigma}$.

It is interesting to note that when studying $\widehat{\boldsymbol{\Sigma}}$ from an asymptotic point of view, the space $\mathcal{C}_{\boldsymbol{\Sigma}}(\boldsymbol{A}) \otimes \mathcal{C}(\boldsymbol{C}')$ is not involved and there is a clear difference between performing non-asymptotic inference and performing asymptotic inference. In some way this indicates that if there are many observations in relation to the number of parameters, there is no point in performing an analysis based on the BRM instead of using a MANOVA model.

4.3 Moments of Estimators of Parameters in the BRM

Throughout this section, as in Corollary 3.1, two matrices, $\boldsymbol{K}$ and $\boldsymbol{L}$, will be used which satisfy $\mathcal{C}(\boldsymbol{K}') \subseteq \mathcal{C}(\boldsymbol{A}')$ and $\mathcal{C}(\boldsymbol{L}) \subseteq \mathcal{C}(\boldsymbol{C})$, respectively. These are the so-called estimability conditions in the BRM in the sense that unique estimators are obtained when these conditions are met. Then, once again,

$$\boldsymbol{K}\widehat{\boldsymbol{B}}\boldsymbol{L} = \boldsymbol{K}(\boldsymbol{A}'\boldsymbol{S}^{-1}\boldsymbol{A})^{-}\boldsymbol{A}'\boldsymbol{S}^{-1}\boldsymbol{X}\boldsymbol{C}'(\boldsymbol{C}\boldsymbol{C}')^{-}\boldsymbol{L}, \tag{4.8}$$

where $\boldsymbol{S} = \boldsymbol{X}(\boldsymbol{I} - \boldsymbol{P}_{C'})\boldsymbol{X}'$. Moments for $\boldsymbol{K}\widehat{\boldsymbol{B}}\boldsymbol{L}$ and $\widehat{\boldsymbol{\Sigma}}$ will now be derived, but there derivation is a rather technical issue. In principle, one needs to combine knowledge from the matrix normal, Wishart and inverse Wishart distributions. As $\boldsymbol{K}$ and $\boldsymbol{L}$, the matrices $\boldsymbol{A}$ and $\boldsymbol{C}$ may be chosen and then, if these matrices are of full rank, i.e. $r(\boldsymbol{A}) = q$ and $r(\boldsymbol{C}) = k$, one may pre-multiply (4.8) by $(\boldsymbol{A}'\boldsymbol{A})^{-1}\boldsymbol{A}'$, post-multiply by $\boldsymbol{C}'(\boldsymbol{C}\boldsymbol{C}')^{-1}$, and obtain

$$\widehat{\boldsymbol{B}} = (\boldsymbol{A}'\boldsymbol{S}^{-1}\boldsymbol{A})^{-1}\boldsymbol{A}'\boldsymbol{S}^{-1}\boldsymbol{X}\boldsymbol{C}'(\boldsymbol{C}\boldsymbol{C}')^{-1}. \tag{4.9}$$

Thus, by studying (4.8) one always obtains complete information about (4.9). When considering the general $\widehat{\boldsymbol{B}}$-expression presented in Corollary 3.1, for each choice of $\boldsymbol{Z}_i$, $i = 1, 2$, we have to treat the estimator separately. If $\boldsymbol{Z}_i$ is non-random, we just have a translation of $\widehat{\boldsymbol{B}}$ and, as will later be seen, we have a biased estimator. If $\boldsymbol{Z}_i$ is random, everything is more complicated and less clear and there is no point discussing this case.

In (4.8) the matrix $\boldsymbol{S}$ is random, and therefore the expression for $\boldsymbol{K}\widehat{\boldsymbol{B}}\boldsymbol{L}$ is quite a complicated non-linear random expression. As noted before, it consists of two parts, namely

$$\boldsymbol{K}(\boldsymbol{A}'\boldsymbol{S}^{-1}\boldsymbol{A})^{-}\boldsymbol{A}'\boldsymbol{S}^{-1} \tag{4.10}$$

and

$$\boldsymbol{X}\boldsymbol{C}'(\boldsymbol{C}\boldsymbol{C}')^{-}\boldsymbol{L}, \tag{4.11}$$

but fortunately $\boldsymbol{S}$ and $\boldsymbol{X}\boldsymbol{C}'$ are independently distributed (see Appendix B, Theorem B.19 (viii)), which will be utilized many times.

The distribution of $\boldsymbol{K}\widehat{\boldsymbol{B}}\boldsymbol{L}$ is a function of $\boldsymbol{S}$ which is used because of the inner product estimation. However, $\boldsymbol{\Sigma}$, which defines the inner product, may be regarded as a nuisance parameter and, therefore, it is of interest to neglect the variation in $\boldsymbol{K}\widehat{\boldsymbol{B}}\boldsymbol{L}$ which is due to $\boldsymbol{S}$ and compare the estimator with the class of estimators proposed by Potthoff and Roy (1964);

$$\boldsymbol{K}\widehat{\boldsymbol{B}}_G\boldsymbol{L} = \boldsymbol{K}(\boldsymbol{A}'\boldsymbol{G}^{-1}\boldsymbol{A})^{-}\boldsymbol{A}'\boldsymbol{G}^{-1}\boldsymbol{X}\boldsymbol{C}'(\boldsymbol{C}\boldsymbol{C}')^{-}\boldsymbol{L}, \tag{4.12}$$

where $\boldsymbol{G}$ is supposed to be a non-random positive definite matrix. One choice is $\boldsymbol{G} = \boldsymbol{I}$. According to Appendix B, Theorem B.19 (i), the distribution of $\boldsymbol{K}\widehat{\boldsymbol{B}}_G\boldsymbol{L}$ is matrix normal. Therefore, it can be valuable to compare the moments of $\boldsymbol{K}\widehat{\boldsymbol{B}}\boldsymbol{L}$ with the corresponding moments of $\boldsymbol{K}\widehat{\boldsymbol{B}}_G\boldsymbol{L}$ in order to understand how the distribution of $\boldsymbol{K}\widehat{\boldsymbol{B}}\boldsymbol{L}$ differs from the normal one. Furthermore, one can use a conditional approach concerning $\boldsymbol{K}\widehat{\boldsymbol{B}}\boldsymbol{L}$, i.e. conditioning with respect to $\boldsymbol{S}$ in $\boldsymbol{K}\widehat{\boldsymbol{B}}\boldsymbol{L}$, since the distribution of $\boldsymbol{S}$ does not involve the parameter $\boldsymbol{B}$.

Now the first two moments for $\boldsymbol{K}\widehat{\boldsymbol{B}}\boldsymbol{L}$ are presented.

Theorem 4.3 *Let $\boldsymbol{K}\widehat{\boldsymbol{B}}\boldsymbol{L}$ be given by (4.8). Then*

(i) $E[\boldsymbol{K}\widehat{\boldsymbol{B}}\boldsymbol{L}] = \boldsymbol{K}\boldsymbol{B}\boldsymbol{L}$;
(ii) *if* $n - r(\boldsymbol{C}) - p + r(\boldsymbol{A}) - 1 > 0$,

$$D[\boldsymbol{K}\widehat{\boldsymbol{B}}\boldsymbol{L}] = \frac{n - r(\boldsymbol{C}) - 1}{n - r(\boldsymbol{C}) - p + r(\boldsymbol{A}) - 1}\boldsymbol{L}'(\boldsymbol{C}\boldsymbol{C}')^{-}\boldsymbol{L} \otimes \boldsymbol{K}(\boldsymbol{A}'\boldsymbol{\Sigma}^{-1}\boldsymbol{A})^{-}\boldsymbol{K}'.$$

Proof Because of independence between $\boldsymbol{S}$ and $\boldsymbol{XC}'$ (see Appendix B, Theorem B.19 (viii)),

$$E[\boldsymbol{K}\widehat{\boldsymbol{B}}\boldsymbol{L}] = E[\boldsymbol{K}(\boldsymbol{A}'\boldsymbol{S}^{-1}\boldsymbol{A})^{-}\boldsymbol{K}'\boldsymbol{S}^{-1}]E[\boldsymbol{XC}'(\boldsymbol{CC}')^{-}\boldsymbol{L}]. \tag{4.13}$$

Since $E[\boldsymbol{X}] = \boldsymbol{ABC}$ implies $E[\boldsymbol{XC}'(\boldsymbol{CC}')^{-}\boldsymbol{L}] = \boldsymbol{ABL}$, the expression in (4.13) is equivalent to

$$\begin{aligned} E[\boldsymbol{K}\widehat{\boldsymbol{B}}\boldsymbol{L}] &= E[\boldsymbol{K}(\boldsymbol{A}'\boldsymbol{S}^{-1}\boldsymbol{A})^{-}\boldsymbol{A}'\boldsymbol{S}^{-1}]\boldsymbol{ABL} \\ &= E[\boldsymbol{K}(\boldsymbol{A}'\boldsymbol{S}^{-1}\boldsymbol{A})^{-}\boldsymbol{A}'\boldsymbol{S}^{-1}\boldsymbol{A}]\boldsymbol{BL} = \boldsymbol{KBL}, \end{aligned}$$

where in the last equality a result from Appendix B, Theorem B.7 (i) has been used.

Continuing with statement (ii), based on the definition of the dispersion matrix,

$$D[\boldsymbol{K}\widehat{\boldsymbol{B}}\boldsymbol{L}] = E[\mathrm{vec}(\boldsymbol{K}(\widehat{\boldsymbol{B}} - \boldsymbol{B})\boldsymbol{L})\mathrm{vec}'(\boldsymbol{K}(\widehat{\boldsymbol{B}} - \boldsymbol{B})\boldsymbol{L})] \tag{4.14}$$

and

$$\boldsymbol{K}(\widehat{\boldsymbol{B}} - \boldsymbol{B})\boldsymbol{L} = \boldsymbol{K}(\boldsymbol{A}'\boldsymbol{S}^{-1}\boldsymbol{A})^{-}\boldsymbol{A}'\boldsymbol{S}^{-1}(\boldsymbol{X} - \boldsymbol{ABC})\boldsymbol{C}'(\boldsymbol{CC}')^{-}\boldsymbol{L}. \tag{4.15}$$

Moreover, since $\mathcal{C}(\boldsymbol{K}') \subseteq \mathcal{C}(\boldsymbol{A}')$, $\boldsymbol{K}' = \boldsymbol{A}'\boldsymbol{H}$, for some $\boldsymbol{H}$. The fact will be utilized that from the uniqueness of the projectors, it follows that

$$\boldsymbol{P}_{A,S} = \boldsymbol{A}(\boldsymbol{A}'\boldsymbol{S}^{-1}\boldsymbol{A})^{-}\boldsymbol{A}'\boldsymbol{S}^{-1} = \underline{\boldsymbol{A}}(\underline{\boldsymbol{A}}'\boldsymbol{S}^{-1}\underline{\boldsymbol{A}})^{-1}\underline{\boldsymbol{A}}'\boldsymbol{S}^{-1} = \boldsymbol{P}_{\underline{A},S}, \tag{4.16}$$

where $\underline{\boldsymbol{A}}$ is any matrix of full rank such that $\mathcal{C}(\boldsymbol{A}) = \mathcal{C}(\underline{\boldsymbol{A}})$.

Put $\boldsymbol{Y} = (\boldsymbol{X} - \boldsymbol{ABC})\boldsymbol{C}'(\boldsymbol{CC}')^{-}\boldsymbol{L}$, which, according to Appendix B, Theorem B.19 (viii), is independent of $\boldsymbol{S}$, and the dispersion of $\boldsymbol{Y}$ equals

$$D[\boldsymbol{Y}] = \boldsymbol{L}'(\boldsymbol{CC}')^{-}\boldsymbol{L} \otimes \boldsymbol{\Sigma}. \tag{4.17}$$

Now,

$$\begin{aligned} D[\boldsymbol{K}\widehat{\boldsymbol{B}}\boldsymbol{L}] &= E[(\boldsymbol{I} \otimes \boldsymbol{H}'\boldsymbol{P}_{\underline{A},S})E[\mathrm{vec}\boldsymbol{Y}\mathrm{vec}'\boldsymbol{Y}](\boldsymbol{I} \otimes \boldsymbol{P}'_{\underline{A},S}\boldsymbol{H})] \\ &= E[(\boldsymbol{I} \otimes \boldsymbol{H}'\boldsymbol{P}_{\underline{A},S})D[\boldsymbol{Y}](\boldsymbol{I} \otimes \boldsymbol{P}'_{\underline{A},S}\boldsymbol{H})] \\ &= \boldsymbol{L}'(\boldsymbol{CC}')^{-}\boldsymbol{L} \otimes E[\boldsymbol{H}'\boldsymbol{P}_{\underline{A},S}\boldsymbol{\Sigma}\boldsymbol{P}'_{\underline{A},S}\boldsymbol{H}]. \end{aligned} \tag{4.18}$$

Therefore, remaining task is to derive $E[\boldsymbol{H}'\boldsymbol{P}_{\underline{A},S}\boldsymbol{\Sigma}\boldsymbol{P}'_{\underline{A},S}\boldsymbol{H}]$, and to derive this expression it is convenient to work with a canonical form. Let (see Appendix B, Theorem B.1 (i))

$$\boldsymbol{A}'\boldsymbol{\Sigma}^{-1/2} = \boldsymbol{T}(\boldsymbol{I}_{r(A)} : \boldsymbol{0})\boldsymbol{\Gamma}', \tag{4.19}$$

where $\boldsymbol{T}$ is non-singular, $\boldsymbol{\Gamma}' = (\boldsymbol{\Gamma}_1' : \boldsymbol{\Gamma}_2')$, $(p \times r(\boldsymbol{A}) : p \times (p - r(\boldsymbol{A}))$, is orthogonal and $\boldsymbol{\Sigma}^{-1/2}$ is a symmetric square root of $\boldsymbol{\Sigma}^{-1}$. Moreover, put

$$\boldsymbol{V} = \boldsymbol{\Gamma}\boldsymbol{\Sigma}^{-1/2}\boldsymbol{S}\boldsymbol{\Sigma}^{-1/2}\boldsymbol{\Gamma}' \sim W_p(\boldsymbol{I}, n - r(\boldsymbol{C})). \tag{4.20}$$

The matrices $\boldsymbol{V}$ and its inverse $\boldsymbol{V}^{-1}$ will be partitioned as follows:

$$\boldsymbol{V} = \begin{pmatrix} \boldsymbol{V}_{11} & \boldsymbol{V}_{12} \\ \boldsymbol{V}_{21} & \boldsymbol{V}_{22} \end{pmatrix} \quad \begin{matrix} r(\boldsymbol{A}) \times r(\boldsymbol{A}) & r(\boldsymbol{A}) \times (p - r(\boldsymbol{A})) \\ (p - r(\boldsymbol{A})) \times r(\boldsymbol{A}) & (p - r(\boldsymbol{A})) \times (p - r(\boldsymbol{A})) \end{matrix}, \tag{4.21}$$

$$\boldsymbol{V}^{-1} = \begin{pmatrix} \boldsymbol{V}^{11} & \boldsymbol{V}^{12} \\ \boldsymbol{V}^{21} & \boldsymbol{V}^{22} \end{pmatrix} \quad \begin{matrix} r(\boldsymbol{A}) \times r(\boldsymbol{A}) & r(\boldsymbol{A}) \times (p - r(\boldsymbol{A})) \\ (p - r(\boldsymbol{A})) \times r(\boldsymbol{A}) & (p - r(\boldsymbol{A})) \times (p - r(\boldsymbol{A})) \end{matrix}. \tag{4.22}$$

Thus, from (4.20) and (4.22) it follows, since $(\boldsymbol{V}^{11})^{-1}\boldsymbol{V}^{12} = -\boldsymbol{V}_{12}\boldsymbol{V}_{22}^{-1}$ (see Appendix B, Theorem B.8 (i)), that

$$\begin{aligned} E[\boldsymbol{P}_{\underline{A},S}\boldsymbol{\Sigma}\boldsymbol{P}_{\underline{A},S}'] &= E[\boldsymbol{\Sigma}^{1/2}\boldsymbol{\Gamma}_1'(\boldsymbol{V}^{11})^{-1}(\boldsymbol{V}^{11} : \boldsymbol{V}^{12})(\boldsymbol{V}^{11} : \boldsymbol{V}^{12})'(\boldsymbol{V}^{11})^{-1}\boldsymbol{\Gamma}_1\boldsymbol{\Sigma}^{1/2}] \\ &= E[\boldsymbol{\Sigma}^{1/2}\boldsymbol{\Gamma}_1'(\boldsymbol{I} : (\boldsymbol{V}^{11})^{-1}\boldsymbol{V}^{12})(\boldsymbol{I} : (\boldsymbol{V}^{11})^{-1}\boldsymbol{V}^{12})'\boldsymbol{\Gamma}_1\boldsymbol{\Sigma}^{1/2}] \\ &= E[\boldsymbol{\Sigma}^{1/2}\boldsymbol{\Gamma}_1'\{\boldsymbol{I} + (\boldsymbol{V}^{11})^{-1}\boldsymbol{V}^{12}\boldsymbol{V}^{21}(\boldsymbol{V}^{11})^{-1}\}\boldsymbol{\Gamma}_1\boldsymbol{\Sigma}^{1/2}] \\ &= \boldsymbol{\Sigma}^{1/2}\boldsymbol{\Gamma}_1'\boldsymbol{\Gamma}_1\boldsymbol{\Sigma}^{1/2} + \boldsymbol{\Sigma}^{1/2}\boldsymbol{\Gamma}_1'E[\boldsymbol{V}_{12}\boldsymbol{V}_{22}^{-1}\boldsymbol{V}_{22}^{-1}\boldsymbol{V}_{21}]\boldsymbol{\Gamma}_1\boldsymbol{\Sigma}^{1/2} \\ &= \boldsymbol{\Sigma}^{1/2}\boldsymbol{\Gamma}_1'\boldsymbol{\Gamma}_1\boldsymbol{\Sigma}^{1/2}(1 + \frac{p - r(\boldsymbol{A})}{n - r(\boldsymbol{C}) - p + r(\boldsymbol{A}) - 1}), \end{aligned} \tag{4.23}$$

where result (vii) of Theorem B.21 in Appendix B has been applied. A remaining task is to express (4.23) in the original matrix $\boldsymbol{A}$, and some calculations yield

$$\boldsymbol{\Sigma}^{1/2}\boldsymbol{\Gamma}_1'\boldsymbol{\Gamma}_1\boldsymbol{\Sigma}^{1/2} = \boldsymbol{A}(\boldsymbol{A}'\boldsymbol{\Sigma}^{-1}\boldsymbol{A})^{-}\boldsymbol{A}'. \tag{4.24}$$

Hence, (4.23) and (4.24) verify statement (ii). □

Corollary 4.1 *Let $\widehat{\boldsymbol{B}}$ be given by (4.9) with $r(\boldsymbol{A}) = q$ and $r(\boldsymbol{C}) = k$. Then*

(i) $E[\widehat{\boldsymbol{B}}] = \boldsymbol{B}$;
(ii) *if* $n - k - p + q - 1 > 0$,

$$D[\widehat{\boldsymbol{B}}] = \frac{n - k - 1}{n - k - p + q - 1}(\boldsymbol{C}\boldsymbol{C}')^{-1} \otimes (\boldsymbol{A}'\boldsymbol{\Sigma}^{-1}\boldsymbol{A})^{-1}.$$

Corollary 4.2 *Let $\widehat{E[\boldsymbol{X}]} = \boldsymbol{A}\widehat{\boldsymbol{B}}\boldsymbol{C}$. Then*

(i) $E[\boldsymbol{A}\widehat{\boldsymbol{B}}\boldsymbol{C}] = \boldsymbol{A}\boldsymbol{B}\boldsymbol{C}$;
(ii) *if* $n - r(\boldsymbol{C}) - p + r(\boldsymbol{A}) - 1 > 0$,

$$D[\widehat{E[\boldsymbol{X}]}] = \frac{n - r(\boldsymbol{C}) - 1}{n - r(\boldsymbol{C}) - p + r(\boldsymbol{A}) - 1}\boldsymbol{C}'(\boldsymbol{C}\boldsymbol{C}')^{-}\boldsymbol{C} \otimes \boldsymbol{A}(\boldsymbol{A}'\boldsymbol{\Sigma}^{-1}\boldsymbol{A})^{-}\boldsymbol{A}'.$$

It is worth noting that the factor

$$\frac{n - r(\boldsymbol{C}) - 1}{n - r(\boldsymbol{C}) - p + r(\boldsymbol{A}) - 1} > 1,$$

which appears in both Theorem 4.3 and Corollary 4.1, shows the contribution to the dispersion due to the random weight $\boldsymbol{S}$. If we had assumed a known covariance matrix, this factor would have been replaced by 1. When $n - r(\boldsymbol{C})$ is somewhat larger than $p - r(\boldsymbol{A})$, the effect of the factor on the dispersion is rather small.

Next for consideration are moments of a higher order and for notational convenience we have chosen to use the moment representation

$$E[(\boldsymbol{K}(\widehat{\boldsymbol{B}} - \boldsymbol{B})\boldsymbol{L})^{\otimes k}].$$

The Kroneckerian power is a convenient way to gather all the possible mixed moments $\mu_{ijk\dots}$, i.e. monomials $(E[x_1^i x_2^j x_3^k \dots])$, as well as operate on them. The drawback is that the same moments $(\mu_{ijk\dots})$ appear in several places in $(\boldsymbol{K}(\widehat{\boldsymbol{B}} - \boldsymbol{B})\boldsymbol{L})^{\otimes k}$ and, therefore, from a computational point of view $(\boldsymbol{K}(\widehat{\boldsymbol{B}} - \boldsymbol{B})\boldsymbol{L})^{\otimes k}$ is not efficient. Different representations and moments of arbitrary order can be studied (see Kollo and von Rosen, 1995), but the technical treatment is rather lengthy and therefore omitted here.

Theorem 4.4 (Kollo and von Rosen, 2005, Theorem 4.2.2) *Let $\boldsymbol{K}\widehat{\boldsymbol{B}}\boldsymbol{L}$ be given by (4.8). Put*

$$\boldsymbol{v}(\boldsymbol{A}) = \mathrm{vec}(\boldsymbol{K}(\boldsymbol{A}'\boldsymbol{\Sigma}^{-1}\boldsymbol{A})^{-}\boldsymbol{K}'),$$
$$\boldsymbol{v}(\boldsymbol{C}') = \mathrm{vec}(\boldsymbol{L}'(\boldsymbol{C}\boldsymbol{C}')^{-}\boldsymbol{L}).$$

In these notations the following statements hold:

(i) *If r is odd, $E[(\boldsymbol{K}(\widehat{\boldsymbol{B}} - \boldsymbol{B})\boldsymbol{L})^{\otimes r}] = \boldsymbol{0}$.*
(ii) *If $n - r(\boldsymbol{C}) - p + r(\boldsymbol{A}) - 1 > 0$, then*

$$E[(\boldsymbol{K}(\widehat{\boldsymbol{B}} - \boldsymbol{B})\boldsymbol{L})^{\otimes 2}] = c_0\boldsymbol{v}(\boldsymbol{A})\boldsymbol{v}'(\boldsymbol{C}'),$$

where

$$c_0 = \frac{n - r(\boldsymbol{C}) - 1}{n - r(\boldsymbol{C}) - p + r(\boldsymbol{A}) - 1}.$$

(iii) *If $n - r(\boldsymbol{C}) - p + r(\boldsymbol{A}) - 3 > 0$, then*

$$\begin{aligned}
E[(\boldsymbol{K}(\widehat{\boldsymbol{B}} - \boldsymbol{B})\boldsymbol{L})^{\otimes 4}] &= (1 + 2c_1)\{\boldsymbol{v}(\boldsymbol{A})\boldsymbol{v}'(\boldsymbol{C}')\}^{\otimes 2} \\
&+ (1 + 2c_1)(\boldsymbol{I}_p \otimes \boldsymbol{K}_{p,p} \otimes \boldsymbol{I}_p)\{\boldsymbol{v}(\boldsymbol{A})\boldsymbol{v}'(\boldsymbol{C}')\}^{\otimes 2}(\boldsymbol{I}_n \otimes \boldsymbol{K}_{n,n} \otimes \boldsymbol{I}_n) \\
&+ (1 + 2c_1)\boldsymbol{K}_{p,p^3}\{\boldsymbol{v}(\boldsymbol{A})\boldsymbol{v}'(\boldsymbol{C}')\}^{\otimes 2}\boldsymbol{K}_{n^3,n} \\
&+ (c_2\boldsymbol{I} + c_3\{(\boldsymbol{I}_p \otimes \boldsymbol{K}_{p,p} \otimes \boldsymbol{I}_p) + \boldsymbol{K}_{p,p^3}\})\{\boldsymbol{v}(\boldsymbol{A})\boldsymbol{v}'(\boldsymbol{C}')\}^{\otimes 2},
\end{aligned}$$

where

$$c_1 = \frac{p-r(\boldsymbol{A})}{n-r(\boldsymbol{C})-p+r(\boldsymbol{A})-1},$$

$$c_2 = \frac{2(p-r(\boldsymbol{A}))(n-r(\boldsymbol{C})-p+r(\boldsymbol{A})-1)+\{2+(n-r(\boldsymbol{C})-p+r(\boldsymbol{A}))(n-r(\boldsymbol{C})-p+r(\boldsymbol{A})-3)\}(p-r(\boldsymbol{A}))^2}{(n-r(\boldsymbol{C})-p+r(\boldsymbol{A}))(n-r(\boldsymbol{C})-p+r(\boldsymbol{A})-1)^2(n-r(\boldsymbol{C})-p+r(\boldsymbol{A})-3)},$$

$$c_3 = \frac{p-r(\boldsymbol{A})}{(n-r(\boldsymbol{C})-p+r(\boldsymbol{A}))(n-r(\boldsymbol{C})-p+r(\boldsymbol{A})-3)} + \frac{(p-r(\boldsymbol{A}))^2}{(n-r(\boldsymbol{C})-p+r(\boldsymbol{A}))(n-r(\boldsymbol{C})-p+r(\boldsymbol{A})-1)(n-r(\boldsymbol{C})-p+r(\boldsymbol{A})-3)}.$$

(iv) *If* $n - r(\boldsymbol{C}) - p + r(\boldsymbol{A}) - 2r + 1 > 0$, *then (for notation see Appendix A, Sect. A.12)*

$$E[(\boldsymbol{K}\widehat{\boldsymbol{B}}\boldsymbol{L})^{\otimes 2r}] = \mathcal{O}(n^{-r}).$$

Proof Because of independence between $\boldsymbol{S}$ and $\boldsymbol{X}\boldsymbol{C}'$ (see Appendix B, Theorem B.19 (viii)),

$$\begin{aligned} E[(\boldsymbol{K}(\widehat{\boldsymbol{B}} - \boldsymbol{B})\boldsymbol{L})^{\otimes r}] &= E[(\boldsymbol{K}(\boldsymbol{A}'\boldsymbol{S}^{-1}\boldsymbol{A})^{-}\boldsymbol{A}'\boldsymbol{S}^{-1})^{\otimes r}] \\ &\quad \times E[(\boldsymbol{X} - \boldsymbol{A}\boldsymbol{B}\boldsymbol{C})^{\otimes r}](\boldsymbol{C}'(\boldsymbol{C}\boldsymbol{C}')^{-}\boldsymbol{L})^{\otimes r}. \end{aligned} \quad (4.25)$$

Due to normality, $E[(\boldsymbol{X} - \boldsymbol{A}\boldsymbol{B}\boldsymbol{C})^{\otimes r}] = \boldsymbol{0}$ for odd r and thus statement (i) is established.

Statement (ii) is just a reorganization of the elements in $D[\boldsymbol{K}\widehat{\boldsymbol{B}}\boldsymbol{L}]$, given in Theorem 4.3 (ii).

Now statement (iii) is considered. In Appendix B, Theorem B.19 (v), the fourth order moments of a variable with a matrix normal distribution with mean $\boldsymbol{0}$ are given. Put

$$\boldsymbol{K}^{1,i} = \boldsymbol{I}_i, \quad \boldsymbol{K}^{2,i} = \boldsymbol{I}_i \otimes \boldsymbol{K}_{i,i} \otimes \boldsymbol{I}_i, \quad \boldsymbol{K}^{3,i} = \boldsymbol{K}_{i,i^3}, \quad (4.26)$$

where the size of the matrices is indicated by i, which in the following equals either p or n. Then some manipulations yield (for details see Kollo and von Rosen, 2005, p. 415)

$$\begin{aligned} &E[(\boldsymbol{K}(\widehat{\boldsymbol{B}} - \boldsymbol{B})\boldsymbol{L})^{\otimes 4}] \\ &= \sum_{j=1}^{3} \boldsymbol{K}^{j,p}\{E[(\mathrm{vec}(\boldsymbol{\Gamma}_1'(\boldsymbol{I} + \boldsymbol{V}_{12}\boldsymbol{V}_{22}^{-1}\boldsymbol{V}_{22}^{-1}\boldsymbol{V}_{21})\boldsymbol{\Gamma}_1))^{\otimes 2}]\boldsymbol{v}'(\boldsymbol{C}')^{\otimes 2}\}\boldsymbol{K}^{j,n'}, \end{aligned} \quad (4.27)$$

where $\boldsymbol{\Gamma}_1$ and $\boldsymbol{V}$ are defined in (4.19) and (4.20), respectively. Expanding (4.27) gives

$$E[(\boldsymbol{K}(\widehat{\boldsymbol{B}}-\boldsymbol{B})\boldsymbol{L})^{\otimes 4}] = \sum_{j=1}^{3}\boldsymbol{K}^{j,p}\Big\{(\mathrm{vec}(\boldsymbol{\Gamma}_1'\boldsymbol{\Gamma}_1))^{\otimes 2}$$
$$+\mathrm{vec}(\boldsymbol{\Gamma}_1'\boldsymbol{\Gamma}_1)\otimes E[\mathrm{vec}(\boldsymbol{\Gamma}_1'\boldsymbol{V}_{12}\boldsymbol{V}_{22}^{-1}\boldsymbol{V}_{22}^{-1}\boldsymbol{V}_{21}\boldsymbol{\Gamma}_1)]$$
$$+E[\mathrm{vec}(\boldsymbol{\Gamma}_1'\boldsymbol{V}_{12}\boldsymbol{V}_{22}^{-1}\boldsymbol{V}_{22}^{-1}\boldsymbol{V}_{21}\boldsymbol{\Gamma}_1)]\otimes \mathrm{vec}(\boldsymbol{\Gamma}_1\boldsymbol{\Gamma}_1')$$
$$+E[(\mathrm{vec}(\boldsymbol{\Gamma}_1'\boldsymbol{V}_{12}\boldsymbol{V}_{22}^{-1}\boldsymbol{V}_{22}^{-1}\boldsymbol{V}_{21}\boldsymbol{\Gamma}_1))^{\otimes 2}]\Big\}\boldsymbol{v}'(\boldsymbol{C}')^{\otimes 2}\boldsymbol{K}^{j,n'}. \tag{4.28}$$

From Appendix B, Theorem B.21 (vii),

$$E[\boldsymbol{\Gamma}_1'\boldsymbol{V}_{12}\boldsymbol{V}_{22}^{-1}\boldsymbol{V}_{22}^{-1}\boldsymbol{V}_{21}\boldsymbol{\Gamma}_1] = c_1\boldsymbol{\Gamma}_1'\boldsymbol{\Gamma}_1,$$
$$E[(\mathrm{vec}(\boldsymbol{\Gamma}_1'\boldsymbol{V}_{12}\boldsymbol{V}_{22}^{-1}\boldsymbol{V}_{22}^{-1}\boldsymbol{V}_{21}\boldsymbol{\Gamma}_1))^{\otimes 2}]$$
$$= c_2(\mathrm{vec}(\boldsymbol{\Gamma}_1'\boldsymbol{\Gamma}_1))^{\otimes 2} + c_3(\boldsymbol{K}^{2,p}+\boldsymbol{K}^{3,p})(\mathrm{vec}(\boldsymbol{\Gamma}_1'\boldsymbol{\Gamma}_1))^{\otimes 2}, \tag{4.29}$$

and together with (4.28) these expressions establish statement (iii) of the theorem.

In order to demonstrate statement (iv) it is first noted that

$$E[(\boldsymbol{K}\widehat{\boldsymbol{B}}\boldsymbol{L})^{\otimes 2r}] = E[(\boldsymbol{K}(\boldsymbol{A}'\boldsymbol{S}^{-1}\boldsymbol{A})^{-}\boldsymbol{A}'\boldsymbol{S}^{-1})^{\otimes 2r}]E[(\boldsymbol{X}\boldsymbol{C}'(\boldsymbol{C}\boldsymbol{C}')^{-}\boldsymbol{L})^{\otimes 2r}].$$

Since one is just interested in the order of magnitude and no explicit expressions of $E[(\boldsymbol{K}\widehat{\boldsymbol{B}}\boldsymbol{L})^{\otimes 2r}]$, it follows from knowledge about moments of the matrix normal distribution that it is sufficient to consider (see Appendix, Theorem B.19 (vi))

$$E[(\mathrm{vec}(\boldsymbol{K}(\boldsymbol{A}'\boldsymbol{S}^{-1}\boldsymbol{A})^{-}\boldsymbol{A}'\boldsymbol{S}^{-1}\boldsymbol{\Sigma}\boldsymbol{S}^{-1}\boldsymbol{A}(\boldsymbol{A}'\boldsymbol{S}^{-1}\boldsymbol{A})^{-}\boldsymbol{K}'))^{\otimes r}].$$

As in (4.29), this expression can be presented in a canonical form,

$$E[(\mathrm{vec}(\boldsymbol{\Gamma}_1'\boldsymbol{V}_{12}\boldsymbol{V}_{22}^{-1}\boldsymbol{V}_{22}^{-1}\boldsymbol{V}_{21}\boldsymbol{\Gamma}))^{\otimes r}] = E[(\boldsymbol{\Gamma}_1'\boldsymbol{V}_{12}\boldsymbol{V}_{22}^{-1/2})^{\otimes 2r}]E[(\mathrm{vec}\boldsymbol{V}_{22}^{-1})^{\otimes r}],$$

where the equality follows from the independence relation given in Appendix B, Theorem B.20 (iv). Furthermore,

$$E[(\mathrm{vec}\boldsymbol{V}_{22}^{-1})^{\otimes r}] = \mathcal{O}(n^{-r}),$$

which is proven in Kollo and von Rosen (2005, p. 417). Furthermore, Theorem B.20 (iv) in Appendix B states that the matrix $\boldsymbol{V}_{12}\boldsymbol{V}_{22}^{-1/2}$ is normally distributed with moments independent of n. Thus, the theorem is established. □

In Theorem 4.3 (ii) and Corollary 4.1 (ii) the dispersion matrices for $\boldsymbol{K}\widehat{\boldsymbol{B}}\boldsymbol{L}$ in (4.8) and $\widehat{\boldsymbol{B}}$ were presented. However, these expressions are of little use if $\boldsymbol{\Sigma}^{-1}$ is not replaced by some appropriate value. If unbiased estimators are of interest, an unbiased estimator of $\boldsymbol{A}(\boldsymbol{A}'\boldsymbol{\Sigma}^{-1}\boldsymbol{A})^{-}\boldsymbol{A}'$ has to be found. This is indeed fairly easy, since Eq. (3.6) stated that

$$n\boldsymbol{A}'\boldsymbol{S}^{-1} = \boldsymbol{A}'\widehat{\boldsymbol{\Sigma}}^{-1},$$

where $\widehat{\boldsymbol{\Sigma}}^{-1}$ is the inverse of the maximum likelihood estimator, and (see Appendix B, Theorem B.20 (v))

$$\begin{aligned}E[\boldsymbol{A}(\boldsymbol{A}'\widehat{\boldsymbol{\Sigma}}^{-1}\boldsymbol{A})^{-}\boldsymbol{A}'] &= 1/nE[\boldsymbol{A}(\boldsymbol{A}'\boldsymbol{S}^{-1}\boldsymbol{A})^{-}\boldsymbol{A}'] \\ &= \frac{n-r(\boldsymbol{C})-p+r(\boldsymbol{A})}{n}\boldsymbol{A}(\boldsymbol{A}'\boldsymbol{\Sigma}^{-1}\boldsymbol{A})^{-}\boldsymbol{A}'.\end{aligned}$$

Hence, the following theorem has been established.

Theorem 4.5 *Consider the BRM presented in Definition 2.1, and let $\widehat{\boldsymbol{\Sigma}}$ be the maximum likelihood estimator. Unbiased estimators of the dispersion matrices for $\boldsymbol{K}\widehat{\boldsymbol{B}}\boldsymbol{L}$ in (4.8) and $\widehat{\boldsymbol{B}}$ are given by the following statements.*

(i) *If $n-r(\boldsymbol{C})-p+r(\boldsymbol{A})-1>0$, then*

$$\widehat{D[\boldsymbol{K}\widehat{\boldsymbol{B}}\boldsymbol{L}]} = \frac{n(n-r(\boldsymbol{C})-1)}{(n-r(\boldsymbol{C})-p+r(\boldsymbol{A})-1)(n-r(\boldsymbol{C})-p+r(\boldsymbol{A}))}\boldsymbol{L}'(\boldsymbol{C}\boldsymbol{C}')^{-}\boldsymbol{L}\otimes\boldsymbol{K}(\boldsymbol{A}'\widehat{\boldsymbol{\Sigma}}^{-1}\boldsymbol{A})^{-}\boldsymbol{K}'.$$

(ii) *If $n-k-p+q-1>0$, and $\boldsymbol{A}$ and $\boldsymbol{C}$ are of full rank*

$$\widehat{D[\widehat{\boldsymbol{B}}]} = \frac{n(n-k-1)}{(n-k-p+q-1)(n-k-p+q)}(\boldsymbol{C}\boldsymbol{C}')^{-1}\otimes(\boldsymbol{A}'\widehat{\boldsymbol{\Sigma}}^{-1}\boldsymbol{A})^{-1}.$$

In the following, the first and second order moments for $\widehat{\boldsymbol{\Sigma}}$ in the BRM are established. The estimator $\widehat{\boldsymbol{\Sigma}}$ was presented in Theorem 3.1, i.e.

$$\begin{aligned}n\widehat{\boldsymbol{\Sigma}} &= \boldsymbol{S}+(\boldsymbol{I}-\boldsymbol{P}_{A,S})\boldsymbol{X}\boldsymbol{P}_{C'}\boldsymbol{X}'(\boldsymbol{I}-\boldsymbol{P}'_{A,S}) \\ &= \boldsymbol{S}+\boldsymbol{P}'_{A^o,S^{-1}}\boldsymbol{X}\boldsymbol{P}_{C'}\boldsymbol{X}'\boldsymbol{P}_{A^o,S^{-1}},\end{aligned} \tag{4.30}$$

where $\boldsymbol{A}^o$ for convenience is chosen to be of full column rank, i.e. $\boldsymbol{A}^o : p\times(p-r(\boldsymbol{A}))$.

Theorem 4.6 (Kollo and von Rosen, 2005, Theorem 4.2.3) *Let $\widehat{\boldsymbol{\Sigma}}$ be as in (4.30).*

(i) *If $n-r(\boldsymbol{C})-p+r(\boldsymbol{A})-1>0$, then*

$$E[\widehat{\boldsymbol{\Sigma}}] = \boldsymbol{\Sigma}-r(\boldsymbol{C})\frac{1}{n}\frac{n-r(\boldsymbol{C})-2(p-r(\boldsymbol{A}))-1}{n-r(\boldsymbol{C})-p+r(\boldsymbol{A})-1}\boldsymbol{A}(\boldsymbol{A}'\boldsymbol{\Sigma}^{-1}\boldsymbol{A})^{-}\boldsymbol{A}'.$$

(ii) *If* $n - r(C) - p + r(A) - 3 > 0$, *then*

$$
\begin{aligned}
D[\widehat{\boldsymbol{\Sigma}}] = {} & d_1(\boldsymbol{I} + \boldsymbol{K}_{p,p})\{(\boldsymbol{A}(\boldsymbol{A}'\boldsymbol{\Sigma}^{-1}\boldsymbol{A})^{-}\boldsymbol{A}') \otimes (\boldsymbol{A}(\boldsymbol{A}'\boldsymbol{\Sigma}^{-1}\boldsymbol{A})^{-}\boldsymbol{A}')\} \\
& + d_2(\boldsymbol{I} + \boldsymbol{K}_{p,p})\{(\boldsymbol{A}(\boldsymbol{A}'\boldsymbol{\Sigma}^{-1}\boldsymbol{A})^{-}\boldsymbol{A}') \otimes (\boldsymbol{\Sigma} - \boldsymbol{A}(\boldsymbol{A}'\boldsymbol{\Sigma}^{-1}\boldsymbol{A})^{-}\boldsymbol{A}')\} \\
& + d_2(\boldsymbol{I} + \boldsymbol{K}_{p,p})\{(\boldsymbol{\Sigma} - \boldsymbol{A}(\boldsymbol{A}'\boldsymbol{\Sigma}^{-1}\boldsymbol{A})^{-}\boldsymbol{A}') \otimes (\boldsymbol{A}(\boldsymbol{A}'\boldsymbol{\Sigma}^{-1}\boldsymbol{A})^{-}\boldsymbol{A}')\} \\
& + \frac{1}{n}(\boldsymbol{I} + \boldsymbol{K}_{p,p})\{(\boldsymbol{\Sigma} - \boldsymbol{A}(\boldsymbol{A}'\boldsymbol{\Sigma}^{-1}\boldsymbol{A})^{-}\boldsymbol{A}') \otimes (\boldsymbol{\Sigma} - \boldsymbol{A}(\boldsymbol{A}'\boldsymbol{\Sigma}^{-1}\boldsymbol{A})^{-}\boldsymbol{A}')\} \\
& + d_3 \mathrm{vec}(\boldsymbol{A}(\boldsymbol{A}'\boldsymbol{\Sigma}^{-1}\boldsymbol{A})^{-}\boldsymbol{A}')\mathrm{vec}'(\boldsymbol{A}(\boldsymbol{A}'\boldsymbol{\Sigma}^{-1}\boldsymbol{A})^{-}\boldsymbol{A}'),
\end{aligned}
$$

where

$$
d_1 = \tfrac{n-r(\boldsymbol{C})}{n^2} + 2r(\boldsymbol{C})\tfrac{p-r(\boldsymbol{A})}{n^2(n-r(\boldsymbol{C})-p+r(\boldsymbol{A})-1)} + r(\boldsymbol{C})\tfrac{2c_1+c_2+c_3}{n^2} + r(\boldsymbol{C})^2\tfrac{c_3}{n^2},
$$

with

$$
\begin{aligned}
c_1 &= \tfrac{p-r(\boldsymbol{A})}{(n-r(\boldsymbol{C})-p+r(\boldsymbol{A})-1)}, \\
c_2 &= \tfrac{2(p-r(\boldsymbol{A}))(n-r(\boldsymbol{C})-p+r(\boldsymbol{A})-1)+\{2+(n-r(\boldsymbol{C})-p+r(\boldsymbol{A}))(n-r(\boldsymbol{C})-p+r(\boldsymbol{A})-3)\}(p-r(\boldsymbol{A}))^2}{(n-r(\boldsymbol{C})-p+r(\boldsymbol{A}))(n-r(\boldsymbol{C})-p+r(\boldsymbol{A})-1)^2(n-r(\boldsymbol{C})-p+r(\boldsymbol{A})-3)}, \\
c_3 &= \tfrac{p-r(\boldsymbol{A})}{(n-r(\boldsymbol{C})-p+r(\boldsymbol{A}))(n-r(\boldsymbol{C})-p+r(\boldsymbol{A})-3)} \\
&\quad + \tfrac{(p-r(\boldsymbol{A}))^2}{(n-r(\boldsymbol{C})-p+r(\boldsymbol{A}))(n-r(\boldsymbol{C})-p+r(\boldsymbol{A})-1)(n-r(\boldsymbol{C})-p+r(\boldsymbol{A})-3)},
\end{aligned}
$$

and

$$
\begin{aligned}
d_2 &= \tfrac{n-p+r(\boldsymbol{A})-1}{n(n-r(\boldsymbol{C})-p+r(\boldsymbol{A})-1)}, \\
d_3 &= \tfrac{2r(\boldsymbol{C})(n-r(\boldsymbol{C})-1)(n-p+r(\boldsymbol{A})-1)(p-r(\boldsymbol{A}))}{n^2(n-r(\boldsymbol{C})-p+r(\boldsymbol{A}))(n-r(\boldsymbol{C})-p+r(\boldsymbol{A})-1)^2(n-r(\boldsymbol{C})-p+r(\boldsymbol{A})-3)}.
\end{aligned}
$$

Proof Only statement (i) will be proven here. For details concerning statement (ii) see Kollo and von Rosen (2005, Theorem 4.2.3). The reason for not giving a proof of the second statement is that it consists of lengthy calculations where most steps in the proof have been applied earlier. Moreover, $D[\widehat{\boldsymbol{\Sigma}}]$ will not be used in the following presentation and is only included for completeness of presentation.

The fact will be utilized that $\boldsymbol{S} \sim W_p(\boldsymbol{\Sigma}, n - r(\boldsymbol{C}))$ and

$$
\boldsymbol{A}^{o'}\boldsymbol{X}\boldsymbol{P}_{\boldsymbol{C}'}\boldsymbol{X}'\boldsymbol{A}^{o} \sim W_{p-r(\boldsymbol{A})}(\boldsymbol{A}^{o'}\boldsymbol{\Sigma}\boldsymbol{A}^{o}, r(\boldsymbol{C}))
$$

are independently distributed (see Appendix B, Theorem B.19 (ix)). From (4.30) and Theorem B.19 (iv), (vii) in Appendix B,

$$\begin{aligned}E[n\widehat{\boldsymbol{\Sigma}}] &= E[\boldsymbol{S}] + E[\boldsymbol{P}'_{\boldsymbol{A}^o,\boldsymbol{S}^{-1}}\boldsymbol{X}\boldsymbol{P}_{\boldsymbol{C}'}\boldsymbol{X}'\boldsymbol{P}_{\boldsymbol{A}^o,\boldsymbol{S}^{-1}} \\ &= E[\boldsymbol{S}] + E[\boldsymbol{S}\boldsymbol{A}^o(\boldsymbol{A}^{o'}\boldsymbol{S}\boldsymbol{A}^o)^- E[\boldsymbol{A}^{o'}\boldsymbol{X}\boldsymbol{C}'(\boldsymbol{C}\boldsymbol{C}')^-\boldsymbol{C}\boldsymbol{X}'\boldsymbol{A}^o](\boldsymbol{A}^{o'}\boldsymbol{S}\boldsymbol{A}^o)^-\boldsymbol{A}^{o'}\boldsymbol{S}] \\ &= (n - r(\boldsymbol{C}))\boldsymbol{\Sigma} + r(\boldsymbol{C})E[\boldsymbol{P}'_{\boldsymbol{A}^o,\boldsymbol{S}^{-1}}\boldsymbol{\Sigma}\boldsymbol{P}_{\boldsymbol{A}^o,\boldsymbol{S}^{-1}}]. \end{aligned} \tag{4.31}$$

Let $\boldsymbol{\Sigma}^{1/2}$ be a symmetric square root of $\boldsymbol{\Sigma}$ and it follows that there exist a non-singular matrix $\boldsymbol{H}$ and an orthogonal matrix $\boldsymbol{\Gamma} = (\boldsymbol{\Gamma}'_1 : \boldsymbol{\Gamma}'_2)'$, where $\boldsymbol{\Gamma}_1 : (p - r(\boldsymbol{A})) \times p$ and $\boldsymbol{\Gamma}_2 : r(\boldsymbol{A}) \times p$, such that (see Appendix B, Theorem B.1 (i))

$$\boldsymbol{A}^{o'} = \boldsymbol{H}(\boldsymbol{I}_{p-r(\boldsymbol{A})} : \boldsymbol{0})\boldsymbol{\Gamma}\boldsymbol{\Sigma}^{-1/2} = \boldsymbol{H}\boldsymbol{\Gamma}_1\boldsymbol{\Sigma}^{-1/2} \tag{4.32}$$

holds. Moreover, similar to (4.20), let

$$\boldsymbol{V} = \boldsymbol{\Gamma}\boldsymbol{\Sigma}^{-1/2}\boldsymbol{S}\boldsymbol{\Sigma}^{-1/2}\boldsymbol{\Gamma}', \tag{4.33}$$

but now with the partition

$$\boldsymbol{V} = \begin{pmatrix}\boldsymbol{V}_{11} & \boldsymbol{V}_{12} \\ \boldsymbol{V}_{21} & \boldsymbol{V}_{22}\end{pmatrix} \quad \begin{matrix}(p - r(\boldsymbol{A})) \times (p - r(\boldsymbol{A})) & (p - r(\boldsymbol{A})) \times r(\boldsymbol{A}) \\ r(\boldsymbol{A}) \times (p - r(\boldsymbol{A})) & r(\boldsymbol{A}) \times r(\boldsymbol{A})\end{matrix}. \tag{4.34}$$

Therefore,

$$\boldsymbol{P}'_{\boldsymbol{A}^o,\boldsymbol{S}^{-1}}\boldsymbol{\Sigma}\boldsymbol{P}_{\boldsymbol{A}^o,\boldsymbol{S}^{-1}} = \boldsymbol{\Sigma}^{-1/2}\boldsymbol{\Gamma}'\begin{pmatrix}\boldsymbol{I} & \boldsymbol{V}_{11}^{-1}\boldsymbol{V}_{12} \\ \boldsymbol{V}_{21}\boldsymbol{V}_{11}^{-1} & \boldsymbol{V}_{21}\boldsymbol{V}_{11}^{-1}\boldsymbol{V}_{11}^{-1}\boldsymbol{V}_{12}\end{pmatrix}\boldsymbol{\Gamma}\boldsymbol{\Sigma}^{-1/2}$$

and

$$E[n\widehat{\boldsymbol{\Sigma}}] = E[\boldsymbol{S}] + r(\boldsymbol{C})\boldsymbol{\Sigma}^{-1/2}\boldsymbol{\Gamma}'E\begin{bmatrix}\boldsymbol{I} & \boldsymbol{V}_{11}^{-1}\boldsymbol{V}_{12} \\ \boldsymbol{V}_{21}\boldsymbol{V}_{11}^{-1} & \boldsymbol{V}_{21}\boldsymbol{V}_{11}^{-1}\boldsymbol{V}_{11}^{-1}\boldsymbol{V}_{12}\end{bmatrix}\boldsymbol{\Gamma}\boldsymbol{\Sigma}^{-1/2}. \tag{4.35}$$

Thus, from Theorem B.20 (ii), (iv), and since $E[\boldsymbol{V}_{21}\boldsymbol{V}_{11}^{-1}] = \boldsymbol{0}$, (4.35) is identical to

$$\begin{aligned}E[n\widehat{\boldsymbol{\Sigma}}] &= (n - r(\boldsymbol{C}))\boldsymbol{\Sigma} + r(\boldsymbol{C})\boldsymbol{\Sigma}^{-1/2}\boldsymbol{\Gamma}'\begin{pmatrix}\boldsymbol{I} & \boldsymbol{0} \\ \boldsymbol{0} & c_1\boldsymbol{I}_{r(\boldsymbol{A})}\end{pmatrix}\boldsymbol{\Gamma}\boldsymbol{\Sigma}^{-1/2} \\ &= (n - r(\boldsymbol{C}))\boldsymbol{\Sigma} + r(\boldsymbol{C})\boldsymbol{\Sigma}^{-1/2}\boldsymbol{\Gamma}'_1\boldsymbol{\Gamma}_1\boldsymbol{\Sigma}^{-1/2} + r(\boldsymbol{C})c_1\boldsymbol{\Sigma}^{-1/2}\boldsymbol{\Gamma}_2\boldsymbol{\Gamma}'_2\boldsymbol{\Sigma}^{-1/2}. \end{aligned} \tag{4.36}$$

Finally, one returns to the original matrices and

$$\boldsymbol{\Sigma}^{1/2}\boldsymbol{\Gamma}'_1\boldsymbol{\Gamma}_1\boldsymbol{\Sigma}^{1/2} = \boldsymbol{\Sigma} - \boldsymbol{A}(\boldsymbol{A}'\boldsymbol{\Sigma}^{-1}\boldsymbol{A})^-\boldsymbol{A}', \quad \boldsymbol{\Sigma}^{1/2}\boldsymbol{\Gamma}'_2\boldsymbol{\Gamma}_2\boldsymbol{\Sigma}^{1/2} = \boldsymbol{A}(\boldsymbol{A}'\boldsymbol{\Sigma}^{-1}\boldsymbol{A})^-\boldsymbol{A}'. \tag{4.37}$$

Thus, the expectations given by (4.36) can be expressed in the original matrices and from (4.37) it follows that (4.36) can be written as

$$E[n\widehat{\boldsymbol{\Sigma}}] = (n - r(\boldsymbol{C}))\boldsymbol{\Sigma} + r(\boldsymbol{C})(\boldsymbol{\Sigma} - \boldsymbol{A}(\boldsymbol{A}'\boldsymbol{\Sigma}^{-1}\boldsymbol{A})^{-}\boldsymbol{A}') + r(\boldsymbol{C})c_1\boldsymbol{A}(\boldsymbol{A}'\boldsymbol{\Sigma}^{-1}\boldsymbol{A})^{-}\boldsymbol{A}', \tag{4.38}$$

which is identical to statement (i) of the theorem. □

It is interesting to devote some thought to the results of Theorem 4.6 (i). Here it is stated that the maximum likelihood estimator of $\boldsymbol{\Sigma}$ is not unbiased. Indeed it follows that $\widehat{\boldsymbol{\Sigma}}$ underestimates $\boldsymbol{\Sigma}$, on average. This was expected, because the MLEs of variances in linear and multivariate linear models are biased estimators. For these estimators, unbiased estimators can always be obtained by rescaling the original estimator. The estimator $\widehat{\boldsymbol{\Sigma}}$ involves $\boldsymbol{A}$ and therefore rescaling is not possible. However, in the next theorem, an unbiased estimator of $\boldsymbol{\Sigma}$ is presented which only is a function of $\widehat{\boldsymbol{\Sigma}}$.

Theorem 4.7 *Let $\widehat{\boldsymbol{\Sigma}}$ be given by (4.30) and*

$$e_1 = r(\boldsymbol{C})\frac{n-r(\boldsymbol{C})-2p+2r(\boldsymbol{A})-1}{(n-r(\boldsymbol{C})-p+r(\boldsymbol{A})-1)(n-r(\boldsymbol{C})-p+r(\boldsymbol{A}))}.$$

Then $\widehat{\boldsymbol{\Sigma}}_U = \widehat{\boldsymbol{\Sigma}} + e_1\boldsymbol{A}(\boldsymbol{A}'\widehat{\boldsymbol{\Sigma}}^{-1}\boldsymbol{A})^{-}\boldsymbol{A}'$ is an unbiased estimator of $\boldsymbol{\Sigma}$.

Proof The proof is based on the fact $\boldsymbol{A}'\widehat{\boldsymbol{\Sigma}}^{-1} = n\boldsymbol{A}'\boldsymbol{S}^{-1}$ and (see Appendix B, Theorem B.20 (v))

$$E[\boldsymbol{A}(\boldsymbol{A}'\boldsymbol{S}^{-1}\boldsymbol{A})^{-}\boldsymbol{A}'] = (n - r(\boldsymbol{C}) - p + r(\boldsymbol{A}))\boldsymbol{A}(\boldsymbol{A}'\boldsymbol{\Sigma}^{-1}\boldsymbol{A})^{-}\boldsymbol{A}'.$$

Hence, from Theorem 4.6 it follows that

$$\begin{aligned} E[\widehat{\boldsymbol{\Sigma}}_U] = \boldsymbol{\Sigma} + \Big\{ -r(\boldsymbol{C})\frac{1}{n}\frac{n - r(\boldsymbol{C}) - 2p + 2r(\boldsymbol{A}) - 1}{n - r(\boldsymbol{C}) - p + r(\boldsymbol{A}) - 1} + r(\boldsymbol{C})e_1\frac{1}{n}(n - r(\boldsymbol{C}) - p + r(\boldsymbol{A}))\Big\} \\ \times\boldsymbol{A}(\boldsymbol{A}'\boldsymbol{\Sigma}^{-1}\boldsymbol{A})^{-}\boldsymbol{A}' = \boldsymbol{\Sigma}. \end{aligned}$$

□

It can be observed that in Theorem 4.7

$$\boldsymbol{A}(\boldsymbol{A}'\widehat{\boldsymbol{\Sigma}}^{-1}\boldsymbol{A})^{-}\boldsymbol{A}' = \boldsymbol{P}_{A,\widehat{\Sigma}}\widehat{\boldsymbol{\Sigma}}\boldsymbol{P}'_{A,\widehat{\Sigma}};$$

i.e. a projection on $\mathcal{C}(\boldsymbol{A})$ takes place. Moreover, one can note that $\frac{1}{n-r(\boldsymbol{C})}\boldsymbol{S}$ also is an unbiased estimator of $\boldsymbol{\Sigma}$. If one compares the estimator $\frac{1}{n-r(\boldsymbol{C})}\boldsymbol{S}$ with the one given by Theorem 3.1, there is in principle only one firm conclusion which can be drawn, namely that the distribution for the estimator $\frac{1}{n-r(\boldsymbol{C})}\boldsymbol{S}$ is a Wishart distribution, whereas the distribution of the maximum-likelihood-based estimator is unknown.

The maximum likelihood estimator $\widehat{\boldsymbol{\Sigma}}$, given by Theorem 3.1, combines the deviation between the observations and the sample mean and the deviation between the sample mean and the estimated model (see also Fig. 3.2). Hence, the maximum likelihood estimator uses two sources of information whereas $\frac{1}{n-r(\boldsymbol{C})}\boldsymbol{S}$ uses only one. Intuitively the maximum likelihood estimator should be preferable, although one must remember that one's choice of estimator depends on the number of observations and the choice of design matrix $\boldsymbol{A}$.

It is possible to compare the two estimators with respect to their variances. Since a comparison can only be made for a given $\boldsymbol{A}$, however, no such comparison will be made. It should, furthermore, be noted that in multivariate analysis the statistic $\frac{1}{n-r(\boldsymbol{C})}\boldsymbol{S}$ is often used as an estimator of $\boldsymbol{\Sigma}$, for example in principal component analysis, canonical correlation analysis and different versions of factor analysis. However, if the mean value is structured as in the BRM, i.e. $E[\boldsymbol{X}] = \boldsymbol{ABC}$, one can very well apply Theorem 4.7.

Next an interesting statement is given which can be proven in the same fashion as several of the previous theorems.

Theorem 4.8 *Let $\boldsymbol{K}\widehat{\boldsymbol{B}}\boldsymbol{L}$ and $\widehat{\boldsymbol{\Sigma}}$ be given by (4.8) and (4.30), respectively. Then*

$$C[\boldsymbol{K}\widehat{\boldsymbol{B}}\boldsymbol{L}, \widehat{\boldsymbol{\Sigma}}] = \boldsymbol{0}.$$

This theorem states that $\boldsymbol{K}\widehat{\boldsymbol{B}}\boldsymbol{L}$ and $\widehat{\boldsymbol{\Sigma}}$ are uncorrelated. However, $\boldsymbol{K}\widehat{\boldsymbol{B}}\boldsymbol{L}$ and $\widehat{\boldsymbol{\Sigma}}$ are not independently distributed, which can be seen from

$$E[\boldsymbol{K}\widehat{\boldsymbol{B}}\boldsymbol{L} \otimes \boldsymbol{K}\widehat{\boldsymbol{B}}\boldsymbol{L} \otimes \widehat{\boldsymbol{\Sigma}}] \neq E[\boldsymbol{K}\widehat{\boldsymbol{B}}\boldsymbol{L} \otimes \boldsymbol{K}\widehat{\boldsymbol{B}}\boldsymbol{L}] \otimes E[\widehat{\boldsymbol{\Sigma}}].$$

To verify this statement, rather lengthy moment calculations have to take place and, therefore, these are omitted here.

This section is ended by showing some calculations when applying the estimators.

Example 4.1 (Continuation of Example 3.1, Potthoff and Roy (1964) data) In Example 3.1 two different models were considered. Now the estimated dispersion of the mean estimators and an unbiased estimator of the dispersion matrices is presented. For details concerning the models the reader is referred to Example 3.1.

Model Ia
According to Corollary 4.1 (ii) and Theorem 4.5 (ii),

$$D[\widehat{\boldsymbol{B}}_1] = 24/22 \begin{pmatrix} 0.09 & 0 \\ 0 & 0.06 \end{pmatrix} \otimes (\boldsymbol{A}_1'\boldsymbol{\Sigma}^{-1}\boldsymbol{A}_1)^{-1},$$

$$\widehat{D[\widehat{\boldsymbol{B}}_1]} = \begin{pmatrix} 0.09 & 0 \\ 0 & 0.06 \end{pmatrix} \otimes \begin{pmatrix} 17.9 & -1.3 \\ -1.3 & 0.1 \end{pmatrix}.$$

It follows from Theorem 4.7 that an unbiased estimator of $\boldsymbol{\Sigma}$ is given by

$$\widehat{\boldsymbol{\Sigma}}_{1U} = \widehat{\boldsymbol{\Sigma}}_1 + \tfrac{2*20}{22*23}\boldsymbol{A}_1(\boldsymbol{A}_1'\widehat{\boldsymbol{\Sigma}}_1^{-1}\boldsymbol{A}_1)^{-}\boldsymbol{A}_1',$$

$$\widehat{\boldsymbol{\Sigma}}_{1Uo} = \begin{pmatrix} 5.4 & 2.7 & 3.8 & 2.7 \\ & 4.2 & 3.0 & 3.3 \\ & & 6.3 & 4.1 \\ & & & 5.0 \end{pmatrix},$$

where $\widehat{\boldsymbol{\Sigma}}_1 = (\boldsymbol{X} - \boldsymbol{A}_1\widehat{\boldsymbol{B}}_1\boldsymbol{C})()'$. For comparison, $\frac{1}{n-r(\boldsymbol{C})}\boldsymbol{S}_o$ is presented as an alternative unbiased estimator of $\boldsymbol{\Sigma}$ which equals

$$\frac{1}{n-r(\boldsymbol{C})}\boldsymbol{S}_o = \frac{1}{n-r(\boldsymbol{C})}\boldsymbol{X}_o(\boldsymbol{I} - \boldsymbol{P}_{\boldsymbol{C}'})\boldsymbol{X}_o' = \begin{pmatrix} 5.4 & 2.7 & 3.9 & 2.7 \\ & 4.2 & 2.9 & 3.3 \\ & & 6.5 & 4.1 \\ & & & 5.0 \end{pmatrix}.$$

It is interesting to note that there are very small differences between $\widehat{\boldsymbol{\Sigma}}_{1Uo}$ and the estimator based on $\boldsymbol{S}_o$.

Model Ib
The dispersion for $\widehat{\boldsymbol{B}}_2 = (\boldsymbol{A}_1'\boldsymbol{A}_1)^{-1}\boldsymbol{A}_1\boldsymbol{X}\boldsymbol{C}'(\boldsymbol{C}\boldsymbol{C}')^{-1}$ can be written as follows:

$$D[\widehat{\boldsymbol{B}}_2] = (\boldsymbol{C}\boldsymbol{C}')^{-1} \otimes (\boldsymbol{A}_1'\boldsymbol{A}_1)^{-1}\boldsymbol{A}_1'\boldsymbol{\Sigma}\boldsymbol{A}_1(\boldsymbol{A}_1'\boldsymbol{A}_1)^{-1}.$$

One way of estimating the dispersion is to replace $\boldsymbol{\Sigma}$ by an unbiased estimator, for example $1/(n - r(\boldsymbol{C}))\boldsymbol{S}$, i.e.

$$\widehat{D[\widehat{\boldsymbol{B}}_2]} = \tfrac{1}{n-r(\boldsymbol{C})}(\boldsymbol{C}\boldsymbol{C}')^{-1} \otimes (\boldsymbol{A}_1'\boldsymbol{A}_1)^{-1}\boldsymbol{A}_1'\boldsymbol{S}\boldsymbol{A}_1(\boldsymbol{A}_1'\boldsymbol{A}_1)^{-1}. \qquad (4.39)$$

The expectation of $\widehat{\boldsymbol{\Sigma}}_2 = (\boldsymbol{X} - \boldsymbol{A}_1\widehat{\boldsymbol{B}}_2\boldsymbol{C})()'$ equals

$$E[\widehat{\boldsymbol{\Sigma}}_2] = \tfrac{n-r(\boldsymbol{C})}{n}\boldsymbol{\Sigma} + \tfrac{r(\boldsymbol{C})}{n}(\boldsymbol{I} - \boldsymbol{P}_{A_1})\boldsymbol{\Sigma}(\boldsymbol{I} - \boldsymbol{P}_{A_1}).$$

Finding an unbiased estimator of $\boldsymbol{\Sigma}$ is performed via the following relation:

$$\widehat{\boldsymbol{\Sigma}}_{2U} = \frac{n}{n-r(\boldsymbol{C})}\widehat{\boldsymbol{\Sigma}}_2 - \frac{r(\boldsymbol{C})}{(n-r(\boldsymbol{C}))^2}(\boldsymbol{I} - \boldsymbol{P}_{A_1})\boldsymbol{S}(\boldsymbol{I} - \boldsymbol{P}_{A_1}). \qquad (4.40)$$

Now explicit calculations of (4.39) and (4.40), respectively, yield

$$\widehat{D[\widehat{\boldsymbol{B}}_2]} = \begin{pmatrix} 0.09 & 0 \\ 0 & 0.06 \end{pmatrix} \otimes \begin{pmatrix} 16.6 & -1.2 \\ -1.2 & 0.1 \end{pmatrix}$$

and

$$\widehat{\boldsymbol{\Sigma}}_{2Uo} = \begin{pmatrix} 5.4 & 2.7 & 3.9 & 2.7 \\ & 4.2 & 3.0 & 3.3 \\ & & 6.3 & 4.2 \\ & & & 5.0 \end{pmatrix}.$$

The difference in performance between Model Ia and Model Ib can be measured by (see Appendix B, Theorem B.9 (v))

$$\widehat{D[\widehat{\boldsymbol{B}}_2]} - \widehat{D[\widehat{\boldsymbol{B}}_1]}$$
$$= (\boldsymbol{C}\boldsymbol{C}')^{-1} \otimes \{\tfrac{1}{n-k}(\boldsymbol{A}_1'\boldsymbol{A}_1)^{-1}\boldsymbol{A}_1'\boldsymbol{S}\boldsymbol{A}_1(\boldsymbol{A}_1'\boldsymbol{A}_1)^{-1} - \tfrac{n-k-1}{(n-k-p+q-1)(n-k-p+q)}(\boldsymbol{A}'\boldsymbol{S}^{-1}\boldsymbol{A})^{-1}\}$$
$$\leq (\tfrac{1}{n-k}\tfrac{(\lambda_1+\lambda_p)^2}{4\lambda_1\lambda_2} - \tfrac{n-k-1}{(n-k-p+q-1)(n-k-p+q)})(\boldsymbol{C}\boldsymbol{C}')^{-1} \otimes (\boldsymbol{A}'\boldsymbol{S}^{-1}\boldsymbol{A})^{-1},$$

where λ_p and λ_1 denote the smallest and largest eigenvalues of $\boldsymbol{S}$, respectively. The inequality is according to the Loewner order (see Appendix A, Sect. A.3). Thus, since $\lambda_1 = 15.3$ and $\lambda_2 = 0.9$,

$$\widehat{D[\widehat{\boldsymbol{B}}_2]} - \widehat{D[\widehat{\boldsymbol{B}}_1]} \leq \begin{pmatrix} 4.9 & -0.4 & 0 & 0 \\ & 0.04 & 0 & 0 \\ & & 3.4 & -0.2 \\ & & & 0.02 \end{pmatrix}.$$

Hence, it can be seen that the upper bound indicates that there might be a difference in the estimated variance between the two approaches. However, we do not know how sharp the upper bound is in reality and one can suspect that it is not very sharp, in particular if the smallest eigenvalue is close to 0.

Model IIa
This model is similar to Model Ia. The difference is that now a second degree polynomial describes the growth instead of a line. The results are as follows:

$$D[\widehat{\boldsymbol{B}}_3] = 24/23 \begin{pmatrix} 0.09 & 0 \\ 0 & 0.06 \end{pmatrix} \otimes (\boldsymbol{A}_2'\boldsymbol{\Sigma}^{-1}\boldsymbol{A}_2)^{-1},$$

$$\widehat{D[\widehat{\boldsymbol{B}}_3]} = \begin{pmatrix} 0.09 & 0 \\ 0 & 0.06 \end{pmatrix} \otimes \begin{pmatrix} 286.7 & -51.0 & 2.2 \\ -51.0 & 9.3 & -0.4 \\ 2.2 & -0.4 & 0.02 \end{pmatrix}.$$

In comparison with Model Ia, the estimated variance of the intercept and slope is much higher. It has indeed become so large that it is difficult to determine whether $\widehat{\boldsymbol{B}}_3$ differs from $\boldsymbol{0}$.

An unbiased estimator of $\mathbf{\Sigma}$ is given by

$$\widehat{\mathbf{\Sigma}}_{3U} = \widehat{\mathbf{\Sigma}}_2 + \tfrac{2*22}{23*24} A_2(A_2'\widehat{\mathbf{\Sigma}}_2^{-1}A_2)^- A_2',$$

$$\mathbf{\Sigma}_{3Uo} = \begin{pmatrix} 5.4 & 2.7 & 3.8 & 2.7 \\ & 4.2 & 3.0 & 3.3 \\ & & 6.3 & 4.1 \\ & & & 5.0 \end{pmatrix}.$$

The estimator of $\mathbf{\Sigma}$ is almost the same as the previously presented unbiased estimators of $\mathbf{\Sigma}$, but, in contrast to that, the estimated dispersion of the mean parameters differs significantly between Model Ia and Model IIa.

Model IIb
This model is an extension of Model Ib and it follows that

$$D[\widehat{\boldsymbol{B}}_4] = (\boldsymbol{C}\boldsymbol{C}')^{-1} \otimes (A_2'A_2)^{-1}A_2'\mathbf{\Sigma}A_2(A_2'A_2)^{-1},$$

$$\widehat{D[\widehat{\boldsymbol{B}}_4]} = \begin{pmatrix} 0.09 & 0 \\ 0 & 0.06 \end{pmatrix} \otimes \begin{pmatrix} 216.6 & -40.4 & 1.8 \\ -40.4 & 7.6 & -0.3 \\ 1.9 & -0.3 & 0.02 \end{pmatrix}.$$

Thus, as for Model IIa there is a relatively large dispersion. An unbiased estimator of $\mathbf{\Sigma}$ is given by

$$\widehat{\mathbf{\Sigma}}_{4Uo} = \begin{pmatrix} 5.4 & 2.7 & 3.9 & 2.7 \\ & 4.1 & 3.0 & 3.3 \\ & & 6.4 & 4.2 \\ & & & 5.0 \end{pmatrix}.$$

The most striking discovery in this example is that when adding a mean parameter to the model, the dispersion of the mean estimators becomes large. Therefore, if in practice one has to choose between a two-parameter linear model and a three-parameter model, the results indicate that a two-parameter model is more relevant to use than a three-parameter model.

The upper bound of the difference $\widehat{D[\widehat{\boldsymbol{B}}_4]} - \widehat{D[\widehat{\boldsymbol{B}}_3]}$ is rather large and computations yield

$$\widehat{D[\widehat{\boldsymbol{B}}_4]} - \widehat{D[\widehat{\boldsymbol{B}}_3]} \leq \begin{pmatrix} 87.7 & -15.6 & 0.7 & 0 & 0 & 0 \\ & 2.8 & -0.1 & 0 & 0 & 0 \\ & & 0.005 & 0 & 0 & 0 \\ & & & 60.3 & -10.7 & 0.46 \\ & & & & 2.0 & -0.08 \\ & & & & & 0.004 \end{pmatrix}.$$

Hence, it can be seen that the upper bound indicates that there can be a difference in the estimated variance between the two approaches. □

Example 4.2 (Continuation of Example 1.5, "Liming Data")

$$\widehat{\boldsymbol{B}}_o = \begin{pmatrix} 7.1 & 7.0 \\ -0.03 & -0.04 \end{pmatrix},$$

$$D[\widehat{\boldsymbol{B}}] = 17/16(\boldsymbol{C}\boldsymbol{C}')^{-1} \otimes (\boldsymbol{A}'\boldsymbol{\Sigma}^{-1}\boldsymbol{A})^{-1},$$

$$\widehat{D[\widehat{\boldsymbol{B}}]} = \begin{pmatrix} 0.1 & 0 \\ 0 & 0.1 \end{pmatrix} \otimes \begin{pmatrix} 0.041 & 0.0010 \\ 0.0010 & 0.00049 \end{pmatrix},$$

$$\widehat{\boldsymbol{\Sigma}}_o = \begin{pmatrix} 0.036 & 0.034 & 0.042 \\ & 0.060 & 0.066 \\ & & 0.088 \end{pmatrix},$$

$$\widehat{\boldsymbol{\Sigma}}_U = \widehat{\boldsymbol{\Sigma}} + \tfrac{2*15}{16*17}\boldsymbol{A}(\boldsymbol{A}'\widehat{\boldsymbol{\Sigma}}^{-1}\boldsymbol{A})^{-1}\boldsymbol{A},$$

$$\widehat{\boldsymbol{\Sigma}}_{Uo} = \begin{pmatrix} 0.040 & 0.038 & 0.047 \\ & 0.067 & 0.073 \\ & & 0.097 \end{pmatrix}.$$

If $\boldsymbol{S}$ in $\widehat{\boldsymbol{B}}$ is considered to be fixed,

$$D[\widehat{\boldsymbol{B}}|\boldsymbol{S}] = (\boldsymbol{C}\boldsymbol{C}')^{-1} \otimes (\boldsymbol{A}'\boldsymbol{S}^{-1}\boldsymbol{A})^{-1}\boldsymbol{A}'\boldsymbol{\Sigma}\boldsymbol{A}(\boldsymbol{A}'\boldsymbol{S}^{-1}\boldsymbol{A})^{-1}$$

with an unbiased estimator $\widehat{D[\widehat{\boldsymbol{B}}|\boldsymbol{S}]} = \frac{16}{17}\widehat{D[\widehat{\boldsymbol{B}}]}$, where $\boldsymbol{\Sigma}$ has been replaced by $\widehat{\boldsymbol{\Sigma}} = \frac{1}{n-r(\boldsymbol{C})}\boldsymbol{S}$. Hence, a conditional approach is fairly relevant to use, in particular since in this case the distribution of $\widehat{\boldsymbol{B}}$ is known. □

4.4 $EBRM_B^3$ and Uniqueness Conditions for MLEs

In order to study the estimators of parameters in the $EBRM_B^3$, the estimators or the bilinear combinations of them have to be unique. If the estimate $\widehat{\boldsymbol{B}}_{io}$ is considered to be unique, it is understood that $\widehat{\boldsymbol{B}}_{io}$ has a unique expression, whereas if the estimator $\widehat{\boldsymbol{B}}_i$ is unique, this means that it has a unique distribution (excluding events with probability mass 0). In the following, however, $\widehat{\boldsymbol{B}}_i$ represents both the estimators and the estimates. It is essential, as for the BRM, to obtain uniqueness conditions, since the conditions reveal whether or not the parameters or bilinear functions of the parameters are estimable. Unfortunately, in comparison with the BRM, there are more parameters for the $EBRM_B^3$ and their estimators are functionally connected. Thus, the handling of the $EBRM_B^3$ is more complex and the technical treatment more complicated. In general the technical details presented in the following will be sparse.

The next theorem presents the uniqueness conditions necessary and sufficient for the estimators of the parameters in the $EBRM_B^3$.

Theorem 4.9 *For the $EBRM_B^3$ presented in Definition 2.2, let $\widehat{\boldsymbol{B}}_i$, $i = 1, 2, 3$, be given in Theorem 3.2 and let $\boldsymbol{K}\widehat{\boldsymbol{B}}_i\boldsymbol{L}$, $i = 1, 2, 3$, be linear combinations of $\widehat{\boldsymbol{B}}_i$; $\boldsymbol{K}$ and $\boldsymbol{L}$ are known matrices of proper sizes. Then the following statements hold:*

(i) $\widehat{\boldsymbol{B}}_3$ *is unique if and only if*

$$r(\boldsymbol{A}_3) = q_3, \quad r(\boldsymbol{C}_3) = k_3, \quad \mathcal{C}(\boldsymbol{A}_3) \cap \mathcal{C}(\boldsymbol{A}_1 : \boldsymbol{A}_2) = \{\boldsymbol{0}\};$$

(ii) $\boldsymbol{K}\widehat{\boldsymbol{B}}_3\boldsymbol{L}$ *is unique if and only if*

$$\mathcal{C}(\boldsymbol{L}) \subseteq \mathcal{C}(\boldsymbol{C}_3), \quad \mathcal{C}(\boldsymbol{K}') \subseteq \mathcal{C}(\boldsymbol{A}_3'(\boldsymbol{A}_1 : \boldsymbol{A}_2)^o);$$

(iii) $\widehat{\boldsymbol{B}}_2$ *is unique if and only if*

$$r(\boldsymbol{A}_2) = q_2, \quad r(\boldsymbol{C}_2) = k_2, \quad \mathcal{C}(\boldsymbol{A}_1) \cap \mathcal{C}(\boldsymbol{A}_2) = \{\boldsymbol{0}\},$$
$$\mathcal{C}(\boldsymbol{A}_1)^\perp \cap \mathcal{C}(\boldsymbol{A}_1 : \boldsymbol{A}_2) \cap \mathcal{C}(\boldsymbol{A}_1 : \boldsymbol{A}_3) = \{\boldsymbol{0}\};$$

(iv) $\boldsymbol{K}\widehat{\boldsymbol{B}}_2\boldsymbol{L}$ *is unique if and only if*

$$\mathcal{C}(\boldsymbol{L}) \subseteq \mathcal{C}(\boldsymbol{C}_2), \quad \mathcal{C}(\boldsymbol{K}') \subseteq \mathcal{C}(\boldsymbol{A}_2'(\boldsymbol{A}_1 : \boldsymbol{A}_3)^o);$$

(v) $\widehat{\boldsymbol{B}}_1$ *is unique if and only if*

$$r(\boldsymbol{A}_1) = q_1, \quad r(\boldsymbol{C}_1) = k_1, \quad \mathcal{C}(\boldsymbol{A}_1) \cap \mathcal{C}(\boldsymbol{A}_2) = \{\boldsymbol{0}\},$$
$$\mathcal{C}(\boldsymbol{A}_2)^\perp \cap \mathcal{C}(\boldsymbol{A}_1 : \boldsymbol{A}_2) \cap \mathcal{C}(\boldsymbol{A}_2 : \boldsymbol{A}_3) = \{\boldsymbol{0}\};$$

(vi) $\boldsymbol{K}\widehat{\boldsymbol{B}}_1\boldsymbol{L}$ *is unique if and only if*

$$\mathcal{C}(\boldsymbol{L}) \subseteq \mathcal{C}(\boldsymbol{C}_1), \quad \mathcal{C}(\boldsymbol{K}') \subseteq \mathcal{C}(\boldsymbol{A}_1'),$$
$$\mathcal{C}(\boldsymbol{A}_3'(\boldsymbol{I} - \boldsymbol{P}_{\boldsymbol{A}_1^o}\boldsymbol{A}_2(\boldsymbol{A}_2'\boldsymbol{P}_{\boldsymbol{A}_1^o}\boldsymbol{A}_2)^-\boldsymbol{A}_2')\boldsymbol{A}_1(\boldsymbol{A}_1'\boldsymbol{A}_1)^-\boldsymbol{K}') \subseteq \mathcal{C}(\boldsymbol{A}_3'(\boldsymbol{A}_1 : \boldsymbol{A}_2)^o),$$
$$\mathcal{C}(\boldsymbol{A}_2'\boldsymbol{A}_1(\boldsymbol{A}_1'\boldsymbol{A}_1)^-\boldsymbol{K}') \subseteq \mathcal{C}(\boldsymbol{A}_2'\boldsymbol{A}_1^o);$$

(vii) *The estimator $\widehat{\boldsymbol{\Sigma}}$ in Theorem 3.2 is always uniquely estimated as well as the estimator $\widehat{E[\boldsymbol{X}]}$ given in Corollary 3.3.*

Proof The proof is based on the expressions given in Theorem 3.2. The estimators will be unique if the expressions do not include the $\boldsymbol{Z}_{ij}$ matrices. Moreover, since the matrix expressions involving $\boldsymbol{Z}_{ij}$ do not include any inner product estimators, the uniqueness conditions will hold irrespective of whether $\boldsymbol{\Sigma}$ is known or unknown;

i.e. in principle the conditions could have been derived from standard linear models theory.

Now the derivations of the statements begin and we start by considering $\widehat{\boldsymbol{B}}_3$, which is unique if $(\boldsymbol{A}_3'\boldsymbol{Q}_2\boldsymbol{Q}_1)^o = \boldsymbol{0}$ and $\boldsymbol{C}_3^o = \boldsymbol{0}$. Note that instead of $\widehat{\boldsymbol{Q}}_2\widehat{\boldsymbol{Q}}_1$ in Theorem 3.2, $\boldsymbol{Q}_2\boldsymbol{Q}_1$ can be used, since the estimate of the inner product, as has been noted above, can be disregarded. Since the derived uniqueness conditions do not depend on the inner product, this fact shortens the derivations significantly. It follows that

$$\mathcal{C}(\boldsymbol{Q}_2\boldsymbol{Q}_1) = \mathcal{C}(\boldsymbol{A}_1 : \boldsymbol{A}_2)^{\perp},$$

and therefore (see Appendix B, Theorem B.5 (iv))

$$r(\boldsymbol{A}_3'\boldsymbol{Q}_2\boldsymbol{Q}_1) = r(\boldsymbol{A}_1 : \boldsymbol{A}_2 : \boldsymbol{A}_3) - r(\boldsymbol{A}_1 : \boldsymbol{A}_2),$$

which implies that $(\boldsymbol{A}_3'\boldsymbol{Q}_2\boldsymbol{Q}_1)^o = \boldsymbol{0}$ is equivalent to

$$\mathcal{C}(\boldsymbol{A}_3) \cap \mathcal{C}(\boldsymbol{A}_1 : \boldsymbol{A}_2) = \{\boldsymbol{0}\}, \quad r(\boldsymbol{A}_3) = q_3.$$

Thus, statement (i) has been verified and statement (ii) can also be obtained from these calculations.

Turning to statement (iii), it follows immediately from Theorem 3.2 that $(\boldsymbol{A}_2'\boldsymbol{Q}_1)^o = \boldsymbol{0}$ and $\boldsymbol{C}_2^o = \boldsymbol{0}$ have to be satisfied. The conditions are equivalent to

$$\mathcal{C}(\boldsymbol{A}_2) \cap \mathcal{C}(\boldsymbol{A}_1) = \{\boldsymbol{0}\}, \quad r(\boldsymbol{A}_2) = q_2, \quad r(\boldsymbol{C}_2) = k_2.$$

Moreover, according to Theorem 3.2, $\boldsymbol{A}_2'\boldsymbol{Q}_1\boldsymbol{\Sigma}^{-1}\boldsymbol{Q}_1'\boldsymbol{A}_3\widehat{\boldsymbol{B}}_3\boldsymbol{C}_3\boldsymbol{C}_2'$ should be unique and using statement (i)

$$\mathcal{C}(\boldsymbol{A}_3'\boldsymbol{Q}_1\boldsymbol{\Sigma}^{-1}\boldsymbol{Q}_1'\boldsymbol{A}_2) \subseteq \mathcal{C}(\boldsymbol{A}_3'(\boldsymbol{A}_1 : \boldsymbol{A}_2)^o) = \mathcal{C}(\boldsymbol{A}_3'\boldsymbol{Q}_1\boldsymbol{Q}_2)$$

should hold. Since $\mathcal{C}(\boldsymbol{\Sigma}^{-1}\boldsymbol{Q}_1'\boldsymbol{A}_2) = \mathcal{C}(\boldsymbol{I} - \boldsymbol{Q}_2)$, this expression is equivalent to

$$\mathcal{C}(\boldsymbol{A}_3'\boldsymbol{Q}_1) \subseteq \mathcal{C}(\boldsymbol{A}_3'\boldsymbol{Q}_1(\boldsymbol{Q}_1\boldsymbol{A}_2)^o).$$

Hence, applying Appendix B, Theorem B.3 (vii), this relation yields

$$\mathcal{C}(\boldsymbol{Q}_1\boldsymbol{A}_3) \cap \mathcal{C}(\boldsymbol{Q}_1\boldsymbol{A}_2) = \{\boldsymbol{0}\},$$

which is an identical statement to statement (iii) of the theorem (see Appendix B, Theorem B.11 (iv)).

Concerning statement (iv), after some reflection, the following relations for a unique expression of $\boldsymbol{K}\widehat{\boldsymbol{B}}_2\boldsymbol{L}$ are obtained from Theorem 3.2:

$$\begin{aligned}
&\mathcal{C}(\boldsymbol{L}) \subseteq \mathcal{C}(\boldsymbol{C}_2),\\
&\mathcal{C}(\boldsymbol{K}') \subseteq \mathcal{C}(\boldsymbol{A}_2'\boldsymbol{A}_1^o), && (4.41)\\
&\mathcal{C}(\boldsymbol{A}_3'\boldsymbol{P}_{A_1^o}\boldsymbol{A}_2(\boldsymbol{A}_2'\boldsymbol{P}_{A_1^o}\boldsymbol{A}_2)^-\boldsymbol{K}') \subseteq \mathcal{C}(\boldsymbol{A}_3'(\boldsymbol{A}_1 : \boldsymbol{A}_2)^o). && (4.42)
\end{aligned}$$

However, further manipulations show that (4.41) and (4.42) jointly can be replaced by

$$\mathcal{C}(\boldsymbol{K}') \subseteq \mathcal{C}(\boldsymbol{A}_2'(\boldsymbol{A}_1 : \boldsymbol{A}_3)^o).$$

Now, $\widehat{\boldsymbol{B}}_1$ is studied very briefly. For details the reader is referred to Kollo and von Rosen (2005, p. 392). From Theorem 3.2 it follows that, in order to have a unique $\widehat{\boldsymbol{B}}_1$, the rank conditions $r(\boldsymbol{A}) = q_1$ and $r(\boldsymbol{C}_1) = k_1$ have to hold, and

$$(\boldsymbol{A}_1'\boldsymbol{A}_1)^{-1}\boldsymbol{A}_1'(\boldsymbol{A}_2\widehat{\boldsymbol{B}}_2\boldsymbol{C}_2 + \boldsymbol{A}_3\widehat{\boldsymbol{B}}_3\boldsymbol{C}_3)\boldsymbol{C}_1'(\boldsymbol{C}_1\boldsymbol{C}_1')^{-1}$$

must be unique. Note that

$$\mathcal{C}(\boldsymbol{A}_2') \subseteq \mathcal{C}(\boldsymbol{A}_2'\boldsymbol{A}_1^o)$$

has to be true and that $\widehat{\boldsymbol{B}}_2$ is a function of $\widehat{\boldsymbol{B}}_3$ which, after some further calculations, leads to the condition

$$\mathcal{C}(\boldsymbol{A}_3'(\boldsymbol{I} - \boldsymbol{P}_{A_1^o}\boldsymbol{A}_2(\boldsymbol{A}_2'\boldsymbol{P}_{A_1^o}\boldsymbol{A}_2)^-\boldsymbol{A}_2')\boldsymbol{A}_1) \subseteq \mathcal{C}(\boldsymbol{A}_3'(\boldsymbol{A}_1 : \boldsymbol{A}_2)^o).$$

This relation can be shown to be equivalent to

$$\mathcal{C}(\boldsymbol{P}_{A_2^o}\boldsymbol{A}_3) \cap \mathcal{C}(\boldsymbol{P}_{A_2^o}\boldsymbol{A}_1) = \{\boldsymbol{0}\},$$

which is identical to (see Appendix B, Theorem B.11 (iv))

$$\mathcal{C}(\boldsymbol{A}_2)^{\perp} \cap \mathcal{C}(\boldsymbol{A}_1 : \boldsymbol{A}_2) \cap \mathcal{C}(\boldsymbol{A}_3 : \boldsymbol{A}_2) = \{\boldsymbol{0}\}.$$

The proof of statement (vi) is omitted because, in addition to being lengthy, the calculations are very similar to those presented above. Finally, it is noted that (see Corollary 3.3)

$$\widehat{E[\boldsymbol{X}]} = \boldsymbol{P}_{A_1,S_1}\boldsymbol{X}\boldsymbol{P}_{C_1'} + \boldsymbol{P}_{\widehat{Q}_1'A_2,\widehat{S}_2}\boldsymbol{X}\boldsymbol{P}_{C_2'} + \boldsymbol{P}_{\widehat{Q}_2'\widehat{Q}_1'A_3,\widehat{S}_3}\boldsymbol{X}\boldsymbol{P}_{C_3'},$$

and instead of this expression it is sufficient to consider

$$\boldsymbol{P}_{A_1,\Sigma}\boldsymbol{X}\boldsymbol{P}_{C_1'} + \boldsymbol{P}_{Q_1'A_2,\Sigma}\boldsymbol{X}\boldsymbol{P}_{C_2'} + \boldsymbol{P}_{Q_2'Q_1'A_3,\Sigma}\boldsymbol{X}\boldsymbol{P}_{C_3'}.$$

Once again, repeating arguments and calculations for proving the other parts of the theorem, it can be shown that $\widehat{E[X]}$ is uniquely estimated. Moreover, it then follows that $\widehat{\boldsymbol{\Sigma}}$ can also be uniquely estimated. □

A general reflection is that the conditions for uniqueness/estimability for the mean parameters are interpretable and useful, whereas when considering $\boldsymbol{K}\widehat{\boldsymbol{B}}_i\boldsymbol{L}$, it is more difficult to understand the relations.

4.5 Asymptotic Properties of Estimators of Parameters in the $EBRM_B^3$

Similar to Lemma 4.1 the next lemma can be established.

Lemma 4.2 *Let S_1, $\widehat{S}_2$, $\widehat{S}_3$, $\widehat{Q}_1$, $\widehat{Q}_2$, Q_1 and Q_2 be defined through Theorem 3.2 and (3.13)–(3.16). Suppose that for large n, $r(\boldsymbol{C}_1) \leq k_1$, and that both $r(\boldsymbol{C}_1) - r(\boldsymbol{C}_2)$ and $r(\boldsymbol{C}_2) - r(\boldsymbol{C}_3)$ are independent of n. Then, as $n \to \infty$,*

(i) $n^{-1}\boldsymbol{S}_1 \xrightarrow{P} \boldsymbol{\Sigma}, \quad n^{-1}\widehat{\boldsymbol{S}}_2 \xrightarrow{P} \boldsymbol{\Sigma}, \quad n^{-1}\widehat{\boldsymbol{S}}_3 \xrightarrow{P} \boldsymbol{\Sigma},$
(ii) $\widehat{\boldsymbol{Q}}_1 \xrightarrow{P} \boldsymbol{Q}_1, \quad \widehat{\boldsymbol{Q}}_2 \xrightarrow{P} \boldsymbol{Q}_2.$

Proof Since the distribution for $\boldsymbol{S}$ (see Lemma 4.1) used in the BRM and the distribution for $\boldsymbol{S}_1$ are the same, $n^{-1}\boldsymbol{S}_1 \xrightarrow{P} \boldsymbol{\Sigma}$ follows from Lemma 4.1, and this is also true for $\widehat{\boldsymbol{Q}}_1 \xrightarrow{P} \boldsymbol{Q}_1$. Then it is noted that $\widehat{\boldsymbol{Q}}_1'\boldsymbol{A}_1 = \boldsymbol{0}$, and hence

$$\widehat{\boldsymbol{S}}_2 = \boldsymbol{S}_1 + \widehat{\boldsymbol{Q}}_1'(\boldsymbol{X} - \boldsymbol{A}_1\boldsymbol{B}_1\boldsymbol{C}_1)(\boldsymbol{P}_{\boldsymbol{C}_1'} - \boldsymbol{P}_{\boldsymbol{C}_2'})(\boldsymbol{X} - \boldsymbol{A}_1\boldsymbol{B}_1\boldsymbol{C}_1)'\widehat{\boldsymbol{Q}}_1. \quad (4.43)$$

From Appendix B, Theorem B.20 (vi) it follows that

$$(\boldsymbol{X} - \boldsymbol{A}_1\boldsymbol{B}_1\boldsymbol{C}_1)(\boldsymbol{P}_{\boldsymbol{C}_1'} - \boldsymbol{P}_{\boldsymbol{C}_2'})(\boldsymbol{X} - \boldsymbol{A}_1\boldsymbol{B}_1\boldsymbol{C}_1)' \sim W_p(\boldsymbol{\Sigma}, r(\boldsymbol{C}_1) - r(\boldsymbol{C}_2)),$$

because $(\boldsymbol{A}_3\boldsymbol{B}_3\boldsymbol{C}_3 + \boldsymbol{A}_2\boldsymbol{B}_2\boldsymbol{C}_2)(\boldsymbol{P}_{\boldsymbol{C}_1'} - \boldsymbol{P}_{\boldsymbol{C}_2'}) = \boldsymbol{0}$. It is assumed that $r(\boldsymbol{C}_1) - r(\boldsymbol{C}_2)$ is fixed for large n, which indeed implies that for large n the Wishart distribution does not depend on the values of n. Hence,

$$\frac{1}{n}(\boldsymbol{X} - \boldsymbol{A}_1\boldsymbol{B}_1\boldsymbol{C}_1)(\boldsymbol{P}_{\boldsymbol{C}_1'} - \boldsymbol{P}_{\boldsymbol{C}_2'})(\boldsymbol{X} - \boldsymbol{A}_1\boldsymbol{B}_1\boldsymbol{C}_1)' \xrightarrow{P} 0,$$

which is precisely what is needed in the following. Thus, (4.43) yields $n^{-1}(\widehat{\boldsymbol{S}}_2 - \boldsymbol{S}_1) \xrightarrow{P} \boldsymbol{0}$, and then $n^{-1}\widehat{\boldsymbol{S}}_2 \xrightarrow{P} \boldsymbol{\Sigma}$. Moreover, $\widehat{\boldsymbol{Q}}_2 \xrightarrow{P} \boldsymbol{Q}_2$ and then copying the above presentation one may show $n^{-1}\widehat{\boldsymbol{S}}_3 \xrightarrow{P} \boldsymbol{\Sigma}$. □

In Lemma 4.2 the most basic relations for a discussion of asymptotically equivalent expressions for $\boldsymbol{K}\widehat{\boldsymbol{B}}_i\boldsymbol{L}$, $i = 1, 2, 3$, have been presented and the derivation of these equivalent expressions begins now.

Starting with $\boldsymbol{K}\widehat{\boldsymbol{B}}_3\boldsymbol{L}$, it is assumed that $\boldsymbol{K}$ and $\boldsymbol{L}$ have been chosen so that $\boldsymbol{K}\widehat{\boldsymbol{B}}_3\boldsymbol{L}$ is unique. Hence, $\boldsymbol{K}\widehat{\boldsymbol{B}}_3\boldsymbol{L}$ equals (see Theorem 3.2)

$$\boldsymbol{K}\widehat{\boldsymbol{B}}_3\boldsymbol{L} = \boldsymbol{K}(\boldsymbol{A}_3'\widehat{\boldsymbol{Q}}_2\widehat{\boldsymbol{Q}}_1\widehat{\boldsymbol{S}}_3^{-1}\widehat{\boldsymbol{Q}}_1'\widehat{\boldsymbol{Q}}_2'\boldsymbol{A}_3)^-\boldsymbol{A}_3'\widehat{\boldsymbol{Q}}_2\widehat{\boldsymbol{Q}}_1\widehat{\boldsymbol{S}}_3^{-1}\boldsymbol{X}\boldsymbol{C}_3'(\boldsymbol{C}_3\boldsymbol{C}_3')^-\boldsymbol{L}. \quad (4.44)$$

From Theorem 4.9 (ii) it is seen that one of the uniqueness conditions is $\mathcal{C}(\boldsymbol{L}) \subseteq \mathcal{C}(\boldsymbol{C}_3)$. This condition depends on the number of columns, n, in $\boldsymbol{C}_3$. Therefore, as for the BRM (see Sect. 4.2), it will be supposed that

$$\mathcal{C}(\boldsymbol{L}) \subseteq \mathcal{C}(\boldsymbol{C}_{3v}), \quad (4.45)$$

for some v, where v is a fixed number and $\boldsymbol{C}_{3v}$ stands for the first v columns of $\boldsymbol{C}_3$.

Let, correspondingly to $D(\boldsymbol{S}, \boldsymbol{\Sigma})$ for the BRM in Sect. 4.2, i.e. (4.5),

$$\begin{aligned} D(\widehat{\boldsymbol{S}}_3, \boldsymbol{\Sigma}) = \boldsymbol{K}((&\boldsymbol{A}_3'\widehat{\boldsymbol{Q}}_2\widehat{\boldsymbol{Q}}_1\widehat{\boldsymbol{S}}_3^{-1}\widehat{\boldsymbol{Q}}_1'\widehat{\boldsymbol{Q}}_2'\boldsymbol{A}_3)^-\boldsymbol{A}_3'\widehat{\boldsymbol{Q}}_2\widehat{\boldsymbol{Q}}_1\widehat{\boldsymbol{S}}_3^{-1} \\ &-(\boldsymbol{A}_3'\boldsymbol{Q}_2\boldsymbol{Q}_1\boldsymbol{\Sigma}^{-1}\boldsymbol{Q}_1'\boldsymbol{Q}_2'\boldsymbol{A}_3)^-\boldsymbol{A}_3'\boldsymbol{Q}_2\boldsymbol{Q}_1\boldsymbol{\Sigma}^{-1}) \end{aligned} \quad (4.46)$$

and put

$$\boldsymbol{K}\boldsymbol{B}_{3\Sigma}\boldsymbol{L} = \boldsymbol{K}(\boldsymbol{A}_3'\boldsymbol{Q}_2\boldsymbol{Q}_1\boldsymbol{\Sigma}^{-1}\boldsymbol{Q}_1'\boldsymbol{Q}_2'\boldsymbol{A}_3)^-\boldsymbol{A}_3'\boldsymbol{Q}_2\boldsymbol{Q}_1\boldsymbol{\Sigma}^{-1}\boldsymbol{X}\boldsymbol{C}_3'(\boldsymbol{C}_3\boldsymbol{C}_3')^-\boldsymbol{L}, \quad (4.47)$$

which is a linear function in the normally distributed matrix $\boldsymbol{X}$. Note that $D(\widehat{\boldsymbol{S}}_3, \boldsymbol{\Sigma})E[\boldsymbol{X}] = \boldsymbol{0}$, as well as

$$D(\widehat{\boldsymbol{S}}_3, \boldsymbol{\Sigma}) \xrightarrow{P} \boldsymbol{0}, \quad n \to \infty. \quad (4.48)$$

Moreover, for any small $\epsilon > 0$,

$$\begin{aligned} &P(||\boldsymbol{K}(\widehat{\boldsymbol{B}}_3 - \boldsymbol{B}_{3\Sigma})\boldsymbol{L}|| > \epsilon) \\ &\quad = P(||D(\widehat{\boldsymbol{S}}_3, \boldsymbol{\Sigma})(\boldsymbol{X} - E[\boldsymbol{X}])\boldsymbol{C}_3'(\boldsymbol{C}_3\boldsymbol{C}_3')^-\boldsymbol{L}|| > \epsilon); \end{aligned} \quad (4.49)$$

the trace distance $|| \bullet ||$ has already been used in (4.3). Now let $\boldsymbol{M}$ be an arbitrary matrix of a proper size. Then

$$\begin{aligned} &P(||D(\widehat{\boldsymbol{S}}_3, \boldsymbol{\Sigma})(\boldsymbol{X} - E[\boldsymbol{X}])\boldsymbol{C}_3'(\boldsymbol{C}_3\boldsymbol{C}_3')^-\boldsymbol{L}|| > \epsilon) \\ &\quad = P(||D(\widehat{\boldsymbol{S}}_3, \boldsymbol{\Sigma})(\boldsymbol{X} - E[\boldsymbol{X}])\boldsymbol{C}_3'(\boldsymbol{C}_3\boldsymbol{C}_3')^-\boldsymbol{L}|| > \epsilon \\ &\qquad\qquad \boldsymbol{M}\boldsymbol{M}' - (\boldsymbol{X} - E[\boldsymbol{X}])\boldsymbol{C}_3'(\boldsymbol{C}_3\boldsymbol{C}_3')^-\boldsymbol{L}\boldsymbol{L}'(\boldsymbol{C}_3\boldsymbol{C}_3')^-\boldsymbol{C}_3 \text{ is p.d.}) \\ &\qquad\quad +P(||D(\widehat{\boldsymbol{S}}_3, \boldsymbol{\Sigma})(\boldsymbol{X} - E[\boldsymbol{X}])\boldsymbol{C}_3'(\boldsymbol{C}_3\boldsymbol{C}_3')^-\boldsymbol{L}|| > \epsilon, \end{aligned}$$

$$
\begin{aligned}
&MM' - (X - E[X])C_3'(C_3C_3')^- LL'(C_3C_3')^- C_3(X - E[X])' \text{ is not p.d.})\\
&\leq P(||D(\widehat{S}_3, \Sigma)M|| > \epsilon,)\\
&\quad +P(\alpha'(X - E[X])C_3'(C_3C_3')^- LL'(C_3C_3')^- C_3(X - E[X])'\alpha \geq \alpha'MM'\alpha),
\end{aligned}
\tag{4.50}
$$

for some specific p-dimensional vector $\boldsymbol{\alpha}$. The first expression in (4.50), based on (4.48), converges to 0, and due to Markov's inequality (see Appendix B, Theorem B.9 (i)) and by choosing M appropriately, the second expression can be made arbitrarily small:

$$
\begin{aligned}
&P(\alpha'(X - E[X])C_3'(C_3C_3')^- LL'(C_3C_3')^- C_3(X - E[X])'\alpha \geq \alpha'MM'\alpha)\\
&\leq \frac{\mathrm{tr}\{L'(C_3C_3')^- L\}}{\alpha'MM'\alpha} \leq \frac{\mathrm{tr}\{L'(C_{3v}C_{3v}')^- L\}}{\alpha'MM'\alpha}.
\end{aligned}
\tag{4.51}
$$

Thus,

$$
K(\widehat{B}_3 - B_{3\Sigma})L \xrightarrow{P} \mathbf{0}. \tag{4.52}
$$

It is worth noting that

$$
KB_{3\Sigma}L \sim N_{r,s}(KB_3L, A_3'Q_1Q_2\Sigma^{-1}Q_2'Q_1'A_3, L'(C_3C_3')^- L), \tag{4.53}
$$

if K has r rows and L has s columns. Thus, for $K\widehat{B}_3L$ there exists an asymptotically equivalent expression which is normally distributed. If Σ had been known, the distribution in (4.53) would have been the natural one to use.

In order to discuss $\widehat{B}_2$ and $\widehat{B}_1$, one needs to reformulate (4.52) somewhat. Let K^n be a sequence of matrices such that for a given n, $\mathcal{C}(K^{n'}) \subseteq \mathcal{C}(A_3'\widehat{Q}_1\widehat{Q}_2)$ and $K^n \xrightarrow{P} K$, for some K. Then

$$
K^n\widehat{B}_3L - KB_{3\Sigma}L \xrightarrow{P} \mathbf{0}. \tag{4.54}
$$

In the following there are also some expressions where L in $K\widehat{B}_3L$ depends on n, i.e. $C_3C_i'(C_iC_i')^- L$, $i = 1, 2$ (here L is different from the above one and does not depend on n), and in particular the following results will be utilized:

$$
\begin{aligned}
&K^n\widehat{B}_3C_3C_2'(C_2C_2')^- L - KB_{3\Sigma}C_3C_2'(C_2C_2')^- L \xrightarrow{P} \mathbf{0},\\
&\mathcal{C}(L) \subseteq \mathcal{C}(C_2), \quad n \to \infty,
\end{aligned}
\tag{4.55}
$$

$$
\begin{aligned}
&K^n\widehat{B}_3C_3C_1'(C_1C_1')^- L - KB_{3\Sigma}C_3C_1'(C_1C_1')^- L \xrightarrow{P} \mathbf{0},\\
&\mathcal{C}(L) \subseteq \mathcal{C}(C_1), \quad n \to \infty.
\end{aligned}
\tag{4.56}
$$

Proceeding by showing $K\widehat{B}_2L$ to be unique, it follows from Theorem 3.2 that

$$K(A_2'\widehat{Q}_1\widehat{S}_2^{-1}\widehat{Q}_1'A_2)^-A_2'\widehat{Q}_1\widehat{S}_2^{-1}\widehat{Q}_1'(X - A_3B_3C_3)C_2'(C_2C_2')^-L \quad (4.57)$$

and

$$K(A_2'\widehat{Q}_1\widehat{S}_2^{-1}\widehat{Q}_1'A_2)^-A_2'\widehat{Q}_1\widehat{S}_2^{-1}\widehat{Q}_1'A_3(\widehat{B}_3 - B_3)C_3C_2'(C_2C_2')^-L \quad (4.58)$$

have to be considered. Analogously to $\mathcal{C}(L) \subseteq \mathcal{C}(C_{3v})$ in the previous case, i.e. (4.45), it is now assumed that $\mathcal{C}(L) \subseteq \mathcal{C}(C_{2v})$ for a matrix C_{2v} which consists of the first v columns of C_2. Put

$$G^n = K(A_2'\widehat{Q}_1'\widehat{S}_2^{-1}\widehat{Q}_1A_2)^-A_2'\widehat{Q}_1'\widehat{S}_2^{-1}$$

and

$$G = K(A_2'Q_1'\Sigma^{-1}Q_1A_2)^-A_2'Q_1'\Sigma^{-1}. \quad (4.59)$$

From Lemma 4.2 it follows that $G^n \xrightarrow{P} G$, $n \to \infty$. Furthermore, $\mathcal{C}(A_3'(G^n)') \subseteq \mathcal{C}(A_3'\widehat{Q}_1\widehat{Q}_2)$. Hence, utilizing (4.53) results in (4.58) converging to $\mathbf{0}$.

Turning to the proof of (4.57), the proof of (4.52) shows that it is sufficient that the next probability can be made arbitrarily small:

$$P(\alpha'(X - E[X])C_2'(C_2C_2')^-LL'(C_2C_2')^-C_2(X - E[X])'\alpha \geq \alpha'MM'\alpha), \quad (4.60)$$

where α is some p-dimensional vector and M is an arbitrary matrix of size $p \times p$. However, choosing M appropriately, via Markov's inequality (see Appendix B, Theorem B.9 (i)), (4.60) can be made arbitrarily small. Therefore,

$$K(A_2'\widehat{Q}_1\widehat{S}_2^{-1}\widehat{Q}_1'A_2)^-A_2'\widehat{Q}_1\widehat{S}_2^{-1}\widehat{Q}_1'XC_2'(C_2C_2)^-L - GXC_2'(C_2C_2)^-L \xrightarrow{P} \mathbf{0},$$
$$n \to \infty, \quad (4.61)$$

where G is given by (4.59). From (4.54) and (4.61), and setting

$$KB_{2\Sigma}L = K(A_2'Q_1\Sigma^{-1}Q_1'A_2)^-A_2'Q_1\Sigma^{-1}Q_1'(X - A_3B_{3\Sigma}C_3)C_2'(C_2C_2)^-L, \quad (4.62)$$

lead to the asymptotic result,

$$K\widehat{B}_2L - KB_{2\Sigma}L \xrightarrow{P} \mathbf{0}, \qquad n \to \infty. \quad (4.63)$$

Moreover, if $\boldsymbol{K}$ has r rows and $\boldsymbol{L}$ has s columns,

$$\boldsymbol{K}\boldsymbol{B}_{2\Sigma}\boldsymbol{L} \sim N_{r,s}(\boldsymbol{K}\boldsymbol{B}_2\boldsymbol{L}, \boldsymbol{K}(\boldsymbol{A}_2'\boldsymbol{Q}_1\boldsymbol{\Sigma}^{-1}\boldsymbol{Q}_1'\boldsymbol{A}_2)^-\boldsymbol{K}', \boldsymbol{L}'(\boldsymbol{C}_2\boldsymbol{C}_2')^-\boldsymbol{L}). \quad (4.64)$$

Next $\boldsymbol{K}\widehat{\boldsymbol{B}}_1\boldsymbol{L}$ is discussed under the condition that it is unique. From Theorem 3.2 it follows that asymptotic expressions for

$$\boldsymbol{K}(\boldsymbol{A}_1'\boldsymbol{S}_1^{-1}\boldsymbol{A}_1)^-\boldsymbol{A}_1'\boldsymbol{S}_1^{-1}\boldsymbol{X}\boldsymbol{C}_1'(\boldsymbol{C}_1\boldsymbol{C}_1')^-\boldsymbol{L}, \quad (4.65)$$

$$\boldsymbol{K}(\boldsymbol{A}_1'\boldsymbol{S}_1^{-1}\boldsymbol{A}_1)^-\boldsymbol{A}_1'\boldsymbol{S}_1^{-1}\boldsymbol{P}_{A_2,S_2,Q_1}\boldsymbol{X}\boldsymbol{P}_{C_2'}\boldsymbol{C}_1'(\boldsymbol{C}_1\boldsymbol{C}_1')^-\boldsymbol{L}, \quad (4.66)$$

$$\boldsymbol{K}(\boldsymbol{A}_1'\boldsymbol{S}_1^{-1}\boldsymbol{A}_1)^-\boldsymbol{A}_1'\boldsymbol{S}_1^{-1}(\boldsymbol{I} - \boldsymbol{P}_{A_2,S_2,Q_1})\boldsymbol{A}_3\widehat{\boldsymbol{B}}_3\boldsymbol{C}_3\boldsymbol{C}_1'(\boldsymbol{C}_1\boldsymbol{C}_1')^-\boldsymbol{L} \quad (4.67)$$

have to be derived. Moreover, for the same reasons as before, $\mathcal{C}(\boldsymbol{L}) = \mathcal{C}(\boldsymbol{C}_{1v})$ is supposed to hold, where v is a fixed number and $\boldsymbol{C}_{1v}$ consists of the first v columns in $\boldsymbol{C}_1$. Copying some of the previous proofs yields that for (4.65)

$$\boldsymbol{K}(\boldsymbol{A}_1'\boldsymbol{S}_1^{-1}\boldsymbol{A}_1)^-\boldsymbol{A}_1'\boldsymbol{S}_1^{-1}\boldsymbol{X}\boldsymbol{C}_1'(\boldsymbol{C}_1\boldsymbol{C}_1')^-\boldsymbol{L} - \boldsymbol{K}(\boldsymbol{A}_1'\boldsymbol{\Sigma}^{-1}\boldsymbol{A}_1)^-\boldsymbol{A}_1'\boldsymbol{\Sigma}^{-1}\boldsymbol{X}\boldsymbol{C}_1'(\boldsymbol{C}_1\boldsymbol{C}_1')^-\boldsymbol{L} \xrightarrow{P} \boldsymbol{0}, \quad n \to \infty, \quad (4.68)$$

and for (4.66)

$$\begin{aligned}&\boldsymbol{K}(\boldsymbol{A}_1'\boldsymbol{S}_1^{-1}\boldsymbol{A}_1)^-\boldsymbol{A}_1'\boldsymbol{S}_1^{-1}\boldsymbol{P}_{A_2,S_2,Q_1}\boldsymbol{X}\boldsymbol{P}_{C_2'}\boldsymbol{C}_1'(\boldsymbol{C}\boldsymbol{C}_1')^-\boldsymbol{L}\\ &\quad -\boldsymbol{K}(\boldsymbol{A}_1'\boldsymbol{\Sigma}^{-1}\boldsymbol{A}_1)^-\boldsymbol{A}_1'\boldsymbol{\Sigma}^{-1}\boldsymbol{P}_{A_2,S_2,Q_1}\boldsymbol{X}\boldsymbol{P}_{C_2'}\boldsymbol{C}_1'(\boldsymbol{C}\boldsymbol{C}_1')^-\boldsymbol{L} \xrightarrow{P} \boldsymbol{0}, \quad n \to \infty, \quad (4.69)\end{aligned}$$

and (4.67) converges to

$$\boldsymbol{K}(\boldsymbol{A}_1'\boldsymbol{\Sigma}^{-1}\boldsymbol{A}_1)^-\boldsymbol{A}_1'\boldsymbol{\Sigma}^{-1}(\boldsymbol{I} - \boldsymbol{P}_{A_2,\Sigma,Q_1})\boldsymbol{A}_3\boldsymbol{B}_{3\Sigma}\boldsymbol{C}_3\boldsymbol{C}_1'(\boldsymbol{C}_1\boldsymbol{C}_1')^-\boldsymbol{L}. \quad (4.70)$$

Set

$$\begin{aligned}\boldsymbol{K}\boldsymbol{B}_{1\Sigma}\boldsymbol{L} &= \boldsymbol{K}(\boldsymbol{A}_1'\boldsymbol{\Sigma}^{-1}\boldsymbol{A}_1)^-\boldsymbol{A}_1'\boldsymbol{\Sigma}^{-1}(\boldsymbol{X} - \boldsymbol{A}_2\boldsymbol{B}_{2\Sigma}\boldsymbol{C}_2 - \boldsymbol{A}_3\boldsymbol{B}_{3\Sigma}\boldsymbol{C}_3)\\ &\quad \times \boldsymbol{C}_1'(\boldsymbol{C}_1\boldsymbol{C}_1')^-\boldsymbol{L}, \quad (4.71)\end{aligned}$$

where the linear combinations of $\boldsymbol{B}_{3\Sigma}$ and $\boldsymbol{B}_{2\Sigma}$ are obtained from (4.47) and (4.62), respectively. Thus, using (4.65)–(4.71) it has been shown that

$$\boldsymbol{K}\widehat{\boldsymbol{B}}_1\boldsymbol{L} - \boldsymbol{K}\boldsymbol{B}_{1\Sigma}\boldsymbol{L} \xrightarrow{P} \boldsymbol{0}, \quad n \to \infty. \quad (4.72)$$

If $\boldsymbol{K}$ has r rows and $\boldsymbol{L}$ has s columns,

$$\boldsymbol{K}\boldsymbol{B}_{1\Sigma}\boldsymbol{L} \sim N_{r,s}(\boldsymbol{K}\boldsymbol{B}_1\boldsymbol{L}, \boldsymbol{K}(\boldsymbol{A}_1'\boldsymbol{\Sigma}^{-1}\boldsymbol{A}_1)^-\boldsymbol{K}', \boldsymbol{L}'(\boldsymbol{C}_1\boldsymbol{C}_1')^-\boldsymbol{L}).$$

Hence, the following theorem has been established, where the last two statements concerning $\widehat{\boldsymbol{\Sigma}}$ follow immediately from Lemma 4.2.

Theorem 4.10 *Let $\widehat{\boldsymbol{B}}_i$ be the maximum likelihood estimators of $\boldsymbol{B}_i$, i=1,2,3, in the $EBRM_B^3$, given in Theorem 3.2.*

(i) *If $\boldsymbol{K}\widehat{\boldsymbol{B}}_3\boldsymbol{L}$ for the specific known matrices $\boldsymbol{K}$ and $\boldsymbol{L}$ is unique for some n, and if additionally there exists a number, v, such that $\mathcal{C}(\boldsymbol{L}) \subseteq \mathcal{C}(\boldsymbol{C}_{3v})$, where $\boldsymbol{C}_{3v}$ is a matrix whose columns are identical to the first v columns in $\boldsymbol{C}_3$, then $\boldsymbol{K}\widehat{\boldsymbol{B}}_3\boldsymbol{L} - \boldsymbol{K}\boldsymbol{B}_{3\Sigma}\boldsymbol{L} \xrightarrow{P} \boldsymbol{0}$, $n \to \infty$, where $\boldsymbol{K}\boldsymbol{B}_{3\Sigma}\boldsymbol{L}$ is given by (4.47).*

(ii) *If $\boldsymbol{K}\widehat{\boldsymbol{B}}_2\boldsymbol{L}$ for the specific known matrices $\boldsymbol{K}$ and $\boldsymbol{L}$ is unique for some n, and if additionally there exists a number, v, such that $\mathcal{C}(\boldsymbol{L}) \subseteq \mathcal{C}(\boldsymbol{C}_{2v})$, where $\boldsymbol{C}_{2v}$ is a matrix whose columns are identical to the first v columns in $\boldsymbol{C}_2$, then $\boldsymbol{K}\widehat{\boldsymbol{B}}_2\boldsymbol{L} - \boldsymbol{K}\boldsymbol{B}_{2\Sigma}\boldsymbol{L} \xrightarrow{P} \boldsymbol{0}$, $n \to \infty$, where $\boldsymbol{K}\boldsymbol{B}_{2\Sigma}\boldsymbol{L}$ is given by (4.62).*

(iii) *If $\boldsymbol{K}\widehat{\boldsymbol{B}}_1\boldsymbol{L}$ for the specific known matrices $\boldsymbol{K}$ and $\boldsymbol{L}$ is unique for some n, and if additionally there exists a number, v, such that $\mathcal{C}(\boldsymbol{L}) \subseteq \mathcal{C}(\boldsymbol{C}_{1v})$, where $\boldsymbol{C}_{1v}$ is a matrix whose columns are identical to the first v columns in $\boldsymbol{C}_1$, then $\boldsymbol{K}\widehat{\boldsymbol{B}}_1\boldsymbol{L} - \boldsymbol{K}\boldsymbol{B}_{1\Sigma}\boldsymbol{L} \xrightarrow{P} \boldsymbol{0}$, $n \to \infty$, where $\boldsymbol{K}\boldsymbol{B}_{1\Sigma}\boldsymbol{L}$ is given by (4.71).*

(iv) *Let $\boldsymbol{X}_v$, $\boldsymbol{C}_{1v}$, $\boldsymbol{C}_{2v}$ and $\boldsymbol{C}_{3v}$ denote the first v columns in $\boldsymbol{X}$, $\boldsymbol{C}_1$, $\boldsymbol{C}_2$ and $\boldsymbol{C}_3$, respectively. Then for $\widehat{E[\boldsymbol{X}_v]} = \sum_{i=1}^{3} \boldsymbol{A}_1\widehat{\boldsymbol{B}}_i\boldsymbol{C}_{iv}$*

$$\widehat{E[\boldsymbol{X}_v]} - (\boldsymbol{A}_1\boldsymbol{B}_{1\Sigma}\boldsymbol{C}_{1v} + \boldsymbol{A}_2\boldsymbol{B}_{2\Sigma}\boldsymbol{C}_{2v} + \boldsymbol{A}_3\boldsymbol{B}_{3\Sigma}\boldsymbol{C}_{3v}) \xrightarrow{P} \boldsymbol{0}, \quad n \to \infty,$$

where $\boldsymbol{A}_1\boldsymbol{B}_{1\Sigma}\boldsymbol{C}_{1v}$ follows from statement (iii) by choosing $\boldsymbol{K} = \boldsymbol{A}_1$ and $\boldsymbol{L} = \boldsymbol{C}_{1v}$, $\boldsymbol{A}_2\boldsymbol{B}_{2\Sigma}\boldsymbol{C}_{2v}$ follows from statement (ii) by choosing $\boldsymbol{K} = \boldsymbol{A}_2$ and $\boldsymbol{L} = \boldsymbol{C}_{2v}$, and $\boldsymbol{A}_1\boldsymbol{B}_{3\Sigma}\boldsymbol{C}_{3v}$ follows from statement (i) by choosing $\boldsymbol{K} = \boldsymbol{A}_3$ and $\boldsymbol{L} = \boldsymbol{C}_{3v}$.

(v) *Let $\boldsymbol{S}_3$, $\boldsymbol{Q}_1$, $\boldsymbol{Q}_2$ and $\boldsymbol{Q}_3$ be defined in (3.13)–(3.16). Then*

$$\widehat{\boldsymbol{\Sigma}} - \frac{1}{n}(\boldsymbol{S}_3 + \boldsymbol{Q}_3\boldsymbol{Q}_2\boldsymbol{Q}_1\boldsymbol{X}\boldsymbol{P}_{\boldsymbol{C}_3'}\boldsymbol{X}'\boldsymbol{Q}_1'\boldsymbol{Q}_2'\boldsymbol{Q}_3') \xrightarrow{P} \boldsymbol{0}, \qquad n \to \infty.$$

(vi) $\widehat{\boldsymbol{\Sigma}} \xrightarrow{P} \boldsymbol{\Sigma}, \qquad n \to \infty.$

4.6 Moments of Estimators of Parameters in the $EBRM_B^3$

For the BRM, the distributions of the maximum likelihood estimators are difficult to find. In Theorem 3.2, the estimators for the $EBRM_B^3$ were given and one can see that the expressions are stochastically much more complicated than the estimators for the BRM. To understand the estimators, moments are useful quantities. For example, approximations of the distributions of the estimators have to take place, and in this book these approximations are based on moments. Before studying

$K\widehat{B}_iL$, $i = 1, 2, 3$, the estimated mean structure $\widehat{E[X]} = \sum_{i=1}^{3} A_i\widehat{B}_iC_i$ and $\widehat{\Sigma}$ are treated. Thereafter, $D[K\widehat{B}_iL]$, $i = 1, 2, 3$, is calculated. The ideas for calculating $D[K\widehat{B}_iL]$ are very similar to the ones presented for obtaining $D[\widehat{E[X]}]$ and $E[\widehat{\Sigma}]$. Some advice is appropriate here. The technical treatment in this section is complicated, although not very difficult. Readers less interested in details are recommended merely to study the results in the given theorems. Moreover, the presentation in different places is not complete due to computational lengthiness. Table 4.1 includes definitions which are used throughout the section.

First it will be shown that in the $EBRM_B^3$, under the uniqueness conditions presented in Theorem 4.9, the maximum likelihood estimators of KB_iL will be unbiased and then it follows that $\widehat{E[X]} = \sum_{i=1}^{m} A_i\widehat{B}_iC_i$ is also unbiased. In Theorem 3.2 the maximum likelihood estimators $\widehat{B}_i$, $i = 1, 2, 3$, were presented. Since $\mathcal{C}(C_3') \subseteq \mathcal{C}(C_2') \subseteq \mathcal{C}(C_1')$, the following facts, which are obtained from Appendix B, Theorem B.19 (ix) and (xi), will be utilized.

Table 4.1 Special definitions used in Sect. 4.6

Notation	Definition	Reference
$A_{1:r}$	$A_{1:r} = (A_1 : A_2 : \cdots : A_r)$	(4.93)
m_r	$m_r = p - r(A_{1:r}) + r(A_{1:r-1})$	(4.78)
c_r	$c_{r-1} = \frac{n-r(C_r)-m_{r-1}-1}{n-r(C_{r-1})-m_{r-1}-1}$	(4.86)
e_r	$e_r = \frac{(p-m_r)(n-r(C_r)-1)}{(n-r(C_r)-m_{r-1}-1)(n-r(C_r)-m_{r-1}+p-m_r-1)}$	(4.91)
f_r	$f_r = \frac{n-r(C_r)-1}{n-r(C_r)-m_r-1}$	(4.92)
$g_{i,j}$	$g_{i,j} = c_ic_{i+1} \times \cdots \times c_{j-1}m_j/(n - r(C_j) - m_j - 1), \quad i < j$ $g_{j,j} = m_j/(n - r(C_j) - m_j - 1)$	(4.118)
G_r	$G_{r+1} = G_r(G_r'A_{r+1})^o, \quad G_0 = I$	(4.73)
W_r	$W_r = X(I - P_{C_r})X'$	(4.74)
Γ_r	$\Gamma_r = (\Gamma_r^{u'} : \Gamma_r^{l'})' \quad \Gamma_r : m_{r-1} \times m_{r-1}, \quad \Gamma_r\Gamma_r' = \Gamma_r'\Gamma_r = I$ $\Gamma_r^u : m_r \times m_{r-1}, \quad \Gamma_0 = I$	(4.75)
V^r	$V^r = \Gamma_r\Gamma_{r-1}^u \times \cdots \times \Gamma_1^u\Sigma^{-1/2}W_r\Sigma^{-1/2}\Gamma_1^{u'}$ $\times \cdots \times \Gamma_1^{u'} \sim W_{m_{r-1}}(I, n - r(C_r))$ $V^1 = \Gamma_1^u\Sigma^{-1/2}W_1\Sigma^{-1/2}\Gamma_1^{u'}$	(4.80)
U^r	$U^r = \Gamma_{r-1}\Gamma_{r-2}^u \times \cdots \times \Gamma_1^u\Sigma^{-1/2}W_r\Sigma^{-1/2}\Gamma_1^{u'}$ $\times \cdots \times \Gamma_{r-2}^{u'}\Gamma_{r-1}' \sim W_{m_{r-2}}(I, n - r(C_r))$ $U^1 = \Sigma^{-1/2}W_1\Sigma^{-1/2}, \quad U^2 = \Gamma_1^u\Sigma^{-1/2}W_2\Sigma^{-1/2}\Gamma_1^{u'}$	(4.81)
M_r	$M_r' = (I : (V_{11}^r)^{-1}V_{12}^r)$	(4.83)
E_r	$E_r = \Gamma_{r-1}^u\Gamma_{r-2}^u \times \cdots \times \Gamma_1^u\Sigma^{-1/2}A_r$	(4.84)
$Z_{r,s}$	$Z_{r,s} = \Gamma_{r-1}^u\Gamma_{r-2}^u \times \cdots \times \Gamma_1^u\Sigma^{-1/2}P'_{G_r,W_r^{-1}}P'_{G_{r+1},W_{r+1}^{-1}}$ $\times \cdots \times P'_{G_s,W_s^{-1}}, \quad 2 \leq r \leq s$ $Z_{1,s} = P'_{G_1,W_1^{-1}}P'_{G_2,W_2^{-1}} \times \cdots \times P'_{G_s,W_s^{-1}}, \quad s \geq 1$ $Z_{r,s} = I, \quad r > s$	(4.107) (4.108)

In this book mostly $r \leq 3$

Facts

(i) S_1 is independent of XC_1', XC_2' and XC_3'.
(ii) $\widehat{Q}_1\widehat{S}_2^{-1}$ is independent of XC_2' and XC_3'.
(iii) $\widehat{Q}_2\widehat{Q}_1\widehat{S}_3^{-1}$ is independent of XC_3'.

These facts will be used throughout this section. Instead of Facts (ii) and (iii), it could be stated that $\widehat{S}_2^{-1}$ is independent of XC_2' and XC_3', and $\widehat{S}_3^{-1}$ is independent of XC_3'. Moreover, it is interesting to note that here there are two nested structures of information which are so linked that explicit moment calculations can take place. On the one hand there is a structure connected to the mean, i.e. $(\{XC_1', XC_2', XC_3'\}, \{XC_2', XC_3'\}, \{XC_3'\})$, and on the other hand there is the residual structure $(\{S_1\}, \{\widehat{Q}_1\widehat{S}_2^{-1}\}, \{\widehat{Q}_2\widehat{Q}_1\widehat{S}_3^{-1}\})$. In the following the notations related to projectors and quadratic forms, presented in Appendix A, Sect. A.7, will frequently be used.

Now, using the expressions presented in Theorem 3.2

$$E[K\widehat{B}_3L] = E[K(A_3'\widehat{Q}_2\widehat{Q}_1\widehat{S}_3^{-1}\widehat{Q}_1'\widehat{Q}_2'A_3)^- A_3'\widehat{Q}_2\widehat{Q}_1\widehat{S}_3^{-1}\widehat{Q}_1'\widehat{Q}_2'] \times E[XC_3'(C_3C_3')^- L]$$

(because XC_3' is independent of $\widehat{S}_3$ and $\widehat{Q}_2\widehat{Q}_1\widehat{S}_3^{-1}$)

$$= E[K(A_3'\widehat{Q}_2\widehat{Q}_1\widehat{S}_3^{-1}\widehat{Q}_1'\widehat{Q}_2'A_3)^- A_3'\widehat{Q}_2\widehat{Q}_1\widehat{S}_3^{-1}\widehat{Q}_1'\widehat{Q}_2']A_3B_3L = KB_3L,$$

$$E[K\widehat{B}_2L] = E[K(A_2'\widehat{Q}_1\widehat{S}_2^{-1}\widehat{Q}_1'A_2)^- A_2'\widehat{Q}_1\widehat{S}_2^{-1}\widehat{Q}_1' (E[X] - A_3\widehat{B}_3C_3)C_2'(C_2C_2')^- L]$$

$$= KB_2L - E[K(A_2'\widehat{Q}_1\widehat{S}_2^{-1}\widehat{Q}_1'A_2)^- A_2'\widehat{Q}_1\widehat{S}_2^{-1} \times \widehat{Q}_1'A_3(\widehat{B}_3 - B_3)C_3C_2'(C_2C_2')^- L]$$

(because XC_3' is independent of $\widehat{Q}_1\widehat{S}_2^{-1}$ and $E[A_3(\widehat{B}_3 - B_3)C_3] = \mathbf{0}$)

$$= KB_2L,$$

$$E[K\widehat{B}_1L] = E[K(A_1'S_1^{-1}A_1)^- A_1'S_1^{-1}(E[X] - A_2\widehat{B}_2C_2 - A_3\widehat{B}_3C_3)C_1'(C_1C_1')^- L]$$

$$= KB_1L$$

$$-E[K(A_1'S_1^{-1}A_1)^- A_1S_1^{-1}(A_2(\widehat{B}_2 - B_2)C_2 + A_3(\widehat{B}_3 - B_3)C_3)C_1'(C_1C_1')^- L]$$

(because XC_3' and XC_2' are independent of S_1 and $E[A_i(\widehat{B}_i - B_i)C_i] = \mathbf{0}$, $i = 1, 2$)

$$= KB_1L.$$

Hence, these calculations have established the following theorem.

Theorem 4.11 *Consider the $EBRM_B^3$ presented in Definition 2.2. Under the uniqueness conditions given in Theorem 4.9, $K\widehat{B}_iL$ is an unbiased estimator of KB_iL, $i = 1, 2, 3$, where $\widehat{B}_i$ is given in Theorem 3.2.*

In the same way as the unbiasedness of $K\widehat{B}_iL$ was verified it can be shown that the sum of profiles $\sum_{i=1}^3 A_i\widehat{B}_iC_i$ is unbiased. The difference is that now we do not have to rely on uniqueness conditions, because $\sum_{i=1}^3 A_i\widehat{B}_iC_i$ is always unique.

Corollary 4.3 *Consider the $EBRM_B^3$ presented in Definition 2.2. The expression $\sum_{i=1}^3 A_i\widehat{B}_iC_i$ is an unbiased estimator of $E[X] = \sum_{i=1}^3 A_iB_iC_i$, where $\widehat{B}_i$, $i = 1, 2, 3$, is given in Theorem 3.2.*

In several of the forthcoming proofs it is indicated how one can handle a model with a mean $E[X] = \sum_{i=1}^m A_iB_iC_i$, $m > 3$, but the comments and explanations concern the model when $m = 3$, since it is only in this case explicit estimators have been presented. The dispersion of $\widehat{E[X]} = \sum_{i=1}^3 A_i\widehat{B}_iC_i$ is studied in some detail, since all the essential steps for carrying out general moment calculations are used. However, before calculations start, in order to shorten the presentation, a number of definitions are provided (see also Table 4.1). Let

$$G_{r+1} = G_r(G_r'A_{r+1})^o, \quad G_0 = I, \tag{4.73}$$

$$W_r = X(I - P_{C_r})X'. \tag{4.74}$$

In particular,

$$\begin{aligned}
&G_1 = A_1^o,\\
&G_2 = G_1(G_1'A_2)^o, \quad \mathcal{C}(G_2) = \mathcal{C}(A_1^o) \cap \mathcal{C}(A_2^o) = \mathcal{C}(A_1 : A_2)^\perp,\\
&G_3 = G_2(G_2'A_3)^o, \quad \mathcal{C}(G_3) = \mathcal{C}(G_2) \cap \mathcal{C}(A_3^o) = \mathcal{C}(A_1 : A_2 : A_3)^\perp.
\end{aligned}$$

For convenience, G_i is supposed to be of full column rank. Moreover, let the non-singular matrix H_r: $m_r \times m_r$, $H_0 = I$, and the orthogonal matrix

$$\Gamma_r = (\Gamma_r^{u'} : \Gamma_r^{l'})', \quad \Gamma_r : m_{r-1} \times m_{r-1}, \quad \Gamma_r^u : m_r \times m_{r-1}, \tag{4.75}$$

be defined through a factorization of $(G_{i-1}'A_i)^o$, i.e.

$$G_1' = A_1^{o'} = H_1(I_{p-r(A)} : 0)\Gamma_1\Sigma^{-1/2} = H_1\Gamma_1^u\Sigma^{-1/2}, \tag{4.76}$$

$$(G_{r-1}'A_r)^{o'}H_{r-1} = H_r(I_{m_r} : 0)\Gamma_r = H_r\Gamma_r^u, \qquad r = 2, 3, \ldots, \tag{4.77}$$

where m_r is a decreasing sequence in r given by

$$m_r = p - r(A_1 : A_2 : \cdots : A_r) + r(A_1 : A_2 : \cdots : A_{r-1}), \quad m_0 = p, \quad m_1 = p - r(A_1). \tag{4.78}$$

Since by definition $\boldsymbol{G}_r = \boldsymbol{G}_{r-1}(\boldsymbol{G}'_{r-1}\boldsymbol{A}_r)^o$, it follows that

$$\boldsymbol{G}'_r = \boldsymbol{H}_r \boldsymbol{\Gamma}^u_r \boldsymbol{\Gamma}^u_{r-1} \times \cdots \times \boldsymbol{\Gamma}^u_1 \boldsymbol{\Sigma}^{-1/2}, \tag{4.79}$$

which is a relation to be used frequently in the following. Moreover, note that the size of $\boldsymbol{G}_r$ is $p \times m_r$. Furthermore, define

$$\begin{aligned}
\boldsymbol{V}^r &= \boldsymbol{\Gamma}_r \boldsymbol{\Gamma}^u_{r-1} \times \cdots \times \boldsymbol{\Gamma}^u_1 \boldsymbol{\Sigma}^{-1/2} \boldsymbol{W}_r \boldsymbol{\Sigma}^{-1/2} \boldsymbol{\Gamma}^{u'}_1 \\
&\quad \times \cdots \times \boldsymbol{\Gamma}^{u'}_{r-1} \boldsymbol{\Gamma}'_r \sim W_{m_{r-1}}(\boldsymbol{I}, n - r(\boldsymbol{C}_r)), \quad r = 2, 3, \ldots, \qquad (4.80)\\
\boldsymbol{V}^1 &= \boldsymbol{\Gamma}^u_1 \boldsymbol{\Sigma}^{-1/2} \boldsymbol{W}_1 \boldsymbol{\Sigma}^{-1/2} \boldsymbol{\Gamma}^{u'}_1 \sim W_{m_1}(\boldsymbol{I}, n - r(\boldsymbol{C}_1)),\\
\boldsymbol{U}^r &= \boldsymbol{\Gamma}_{r-1} \boldsymbol{\Gamma}^u_{r-2} \times \cdots \times \boldsymbol{\Gamma}^u_1 \boldsymbol{\Sigma}^{-1/2} \boldsymbol{W}_r \boldsymbol{\Sigma}^{-1/2} \boldsymbol{\Gamma}^{u'}_1 \\
&\quad \times \cdots \times \boldsymbol{\Gamma}^{u'}_{r-2} \boldsymbol{\Gamma}'_{r-1} \sim W_{m_{r-2}}(\boldsymbol{I}, n - r(\boldsymbol{C}_r)), \quad r = 3, 4, \ldots, \qquad (4.81)\\
\boldsymbol{U}^1 &= \boldsymbol{\Sigma}^{-1/2} \boldsymbol{W}_1 \boldsymbol{\Sigma}^{-1/2} \sim W_p(\boldsymbol{I}, n - r(\boldsymbol{C}_1)),\\
\boldsymbol{U}^2 &= \boldsymbol{\Gamma}^u_1 \boldsymbol{\Sigma}^{-1/2} \boldsymbol{W}_2 \boldsymbol{\Sigma}^{-1/2} \boldsymbol{\Gamma}^{u'}_1 \sim W_{m_1}(\boldsymbol{I}, n - r(\boldsymbol{C}_2)),
\end{aligned}$$

and

$$\boldsymbol{V}^r_{11} = (\boldsymbol{I}_{m_r} : \boldsymbol{0}) \boldsymbol{V}^r (\boldsymbol{I}_{m_r} : \boldsymbol{0})', \qquad \boldsymbol{U}^r_{11} = (\boldsymbol{I}_{m_{r-1}} : \boldsymbol{0}) \boldsymbol{U}^r (\boldsymbol{I}_{m_{r-1}} : \boldsymbol{0})'. \tag{4.82}$$

In particular, many of the forthcoming moment relations will be based on calculations involving $\boldsymbol{V}^r_{11}$ and $\boldsymbol{U}^r_{11}$, given in (4.82). Connected to these matrices are

$$\boldsymbol{M}'_r = \left(\boldsymbol{I} : (\boldsymbol{V}^r_{11})^{-1} \boldsymbol{V}^r_{12}\right), \tag{4.83}$$

$$\boldsymbol{E}_r = \boldsymbol{\Gamma}^u_{r-1} \boldsymbol{\Gamma}^u_{r-2} \times \cdots \times \boldsymbol{\Gamma}^u_1 \boldsymbol{\Sigma}^{-1/2} \boldsymbol{A}_r, \tag{4.84}$$

where specially it is noted that

$$r(\boldsymbol{E}_r) = r(\boldsymbol{G}_{r-1} \boldsymbol{A}_r) = p - m_r. \tag{4.85}$$

One of the main tricks when deriving the moment expressions is to use the observation presented in the next lemma.

Lemma 4.3 *Let $\boldsymbol{V}^r_{11}$ and $\boldsymbol{U}^r_{11}$ be given by (4.82) and let $\boldsymbol{h}(\bullet)$ be any measurable function of $(\boldsymbol{U}^r_{11})^{-1}$ of proper size. Then*

$$E[(\boldsymbol{V}^{r-1}_{11})^{-1} \boldsymbol{h}(\boldsymbol{U}^r_{11})] = c_{r-1} E[(\boldsymbol{U}^r_{11})^{-1} \boldsymbol{h}(\boldsymbol{U}^r_{11})], \quad r = 2, 3,$$

where

$$c_{r-1} = \frac{n - r(\boldsymbol{C}_r) - m_{r-1} - 1}{n - r(\boldsymbol{C}_{r-1}) - m_{r-1} - 1} = 1 + \frac{r(\boldsymbol{C}_{r-1}) - r(\boldsymbol{C}_r)}{n - r(\boldsymbol{C}_{r-1}) - m_{r-1} - 1}. \quad (4.86)$$

Proof According to the definitions of $\boldsymbol{V}_{11}^{r-1}$ and $\boldsymbol{U}_{11}^r$, and Theorem B.22 (i) in Appendix B, there exists a unique lower triangular matrix $\boldsymbol{T}$ such that

$$\boldsymbol{U}_{11}^r = \boldsymbol{T}\boldsymbol{T}', \quad \boldsymbol{V}_{11}^{r-1} = \boldsymbol{T}\boldsymbol{F}\boldsymbol{T}', \quad (4.87)$$

where $\boldsymbol{F} \sim M\beta_I(m_{r-1}, n-r(\boldsymbol{C}_{r-1}), r(\boldsymbol{C}_{r-1})-r(\boldsymbol{C}_r))$ (see Appendix A, Sect. A.9 for a definition of the multivariate β-distribution) is independent of $\boldsymbol{T}$. Since (see Appendix B, Theorem B.22 (iii))

$$E[\boldsymbol{F}^{-1}] = c_{r-1}\boldsymbol{I},$$

the lemma is established. □

The result in (4.87) is of special interest, in particular the fact that $\boldsymbol{F}$ is independent of $\boldsymbol{T}$, which follows from the derivation of the $M\beta_I(\bullet, \bullet, \bullet)$ distribution (e.g. see Kollo and von Rosen, 2005, pp. 248–249). One should note that $\boldsymbol{U}_{11}^r = \boldsymbol{V}_{11}^{r-1} + \boldsymbol{W}$, where $\boldsymbol{U}_{11}^r$, $\boldsymbol{V}_{11}^{r-1}$ and $\boldsymbol{W} \sim W_{m_{r-1}}(\boldsymbol{I}, r(\boldsymbol{C}_{r-1}) - r(\boldsymbol{C}_r))$ are Wishart-distributed, and $\boldsymbol{W}$ is independent of $\boldsymbol{V}_{11}^{r-1}$.

Another important result which will also be used repeatedly is the following lemma.

Lemma 4.4 *Let $\boldsymbol{M}_r$ be given by (4.83) and let $\boldsymbol{Q}$ be an arbitrary non-random matrix of a proper size. Then*

$$E[\boldsymbol{M}_r\boldsymbol{Q}\boldsymbol{M}_r'] = E[\begin{pmatrix} \boldsymbol{I} \\ \boldsymbol{V}_{21}^r(\boldsymbol{V}_{11}^r)^{-1} \end{pmatrix} \boldsymbol{Q} \begin{pmatrix} \boldsymbol{I} & (\boldsymbol{V}_{11}^r)^{-1}\boldsymbol{V}_{12}^r \end{pmatrix}]$$
$$= \begin{pmatrix} \boldsymbol{Q} & \boldsymbol{0} \\ \boldsymbol{0} & E[\mathrm{tr}\{(\boldsymbol{V}_{11}^r)^{-1}\boldsymbol{Q}\}]\boldsymbol{I} \end{pmatrix}.$$

Proof Since $\boldsymbol{V}^r$ is Wishart-distributed, there exists an $\boldsymbol{N} \sim N_{m_{r-1}, n-r(\boldsymbol{C}_r)}(\boldsymbol{0}, \boldsymbol{I}, \boldsymbol{I})$ such that $\boldsymbol{V}^r = \boldsymbol{N}\boldsymbol{N}'$. Corresponding to the $\boldsymbol{V}_{11}^r$ partition $\boldsymbol{N}' = (\boldsymbol{N}_1' : \boldsymbol{N}_2')$, i.e. $\boldsymbol{V}_{11}^r = \boldsymbol{N}_1\boldsymbol{N}_1'$, and it is noted that $\boldsymbol{N}_2$ is independent of $\boldsymbol{N}_1$. Then the proof follows by an application of Appendix B, Theorem B.19 (iv). □

In Corollary 3.3 $\widehat{E[\boldsymbol{X}]}$ was presented as a sum of three random variables:

$$\widehat{E[\boldsymbol{X}]} = \sum_{i=1}^{3} \boldsymbol{A}_i\widehat{\boldsymbol{B}}_i\boldsymbol{C}_i = \boldsymbol{P}_{A_1,S_1}\boldsymbol{X}\boldsymbol{P}_{C_1'} + \boldsymbol{P}_{\widehat{Q}_1'A_2,\widehat{S}_2}\boldsymbol{X}\boldsymbol{P}_{C_2'} + \boldsymbol{P}_{\widehat{Q}_2'\widehat{Q}_1'A_3,\widehat{S}_3}\boldsymbol{X}\boldsymbol{P}_{C_3'}, \quad (4.88)$$

where

$$\widehat{P}_1 = P_{A_1,S_1}, \quad \widehat{P}_2 = P_{\widehat{Q}_1' A_2,\widehat{S}_2}, \quad \widehat{P}_3 = P_{\widehat{Q}_2'\widehat{Q}_1' A_3,\widehat{S}_3}, \tag{4.89}$$

$$\widehat{Q}_1 = I - \widehat{P}_1', \quad \widehat{Q}_2 = I - \widehat{P}_2'. \tag{4.90}$$

The variables in (4.88) are of the same type as $\widehat{E[X]}$ in the BRM but unfortunately the variables are not independently distributed. Now it will be shown how to derive the dispersion matrix $D[\widehat{E[X]}]$. Note that $E[\widehat{E[X]}] = E[X]$ and

$$D[\widehat{E[X]}] = D[\widehat{E[X]} - E[X]] = D[\sum_{i=1}^{3} \widehat{P}_i(X - E[X])P_{C_i'}].$$

This means that in order to find $D[\widehat{E[X]}]$, it is sufficient to consider the dispersion

$$D[\widehat{P}_r(X - E[X])P_{C_r'}], \quad r = 1, 2, 3,$$

and the covariance

$$C[\widehat{P}_r(X - E[X])P_{C_r'}, \widehat{P}_s(X - E[X])P_{C_s'}], \quad 1 \leq r < s \leq 3.$$

By summing all the necessary dispersion and covariance matrices, $D[\widehat{E[X]}]$ is obtained. In the next theorem the dispersion is studied, whereas the covariance is treated in Theorem 4.13. The final expression for $D[\widehat{E[X]}]$ is presented in Theorem 4.14.

Theorem 4.12 *Consider the $EBRM_B^3$ presented in Definition 2.2. Let m_r and c_r be defined by (4.78) and (4.86), respectively. Put*

$$d_{1,2} = c_1 e_2, \quad d_{1,3} = c_1 c_2 e_3, \quad d_{2,3} = c_2 e_3,$$

where

$$e_r = \frac{(p - m_r)(n - r(C_r) - 1)}{(n - r(C_r) - m_{r-1} - 1)(n - r(C_r) - m_{r-1} + p - m_r - 1)}, \quad r = 2, 3, \tag{4.91}$$

and

$$f_r = \frac{n - r(C_r) - 1}{n - r(C_r) - m_r - 1}, \quad r = 1, 2, 3. \tag{4.92}$$

Furthermore, let

$$A_{1:i} = (A_1 : A_2 : \cdots : A_i), \quad A_{1:0} = 0 \tag{4.93}$$

and define

$$\begin{aligned} K_i &= \Sigma(P_{G_{i-1},\Sigma^{-1}} - P_{G_i,\Sigma^{-1}}) \\ &= A_{1:i}(A'_{1:i}\Sigma^{-1}A_{1:i})^{-}A'_{1:i} - A_{1:i-1}(A'_{1:i-1}\Sigma^{-1}A_{1:i-1})^{-}A'_{1:i-1}, \end{aligned}$$

where in particular

$$\begin{aligned} K_1 &= A_1(A'_1\Sigma^{-1}A_1)^{-}A'_1, \\ K_2 &= A_{1:2}(A'_{1:2}\Sigma^{-1}A_{1:2})^{-}A'_{1:2} - A_1(A'_1\Sigma^{-1}A_1)^{-}A'_1, \\ K_3 &= A_{1:3}(A'_{1:3}\Sigma^{-1}A_{1:3})^{-}A'_{1:3} - A_{1:2}(A'_{1:2}\Sigma^{-1}A_{1:2})^{-}A'_{1:2}. \end{aligned}$$

Then, if e_r and f_r are finite and positive,

$$\begin{aligned} D[P_{A_1,S_1}(X - E[X])P_{C'_1}] &= f_1 P_{C'_1} \otimes K_1, \qquad (4.94) \\ D[P_{\widehat{Q}'_1 A_2,\widehat{S}_2}(X - E[X])P_{C'_2}] &= P_{C'_2} \otimes (d_{1,2}K_1 + f_2K_2), \\ D[P_{\widehat{Q}'_2\widehat{Q}'_1 A_3,\widehat{S}_3}(X - E[X])P_{C'_3}] &= P_{C'_3} \otimes (d_{1,3}K_1 + d_{2,3}K_2 + f_3K_3), \end{aligned}$$

where $\widehat{Q}_r$, $r = 1, 2$, is defined in (4.90).

Proof It follows that the proof in principle holds for an arbitrary r, which, however, will not be highlighted. Due to independence between the "mean" and the "residuals"

$$D[\widehat{P}_r(X - E[X])P_{C'_r}] = P_{C'_r} \otimes E[\widehat{P}_r\Sigma\widehat{P}'_r], \quad r = 1, 2, 3, \tag{4.95}$$

where for notational convenience $\widehat{P}_r$ in (4.89) is used, and therefore the crucial quantity to consider is

$$E[\widehat{P}_r\Sigma\widehat{P}'_r].$$

When $r = 1$, relation (4.95) is immediately obtained from Theorem 4.3 (ii), since the expressions which have to be calculated have the same form as those used when calculating the dispersion for the dispersion of $\widehat{B}$ in the BRM, i.e.

$$E[\widehat{P}_1\Sigma\widehat{P}'_1] = f_1K_1, \tag{4.96}$$

where f_1 is given by (4.92).

Before starting the derivation of $E[\widehat{\boldsymbol{P}}_r\boldsymbol{\Sigma}\widehat{\boldsymbol{P}}_r']$, $r = 2, 3$, some preparatory results are stated without proofs. For $r = 2$ the "open sesame" relation

$$\widehat{\boldsymbol{Q}}_1\widehat{\boldsymbol{S}}_2^{-1}\widehat{\boldsymbol{Q}}_1' = \widehat{\boldsymbol{Q}}_1\widehat{\boldsymbol{S}}_2^{-1} = \boldsymbol{G}_1(\boldsymbol{G}_1'\boldsymbol{W}_2\boldsymbol{G}_1)^{-1}\boldsymbol{G}_1' \tag{4.97}$$

will be used, where $\boldsymbol{G}_1$ and $\boldsymbol{W}_2$ are defined in (4.73) and (4.74), respectively. This relation and a similar one given below in (4.101) are two of the most important relations for treating the $EBRM_B^3$ theoretically, since, for example, the right-hand side of (4.97) shows that $\widehat{\boldsymbol{Q}}_1\widehat{\boldsymbol{S}}_2^{-1}\widehat{\boldsymbol{Q}}_1' = \widehat{\boldsymbol{Q}}_1\widehat{\boldsymbol{S}}_2^{-1}$ is inverted Wishart-distributed, and therefore moments are also available. Moreover, with $\boldsymbol{M}_1$ as defined in (4.83)

$$\widehat{\boldsymbol{P}}_2 = \widehat{\boldsymbol{Q}}_1'\boldsymbol{P}_{A_2,G_1'W_2G_1,G_1} = \boldsymbol{P}'_{G_1,W_1^{-1}}\boldsymbol{P}_{A_2,G_1'W_2G_1,G_1} = \boldsymbol{\Sigma}^{1/2}\boldsymbol{\Gamma}_1'\boldsymbol{M}_1\boldsymbol{H}_1^{-1}\boldsymbol{P}_{G_1'A_2,G_1'W_2G_1}\boldsymbol{G}_1' \tag{4.98}$$

yields

$$\widehat{\boldsymbol{P}}_2\boldsymbol{\Sigma}\widehat{\boldsymbol{P}}_2' = \boldsymbol{\Sigma}^{1/2}\boldsymbol{\Gamma}_1'\boldsymbol{M}_1\boldsymbol{P}_{E_2,U_{11}^2}\boldsymbol{P}'_{E_2,U_{11}^2}\boldsymbol{M}_1'\boldsymbol{\Gamma}_1\boldsymbol{\Sigma}^{1/2},$$

where $\boldsymbol{E}_2$ is defined in (4.84). Then, because $\boldsymbol{V}^1$ is Wishart distributed, $\boldsymbol{V}^1 = \boldsymbol{N}\boldsymbol{N}'$ and $\boldsymbol{V}_{12}^1 = \boldsymbol{N}_1\boldsymbol{N}_2'$ for some normally distributed

$$\boldsymbol{N} = (\boldsymbol{N}_1' : \boldsymbol{N}_2')' \sim N_{p,n-r(C_1)}(\boldsymbol{0}, \boldsymbol{I}, \boldsymbol{I}),$$

implying, among other things, that $\boldsymbol{N}_2$ is independent of $\boldsymbol{N}_1$ and $\boldsymbol{U}_{11}^2 = \boldsymbol{V}_{11}^1 + \boldsymbol{W}$, where $\boldsymbol{W} \sim W_{p-r(\boldsymbol{A})}(\boldsymbol{I}, r(\boldsymbol{C}_1) - r(\boldsymbol{C}_2))$ is independent of $\boldsymbol{V}_{11}^1$. It follows, by using Lemma 4.4, that

$$E[\widehat{\boldsymbol{P}}_2\boldsymbol{\Sigma}\widehat{\boldsymbol{P}}_2'] = \boldsymbol{\Sigma}^{1/2}\boldsymbol{\Gamma}_1^{u'}E[\boldsymbol{P}_{E_2,U_{11}^2}\boldsymbol{P}'_{E_2,U_{11}^2}]\boldsymbol{\Gamma}_1^u\boldsymbol{\Sigma}^{1/2}$$
$$+\boldsymbol{\Sigma}^{1/2}\boldsymbol{\Gamma}_1^{l'}\boldsymbol{\Gamma}_1^l\boldsymbol{\Sigma}^{1/2}E[\mathrm{tr}\{(\boldsymbol{V}_{11}^1)^{-1}\boldsymbol{P}_{E_2,U_{11}^2}\boldsymbol{P}'_{E_2,U_{11}^2}\}].$$

Using Lemma 4.3 and Theorem B.26 (i) in Appendix B, the expectations can be calculated:

$$E[\boldsymbol{P}_{E_2,U_{11}^2}\boldsymbol{P}'_{E_2,U_{11}^2}] = f_2\boldsymbol{P}_{E_2},$$

$$E[\mathrm{tr}\{(\boldsymbol{V}_{11}^1)^{-1}\boldsymbol{P}_{E_2,U_{11}^2}\boldsymbol{P}'_{E_2,U_{11}^2}\}] = c_1E[\mathrm{tr}\{(\boldsymbol{U}_{11}^2)^{-1}\boldsymbol{P}_{E_2,U_{11}^2}\boldsymbol{P}'_{E_2,U_{11}^2}\}]$$
$$= c_1E[\mathrm{tr}\{(\boldsymbol{U}_{11}^2)^{-1}\boldsymbol{P}_{E_2,U_{11}^2}\}] = d_{1,2}, \tag{4.99}$$

defined in the statement of the theorem. Furthermore, it can be shown that $\boldsymbol{K}_1$ and $\boldsymbol{K}_2$, also given in the statement of the theorem, satisfy

$$\boldsymbol{K}_1 = \boldsymbol{\Sigma}^{1/2}\boldsymbol{\Gamma}_1^{l\prime}\boldsymbol{\Gamma}_1^l\boldsymbol{\Sigma}^{1/2},$$
$$\boldsymbol{K}_2 = \boldsymbol{\Sigma}^{1/2}\boldsymbol{\Gamma}_1^{u\prime}\boldsymbol{P}_{E_2}\boldsymbol{\Gamma}_1^u\boldsymbol{\Sigma}^{1/2},$$

respectively, and hence

$$E[\widehat{\boldsymbol{P}}_2\boldsymbol{\Sigma}\widehat{\boldsymbol{P}}_2'] = d_{1,2}\boldsymbol{K}_1 + f_2\boldsymbol{K}_2 \tag{4.100}$$

has been determined.

Next $r = 3$ is considered and the derivation follows the previous case when $r = 2$. Instead of (4.97), the following equations now appear:

$$\widehat{\boldsymbol{Q}}_2\widehat{\boldsymbol{Q}}_1\widehat{\boldsymbol{S}}_3^{-1}\widehat{\boldsymbol{Q}}_1'\widehat{\boldsymbol{Q}}_2' = \widehat{\boldsymbol{Q}}_2\widehat{\boldsymbol{Q}}_1\widehat{\boldsymbol{S}}_3^{-1} = \boldsymbol{G}_2(\boldsymbol{G}_2'\boldsymbol{W}_3\boldsymbol{G}_2)^{-1}\boldsymbol{G}_2' \tag{4.101}$$

and

$$\begin{aligned}\widehat{\boldsymbol{P}}_3 &= \widehat{\boldsymbol{Q}}_2'\widehat{\boldsymbol{Q}}_1'\boldsymbol{P}_{A_3,G_2'W_3G_2,G_2} = \boldsymbol{P}'_{G_1,W_1^{-1}}\boldsymbol{P}'_{G_2,W_2^{-1}}\boldsymbol{P}_{A_3,G_2'W_3G_2,G_2}\\ &= \boldsymbol{\Sigma}^{1/2}\boldsymbol{\Gamma}_1'\boldsymbol{M}_1\boldsymbol{\Gamma}_2'\boldsymbol{M}_2\boldsymbol{H}_2^{-1}\boldsymbol{P}_{G_2'A_3,G_2'W_3G_2}\boldsymbol{G}_2',\end{aligned} \tag{4.102}$$

as well as

$$\widehat{\boldsymbol{P}}_3\boldsymbol{\Sigma}\widehat{\boldsymbol{P}}_3' = \boldsymbol{\Sigma}^{1/2}\boldsymbol{\Gamma}_1'\boldsymbol{M}_1\boldsymbol{\Gamma}_2'\boldsymbol{M}_2\boldsymbol{P}_{E_3,U_{11}^3}\boldsymbol{P}'_{E_3,U_{11}^3}\boldsymbol{M}_2'\boldsymbol{\Gamma}_2\boldsymbol{M}_1'\boldsymbol{\Gamma}_1\boldsymbol{\Sigma}^{1/2}.$$

Then, once again applying Lemma 4.4 and using $\boldsymbol{V}_{12}^1 = \boldsymbol{N}_1\boldsymbol{N}_2'$ for some normally distributed $\boldsymbol{N}' = (\boldsymbol{N}_1' : \boldsymbol{N}_2')$, where $\boldsymbol{N}_2$ is uncorrelated with $\boldsymbol{N}_1$, $\boldsymbol{M}_2$ and $\boldsymbol{U}_{11}^3$,

$$E[\widehat{\boldsymbol{P}}_3\boldsymbol{\Sigma}\widehat{\boldsymbol{P}}_3'] = \boldsymbol{\Sigma}^{1/2}\boldsymbol{\Gamma}_1^{u\prime}\boldsymbol{\Gamma}_2'E[\boldsymbol{M}_2\boldsymbol{P}_{E_3,U_{11}^3}\boldsymbol{P}'_{E_3,U_{11}^3}\boldsymbol{M}_2']\boldsymbol{\Gamma}_2\boldsymbol{\Gamma}_1^u\boldsymbol{\Sigma}^{1/2} \tag{4.103}$$
$$+ \boldsymbol{\Sigma}^{1/2}\boldsymbol{\Gamma}_1^{l\prime}\boldsymbol{\Gamma}_1^l\boldsymbol{\Sigma}^{1/2}E[\mathrm{tr}\{(\boldsymbol{V}_{11}^1)^{-1}\boldsymbol{\Gamma}_2\boldsymbol{M}_2\boldsymbol{P}_{E_3,U_{11}^3}\boldsymbol{P}'_{E_3,U_{11}^3}\boldsymbol{M}_2'\boldsymbol{\Gamma}_2'\}]. \tag{4.104}$$

It is observed that $E[\boldsymbol{M}_2\boldsymbol{P}_{E_3,U_{11}^3}\boldsymbol{P}'_{E_3,U_{11}^3}\boldsymbol{M}_2']$ has the same stochastic structure as $E[\widehat{\boldsymbol{P}}_2\boldsymbol{\Sigma}\widehat{\boldsymbol{P}}_2']$ and therefore the right-hand side of (4.103) equals

$$\begin{aligned}&\boldsymbol{\Sigma}^{1/2}\boldsymbol{\Gamma}_1^{u\prime}\boldsymbol{\Gamma}_2'E[\boldsymbol{M}_2\boldsymbol{P}_{E_3,U_{11}^3}\boldsymbol{P}'_{E_3,U_{11}^3}\boldsymbol{M}_2']\boldsymbol{\Gamma}_2\boldsymbol{\Gamma}_1^u\boldsymbol{\Sigma}^{1/2}\\ &\quad= \boldsymbol{\Sigma}^{1/2}\boldsymbol{\Gamma}_1^{u\prime}\boldsymbol{\Gamma}_2^{u\prime}E[\boldsymbol{P}_{E_3,U_{11}^3}\boldsymbol{P}'_{E_3,U_{11}^3}]\boldsymbol{\Gamma}_2^u\boldsymbol{\Gamma}_1^u\boldsymbol{\Sigma}^{1/2}\\ &\quad+\boldsymbol{\Sigma}^{1/2}\boldsymbol{\Gamma}_1^{u\prime}\boldsymbol{\Gamma}_2^{l\prime}\boldsymbol{\Gamma}_2^l\boldsymbol{\Gamma}_1^u\boldsymbol{\Sigma}^{1/2}E[\mathrm{tr}\{(\boldsymbol{V}_{11}^2)^{-1}\boldsymbol{P}_{E_3,U_{11}^3}\boldsymbol{P}'_{E_3,U_{11}^3}\}].\end{aligned}$$

Now Lemma 4.3 and Theorem B.26 (i) in Appendix B, yield

$$\begin{aligned} E[\boldsymbol{P}_{E_3,U_{11}^3}\boldsymbol{P}'_{E_3,U_{11}^3}] &= f_3\boldsymbol{P}_{E_3}, \\ E[\mathrm{tr}\{(\boldsymbol{V}_{11}^2)^{-1}\boldsymbol{P}_{E_3,U_{11}^3}\boldsymbol{P}'_{E_3,U_{11}^3}\}] &= c_2E[\mathrm{tr}\{(\boldsymbol{U}_{11}^3)^{-1}\boldsymbol{P}_{E_3,U_{11}^3}\boldsymbol{P}'_{E_3,U_{11}^3}\}] \\ &= c_2E[\mathrm{tr}\{(\boldsymbol{U}_{11}^3)^{-1}\boldsymbol{P}_{E_3,U_{11}^3}\}] = d_{2,3}, \end{aligned} \tag{4.105}$$

where f_3 and c_2 are given in Table 4.1 and $d_{2,3}$ is defined in the beginning of the theorem. Finally, (4.104) is considered:

$$\begin{aligned} &\boldsymbol{\Sigma}^{1/2}\boldsymbol{\Gamma}_1^{l'}\boldsymbol{\Gamma}_1^l\boldsymbol{\Sigma}^{1/2}E[\mathrm{tr}\{(\boldsymbol{V}_{11}^1)^{-1}\boldsymbol{\Gamma}_2'\boldsymbol{M}_2\boldsymbol{P}_{E_3,U_{11}^3}\boldsymbol{P}'_{E_3,U_{11}^3}\boldsymbol{M}_2'\boldsymbol{\Gamma}_2\}] \\ &= \boldsymbol{\Sigma}^{1/2}\boldsymbol{\Gamma}_1^{l'}\boldsymbol{\Gamma}_1^l\boldsymbol{\Sigma}^{1/2}c_1E[\mathrm{tr}\{(\boldsymbol{U}_{11}^2)^{-1}\boldsymbol{\Gamma}_2'\boldsymbol{M}_2\boldsymbol{P}_{E_3,U_{11}^3}\boldsymbol{P}'_{E_3,U_{11}^3}\boldsymbol{M}_2'\boldsymbol{\Gamma}_2\}] \\ &= \boldsymbol{\Sigma}^{1/2}\boldsymbol{\Gamma}_1^{l'}\boldsymbol{\Gamma}_1^l\boldsymbol{\Sigma}^{1/2} \\ &\quad\times c_1E[\mathrm{tr}\{(\boldsymbol{U}_{11}^2)^{-1}\boldsymbol{\Gamma}_2'\boldsymbol{V}^2\boldsymbol{\Gamma}_2\boldsymbol{\Gamma}_2^{u'}(\boldsymbol{V}_{11}^2)^{-1}\boldsymbol{P}_{E_3,U_{11}^3}\boldsymbol{P}'_{E_3,U_{11}^3}(\boldsymbol{V}_{11}^2)^{-1}\boldsymbol{\Gamma}_2^u\boldsymbol{\Gamma}_2'\boldsymbol{V}^2\boldsymbol{\Gamma}_2\}] \\ &= \boldsymbol{\Sigma}^{1/2}\boldsymbol{\Gamma}_1^{l'}\boldsymbol{\Gamma}_1^l\boldsymbol{\Sigma}^{1/2}c_1E[\mathrm{tr}\{\boldsymbol{\Gamma}_2^{u'}(\boldsymbol{V}_{11}^2)^{-1}\boldsymbol{P}_{E_3,U_{11}^3}\boldsymbol{P}'_{E_3,U_{11}^3}(\boldsymbol{V}_{11}^2)^{-1}\boldsymbol{\Gamma}_2^u\boldsymbol{U}_{11}^2\}] \\ &= \boldsymbol{\Sigma}^{1/2}\boldsymbol{\Gamma}_1^{l'}\boldsymbol{\Gamma}_1^l\boldsymbol{\Sigma}^{1/2}c_1E[\mathrm{tr}\{(\boldsymbol{V}_{11}^2)^{-1}\boldsymbol{P}_{E_3,U_{11}^3}\boldsymbol{P}'_{E_3,U_{11}^3}\}], \end{aligned}$$

since $\boldsymbol{\Gamma}_2'\boldsymbol{V}^2\boldsymbol{\Gamma}_2 = \boldsymbol{U}_{11}^2$ and $\boldsymbol{\Gamma}_2^u\boldsymbol{U}_{11}^2\boldsymbol{\Gamma}_2^{u'} = \boldsymbol{V}_{11}^2$. Thus, the last expression has the same form as the left-hand side of (4.99) and, therefore, the expectation in (4.104) equals

$$E[\mathrm{tr}\{(\boldsymbol{V}_{11}^1)^{-1}\boldsymbol{\Gamma}_2'\boldsymbol{M}_2\boldsymbol{P}_{E_3,U_{11}^3}\boldsymbol{P}'_{E_3,U_{11}^3}\boldsymbol{M}_2'\boldsymbol{\Gamma}_2\}] = d_{1,3}.$$

The statement of the theorem concerning $r = 3$ is verified by observing that

$$\begin{aligned} \boldsymbol{K}_2 &= \boldsymbol{\Sigma}^{1/2}\boldsymbol{\Gamma}_1^{u'}\boldsymbol{\Gamma}_2^{l'}\boldsymbol{\Gamma}_2^l\boldsymbol{\Gamma}_1^u\boldsymbol{\Sigma}^{1/2}, \\ \boldsymbol{K}_3 &= \boldsymbol{\Sigma}^{1/2}\boldsymbol{\Gamma}_1^{u'}\boldsymbol{\Gamma}_2^{u'}\boldsymbol{P}_{E_3}\boldsymbol{\Gamma}_2^u\boldsymbol{\Gamma}_1^u\boldsymbol{\Sigma}^{1/2}. \end{aligned} \tag{4.106}$$

□

It is of interest to reflect on how the proof was carried out and understand that the main parts consist of two recursive relations, and in particular to understand when and why Lemmas 4.3 and 4.4 were applied. Now the covariance between the terms in

$$\widehat{E[\boldsymbol{X}]} = \boldsymbol{P}_{A_1,S_1}\boldsymbol{X}\boldsymbol{P}_{C_1'} + \boldsymbol{P}_{\widehat{Q}_1'A_2,\widehat{S}_2}\boldsymbol{X}\boldsymbol{P}_{C_2'} + \boldsymbol{P}_{\widehat{Q}_2'\widehat{Q}_1'A_3,\widehat{S}_3}\boldsymbol{X}\boldsymbol{P}_{C_3'}$$

is studied.

Theorem 4.13 *Let $r < s \leq 3$ and let the notation be the same as in Theorem 4.12 and its proof. Then, for the $EBRM_B^3$ presented in Definition 2.2, if e_r, given in Theorem 4.12, is finite and positive,*

$$
C[\widehat{\boldsymbol{P}}_r(\boldsymbol{X} - E[\boldsymbol{X}])\boldsymbol{P}_{C'_r}, \widehat{\boldsymbol{P}}_s(\boldsymbol{X} - E[\boldsymbol{X}])\boldsymbol{P}_{C'_s}]
$$

$$
= \begin{cases} -\boldsymbol{P}_{C'_3} \otimes d_{2,3}\boldsymbol{K}_2, & \text{if } r > 1, \\ \boldsymbol{P}_{C'_s} \otimes (d_{1,s}\boldsymbol{K}_1 + \boldsymbol{K}_s), & \text{if } r = 1. \end{cases}
$$

Proof The following proof indicates that the result holds for a general $m > 3$ in an $EBRM_B^m$, if MLEs have been derived. The matrices $\boldsymbol{M}_r$ and $\boldsymbol{E}_r$ given by (4.83) and (4.84) will be used. Additionally, a matrix $\boldsymbol{Z}_{r,s}$ simplifies the presentation as follows:

$$
\boldsymbol{Z}_{r,s} = \boldsymbol{\Gamma}^u_{r-1}\boldsymbol{\Gamma}^u_{r-2} \times \cdots \times \boldsymbol{\Gamma}^u_1\boldsymbol{\Sigma}^{-1/2}\boldsymbol{P}'_{G_r,W_r^{-1}}\boldsymbol{P}'_{G_{r+1},W_{r+1}^{-1}} \times \cdots \times \boldsymbol{P}'_{G_s,W_s^{-1}},
$$

$$
2 \leq r \leq s, \tag{4.107}
$$

$$
\boldsymbol{Z}_{1,s} = \boldsymbol{P}'_{G_1,W_1^{-1}}\boldsymbol{P}'_{G_2,W_2^{-1}} \times \cdots \times \boldsymbol{P}'_{G_s,W_s^{-1}}, \quad s \geq 1, \tag{4.108}
$$

$$
\boldsymbol{Z}_{r,s} = \boldsymbol{I}, \quad r > s.
$$

First consider the case $r = 1$:

$$
\begin{aligned}
E[\widehat{\boldsymbol{P}}_1\boldsymbol{\Sigma}\widehat{\boldsymbol{P}}'_s] &= E[\boldsymbol{\Sigma}^{1/2}\boldsymbol{\Gamma}'_1\boldsymbol{M}_1\boldsymbol{\Gamma}^u_1\boldsymbol{\Sigma}^{1/2}\boldsymbol{P}'_{A_s,G'_{s-1}W_sG_{s-1},G_s}\boldsymbol{Z}'_{1,s-1}] \\
&= \boldsymbol{\Sigma}^{1/2}\boldsymbol{\Gamma}^{u'}_1 E[\boldsymbol{\Gamma}^u_1\boldsymbol{\Sigma}^{1/2}\boldsymbol{P}'_{A_s,G'_{s-1}W_sG_{s-1},G_s}\boldsymbol{Z}'_{2,s-1}]\boldsymbol{\Gamma}^u_1\boldsymbol{\Sigma}^{1/2} \\
&\quad + E[\mathrm{tr}\{(\boldsymbol{V}^1_{11})^{-1}\boldsymbol{\Gamma}^u_1\boldsymbol{\Sigma}^{-1/2}\boldsymbol{\Sigma}\boldsymbol{P}'_{A_s,G'_{s-1}W_sG_{s-1},G_s}\boldsymbol{Z}'_{2,s-1}\}]\boldsymbol{\Sigma}^{1/2}\boldsymbol{\Gamma}^{l'}_1\boldsymbol{\Gamma}^l_1\boldsymbol{\Sigma}^{1/2} \\
&= \boldsymbol{\Sigma}^{1/2}\boldsymbol{\Gamma}^{u'}_1\boldsymbol{\Gamma}^u_1\boldsymbol{\Sigma}^{-1/2}\boldsymbol{\Sigma}E[\boldsymbol{\Sigma}^{-1/2}\boldsymbol{\Gamma}^{u'}_1 \times \cdots \times \boldsymbol{\Gamma}^{u'}_{s-1}\boldsymbol{P}'_{E_s,U^{s-1}_{11}}] \qquad (4.109) \\
&\quad \times\boldsymbol{\Gamma}^u_{s-1} \times \cdots \times \boldsymbol{\Gamma}^u_1\boldsymbol{\Sigma}^{1/2} + d_{1,s}\boldsymbol{K}_1 \qquad (4.110) \\
&= \boldsymbol{\Sigma}^{1/2}\boldsymbol{\Gamma}^{u'}_1\boldsymbol{\Gamma}^u_1\boldsymbol{\Sigma}^{-1/2}\boldsymbol{\Sigma}\boldsymbol{\Sigma}^{-1/2}\boldsymbol{\Gamma}^{u'}_1 \times \cdots \times \boldsymbol{\Gamma}^{u'}_{s-1}\boldsymbol{P}_{E_s}\boldsymbol{\Gamma}^u_{s-1} \times \cdots \times \boldsymbol{\Gamma}^u_1\boldsymbol{\Sigma}^{1/2} + d_{1,s}\boldsymbol{K}_1 \\
&= \boldsymbol{K}_s + d_{1,s}\boldsymbol{K}_1, \qquad (4.111)
\end{aligned}
$$

where, among other used results, Lemma 4.4 has been applied.

Now suppose $r = 2$ and $s = 3$. Note that $(\boldsymbol{X} - E[\boldsymbol{X}])\boldsymbol{P}_{C'_2}$ can be written as

$$
(\boldsymbol{X} - E[\boldsymbol{X}])\boldsymbol{P}_{C'_2} = (\boldsymbol{X} - E[\boldsymbol{X}])(\boldsymbol{P}_{C'_3} + \boldsymbol{P}_{C'_2} - \boldsymbol{P}_{C'_3}),
$$

where $(\boldsymbol{X} - E[\boldsymbol{X}])\boldsymbol{P}_{C'_3}$ is independent of $\widehat{\boldsymbol{P}}_2$, $\widehat{\boldsymbol{P}}_3$ and $(\boldsymbol{X} - E[\boldsymbol{X}])(\boldsymbol{P}_{C'_2} - \boldsymbol{P}_{C'_3})$. Hence,

$$
C[\widehat{\boldsymbol{P}}_2(\boldsymbol{X} - E[\boldsymbol{X}])\boldsymbol{P}_{C'_2}, \widehat{\boldsymbol{P}}_3(\boldsymbol{X} - E[\boldsymbol{X}])\boldsymbol{P}_{C'_3}] = \boldsymbol{P}_{C'_3} \otimes E[\widehat{\boldsymbol{P}}_2\boldsymbol{\Sigma}\widehat{\boldsymbol{P}}'_3].
$$

Thus, from now on $E[\widehat{\boldsymbol{P}}_2\boldsymbol{\Sigma}\widehat{\boldsymbol{P}}_3']$ is discussed in a manner similar to the way in which we discussed the case when $r = s$, and it turns out that there exists a recurrence property which is somewhat easier to handle than when $r = s$, as in Theorem 4.12. It can be shown, using the same arguments as were used when (4.103) and (4.104) were obtained, that if one assumes that

$$E\Big[\mathrm{tr}\{(\boldsymbol{V}_{11}^1)^{-1}\boldsymbol{\Gamma}_1^u\boldsymbol{\Sigma}^{-1/2}\boldsymbol{P}_{A_2,G_1'W_2G_1,G_1}\boldsymbol{\Sigma}\boldsymbol{P}'_{A_3,G_2'W_3G_2,G_2}$$
$$\times\boldsymbol{G}_2(\boldsymbol{G}_2'\boldsymbol{W}_2\boldsymbol{G}_2)^{-1}\boldsymbol{G}_2'\boldsymbol{W}_2\boldsymbol{\Sigma}^{-1/2}\boldsymbol{\Gamma}_1^{u'}\}\Big] = 0, \tag{4.112}$$

then

$$\begin{aligned}E[\widehat{\boldsymbol{P}}_2\boldsymbol{\Sigma}\widehat{\boldsymbol{P}}_3'] &= E[\boldsymbol{Z}_{1,1}\boldsymbol{P}_{A_2,G_1'W_2G_1,G_1}\boldsymbol{\Sigma}\boldsymbol{P}'_{A_3,G_2'W_3G_2,G_2}\boldsymbol{Z}_{1,2}']\\ &= \boldsymbol{\Sigma}^{1/2}\boldsymbol{\Gamma}_1'E[\boldsymbol{M}_1\boldsymbol{\Gamma}_1^u\boldsymbol{\Sigma}^{-1/2}\boldsymbol{P}_{A_2,G_1'W_2G_1,G_1}\boldsymbol{\Sigma}\boldsymbol{P}'_{A_3,G_2'W_3G_2,G_2}\boldsymbol{Z}_{2,2}'\boldsymbol{M}_1']\boldsymbol{\Gamma}_1\boldsymbol{\Sigma}^{1/2}\\ &= \boldsymbol{\Sigma}^{1/2}\boldsymbol{\Gamma}_1^{u'}\boldsymbol{\Gamma}_1^u\boldsymbol{\Sigma}^{-1/2}E[\boldsymbol{P}_{A_2,G_1'W_2G_1,G_1}\boldsymbol{\Sigma}\boldsymbol{P}'_{A_3,G_2'W_3G_2,G_2}\boldsymbol{Z}_{2,2}']\boldsymbol{\Gamma}_1^u\boldsymbol{\Sigma}^{1/2}.\end{aligned} \tag{4.113}$$

To verify (4.112), Lemma 4.3 together with some calculations are used. The left-hand side equals

$$\begin{aligned}&c_1E[\mathrm{tr}\{(\boldsymbol{U}_{11}^2)^{-1}\boldsymbol{\Gamma}_1^u\boldsymbol{\Sigma}^{-1/2}\boldsymbol{P}_{A_2,G_1'W_2G_1,G_1}\boldsymbol{\Sigma}\boldsymbol{P}'_{A_3,G_2'W_3G_2,G_2}\\ &\qquad\times\boldsymbol{G}_2(\boldsymbol{G}_2'\boldsymbol{W}_2\boldsymbol{G}_2)^{-1}\boldsymbol{G}_2'\boldsymbol{W}_2\boldsymbol{\Sigma}^{-1/2}\boldsymbol{\Gamma}_1^{u'}\}]\\ &\quad= c_1E[\mathrm{tr}\{\boldsymbol{\Gamma}_1^u\boldsymbol{\Sigma}^{-1/2}\boldsymbol{P}_{A_2,G_1'W_2G_1,G_1}\boldsymbol{\Sigma}\boldsymbol{P}'_{A_3,G_2'W_3G_2,G_2}\boldsymbol{G}_2(\boldsymbol{G}_2'\boldsymbol{W}_2\boldsymbol{G}_2)^{-1}\boldsymbol{H}_2\boldsymbol{\Gamma}_2^u\}]\\ &\quad= c_1E[\mathrm{tr}\{\boldsymbol{G}_2'\boldsymbol{P}_{A_2,G_1'W_2G_1,G_1}\boldsymbol{\Sigma}\boldsymbol{P}'_{A_3,G_2'W_3G_2,G_2}\boldsymbol{G}_2(\boldsymbol{G}_2'\boldsymbol{W}_2\boldsymbol{G}_2)^{-1}\}] = 0,\end{aligned}$$

since according to the definition of $\boldsymbol{G}_2$, given in (4.79), $\boldsymbol{G}_2'\boldsymbol{A}_2 = \boldsymbol{0}$, which implies that

$$\boldsymbol{G}_2'\boldsymbol{P}_{A_2,G_1'W_2G_1,G_1} = \boldsymbol{0}.$$

Continuing with (4.113), by the definition of $\boldsymbol{P}_{A_2,G_1'W_2G_1,G_1}$, it is obtained that (4.113) equals (in particular using (4.79))

$$\boldsymbol{\Sigma}^{1/2}\boldsymbol{\Gamma}_1^{u'}\boldsymbol{\Gamma}_1^u\boldsymbol{\Sigma}^{-1/2}E[(\boldsymbol{I}-\boldsymbol{P}'_{G_2,W_2^{-1}})\boldsymbol{\Sigma}\boldsymbol{P}'_{A_3,G_2'W_3G_2,G_2}\boldsymbol{Z}_{2,2}']\boldsymbol{\Gamma}_1^u\boldsymbol{\Sigma}^{1/2}, \tag{4.114}$$

which consists of a difference of two moment expressions. Concerning the first expression, it follows that:

$$\begin{aligned}&\boldsymbol{\Sigma}^{1/2}\boldsymbol{\Gamma}_1^{u'}\boldsymbol{\Gamma}_1^u\boldsymbol{\Sigma}^{1/2}E[\boldsymbol{P}'_{A_3,G_2'W_3G_2,G_2}\boldsymbol{Z}_{2,2}]\boldsymbol{\Gamma}_1^u\boldsymbol{\Sigma}^{1/2}\\ &\quad= \boldsymbol{\Sigma}^{1/2}\boldsymbol{\Gamma}_1^{u'}\boldsymbol{\Gamma}_1^u\boldsymbol{\Sigma}^{1/2}E[\boldsymbol{P}'_{A_3,G_2'W_3G_2,G_2}]\boldsymbol{\Sigma}^{-1/2}\boldsymbol{\Gamma}_1^{u'}\boldsymbol{\Gamma}_2^{u'}\boldsymbol{\Gamma}_2^u\boldsymbol{\Gamma}_1^u\boldsymbol{\Sigma}^{1/2},\end{aligned} \tag{4.115}$$

since

$$\begin{aligned}Z'_{2,2}\Gamma_1^u\Sigma^{1/2} &= P_{G_2,W_2^{-1}}\Sigma^{-1/2}\Gamma_1^{u'}\Gamma_1^u\Sigma^{1/2}\\ &= \Sigma^{-1/2}\Gamma_1^{u'}\Gamma_2^{u'}(V_{11}^2)^{-1}(V_{11}^2 : V_{12}^2)\Gamma_2\Gamma_1^u\Sigma^{1/2},\end{aligned}$$

and when in (4.115) the expectation is taken, the expression including V_{12}^2 is cancelled. Because for some normally distributed $N = (N_1' : N_2')' \sim N_{m_1,n-r(C_2)}(\mathbf{0}, I, I)$, i.e. N has independent elements and a zero mean, $V_{12}^2 = N_1N_2'$ and in particular N_2 is independent of the other random quantities in (4.115). It appears from the following that it is not necessary to express $E[P'_{A_3,G_2'W_3G_2,G_2}]$ in (4.115).

When studying the second expression in (4.114), it can be observed that

$$\begin{aligned}&\Sigma^{1/2}\Gamma_1^{u'}\Gamma_1^u\Sigma^{-1/2}E[P_{G_2,W_2^{-1}}\Sigma P'_{A_3,G_2'W_3G_2,G_2}Z_{2,2}]\Gamma_1^u\Sigma^{1/2}\\ &= \Sigma^{1/2}\Gamma_1^{u'}\Gamma_2^{u'}\Gamma_2^u\Gamma_1^u\Sigma^{1/2}E[P'_{A_3,G_2'W_3G_2,G_2}]\Sigma^{-1/2}\Gamma_1^{u'}\Gamma_2^{u'}\Gamma_2^u\Gamma_1^u\Sigma^{1/2} \qquad (4.116)\\ &\quad+\Sigma^{1/2}\Gamma_1^{u'}\Gamma_2^{l'}\Gamma_2^l\Gamma_1^u\Sigma^{1/2}E[\mathrm{tr}\{(V_{11}^2)^{-1}\Gamma_2^u\Gamma_1^u\Sigma^{1/2}P'_{A_3,G_2'W_3G_2,G_2}\Sigma^{-1/2}\Gamma_1^{u'}\Gamma_1^{l'}\}], \qquad (4.117)\end{aligned}$$

since

$$\begin{aligned}&\Sigma^{1/2}\Gamma_1^{u'}\Gamma_1^u\Sigma^{-1/2}P'_{G_2,W_2^{-1}}\Sigma P'_{A_3,G_2'W_3G_2,G_2}Z_{2,2}\Gamma_1^u\Sigma^{1/2}\\ &= \Sigma^{1/2}\Gamma_1^{u'}\Gamma_1^u\Sigma^{-1/2}P'_{G_2,W_2^{-1}}\Sigma P'_{A_3,G_2'W_3G_2,G_2}P_{G_2,W_2^{-1}}\Sigma^{-1/2}G_1^1\Gamma_1^{u'}\Gamma_1^u\Sigma^{1/2}\\ &= \Sigma^{1/2}\Gamma_1^{u'}\Gamma_2^{u'}M_2\Gamma_2^u\Gamma_1^u\Sigma^{1/2}P'_{A_3,G_2'W_3G_2,G_2}\Sigma^{-1/2}\Gamma_1^{u'}\Gamma_2^{u'}M_2'\Gamma_2\Gamma_1^u\Sigma^{1/2},\end{aligned}$$

and if one calculates the expected value of this expression, one obtains the sum of (4.116) and (4.117). However, (4.116) is identical to (4.115), since

$$\Sigma^{1/2}\Gamma_1^{u'}\Gamma_2^{u'}\Gamma_2^u\Gamma_1^u\Sigma^{1/2}G_2 = \Sigma^{1/2}\Gamma_1^{u'}\Gamma_1^u\Sigma^{1/2}G_2 = \Sigma G_2.$$

Hence,

$$\begin{aligned}E[\widehat{P}_2\Sigma\widehat{P}_3'] = &-\Sigma^{1/2}\Gamma_1^{u'}\Gamma_2^{l'}\Gamma_2^l\Gamma_1^u\Sigma^{1/2}\\ &\times E[\mathrm{tr}\{(V_{11}^2)^{-1}\Gamma_2^u\Gamma_1^u\Sigma^{1/2}P'_{A_3,G_2'W_3G_2,G_2}\Sigma^{-1/2}\Gamma_1^{u'}\Gamma_2^{l'}\}].\end{aligned}$$

Finally, it is noted that, according to (4.106), $K_2 = \Sigma^{1/2}\Gamma_1^{u'}\Gamma_2^{l'}\Gamma_2^{l}\Gamma_1^{u}\Sigma^{1/2}$ and using Lemma 4.3

$$\begin{aligned}
&E[\mathrm{tr}\{(V_{11}^2)^{-1}\Gamma_2^u\Gamma_1^u\Sigma^{1/2}P'_{A_3,G_2'W_3G_2,G_2}\Sigma^{-1/2}\Gamma_1^{u'}\Gamma_2^{u'}\}]\\
&= c_2E[\mathrm{tr}\{(U_{11}^3)^{-1}\Gamma_2^u\Gamma_1^u\Sigma^{1/2}P'_{A_3,G_2'W_3G_2,G_2}\Sigma^{-1/2}\Gamma_1^{u'}\Gamma_1^{u'}\}]\\
&= c_2E[\mathrm{tr}\{(U_{11}^3)^{-1}P_{E_3,U_{11}^3}\}] = d_{2,3},
\end{aligned}$$

where E_3 is given by (4.84) and the last equality follows from (4.105). All these calculations establish the theorem. □

Theorems 4.12 and 4.13 imply the next result.

Theorem 4.14 *Consider the $EBRM_B^3$ presented in Definition 2.2 and apply the notation used in Theorems 4.12 and 4.13. Then*

$$\begin{aligned}
D[\widehat{E[X]}] &= D[\sum_{i=1}^{3} A_i\widehat{B}_iC_i]\\
&= D[P_{A_1,S_1}XP_{C_1'} + P_{\widehat{Q}_1'A_2,\widehat{S}_2}XP_{C_2'} + P_{\widehat{Q}_2'\widehat{Q}_1'A_3,\widehat{S}_3}XP_{C_3'}]\\
&= D[P_{A_1,S_1}XP_{C_1'}] + D[P_{\widehat{Q}_1'A_2,\widehat{S}_2}XP_{C_2'}] + D[P_{\widehat{Q}_2'\widehat{Q}_1'A_3,\widehat{S}_3}XP_{C_3'}]\\
&\quad +2C[P_{A_1,S_1}XP_{C_1'}, P_{\widehat{Q}_1'A_2,\widehat{S}_2}XP_{C_2'}]\\
&\quad +2C[P_{A_1,S_1}XP_{C_1'}, P_{\widehat{Q}_2'\widehat{Q}_1'A_3,\widehat{S}_3}XP_{C_3'}]\\
&\quad +2C[P_{\widehat{Q}_1'A_2,\widehat{S}_2}XP_{C_2'}, P_{\widehat{Q}_2'\widehat{Q}_1'A_3,\widehat{S}_3}XP_{C_3'}]\\
&= f_1P_{C_1'}\otimes K_1 + P_{C_2'}\otimes(3d_{1,2}K_1 + (f_2+2)K_2)\\
&\quad +P_{C_3'}\otimes(3d_{1,3}K_1 - d_{2,3}K_2 + (f_3+2)K_3).
\end{aligned}$$

Now the expectation of $\widehat{\Sigma}$ is considered (see Theorem 3.2 for a presentation of $\widehat{\Sigma}$). The necessary calculations will be similar, but easier than those presented above, because certain random matrices are not included in the expressions given below.

Theorem 4.15 *Let K_i be defined in Theorem 4.12 and let m_r and c_r be defined by (4.78) and (4.86), respectively. Put*

$$g_{i,j} = c_ic_{i+1}\times\cdots\times c_{j-1}m_j/(n - r(C_j) - m_j - 1), \qquad i < j \leq 3, \tag{4.118}$$

$$g_{j,j} = m_j/(n - r(C_j) - m_j - 1),$$

which are supposed to be finite and positive. For the $EBRM_B^3$, let $\widehat{\boldsymbol{\Sigma}}$ be as in Theorem 3.2, i.e.

$$n\widehat{\boldsymbol{\Sigma}} = \boldsymbol{X}(\boldsymbol{I} - \boldsymbol{P}_{C_1'})\boldsymbol{X}' + \widehat{\boldsymbol{Q}}_1'\boldsymbol{X}(\boldsymbol{P}_{C_1'} - \boldsymbol{P}_{C_2'})\boldsymbol{X}'\widehat{\boldsymbol{Q}}_1$$
$$+\widehat{\boldsymbol{Q}}_2'\widehat{\boldsymbol{Q}}_1'\boldsymbol{X}(\boldsymbol{P}_{C_2'} - \boldsymbol{P}_{C_3'})\boldsymbol{X}'\widehat{\boldsymbol{Q}}_1\widehat{\boldsymbol{Q}}_2 + \widehat{\boldsymbol{Q}}_3'\widehat{\boldsymbol{Q}}_2'\widehat{\boldsymbol{Q}}_1'\boldsymbol{X}\boldsymbol{P}_{C_3'}\boldsymbol{X}'\widehat{\boldsymbol{Q}}_1\widehat{\boldsymbol{Q}}_2\widehat{\boldsymbol{Q}}_3, \quad (4.119)$$

where $\widehat{\boldsymbol{Q}}_i$ is defined in Theorem 3.2. Then

$$E[n\widehat{\boldsymbol{\Sigma}}] = (n - r(\boldsymbol{C}_1))\boldsymbol{\Sigma} + \sum_{j=2}^{3}(r(\boldsymbol{C}_{j-1}) - r(\boldsymbol{C}_j))$$
$$\times(\sum_{i=1}^{j-1} g_{i,j-1}\boldsymbol{K}_i + \boldsymbol{\Sigma}\boldsymbol{G}_{j-1}(\boldsymbol{G}_{j-1}'\boldsymbol{\Sigma}\boldsymbol{G}_{j-1})^{-1}\boldsymbol{G}_{j-1}'\boldsymbol{\Sigma})$$
$$+r(\boldsymbol{C}_3)(\sum_{i=1}^{3} g_{i,3}\boldsymbol{K}_i + \boldsymbol{\Sigma}\boldsymbol{G}_3(\boldsymbol{G}_3'\boldsymbol{\Sigma}\boldsymbol{G}_3)^{-1}\boldsymbol{G}_3'\boldsymbol{\Sigma}).$$

Proof The proof of the theorem could be based on many of the calculations and established relations which were used when verifying Theorems 4.12 and 4.13. However, since the problem is now somewhat simpler, the proof will mainly rest on taking the expectations of squares of $\boldsymbol{Z}_{r,s}$, defined in (4.107) and (4.108). From the given expression of $n\widehat{\boldsymbol{\Sigma}}$, it follows that the expectations of $\boldsymbol{X}(\boldsymbol{I} - \boldsymbol{P}_{C_1'})\boldsymbol{X}'$, $\widehat{\boldsymbol{Q}}_1'\boldsymbol{X}(\boldsymbol{P}_{C_1'} - \boldsymbol{P}_{C_2'})\boldsymbol{X}'\widehat{\boldsymbol{Q}}_1$, $\widehat{\boldsymbol{Q}}_2'\widehat{\boldsymbol{Q}}_1'\boldsymbol{X}(\boldsymbol{P}_{C_2'} - \boldsymbol{P}_{C_3'})\boldsymbol{X}'\widehat{\boldsymbol{Q}}_1\widehat{\boldsymbol{Q}}_2$ and $\widehat{\boldsymbol{Q}}_3'\widehat{\boldsymbol{Q}}_2'\widehat{\boldsymbol{Q}}_1'\boldsymbol{X}\boldsymbol{P}_{C_3'}\boldsymbol{X}'\widehat{\boldsymbol{Q}}_1\widehat{\boldsymbol{Q}}_2\widehat{\boldsymbol{Q}}_3$ are needed. When obtaining the moments, Facts (i)–(iii) presented at the beginning of Sect. 4.6 will be utilized. The following moment expressions will be used:

$$E[\boldsymbol{X}(\boldsymbol{I} - \boldsymbol{P}_{C_1'})\boldsymbol{X}'] = (n - r(\boldsymbol{C}_1))\boldsymbol{\Sigma},$$
$$E[\boldsymbol{X}(\boldsymbol{P}_{C_{j-1}'} - \boldsymbol{P}_{C_j'})\boldsymbol{X}'] = (r(\boldsymbol{C}_{j-1}) - r(\boldsymbol{C}_j))\boldsymbol{\Sigma}, \qquad j = 2, 3,$$
$$E[\boldsymbol{X}\boldsymbol{P}_{C_3'}\boldsymbol{X}'] = r(\boldsymbol{C}_3)\boldsymbol{\Sigma}.$$

Then it follows from (4.119) that the theorem is verified if it is shown that

$$E[\widehat{\boldsymbol{Q}}_1'\boldsymbol{\Sigma}\widehat{\boldsymbol{Q}}_1] = g_{1,1}\boldsymbol{K}_1 + \boldsymbol{\Sigma}\boldsymbol{G}_1(\boldsymbol{G}_1'\boldsymbol{\Sigma}\boldsymbol{G}_1)^{-1}\boldsymbol{G}_1'\boldsymbol{\Sigma}, \quad (4.120)$$

$$E[\widehat{\boldsymbol{Q}}_2'\widehat{\boldsymbol{Q}}_1'\boldsymbol{\Sigma}\widehat{\boldsymbol{Q}}_1\widehat{\boldsymbol{Q}}_2] = g_{1,2}\boldsymbol{K}_1 + g_{2,2}\boldsymbol{K}_2 + \boldsymbol{\Sigma}\boldsymbol{G}_2(\boldsymbol{G}_2'\boldsymbol{\Sigma}\boldsymbol{G}_2)^{-1}\boldsymbol{G}_2'\boldsymbol{\Sigma}, \quad (4.121)$$

$$E[\widehat{\boldsymbol{Q}}_3'\widehat{\boldsymbol{Q}}_2'\widehat{\boldsymbol{Q}}_1'\boldsymbol{\Sigma}\widehat{\boldsymbol{Q}}_1\widehat{\boldsymbol{Q}}_2\widehat{\boldsymbol{Q}}_3] = g_{1,3}\boldsymbol{K}_1 + g_{2,3}\boldsymbol{K}_2 + g_{3,3}\boldsymbol{K}_3$$
$$+ \boldsymbol{\Sigma}\boldsymbol{G}_3(\boldsymbol{G}_3'\boldsymbol{\Sigma}\boldsymbol{G}_3)^{-1}\boldsymbol{G}_3'\boldsymbol{\Sigma}. \quad (4.122)$$

Expression (4.120) is true, since

$$
\begin{aligned}
E[\widehat{\boldsymbol{Q}}_1'\boldsymbol{\Sigma}\widehat{\boldsymbol{Q}}_1] &= E[\boldsymbol{Z}_{1,1}\boldsymbol{\Sigma}\boldsymbol{Z}_{1,1}'] = \boldsymbol{\Sigma}^{1/2}\boldsymbol{\Gamma}_1' E[\boldsymbol{M}_1\boldsymbol{M}_1']\boldsymbol{\Gamma}_1\boldsymbol{\Sigma}^{1/2} \\
&= \boldsymbol{\Sigma}^{1/2}\boldsymbol{\Gamma}_1^{u'}\boldsymbol{\Gamma}_1^{u}\boldsymbol{\Sigma}^{1/2} + \boldsymbol{\Sigma}^{1/2}\boldsymbol{\Gamma}_1^{l'}\boldsymbol{\Gamma}_1^{l}\boldsymbol{\Sigma}^{1/2}E[\mathrm{tr}\{(\boldsymbol{V}_{11}^1)^{-1}\}] \\
&= \boldsymbol{\Sigma}\boldsymbol{G}_1(\boldsymbol{G}_1'\boldsymbol{\Sigma}\boldsymbol{G}_1)^{-1}\boldsymbol{G}_1'\boldsymbol{\Sigma} + g_{1,1}\boldsymbol{K}_1,
\end{aligned}
$$

where $\boldsymbol{M}_r$ is defined in (4.83), $r = 1$, and $E[\mathrm{tr}\{(\boldsymbol{V}_{11}^1)^{-1}\}]$ follows from Appendix B, Theorem B.21 (i).

Concerning (4.121),

$$
\begin{aligned}
E[\widehat{\boldsymbol{Q}}_2'\widehat{\boldsymbol{Q}}_1'\boldsymbol{\Sigma}\widehat{\boldsymbol{Q}}_1\widehat{\boldsymbol{Q}}_2] &= E[\boldsymbol{Z}_{1,2}\boldsymbol{\Sigma}\boldsymbol{Z}_{1,2}'] = \boldsymbol{\Sigma}^{1/2}\boldsymbol{\Gamma}_1' E[\boldsymbol{M}_1\boldsymbol{Z}_{2,2}\boldsymbol{\Sigma}\boldsymbol{Z}_{2,2}'\boldsymbol{M}_1']\boldsymbol{\Gamma}_1\boldsymbol{\Sigma}^{1/2} \\
&= \boldsymbol{\Sigma}^{1/2}\boldsymbol{\Gamma}_1^{u'}E[\boldsymbol{Z}_{2,2}\boldsymbol{\Sigma}\boldsymbol{Z}_{2,2}']\boldsymbol{\Gamma}_1^{u}\boldsymbol{\Sigma}^{1/2} + \boldsymbol{\Sigma}^{1/2}\boldsymbol{\Gamma}_1^{l'}\boldsymbol{\Gamma}_1^{l}\boldsymbol{\Sigma}^{1/2}E[\mathrm{tr}\{(\boldsymbol{V}_{11}^1)^{-1}\boldsymbol{Z}_{2,2}\boldsymbol{\Sigma}\boldsymbol{Z}_{2,2}'\}] \\
&= \boldsymbol{\Sigma}^{1/2}\boldsymbol{\Gamma}_1^{u'}\boldsymbol{\Gamma}_2'E[\boldsymbol{M}_2\boldsymbol{M}_2']\boldsymbol{\Gamma}_2\boldsymbol{\Gamma}_1^{u}\boldsymbol{\Sigma}^{1/2} + c_1\boldsymbol{\Sigma}^{1/2}\boldsymbol{\Gamma}_1^{l'}\boldsymbol{\Gamma}_1^{l}\boldsymbol{\Sigma}^{1/2}E[\mathrm{tr}\{(\boldsymbol{U}_{11}^2)^{-1}\boldsymbol{Z}_{2,2}\boldsymbol{\Sigma}\boldsymbol{Z}_{2,2}'\}] \\
&= \boldsymbol{\Sigma}^{1/2}\boldsymbol{\Gamma}_1^{u'}\boldsymbol{\Gamma}_2^{u'}\boldsymbol{\Gamma}_2^{u}\boldsymbol{\Gamma}_1^{u}\boldsymbol{\Sigma}^{1/2} + \boldsymbol{\Sigma}^{1/2}\boldsymbol{\Gamma}_1^{u'}\boldsymbol{\Gamma}_2^{l'}\boldsymbol{\Gamma}_2^{l}\boldsymbol{\Gamma}_1^{u}\boldsymbol{\Sigma}^{1/2}E[\mathrm{tr}\{(\boldsymbol{V}_{11}^2)^{-1}\}] \\
&\quad + c_1\boldsymbol{\Sigma}^{1/2}\boldsymbol{\Gamma}_1^{l'}\boldsymbol{\Gamma}_1^{l}\boldsymbol{\Sigma}^{1/2}E[\mathrm{tr}\{(\boldsymbol{V}_{11}^2)^{-1}\}] \\
&= \boldsymbol{\Sigma}\boldsymbol{G}_2(\boldsymbol{G}_2'\boldsymbol{\Sigma}\boldsymbol{G}_2)^{-1}\boldsymbol{G}_2'\boldsymbol{\Sigma} + g_{1,2}\boldsymbol{K}_1 + g_{2,2}\boldsymbol{K}_2.
\end{aligned}
$$

Finally, (4.122) is presented and the ideas for proving the result are similar to those used when calculating (4.120) and (4.121):

$$
\begin{aligned}
E[\widehat{\boldsymbol{Q}}_3'\widehat{\boldsymbol{Q}}_2'\widehat{\boldsymbol{Q}}_1'\boldsymbol{\Sigma}\widehat{\boldsymbol{Q}}_1\widehat{\boldsymbol{Q}}_2\widehat{\boldsymbol{Q}}_3] &= E[\boldsymbol{Z}_{1,3}\boldsymbol{\Sigma}\boldsymbol{Z}_{1,3}'] \\
&= \boldsymbol{\Sigma}\boldsymbol{G}_3(\boldsymbol{G}_3'\boldsymbol{\Sigma}\boldsymbol{G}_3)^{-1}\boldsymbol{G}_3'\boldsymbol{\Sigma} + g_{3,3}\boldsymbol{K}_3 + g_{1,3}\boldsymbol{K}_1 + g_{2,3}\boldsymbol{K}_2.
\end{aligned}
$$

Hence, based on the above-derived formulas, it is straightforward to obtain $E[\boldsymbol{X}(\boldsymbol{I} - \boldsymbol{P}_{\boldsymbol{C}_1'})\boldsymbol{X}']$, $E[\widehat{\boldsymbol{Q}}_1'\boldsymbol{X}(\boldsymbol{P}_{\boldsymbol{C}_1'} - \boldsymbol{P}_{\boldsymbol{C}_2'})\boldsymbol{X}'\widehat{\boldsymbol{Q}}_1]$, $E[\widehat{\boldsymbol{Q}}_2'\widehat{\boldsymbol{Q}}_1'\boldsymbol{X}(\boldsymbol{P}_{\boldsymbol{C}_2'} - \boldsymbol{P}_{\boldsymbol{C}_3'})\boldsymbol{X}'\widehat{\boldsymbol{Q}}_1\widehat{\boldsymbol{Q}}_2]$ and $E[\widehat{\boldsymbol{Q}}_3'\widehat{\boldsymbol{Q}}_2'\widehat{\boldsymbol{Q}}_1'\boldsymbol{X}\boldsymbol{P}_{\boldsymbol{C}_3'}\boldsymbol{X}'\widehat{\boldsymbol{Q}}_1\widehat{\boldsymbol{Q}}_2\widehat{\boldsymbol{Q}}_3]$, and then the theorem is established. □

As shown in Theorem 4.15, the estimator $\widehat{\boldsymbol{\Sigma}}$ is not an unbiased estimator. This is by no means unexpected, because this fact has already been observed when $m = 1$ in the $EBRM_B^m$, i.e. the BRM. It can be shown that

$$
\begin{aligned}
E[n\widehat{\boldsymbol{\Sigma}}] &= n\boldsymbol{\Sigma} \\
&\quad + \sum_{j=2}^{3}\sum_{i=1}^{j-1}(r(\boldsymbol{C}_{j-1}) - r(\boldsymbol{C}_j))(g_{i,j-1} - 1)\boldsymbol{K}_i + r(\boldsymbol{C}_3)\sum_{i=1}^{3}(g_{i,3} - 1)\boldsymbol{K}_i,
\end{aligned}
$$

where $K_i, i = 1, 2, 3$, are given in Theorem 4.12. Therefore, if unbiased estimators of $K_i, i = 1, 2, 3$, can be found, an unbiased estimator of $\widehat{\Sigma}$ is available. Copying previous calculations yields

$$E[A_1(A_1'\widehat{\Sigma}^{-1}A_1)^- A_1'] = E[A_1(A_1'S_1^{-1}A_1)^- A_1'] = (n - r(C_1) - m_1)K_1,$$

$$E[\widehat{Q}_1'A_2(A_2'\widehat{Q}_1\widehat{\Sigma}^{-1}\widehat{Q}_1'A_2)^- A_2'\widehat{Q}_1] = E[\widehat{Q}_1'A_2(A_2'\widehat{Q}_1\widehat{S}_2^{-1}\widehat{Q}_1'A_2)^- A_2'\widehat{Q}_1]$$
$$= (n - r(C_2) - m_1 + p - m_2)K_2 + c_1(p - m_2)K_1,$$

$$E[\widehat{Q}_1'\widehat{Q}_2'A_3(A_3'\widehat{Q}_2\widehat{Q}_1\widehat{\Sigma}^{-1}\widehat{Q}_1'\widehat{Q}_2'A_3)^- A_3'\widehat{Q}_2\widehat{Q}_1]$$
$$= E[\widehat{Q}_1'\widehat{Q}_2'A_3(A_3'\widehat{Q}_2\widehat{Q}_1\widehat{S}_3^{-1}\widehat{Q}_1'\widehat{Q}_2'A_3)^- A_3'\widehat{Q}_2\widehat{Q}_1]$$
$$= (n - r(C_3) - m_2 + p - m_3)K_3 + c_1(p - m_3)K_2 + c_1c_2(p - m_3)K_1.$$

From these expressions unbiased estimators of $K_i, i = 1, 2, 3$, let us say $\widehat{K}_i$, can be obtained which are pure functions of the MLE of Σ. Hence, the next theorem has been established.

Theorem 4.16 *With $\widehat{\Sigma}$ as presented in Theorem 4.15, an unbiased estimator of Σ in the $EBRM_B^3$, presented in Definition 2.2, is given by*

$$\widehat{\Sigma}_U = \widehat{\Sigma} - \frac{1}{n}\sum_{j=2}^{3}\sum_{i=1}^{j-1}(r(C_{j-1}) - r(C_j))(g_{i,j-1} - 1)\widehat{K}_i - \frac{1}{n}r(C_3)(\sum_{i=1}^{3}(g_{i,3} - 1)\widehat{K}_i,$$

where

$$\widehat{K}_1 = \frac{1}{n - r(C_1) - m_1}A_1(A_1'\widehat{\Sigma}^{-1}A_1)^- A_1',$$

$$\widehat{K}_2 = \frac{1}{n - r(C_2) - m_1 + p - m_2}\widehat{Q}_1'A_2(A_2'\widehat{Q}_1\widehat{\Sigma}^{-1}\widehat{Q}_1'A_2)^- A_2'\widehat{Q}_1$$
$$- \frac{c_1(p - m_2)}{n - r(C_2) - m_1 + p - m_2}\widehat{K}_1,$$

$$\widehat{K}_3 = \frac{1}{n - r(C_3) - m_2 + p - m_3}\widehat{Q}_1'\widehat{Q}_2'A_3(A_3'\widehat{Q}_2\widehat{Q}_1\widehat{\Sigma}^{-1}\widehat{Q}_1'\widehat{Q}_2'A_3)^- A_3'\widehat{Q}_2\widehat{Q}_1$$
$$- \frac{c_1(p - m_3)}{n - r(C_3) - m_2 + p - m_3}\widehat{K}_2 - \frac{c_1c_2(p - m_3)}{n - r(C_3) - m_2 + p - m_3}\widehat{K}_1.$$

In the rest of this section $D[\widehat{B}_i]$ and $\widehat{D[\widehat{B}_i]}$, $i = 1, 2, 3$, will be considered. For $\widehat{B}_3$ it follows from Theorem 3.2 that

$$\widehat{B}_3 = (A_3'G_2(G_2'W_3G_2)^{-1}G_2'A_3)^{-1}A_3'G_2(G_2'W_3G_2)^{-1}G_2'XC_3'(C_3C_3')^{-1}, \tag{4.123}$$

where G_2 and W_3 are given by (4.73) and (4.74), respectively. Thus, from Corollary 4.1 (ii), if $n - k_3 - m_2 + q_3 - 1 > 0$,

$$D[\widehat{B}_3] = \frac{n - k_3 - 1}{n - k_3 - m_2 + q_3 - 1}(C_3C_3')^{-1} \otimes (A_3'G_2(G_2'\Sigma G_2)^{-1}G_2'A_3)^{-1}.$$

It is now shown how to obtain the dispersion matrix for $\widehat{B}_2$. Because of the assumption of uniqueness, given in Theorem 4.9 (iii),

$$G_1'A_2\widehat{B}_2C_2$$

can be studied, since

$$(A_2'G_1G_1'A_2)^{-1}A_2'G_1G_1'A_2\widehat{B}_2C_2C_2'(C_2C_2')^{-1} = \widehat{B}_2.$$

It has already been shown that $\widehat{B}_2$ is an unbiased estimator and therefore

$$G_1'A_2(\widehat{B}_2 - B_2)C_2 \tag{4.124}$$

is treated. The expression in (4.124) can be rewritten as

$$\begin{aligned}
G_1'A_2(\widehat{B}_2 - B_2)C_2 &= P_{G_1'A_2,G_1'W_2G_1}G_1'(X - E[X] - A_3(\widehat{B}_3 - B_3)C_3)P_{C_2'} \\
&= P_{G_1'A_2,G_1'W_2G_1}G_1'\{(X - E[X])(P_{C_2'} - P_{C_3'}) + (X - E[X])P_{C_3'} \\
&\quad -P_{A_3,G_2'W_3G_2,G_2}(X - E[X])P_{C_3'}\} \\
&= P_{G_1'A_2,G_1'W_2G_1}G_1'(X - E[X])(P_{C_2'} - P_{C_3'}) \\
&\quad +P_{G_1'A_2,G_1'W_2G_1}G_1'(I - P_{A_3,G_2'W_3G_2,G_2})(X - E[X])P_{C_3'}.
\end{aligned} \tag{4.125}$$

The idea behind the decomposition of $G_1'A_2(\widehat{B}_2 - B_2)C_2$ is that the components are partly independent: $(X - E[X])P_{C_3'}$ is independent of $(X - E[X])(P_{C_2'} - P_{C_3'})$, $P_{G_1'A_2,G_1'W_2G_1}G_1'$ and $P_{A_3,G_2'W_3G_2,G_2}$, because W_2 and W_3 are independent of $XP_{C_3'}$. Hence,

$$C\Big[P_{G_1'A_2,G_1'W_2G_1}G_1'(X - E[X])(P_{C_2'} - P_{C_3'}), \\
P_{G_1'A_2,G_1'W_2G_1}(I - P_{A_3,G_2'W_3G_2,G_2})(X - E[X])P_{C_3'}\Big] = 0$$

and therefore

$$\begin{aligned}
&D[G_1'A_2(\widehat{B}_2 - B_2)C_2] \\
&\quad = D[P_{G_1'A_2,G_1'W_2G_1}G_1'(X - E[X])(P_{C_2'} - P_{C_3'})] &(4.126)\\
&\quad +D[P_{G_1'A_2,G_1'W_2G_1}(I - P_{A_3,G_2'W_3G_2,G_2})(X - E[X])P_{C_3'}]. &(4.127)
\end{aligned}$$

The two expressions given by (4.126) and (4.127) are now treated separately. Firstly,

$$D[\boldsymbol{P}_{G_1'A_2,G_1'W_2G_1}\boldsymbol{G}_1'(\boldsymbol{X}-E[\boldsymbol{X}])(\boldsymbol{P}_{C_2'}-\boldsymbol{P}_{C_3'})]$$
$$=(\boldsymbol{P}_{C_2'}-\boldsymbol{P}_{C_3'})\otimes E[\boldsymbol{P}_{G_1'A_2,G_1'W_2G_1}\boldsymbol{G}_1'\boldsymbol{\Sigma}\boldsymbol{G}_1\boldsymbol{P}'_{G_1'A_2,G_1'W_2G_1}]$$

and the rest follows from the treatment of the BRM, e.g. see (4.23). Thus, (4.126) equals

$$D[\boldsymbol{P}_{G_1'A_2,G_1'W_2G_1}\boldsymbol{G}_1'(\boldsymbol{X}-E[\boldsymbol{X}])(\boldsymbol{P}_{C_2'}-\boldsymbol{P}_{C_3'})]=(\boldsymbol{P}_{C_2'}-\boldsymbol{P}_{C_3'})$$
$$\otimes\frac{n-r(\boldsymbol{C}_2)-1}{n-r(\boldsymbol{C}_1)-m_1+r(\boldsymbol{G}_1'\boldsymbol{A}_2)-1}\boldsymbol{P}_{G_1'A_2,G_1'\Sigma G_1}\boldsymbol{G}_1'\boldsymbol{\Sigma}\boldsymbol{G}_1. \quad (4.128)$$

Secondly, the expression (4.127) is treated, which is somewhat more complicated to handle. Note that

$$D[\boldsymbol{P}_{G_1'A_2,G_1'W_2G_1}\boldsymbol{G}_1'(\boldsymbol{I}-\boldsymbol{P}_{A_3,G_2'W_3G_2,G_2})(\boldsymbol{X}-E[\boldsymbol{X}])\boldsymbol{P}_{C_3'}]=\boldsymbol{P}_{C_3'}\otimes$$
$$E[\boldsymbol{P}_{G_1'A_2,G_1'W_2G_1}\boldsymbol{G}_1'(\boldsymbol{I}-\boldsymbol{P}_{A_3,G_2'W_3G_2,G_2})\boldsymbol{\Sigma}(\boldsymbol{I}-\boldsymbol{P}'_{A_3,G_2'W_3G_2,G_2})\boldsymbol{G}_1\boldsymbol{P}'_{G_1'A_2,G_1'W_2G_1}]$$

and

$$\boldsymbol{P}_{G_1'A_2,G_1'W_2G_1}\boldsymbol{G}_1'=\boldsymbol{H}_1\boldsymbol{\Gamma}_2^{l'}\boldsymbol{\Gamma}_2^{l}\boldsymbol{\Gamma}_1^{u}\boldsymbol{\Sigma}^{-1/2}-\boldsymbol{H}_1\boldsymbol{\Gamma}_2^{l'}\boldsymbol{V}_{21}^2(\boldsymbol{V}_{11}^2)^{-1}\boldsymbol{\Gamma}_2^{u}\boldsymbol{\Gamma}_1^{u}\boldsymbol{\Sigma}^{-1/2}, \quad (4.129)$$

where $\boldsymbol{\Gamma}_1$, $\boldsymbol{\Gamma}_2$ and $\boldsymbol{H}_1$ are defined in (4.75) and (4.76). Then, because $E[\boldsymbol{V}_{21}^2(\boldsymbol{V}_{11}^2)^{-1}]=\boldsymbol{0}$,

$$E[\boldsymbol{P}_{G_1'A_2,G_1'W_2G_1}\boldsymbol{G}_1'(\boldsymbol{I}-\boldsymbol{P}_{A_3,G_2'W_3G_2,G_2})\boldsymbol{\Sigma}(\boldsymbol{I}-\boldsymbol{P}'_{A_3,G_2'W_3G_2,G_2})\boldsymbol{G}_1\boldsymbol{P}'_{G_1'A_2,G_1'W_2G_1}]$$
$$=E[\boldsymbol{H}_1\boldsymbol{\Gamma}_2^{l'}\boldsymbol{\Gamma}_2^{l}\boldsymbol{\Gamma}_1^{u}\boldsymbol{\Sigma}^{-1/2}(\boldsymbol{I}-\boldsymbol{P}_{A_3,G_2'W_3G_2,G_2})\boldsymbol{\Sigma}(\boldsymbol{I}-\boldsymbol{P}_{A_3,G_2'W_3G_2,G_2})\boldsymbol{\Sigma}^{-1/2}\boldsymbol{\Gamma}_1^{u'}\boldsymbol{\Gamma}_2^{l'}\boldsymbol{\Gamma}_2^{l}\boldsymbol{H}_1']$$
$$+E\Big[\boldsymbol{H}_1\boldsymbol{\Gamma}_2^{l'}\boldsymbol{V}_{21}^2(\boldsymbol{V}_{11}^2)^{-1}\boldsymbol{\Gamma}_2^{u}\boldsymbol{\Gamma}_1^{u}\boldsymbol{\Sigma}^{-1/2}(\boldsymbol{I}-\boldsymbol{P}_{A_3,G_2'W_3G_2,G_2})\boldsymbol{\Sigma}(\boldsymbol{I}-\boldsymbol{P}'_{A_3,G_2'W_3G_2,G_2})$$
$$\times\boldsymbol{\Sigma}^{-1/2}\boldsymbol{\Gamma}_1^{u'}\boldsymbol{\Gamma}_2^{u'}(\boldsymbol{V}_{11}^2)^{-1}\boldsymbol{V}_{12}^2\boldsymbol{\Gamma}_2^{l}\boldsymbol{H}_1'\Big]. \quad (4.130)$$

The two expressions on the right-hand side of (4.130) will from now on be considered separately. The difference between obtaining moments for the mean parameters and obtaining moments for $\widehat{E[\boldsymbol{X}]}$ or $\widehat{\boldsymbol{\Sigma}}$ is that in the latter cases one has not to rely on uniqueness for the mean parameters. Concerning $\widehat{\boldsymbol{B}}_2$, it follows from the proof of Theorem 4.9 (iii) that in order for $\widehat{\boldsymbol{B}}_2$ to be unique, $\mathcal{C}(\boldsymbol{A}_3'\boldsymbol{G}_1)=\mathcal{C}(\boldsymbol{A}_3'\boldsymbol{G}_2)$ has to be true. Thus, utilizing (4.79),

$$\boldsymbol{\Gamma}_1^{u}\boldsymbol{\Sigma}^{-1/2}\boldsymbol{A}_3=\boldsymbol{Z}\boldsymbol{\Gamma}_2^{u}\boldsymbol{\Gamma}_1^{u}\boldsymbol{\Sigma}^{-1/2}\boldsymbol{A}_3$$

for some matrix $\mathbf{Z}$, and

$$\boldsymbol{\Gamma}_1^u\boldsymbol{\Sigma}^{-1/2}(\boldsymbol{I}-\boldsymbol{P}_{A_3,G_2'W_3G_2,G_2})$$
$$=\boldsymbol{\Gamma}_1^u\boldsymbol{\Sigma}^{-1/2}-\boldsymbol{Z}\boldsymbol{\Gamma}_3^{l'}\boldsymbol{\Gamma}_3^l\boldsymbol{\Gamma}_2^u\boldsymbol{\Gamma}_1^u\boldsymbol{\Sigma}^{-1/2}+\boldsymbol{Z}\boldsymbol{\Gamma}_3^{l'}\boldsymbol{V}_{21}^3(\boldsymbol{V}_{11}^3)^{-1}\boldsymbol{\Gamma}_3^u\boldsymbol{\Gamma}_2^u\boldsymbol{\Gamma}_1^u\boldsymbol{\Sigma}^{-1/2}.$$

Then, since $E[\boldsymbol{V}_{21}^3(\boldsymbol{V}_{11}^3)^{-1}]=\mathbf{0}$ and $\boldsymbol{\Gamma}_2^l\boldsymbol{\Gamma}_2^{u'}=\mathbf{0}$,

$$E[\boldsymbol{H}_1\boldsymbol{\Gamma}_2^{l'}\boldsymbol{\Gamma}_2^l\boldsymbol{\Gamma}_1^u\boldsymbol{\Sigma}^{-1/2}(\boldsymbol{I}-\boldsymbol{P}_{A_3,G_2'W_3G_2,G_2})\boldsymbol{\Sigma}(\boldsymbol{I}-\boldsymbol{P}'_{A_3,G_2'W_3G_2,G_2})\boldsymbol{\Sigma}^{-1/2}\boldsymbol{\Gamma}_1^{u'}\boldsymbol{\Gamma}_2^{l'}\boldsymbol{\Gamma}_2^l\boldsymbol{H}_1']$$
$$=\boldsymbol{H}_1\boldsymbol{\Gamma}_2^{l'}\boldsymbol{\Gamma}_2^l\boldsymbol{H}_1'+\frac{n-r(\boldsymbol{C}_3)-1}{n-r(\boldsymbol{C}_3)-m_3-1}\boldsymbol{H}_1\boldsymbol{\Gamma}_2^{l'}\boldsymbol{\Gamma}_2^l\boldsymbol{Z}\boldsymbol{\Gamma}_3^{l'}\boldsymbol{\Gamma}_3^l\boldsymbol{Z}'\boldsymbol{\Gamma}_2^{l'}\boldsymbol{\Gamma}_2^l\boldsymbol{H}_1',$$

where $\boldsymbol{H}_1\boldsymbol{\Gamma}_2^{l'}\boldsymbol{\Gamma}_2^l\boldsymbol{H}_1'$ and $\boldsymbol{H}_1\boldsymbol{\Gamma}_2^{l'}\boldsymbol{\Gamma}_2^l\boldsymbol{Z}\boldsymbol{\Gamma}_3^{l'}\boldsymbol{\Gamma}_3^l\boldsymbol{Z}'\boldsymbol{\Gamma}_2^{l'}\boldsymbol{\Gamma}_2^l\boldsymbol{H}_1'$ now have to be expressed in the original matrices. A few calculations show that

$$\boldsymbol{\Gamma}_3^{l'}\boldsymbol{\Gamma}_3^l=\boldsymbol{\Gamma}_2^u\boldsymbol{\Gamma}_1^u\boldsymbol{\Sigma}^{-1/2}\boldsymbol{A}_3(\boldsymbol{A}_3'\boldsymbol{G}_2(\boldsymbol{G}_2'\boldsymbol{\Sigma}\boldsymbol{G}_2)^{-1}\boldsymbol{G}_2'\boldsymbol{A}_3)^-\boldsymbol{A}_3'\boldsymbol{\Sigma}^{-1/2}\boldsymbol{\Gamma}_1^{u'}\boldsymbol{\Gamma}_2^{u'},\tag{4.131}$$
$$\boldsymbol{\Gamma}_2^{l'}\boldsymbol{\Gamma}_2^l=\boldsymbol{\Gamma}_1^u\boldsymbol{\Sigma}^{-1/2}\boldsymbol{A}_2(\boldsymbol{A}_2'\boldsymbol{G}_1(\boldsymbol{G}_1'\boldsymbol{\Sigma}\boldsymbol{G}_1)^{-1}\boldsymbol{G}_1'\boldsymbol{A}_2)^-\boldsymbol{A}_2'\boldsymbol{\Sigma}^{-1/2}\boldsymbol{\Gamma}_1^{u'},\tag{4.132}$$
$$\boldsymbol{\Gamma}_1^{u'}\boldsymbol{\Gamma}_1^u=\boldsymbol{\Sigma}^{1/2}\boldsymbol{G}_1(\boldsymbol{G}_1'\boldsymbol{\Sigma}\boldsymbol{G}_1)^{-1}\boldsymbol{G}_1'\boldsymbol{\Sigma}^{1/2},\tag{4.133}$$

and then (4.132) implies the relation

$$\boldsymbol{H}_1\boldsymbol{\Gamma}_2^{l'}\boldsymbol{\Gamma}_2^l=\boldsymbol{G}_1\boldsymbol{A}_2(\boldsymbol{A}_2'\boldsymbol{G}_1(\boldsymbol{G}_1'\boldsymbol{\Sigma}\boldsymbol{G}_1)^{-1}\boldsymbol{G}_1'\boldsymbol{A}_2)^-\boldsymbol{A}_2'\boldsymbol{\Sigma}^{-1/2}\boldsymbol{\Gamma}_1^{u'}$$

and (4.131) implies that

$$\boldsymbol{Z}\boldsymbol{\Gamma}_3^{l'}\boldsymbol{\Gamma}_3^l\boldsymbol{Z}'=\boldsymbol{\Gamma}_1^u\boldsymbol{\Sigma}^{-1/2}\boldsymbol{A}_3(\boldsymbol{A}_3'\boldsymbol{G}_2(\boldsymbol{G}_2'\boldsymbol{\Sigma}\boldsymbol{G}_2)^{-1}\boldsymbol{G}_2'\boldsymbol{A}_3)^-\boldsymbol{A}_3'\boldsymbol{\Sigma}^{-1/2}\boldsymbol{\Gamma}_1^{u'}.$$

Moreover, using (4.133) the first expression on the right-hand side of (4.130) equals

$$E[\boldsymbol{H}_1\boldsymbol{\Gamma}_2^{l'}\boldsymbol{\Gamma}_2^l\boldsymbol{\Gamma}_1^u\boldsymbol{\Sigma}^{-1/2}(\boldsymbol{I}-\boldsymbol{P}_{A_3,G_2'W_3G_2,G_2})\boldsymbol{\Sigma}(\boldsymbol{I}-\boldsymbol{P}'_{A_3,G_2'W_3G_2,G_2})\boldsymbol{\Sigma}^{-1/2}\boldsymbol{\Gamma}_1^{u'}\boldsymbol{\Gamma}_2^{l'}\boldsymbol{\Gamma}_2^l\boldsymbol{H}_1']$$
$$=\tfrac{n-r(\boldsymbol{C}_3)-1}{n-r(\boldsymbol{C}_3)-m_3-1}\boldsymbol{P}_{G_1'A_2,G_1'\Sigma G_1}\boldsymbol{G}_1'\boldsymbol{A}_3(\boldsymbol{A}_3'\boldsymbol{G}_2(\boldsymbol{G}_2'\boldsymbol{\Sigma}\boldsymbol{G}_2)^{-1}\boldsymbol{G}_2'\boldsymbol{A}_3)^-\boldsymbol{A}_3'\boldsymbol{G}_1\boldsymbol{P}'_{G_1'A_2,G_1'\Sigma G_1}$$
$$+\boldsymbol{P}_{G_1'A_2,G_1'\Sigma G_1}\boldsymbol{G}_1'\boldsymbol{\Sigma}\boldsymbol{G}_1.\tag{4.134}$$

The second term on the right-hand side of (4.130) can after some calculations be shown to equal

$$E\Big[\boldsymbol{H}_1\boldsymbol{\Gamma}_2^{l'}\boldsymbol{V}_{21}^2(\boldsymbol{V}_{11}^2)^{-1}\boldsymbol{\Gamma}_2^u\boldsymbol{\Gamma}_1^u\boldsymbol{\Sigma}^{-1/2}(\boldsymbol{I}-\boldsymbol{P}_{A_3,G_2'W_3G_2,G_2})\boldsymbol{\Sigma}(\boldsymbol{I}-\boldsymbol{P}'_{A_3,G_2'W_3G_2,G_2})\boldsymbol{\Sigma}^{-1/2}\boldsymbol{\Gamma}_1^{u'}\boldsymbol{\Gamma}_2^{u'}$$
$$\times(\boldsymbol{V}_{11}^2)^{-1}\boldsymbol{V}_{12}^2\boldsymbol{\Gamma}_2^l\boldsymbol{H}_1'\Big]$$
$$=\boldsymbol{H}_1\boldsymbol{\Gamma}_2^{l'}\boldsymbol{\Gamma}_2^l\boldsymbol{H}_1'E[\mathrm{tr}\{(\boldsymbol{V}_{11}^2)^{-1}\boldsymbol{\Gamma}_2^u\boldsymbol{\Gamma}_1^u\boldsymbol{\Sigma}^{-1/2}(\boldsymbol{I}-\boldsymbol{P}_{A_3,G_2'W_3G_2,G_2}\boldsymbol{\Sigma}(\boldsymbol{I}-\boldsymbol{P}'_{A_3,G_2'W_3G_2,G_2})$$
$$\times\boldsymbol{\Sigma}^{-1/2}\boldsymbol{\Gamma}_1^{u'}\boldsymbol{\Gamma}_2^{u'}\}],\tag{4.135}$$

and the remaining task is to obtain the expectation of the trace function in (4.135). However, the necessary calculations have by now been repeated several times and therefore, without showing any details, it is stated that

$$
\begin{aligned}
&E[\mathrm{tr}\{(\boldsymbol{V}_{11}^2)^{-1}\boldsymbol{\Gamma}_2^u\boldsymbol{\Gamma}_1^u\boldsymbol{\Sigma}^{-1/2}(\boldsymbol{I}-\boldsymbol{P}_{A_3,G_2'W_3G_2,G_2})\boldsymbol{\Sigma}(\boldsymbol{I}-\boldsymbol{P}'_{A_3,G_2'W_3G_2,G_2})\boldsymbol{\Sigma}^{-1/2}\boldsymbol{\Gamma}_1^{u'}\boldsymbol{\Gamma}_2^{u'}\}]\\
&\quad = c_2E[\mathrm{tr}\{(\boldsymbol{U}_{11}^3)^{-1}\boldsymbol{U}_{11}^3\boldsymbol{\Gamma}_3^{u'}(\boldsymbol{V}_{11}^3)^{-1}(\boldsymbol{V}_{11}^3)^{-1}\boldsymbol{\Gamma}_3^u\boldsymbol{U}_{11}^3\}]\\
&\quad = c_2E[\mathrm{tr}\{(\boldsymbol{V}_{11}^3)^{-1}\}] = c_2\frac{m_3}{n-r(\boldsymbol{C}_3)-m_3-1},
\end{aligned}
\tag{4.136}
$$

where $\boldsymbol{U}_{11}^3$ is defined in (4.82).

Hence, by using (4.126)–(4.130), (4.134)–(4.136), $D[\boldsymbol{G}_1'\boldsymbol{A}_2(\widehat{\boldsymbol{B}}_2-\boldsymbol{B}_2)\boldsymbol{C}_2]$, can be obtained and after a discussion of $D[\widehat{\boldsymbol{B}}_1]$, a forthcoming Theorem 4.17 will be presented where, among other things, a complete expression for $D[\widehat{\boldsymbol{B}}_2]$ is given.

Concerning $D[\widehat{\boldsymbol{B}}_1]$, it should be noted that the treatment of $D[\widehat{\boldsymbol{B}}_1]$ is similar to the treatment of $D[\widehat{\boldsymbol{B}}_2]$, although some additional arguments are needed. If $\widehat{\boldsymbol{B}}_1$ is to be unique, it follows from Theorem 4.9 that $\boldsymbol{A}_1$ and $\boldsymbol{C}_1$ must be of full rank and, therefore, instead of $\widehat{\boldsymbol{B}}_1$, the linear combinations $\boldsymbol{A}_1(\widehat{\boldsymbol{B}}_1-\boldsymbol{B}_1)\boldsymbol{C}_1$, with expectation $\boldsymbol{0}$, will be studied.

As when treating (4.124), $\boldsymbol{A}_1(\widehat{\boldsymbol{B}}_1-\boldsymbol{B}_1)\boldsymbol{C}_1$ will be decomposed, i.e.

$$
\begin{aligned}
&\boldsymbol{A}_1(\widehat{\boldsymbol{B}}_1-\boldsymbol{B}_1)\boldsymbol{C}_1\\
&\qquad = \boldsymbol{P}_{A_1,W_1}(\boldsymbol{X}-E[\boldsymbol{X}])(\boldsymbol{P}_{C_1'}-\boldsymbol{P}_{C_2'})\\
&\qquad\quad +\boldsymbol{P}_{A_1,W_1}(\boldsymbol{I}-\boldsymbol{P}_{A_2,G_1'W_2G_1,G_1})(\boldsymbol{X}-E[\boldsymbol{X}])(\boldsymbol{P}_{C_2'}-\boldsymbol{P}_{C_3'})\\
&\qquad\quad +\boldsymbol{P}_{A_1,W_1}(\boldsymbol{I}-\boldsymbol{P}_{A_2,G_1'W_2G_1,G_1})(\boldsymbol{I}-\boldsymbol{P}_{A_3,G_2'W_3G_2,G_2})(\boldsymbol{X}-E[\boldsymbol{X}])\boldsymbol{P}_{C_3'}.
\end{aligned}
\tag{4.137}
$$

Due to independence among the terms

$$
\begin{aligned}
&D[\boldsymbol{A}_1(\widehat{\boldsymbol{B}}_1-\boldsymbol{B}_1)\boldsymbol{C}_1]\\
&\quad = D[\boldsymbol{P}_{A_1,W_1}(\boldsymbol{X}-E[\boldsymbol{X}])(\boldsymbol{P}_{C_1'}-\boldsymbol{P}_{C_2'})]\\
&\quad\quad +D[\boldsymbol{P}_{A_1,W_1}(\boldsymbol{I}-\boldsymbol{P}_{A_2,G_1'W_2G_1,G_1})(\boldsymbol{X}-E[\boldsymbol{X}])(\boldsymbol{P}_{C_2'}-\boldsymbol{P}_{C_3'})]\\
&\quad\quad +D[\boldsymbol{P}_{A_1,W_1}(\boldsymbol{I}-\boldsymbol{P}_{A_2,G_1'W_2G_1,G_1})(\boldsymbol{I}-\boldsymbol{P}_{A_3,G_2'W_3G_2,G_2})(\boldsymbol{X}-E[\boldsymbol{X}])\boldsymbol{P}_{C_3'}].
\end{aligned}
\tag{4.138}
$$

The three terms on the right-hand side of (4.138) are now treated one by one. Using the independence between $\boldsymbol{P}_{A_1,W_1}$ and $(\boldsymbol{X}-E[\boldsymbol{X}])(\boldsymbol{P}_{C_1'}-\boldsymbol{P}_{C_2'})$,

$$
D[\boldsymbol{P}_{A_1,W_1}(\boldsymbol{X}-E[\boldsymbol{X}])(\boldsymbol{P}_{C_1'}-\boldsymbol{P}_{C_2'})] = (\boldsymbol{P}_{C_1'}-\boldsymbol{P}_{C_2'})\otimes E[\boldsymbol{P}_{A_1,W_1}\boldsymbol{\Sigma}\boldsymbol{P}'_{A_1,W_1}],
$$

and knowledge about the BRM yields

$$
E[\boldsymbol{P}_{A_1,W_1}\boldsymbol{\Sigma}\boldsymbol{P}'_{A_1,W_1}] = \frac{n-k_1-1}{n-k_1-p+q_1-1}\boldsymbol{A}_1(\boldsymbol{A}_1'\boldsymbol{\Sigma}^{-1}\boldsymbol{A}_1)^{-1}\boldsymbol{A}_1'. \tag{4.139}
$$

Concerning the second expression, it is noted that $(X - E[X])(P_{C_2'} - P_{C_3'})$ is independent of P_{A_1,W_1} and $P_{A_2,G_1'W_2G_1,G_1}$. Hence,

$$\begin{aligned}
&D[P_{A_1,W_1}(I - P_{A_2,G_1'W_2G_1,G_1})(X - E[X])(P_{C_2'} - P_{C_3'})] \\
&= (P_{C_2'} - P_{C_3'}) \otimes E[P_{A_1,W_1}(I - P_{A_2,G_1'W_2G_1,G_1})\Sigma(I - P'_{A_2,G_1'W_2G_1,G_1})P'_{A_1,W_1}].
\end{aligned} \tag{4.140}$$

In order to find an explicit expression of (4.140), the approach to finding the expectation in (4.130) is copied. Rewriting P_{A_1,W_1} and $P_{A_2,G_1'W_2G_1,G_1}$ in a canonical form, one obtains:

$$P_{A_1,W_1} = \Sigma^{1/2}\Gamma_1^{l'}\Gamma_1^{l}\Sigma^{-1/2} - \Sigma^{1/2}\Gamma_1^{l'}V_{21}^1(V_{11}^1)^{-1}\Gamma_1^{u}\Sigma^{-1/2}$$

and

$$P_{A_2,G_1'W_2G_1,G_1} = Z_1H_1\Gamma_2^{l'}\Gamma_2^{l}\Gamma_1^{u}\Sigma^{-1/2} - Z_1H_1\Gamma_2^{l'}V_{21}^2(V_{11}^2)^{-1}\Gamma_2^{u}\Gamma_1^{u}\Sigma^{-1/2},$$

where Z_1 is defined based on the fact that the uniqueness of $\widehat{B}_1$ implies $\mathcal{C}(A_2') = \mathcal{C}(A_2'G_1)$: hence a Z_1 exists such that

$$A_2 = Z_1G_1'A_2.$$

Applying the same techniques as before gives

$$\begin{aligned}
&E[P_{A_1,W_1}(I - P_{A_2,G_1'W_2G_1,G_1})\Sigma(I - P'_{A_2,G_1'W_2G_1,G_1})P'_{A_1,W_1}] \\
&= (1 + c_1\frac{m_2}{n - r(C_2) - m_2 - 1})A_1(A_1'\Sigma^{-1}A_1)^{-1}A_1' \\
&\quad + \frac{n - r(C_2) - 1}{n - r(C_2) - m_2 - 1}P_{A_1,\Sigma}A_2(A_2'G_1(G_1'\Sigma G_1)^{-1}G_1'A_2)^{-}A_2'P'_{A_1,\Sigma}.
\end{aligned}$$

Finally, the third term in (4.138) can be written as follows:

$$\begin{aligned}
&D[P_{A_1,W_1}(I - P_{A_2,G_1'W_2G_1,G_1})(I - P_{A_3,G_2'W_3G_2,G_2})(X - E[X])P_{C_3'}] \\
&= P_{C_3'} \otimes E\Big[P_{A_1,W_1}(I - P_{A_2,G_1'W_2G_1,G_1})(I - P_{A_3,G_2'W_3G_2,G_2})\Sigma \\
&\quad \times (I - P'_{A_3,G_2'W_3G_2,G_2})(I - P'_{A_2,G_1'W_2G_1,G_1})P'_{A_1,W_1}\Big].
\end{aligned}$$

It can be shown that the expectation equals

$$E[\boldsymbol{\Sigma}^{1/2}\boldsymbol{\Gamma}_1^{u\prime}\boldsymbol{\Gamma}_1^{u}\boldsymbol{\Sigma}^{-1/2}(\boldsymbol{I}-\boldsymbol{P}_{A_2,G_1'W_2G_1,G_1})(\boldsymbol{I}-\boldsymbol{P}_{A_3,G_2'W_3G_2,G_2})\boldsymbol{\Sigma}$$
$$\times(\boldsymbol{I}-\boldsymbol{P}'_{A_3,G_2'W_3G_2,G_2})(\boldsymbol{I}-\boldsymbol{P}'_{A_2,G_1'W_2G_1,G_1})\boldsymbol{\Sigma}^{-1/2}\boldsymbol{\Gamma}_1^{l\prime}\boldsymbol{\Gamma}_1^{l}\boldsymbol{\Sigma}^{1/2}]$$
$$+E\Big[\boldsymbol{\Sigma}^{1/2}\boldsymbol{\Gamma}_1^{l\prime}\boldsymbol{V}_{21}^1(\boldsymbol{V}_{11}^1)^{-1}\boldsymbol{\Gamma}_1^{u}\boldsymbol{\Sigma}^{-1/2}(\boldsymbol{I}-\boldsymbol{P}_{A_2,G_1'W_2G_1,G_1})(\boldsymbol{I}-\boldsymbol{P}_{A_3,G_2'W_3G_2,G_2})\boldsymbol{\Sigma}$$
$$\times(\boldsymbol{I}-\boldsymbol{P}'_{A_3,G_2'W_3G_2,G_2})(\boldsymbol{I}-\boldsymbol{P}'_{A_2,G_1'W_2G_1,G_1})\boldsymbol{\Sigma}^{-1/2}\boldsymbol{\Gamma}_1^{u\prime}(\boldsymbol{V}_{11}^1)^{-1}\boldsymbol{V}_{12}^1\boldsymbol{\Gamma}_1^{u}\boldsymbol{\Sigma}^{1/2}\Big], \tag{4.141}$$

where

$$E\Big[\boldsymbol{\Sigma}^{1/2}\boldsymbol{\Gamma}_1^{u\prime}\boldsymbol{\Gamma}_1^{u}\boldsymbol{\Sigma}^{-1/2}(\boldsymbol{I}-\boldsymbol{P}_{A_2,G_1'W_2G_1,G_1})(\boldsymbol{I}-\boldsymbol{P}_{A_3,G_2'W_3G_2,G_2})\boldsymbol{\Sigma}$$
$$\times(\boldsymbol{I}-\boldsymbol{P}'_{A_3,G_2'W_3G_2,G_2})(\boldsymbol{I}-\boldsymbol{P}'_{A_2,G_1'W_2G_1,G_1})\boldsymbol{\Sigma}^{-1/2}\boldsymbol{\Gamma}_1^{l\prime}\boldsymbol{\Gamma}_1^{l}\boldsymbol{\Sigma}^{1/2}\Big]$$
$$=\boldsymbol{P}_{A_1,\Sigma}\boldsymbol{\Sigma}+\boldsymbol{P}_{A_1,\Sigma}\boldsymbol{A}_2(\boldsymbol{A}_2'\boldsymbol{G}_1(\boldsymbol{G}_1'\boldsymbol{\Sigma}\boldsymbol{G}_1)^{-1}\boldsymbol{G}_1'\boldsymbol{A}_2)^{-}\boldsymbol{A}_2'\boldsymbol{P}'_{A_1,\Sigma}$$
$$+\tfrac{n-r(C_3)-1}{n-r(C_3)-m_3-1}\boldsymbol{P}_{A_1,\Sigma}(\boldsymbol{I}-\boldsymbol{P}_{A_2,G_1'\Sigma G_1,G_1})$$
$$\times\boldsymbol{A}_3(\boldsymbol{A}_3'\boldsymbol{G}_2(\boldsymbol{G}_2'\boldsymbol{\Sigma}\boldsymbol{G}_2)^{-1}\boldsymbol{G}_2'\boldsymbol{A}_3)^{-}\boldsymbol{A}_3'(\boldsymbol{I}-\boldsymbol{P}_{A_2,G_1'\Sigma G_1,G_1})'\boldsymbol{P}'_{A_1,\Sigma} \tag{4.142}$$

and

$$E\Big[\boldsymbol{\Sigma}^{1/2}\boldsymbol{\Gamma}_1^{l\prime}\boldsymbol{V}_{21}^1(\boldsymbol{V}_{11}^1)^{-1}\boldsymbol{\Gamma}_1^{u}\boldsymbol{\Sigma}^{-1/2}(\boldsymbol{I}-\boldsymbol{P}_{A_2,G_1'W_2G_1,G_1})(\boldsymbol{I}-\boldsymbol{P}_{A_3,G_2'W_3G_2,G_2})\boldsymbol{\Sigma}$$
$$\times(\boldsymbol{I}-\boldsymbol{P}'_{A_3,G_2'W_3G_2,G_2})(\boldsymbol{I}-\boldsymbol{P}'_{A_2,G_1'W_2G_1,G_1})\boldsymbol{\Sigma}^{-1/2}(\boldsymbol{\Gamma}_1^1)'(\boldsymbol{V}_{11}^1)^{-1}\boldsymbol{V}_{12}^1\boldsymbol{\Gamma}_1^{u}\boldsymbol{\Sigma}^{1/2}\Big]$$
$$=\boldsymbol{A}_1(\boldsymbol{A}_1'\boldsymbol{\Sigma}^{-1}\boldsymbol{A}_1)^{-1}\boldsymbol{A}_1'c_1c_2\frac{m_3}{n-r(C_3)-m_3-1}. \tag{4.143}$$

In the next theorem $\boldsymbol{D}[\widehat{\boldsymbol{B}}_i]$, $i=1,2,3$, are stated explicitly.

Theorem 4.17 *Consider the* $EBRM_B^3$ *presented in Definition 2.2. Let* $\widehat{\boldsymbol{B}}_i$, $i=1,2,3$, *be given in Theorem 3.2 and suppose that for each* $\widehat{\boldsymbol{B}}_i$ *the uniqueness conditions in Theorem 4.9 are satisfied. Let* $\boldsymbol{G}_i$, m_i *and* c_i *be defined by (4.73), (4.78) and (4.86), respectively. Then, if the dispersion matrices are supposed to exist,*

(i) *if* $n-k_3-m_2+q_3-1>0$,

$$D[\widehat{\boldsymbol{B}}_3]=\tfrac{n-k_3-1}{n-k_3-m_2+q_3-1}(\boldsymbol{C}_3\boldsymbol{C}_3')^{-1}\otimes(\boldsymbol{A}_3'\boldsymbol{G}_2(\boldsymbol{G}_2'\boldsymbol{\Sigma}\boldsymbol{G}_2)^{-1}\boldsymbol{G}_2'\boldsymbol{A}_3)^{-1};$$

(ii) *if* $n - r(C_3) - m_3 - 1 > 0$ *and* $n - r(C_1) - m_1 + q_2 - 1 > 0$,

$$
\begin{aligned}
D[\widehat{B}_2] = {} & D\Big[(A_2'G_1G_1'A_2)^{-1}A_2'G_1P_{G_1'A_2,G_1'W_2G_1}G_1'(X - E[X]) \\
& \times(P_{C_2'} - P_{C_3'})C_2'(C_2C_2')^{-1}\Big] \\
& +D\Big[(A_2'G_1G_1'A_2)^{-1}A_2'G_1P_{G_1'A_2,G_1'W_2G_1}G_1'(I - P_{A_3,G_2'W_3G_2,G_2}) \\
& \times(X - E[X])P_{C_3'}C_2'(C_2C_2')^{-1}\Big],
\end{aligned}
$$

where

$$
\begin{aligned}
& D[(A_2'G_1G_1'A_2)^{-1}A_2'G_1P_{G_1'A_2,G_1'W_2G_1}G_1'(X - E[X])(P_{C_2'} - P_{C_3'})C_2'(C_2C_2')^{-1}] \\
& \quad = (C_2C_2')^{-1}C_2(I - P_{C_3'})C_2'(C_2C_2')^{-1} \\
& \qquad \otimes\tfrac{n-k_2-1}{n-r(C_1)-m_1+q_2-1}(A_2'G_1(G_1'\Sigma G_1)^{-1}G_1'A_2)^{-1},
\end{aligned}
$$

and

$$
\begin{aligned}
& D\Big[(A_2'G_1G_1'A_2)^{-1}A_2'G_1P_{G_1'A_2,G_1'W_2G_1}G_1'(I - P_{A_3,G_2'W_3G_2,G_2})(X - E[X]) \\
& \qquad \times P_{C_3'}C_2'(C_2C_2')^{-1}\Big] \\
& \quad = (C_2C_2')^{-1}C_2P_{C_3'}C_2'(C_2C_2')^{-1} \\
& \qquad \otimes\Big\{\tfrac{n-r(C_3)-1}{n-r(C_3)-m_3-1}F_1A_3(A_3'G_2(G_2'\Sigma G_2)^{-1}G_2'A_3)^{-}A_3'F_1' \\
& \qquad\quad +(1 + c_2\tfrac{m_3}{n-r(C_3)-m_3-1})(A_2'G_1(G_1'\Sigma G_1)^{-1}G_1'A_2)^{-1}\Big\},
\end{aligned}
$$

where

$$
F_1 = (A_2'A_2)^{-1}A_2'P_{A_2,G_1'\Sigma G_1,G_1};
$$

(iii) *if* $n-k_1-p+q_1-1 > 0$, $n-r(C_2)-m_2-1 > 0$ *and* $n-r(C_3)-m_3-1 > 0$,

$$
\begin{aligned}
D[\widehat{B}_1] = {} & D[(A_1'A_1)^{-1}A_1'P_{A_1,W_1}(X - E[X])(P_{C_1'} - P_{C_2'})C_1'(C_1C_1')^{-1}] \\
& +D\Big[(A_1'A_1)^{-1}A_1'P_{A_1,W_1}(I - P_{A_2,G_1'W_2G_1,G_1})(X - E[X]) \\
& \times(P_{C_2'} - P_{C_3'})C_1'(C_1C_1')^{-1}\Big] \\
& +D\Big[(A_1'A_1)^{-1}A_1'P_{A_1,W_1}(I - P_{A_2,G_1'W_2G_1,G_1})(I - P_{A_3,G_2'W_3G_2,G_2}) \\
& \times(X - E[X])P_{C_3'}C_1'(C_1C_1')^{-1}\Big],
\end{aligned}
$$

where

$$D[(A_1'A_1)^{-1}A_1'P_{A_1,W_1}(X-E[X])(P_{C_1'}-P_{C_2'})C_1'(C_1C_1')^{-1}]$$
$$=(C_1C_1')^{-1}C_1(I-P_{C_2'})C_1'(C_1C_1')^{-1}\otimes\tfrac{n-k_1-1}{n-k_1-p+q_1-1}(A_1'\Sigma^{-1}A_1)^{-1},$$

$$D[(A_1'A_1)^{-1}A_1P_{A_1,W_1}(I-P_{A_2,G_1'W_2G_1,G_1})(X-E[X])(P_{C_2'}-P_{C_3'})C_1'(C_1C_1')^{-1}]$$
$$=(C_1C_1')^{-1}C_1(P_{C_2'}-P_{C_3'})C_1'(C_1C_1')^{-1}$$
$$\otimes\Big\{(1+c_1\tfrac{m_2}{n-r(C_2)-m_2-1})(A_1'\Sigma^{-1}A_1)^{-1}$$
$$+\tfrac{n-r(C_2)-1}{n-r(C_2)-m_2-1}F_2A_2(A_2'G_1(G_1'\Sigma G_1)^{-1}G_1'A_2)^{-}A_2'F_2'\Big\}$$

with

$$F_2=(A_1'A_1)^{-1}A_1'P_{A_1,\Sigma} \tag{4.144}$$

and

$$D\Big[(A_1'A_1)^{-1}A_1'P_{A_1,W_1}(I-P_{A_2,G_1'W_2G_1,G_1})(I-P_{A_3,G_2'W_3G_2,G_2})$$
$$\times(X-E[X])P_{C_3'}C_1'(C_1C_1')^{-1}\Big]$$
$$=(C_1C_1')^{-1}C_1P_{C_3'}C_1'(C_1C_1')^{-1}$$
$$\otimes\Big\{(1+c_1c_2\tfrac{m_3}{n-r(C_3)-m_3-1})(A_1'\Sigma^{-1}A_1)^{-1}$$
$$+F_2A_2(A_2'G_1(G_1'\Sigma G_1)^{-1}G_1'A_2)^{-}A_2'F_2'$$
$$+\tfrac{n-r(C_3)-1}{n-r(C_3)-m_3-1}F_3A_3(A_3'G_2(G_2'\Sigma G_2)^{-1}G_2'A_3)^{-}A_3'F_3'\Big\},$$

where

$$F_3=(A_1'A_1)^{-1}A_1'P_{A_1,\Sigma}(I-P_{A_2,G_1'\Sigma G_1,G_1}). \tag{4.145}$$

In Theorem 4.17 $D[\widehat{B}_i]$, $i=1,2,3$, was presented. However, in order to apply the results, estimators of these quantities are needed. Now estimators based on the

MLEs are derived, and according to Theorem 4.17, these estimators are immediately obtained if unbiased estimators of $L_1 - L_6$, given below, are found:

$$L_1 = (A_3'G_2(G_2'\Sigma G_2)^{-1}G_2'A_3)^{-1}, \quad L_2 = (A_2'G_1(G_1'\Sigma G_1)^{-1}G_1'A_2)^{-1},$$
$$L_3 = (A_1'\Sigma^{-1}A_1)^{-1}, \quad L_4 = F_1A_3(A_3'G_2(G_2'\Sigma G_2)^{-1}G_2'A_3)^{-}A_3'F_1',$$
$$L_5 = F_2A_2(A_2'G_1(G_1'\Sigma G_1)^{-1}G_1'A_2)^{-}A_2'F_2',$$
$$L_6 = F_3A_3(A_3'G_2(G_2'\Sigma G_2)^{-1}G_2'A_3)^{-}A_3'F_3'.$$

An unbiased estimator of L_1, let us say $\widehat{L}_1$, is given by

$$\widehat{L}_1 = \frac{n}{n - r(C_3) - m_2 + r(A_3'G_2)}(A_3'\widehat{Q}_2\widehat{Q}_1\widehat{\Sigma}^{-1}\widehat{Q}_1'\widehat{Q}_2'A_3)^{-1}, \quad (4.146)$$

since $\widehat{Q}_2\widehat{Q}_1(n\widehat{\Sigma})^{-1}\widehat{Q}_1'\widehat{Q}_2' = G_2(G_2'W_3G_2)^{-1}G_2'$, $G_2'W_3G_2 \sim W_{m_2}(G_2'\Sigma G_2, n-r(C_3))$, and then Appendix B, Theorem B.21 (i) gives the result.

For the same reasons, an unbiased estimator of L_2 equals

$$\widehat{L}_2 = \frac{n}{n - r(C_2) - m_1 + r(A_2'G_1)}(A_2'\widehat{Q}_1\widehat{\Sigma}^{-1}\widehat{Q}_1'A_2)^{-1}, \quad (4.147)$$

since $\widehat{Q}_1(n\widehat{\Sigma})^{-1}\widehat{Q}_1' = G_1(G_1'W_2G_1)^{-1}G_1'$, $G_1'W_2G_1 \sim W_{m_1}(G_1'\Sigma G_1, n - r(C_2))$, and once again Theorem B.21 (i) in Appendix B gives the result. Moreover, since

$$E[(A_1'(n\widehat{\Sigma})^{-1}A_1)^{-1}] = E[(A_1'S_1^{-1}A_1)^{-1}] = (n - r(C_1) - p + r(A_1))$$
$$\times(A_1'\Sigma^{-1}A_1)^{-1},$$

$$\widehat{L}_3 = \frac{n}{n - r(C_1) - p + r(A_1)}(A_1'\widehat{\Sigma}^{-1}A_1)^{-1}. \quad (4.148)$$

Concerning L_4–L_6 the situation is slightly more complicated. Details of how to obtain $\widehat{L}_4$ are presented, whereas the other estimators are only listed. Inspired by the handling of (4.127),

$$E[P_{G_1'A_2,G_1'W_2G_1}G_1'A_3(A_3'G_2(G_2'W_3G_2)^{-1}A_3'G_1P'_{G_1'A_2,G_1'W_2G_1}] \quad (4.149)$$

is now studied. From (4.129) it follows that the expectation in (4.149) equals

$$H_1\Gamma_2^{l'}\Gamma_2^{l}\Gamma_1^{u}\Sigma^{-1/2}A_3E[(A_3G_2(G_2'W_3G_2)^{-1}G_2'A_3)^{-1}]A_3'\Sigma^{-1/2}\Gamma_1^{u'}\Gamma_2^{l'}\Gamma_2^{l}H_1'$$
$$+H_1\Gamma_2^{l'}\Gamma_2^{l}H_1'E[\mathrm{tr}\{(V_{11}^2)^{-1}E_3(E_3'(U_{11}^3)^{-1}E_3)^{-1}E_3'\}],$$

where $\boldsymbol{H}_1, \boldsymbol{\Gamma}_1, \boldsymbol{\Gamma}_2$ are defined in (4.75) and (4.76), and $\boldsymbol{E}_3$ is defined in (4.84). The formula comprises two expectations which have been calculated before; i.e. they are given by

$$
\begin{aligned}
&(n - r(\boldsymbol{C}_3) - m_2 - r(\boldsymbol{A}_3'\boldsymbol{G}_2))\boldsymbol{H}_1\boldsymbol{\Gamma}_2^{l'}\boldsymbol{\Gamma}_2^{l}\boldsymbol{\Gamma}_1^{u}\boldsymbol{\Sigma}^{-1/2}\boldsymbol{A}_3(\boldsymbol{A}_3\boldsymbol{G}_2(\boldsymbol{G}_2'\boldsymbol{\Sigma}\boldsymbol{G}_2)^{-1}\boldsymbol{G}_2'\boldsymbol{A}_3)^{-1}\\
&\quad\times\boldsymbol{A}_3'\boldsymbol{\Sigma}^{-1/2}\boldsymbol{\Gamma}_1^{u'}\boldsymbol{\Gamma}_2^{l'}\boldsymbol{\Gamma}_2^{l}\boldsymbol{H}_1'\\
&= (n - r(\boldsymbol{C}_3) - m_2 + r(\boldsymbol{A}_3'\boldsymbol{G}_2))\boldsymbol{P}_{G_1'A_2, G_1'\Sigma G_1}\boldsymbol{G}_1(\boldsymbol{A}_3\boldsymbol{G}_2(\boldsymbol{G}_2'\boldsymbol{\Sigma}\boldsymbol{G}_2)^{-1}\boldsymbol{G}_2'\boldsymbol{A}_3)^{-1}\\
&\quad\times\boldsymbol{A}_3'\boldsymbol{G}_2\boldsymbol{P}'_{G_1'A_2, G_1'\Sigma G_1}
\end{aligned}
$$

and

$$
c_2(p - m_3)\boldsymbol{H}_1\boldsymbol{\Gamma}_2^{l'}\boldsymbol{\Gamma}_2^{l}\boldsymbol{H}_1' = c_2(p - m_3)\boldsymbol{P}_{G_1'A_2, G_1'\Sigma G_1}\boldsymbol{G}_1'\boldsymbol{\Sigma}\boldsymbol{G}_1,
$$

respectively. Hence, once again using

$$
\boldsymbol{G}_2(\boldsymbol{G}_2'\boldsymbol{W}_3\boldsymbol{G}_2)^{-1}\boldsymbol{G}_2' = \widehat{\boldsymbol{Q}}_2\widehat{\boldsymbol{Q}}_1(n\widehat{\boldsymbol{\Sigma}})^{-1}\widehat{\boldsymbol{Q}}_1'\widehat{\boldsymbol{Q}}_2', \tag{4.150}
$$

$$
\boldsymbol{G}_1(\boldsymbol{G}_1'\boldsymbol{W}_2\boldsymbol{G}_1)^{-1}\boldsymbol{G}_1' = \widehat{\boldsymbol{Q}}_1(n\widehat{\boldsymbol{\Sigma}})^{-1}\widehat{\boldsymbol{Q}}_1', \tag{4.151}
$$

it can be shown that

$$
\begin{aligned}
\widehat{\boldsymbol{L}}_4 &= (n - r(\boldsymbol{C}_3) - m_2 + r(\boldsymbol{A}_3'\boldsymbol{G}_2))^{-1}(\boldsymbol{A}_2'\boldsymbol{G}_1\boldsymbol{G}_1'\boldsymbol{A}_2)^{-1}\boldsymbol{A}_2'\boldsymbol{G}_1\boldsymbol{P}_{G_1'A_2, G_1'W_2G_1}\\
&\quad\times\boldsymbol{G}_1'\boldsymbol{A}_3(\boldsymbol{A}_3'\boldsymbol{G}_2(\boldsymbol{G}_2'\boldsymbol{W}_3\boldsymbol{G}_2)^{-1}\boldsymbol{G}_2'\boldsymbol{A}_3)^{-1}\boldsymbol{A}_3'\boldsymbol{G}_1\boldsymbol{P}'_{G_1'A_2, G_1'W_2G_1}\boldsymbol{G}_1'\boldsymbol{A}_2(\boldsymbol{A}_2'\boldsymbol{G}_1\boldsymbol{G}_1'\boldsymbol{A}_2)^{-1}\\
&\quad-c_2(p - m_3)(n - r(\boldsymbol{C}_3) - m_2 + r(\boldsymbol{A}_3'\boldsymbol{G}_2))^{-1}\widehat{\boldsymbol{L}}_2
\end{aligned} \tag{4.152}
$$

is an unbiased estimator of $\boldsymbol{L}_4$. Note that in the above relation, if one uses (4.150) and (4.151), $\widehat{\boldsymbol{L}}_4$ is explicitly expressible as a function of $\widehat{\boldsymbol{\Sigma}}$.

Similar calculations yield that an unbiased estimator of $\boldsymbol{L}_5$ is given by

$$
\begin{aligned}
\widehat{\boldsymbol{L}}_5 &= (n - r(\boldsymbol{C}_2) - m_1 + r(\boldsymbol{A}_2'\boldsymbol{G}_1))^{-1}(\boldsymbol{A}_1'\boldsymbol{A}_1)^{-1}\boldsymbol{A}_1'\boldsymbol{P}_{A_1, S_1}\\
&\quad\times\boldsymbol{A}_2(\boldsymbol{A}_2'\boldsymbol{G}_1(\boldsymbol{G}_1'\boldsymbol{W}_2\boldsymbol{G}_1)^{-1}\boldsymbol{G}_1'\boldsymbol{A}_2)^{-}\boldsymbol{A}_2'\boldsymbol{G}_1\boldsymbol{P}'_{G_1'A_2, G_1'W_2G_1}\boldsymbol{P}_{A_1, S_1}\boldsymbol{A}_1(\boldsymbol{A}_1'\boldsymbol{A}_1)^{-1}\\
&\quad-c_1(p - m_2)(n - r(\boldsymbol{C}_2) - m_1 + r(\boldsymbol{A}_2'\boldsymbol{G}_1))^{-1}\widehat{\boldsymbol{L}}_3,
\end{aligned} \tag{4.153}
$$

which is expressible as a function of $\widehat{\boldsymbol{\Sigma}}$ via (4.151). Concerning $\boldsymbol{L}_6$, an unbiased estimator equals

$$
\begin{aligned}
\widehat{\boldsymbol{L}}_6 &= (n - r(\boldsymbol{C}_3) - m_2 + r(\boldsymbol{A}_3'\boldsymbol{G}_2))^{-1}(\boldsymbol{A}_1'\boldsymbol{A}_1)^{-1}\boldsymbol{A}_1'\boldsymbol{P}_{A_1, S_1}(\boldsymbol{I} - \boldsymbol{P}_{A_2, G_1'W_2G_1, G_1})\\
&\quad\times\boldsymbol{A}_3(\boldsymbol{A}_3'\boldsymbol{G}_2(\boldsymbol{G}_2'\boldsymbol{W}_3\boldsymbol{G}_2)^{-1}\boldsymbol{G}_2'\boldsymbol{A}_3)^{-}\boldsymbol{A}_3'(\boldsymbol{I} - \boldsymbol{P}_{A_2, G_1'W_2G_1, G_1})'\boldsymbol{P}_{A_1, S_1}\boldsymbol{A}_1(\boldsymbol{A}_1'\boldsymbol{A}_1)^{-1}\\
&\quad-c_1(p - m_3)(\boldsymbol{A}_1'\boldsymbol{A}_1)^{-1}\boldsymbol{A}_1'(\widehat{\boldsymbol{L}}_5 - c_2\widehat{\boldsymbol{L}}_3)\boldsymbol{A}_1(\boldsymbol{A}_1'\boldsymbol{A}_1)^{-1},
\end{aligned} \tag{4.154}
$$

where (4.150) and (4.151) can be used to express the estimator through $\widehat{\boldsymbol{\Sigma}}$.

Theorem 4.18 *Consider the $EBRM_B^3$ presented in Definition 2.2. Let $D[\widehat{\boldsymbol{B}}_i]$, $i = 1, 2, 3$, be given in Theorem 4.17 and suppose that for each $\widehat{\boldsymbol{B}}_i$ the uniqueness conditions in Theorem 4.9 are satisfied. Let for i=1,2,3, $\boldsymbol{G}_i$, m_i and c_i be defined by (4.73), (4.78) and (4.86), respectively, and let $\widehat{\boldsymbol{L}}_i$, $i = 1, 2, 3, 4, 5, 6$, be defined by (4.146)–(4.148), (4.152)–(4.154). Then, if the estimators exist:*

(i)

$$\widehat{D[\widehat{\boldsymbol{B}}_3]} = \tfrac{n-k_3-1}{n-k_3-m_2+q_3-1}(\boldsymbol{C}_3\boldsymbol{C}_3')^{-1} \otimes \widehat{\boldsymbol{L}}_1;$$

(ii)

$$\begin{aligned}\widehat{D[\widehat{\boldsymbol{B}}_2]} = \widehat{D}\Big[&(\boldsymbol{A}_2'\boldsymbol{G}_1\boldsymbol{G}_1'\boldsymbol{A}_2)^{-1}\boldsymbol{A}_2'\boldsymbol{G}_1\boldsymbol{P}_{G_1'A_2,G_1'W_2G_1}\boldsymbol{G}_1'(\boldsymbol{X} - E[\boldsymbol{X}])\\ &\times(\boldsymbol{P}_{C_2'} - \boldsymbol{P}_{C_3'})\boldsymbol{C}_2'(\boldsymbol{C}_2\boldsymbol{C}_2')^{-1}\Big]\\ &+\widehat{D}\Big[(\boldsymbol{A}_2'\boldsymbol{G}_1\boldsymbol{G}_1'\boldsymbol{A}_2)^{-1}\boldsymbol{A}_2'\boldsymbol{G}_1\boldsymbol{P}_{G_1'A_2,G_1'W_2G_1}\boldsymbol{G}_1'(\boldsymbol{I} - \boldsymbol{P}_{A_3,G_2'W_3G_2,G_2})\\ &\times(\boldsymbol{X} - E[\boldsymbol{X}])\boldsymbol{P}_{C_3'}\boldsymbol{C}_2'(\boldsymbol{C}_2\boldsymbol{C}_2')^{-1}\Big],\end{aligned}$$

where

$$\begin{aligned}&\widehat{D}\Big[(\boldsymbol{A}_2'\boldsymbol{G}_1\boldsymbol{G}_1'\boldsymbol{A}_2)^{-1}\boldsymbol{A}_2'\boldsymbol{G}_1\boldsymbol{P}_{G_1'A_2,G_1'W_2G_1}\boldsymbol{G}_1'(\boldsymbol{X} - E[\boldsymbol{X}])\\ &\quad\times(\boldsymbol{P}_{C_2'} - \boldsymbol{P}_{C_3'})\boldsymbol{C}_2'(\boldsymbol{C}_2\boldsymbol{C}_2')^{-1}\Big]\\ &= (\boldsymbol{C}_2\boldsymbol{C}_2')^{-1}\boldsymbol{C}_2(\boldsymbol{P}_{C_2'} - \boldsymbol{P}_{C_3'})\boldsymbol{C}_2'(\boldsymbol{C}_2\boldsymbol{C}_2')^{-1} \otimes \tfrac{n-k_2-1}{n-r(\boldsymbol{C}_1)-m_1+q_2-1}\widehat{\boldsymbol{L}}_2,\end{aligned}$$

and

$$\begin{aligned}&\widehat{D}\Big[(\boldsymbol{A}_2'\boldsymbol{G}_1\boldsymbol{G}_1'\boldsymbol{A}_2)^{-1}\boldsymbol{A}_2'\boldsymbol{G}_1\boldsymbol{P}_{G_1'A_2,G_1'W_2G_1}\boldsymbol{G}_1'(\boldsymbol{I} - \boldsymbol{P}_{A_3,G_2'W_3G_2,G_2})(\boldsymbol{X} - E[\boldsymbol{X}])\\ &\quad\times\boldsymbol{P}_{C_3'}\boldsymbol{C}_2'(\boldsymbol{C}_2\boldsymbol{C}_2')^{-1}\Big]\\ &= (\boldsymbol{C}_2\boldsymbol{C}_2')^{-1}\boldsymbol{C}_2\boldsymbol{P}_{C_3'}\boldsymbol{C}_2'(\boldsymbol{C}_2\boldsymbol{C}_2')^{-1}\\ &\quad\otimes\{\tfrac{n-r(\boldsymbol{C}_3)-1}{n-r(\boldsymbol{C}_3)-m_3-1}\widehat{\boldsymbol{L}}_4 + (1 + c_2\tfrac{m_3}{n-r(\boldsymbol{C}_3)-m_3-1})\widehat{\boldsymbol{L}}_2\};\end{aligned}$$

(iii)

$$
\begin{aligned}
\widehat{D[\widehat{B}_1]} = &\widehat{D}[(A_1'A_1)^{-1}A_1'P_{A_1,W_1}(X - E[X])(P_{C_1'} - P_{C_2'})C_1'(C_1C_1')^{-1}] \\
&+\widehat{D}\Big[(A_1'A_1)^{-1}A_1'P_{A_1,W_1}(I - P_{A_2,G_1'W_2G_1,G_1})(X - E[X]) \\
&\quad\times(P_{C_2'} - P_{C_3'})C_1'(C_1C_1')^{-1}\Big] \\
&+\widehat{D}\Big[(A_1'A_1)^{-1}A_1'P_{A_1,W_1}(I - P_{A_2,G_1'W_2G_1,G_1})(I - P_{A_3,G_2'W_3G_2,G_2}) \\
&\quad\times(X - E[X])P_{C_3'}C_1'(C_1C_1')^{-1}\Big],
\end{aligned}
$$

where

$$
\begin{aligned}
&\widehat{D}[(A_1'A_1)^{-1}A_1'P_{A_1,W_1}(X - E[X])(P_{C_1'} - P_{C_2'})C_1'(C_1C_1')^{-1}] \\
&= (C_1C_1')^{-1}C_1(P_{C_1'} - P_{C_2'})C_1'(C_1C_1')^{-1} \otimes \tfrac{n-k_1-1}{n-k_1-p+q_1-1}\widehat{L}_3,
\end{aligned}
$$

$$
\begin{aligned}
&\widehat{D}[(A_1'A_1)^{-1}A_1R_0(I - P_{A_3,G_2'W_3G_2,G_2})(X - E[X])(P_{C_2'} - P_{C_3'})C_1'(C_1C_1')^{-1}] \\
&= (C_1C_1')^{-1}C_1(P_{C_2'} - P_{C_3'})C_1'(C_1C_1')^{-1} \\
&\qquad\otimes\{(1 + c_1\tfrac{m_2}{n-r(C_2)-m_2-1})\widehat{L}_3\tfrac{n-r(C_2)-1}{n-r(C_2)-m_2-1}\widehat{L}_5\}
\end{aligned}
$$

and

$$
\begin{aligned}
&\widehat{D}\Big[(A_1'A_1)^{-1}A_1'P_{A_1,W_1}(I - P_{A_2,G_1'W_2G_1,G_1})(I - P_{A_3,G_2'W_3G_2,G_2}) \\
&\qquad\times(X - E[X])P_{C_3'}C_1'(C_1C_1')^{-1}\Big] \\
&= (C_1C_1')^{-1}C_1P_{C_3'}C_1'(C_1C_1')^{-1} \\
&\qquad\otimes\{(1 + c_1c_2\tfrac{m_3}{n-r(C_3)-m_3-1})\widehat{L}_3 + \widehat{L}_5 + \tfrac{n-r(C_3)-1}{n-r(C_3)-m_3-1}\widehat{L}_6\}.
\end{aligned}
$$

4.7 $EBRM_W^3$ and Uniqueness Conditions for MLEs

The $EBRM_W^3$ is presented in Definition 2.3 and our study of this model in this section and the following sections includes fewer details than were provided for the $EBRM_B^3$ in the previous section. For definitions of the matrices used in Sects. 4.7–4.9 the reader is referred to Chap. 3. The difference between the treatments of the two models will be highlighted, but usually only theorems containing the results are stated without proofs. Indeed, if one has followed the treatment of the $EBRM_B^3$, the proofs can be considered as classroom exercises. Estimators for the parameters of the $EBRM_W^3$ were given in Theorem 3.3, and in Corollary 3.4 the estimator $\widehat{E[X]}$ was presented. As before, $\widehat{E[X]}$ and $\widehat{\boldsymbol{\Sigma}}$ are always unique. When treating the $EBRM_B^3$, it was noted that the uniqueness of estimators is independent of the estimated inner product. Thus, by assuming $\boldsymbol{\Sigma} = \boldsymbol{I}$, the next theorem can be verified by transposing the matrices in the $EBRM_B^3$ and applying Theorem 4.9.

Theorem 4.19 *Consider the $EBRM_W^3$ presented in Definition 2.3. Let $\widehat{\boldsymbol{B}}_i$, $i = 1, 2, 3$, be given in Theorem 3.3 and let $\boldsymbol{K}\widehat{\boldsymbol{B}}_i\boldsymbol{L}$, $i = 1, 2, 3$, be linear combinations of $\widehat{\boldsymbol{B}}_i$; $\boldsymbol{K}$ and $\boldsymbol{L}$ are known matrices of proper sizes. Then the following statements hold:*

(i) $\widehat{\boldsymbol{B}}_3$ *is unique if and only if*

$$r(\boldsymbol{A}_3) = q_3, \quad r(\boldsymbol{C}_3) = k_3, \quad \mathcal{C}(\boldsymbol{C}_3') \cap \mathcal{C}(\boldsymbol{C}_1' : \boldsymbol{C}_2') = \{\boldsymbol{0}\};$$

(ii) $\boldsymbol{K}\widehat{\boldsymbol{B}}_3\boldsymbol{L}$ *is unique if and only if*

$$\mathcal{C}(\boldsymbol{K}') \subseteq \mathcal{C}(\boldsymbol{A}_3'), \quad \mathcal{C}(\boldsymbol{L}') \subseteq \mathcal{C}(\boldsymbol{C}_3(\boldsymbol{C}_1' : \boldsymbol{C}_2')^o);$$

(iii) $\widehat{\boldsymbol{B}}_2$ *is unique if and only if*

$$r(\boldsymbol{A}_2) = q_2, \quad r(\boldsymbol{C}_2) = k_2, \quad \mathcal{C}(\boldsymbol{C}_1') \cap \mathcal{C}(\boldsymbol{C}_2') = \{\boldsymbol{0}\},$$
$$\mathcal{C}(\boldsymbol{C}_1')^{\perp} \cap \mathcal{C}(\boldsymbol{C}_1' : \boldsymbol{C}_2') \cap \mathcal{C}(\boldsymbol{C}_1' : \boldsymbol{C}_3') = \{\boldsymbol{0}\};$$

(iv) $\boldsymbol{K}\widehat{\boldsymbol{B}}_2\boldsymbol{L}$ *is unique if and only if*

$$\mathcal{C}(\boldsymbol{K}') \subseteq \mathcal{C}(\boldsymbol{A}_2'), \quad \mathcal{C}(\boldsymbol{L}) \subseteq \mathcal{C}(\boldsymbol{C}_2(\boldsymbol{C}_1' : \boldsymbol{C}_3')^o);$$

(v) $\widehat{\boldsymbol{B}}_1$ *is unique if and only if*

$$r(\boldsymbol{A}_1) = q_1, \quad r(\boldsymbol{C}_1) = k_1, \quad \mathcal{C}(\boldsymbol{C}_1') \cap \mathcal{C}(\boldsymbol{C}_2') = \{\boldsymbol{0}\},$$
$$\mathcal{C}(\boldsymbol{C}_2')^{\perp} \cap \mathcal{C}(\boldsymbol{C}_1' : \boldsymbol{C}_2') \cap \mathcal{C}(\boldsymbol{C}_2' : \boldsymbol{C}_3') = \{\boldsymbol{0}\};$$

(vi) $\boldsymbol{K}\widehat{\boldsymbol{B}}_1\boldsymbol{L}$ *is unique if and only if*

$$\mathcal{C}(\boldsymbol{K}') \subseteq \mathcal{C}(\boldsymbol{A}_1'), \quad \mathcal{C}(\boldsymbol{L}) \subseteq \mathcal{C}(\boldsymbol{C}_1),$$
$$\mathcal{C}(\boldsymbol{C}_3(\boldsymbol{I} - \boldsymbol{P}_{(\boldsymbol{C}_1')^o}\boldsymbol{C}_2'(\boldsymbol{C}_2\boldsymbol{P}_{(\boldsymbol{C}_1')^o}\boldsymbol{C}_2')^-\boldsymbol{C}_2)\boldsymbol{C}_1'(\boldsymbol{C}_1\boldsymbol{C}_1')^-\boldsymbol{L}) \subseteq \mathcal{C}(\boldsymbol{C}_3(\boldsymbol{C}_1' : \boldsymbol{C}_2')^o),$$
$$\mathcal{C}(\boldsymbol{C}_2\boldsymbol{C}_1'(\boldsymbol{C}_1\boldsymbol{C}_1')^-\boldsymbol{L}) \subseteq \mathcal{C}(\boldsymbol{C}_2(\boldsymbol{C}_1')^o).$$

4.8 Asymptotic Properties of Estimators of Parameters in the $EBRM_W^3$

Concerning asymptotic properties we can once again rely completely on the approach and results for the $EBRM_B^3$. Correspondingly to Lemma 4.2 the next lemma can be stated, whose proof follows directly from the proof of Lemma 4.2.

Lemma 4.5 *Let $\boldsymbol{S}_1$, $\widehat{\boldsymbol{S}}_2$ and $\widehat{\boldsymbol{S}}_3$ be as in Theorem 3.3. Suppose that for large n, $r(\boldsymbol{C}_1) \leq k_1$, and that both $r(\boldsymbol{C}_1 : \boldsymbol{C}_2 : \boldsymbol{C}_3) - r(\boldsymbol{C}_1 : \boldsymbol{C}_2)$ and $r(\boldsymbol{C}_1 : \boldsymbol{C}_2) - r(\boldsymbol{C}_1)$ do not depend on n. Then, if $n \to \infty$,*

$$n^{-1}\boldsymbol{S}_1 \overset{P}{\to} \boldsymbol{\Sigma}, \quad n^{-1}\widehat{\boldsymbol{S}}_2 \overset{P}{\to} \boldsymbol{\Sigma}, \quad n^{-1}\widehat{\boldsymbol{S}}_3 \overset{P}{\to} \boldsymbol{\Sigma}.$$

The following limiting quantities will be used:

$$\boldsymbol{K}\boldsymbol{B}_{3\Sigma}\boldsymbol{L} = \boldsymbol{K}(\boldsymbol{A}_3'\boldsymbol{\Sigma}\boldsymbol{A}_3)^-\boldsymbol{A}_3'\boldsymbol{\Sigma}\boldsymbol{X}\boldsymbol{Q}_2\boldsymbol{C}_3'(\boldsymbol{C}_3\boldsymbol{Q}_2\boldsymbol{C}_3')^-\boldsymbol{L}, \tag{4.155}$$

$$\boldsymbol{K}\boldsymbol{B}_{2\Sigma}\boldsymbol{L} = \boldsymbol{K}(\boldsymbol{A}_2'\boldsymbol{\Sigma}^{-1}\boldsymbol{A}_2)^-\boldsymbol{A}_2'\boldsymbol{\Sigma}^{-1}(\boldsymbol{X} - \boldsymbol{A}_3\boldsymbol{B}_{3\Sigma}\boldsymbol{C}_3)\boldsymbol{Q}_1\boldsymbol{C}_2'(\boldsymbol{C}_2\boldsymbol{Q}_1\boldsymbol{C}_2')^-\boldsymbol{L}, \tag{4.156}$$

$$\boldsymbol{K}\boldsymbol{B}_{1\Sigma}\boldsymbol{L} = \boldsymbol{K}(\boldsymbol{A}_1'\boldsymbol{\Sigma}^{-1}\boldsymbol{A}_1)^-\boldsymbol{A}_1'\boldsymbol{\Sigma}^{-1}(\boldsymbol{X} - \boldsymbol{A}_2\boldsymbol{B}_{2\Sigma}\boldsymbol{C}_2 - \boldsymbol{A}_3\boldsymbol{B}_{3\Sigma}\boldsymbol{C}_3)\boldsymbol{C}_1'(\boldsymbol{C}_1\boldsymbol{C}_1')^-\boldsymbol{L}, \tag{4.157}$$

which all are normally distributed, and where it is supposed that $\boldsymbol{K}$ and $\boldsymbol{L}$ are so chosen that (4.155)–(4.157) do not depend on the choice of g-inverses, i.e. are unique. The matrices $\boldsymbol{Q}_1$ and $\boldsymbol{Q}_2$ are defined in (3.27), i.e. $\boldsymbol{Q}_1 = \boldsymbol{I} - \boldsymbol{P}_{C_1'}$ and $\boldsymbol{Q}_2 = \boldsymbol{I} - \boldsymbol{P}_{C_1':C_2'}$.

Correspondingly to Theorem 4.10, where the $EBRM_B^3$ was considered, the next theorem can be verified.

Theorem 4.20 *Consider the $EBRM_W^3$ presented in Definition 2.3. Let for i=1,2,3, $\widehat{\boldsymbol{B}}_i$ and $\widehat{\boldsymbol{\Sigma}}$ be the maximum likelihood estimators of $\boldsymbol{B}_i$ and $\boldsymbol{\Sigma}$ in the $EBRM_W^3$, given in Theorem 3.3.*

(i) *If $\boldsymbol{K}\widehat{\boldsymbol{B}}_3\boldsymbol{L}$ for the specific known matrices $\boldsymbol{K}$ and $\boldsymbol{L}$ is unique for some n, and if additionally there exists a number, v, such that $\mathcal{C}(\boldsymbol{L}) \subseteq \mathcal{C}(\boldsymbol{C}_3\boldsymbol{Q}_{2v})$, where $\boldsymbol{C}_3\boldsymbol{Q}_{2v}$ is a matrix whose columns are identical to the first v columns in $\boldsymbol{C}_3\boldsymbol{Q}_2$, then $\boldsymbol{K}\widehat{\boldsymbol{B}}_3\boldsymbol{L} - \boldsymbol{K}\boldsymbol{B}_{3\Sigma}\boldsymbol{L} \overset{P}{\to} \boldsymbol{0}$, $n \to \infty$, where $\boldsymbol{K}\boldsymbol{B}_{3\Sigma}\boldsymbol{L}$ is given by (4.155).*

(ii) *If $\boldsymbol{K}\widehat{\boldsymbol{B}}_2\boldsymbol{L}$ for the specific known matrices $\boldsymbol{K}$ and $\boldsymbol{L}$ is unique for some n, and if additionally there exists a number, v, such that $\mathcal{C}(\boldsymbol{L}) \subseteq \mathcal{C}(\boldsymbol{C}_2\boldsymbol{Q}_{1v})$, where $\boldsymbol{C}_2\boldsymbol{Q}_{1v}$ is a matrix whose columns are identical to the first v columns in $\boldsymbol{C}_2\boldsymbol{Q}_1$, then $\boldsymbol{K}\widehat{\boldsymbol{B}}_2\boldsymbol{L} - \boldsymbol{K}\boldsymbol{B}_{2\Sigma}\boldsymbol{L} \overset{P}{\to} \boldsymbol{0}$, $n \to \infty$, where $\boldsymbol{K}\boldsymbol{B}_{2\Sigma}\boldsymbol{L}$ is given by (4.156).*

(iii) *If $\boldsymbol{K}\widehat{\boldsymbol{B}}_1\boldsymbol{L}$ for the specific known matrices $\boldsymbol{K}$ and $\boldsymbol{L}$ is unique for some n, and if additionally there exists a number, v, such that $\mathcal{C}(\boldsymbol{L}) \subseteq \mathcal{C}(\boldsymbol{C}_{1v})$, where $\boldsymbol{C}_{1v}$*

is a matrix whose columns are identical to the first v *columns in* $\boldsymbol{C}_1$*, then* $\boldsymbol{K}\widehat{\boldsymbol{B}}_1\boldsymbol{L} - \boldsymbol{K}\boldsymbol{B}_{1\Sigma}\boldsymbol{L} \xrightarrow{P} \mathbf{0}$*,* $n \to \infty$*, where* $\boldsymbol{K}\boldsymbol{B}_{1\Sigma}\boldsymbol{L}$ *is given by (4.157).*

(iv) *Let* $\boldsymbol{X}_v$*,* $\boldsymbol{C}_{1v}$*,* $\boldsymbol{C}_{2v}$ *and* $\boldsymbol{C}_{3v}$ *denote the first* v *columns in* $\boldsymbol{X}$*,* $\boldsymbol{C}_1$*,* $\boldsymbol{C}_2$ *and* $\boldsymbol{C}_3$*, respectively. Then for* $\widehat{E[\boldsymbol{X}_v]} = \sum_{i=1}^{3} \boldsymbol{A}_i\widehat{\boldsymbol{B}}_i\boldsymbol{C}_{iv}$

$$\widehat{E[\boldsymbol{X}_v]} - (\boldsymbol{A}_1\boldsymbol{B}_{1\Sigma}\boldsymbol{C}_{1v} + \boldsymbol{A}_2\boldsymbol{B}_{2\Sigma}\boldsymbol{C}_{2v} + \boldsymbol{A}_3\boldsymbol{B}_{3\Sigma}\boldsymbol{C}_{3v}) \xrightarrow{P} \mathbf{0}, \quad n \to \infty,$$

where $\boldsymbol{A}_1\boldsymbol{B}_{1\Sigma}\boldsymbol{C}_{1v}$ *follows from statement* (iii) *by choosing* $\boldsymbol{K} = \boldsymbol{A}_1$ *and* $\boldsymbol{L} = \boldsymbol{C}_{1v}$*,* $\boldsymbol{A}_2\boldsymbol{B}_{2\Sigma}\boldsymbol{C}_{2v}$ *follows from statement* (ii) *by choosing* $\boldsymbol{K} = \boldsymbol{A}_2$ *and* $\boldsymbol{L} = \boldsymbol{C}_{2v}$*, and* $\boldsymbol{A}_1\boldsymbol{B}_{3\Sigma}\boldsymbol{C}_{3v}$ *follows from statement* (i) *by choosing* $\boldsymbol{K} = \boldsymbol{A}_3$ *and* $\boldsymbol{L} = \boldsymbol{C}_{3v}$*.*

(v) *Let* $\boldsymbol{S}_3 = \boldsymbol{S}_1 + \boldsymbol{P}'_{A_3^o,\Sigma^{-1}}\boldsymbol{X}\boldsymbol{P}_3\boldsymbol{X}'\boldsymbol{P}_{A_3^o,\Sigma^{-1}} + \boldsymbol{P}'_{A_2^o,\Sigma^{-1}}\boldsymbol{X}\boldsymbol{P}_2\boldsymbol{X}'\boldsymbol{P}_{A_2^o,\Sigma^{-1}}$ *with* $\boldsymbol{P}_3$ *and* $\boldsymbol{P}_2$ *defined in (3.27). Then*

$$\widehat{\boldsymbol{\Sigma}} - \frac{1}{n}(\boldsymbol{S}_3 + \boldsymbol{P}'_{A_1^o,\Sigma^{-1}}\boldsymbol{X}\boldsymbol{P}_{C_1'}\boldsymbol{X}'\boldsymbol{P}_{A_1^o,\Sigma^{-1}}) \xrightarrow{P} \mathbf{0}, \qquad n \to \infty.$$

(vi) $\widehat{\boldsymbol{\Sigma}} \xrightarrow{P} \boldsymbol{\Sigma}, \qquad n \to \infty.$

4.9 Moments of Estimators of Parameters in the $EBRM_W^3$

Let, as in Theorem 3.3, $\boldsymbol{S}_1$, $\widehat{\boldsymbol{S}}_2$ and $\widehat{\boldsymbol{S}}_3$ be defined by

$$\boldsymbol{S}_1 = \boldsymbol{X}(\boldsymbol{I} - \boldsymbol{P}_{C_1':C_2':C_3'})\boldsymbol{X}', \quad \widehat{\boldsymbol{S}}_2 = \boldsymbol{S}_1 + \boldsymbol{P}'_{A_3^o,S_1^{-1}}\boldsymbol{X}\boldsymbol{P}_{Q_2C_3'}\boldsymbol{X}'\boldsymbol{P}_{A_3^o,S_1^{-1}},$$

$$\widehat{\boldsymbol{S}}_3 = \widehat{\boldsymbol{S}}_2 + \boldsymbol{P}'_{A_2^o,\widehat{S}_2^{-1}}\boldsymbol{X}\boldsymbol{P}_{Q_1C_2'}\boldsymbol{X}'\boldsymbol{P}_{A_2^o,\widehat{S}_2^{-1}},$$

where the projections $\boldsymbol{Q}_1 = \boldsymbol{I} - \boldsymbol{P}_{C_1'}$ and $\boldsymbol{Q}_2 = \boldsymbol{I} - \boldsymbol{P}_{C_1':C_2'}$. Similar to the facts for the estimators in the $EBRM_B^3$, stated at the beginning of Sect. 4.6, the following facts now hold.

Facts

(i) $\boldsymbol{X}\boldsymbol{C}_1'$ is independent of $\boldsymbol{X}\boldsymbol{Q}_1\boldsymbol{C}_2'$ and $\boldsymbol{X}\boldsymbol{Q}_2\boldsymbol{C}_3'$.
(ii) $\boldsymbol{X}\boldsymbol{Q}_1\boldsymbol{C}_2'$ is independent of $\boldsymbol{X}\boldsymbol{Q}_2\boldsymbol{C}_3'$.
(iii) $\boldsymbol{S}_1$ is independent of $\boldsymbol{X}\boldsymbol{Q}_2\boldsymbol{C}_3'$, $\boldsymbol{X}\boldsymbol{Q}_1\boldsymbol{C}_2'$ and $\boldsymbol{X}\boldsymbol{C}_1'$.
(iv) $\widehat{\boldsymbol{S}}_2$ is independent of $\boldsymbol{X}\boldsymbol{Q}_1\boldsymbol{C}_2'$ and $\boldsymbol{X}\boldsymbol{C}_1'$.
(v) $\widehat{\boldsymbol{S}}_3$ is independent of $\boldsymbol{X}\boldsymbol{C}_1'$.

Using these statements, correspondingly to Theorem 4.11, the next theorem can be stated concerning the unbiasedness of the mean parameter estimators in the $EBRM_W^3$.

Theorem 4.21 *Consider the $EBRM_W^3$ presented in Definition 2.3. Under the uniqueness conditions given in Theorem 4.19, $\boldsymbol{K}\widehat{\boldsymbol{B}}_i\boldsymbol{L}$ is an unbiased estimator of $\boldsymbol{K}\boldsymbol{B}_i\boldsymbol{L}$, $i = 1, 2, 3$, where $\widehat{\boldsymbol{B}}_i$ is given in Theorem 3.3.*

Corollary 4.4 *The expression $\sum_{i=1}^{3} \boldsymbol{A}_i\widehat{\boldsymbol{B}}_i\boldsymbol{C}_i$ is an unbiased estimator of $E[\boldsymbol{X}] = \sum_{i=1}^{3} \boldsymbol{A}_i\boldsymbol{B}_i\boldsymbol{C}_i$, where $\widehat{\boldsymbol{B}}_i$ is given in Theorem 3.3.*

Many of the following moment expressions rest on the next lemma, for example when considering $E[n\widehat{\boldsymbol{\Sigma}}]$ and $D[\boldsymbol{K}\widehat{\boldsymbol{B}}_i\boldsymbol{L}]$, $i = 1, 2, 3$.

Lemma 4.6 *Let all the matrices be as in Theorem 3.3. Then,*

(i) *if $n - r(\boldsymbol{C}_1' : \boldsymbol{C}_2' : \boldsymbol{C}_3') - 1 > 0$,*

$$E[\boldsymbol{P}_{A_3,S_1}\boldsymbol{\Sigma}\boldsymbol{P}_{A_3,S_1}'] = \frac{n-r(\boldsymbol{C}_1':\boldsymbol{C}_2':\boldsymbol{C}_3')-1}{n-r(\boldsymbol{C}_1':\boldsymbol{C}_2':\boldsymbol{C}_3')-p+r(\boldsymbol{A}_3)-1}\boldsymbol{A}_3(\boldsymbol{A}_3'\boldsymbol{\Sigma}^{-1}\boldsymbol{A}_3)^-\boldsymbol{A}_3';$$

(ii) *if $0 < c_i < \infty$, $i = 1, 2$, where*

$$c_1 = \frac{p-r(\boldsymbol{A}_2)}{n-r(\boldsymbol{C}_1':\boldsymbol{C}_2')-p+r(\boldsymbol{A}_2)-1}, \qquad c_2 = \frac{n-r(\boldsymbol{C}_1':\boldsymbol{C}_2')-p+r(\boldsymbol{A}_3)-1}{n-r(\boldsymbol{C}_1':\boldsymbol{C}_2':\boldsymbol{C}_3')-p+r(\boldsymbol{A}_3)-1},$$

$$\begin{aligned}E[\boldsymbol{P}_{A_2,\widehat{S}_2}\boldsymbol{\Sigma}\boldsymbol{P}_{A_2,\widehat{S}_2}'] &= \boldsymbol{A}_2(\boldsymbol{A}_2'\boldsymbol{\Sigma}^{-1}\boldsymbol{A}_2)^-\boldsymbol{A}_2' + c_1\boldsymbol{P}_{A_3^o,\boldsymbol{\Sigma}^{-1}}'\boldsymbol{A}_2(\boldsymbol{A}_2'\boldsymbol{\Sigma}^{-1}\boldsymbol{A}_2)^-\boldsymbol{A}_2'\boldsymbol{P}_{A_3^o,\boldsymbol{\Sigma}^{-1}}\\&\quad+c_1c_2\boldsymbol{A}_3(\boldsymbol{A}_3'\boldsymbol{\Sigma}^{-1}\boldsymbol{A}_3)^-\boldsymbol{A}_3'\\&= (1+c_1)\boldsymbol{A}_2(\boldsymbol{A}_2'\boldsymbol{\Sigma}^{-1}\boldsymbol{A}_2)^-\boldsymbol{A}_2' + c_1(c_2-1)\boldsymbol{A}_3(\boldsymbol{A}_3'\boldsymbol{\Sigma}^{-1}\boldsymbol{A}_3)^-\boldsymbol{A}_3';\end{aligned}$$

(iii) *if $0 < d_i < \infty$, $i = 1, 2$, where*

$$d_1 = \frac{p-r(\boldsymbol{A}_1)}{n-r(\boldsymbol{C}_1)-p+r(\boldsymbol{A}_1)-1}, \qquad d_2 = \frac{n-r(\boldsymbol{C}_1)-p+r(\boldsymbol{A}_2)-1}{n-r(\boldsymbol{C}_1':\boldsymbol{C}_2')-p+r(\boldsymbol{A}_2)-1},$$

and if $0 < c_2 < \infty$,

$$\begin{aligned}E[\boldsymbol{P}_{A_1,\widehat{S}_3}\boldsymbol{\Sigma}\boldsymbol{P}_{A_1,\widehat{S}_3}'] &= (1+d_1)\boldsymbol{A}_1(\boldsymbol{A}_1'\boldsymbol{\Sigma}^{-1}\boldsymbol{A}_1)^-\boldsymbol{A}_1' + d_2(d_2-1)\boldsymbol{A}_2(\boldsymbol{A}_2'\boldsymbol{\Sigma}^{-1}\boldsymbol{A}_2)^-\boldsymbol{A}_2'\\&\quad+d_2d_1(c_2-1)\boldsymbol{A}_3(\boldsymbol{A}_3'\boldsymbol{\Sigma}^{-1}\boldsymbol{A}_3)^-\boldsymbol{A}_3'.\end{aligned}$$

Proof Statement (i) is almost identical to the moment expression in (4.96), which in turn followed from calculations used when proving Theorem 4.3 (ii). The difference is that in Theorem 4.3, $\boldsymbol{S} \sim W_p(\boldsymbol{\Sigma}, n - r(\boldsymbol{C}_1))$, whereas now $\boldsymbol{S}_1 \sim W_p(\boldsymbol{\Sigma}, n - r(\boldsymbol{C}_1' : \boldsymbol{C}_2' : \boldsymbol{C}_3'))$.

Proving statement (ii) turns out to be much more complicated than proving statement (i). This stems from the fact that $\widehat{\boldsymbol{S}}_2$ is not Wishart-distributed. Because it is easier to work with $\boldsymbol{P}_{A_2^o,\widehat{S}_2^{-1}}$ instead of $\boldsymbol{P}_{A_2,\widehat{S}_2}$, the following relation will be used:

$$E[\boldsymbol{P}_{A_2,\widehat{S}_2}\boldsymbol{\Sigma}\boldsymbol{P}_{A_2,\widehat{S}_2}'] = E[(\boldsymbol{I}-\boldsymbol{P}_{A_2^o,\widehat{S}_2^{-1}}')\boldsymbol{\Sigma}(\boldsymbol{I}-\boldsymbol{P}_{A_2^o,\widehat{S}_2^{-1}})], \qquad (4.158)$$

and after expansion the terms on the right-hand side of (4.158) will be considered in detail. It appears that $E[\boldsymbol{P}'_{A_2^o,\widehat{S}_2^{-1}}\boldsymbol{\Sigma}]$ is symmetric and, therefore, in order to determine (4.158), it suffices to consider

$$E[\boldsymbol{P}'_{A_2^o,\widehat{S}_2^{-1}}\boldsymbol{\Sigma}], \tag{4.159}$$

$$E[\boldsymbol{P}'_{A_2^o,\widehat{S}_2^{-1}}\boldsymbol{\Sigma}\boldsymbol{P}_{A_2^o,\widehat{S}_2^{-1}}]. \tag{4.160}$$

In several places the following trick of multiplying by projectors, decomposing the whole space, will be used. It is noted that since $\boldsymbol{I} = \boldsymbol{P}'_{A_3^o,\Sigma^{-1}} + \boldsymbol{P}_{A_3,\Sigma}$ (see Appendix B, Theorem B.11 (v)), (4.159) is identical to

$$E[(\boldsymbol{P}'_{A_3^o,\Sigma^{-1}} + \boldsymbol{P}_{A_3,\Sigma})\boldsymbol{P}'_{A_2^o,\widehat{S}_2^{-1}}\boldsymbol{\Sigma}] = E[\boldsymbol{P}'_{A_3^o,\Sigma^{-1}}\boldsymbol{P}'_{A_2^o,\widehat{S}_2^{-1}}\boldsymbol{\Sigma}]. \tag{4.161}$$

Note that the expression $\boldsymbol{A}_3'\boldsymbol{\Sigma}^{-1}\boldsymbol{X}(\boldsymbol{I}-\boldsymbol{P}_{C_1':C_2':C_3'})$ is independent of $\boldsymbol{A}_2^{o'}\boldsymbol{X}$ and $\boldsymbol{A}_3^{o'}\boldsymbol{X}$, and $E[\boldsymbol{A}_3'\boldsymbol{\Sigma}^{-1}\boldsymbol{X}(\boldsymbol{I} - \boldsymbol{P}_{C_1':C_2':C_3'})] = \boldsymbol{0}$, and therefore in (4.161)

$$E[\boldsymbol{P}_{A_3,\Sigma}\boldsymbol{P}'_{A_2^o,\widehat{S}_2^{-1}}\boldsymbol{\Sigma}] = \boldsymbol{0}.$$

Moreover, put

$$\boldsymbol{W} = \boldsymbol{S}_1 + \boldsymbol{X}\boldsymbol{P}_{Q_2C_3'}\boldsymbol{X}' \sim W_p(\boldsymbol{\Sigma}, n - r(\boldsymbol{C}_1' : \boldsymbol{C}_2')) \tag{4.162}$$

and then the important relations

$$\boldsymbol{A}_2^{o'}\widehat{\boldsymbol{S}}_2\boldsymbol{A}_2^o = \boldsymbol{A}_2^{o'}\boldsymbol{W}\boldsymbol{A}_2^o, \tag{4.163}$$

$$\boldsymbol{A}_3^{o'}\widehat{\boldsymbol{S}}_2\boldsymbol{A}_2^o = \boldsymbol{A}_3^{o'}\boldsymbol{W}\boldsymbol{A}_2^o \tag{4.164}$$

can be obtained, meaning that $\boldsymbol{A}_3^{o'}\boldsymbol{P}'_{A_2^o,\widehat{S}_2^{-1}}$ is solely a function of a Wishart variable $\boldsymbol{W}$ and

$$\begin{aligned} E[\boldsymbol{P}'_{A_3^o,\Sigma^{-1}}\boldsymbol{P}'_{A_2^o,\widehat{S}_2^{-1}}\boldsymbol{\Sigma}] &= E[\boldsymbol{P}'_{A_3^o,\Sigma^{-1}}\boldsymbol{P}'_{A_2^o,W^{-1}}\boldsymbol{\Sigma}] = \boldsymbol{P}'_{A_3^o,\Sigma^{-1}}\boldsymbol{P}'_{A_2^o,\Sigma^{-1}}\boldsymbol{\Sigma} \\ &= \boldsymbol{P}'_{A_2^o,\Sigma^{-1}}\boldsymbol{\Sigma} = \boldsymbol{\Sigma} - \boldsymbol{A}_2(\boldsymbol{A}_2'\boldsymbol{\Sigma}^{-1}\boldsymbol{A}_2)^-\boldsymbol{A}_2', \end{aligned} \tag{4.165}$$

where Appendix B, Theorem B.20 (ix) has been applied.

Next (4.160) is considered and following the above ideas it is noted that (4.160) equals

$$\boldsymbol{P}_{A_3,\Sigma}E[\boldsymbol{P}'_{A_2^o,\widehat{S}_2^{-1}}\boldsymbol{\Sigma}\boldsymbol{P}_{A_2^o,\widehat{S}_2^{-1}}]\boldsymbol{P}'_{A_3,\Sigma} + \boldsymbol{P}'_{A_3^o,\Sigma^{-1}}E[\boldsymbol{P}'_{A_2^o,\widehat{S}_2^{-1}}\boldsymbol{\Sigma}\boldsymbol{P}_{A_2^o,\widehat{S}_2^{-1}}]\boldsymbol{P}_{A_3^o,\Sigma^{-1}}. \tag{4.166}$$

This is true since $\boldsymbol{P}_{A_3,\Sigma}E[\boldsymbol{P}'_{A_2^o,\widehat{S}_2^{-1}}\boldsymbol{\Sigma}\boldsymbol{P}_{A_2^o,\widehat{S}_2^{-1}}]\boldsymbol{P}_{A_3^o,\Sigma^{-1}} = \mathbf{0}$, which holds because $\boldsymbol{A}_3'\boldsymbol{\Sigma}^{-1}\boldsymbol{X}(\boldsymbol{I}-\boldsymbol{P}_{C_1':C_2':C_3'})$ is independent of $\boldsymbol{A}_2^{o'}\boldsymbol{X}$ and $\boldsymbol{A}_3^{o'}\boldsymbol{X}$, and

$$E[\boldsymbol{A}_3'\boldsymbol{\Sigma}^{-1}\boldsymbol{X}(\boldsymbol{I}-\boldsymbol{P}_{C_1':C_2':C_3'})] = \mathbf{0}.$$

Now, due to (4.163) and (4.164)

$$\begin{aligned}\boldsymbol{P}'_{A_3^o,\Sigma^{-1}}E[\boldsymbol{P}'_{A_2^o,\widehat{S}_2^{-1}}\boldsymbol{\Sigma}\boldsymbol{P}_{A_2^o,\widehat{S}_2^{-1}}]\boldsymbol{P}_{A_3^o,\Sigma^{-1}} &= \boldsymbol{P}'_{A_3^o,\Sigma^{-1}}E[\boldsymbol{P}'_{A_2^o,W^{-1}}\boldsymbol{\Sigma}\boldsymbol{P}_{A_2^o,W^{-1}}]\boldsymbol{P}_{A_3^o,\Sigma^{-1}}\\ &= \boldsymbol{\Sigma} - \boldsymbol{A}_2(\boldsymbol{A}_2'\boldsymbol{\Sigma}^{-1}\boldsymbol{A}_2)^-\boldsymbol{A}_2' + c_1\boldsymbol{P}'_{A_3^o,\Sigma^{-1}}\boldsymbol{A}_2(\boldsymbol{A}_2'\boldsymbol{\Sigma}^{-1}\boldsymbol{A}_2)^-\boldsymbol{A}_2'\boldsymbol{P}_{A_3^o,\Sigma^{-1}};\end{aligned} \quad (4.167)$$

c_1 in this equation and in the formulation of the lemma is determined by following the proof of Theorem 4.6 (i) and, in particular, by making a comparison with the derivation of (4.31), as well as by performing some calculations.

In order to complete the proof of statement (ii), the remaining task is to discuss

$$\boldsymbol{P}_{A_3,\Sigma}E[\boldsymbol{P}'_{A_2^o,\widehat{S}_2^{-1}}\boldsymbol{\Sigma}\boldsymbol{P}_{A_2^o,\widehat{S}_2^{-1}}]\boldsymbol{P}'_{A_3,\Sigma}. \quad (4.168)$$

Now another trick is applied. Note that $\boldsymbol{I} = \boldsymbol{P}_{A_3,S_1}+\boldsymbol{P}'_{A_3^o,S_1^{-1}}$ and $\boldsymbol{A}_3\boldsymbol{S}_1^{-1}\boldsymbol{S}_2\boldsymbol{A}_2^o = \mathbf{0}$. Therefore (4.168) is identical to

$$\begin{aligned}&\boldsymbol{P}_{A_3,\Sigma}E[\boldsymbol{P}'_{A_3^o,S_1^{-1}}\boldsymbol{P}'_{A_2^o,\widehat{S}_2^{-1}}\boldsymbol{\Sigma}\boldsymbol{P}_{A_2^o,\widehat{S}_2^{-1}}\boldsymbol{P}_{A_3^o,S_1^{-1}}]\boldsymbol{P}'_{A_3,\Sigma}\\ &\quad= \boldsymbol{P}_{A_3,\Sigma}E[\boldsymbol{P}'_{A_3^o,S_1^{-1}}\boldsymbol{P}'_{A_2^o,W^{-1}}\boldsymbol{\Sigma}\boldsymbol{P}_{A_2^o,W^{-1}}\boldsymbol{P}_{A_3^o,S_1^{-1}}]\boldsymbol{P}'_{A_3,\Sigma}.\end{aligned} \quad (4.169)$$

The reason for including $\boldsymbol{P}_{A_3^o,S_1^{-1}}$ in (4.168) is that $\widehat{\boldsymbol{S}}_2$ is not Wishart-distributed, whereas (4.169) is a function of Wishart matrices, i.e. $\boldsymbol{S}_1 \sim W_p(\boldsymbol{\Sigma}, n-r(\boldsymbol{C}_1':\boldsymbol{C}_2':\boldsymbol{C}_3'))$ and $\boldsymbol{W} \sim W_p(\boldsymbol{\Sigma}, n-r(\boldsymbol{C}_1':\boldsymbol{C}_2'))$, which therefore is relatively easy to treat. Moreover, since $\boldsymbol{A}_3'\boldsymbol{\Sigma}^{-1}\boldsymbol{X}(\boldsymbol{I}-\boldsymbol{P}_{C_1':C_2':C_3'})$ is independent of $\boldsymbol{A}_3^{o'}\boldsymbol{X}$ and $\boldsymbol{A}_2^{o'}\boldsymbol{X}$, and hence also independent of $\boldsymbol{A}_3^{o'}\boldsymbol{W}\boldsymbol{A}_3^o$ and $\boldsymbol{A}_2^{o'}\boldsymbol{W}\boldsymbol{A}_2^o$, (4.169) equals

$$\boldsymbol{P}_{A_3,\Sigma}\boldsymbol{\Sigma}\boldsymbol{P}'_{A_3,\Sigma}E[\mathrm{tr}\{\boldsymbol{P}'_{A_2^o,W^{-1}}\boldsymbol{\Sigma}\boldsymbol{P}_{A_2^o,W^{-1}}\boldsymbol{A}_3^o(\boldsymbol{A}_3^{o'}\boldsymbol{S}_1\boldsymbol{A}_3^o)^{-1}\boldsymbol{A}_3^{o'}\}]. \quad (4.170)$$

For the derivation of moments of estimators in the $EBRM_B^3$, Lemma 4.3 has turned out to be crucial and this will also be the case when exploiting the expectation of the trace function in (4.170). Let

$$\begin{aligned}\boldsymbol{V} &= \boldsymbol{\Sigma}^{-1/2}\boldsymbol{S}_1\boldsymbol{\Sigma}^{-1/2} \sim W_p(\boldsymbol{I}, n-r(\boldsymbol{C}_1':\boldsymbol{C}_2':\boldsymbol{C}_3')),\\ \boldsymbol{V}_{11} &= (\boldsymbol{I}_{r(A_3^o)}, \mathbf{0})\boldsymbol{V}(\boldsymbol{I}_{r(A_3^o)}, \mathbf{0})' \sim W_{p-r(A_3)}(\boldsymbol{I}, n-r(\boldsymbol{C}_1':\boldsymbol{C}_2':\boldsymbol{C}_3')).\end{aligned}$$

Since $\mathcal{C}(A_2^o) \subseteq \mathcal{C}(A_3^o)$, according to the definition of W, $A_3^{o'} P'_{A_2^o, W^{-1}} \Sigma P_{A_2^o, W^{-1}} A_3^o$ is a function of V_{11} and a random quantity which is independent of $A_3^{o'} S_1 A_3^o$. Therefore, applying Lemma 4.3 yields

$$\begin{aligned}
&E[\mathrm{tr}\{P'_{A_2^o, W^{-1}} \Sigma P_{A_2^o, W^{-1}} A_3^o (A_3^{o'} S_1 A_3^o)^{-1} A_3^{o'}\}] \\
&= c_2 E[\mathrm{tr}\{P'_{A_2^o, W^{-1}} \Sigma P_{A_2^o, W^{-1}} A_3^o (A_3^{o'} W A_3^o)^{-1} A_3^{o'}\}] \\
&= c_2 E[\mathrm{tr}\{\Sigma A_2^o (A_2^{o'} W A_2^o)^{-1} A_2^{o'}\}],
\end{aligned}$$

where c_2 is given in the statement of the lemma. Furthermore, it can be shown (Theorem B.21 (i) in Appendix B) that $c_1 = E[\mathrm{tr}\{\Sigma A_2^o (A_2^{o'} W A_2^o)^{-1} A_2^{o'}\}]$. Thus, (4.170) equals

$$c_1 c_2 A_3 (A_3' \Sigma^{-1} A_3)^{-} A_3', \tag{4.171}$$

and (4.159) and (4.160) have been determined. By expanding (4.158) and then using (4.165)–(4.167) and (4.171), statement (ii) of the lemma has been verified.

Now the proof of statement (iii) is briefly described. The first observation is that the expectation in statement (iii) equals

$$E[(I - P'_{A_1^o, \widehat{S}_3^{-1}}) \Sigma (I - P_{A_1^o, \widehat{S}_3^{-1}})] \tag{4.172}$$

and therefore

$$E[P'_{A_1^o, \widehat{S}_3^{-1}} \Sigma], \tag{4.173}$$

$$E[P'_{A_1^o, \widehat{S}_3^{-1}} \Sigma P_{A_1^o, \widehat{S}_3^{-1}}] \tag{4.174}$$

are of interest. When proving statement (ii), the decomposition $\mathcal{C}(A_3) \boxplus \mathcal{C}(A_3)^{\perp}$ was used. For statement (iii), let A_{23} be any matrix generating $\mathcal{C}(A_2) \cap \mathcal{C}(A_3)^{\perp}$. Thus,

$$\mathcal{C}(A_3) \boxplus \mathcal{C}(A_2) \cap \mathcal{C}(A_3)^{\perp} \boxplus \mathcal{C}(A_2)^{\perp} = \mathcal{C}(A_3) \boxplus \mathcal{C}(A_{23}) \boxplus \mathcal{C}(A_2)^{\perp},$$

and (4.173) is identical to

$$(P'_{A_2^o, \Sigma^{-1}} + P_{A_{23}, \Sigma} + P_{A_3, \Sigma}) E[P'_{A_1^o, \widehat{S}_3^{-1}} \Sigma] = E[P'_{A_2^o, \Sigma^{-1}} P'_{A_1^o, \widehat{S}_3^{-1}} \Sigma],$$

since $(P_{A_{23}, \Sigma} + P_{A_3, \Sigma}) E[P'_{A_1^o, \widehat{S}_3^{-1}} \Sigma] = \mathbf{0}$. Furthermore, put

$$W_1 = W + X P_{Q_1 C_2'} X' \sim W_p(\Sigma, n - r(C_1)),$$

and then

$$A_1^{o'}\widehat{S}_3 A_1^o = A_1^{o'} W_1 A_1^o, \tag{4.175}$$

$$A_2^{o'}\widehat{S}_3 A_1^o = A_2^{o'} W_1 A_1^o. \tag{4.176}$$

Hence,

$$E[P'_{A_2^o,\Sigma^{-1}} P'_{A_1^o,\widehat{S}_3^{-1}}\Sigma] = E[P'_{A_2^o,\Sigma^{-1}} P'_{A_1^o,W_1^{-1}}\Sigma]$$
$$= P'_{A_2^o,\Sigma^{-1}} P'_{A_1^o,\Sigma^{-1}}\Sigma = P'_{A_1^o,\Sigma^{-1}}\Sigma. \tag{4.177}$$

Since (4.177) is a symmetric expression, $E[\Sigma P_{A_1^o,\widehat{S}_3^{-1}}]$ takes the same value as the moment expression in (4.173).

Now $E[P'_{A_1^o,\widehat{S}_3^{-1}}\Sigma P_{A_1^o,\widehat{S}_3^{-1}}]$ in (4.174) is derived. The first observation is that the expectation equals

$$P'_{A_2^o,\Sigma^{-1}} E[P'_{A_1^o,\widehat{S}_3^{-1}}\Sigma P_{A_1^o,\widehat{S}_3^{-1}}] P_{A_2^o,\Sigma^{-1}} \tag{4.178}$$
$$+ P_{A_{23},\Sigma} E[P'_{A_1^o,\widehat{S}_3^{-1}}\Sigma P_{A_1^o,\widehat{S}_3^{-1}}] P'_{A_{23},\Sigma} \tag{4.179}$$
$$+ P_{A_3,\Sigma} E[P'_{A_1^o,\widehat{S}_3^{-1}}\Sigma P_{A_1^o,\widehat{S}_3^{-1}}] P'_{A_3,\Sigma}, \tag{4.180}$$

which is true since $P'_{A_2^o,\Sigma^{-1}} E[P'_{A_1^o,\widehat{S}_3^{-1}}\Sigma P_{A_1^o,\widehat{S}_3^{-1}}] P_{A_2,\Sigma} = \mathbf{0}$ and $\mathcal{C}(A_2) = \mathcal{C}(A_3) \boxplus \mathcal{C}(A_{23})$. The expectations (4.178)–(4.180) are derived separately and one starts with (4.178), which equals (see (4.167) for hints about calculations)

$$\Sigma - A_1(A_1'\Sigma^{-1}A_1)^- A_1' + d_1 P'_{A_2^o,\Sigma^{-1}} A_1(A_1'\Sigma^{-1}A_1)^- A_1' P_{A_2^o,\Sigma^{-1}}, \tag{4.181}$$

where d_1 is given in statement (iii) of the lemma. Since $A_2'\widehat{S}_2^{-1}\widehat{S}_3 A_1^o = \mathbf{0}$, (4.179) can be written as follows:

$$P_{A_{23},\Sigma} E[P'_{A_2^o,\widehat{S}_2^{-1}} P'_{A_1^o,\widehat{S}_3^{-1}}\Sigma P_{A_1^o,\widehat{S}_3^{-1}} P_{A_2^o,\widehat{S}_2^{-1}}] P'_{A_{23},\Sigma}$$
$$= P_{A_{23},\Sigma} E[P'_{A_2^o,W^{-1}} P'_{A_1^o,W_1^{-1}}\Sigma P_{A_1^o,W_1^{-1}} P_{A_2^o,W^{-1}}] P'_{A_{23},\Sigma}$$
$$= P_{A_{23},\Sigma}\Sigma P'_{A_{23},\Sigma} E[\mathrm{tr}\{P'_{A_1^o,W_1^{-1}}\Sigma P_{A_1^o,W_1^{-1}} A_2^o(A_2^{o'} W A_2^o)^{-1} A_2^{o'}\}]. \tag{4.182}$$

However, since $\mathcal{C}(A_1^o) \subseteq \mathcal{C}(A_2^o)$, it follows from Lemma 4.3 that (4.182) equals

$$d_1 A_{23}(A_{23}'\Sigma^{-1}A_{23})^- A_{23}' E[\mathrm{tr}\{P'_{A_1^o,W_1^{-1}}\Sigma P_{A_1^o,W_1^{-1}} A_2^o(A_2^{o'} W_1 A_2^o)^{-1} A_2^{o'}\}]$$
$$= d_1 A_{23}(A_{23}'\Sigma^{-1}A_{23})^- A_{23}' E[\mathrm{tr}\{\Sigma A_1^o(A_1^{o'} W_1 A_1^o)^{-1} A_1^{o'}\}]$$
$$= d_2 d_1 (A_2(A_2'\Sigma^{-1}A_2)^- A_2' - A_3(A_3'\Sigma^{-1}A_3)^- A_3'), \tag{4.183}$$

where d_2 is given in statement (iii) of the lemma and

$$A_{23}(A_{23}'\Sigma^{-1}A_{23})^- A_{23}' = A_2(A_2'\Sigma^{-1}A_2)^- A_2' - A_3(A_3'\Sigma^{-1}A_3)^- A_3'.$$

Finally, the expression for (4.180) is obtained. Since both $A_3'\widehat{S}_1^{-1}\widehat{S}_3 A_1^o = 0$ and $A_2'\widehat{S}_2^{-1}\widehat{S}_3 A_1^o = 0$, (4.180) is identical to

$$\begin{aligned}
&P_{A_3,\Sigma} E[P'_{A_3^o,S_1^{-1}} P'_{A_2^o,\widehat{S}_2^{-1}} P'_{A_1^o,\widehat{S}_3^{-1}} \Sigma P_{A_1^o,\widehat{S}_3^{-1}} P_{A_2^o,\widehat{S}_2^{-1}} P_{A_3^o,S_1^{-1}}] P'_{A_3,\Sigma}\\
&= P_{A_3,\Sigma} E[P'_{A_3^o,S_1^{-1}} P'_{A_2^o,W^{-1}} P'_{A_1^o,W_1^{-1}} \Sigma P_{A_1^o,W_1^{-1}} P_{A_2^o,W^{-1}} P_{A_3^o,S_1^{-1}}] P'_{A_3,\Sigma}
\end{aligned}$$

and the following chain of calculations holds, i.e. (4.180) equals

$$\begin{aligned}
&P_{A_3,\Sigma}\Sigma P'_{A_3,\Sigma} E[\mathrm{tr}\{P'_{A_2^o,W^{-1}} P'_{A_1^o,W_1^{-1}} \Sigma P_{A_1^o,W_1^{-1}} P_{A_2^o,W^{-1}} A_3^o(A_3^{o'} S_1 A_3^o)^{-1} A_3^{o'}\}]\\
&= c_2 A_3(A_3'\Sigma^{-1}A_3)^- A_3' E[\mathrm{tr}\{P'_{A_1^o,W_1^{-1}} \Sigma P_{A_1^o,W_1^{-1}} A_2^o(A_2^{o'} W A_2^o)^{-1} A_2^{o'}\}]\\
&= c_2 d_1 A_3(A_3'\Sigma^{-1}A_3)^- A_3' E[\mathrm{tr}\{\Sigma A_1^o(A_1^{o'} W_1 A_1^o)^{-1} A_3^{o'}\}]\\
&= c_2 d_1 d_2 A_3(A_3'\Sigma^{-1}A_3)^- A_3'. \qquad (4.184)
\end{aligned}$$

Thus, by combining (4.172)–(4.174), (4.177), (4.183) and (4.184), the expression for statement (iii) of the lemma is obtained. □

In Lemma 4.6, necessary preparatory results were presented. Next they will be used when deriving $D[\widehat{E[X]}]$, where

$$\begin{aligned}
\widehat{E[X]} - E[X] = &P_{A_1,\widehat{S}_3}(X - E[X])P_{C_1'} + P_{A_2,\widehat{S}_2}(X - E[X])P_{Q_1 C_2'}\\
&+ P_{A_3,S_1}(X - E[X])P_{Q_2 C_3'}. \qquad (4.185)
\end{aligned}$$

Due to independence (see Facts (i)–(iii) at the beginning of this section), the covariances between the terms in (4.185) equal 0, i.e.

$$\begin{aligned}
&C[P_{A_1,\widehat{S}_3}(X - E[X])P_{C_1'}, P_{A_2,\widehat{S}_2}(X - E[X])P_{Q_1 C_2'}] = 0,\\
&C[P_{A_1,\widehat{S}_3}(X - E[X])P_{C_1'}, P_{A_3,S_1}(X - E[X])P_{Q_2 C_3'}] = 0,\\
&C[P_{A_2,\widehat{S}_2}(X - E[X])P_{Q_1 C_2'}, P_{A_3,S_1}(X - E[X])P_{Q_2 C_3'}] = 0.
\end{aligned}$$

In comparison with $\widehat{E[X]}$ for the $EBRM_B^3$, where the covariances between the terms differed from 0, the situation for the $EBRM_W^3$ is somewhat simpler. Without a proof we state the next theorem.

Theorem 4.22 *Consider the $EBRM_W^3$ presented in Definition 2.3, and apply the notation used in Lemma 4.6. Then*

$$\begin{aligned}D[\widehat{E[X]}] &= D[P_{A_1,\widehat{S}_3}(X - E[X])P_{C_1'}] + D[P_{A_2,\widehat{S}_2}(X - E[X])P_{Q_1C_2'}]\\ &\quad + D[P_{A_3,S_1}(X - E[X])P_{Q_2C_3'}]\\ &= P_{C_1'} \otimes E[P_{A_1,\widehat{S}_3}\Sigma P'_{A_1,\widehat{S}_3}] + P_{Q_1C_2'} \otimes E[P_{A_2,\widehat{S}_2}\Sigma P'_{A_2,\widehat{S}_2}]\\ &\quad + P_{Q_2C_3'} \otimes E[P_{A_3,S_1}\Sigma P'_{A_3,S_1}],\end{aligned}$$

where $E[P_{A_1,\widehat{S}_3}\Sigma P'_{A_1,\widehat{S}_3}]$, $E[P_{A_2,\widehat{S}_2}\Sigma P'_{A_2,\widehat{S}_2}]$ and $E[P_{A_3,S_1}\Sigma P'_{A_3,S_1}]$ are all given in Lemma 4.6.

The estimated dispersion was presented in Theorem 3.3, i.e.

$$n\widehat{\Sigma} = \widehat{S}_3 + P'_{A_1^o,\widehat{S}_3^{-1}} X P_{C_1'} X' P_{A_1^o,\widehat{S}_3^{-1}}. \tag{4.186}$$

Calculating the expectation of $\widehat{\Sigma}$ is relatively straightforward since the necessary moment expressions were used in the proof of Lemma 4.6. Note that $XP_{C_1'}$ is independent of $\widehat{S}_3$, $XP_{Q_1C_2'}$ is independent of $\widehat{S}_2$ and $XP_{Q_2C_3'}$ is independent of S_1, and that $E[P'_{A_1^o,\widehat{S}_3^{-1}}\Sigma P_{A_1^o,\widehat{S}_3^{-1}}]$, $E[P'_{A_2^o,\widehat{S}_2^{-1}}\Sigma P_{A_2^o,\widehat{S}_2^{-1}}]$ and $E[P'_{A_3^o,S_1^{-1}}\Sigma P_{A_3^o,S_1^{-1}}]$ are obtained in the proof of Lemma 4.6.

Theorem 4.23 *Consider the $EBRM_W^3$ presented in Definition 2.3, and apply the notation used in Lemma 4.6. Then*

$$\begin{aligned}E[n\widehat{\Sigma}] &= E[S_1] + r(Q_2C_3')E[P'_{A_3^o,S_1^{-1}}\Sigma P_{A_3^o,S_1^{-1}}]\\ &\quad + r(Q_1C_2')E[P'_{A_2^o,\widehat{S}_2^{-1}}\Sigma P_{A_2^o,\widehat{S}_2^{-1}}] + r(C_1)E[P'_{A_1^o,\widehat{S}_3^{-1}}\Sigma P_{A_1^o,\widehat{S}_3^{-1}}],\end{aligned}$$

where

$$\begin{aligned}E[S_1] &= (n - r(C_1' : C_2' : C_3'))\Sigma,\\ E[P'_{A_3^o,S_1^{-1}}\Sigma P_{A_3^o,S_1^{-1}}] &= \tfrac{p-r(A_3)}{n-r(C_1':C_2':C_3')-p+r(A_3)-1} A_3(A_3'\Sigma^{-1}A_3)^- A_3'\\ &\quad + A_3^o(A_3^{o'}\Sigma A_3^o)^{-1}A_3^{o'},\\ E[P'_{A_2^o,\widehat{S}_2^{-1}}\Sigma P_{A_2^o,\widehat{S}_2^{-1}}] &= A_2^o(A_2^{o'}\Sigma A_2^o)^{-1}A_2^{o'} + A_3(A_3'\Sigma^{-1}A_3)^- A_3'\\ &\quad + c_1 P'_{A_3^o,\Sigma^{-1}} A_2(A_2'\Sigma^{-1}A_2)^{-1}A_2' P_{A_3^o,\Sigma^{-1}}\\ &\quad + c_1c_2 A_3(A_3'\Sigma^{-1}A_3)^- A_3',\end{aligned}$$

$$E[\boldsymbol{P}'_{\boldsymbol{A}_1^o,\widehat{\boldsymbol{S}}_3^{-1}}\boldsymbol{\Sigma}\boldsymbol{P}_{\boldsymbol{A}_1^o,\widehat{\boldsymbol{S}}_3^{-1}}] = \boldsymbol{A}_1^o(\boldsymbol{A}_1^{o'}\boldsymbol{\Sigma}\boldsymbol{A}_1^o)^{-1}\boldsymbol{A}_1^{o'} + d_1\boldsymbol{P}'_{\boldsymbol{A}_2^o,\boldsymbol{\Sigma}^{-1}}\boldsymbol{A}_1(\boldsymbol{A}_1'\boldsymbol{\Sigma}^{-1}\boldsymbol{A}_1)^- \times\boldsymbol{A}_1'\boldsymbol{P}_{\boldsymbol{A}_2^o,\boldsymbol{\Sigma}^{-1}} + d_1d_2\boldsymbol{A}_{23}(\boldsymbol{A}_{23}'\boldsymbol{\Sigma}^{-1}\boldsymbol{A}_{23})^-\boldsymbol{A}_{23}' + c_2d_1d_2\boldsymbol{A}_3(\boldsymbol{A}_3'\boldsymbol{\Sigma}^{-1}\boldsymbol{A}_3)^-\boldsymbol{A}_3',$$

and

$$r(\boldsymbol{Q}_2\boldsymbol{C}_3') = r(\boldsymbol{C}_1' : \boldsymbol{C}_2' : \boldsymbol{C}_3') - r(\boldsymbol{C}_1' : \boldsymbol{C}_2'), \quad r(\boldsymbol{Q}_1\boldsymbol{C}_2') = r(\boldsymbol{C}_1' : \boldsymbol{C}_2') - r(\boldsymbol{C}_1).$$

The next task is to find an unbiased estimator of $\boldsymbol{\Sigma}$, which, according to Theorem 4.23, can be achieved if unbiased estimators of $E[\boldsymbol{P}'_{\boldsymbol{A}_1^o,\widehat{\boldsymbol{S}}_3^{-1}}\boldsymbol{\Sigma}\boldsymbol{P}_{\boldsymbol{A}_1^o,\widehat{\boldsymbol{S}}_3^{-1}}]$, $E[\boldsymbol{P}'_{\boldsymbol{A}_2^o,\widehat{\boldsymbol{S}}_2^{-1}}\boldsymbol{\Sigma}\boldsymbol{P}_{\boldsymbol{A}_2^o,\widehat{\boldsymbol{S}}_2^{-1}}]$ and $E[\boldsymbol{P}'_{\boldsymbol{A}_3^o,\boldsymbol{S}_1^{-1}}\boldsymbol{\Sigma}\boldsymbol{P}_{\boldsymbol{A}_3^o,\boldsymbol{S}_1^{-1}}]$ are established. Thus, unbiased estimators of $\boldsymbol{A}_i(\boldsymbol{A}_i'\boldsymbol{\Sigma}^{-1}\boldsymbol{A}_i)^-\boldsymbol{A}_i'$ and $\boldsymbol{A}_i^o(\boldsymbol{A}_i^{o'}\boldsymbol{\Sigma}\boldsymbol{A}_i^o)^{-1}\boldsymbol{A}_i^{o'}$, $i = 1,2,3$, solve the problem. One strategy for finding these unbiased estimators is to replace $\boldsymbol{\Sigma}$ by its MLE and then, after rather lengthy calculations, to find an estimator which is solely a function of the MLE. This procedure was carried out for the $EBRM_B^3$ and the result was presented in Theorem 4.16. However, there are many alternatives and an easy method is to apply Appendix B, Theorems B.20 (v) and B.21 (i) to $\boldsymbol{S}_1$ and $(\boldsymbol{A}_i^{o'}\boldsymbol{S}_1\boldsymbol{A}_i^o)^{-1}$, i.e.

$$\boldsymbol{A}_i(\boldsymbol{A}_i'\boldsymbol{S}_1^{-1}\boldsymbol{A}_i)^-\boldsymbol{A}_i' \sim W_p(\boldsymbol{A}_i(\boldsymbol{A}_i'\boldsymbol{\Sigma}^{-1}\boldsymbol{A}_i)^-\boldsymbol{A}_i', n - r(\boldsymbol{C}_1' : \boldsymbol{C}_2' : \boldsymbol{C}_3') - p + r(\boldsymbol{A}_i)),$$
$$E[\boldsymbol{A}_i(\boldsymbol{A}_i'\boldsymbol{S}_1^{-1}\boldsymbol{A}_i)^-\boldsymbol{A}_i'] = (n - r(\boldsymbol{C}_1' : \boldsymbol{C}_2' : \boldsymbol{C}_3') - p + r(\boldsymbol{A}_i))\boldsymbol{A}_i(\boldsymbol{A}_i'\boldsymbol{\Sigma}^{-1}\boldsymbol{A}_i)^-\boldsymbol{A}_i',$$

and if $n - r(\boldsymbol{C}_1' : \boldsymbol{C}_2' : \boldsymbol{C}_3') - p + r(\boldsymbol{A}_i) - 1 > 0$

$$E[\boldsymbol{A}_i^o(\boldsymbol{A}_i^{o'}\boldsymbol{S}_1\boldsymbol{A}_i^o)^{-1}\boldsymbol{A}_i^{o'}] = \frac{1}{n-r(\boldsymbol{C}_1':\boldsymbol{C}_2':\boldsymbol{C}_3')-p+r(\boldsymbol{A}_i)-1}\boldsymbol{A}_i^o(\boldsymbol{A}_i^{o'}\boldsymbol{\Sigma}\boldsymbol{A}_i^o)^{-1}\boldsymbol{A}_i^{o'}.$$

Via these relations the next lemma can be proved.

Lemma 4.7 *Let* $\boldsymbol{S}_1$, $\widehat{\boldsymbol{S}}_2$ *and* $\widehat{\boldsymbol{S}}_3$ *be as in Theorem 3.3 and put*

$$h_{11} = \frac{1}{n-r(\boldsymbol{C}_1':\boldsymbol{C}_2':\boldsymbol{C}_3')-p+r(\boldsymbol{A}_3)}\frac{p-r(\boldsymbol{A}_3)}{n-r(\boldsymbol{C}_1':\boldsymbol{C}_2':\boldsymbol{C}_3')-p+r(\boldsymbol{A}_3)-1},$$
$$h_{12} = n - r(\boldsymbol{C}_1' : \boldsymbol{C}_2' : \boldsymbol{C}_3') - p + r(\boldsymbol{A}_3) - 1,$$
$$h_{21} = n - r(\boldsymbol{C}_1' : \boldsymbol{C}_2' : \boldsymbol{C}_3') - p + r(\boldsymbol{A}_2) - 1,$$
$$h_{22} = \frac{1}{n-r(\boldsymbol{C}_1':\boldsymbol{C}_2':\boldsymbol{C}_3')-p+r(\boldsymbol{A}_3)}, \quad h_{23} = \frac{1}{n-r(\boldsymbol{C}_1':\boldsymbol{C}_2':\boldsymbol{C}_3')-p+r(\boldsymbol{A}_2)},$$
$$h_{31} = n - r(\boldsymbol{C}_1' : \boldsymbol{C}_2' : \boldsymbol{C}_3') - p + r(\boldsymbol{A}_1) - 1,$$
$$h_{32} = \frac{1}{n-r(\boldsymbol{C}_1':\boldsymbol{C}_2':\boldsymbol{C}_3')-p+r(\boldsymbol{A}_1)}, \quad h_{33} = \frac{1}{n-r(\boldsymbol{C}_1':\boldsymbol{C}_2':\boldsymbol{C}_3')-p+r(\boldsymbol{A}_{23})}.$$

Then

$$E[\boldsymbol{P}'_{A_3^o,S_1^{-1}}\widehat{\boldsymbol{\Sigma P}}_{A_3^o,S_1^{-1}}] = h_{11}\boldsymbol{A}_3(\boldsymbol{A}_3'\boldsymbol{S}_1^{-1}\boldsymbol{A}_3)^-\boldsymbol{A}_3' + h_{12}\boldsymbol{A}_3^o(\boldsymbol{A}_3^{o'}\boldsymbol{S}_1\boldsymbol{A}_3^o)^{-1}\boldsymbol{A}_3^{o'},$$

$$E[\boldsymbol{P}'_{A_2^o,\widehat{S}_2^{-1}}\widehat{\boldsymbol{\Sigma P}}_{A_2^o,\widehat{S}_2^{-1}}] = h_{21}\boldsymbol{A}_2^o(\boldsymbol{A}_2^{o'}\boldsymbol{S}_1\boldsymbol{A}_2^o)^{-1}\boldsymbol{A}_2^{o'} + h_{22}\boldsymbol{A}_3(\boldsymbol{A}_3'\boldsymbol{S}_1^{-1}\boldsymbol{A}_3)^-\boldsymbol{A}_3'$$
$$+h_{23}c_1\boldsymbol{A}_2(\boldsymbol{A}_2'\boldsymbol{S}_1^{-1}\boldsymbol{A}_2)^{-1}\boldsymbol{A}_2' - h_{22}c_1\boldsymbol{A}_3(\boldsymbol{A}_3'\boldsymbol{S}_1^{-1}\boldsymbol{A}_3)^{-1}\boldsymbol{A}_3'$$
$$+h_{22}c_1c_2\boldsymbol{A}_3(\boldsymbol{A}_3'\boldsymbol{S}_1^{-1}\boldsymbol{A}_3)^-\boldsymbol{A}_3',$$

$$E[\boldsymbol{P}'_{A_1^o,\widehat{S}_3^{-1}}\widehat{\boldsymbol{\Sigma P}}_{A_1^o,\widehat{S}_3^{-1}}] = h_{31}\boldsymbol{A}_1^o(\boldsymbol{A}_1^{o'}\boldsymbol{S}_1\boldsymbol{A}_1^o)^{-1}\boldsymbol{A}_1^{o'} + h_{32}d_1\boldsymbol{A}_1(\boldsymbol{A}_1'\boldsymbol{S}_1^{-1}\boldsymbol{A}_1)^-\boldsymbol{A}_1'$$
$$-h_{23}c_1\boldsymbol{A}_2(\boldsymbol{A}_2'\boldsymbol{S}_1^{-1}\boldsymbol{A}_2)^{-1}\boldsymbol{A}_2'$$
$$+h_{33}d_1d_2\boldsymbol{A}_{23}(\boldsymbol{A}_{23}'\boldsymbol{S}_1^{-1}\boldsymbol{A}_{23})^-\boldsymbol{A}_{23}' + h_{22}c_2d_1d_2\boldsymbol{A}_3(\boldsymbol{A}_3'\boldsymbol{S}_1^{-1}\boldsymbol{A}_3)^-\boldsymbol{A}_3'.$$

Using Lemma 4.7 the following theorem is established.

Theorem 4.24 *Let $\widehat{\boldsymbol{\Sigma}}$ be as in Theorem 3.3. Then, for the $EBRM_W^3$ presented in Definition 2.3, an unbiased estimator of $\boldsymbol{\Sigma}$ is given by*

$$\widehat{\boldsymbol{\Sigma}}_U = \widehat{\boldsymbol{\Sigma}} + \frac{r(\boldsymbol{C}_1':\boldsymbol{C}_2':\boldsymbol{C}_3')}{n(n-r(\boldsymbol{C}_1':\boldsymbol{C}_2':\boldsymbol{C}_3'))}\boldsymbol{S}_1 - \frac{r(\boldsymbol{Q}_2\boldsymbol{C}_3')}{n}E[\boldsymbol{P}'_{A_3^o,S_1^{-1}}\widehat{\boldsymbol{\Sigma P}}_{A_3^o,S_1^{-1}}]$$
$$-\frac{r(\boldsymbol{Q}_1\boldsymbol{C}_2')}{n}E[\boldsymbol{P}'_{A_2^o,\widehat{S}_2^{-1}}\widehat{\boldsymbol{\Sigma P}}_{A_2^o,\widehat{S}_2^{-1}}] - \frac{r(\boldsymbol{C}_1)}{n}E[\boldsymbol{P}'_{A_1^o,\widehat{S}_3^{-1}}\widehat{\boldsymbol{\Sigma P}}_{A_1^o,\widehat{S}_3^{-1}}],$$

where $E[\boldsymbol{P}'_{A_3^o,S_1^{-1}}\widehat{\boldsymbol{\Sigma P}}_{A_3^o,S_1^{-1}}]$, $E[\boldsymbol{P}'_{A_2^o,\widehat{S}_2^{-1}}\widehat{\boldsymbol{\Sigma P}}_{A_2^o,\widehat{S}_2^{-1}}]$ and $E[\boldsymbol{P}'_{A_1^o,\widehat{S}_3^{-1}}\widehat{\boldsymbol{\Sigma P}}_{A_1^o,\widehat{S}_3^{-1}}]$ are all presented in Lemma 4.7.

Now $D[\boldsymbol{K}\widehat{\boldsymbol{B}}_i\boldsymbol{L}]$, $i = 1, 2, 3$, will be obtained for known $\boldsymbol{K}$ and $\boldsymbol{L}$ under the assumption that $\boldsymbol{K}\widehat{\boldsymbol{B}}_i\boldsymbol{L}$ is unique.

Theorem 4.25 *Let $\widehat{\boldsymbol{B}}_i$, $i = 1, 2, 3$, be given in Theorem 3.3 and suppose that for each $\boldsymbol{K}\widehat{\boldsymbol{B}}_i\boldsymbol{L}$, $i = 1, 2, 3$, the uniqueness conditions presented in Theorem 4.19 are satisfied. Then, if the dispersion matrices are supposed to exist,*

(i)

$$D[\boldsymbol{K}\widehat{\boldsymbol{B}}_3\boldsymbol{L}] = \frac{n-r(\boldsymbol{C}_1':\boldsymbol{C}_2':\boldsymbol{C}_3')-1}{n-r(\boldsymbol{C}_1':\boldsymbol{C}_2':\boldsymbol{C}_3')-p+r(\boldsymbol{A}_3)-1}\boldsymbol{L}'(\boldsymbol{C}_3\boldsymbol{Q}_2\boldsymbol{C}_3')^-\boldsymbol{L}\otimes\boldsymbol{K}(\boldsymbol{A}_3'\boldsymbol{\Sigma}^{-1}\boldsymbol{A}_3)^-\boldsymbol{K}';$$

(ii)

$$D[\boldsymbol{K}\widehat{\boldsymbol{B}}_2\boldsymbol{L}] = D[\boldsymbol{K}(\boldsymbol{A}_2'\widehat{\boldsymbol{S}}_2^{-1}\boldsymbol{A}_2)^-\boldsymbol{A}_2'\widehat{\boldsymbol{S}}_2^{-1}(\boldsymbol{X}-E[\boldsymbol{X}])\boldsymbol{Q}_1\boldsymbol{C}_2'(\boldsymbol{C}_2\boldsymbol{Q}_1\boldsymbol{C}_2')^-\boldsymbol{L}]$$
$$+D[\boldsymbol{K}(\boldsymbol{A}_2'\boldsymbol{A}_2)^-\boldsymbol{A}_2'\boldsymbol{A}_3(\widehat{\boldsymbol{B}}_3-\boldsymbol{B}_3)\boldsymbol{C}_3\boldsymbol{Q}_1\boldsymbol{C}_2'(\boldsymbol{C}_2\boldsymbol{Q}_1\boldsymbol{C}_2')^-\boldsymbol{L}],$$

where $D[K(A_2'\widehat{S}_2^{-1}A_2)^-A_2'\widehat{S}_2^{-1}(X - E[X])Q_1C_2'(C_2Q_1C_2')^-L]$ *is obtained by applying Lemma 4.6 (ii) and* $D[K(A_2'A_2)^-A_2'A_3(\widehat{B}_3 - B_3)C_3Q_1C_2'(C_2Q_1C_2')^-L]$ *follows from statement (i) of this theorem;*

(iii)

$$
\begin{aligned}
D[K\widehat{B}_1L] = {} & D[K(A_1'\widehat{S}_3^{-1}A_1)^-A_1'\widehat{S}_3^{-1}(X - E[X])C_1'(C_1C_1')^-L] \\
& + D[K(A_1'A_1)^-A_1'P_{A_2,\widehat{S}_2}XQ_1C_2'(C_2Q_1C_2')^-C_2C_1'(C_1C_1')^-L] \\
& + D[K(A_1'A_1)^-A_1'A_3(\widehat{B}_3 - B_3)C_3(I - Q_1C_2'(C_2Q_1C_2')^-C_2)C_1'(C_1C_1')^-L],
\end{aligned}
$$

where

$$D[K(A_1'\widehat{S}_3^{-1}A_1)^-A_1'\widehat{S}_3^{-1}(X - E[X])C_1'(C_1C_1')^-L]$$

and

$$D[K(A_1'A_1)^-A_1'P_{A_2,\widehat{S}_2}XQ_1C_2'(C_2Q_1C_2')^-C_2C_1'(C_1C_1')^-L]$$

are obtained by applying Lemma 4.6 (ii) and (iii), and

$$D[K(A_1'A_1)^-A_1'A_3(\widehat{B}_3 - B_3)C_3(I - Q_1C_2'(C_2Q_1C_2')^-C_2)C_1'(C_1C_1')^-L]$$

follows from statement (i).

Proof Note that $D[K\widehat{B}_3L]$ has the same structure as $D[K\widehat{B}L]$ in the BRM (see Theorem 4.3 (ii)); i.e. the result for statement (i) follows from Theorem 4.3 (ii).

For $K\widehat{B}_2L$ in statement (ii) the moments are more difficult to obtain than those for $K\widehat{B}_3L$ in statement (i). It follows from the facts presented at the beginning of Sect. 4.9 that XQ_1C_2' is independent of S_1 and $\widehat{S}_2$, as well as XQ_2C_3'. Hence

$$K(A_2'\widehat{S}_2^{-1}A_2)^-A_2'\widehat{S}_2^{-1}(X - E[X])Q_1C_2'(C_2Q_1C_2')^-L$$

and

$$K(A_2'A_2)^-A_2'A_3(\widehat{B}_3 - B_3)C_3Q_1C_2'(C_2Q_1C_2')^-L$$

are uncorrelated. Moreover, due to assumptions about K and the fact that $\mathcal{C}(A_3) \subseteq \mathcal{C}(A_2)$,

$$K(A_2'\widehat{S}_2^{-1}A_2)^-A_2'\widehat{S}_2^{-1}A_3 = K(A_2'A_2)^-A_2'A_3$$

and therefore Lemma 4.6 (ii), together with statement (i) of this theorem, establishes statement (ii).

Similar arguments to those used for the proof of $D[K\widehat{B}_2L]$ also apply to $D[K\widehat{B}_1L]$ in statement (iii), but these arguments are omitted here. □

When performing inference about parameters in a model, it is important to understand how the estimators of these parameters are correlated. Ideally the estimators should be independently distributed, but uncorrelated estimators or estimators with low correlations are to be preferred to highly related estimators. For the BRM and its extensions, usually only statements about correlation can take place. In the next theorem the covariances between $\widehat{B}_1$, $\widehat{B}_2$ and $\widehat{B}_3$ are presented. The proof is based on the facts presented at the beginning of this section, i.e. Sect. 4.9, and, since the technical treatment follows the one used when verifying the previous theorem, it is omitted here.

Theorem 4.26 *Consider the $EBRM_W^3$ presented in Definition 2.3. Let $\widehat{B}_i$, $i = 1, 2, 3$, be given in Theorem 3.3 and suppose that for each $\widehat{B}_i$, $i = 1, 2, 3$, the uniqueness conditions given in Theorem 4.19 are satisfied. Then, if the dispersion matrices are supposed to exist,*

(i)

$$C[\widehat{B}_2, \widehat{B}_3] = -((C_2Q_1C_2')^{-1}C_2Q_1C_3' \otimes (A_2'A_2)^{-1}A_2'A_3)D[\widehat{B}_3],$$

where $D[\widehat{B}_3]$ is presented in Theorem 4.25 (i);

(ii)

$$\begin{aligned} C[\widehat{B}_1, \widehat{B}_3] = &-((C_1C_1')^{-1}C_1C_2' \otimes (A_1'A_1)^{-1}A_1'A_2)C[\widehat{B}_2, \widehat{B}_3] \\ &-((C_1C_1')^{-1}C_1C_3' \otimes (A_1'A_1)^{-1}A_1'A_3)D[\widehat{B}_3], \end{aligned}$$

where $C[\widehat{B}_2, \widehat{B}_3]$ follows from statement (i), and $D[\widehat{B}_3]$ follows from Theorem 4.25 (i);

(iii)

$$\begin{aligned} C[\widehat{B}_1, \widehat{B}_2] = &-((C_1C_1')^{-1}C_1C_3' \otimes (A_1'A_1)^{-1}A_1'A_3)C[\widehat{B}_2, \widehat{B}_3] \\ &-((C_1C_1')^{-1}C_1C_2' \otimes (A_1'A_1)^{-1}A_1'A_2)D[\widehat{B}_2], \end{aligned}$$

where $C[\widehat{B}_2, \widehat{B}_3]$ follows from statement (i), and $D[\widehat{B}_2]$ follows from Theorem 4.25 (ii).

Corollary 4.5 *Let $\widehat{B}_i$, i=1,2,3, be given in Corollary 3.5, where it is supposed that $\mathcal{C}(C_1')$ is orthogonal to $\mathcal{C}(C_2' : C_3')$ and $\mathcal{C}(C_2')$ is orthogonal to $\mathcal{C}(C_1' : C_3')$. Then $C[\widehat{B}_1, \widehat{B}_2] = \mathbf{0}$, $C[\widehat{B}_1, \widehat{B}_3] = \mathbf{0}$ and $C[\widehat{B}_2, \widehat{B}_3] = \mathbf{0}$.*

Problems

1 Consider the BRM presented in Definition 2.1. Use simulations to indicate that the MLE $\widehat{\boldsymbol{B}}$ is unbiased. For a given data set estimate $D[\widehat{\boldsymbol{B}}]$. Moreover, show via simulations that $\widehat{\boldsymbol{B}}$ is not normally distributed.

2 Consider the $EBRM_W^2$ presented in Definition 2.3. Show that the MLE $\widehat{\boldsymbol{\Sigma}}$ is not an unbiased estimator. Derive three different unbiased estimators of $\boldsymbol{\Sigma}$.

3 (*GMANOVA* + *MANOVA*, continuation of Problem 2 of Chap. 3) Let

$$\boldsymbol{X} = \boldsymbol{A}\boldsymbol{B}_1\boldsymbol{C}_1 + \boldsymbol{B}_2\boldsymbol{C}_2 + \boldsymbol{E},$$

where all matrices are given in Problem 2 of Chap. 3. Consider the MLEs and show their consistency, and that the estimators of the mean parameters are unbiased. Moreover, find the dispersion of the estimators of the mean parameters and $E[\widehat{\boldsymbol{\Sigma}}]$.

4 Show the relations presented in (4.97).

5 In Example 3.1 the MLE and an "unweighted" estimator of $\boldsymbol{B}$ were presented. Moreover, an upper bound (which due to randomness is not a real upper bound) between the differences of the corresponding dispersion matrices was shown. Try to find out via simulations how sharp this upper bound is.

6 Let $\boldsymbol{X} \sim N_{p,n}(\boldsymbol{\mu}, \boldsymbol{\Sigma}, \boldsymbol{\Psi})$. Find $E[\mathrm{tr}\{\boldsymbol{X}\boldsymbol{X}'\}]$ and $D[\mathrm{tr}\{\boldsymbol{X}\boldsymbol{X}'\}]$.

7 Consider the $EBRM_W^2$ presented in Definition 2.3. Show that $\sum_{i=1}^{2} \boldsymbol{A}_i\widehat{\boldsymbol{B}}_i\boldsymbol{C}_i$, where $\widehat{\boldsymbol{B}}_i$ is the MLE of $\boldsymbol{B}_i$, $i = 1, 2$, is an unbiased estimator of $E[\boldsymbol{X}]$ and derive its dispersion matrix.

8 Let $\boldsymbol{X} \sim N_{p,n}(\boldsymbol{A}_1\boldsymbol{B}_1\boldsymbol{C}_1 + \boldsymbol{A}_2\boldsymbol{B}_2\boldsymbol{C}_2 + \boldsymbol{A}_3\boldsymbol{B}_3\boldsymbol{C}_3, \boldsymbol{\Sigma}, \boldsymbol{I})$, where $\boldsymbol{B}_i$, $i = 1, 2, 3$, and $\boldsymbol{\Sigma}$ are the unknown parameters,

$$\boldsymbol{A}_1 = \begin{pmatrix} \boldsymbol{I}_{p_1} \\ \boldsymbol{0} \\ \boldsymbol{0} \end{pmatrix}, \quad \boldsymbol{A}_2 = \begin{pmatrix} \boldsymbol{0} \\ \boldsymbol{I}_{p_2} \\ \boldsymbol{0} \end{pmatrix}, \quad \boldsymbol{A}_3 = \begin{pmatrix} \boldsymbol{0} \\ \boldsymbol{0} \\ \boldsymbol{I}_{p_3} \end{pmatrix},$$

where $p_1 + p_2 + p_3 = p$, and $\mathcal{C}(\boldsymbol{C}_3') \subseteq \mathcal{C}(\boldsymbol{C}_2') \subseteq \mathcal{C}(\boldsymbol{C}_1')$. Find the MLEs of the parameters, as well as their asymptotic distributions.

9 In the BRM presented in Definition 2.1, suppose that $\boldsymbol{F}\boldsymbol{B} = \boldsymbol{0}$ and $\boldsymbol{B}\boldsymbol{G} = \boldsymbol{0}$ hold, where $\boldsymbol{F}$: $s \times q$ and $\boldsymbol{G}$: $k \times t$ are known matrices. Give conditions when the MLE for $\boldsymbol{B}$ is unique.

10 In the BRM presented in Definition 2.1, suppose that $\boldsymbol{F}\boldsymbol{B}\boldsymbol{G} = \boldsymbol{0}$ holds, where $\boldsymbol{F}$: $s \times q$ and $\boldsymbol{G}$: $k \times t$ are known matrices. Find $E[\widehat{\boldsymbol{\Sigma}}]$, where $\widehat{\boldsymbol{\Sigma}}$ is the MLE of $\boldsymbol{\Sigma}$.

Literature

Asymptotics for linear models (including regression models), constitutes in fact the basis for the asymptotic results for the BRM and the $EBRM_{\bullet}^m$ and was presented by Eicker (1963, 1966) (see also Drygas, 1971). Another way of contemplating asymptotic inference is, when the inference is based on an assumption about normality of errors, as in this book, to view it in the light of classical likelihood theory modified to handle non-identically distributed observations. Since this book contains explicit estimators, one can adopt some approach based on working with the estimators directly. An alternative approach is first to study an appropriate sequence of criteria functions (loss functions, likelihood functions) and determine that they converge for large n, i.e. many independent observations, and thereafter to utilize that the estimators obtained through minimization/maximization of the criteria function also converge (e.g. see van der Vaart, 1998).

Essential for the interpretation of results for the BRM and the $EBRM_{\bullet}^m$ is the concept of estimability. Bose (1944) formally introduced the concept and its importance is highlighted in classical Gauss-Markov theory (e.g. see Rao, 1973; Wang and Chow, 1994). However, Thiele (1889) had already considered the estimability problem in remarkable detail (see Hald, 1981). Essential for the asymptotics applied to dispersion are the results for the sample dispersion matrix which is proportional to $\boldsymbol{S} = \boldsymbol{X}(\boldsymbol{I} - \boldsymbol{P}_{C'})\boldsymbol{X}'$ (following the notation of the book). An early work which treated the results of Lemma 4.1 is the monograph by Anderson (1958). A useful trick when obtaining asymptotically equivalent expression for the MLEs of the BRM and the $EBRM_{\bullet}^m$ is to apply the Cramér-Slutsky theorem (see Rao, 1973; Gut, 2013). The estimator $n^{-1}\boldsymbol{S}$ in the projection operators converges in probability to $\boldsymbol{\Sigma}$, and the remaining parts of the MLEs of the mean parameters and their approximating quantities are equal in distribution. Thus, results about asymptotically equivalent expressions are easily obtained via the Cramér-Slutsky theorem.

Moments are used in this book to understand estimators and perform density approximations (see Chap. 5) called Edgeworth-type approximations. These moments are based on moments of the normal distribution, i.e. the multivariate normal distribution and the matrix normal distribution (see Holmquist, 1988; von Rosen, 1988a), and moments from the Wishart distribution (Holmquist, 1985; Lu and Richards, 2001; Letac and Massam, 2004; Graczyk et al., 2005; Collins et al., 2014). For the most commonly used definition of the Wishart matrix ($\boldsymbol{X}\boldsymbol{X}'$, where $\boldsymbol{X}$ is matrix normally distributed) these results can be obtained from the moments of the matrix normal distribution. Moreover, moments from the inverse Wishart distribution (Haff, 1982; von Rosen, 1988b, 1997; Letac and Massam, 2004; Matsumoto, 2012; Collins et al., 2014), and sometimes moments for the multivariate β-distribution of type I and the multivariate β-distribution of type II (see Kollo and von Rosen, 2005, Subsection 2.4.5) are needed when working with the BRM or its extensions. Many of the above-cited references on Wishart moments and inverse Wishart moments are fairly mathematical and often based on combinatorial theory. Wong and Hua (2000) solved some of the combinatorial problems via differentiation. However, if one is only interested in the mean and dispersion, i.e. the first and second order moments, these moments have for a long time been available in many texts on multivariate analysis (e.g. see Srivastava and Khatri, 1979; Kollo and von Rosen, 2005). When looking for moment relations for the symmetric Wishart matrix, it is important to clarify which object the moments are being derived for, i.e. whether they are being derived for the upper or lower triangular of the Wishart matrix, $\boldsymbol{W}$, for all elements in $\boldsymbol{W}$ or for the object $\boldsymbol{W}$ which belongs to the space of symmetric matrices. It is also advisable to distinguish clearly between real valued and complex valued vectors/matrices. Moreover, sometimes expectations of the trace of a Wishart matrix or an inverse Wishart matrix are needed and both categories of expectations can be obtained via moments of hypergeometric function with Wishart arguments (e.g. see Muirhead, 1982; Watamori, 1990; Lu and Richards, 2001) or by applying some of the results derived by Letac and Massam (2004), among others.

Moments for the mean and dispersion for the BRM were first presented by Grizzle and Allen (1969) who also referred to Rao (1967) and other authors where similar calculations had been performed. The other moment expressions presented in Theorems 4.6–4.11 follow from results in von Rosen (1990) (see also Kollo and von Rosen, 2005, Chap. 4). The moment results for the $EBRM_B^3$ mostly stem from von Rosen (1990) and for the corresponding results for the $EBRM_W^3$, the reader is referred to Filipiak von Rosen (2012).

References

Anderson, T. W. (1958). *An introduction to multivariate statistical analysis*. New York/London: Wiley/Chapman & Hall.

Bose, R. C. (1944). The fundamental theorem of linear estimation. In *Proceedings of 31st Indian Science Congress, Part III* (pp. 4–5).

Collins, B., Matsumoto, S., & Saad, N. (2014). Integration of invariant matrices and moments of inverses of Ginibre and Wishart matrices. *Journal of Multivariate Analysis, 126*, 1–13.

Drygas, H. (1971). Consistency of the least squares and Gauss-Markov estimators in regression models. *Zeitschrift für Wahrscheinlichkeitstheorie und Verwandte Gebiete, 17*, 309–326.

Eicker, F. (1963). Asymptotic normality and consistency of the least squares estimators for families of linear regressions. *Annals of Mathematical Statistics, 34*, 447–456.

Eicker, F. (1966). A multivariate central limit theorem for random linear vector forms. *Annals of Mathematical Statistics, 37*, 1825–1828.

Filipiak, K., & von Rosen, D. (2012). On MLEs in an extended multivariate linear growth curve model. *Metrika, 75*, 1069–1092.

Graczyk, P., Letac, G., & Massam, H. (2005). The hyperoctahedral group, symmetric group representations and the moments of the real Wishart distribution. *Journal of Theoretical Probability, 18*, 1–42.

Grizzle, J. E., & Allen, D. M. (1969). Analysis of growth and dose response curves. *Biometrics, 25*, 357–381.

Gut, A. (2013). *Probability: A graduate course. Springer texts in statistics* (2nd ed.). New York: Springer.

Haff, L. R. (1982). Identities for the inverse Wishart distribution with computational results in linear and quadratic discrimination. *Sankhyā, Series A, 44*, 245–258.

Hald, A. (1981). T.N. Thiele's contributions to statistics. *International Statistical Review, 49*, 1–20.

Holmquist, B. (1985). *Moments and cumulants from generating functions of Hilbert space-valued random variables and an application to the Wishart distribution*. University of Lund, Statistical Research Report 1985:3.

Holmquist, B. (1988). Moments and cumulants of the multivariate normal distribution. *Stochastic Analysis and Applications, 6*, 273–278.

Kollo, T., & von Rosen, D. (1995). Minimal moments and cumulants of symmetric matrices: An application to the Wishart distribution. *Journal of Multivariate Analysis, 55*, 149–164.

Kollo, T., & von Rosen, D. (2005). *Advanced multivariate statistics with matrices. Mathematics and its applications* (Vol. 579). Dordrecht: Springer.

Letac, G., & Massam, H. (2004). All invariant moments of the Wishart distribution. *Scandinavian Journal of Statistics, 31*, 295–318.

Li, Y., Udén, P., & von Rosen, D. (2015). A two-step estimation method for grouped data with connections to the extended growth curve model and partial least squares regression. *Journal of Multivariate Analysis, 139*, 347–359.

Lu, I.-Li., & Richards, D. St. P. (2001). MacMahon's master theorem, representation theory, and moments of Wishart distributions. Special issue in honor of Dominique Foata's 65th birthday (Philadelphia, PA, 2000). *Advances in Applied Mathematics*, **27**, 531–547.

Matsumoto, S. (2012). General moments of the inverse real Wishart distribution and orthogonal Weingarten functions. *Journal of Theoretical Probability, 25*, 798–822.

Muirhead, R. J. (1982). *Aspects of multivariate statistical theory*. New York: Wiley.

Potthoff, R. F., & Roy, S. N. (1964). A generalized multivariate analysis of variance model useful especially for growth curve problems. *Biometrika, 51*, 313–326.

Rao, C. R. (1967). Least squares theory using an estimated dispersion matrix and its application to measurement of signals. In *Proceedings of Fifth Berkeley Symposium on Mathematical Statistics and Probability (Berkeley, CA, 1965/66)* (Vol. I). *Statistics* (pp. 355–372). Berkeley: University of California Press.

Rao, C. R. (1973). *Linear statistical inference and its applications. Wiley series in Probability and mathematical statistics* (2nd ed.). New York: Wiley.

Srivastava, M. S., & Khatri, C. G. (1979). *An introduction to multivariate statistics*. New York: North-Holland.

Thiele, T. N. (1889). *Forelæsninger over Almindelig Iagttagelseslære: Sandsynlighedsregning og Mindste Kvadraters Methode*. København: Reitzel (in Danish).

van der Vaart, A. W. (1998). *Asymptotic statistics. Cambridge series in statistical and probabilistic mathematics* (Vol. 3). Cambridge: Cambridge University Press.

von Rosen, D. (1988a). Moments for matrix normal variables. *Statistics, 19*, 575–583.

von Rosen, D. (1988b). Moments for the inverted Wishart distribution. *Scandinavian Journal of Statistics, 15*, 97–109.

von Rosen, D. (1990). Moments for a multivariate linear model with an application to the growth curve model. *Journal of Multivariate Analysis, 35*, 243–259.

von Rosen, D. (1997). On moments of the inverted Wishart distribution. *Statistics, 30*, 259–278.

Wang, S. G., & Chow, S.-C. (1994). *Advanced linear models. Theory and applications. Statistics: Textbooks and monographs* (Vol. 141). New York: Marcel Dekker.

Watamori, Y. (1990). On the moments of traces of Wishart and inverted Wishart matrices. *South African Statistical Journal, 24*, 153–176.

Wong, C. S., & Hua, C. (2000). Evaluating matrix-variate moments through higher-order differential forms and combinatorial algorithms. *Journal of Statistical Planning and Inference, 91*, 1–21.

Chapter 5
Density Approximations

5.1 Introduction

In the previous section some of the most elementary properties, i.e. moments, of the MLEs in the BRM, $EBRM_B^3$ and $EBRM_W^3$ were derived. In these models the exact distribution of the MLEs is difficult to obtain in a useful form. Thus, one needs to rely on either simulations or approximations. In general, simulations may be useful in some particular cases, but can often become computationally demanding, for example when used to solve distributional problems connected to high-dimensional statistical problems.

When finding approximations of distributions, it may be advisable to start from the asymptotic distribution under the assumption of a large number of independent observations. It is a fairly natural approximation strategy that one should let the asymptotic result direct the approximation. For example, if the distribution of a statistic converges to the normal distribution, it is natural to approximate with a normal distribution. The art in this connection resides in the correction of the approximation for the finite number of independent observations concerned. Moreover, in any serious context it is always of interest to indicate the error of the approximation and the best approach here is to find a sharp upper bound of the error.

Distributions of a statistic can be approximated in many ways, for example, by approximating the statistic itself, by approximating the characteristic function before transforming it back into a density, by approximating the density function or by directly approximating the distribution function. In this section a special type of density approximation will be considered which is termed Edgeworth-type expansion. From the derivation of this type of approximation it follows that one approximates the characteristic function by excluding higher terms in a Taylor series expansion of the characteristic function. At this stage the knowledge of moments and cumulants is crucial. Thereafter an inverse transform is applied to obtain the density approximation. The reason for calling this type of approximation

D. von Rosen, *Bilinear Regression Analysis*, Lecture Notes in Statistics 220,
https://doi.org/10.1007/978-3-319-78784-8_5

an Edgeworth-type expansion is that it is based on the normal distribution. However, the correct term is Gram-Charlier A series expansion. Usually the difference between Edgeworth and Gram-Charlier expansions lies in the organization of terms in the expansion, which then affects the approximation when series are truncated. The reason for choosing the term "Edgeworth-type expansion" is that in our approach we do not have to distinguish between the Gram-Charlier and Edgeworth expansions, and at the same time, the term "Gram-Charlier expansion" is incorrect from a historical perspective (see Hald, 2002).

This chapter focuses mainly on the approximation of the distribution of the maximum likelihood estimators of the mean parameters. Here the results are unexpectedly beautiful. The same approach could be adopted for the estimators of the dispersion estimators, but in this case it is not possible to bound the errors of the approximations and therefore no results will be presented.

5.2 Preparation

Let $\boldsymbol{Y}$ be a random matrix variable with density $f_{\boldsymbol{Y}}(\boldsymbol{Y}_o)$. The density $f_{\boldsymbol{Y}}(\boldsymbol{Y}_o)$ should be approximated via another random variable $\boldsymbol{X}$ and its density $f_{\boldsymbol{X}}(\boldsymbol{Y}_o)$, and knowledge about the cumulants for both distributions. Moreover, the approximating density and the characteristic functions are going to be differentiated several times and this will be based on the following matrix derivative.

Definition 5.1 Let $\boldsymbol{Y}$ be a function of $\boldsymbol{X}$. The kth matrix derivative is defined by

$$\frac{d^k \boldsymbol{Y}}{d\,\boldsymbol{X}^k} = \frac{d}{\boldsymbol{X}} \frac{d^{k-1} \boldsymbol{Y}}{d\,\boldsymbol{X}^{k-1}}, \qquad k = 1, 2, \ldots,$$

and

$$\frac{d\,\boldsymbol{Y}}{d\,\boldsymbol{X}} = \frac{d\,\mathrm{vec}'\boldsymbol{Y}}{d\,\mathrm{vec}\boldsymbol{X}}, \qquad \frac{d^0\,\boldsymbol{Y}}{d\,\boldsymbol{X}^0} = \boldsymbol{Y},$$

where, if $\boldsymbol{X} \in \mathbb{R}^{p\times q}$,

$$\frac{d}{d\,\boldsymbol{X}} = \left(\frac{d}{d\,x_{11}}, \ldots \frac{d}{d\,x_{p1}}, \frac{d}{d\,x_{12}}, \ldots, \frac{d}{d\,x_{p2}}, \ldots, \frac{d}{d\,x_{1q}}, \ldots, \frac{d}{d\,x_{pq}}\right)'.$$

Note that a more precise, but clumsy, notation would have been $\frac{d^k \boldsymbol{Y}}{(d\,\boldsymbol{X})^k}$ or $\frac{d^k \boldsymbol{Y}}{d\,\boldsymbol{X} d\,\boldsymbol{X} \ldots d\,\boldsymbol{X}}$; i.e. here in Definition 5.1, $\boldsymbol{X}^k$ does not denote the matrix power.

Since the Edgeworth-type expansion is based on knowledge about multivariate cumulants, it is necessary to define them. Let $\varphi_{\boldsymbol{X}}(\boldsymbol{T})$ denote the characteristic function (Fourier transform),

$$\varphi_X(T) = E[e^{i\mathrm{tr}(T'X)}],$$

where i is the imaginary unit, and then the kth cumulant $c_k[X]$ is presented in the next definition.

Definition 5.2 Let X be a random matrix. Supposing the existence of cumulants of X, the kth cumulant of X is given by

$$c_k[X] = \frac{1}{i^k}\frac{d^k \ln \varphi_X(T)}{dT^k}\bigg|_{T=0}, \qquad k = 1, 2, \ldots.$$

In particular, $c_1[X] = E[\mathrm{vec}X]$ and $c_2[X] = D[X]$ (see Appendix B, Theorem B.16 (iii)). Since $\frac{dY}{dX} = \frac{d\,\mathrm{vec}'Y}{dX}$, it follows that $c_k[X] = c_k[\mathrm{vec}X]$, which is sometimes useful to note. There exist one-to-one relations between cumulants of an arbitrary order and moments of an arbitrary order. Moreover, for normally distributed variables cumulants of an order > 2 equal $\mathbf{0}$. In the following the kth derivative of a density $f_X(X_o)$ will be denoted by $f_X^k(X_o)$ and $f_X^0(X_o) = f_X(X_o)$, where the derivative is given in Definition 5.1. Now necessary notations have been introduced and it is time to present a result concerning multivariate Edgeworth-type expansions.

Theorem 5.1 *Let Y and X be two random matrices of the same size with densities $f_Y(X_o)$ and $f_X(X_o)$, respectively, both evaluated at X_o. Then*

$$\begin{aligned}
f_Y(X_o) &= f_X(X_o) - \mathrm{vec}'(E[Y] - E[X])f_X^1(X_o)\\
&\quad + \frac{1}{2}\mathrm{vec}'(D[Y] - D[X] + \mathrm{vec}(E[Y] - E[X])\mathrm{vec}'(E[Y] - E[X]))\mathrm{vec}\, f_X^2(X_o)\\
&\quad - \frac{1}{6}\Big(\mathrm{vec}'(c_3[Y] - c_3[X]) + 3\mathrm{vec}'(D[Y] - D[X]) \otimes \mathrm{vec}'(E[Y] - E[X])\\
&\quad + \mathrm{vec}'(E[Y] - E[X])^{\otimes 3}\Big)\mathrm{vec}\, f_X^3(X_o) + \ldots.
\end{aligned}$$

Proof Consider the trivial identity

$$\varphi_Y(T) = \frac{\varphi_Y(T)}{\varphi_X(T)}\varphi_X(T) = \varphi_X(T)\exp\{\ln \varphi_Y(T) - \ln \varphi_X(T)\}.$$

Now $\ln \varphi_Y(T) - \ln \varphi_X(T)$ is, according to the above definition given in Definition 5.2 of cumulants, expanded as

$$\ln \varphi_Y(T) - \ln \varphi_X(T) = \sum_{k=1}^{\infty} \tfrac{i^k}{k!} t'(c_k[Y] - c_k[X])t^{\otimes k-1},$$

where $t = \text{vec}T$. Thus,

$$\varphi_Y(t) = \varphi_X(t) \prod_{k=1}^{\infty} \exp\{\tfrac{1}{k!} it'(c_k[Y] - c_k[X])(it)^{\otimes k-1}\}.$$

Ordering the terms in a series expansion, according to $t^{\otimes k}$, this relation yields

$$\begin{aligned}
\varphi_Y(T) = \varphi_X(T)\Big\{ & 1 + i(c_1[Y] - c_1[X])'t \\
& + \tfrac{i^2}{2}\text{vec}'\{c_2[Y] - c_2[X] + (c_1[Y] - c_1[X])(c_1[Y] - c_1[X])'\}t^{\otimes 2} \\
& + \tfrac{i^3}{6}\Big(\text{vec}'(c_3[Y] - c_3[X]) + 3\text{vec}'(c_2[Y] - c_2[X]) \otimes (c_1[Y] - c_1[X])' \\
& \quad + (c_1[Y] - c_1[X])'^{\otimes 3}\Big)t^{\otimes 3} + \cdots \Big\}.
\end{aligned}$$

Next this expression is inverted via the inverse Fourier transform; i.e. the following relation is utilized:

$$(-1)^k a' \text{vec} f_X^k(X) = (2\pi)^{-pq} \int_{\mathcal{R}^{pq}} \varphi_X(T) a'(it)^{\otimes k} e^{-i\text{tr}(T'X)} dT, \; k = 0, 1, 2, \ldots, \tag{5.1}$$

where a is an arbitrary constant $(pq)^k$-vector, which establishes the theorem. □

The theorem shows how one density is approximated using another density via knowledge about cumulants and derivatives of the approximating density. The approximation is point-wise and the approximating density does not necessarily have to be a real density, i.e. positive, and when integrating the approximation over all the values of X, it equals 1.

From Theorem 5.1 it follows that derivatives of densities are needed. Thus, if the matrix normal distribution is used, the derivatives of the corresponding normal density are needed; i.e. the Hermite polynomials have to be expressed, and they are presented now in the next lemma (see Appendix A, Sect. A.13 for a definition of Hermite polynomials).

Lemma 5.1 *Let $X \sim N_{p,n}(\mu, \Sigma, \Psi)$. Then the generalized Hermite polynomials of an order up to 3 equal*

$$H_0(X, \mu, \Sigma, \Psi) = 1, \tag{5.2}$$

$$H_1(X, \mu, \Sigma, \Psi) = \text{vec}(\Sigma^{-1}(X - \mu)\Psi^{-1}), \tag{5.3}$$

$$\begin{aligned} H_2(X, \mu, \Sigma, \Psi) = & \text{vec}(\Sigma^{-1}(X - \mu)\Psi^{-1})\text{vec}'(\Sigma^{-1}(X - \mu)\Psi^{-1}) \\ & - \Psi^{-1} \otimes \Sigma^{-1}, \end{aligned} \tag{5.4}$$

$$
\begin{aligned}
\boldsymbol{H}_3(\boldsymbol{X},\boldsymbol{\mu},\boldsymbol{\Sigma},\boldsymbol{\Psi}) = {} & \mathrm{vec}(\boldsymbol{\Sigma}^{-1}(\boldsymbol{X}-\boldsymbol{\mu})\boldsymbol{\Psi}^{-1})(\mathrm{vec}'(\boldsymbol{\Sigma}^{-1}(\boldsymbol{X}-\boldsymbol{\mu})\boldsymbol{\Psi}^{-1}))^{\otimes 2}\\
& -\mathrm{vec}(\boldsymbol{\Sigma}^{-1}(\boldsymbol{X}-\boldsymbol{\mu})\boldsymbol{\Psi}^{-1})\mathrm{vec}'(\boldsymbol{\Psi}^{-1}\otimes\boldsymbol{\Sigma}^{-1})\\
& -\mathrm{vec}'(\boldsymbol{\Sigma}^{-1}(\boldsymbol{X}-\boldsymbol{\mu})\boldsymbol{\Psi}^{-1})\otimes\boldsymbol{\Psi}^{-1}\otimes\boldsymbol{\Sigma}^{-1}\\
& -\boldsymbol{\Psi}^{-1}\otimes\boldsymbol{\Sigma}^{-1}\otimes\mathrm{vec}'(\boldsymbol{\Sigma}^{-1}(\boldsymbol{X}-\boldsymbol{\mu})\boldsymbol{\Psi}^{-1}).
\end{aligned} \tag{5.5}
$$

In Theorem 5.1 no errors were presented. Next a special case is considered for which not only are errors presented, but also an upper bound of the error is given. Let in the next theorem $|\bullet|$ denote the absolute value (modulus) of a real (complex) number.

Theorem 5.2 *Let $\boldsymbol{Y}$ and $\boldsymbol{X}$ be two random matrices of the same size, $p \times q$, with densities $f_{\boldsymbol{Y}}(\boldsymbol{X}_o)$ and $f_{\boldsymbol{X}}(\boldsymbol{X}_o)$, respectively, both evaluated at $\boldsymbol{X}_o$. Moreover, suppose that*

$$
\boldsymbol{Y} = \boldsymbol{X} - \boldsymbol{U}, \tag{5.6}
$$

where $\boldsymbol{X}$ and $\boldsymbol{U}$ are independently distributed, and let $\boldsymbol{u} = \mathrm{vec}\boldsymbol{U}$ and $\boldsymbol{t} = \mathrm{vec}\boldsymbol{T}$. Then, if $m+1$ is even,

$$
f_{\boldsymbol{Y}}(\boldsymbol{X}_o) = f_{\boldsymbol{X}}(\boldsymbol{X}_o) + \sum_{k=1}^{m} \frac{1}{k!}\mathrm{vec}' E[\boldsymbol{u}^{\otimes k}]\mathrm{vec} \boldsymbol{f}^k_{\boldsymbol{X}}(\boldsymbol{X}_o) + r^{\star}_m,
$$

where

$$
|r^{\star}_m| \leq (2\pi)^{-pq}\frac{1}{(m+1)!}E[(\boldsymbol{u}')^{\otimes m+1}]\int_{\mathcal{R}^{pq}} \boldsymbol{t}^{\otimes m+1}|\varphi_{\boldsymbol{X}}(\boldsymbol{T})|d\boldsymbol{t}.
$$

Proof The proof is in principle a copy of the proof of Theorem 5.1. However, due to the assumption $\boldsymbol{Y} = \boldsymbol{X} - \boldsymbol{U}$, where $\boldsymbol{X}$ and $\boldsymbol{U}$ are independently distributed, the equations of the proof look somewhat different from those in the proof of the previous theorem. Now let us begin to work with the trivial identity

$$
\begin{aligned}
\varphi_{\boldsymbol{Y}}(\boldsymbol{T}) &= \frac{\varphi_{\boldsymbol{Y}}(\boldsymbol{T})}{\varphi_{\boldsymbol{X}}(\boldsymbol{T})}\varphi_{\boldsymbol{X}}(\boldsymbol{T}) = \varphi_{-\boldsymbol{U}}(\boldsymbol{T})\varphi_{\boldsymbol{X}}(\boldsymbol{T})\\
&= \varphi_{\boldsymbol{X}}(\boldsymbol{T})(1+\sum_{k=1}^{m}\frac{(-i)^k}{k!}\boldsymbol{t}'\boldsymbol{m}_k[\boldsymbol{u}]\boldsymbol{t}^{\otimes(k-1)} + r_m(\boldsymbol{T})),
\end{aligned} \tag{5.7}
$$

$$
r_m(\boldsymbol{T}) = \frac{1}{(m+1)!}\boldsymbol{t}'\boldsymbol{\varphi}^{m+1}_{-\boldsymbol{U}}(\boldsymbol{\Theta}\odot\boldsymbol{T})\boldsymbol{t}^{\otimes m}, \tag{5.8}
$$

where $\boldsymbol{\varphi}^{m+1}_{-\boldsymbol{U}}(\boldsymbol{\Theta}\odot\boldsymbol{T})$ is the $m+1$ derivative of $\varphi_{-\boldsymbol{U}}(\boldsymbol{\Theta}\odot\boldsymbol{T})$ evaluated at $\boldsymbol{\Theta}\odot\boldsymbol{T}$, $\odot$ is the Hadamard product (element-wise product, see Appendix A, Sect. A.6) and $\boldsymbol{\Theta}$ is a $p\times q$ matrix whose elements have values between 0 and 1.

Next the inverse Fourier transform given in (5.1) is applied to (5.7) and (5.8). Thus, the density presented in the theorem is found and a remaining task is to find the upper bound of

$$r_m^\star = (2\pi)^{-pq}\frac{1}{(m+1)!}\int_{\mathcal{R}^{pq}} \mathrm{vec}'\boldsymbol{\varphi}_{-U}^{m+1}(\boldsymbol{\Theta}\odot \boldsymbol{T})\boldsymbol{t}^{\otimes m+1}\exp(-i\mathrm{tr}\{\boldsymbol{T}'\boldsymbol{X}_o\})\varphi_{\boldsymbol{X}}(\boldsymbol{T})d\boldsymbol{t}.$$

Then

$$\begin{aligned}|r_m^\star| &\le (2\pi)^{-pq}\frac{1}{(m+1)!}\int_{\mathcal{R}^{pq}} |\mathrm{vec}'\boldsymbol{\varphi}_{-U}^{m+1}(\boldsymbol{\Theta}\odot \boldsymbol{T})\boldsymbol{t}^{\otimes m+1}||\varphi_{\boldsymbol{X}}(\boldsymbol{T})|d\boldsymbol{t}\\ &\le (2\pi)^{-pq}\frac{1}{(m+1)!}\int_{\mathcal{R}^{pq}} E[(\boldsymbol{u}')^{\otimes m+1}]\boldsymbol{t}^{\otimes m+1}|\varphi_{\boldsymbol{X}}(\boldsymbol{T})|d\boldsymbol{t},\end{aligned}$$

which is identical to the statement of the theorem. □

It is interesting to note that if $E[(\boldsymbol{u}')^{\otimes m+1}]$ and $\int_{\mathbb{R}^{pq}} \boldsymbol{t}^{\otimes m+1}|\varphi_{\boldsymbol{X}}(\boldsymbol{T})|d\boldsymbol{t}$ can be calculated, an upper bound of the error has been found. However, this does not mean that the proposed boundary is sharp. In special cases one can probably find better bounds.

An important approximating distribution is the normal distribution with a mean equal to $\boldsymbol{0}$. If $\boldsymbol{X} \sim N_{p,n}(\boldsymbol{0}, \boldsymbol{\Sigma}, \boldsymbol{\Psi})$, then

$$\varphi_{\boldsymbol{X}}(\boldsymbol{T}) = \exp(-\tfrac{1}{2}\mathrm{tr}\{\boldsymbol{\Sigma}\boldsymbol{T}\boldsymbol{\Psi}\boldsymbol{T}'\}),$$

which is real-valued. Moreover, this expression, as a function in $\boldsymbol{T}$, is proportional to the normal density and therefore the next corollary can be stated. The normal distribution is, however, not the only possible choice of density.

Corollary 5.1 *Let $\boldsymbol{Y}$ and $\boldsymbol{X}$ be two random matrices of the same size, $p \times q$, with densities $f_{\boldsymbol{Y}}(\boldsymbol{X}_o)$ and the matrix normal density (see Appendix A, Sect. A.10)*

$$f_{\boldsymbol{X}}(\boldsymbol{X}_o) = (2\pi)^{-pq/2}|\boldsymbol{\Psi}|^{-p/2}|\boldsymbol{\Sigma}|^{-q/2}\exp(-\tfrac{1}{2}\mathrm{tr}\{\boldsymbol{\Sigma}^{-1}\boldsymbol{X}_o\boldsymbol{\Psi}^{-1}\boldsymbol{X}_o'\}),$$

respectively, both evaluated at $\boldsymbol{X}_o$; it is supposed that both $\boldsymbol{\Sigma}$ and $\boldsymbol{\Psi}$ are p.d., and $E[\boldsymbol{X}] = E[\boldsymbol{Y}] = \boldsymbol{0}$. Suppose that

$$\boldsymbol{Y} = \boldsymbol{X} - \boldsymbol{U}, \tag{5.9}$$

where $\boldsymbol{X}$ and $\boldsymbol{U}$ are independently distributed and let $\boldsymbol{u} = \mathrm{vec}\boldsymbol{U}$. Then

$$f_{\boldsymbol{Y}}(\boldsymbol{X}_o) = f_{\boldsymbol{X}}(\boldsymbol{X}_o) + \sum_{k=1}^{3}\frac{1}{k!}(-1)^k E[(\boldsymbol{u}')^{\otimes k}]\mathrm{vec}\boldsymbol{H}_k(\boldsymbol{X}_o, \boldsymbol{0}, \boldsymbol{\Sigma}, \boldsymbol{\Psi})f_{\boldsymbol{X}}(\boldsymbol{X}_o) + r_3^\star,$$

where $\boldsymbol{H}_k(\boldsymbol{X}_o, \mathbf{0}, \boldsymbol{\Sigma}, \boldsymbol{\Psi})$ *follows from Lemma 5.1 and*

$$|r_3^\star| \leq (2\pi)^{-pq}\frac{1}{4!}|\boldsymbol{\Sigma}|^{-q/2}|\boldsymbol{\Psi}|^{-p/2}E[(\boldsymbol{u}')^{\otimes 4}]E[z^{\otimes 4}]$$

with $z \sim N_{pq}(\mathbf{0}, \boldsymbol{\Psi}^{-1} \otimes \boldsymbol{\Sigma}^{-1})$.

It follows from the corollary that the precision of the density approximation mainly depends on $E[(\text{vec}\boldsymbol{U})^{\otimes 4}]$, which in our application can be made small when the number of independent observations becomes large. Indeed, $\boldsymbol{U}$ can be thought of as an error term when approximating $\boldsymbol{Y}$ using $\boldsymbol{X}$. However, at the same time the eigenvalues of $\boldsymbol{\Sigma}$ and $\boldsymbol{\Psi}$, and $E[z^{\otimes 4}]$ play a role. The expression $E[z^{\otimes 4}]$ is given in Appendix B, Theorem B.19 (v). Thus, if it is possible to choose a structure for $\boldsymbol{\Sigma}$ and $\boldsymbol{\Psi}$, this can be utilized when planning experiments so that, before the experiment is carried out, there is some guarantee that an approximation of the density will work.

Moreover, when calculating the error term of the approximation, the mean can very well differ from $\mathbf{0}$ since under normality $|\varphi_{\boldsymbol{X}}(\boldsymbol{T})|$ is not affected by the mean. Thus, Corollary 5.1 can immediately be extended by replacing $f_{\boldsymbol{X}}(\boldsymbol{X}_o)$ and $\boldsymbol{H}_k(\boldsymbol{X}_o, \mathbf{0}, \boldsymbol{\Sigma}, \boldsymbol{\Psi})$ by

$$(2\pi)^{-pq/2}|\boldsymbol{\Psi}|^{-p/2}|\boldsymbol{\Sigma}|^{-q/2}\exp(-\tfrac{1}{2}\text{tr}\{\boldsymbol{\Sigma}^{-1}(\boldsymbol{X}_o - \boldsymbol{\mu})\boldsymbol{\Psi}^{-1}(\boldsymbol{X}_o - \boldsymbol{\mu})'\})$$

and

$$\boldsymbol{H}_k(\boldsymbol{X}_o, \boldsymbol{\mu}, \boldsymbol{\Sigma}, \boldsymbol{\Psi}),$$

respectively. Under these assumptions the error is still the same as in Corollary 5.1.

In Corollary 5.1 it was assumed that $\boldsymbol{X}$ followed a matrix normal distribution with mean $\mathbf{0}$. Next it is assumed that for vectors $\boldsymbol{y}$, $\boldsymbol{x}$ and $\boldsymbol{u}$, the relation $\boldsymbol{y} = \boldsymbol{x} - \boldsymbol{u}$ holds, where $\boldsymbol{u}$ is independent of the normally distributed $\boldsymbol{x}$ and, in addition, symmetrically distributed with a mean equal to $\mathbf{0}$. Then

$$E[\boldsymbol{u}^{\otimes 2}] = vec(D[\boldsymbol{y}] - D[\boldsymbol{x}]).$$

Furthermore, noting that

$$\boldsymbol{H}_2(\boldsymbol{x}_o, \boldsymbol{\mu}, \boldsymbol{\Sigma}, 1) = \boldsymbol{\Sigma}^{-1}(\boldsymbol{x}_o - \boldsymbol{\mu})(\boldsymbol{x}_o - \boldsymbol{\mu})'\boldsymbol{\Sigma}^{-1} - \boldsymbol{\Sigma}^{-1},$$

the next corollary can be established.

Corollary 5.2 *Let* $\boldsymbol{y}$ *and* $\boldsymbol{x}$ *be two random vectors of size* p *with densities* $f_{\boldsymbol{y}}(\boldsymbol{x}_o)$ *and*

$$f_{\boldsymbol{x}}(\boldsymbol{x}_o) = (2\pi)^{-p/2}|\boldsymbol{\Sigma}|^{-1/2}\exp(-\tfrac{1}{2}\text{tr}\{\boldsymbol{\Sigma}^{-1}(\boldsymbol{x}_o - \boldsymbol{\mu})(\boldsymbol{x}_o - \boldsymbol{\mu})'\}),$$

respectively, both evaluated at $\boldsymbol{x}_o$*; it is supposed that* $\boldsymbol{\Sigma}$ *is p.d. Moreover, suppose that*

$$\boldsymbol{y} = \boldsymbol{x} - \boldsymbol{u}, \tag{5.10}$$

where $\boldsymbol{u}$ *is independent of* $\boldsymbol{x}$ *and symmetrically distributed with mean* $\mathbf{0}$*. Then*

$$\begin{aligned} f_{\boldsymbol{y}}(\boldsymbol{x}_o) &= f_{\boldsymbol{x}}(\boldsymbol{x}_o) \\ &\quad + \tfrac{1}{2}\mathrm{tr}\{(D[\boldsymbol{y}] - \boldsymbol{\Sigma})(\boldsymbol{\Sigma}^{-1}(\boldsymbol{x}_o - \boldsymbol{\mu})(\boldsymbol{x}_o - \boldsymbol{\mu})'\boldsymbol{\Sigma}^{-1} - \boldsymbol{\Sigma}^{-1})\} f_{\boldsymbol{x}}(\boldsymbol{x}_o) + r_3^\star \\ &= (1 - \tfrac{1}{2}\mathrm{tr}\{D[\boldsymbol{y}]\boldsymbol{\Sigma}^{-1}\boldsymbol{I}\}) f_{\boldsymbol{x}}(\boldsymbol{x}_o) \\ &\quad + \tfrac{1}{2}\mathrm{tr}\{(D[\boldsymbol{y}]\boldsymbol{\Sigma}^{-1} - \boldsymbol{I})(\boldsymbol{x}_o - \boldsymbol{\mu})(\boldsymbol{x}_o - \boldsymbol{\mu})'\boldsymbol{\Sigma}^{-1}\} f_{\boldsymbol{x}}(\boldsymbol{x}_o) + r_3^\star, \end{aligned}$$

where

$$|r_3^\star| \leq (2\pi)^{-p}\frac{1}{4!}|\boldsymbol{\Sigma}|^{-1/2}E[(\boldsymbol{u}')^{\otimes 4}]E[\boldsymbol{z}^{\otimes 4}]$$

with $\boldsymbol{z} \sim N_p(\mathbf{0}, \boldsymbol{\Sigma}^{-1})$.

Later Corollary 5.2 will be applied when $D[\boldsymbol{y}]$ is proportional to $\boldsymbol{\Sigma}$ and then the expressions of the corollary can be simplified further. The difference $D[\boldsymbol{y}] - \boldsymbol{\Sigma}$ is positive definite. Moreover, note the following interesting fact. When integrating the approximation over $\boldsymbol{x}_o$, i.e. omitting the error term in the expansion, the integral equals 1, meaning that if the approximating density is positive, the approximating density is also a proper density, which is very uncommon when applying Edgeworth-type approximations. A second interesting fact appears when, instead of independence in (5.10), only uncorrelatedness holds.

Corollary 5.3 *Let* $\boldsymbol{y}$ *and* $\boldsymbol{x}$ *be two random vectors of size* p *with densities* $f_{\boldsymbol{y}}(\boldsymbol{x}_o)$ *and*

$$f_{\boldsymbol{x}}(\boldsymbol{x}_o) = (2\pi)^{-p/2}|\boldsymbol{\Sigma}|^{-1/2}\exp(-\tfrac{1}{2}\mathrm{tr}\{\boldsymbol{\Sigma}^{-1}(\boldsymbol{x}_o - \boldsymbol{\mu})(\boldsymbol{x}_o - \boldsymbol{\mu})'\}),$$

respectively, both evaluated at $\boldsymbol{x}_o$*; it is supposed that* $\boldsymbol{\Sigma}$ *is p.d. Moreover, suppose that*

$$\boldsymbol{y} = \boldsymbol{x} - \boldsymbol{u}, \tag{5.11}$$

where $C[\boldsymbol{u}, \boldsymbol{x}] = \mathbf{0}$ *and* $\boldsymbol{u}$ *is symmetrically distributed with mean* $\mathbf{0}$*. Then an Edgeworth-type approximation of* $f_{\boldsymbol{y}}(\boldsymbol{x}_o)$*, which also is a density, is given by*

$$f_{\boldsymbol{x}}(\boldsymbol{x}_o) + \tfrac{1}{2}\mathrm{tr}\{(D[\boldsymbol{y}] - \boldsymbol{\Sigma})(\boldsymbol{\Sigma}^{-1}(\boldsymbol{x}_o - \boldsymbol{\mu})(\boldsymbol{x}_o - \boldsymbol{\mu})'\boldsymbol{\Sigma}^{-1} - \boldsymbol{\Sigma}^{-1})\} f_{\boldsymbol{x}}(\boldsymbol{x}_o),$$

provided that the approximating function is ≥ 0 *for all* $\boldsymbol{x}_o$.

5.3 Density Approximation for the Mean Parameter in the BRM

For the BRM, presented in Definition 2.1, the density of $\widehat{\boldsymbol{B}} - \boldsymbol{B}$ is now approximated. It is assumed that $\widehat{\boldsymbol{B}}$ is unique, i.e. the matrices $\boldsymbol{A}$ and $\boldsymbol{C}$ are of full rank, and therefore (see Corollary 3.1)

$$\widehat{\boldsymbol{B}} - \boldsymbol{B} = (\boldsymbol{A}'\boldsymbol{S}^{-1}\boldsymbol{A})^{-1}\boldsymbol{A}'\boldsymbol{S}^{-1}(\boldsymbol{X} - \boldsymbol{ABC})\boldsymbol{C}'(\boldsymbol{CC}')^{-1} \tag{5.12}$$

is discussed, where $\boldsymbol{S} \sim W_p(\boldsymbol{\Sigma}, n-k)$. Since (see Appendix B, Theorem B.18 (ii))

$$\frac{1}{n-k}\boldsymbol{S} \stackrel{P}{\to} \boldsymbol{\Sigma}, \qquad n \to \infty,$$

a natural approximating quantity is

$$\boldsymbol{B}_\Sigma - \boldsymbol{B} = (\boldsymbol{A}'\boldsymbol{\Sigma}^{-1}\boldsymbol{A})^{-1}\boldsymbol{A}'\boldsymbol{\Sigma}^{-1}(\boldsymbol{X} - \boldsymbol{ABC})\boldsymbol{C}'(\boldsymbol{CC}')^{-1}. \tag{5.13}$$

Moreover, $\boldsymbol{B}_\Sigma$ is normally distributed and

$$E[\widehat{\boldsymbol{B}} - \boldsymbol{B}] = E[\boldsymbol{B}_\Sigma - \boldsymbol{B}] = \boldsymbol{0},$$

$$D[\widehat{\boldsymbol{B}}] - D[\boldsymbol{B}_\Sigma] = \frac{p-q}{n-k-p+q-1}(\boldsymbol{CC}')^{-1} \otimes (\boldsymbol{A}'\boldsymbol{\Sigma}^{-1}\boldsymbol{A})^{-1}, \tag{5.14}$$

where (5.14) is obtained from $D[\widehat{\boldsymbol{B}}]$, presented in Corollary 4.1 (ii), and $D[\boldsymbol{B}_\Sigma]$ is established with the help of Appendix B, Theorem B.19 (iii). In many natural applications $(\boldsymbol{CC}')^{-1}$ will become small, or at least its elements are bounded when $n \to \infty$, and therefore the first two moments (cumulants) of $\widehat{\boldsymbol{B}}$ and $\boldsymbol{B}_\Sigma$ are close to each other. We also know that $\widehat{\boldsymbol{B}} - \widehat{\boldsymbol{B}}_\Sigma \stackrel{P}{\to} \boldsymbol{0}$ as $n \to \infty$ (see the proof of Theorem 4.1). Hence, many properties of $\widehat{\boldsymbol{B}}$ support the idea of approximating the density of $\widehat{\boldsymbol{B}} - \boldsymbol{B}$ with the density of $\boldsymbol{B}_\Sigma - \boldsymbol{B}$. The consequences of this approach are studied now and our starting point is the next important observation:

$$\widehat{\boldsymbol{B}} - \boldsymbol{B} = \boldsymbol{B}_\Sigma - \boldsymbol{B} - \boldsymbol{U},$$

where

$$\boldsymbol{U} = (\boldsymbol{A}'\boldsymbol{S}^{-1}\boldsymbol{A})^{-1}\boldsymbol{A}'\boldsymbol{S}^{-1}(\boldsymbol{P}_{A,\Sigma} - \boldsymbol{I})(\boldsymbol{X} - \boldsymbol{ABC})\boldsymbol{C}'(\boldsymbol{CC}')^{-1}.$$

Now $(\boldsymbol{A}'\boldsymbol{\Sigma}^{-1}\boldsymbol{A})^{-1}\boldsymbol{A}'\boldsymbol{\Sigma}^{-1}\boldsymbol{XC}'(\boldsymbol{CC}')^{-1}$ and $(\boldsymbol{P}_{A,\Sigma} - \boldsymbol{I})\boldsymbol{XC}'(\boldsymbol{CC}')^{-1}$ are independent (see Appendix B, Theorem B.19 (x)) and $\boldsymbol{XC}'(\boldsymbol{CC}')^{-1}$ is independent of $\boldsymbol{S}$ (see Appendix B, Theorem B.19 (viii)). Therefore, $\boldsymbol{B}_\Sigma$ and $\boldsymbol{U}$ are independently distributed. Hence, Theorem 5.2 can be applied and the following quantities are needed if $m = 3$ is chosen in Theorem 5.2:

$$\boldsymbol{B}_\Sigma - \boldsymbol{B} \sim N_{q,k}(\boldsymbol{0}, (\boldsymbol{A}'\boldsymbol{\Sigma}^{-1}\boldsymbol{A})^{-1}, (\boldsymbol{C}\boldsymbol{C}')^{-1}),$$

$$E[\boldsymbol{U}] = \boldsymbol{0}, \qquad E[\boldsymbol{u}^{\otimes 3}] = \boldsymbol{0}, \quad (\boldsymbol{u} = \mathrm{vec}\boldsymbol{U}),$$

$$E[\boldsymbol{u}^{\otimes 2}] = \mathrm{vec}(D[\widehat{\boldsymbol{B}}] - D[\boldsymbol{B}_\Sigma]) = \frac{p-q}{n-k-p+q-1}\mathrm{vec}((\boldsymbol{C}\boldsymbol{C}')^{-1} \otimes (\boldsymbol{A}'\boldsymbol{\Sigma}^{-1}\boldsymbol{A})^{-1}).$$

The last expression above is a vectorized version of (5.14). Moreover, in order to obtain the error bound of the approximation $E[\boldsymbol{u}^{\otimes 4}]$ has to be considered. Although it is not difficult to derive $E[\boldsymbol{u}^{\otimes 4}]$ explicitly, it makes sense only to consider the order of the error without presenting any details involving $\boldsymbol{A}$ and $\boldsymbol{C}$. The important observation is that

$$\boldsymbol{U}|\boldsymbol{S} \sim N_{q,k}(\boldsymbol{0}, (\boldsymbol{A}'\boldsymbol{S}^{-1}\boldsymbol{A})^{-1}\boldsymbol{A}'\boldsymbol{S}^{-1}\boldsymbol{\Sigma}\boldsymbol{S}^{-1}\boldsymbol{A}(\boldsymbol{A}'\boldsymbol{S}^{-1}\boldsymbol{A})^{-1} - (\boldsymbol{A}'\boldsymbol{\Sigma}^{-1}\boldsymbol{A})^{-1}, (\boldsymbol{C}\boldsymbol{C}')^{-1}). \tag{5.15}$$

Now, using $\boldsymbol{T}$ and $\boldsymbol{V}$, given in (4.19) and (4.20), respectively,

$$(\boldsymbol{A}'\boldsymbol{S}^{-1}\boldsymbol{A})^{-1}\boldsymbol{A}'\boldsymbol{S}^{-1}\boldsymbol{\Sigma}\boldsymbol{S}^{-1}\boldsymbol{A}(\boldsymbol{A}'\boldsymbol{S}^{-1}\boldsymbol{A})^{-1} - (\boldsymbol{A}'\boldsymbol{\Sigma}^{-1}\boldsymbol{A})^{-1} = (\boldsymbol{T}')^{-1}\boldsymbol{V}_{12}\boldsymbol{V}_{22}^{-1}\boldsymbol{V}_{22}^{-1}\boldsymbol{V}_{21}\boldsymbol{T}^{-1}.$$

However,

$$\boldsymbol{Z} = \boldsymbol{V}_{12}\boldsymbol{V}_{22}^{-1/2}$$

is independent of $\boldsymbol{V}_{22}$ (see Appendix B, Theorem B.20 (iv)), and instead of (5.15)

$$\boldsymbol{U}|\boldsymbol{Z}, \boldsymbol{V}_{22} \sim N_{q,k}(\boldsymbol{0}, (\boldsymbol{T}')^{-1}\boldsymbol{Z}\boldsymbol{V}_{22}^{-1}\boldsymbol{Z}'\boldsymbol{T}^{-1}, (\boldsymbol{C}\boldsymbol{C}')^{-1})$$

can be studied. It follows that $E[\boldsymbol{u}^{\otimes 4}|\boldsymbol{Z}, \boldsymbol{V}_{22}]$ is a linear function in $\boldsymbol{Z}\boldsymbol{V}_{22}^{-1}\boldsymbol{Z}' \otimes \boldsymbol{Z}\boldsymbol{V}_{22}^{-1}\boldsymbol{Z}'$, and since (see Appendix B, Theorem B.19 (vii) and Theorem B.21 (iii)) in the sense of the Loewner order (see Appendix A, Sect. A.3)

$$E[(\boldsymbol{Z}\boldsymbol{V}_{22}^{-1}\boldsymbol{Z}')^{\otimes 2}] \leq \frac{c}{n^2}\boldsymbol{I}$$

for some specific constant c, depending on $\boldsymbol{A}$ and $\boldsymbol{C}$, the following theorem has been established.

Theorem 5.3 *For the BRM presented in Definition 2.1, suppose that $r(\boldsymbol{A}) = q$ and $r(\boldsymbol{C}) = k$, and that*

$$\widehat{\boldsymbol{B}} = (\boldsymbol{A}'\boldsymbol{S}^{-1}\boldsymbol{A})^{-1}\boldsymbol{A}'\boldsymbol{S}^{-1}\boldsymbol{X}\boldsymbol{C}'(\boldsymbol{C}\boldsymbol{C}')^{-1}.$$

Let

$$B_{\Sigma} = (A'\Sigma^{-1}A)^{-1}A'\Sigma^{-1}XC'(CC')^{-1} \sim N_{q,k}(B, (A'\Sigma^{-1}A)^{-1}, (CC')^{-1}).$$

Then an Edgeworth-type expansion of the density of $\widehat{B}$ *equals*

$$f_{\widehat{B}}(B_o) = f_{B_E}(B_o) + r_3^{\star},$$

where

$$f_{B_E}(B_o) = \{1 - \tfrac{1}{2}skq + \tfrac{1}{2}s\mathrm{tr}\{A'\Sigma^{-1}A(B_o - B)CC'(B_o - B)'\}\}f_{B_{\Sigma}}(B_o),$$

$$s = \frac{p-q}{n-k-p+q-1}, \qquad n-k-p+q-1 > 0,$$

and

$$|r_3^{\star}| \leq \frac{c}{n^2},$$

for some fixed constant c which is a function of A *and* C*.*

In general the sum of the first terms in an Edgeworth-type expansion is not a density. However, as was also observed after Corollary 5.2, the density approximation for $\widehat{B}$ given in Theorem 5.3 works unusually well.

Theorem 5.4 *The function* $f_{B_E}(B_o)$ *given in Theorem 5.3 is a density if* $0 < 1 - \frac{1}{2}skq$*.*

Proof If $0 < 1 - \frac{1}{2}skq$, then $f_{B_E}(B_o) \geq 0$. Hence, it has to be shown that the integral of $f_{B_E}(B_o)$ over the whole space equals 1, i.e.

$$\int_{\mathcal{R}^{q\times k}} f_{B_E}(B_o)dB_o = 1 - \tfrac{1}{2}skq + \tfrac{1}{2}sE[\mathrm{tr}\{A'\Sigma^{-1}A(B_{\Sigma} - B)CC'(B_{\Sigma} - B)'\}] = 1,$$

where the expectation is taken with respect to $B_{\Sigma} \sim N_{qk}(B, (A'\Sigma^{-1}A)^{-1}, (CC')^{-1})$ and equals kq. □

The density function

$$f_Y(Y_o) = c|\Sigma|^{-n/2}|\Psi|^{-p/2}g(\mathrm{tr}\{\Sigma^{-1}(Y_o - \mu)\Psi^{-1}(Y_o - \mu)'\}),$$

where c is a standardization constant, is of the form $g(u) = u\exp(-u/2)$, Y: $p \times n$, μ: $p \times n$, $\Sigma > 0$: $p \times p$, $\Psi > 0$: $n \times n$, and is the density function of a random variable Y with a matrix Kotz-type distribution (see Nadarajah, 2003 and Appendix A, Sect. A.10 for a definition of the Kotz-type distribution).

Theorem 5.5 *The distribution of* $\boldsymbol{B}_E$ *with density* $f_{\boldsymbol{B}_E}(\boldsymbol{B}_o)$, *given in Theorem 5.3 is a mixture of a normal distribution and a matrix Kotz-type distribution with weights* $1 - \frac{1}{2}skq$ *and* $\frac{1}{2}skq$, *respectively, assuming that* $1 - \frac{1}{2}skq > 0$.

A consequence of this theorem is that the distribution of $\boldsymbol{B}_E$ may be multimodal, which is an undesirable feature in that it makes it more difficult to interpret extreme observations. However, it can be shown that if

$$s < \frac{2}{2 + pq}, \tag{5.16}$$

the distribution is unimodal. This means that if p is large in relation to n, i.e. the dimension in relation to the number of independent observations is large, one may run into problems when interpreting estimators via the approximation. Broadly speaking, if the approximating distribution deviates to a large extent from the normal distribution, then the conclusions should be carefully evaluated. However, if condition (5.16) holds, we can be reasonable confident in the validity of our conclusions.

When showing the independence between $\boldsymbol{B}_N$ and $\boldsymbol{U}$, the bilinear structure of the model was indeed used. The matrix $\boldsymbol{U}$ is a function of $\boldsymbol{S}$ and $\boldsymbol{X}\boldsymbol{C}'(\boldsymbol{C}\boldsymbol{C}')^{-1}$, whereas $\boldsymbol{B}_N$ is a function of $\boldsymbol{X}\boldsymbol{C}'(\boldsymbol{C}\boldsymbol{C}')^{-1}$. The spaces which are involved are $\mathcal{R}^n \otimes \mathcal{R}^p$, and its decomposition, i.e. $(\mathcal{C}(\boldsymbol{C}') \boxplus \mathcal{C}(\boldsymbol{C}')^{\perp}) \otimes (\mathcal{C}_{\Sigma}(\boldsymbol{A}) \boxplus \mathcal{C}_{\Sigma}(\boldsymbol{A})^{\perp})$, and the projections on these spaces: $\boldsymbol{P}_{C'}$, $\boldsymbol{I} - \boldsymbol{P}_{C'}$, $\boldsymbol{P}_{A,\Sigma}$ and $\boldsymbol{I} - \boldsymbol{P}_{A,\Sigma}$. When projecting $\boldsymbol{X}$ on these spaces, four independent quantities are obtained: $\boldsymbol{P}_{A,\Sigma}\boldsymbol{X}\boldsymbol{P}_{C'}$, $\boldsymbol{P}_{A,\Sigma}\boldsymbol{X}(\boldsymbol{I} - \boldsymbol{P}_{C'})$, $(\boldsymbol{I} - \boldsymbol{P}_{A,\Sigma})\boldsymbol{X}\boldsymbol{P}_{C'}$ and $(\boldsymbol{I} - \boldsymbol{P}_{A,\Sigma})\boldsymbol{X}(\boldsymbol{I} - \boldsymbol{P}_{C'})$. Since $\boldsymbol{A}\boldsymbol{B}_N\boldsymbol{C} = \boldsymbol{P}_{A,\Sigma}\boldsymbol{X}\boldsymbol{P}_{C'}$ and $\boldsymbol{U}$ is a function of $(\boldsymbol{I} - \boldsymbol{P}_{A,\Sigma})\boldsymbol{X}$ and $\boldsymbol{X}(\boldsymbol{I} - \boldsymbol{P}_{C'})$, the variables $\boldsymbol{B}_N$ and $\boldsymbol{U}$ are independently distributed. Hence, vector space decomposition is also essential for the Edgeworth-type expansion of the mean estimator in the BRM, and one should apply knowledge concerning the tensor space $\mathcal{R}^n \otimes \mathcal{R}^p$ in a manner similar to that used when estimating parameters. Moreover, an interesting technical observation is that projecting $\boldsymbol{X}$ on $\mathcal{C}_{\Sigma}(\boldsymbol{A})^{\perp}$ with an estimated inner product, i.e. $(\boldsymbol{I} - \boldsymbol{P}_{A,S})\boldsymbol{X}$, is the same as first projecting $\boldsymbol{X}$ on $\mathcal{C}_{\Sigma}(\boldsymbol{A})^{\perp}$ and then performing a second projection on $\mathcal{C}_S(\boldsymbol{A})^{\perp}$.

If one's intention is to perform the inference marginally on the elements of $\boldsymbol{B}$, then the marginal distribution will also be a mixture of a Kotz-type distribution and a normal distribution, but the influence of the Kotz part will be less in this case compared to the case where simultaneous inference on the elements of $\boldsymbol{B}$ is taking place. Without a proof, Theorem 5.3 is now generalized as follows.

Theorem 5.6 *For the* BRM, *suppose that* $\mathcal{C}(\boldsymbol{K}') \subseteq \mathcal{C}(\boldsymbol{A}')$ *and* $\mathcal{C}(\boldsymbol{L}) \subseteq \mathcal{C}(\boldsymbol{C})$, *and*

$$\boldsymbol{K}\widehat{\boldsymbol{B}}\boldsymbol{L} = \boldsymbol{K}(\boldsymbol{A}'\boldsymbol{S}^{-1}\boldsymbol{A})^{-}\boldsymbol{A}'\boldsymbol{S}^{-1}\boldsymbol{X}\boldsymbol{C}'(\boldsymbol{C}\boldsymbol{C}')^{-}\boldsymbol{L}.$$

Let

$$\begin{aligned}\boldsymbol{K}\boldsymbol{B}_{\Sigma}\boldsymbol{L} &= \boldsymbol{K}(\boldsymbol{A}'\boldsymbol{\Sigma}^{-1}\boldsymbol{A})^{-}\boldsymbol{A}'\boldsymbol{\Sigma}^{-1}\boldsymbol{X}\boldsymbol{C}'(\boldsymbol{C}\boldsymbol{C}')^{-}\boldsymbol{L}\\ &\sim N_{\bullet,\bullet}(\boldsymbol{K}\boldsymbol{B}\boldsymbol{L}, \boldsymbol{K}(\boldsymbol{A}'\boldsymbol{\Sigma}^{-1}\boldsymbol{A})^{-}\boldsymbol{K}', \boldsymbol{L}(\boldsymbol{C}\boldsymbol{C}')^{-}\boldsymbol{L}').\end{aligned}$$

Then an Edgeworth-type expansion of the density of $\boldsymbol{K}\widehat{\boldsymbol{B}}\boldsymbol{L}$ *equals*

$$f_{\boldsymbol{K}\widehat{\boldsymbol{B}}\boldsymbol{L}}(\boldsymbol{B}_o) = f_{\boldsymbol{K}\boldsymbol{B}_E\boldsymbol{L}}(\boldsymbol{B}_o) + r_3^\star,$$

where

$$f_{\boldsymbol{K}\boldsymbol{B}_E\boldsymbol{L}}(\boldsymbol{B}_o) = \{1 - \tfrac{1}{2}s_1 r(\boldsymbol{K})r(\boldsymbol{L}) + \tfrac{1}{2}s_1 \mathrm{tr}\{\boldsymbol{K}'(\boldsymbol{K}(\boldsymbol{A}'\boldsymbol{\Sigma}^{-1}\boldsymbol{A})^-\boldsymbol{K}')^-\boldsymbol{K}$$
$$\times (\boldsymbol{B}_o - \boldsymbol{B})\boldsymbol{L}(\boldsymbol{L}'(\boldsymbol{C}\boldsymbol{C}')^-\boldsymbol{L})^-\boldsymbol{L}'(\boldsymbol{B}_o - \boldsymbol{B})'\}\} f_{\boldsymbol{K}\boldsymbol{B}_\Sigma\boldsymbol{L}}(\boldsymbol{B}_o),$$

$$s_1 = \frac{p - r(\boldsymbol{A})}{n - r(\boldsymbol{C}) - p + r(\boldsymbol{A}) - 1}, \qquad n - r(\boldsymbol{C}) - p + r(\boldsymbol{A}) - 1 > 0,$$

and

$$|r_3^\star| \le \frac{c}{n^2},$$

for some fixed constant c which is a function of $\boldsymbol{A}$ *and* $\boldsymbol{C}$.

Example 5.1 In Example 3.1 different estimates of $\boldsymbol{B}$ in the *BRM* were presented, for example the maximum likelihood estimate (Model Ia)

$$\widehat{\boldsymbol{B}}_{1o} = (\boldsymbol{A}'\boldsymbol{S}_o^{-1}\boldsymbol{A})^{-1}\boldsymbol{A}'\boldsymbol{S}_o^{-1}\boldsymbol{X}_o\boldsymbol{C}'(\boldsymbol{C}\boldsymbol{C}')^{-1} = \begin{pmatrix} 17.4 & 15.8 \\ 0.48 & 0.83 \end{pmatrix} \tag{5.17}$$

and an unweighted estimate (Model Ib),

$$\widehat{\boldsymbol{B}}_{2o} = (\boldsymbol{A}'\boldsymbol{A})^{-1}\boldsymbol{A}'\boldsymbol{X}_o\boldsymbol{C}'(\boldsymbol{C}\boldsymbol{C}')^{-1} = \begin{pmatrix} 17.4 & 16.3 \\ 0.48 & 0.78 \end{pmatrix}. \tag{5.18}$$

These estimates are very close to each other and one wish to ascertain which of the corresponding estimators is to be preferred. A natural means of determining this is to compare their distributions. The unweighted estimator has a matrix normal distribution and now Theorem 5.6 provides a density approximation which, according to the theory, is fairly accurate, i.e. $\mathcal{O}_p(n^{-2})$ (see Appendix A, Sect. A.12 for a definition of $\mathcal{O}_p(\bullet)$).

In Fig. 5.1 the approximate distribution of $\widehat{\boldsymbol{B}}_1$ and the distribution of $\widehat{\boldsymbol{B}}_2$ are compared. Since there are four elements in $\widehat{\boldsymbol{B}}_i$, $i = 1, 2$, the distribution is presented via the following pairs: $(\widehat{b}_{i11}, \widehat{b}_{i21})$, the estimated intercept and slope for girls; $(\widehat{b}_{i11}, \widehat{b}_{i12})$, the estimated intercepts for girls and boys; $(\widehat{b}_{i12}, \widehat{b}_{i22})$, the estimated intercept and slope for boys; and $(\widehat{b}_{i21}, \widehat{b}_{i22})$, the estimated slopes for boys and girls.

The overall conclusion when inspecting Fig. 5.1 is that there is almost no difference between the distributions of the estimators $\widehat{\boldsymbol{B}}_1$ and $\widehat{\boldsymbol{B}}_2$. Note that the different shapes in **(a)**–**(d)** are due to scaling and are not of any particular interest. Thus, from now on one can completely rely on $\widehat{\boldsymbol{B}}_2$, which, due to its well-known distribution, is

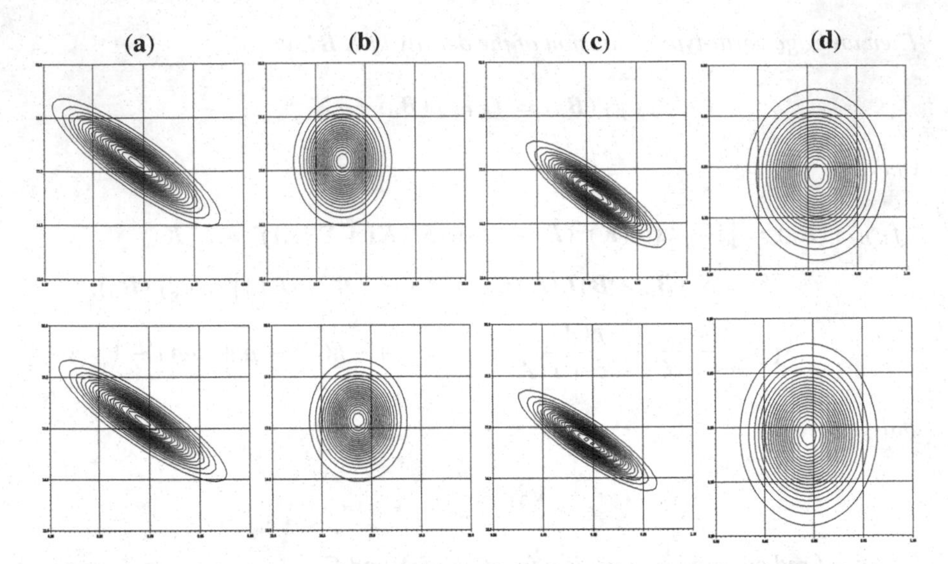

Fig. 5.1 Illustration of the distributions in Example 5.2. The first row shows for the MLE, $\widehat{\boldsymbol{B}}_1 = (\boldsymbol{A}'\boldsymbol{S}^{-1}\boldsymbol{A})^{-1}\boldsymbol{A}'\boldsymbol{S}^{-1}\boldsymbol{X}\boldsymbol{C}'(\boldsymbol{C}\boldsymbol{C}')^{-1}$, given in (5.17), the bivariate densities for the following pairs: $(\widehat{b}_{11}, \widehat{b}_{21})$, given under (**a**), $(\widehat{b}_{11}, \widehat{b}_{12})$, given under (**b**), $(\widehat{b}_{12}, \widehat{b}_{22})$, given under (**c**), and $(\widehat{b}_{21}, \widehat{b}_{22})$, given under (**d**). The second row shows the corresponding densities for the unweighted estimator $\widehat{\boldsymbol{B}}_2 = (\boldsymbol{A}'\boldsymbol{A})^{-1}\boldsymbol{A}'\boldsymbol{X}\boldsymbol{C}'(\boldsymbol{C}\boldsymbol{C}')^{-1}$, given in (5.18)

easier to handle than $\widehat{\boldsymbol{B}}_1$, for example when constructing tests concerning $\boldsymbol{B}$. Hence, an estimator is chosen which is not the maximum likelihood estimator and thus is not asymptotically the best estimator. Moreover, redirecting the discussion one can conclude that the density approximation presented in Theorem 5.3 seems to work well. □

Finally, an example is presented where there are some differences between the MLE and an unweighted estimator of the mean parameters.

Example 5.2 Artificial data have been generated according to

$$\boldsymbol{X} = \boldsymbol{A}\boldsymbol{B}\boldsymbol{C} + \boldsymbol{E}, \qquad \boldsymbol{E} \sim N_{p,n}(\boldsymbol{0}, \boldsymbol{\Sigma}, \boldsymbol{I}),$$

where

$$\boldsymbol{A} = \begin{pmatrix} 1 & 8 \\ 1 & 12 \\ 1 & 16 \\ 1 & 20 \\ 1 & 24 \end{pmatrix}, \quad \boldsymbol{B} = \begin{pmatrix} 1 & 3 \\ 2 & 3 \end{pmatrix}, \quad \boldsymbol{C} = \left(\boldsymbol{1}'_{14} \otimes \begin{pmatrix} 1 \\ 0 \end{pmatrix} : \boldsymbol{1}'_{14} \otimes \begin{pmatrix} 0 \\ 1 \end{pmatrix}\right),$$

$$\boldsymbol{\Sigma} = \begin{pmatrix} 2 & 1.6 & 0.9 & 1.5 & 0.9 \\ 1.6 & 4 & 1.9 & 3.0 & 1.9 \\ 0.9 & 1.9 & 2 & 1.9 & 0.9 \\ 1.5 & 3.0 & 1.9 & 4 & 1.5 \\ 0.9 & 1.9 & 0.9 & 1.5 & 2 \end{pmatrix}.$$

The correlations among the variables are medium-sized, i.e. they vary between 0.45 and 0.75. If one generates data with correlations around 0.90, the estimators, due to collinearity, start to perform poorly. With the above choice of matrices, the following data were generated:

$$\boldsymbol{X} = \begin{pmatrix} 15.7 & 17.6 & 18.3 & 19.5 & 19.2 & 16.9 & 18.1 & 19.0 & 16.0 & 16.6 & 15.3 & 16.8 & 17.9 & 16.8, \\ 26.9 & 29.7 & 28.4 & 24.4 & 23.9 & 25.3 & 26.2 & 27.8 & 26.5 & 27.4 & 29.4 & 25.0 & 27.3 & 26.8 \\ 19.3 & 26.9 & 24.9 & 27.4 & 24.7 & 25.7 & 23.6 & 24.3 & 23.6 & 26.2 & 22.1 & 24.5 & 27.3 & 26.0, \\ 42.1 & 41.8 & 39.2 & 33.4 & 37.4 & 39.4 & 39.9 & 40.4 & 36.4 & 42.0 & 41.0 & 37.8 & 40.9 & 42.0 \\ 30.0 & 34.7 & 31.7 & 34.0 & 33.4 & 33.0 & 32.5 & 32.0 & 31.5 & 31.7 & 30.9 & 33.5 & 33.6 & 34.4, \\ 52.9 & 53.2 & 48.6 & 46.9 & 51.3 & 52.2 & 49.4 & 52.2 & 49.6 & 53.4 & 50.5 & 49.4 & 51.0 & 50.7 \\ 36.3 & 43.4 & 42.2 & 43.4 & 41.0 & 40.8 & 39.2 & 39.5 & 40.0 & 40.7 & 39.0 & 42.0 & 43.5 & 40.5, \\ 63.7 & 63.9 & 60.1 & 58.5 & 63.0 & 63.0 & 62.7 & 62.5 & 59.9 & 64.4 & 61.8 & 61.2 & 62.7 & 63.7 \\ 44.3 & 49.1 & 48.6 & 52.3 & 48.2 & 49.1 & 50.7 & 49.0 & 47.8 & 48.1 & 46.1 & 48.6 & 49.9 & 49.26, \\ 76.8 & 77.1 & 75.4 & 72.6 & 73.8 & 72.8 & 74.6 & 75.8 & 73.6 & 76.4 & 75.6 & 72.1 & 78.3 & 75.0 \end{pmatrix}.$$

Note that each row in $\boldsymbol{X}$: 5×28 is represented by two lines. The data produced

$$\widehat{\boldsymbol{B}}_{1o} = (\boldsymbol{A}'\boldsymbol{S}_o^{-1}\boldsymbol{A})^{-1}\boldsymbol{A}'\boldsymbol{S}_o^{-1}\boldsymbol{X}_o\boldsymbol{C}'(\boldsymbol{C}\boldsymbol{C}')^{-1} = \begin{pmatrix} 1.63 & 2.45 \\ 1.97 & 2.97 \end{pmatrix}, \tag{5.19}$$

$$\widehat{\boldsymbol{B}}_{2o} = (\boldsymbol{A}'\boldsymbol{A})^{-1}\boldsymbol{A}'\boldsymbol{X}_o\boldsymbol{C}'(\boldsymbol{C}\boldsymbol{C}')^{-1} = \begin{pmatrix} 1.43 & 3.23 \\ 1.96 & 2.98 \end{pmatrix}. \tag{5.20}$$

Moreover, the estimated dispersion matrices for the weighted and unweighted approach equal

$$\widehat{\boldsymbol{\Sigma}}_{1o} = (\boldsymbol{X} - \boldsymbol{A}\widehat{\boldsymbol{B}}_{1o}\boldsymbol{C})()'/28 = \begin{pmatrix} 2.39 & 2.50 & 1.23 & 1.11 & 2.29 \\ 2.50 & 6.46 & 3.61 & 3.91 & 4.21 \\ 1.23 & 3.61 & 3.08 & 2.57 & 2.42 \\ 1.11 & 3.91 & 2.57 & 3.37 & 2.33 \\ 2.29 & 4.21 & 2.42 & 2.33 & 4.13 \end{pmatrix},$$

$$\widehat{\boldsymbol{\Sigma}}_{2o} = (\boldsymbol{X} - \boldsymbol{A}\widehat{\boldsymbol{B}}_{2o}\boldsymbol{C})()'/28 = \begin{pmatrix} 2.29 & 1.96 & 0.96 & 1.09 & 1.88 \\ 1.96 & 5.43 & 2.83 & 3.37 & 3.25 \\ 0.96 & 2.83 & 2.59 & 2.34 & 1.76 \\ 1.09 & 3.37 & 2.34 & 3.43 & 1.96 \\ 1.88 & 3.25 & 1.76 & 1.96 & 3.29 \end{pmatrix}.$$

Both dispersion estimators are fairly far away from the true values, but this is not completely unexpected since the estimators according to the theory are biased. The estimator based on the unweighted mean is less biased. In Fig. 5.2 the approximate

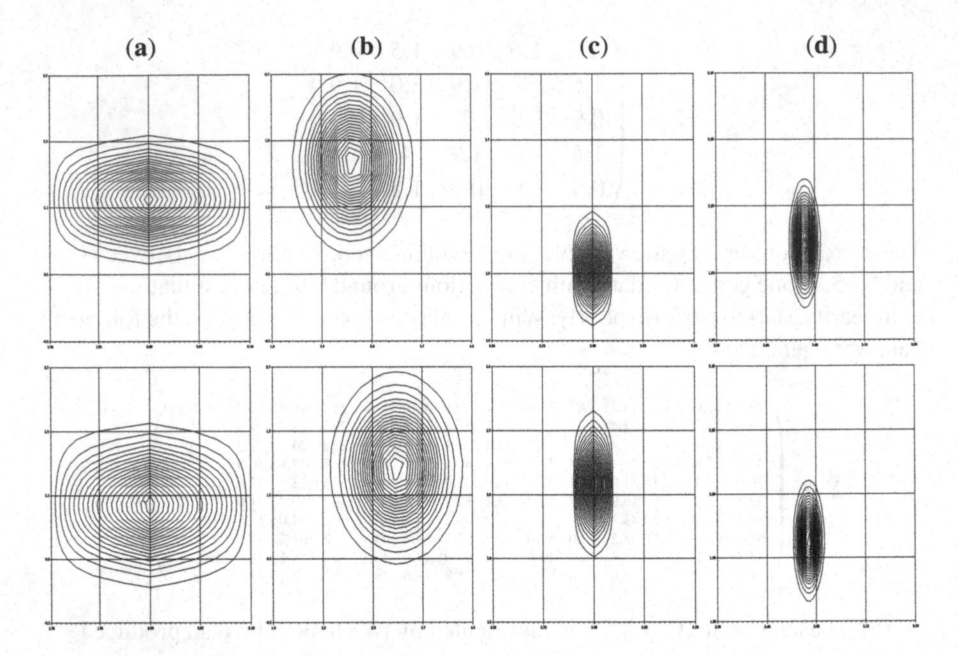

Fig. 5.2 Illustration of the distributions in Example 5.2. The first row shows, for the MLE, $\widehat{\boldsymbol{B}}_1 = (\boldsymbol{A}'\boldsymbol{S}^{-1}\boldsymbol{A})^{-1}\boldsymbol{A}'\boldsymbol{S}^{-1}\boldsymbol{X}\boldsymbol{C}'(\boldsymbol{C}\boldsymbol{C}')^{-1}$, given in (5.19), the bivariate densities for the following pairs: $(\widehat{b}_{11}, \widehat{b}_{21})$, given under (**a**); $(\widehat{b}_{11}, \widehat{b}_{12})$, given under (**b**); $(\widehat{b}_{12}, \widehat{b}_{22})$, given under (**c**); and $(\widehat{b}_{21}, \widehat{b}_{22})$, given under (**d**). The second row shows the corresponding densities for the unweighted estimator $\widehat{\boldsymbol{B}}_2 = (\boldsymbol{A}'\boldsymbol{A})^{-1}\boldsymbol{A}'\boldsymbol{X}\boldsymbol{C}'(\boldsymbol{C}\boldsymbol{C}')^{-1}$, given in (5.20)

distribution of the MLE and the exact distribution of the unweighted estimator are presented. Small differences between the weighted and the unweighted estimator can be observed. With more parameters describing the mean, it would be possible to show larger differences.

□

5.4 Density Approximation for the Mean Parameter Estimators in the $EBRM_B^3$

For the BRM, the results possess a certain degree of mathematical beauty. Now the more complicated $EBRM_B^3$, presented in Definition 2.2, is considered. Once again, only the densities of the maximum likelihood estimators of the mean parameters will be treated. Since moments for these estimators were derived in Chap. 4, it is clear that an Edgeworth-type expansion can be performed. However, it is of interest to know what can be stated concerning the error of the approximation. For $\widehat{\boldsymbol{B}}$ in the BRM it was shown that the estimator was a sum of a normally distributed variable $\boldsymbol{B}_\Sigma$ and a random variable $(-\boldsymbol{U})$ which was independent of $\boldsymbol{B}_\Sigma$, and it is now investigated if this also takes place for $\boldsymbol{B}_i$, $i = 1, 2, 3$, in the $EBRM_B^3$. It is always supposed that the conditions for uniqueness of the estimators are satisfied, which, as has been shown in Theorem 4.9, depend on which $\widehat{\boldsymbol{B}}_i$ is being studied.

Let us start with $\widehat{\boldsymbol{B}}_3$ and the expression presented in (4.123) is used:

$$\widehat{\boldsymbol{B}}_3 = (\boldsymbol{A}_3'\boldsymbol{G}_2(\boldsymbol{G}_2'\boldsymbol{W}_3\boldsymbol{G}_2)^{-1}\boldsymbol{G}_2'\boldsymbol{A}_3)^{-1}\boldsymbol{A}_3'\boldsymbol{G}_2(\boldsymbol{G}_2'\boldsymbol{W}_3\boldsymbol{G}_2)^{-1}\boldsymbol{G}_2'\boldsymbol{X}\boldsymbol{C}_3'(\boldsymbol{C}_3\boldsymbol{C}_3')^{-1}. \tag{5.21}$$

Then, as was also noted when obtaining its dispersion, the estimator has the same form as $\widehat{\boldsymbol{B}}$ in the BRM. Therefore,

$$\widehat{\boldsymbol{B}}_3 - \boldsymbol{B}_3 = \boldsymbol{B}_{3N} - \boldsymbol{B}_3 - \boldsymbol{U}_3,$$

where the normally distributed variable $\boldsymbol{B}_{3N}$ satisfies

$$\begin{aligned}\boldsymbol{B}_{3N} - \boldsymbol{B}_3 =& (\boldsymbol{A}_3'\boldsymbol{G}_2(\boldsymbol{G}_2'\boldsymbol{\Sigma}\boldsymbol{G}_2)^{-1}\boldsymbol{G}_2'\boldsymbol{A}_3)^{-1}\boldsymbol{A}_3'\boldsymbol{G}_2(\boldsymbol{G}_2'\boldsymbol{\Sigma}\boldsymbol{G}_2)^{-1}\boldsymbol{G}_2'\\ &\times(\boldsymbol{X} - \boldsymbol{A}_3\boldsymbol{B}_3\boldsymbol{C}_3)\boldsymbol{C}_3'(\boldsymbol{C}_3\boldsymbol{C}_3')^{-1}\end{aligned} \tag{5.22}$$

and

$$\begin{aligned}\boldsymbol{U}_3 =& (\boldsymbol{A}_3'\boldsymbol{G}_2(\boldsymbol{G}_2'\boldsymbol{W}_3\boldsymbol{G}_2)^{-1}\boldsymbol{G}_2'\boldsymbol{A}_3)^{-1}\boldsymbol{A}_3'\boldsymbol{G}_2(\boldsymbol{G}_2'\boldsymbol{W}_3\boldsymbol{G}_2)^{-1}\\ &\times(\boldsymbol{P}_{G_2'A_3, G_2'\Sigma G_2} - \boldsymbol{I})\boldsymbol{G}_2'\boldsymbol{X}\boldsymbol{C}_3'(\boldsymbol{C}_3\boldsymbol{C}_3')^{-1}.\end{aligned} \tag{5.23}$$

According to Appendix B, Theorem B.19 (viii), the matrix $\boldsymbol{X}\boldsymbol{C}_3'(\boldsymbol{C}_3\boldsymbol{C}_3')^{-1}$ is independent of $\boldsymbol{W}_3$ and $\boldsymbol{A}_3'\boldsymbol{G}_2(\boldsymbol{G}_2'\boldsymbol{\Sigma}\boldsymbol{G}_2)^{-1}\boldsymbol{G}_2'\boldsymbol{X}$ is independent of (see Appendix B, Theorem B.19 (xi))

$$(\boldsymbol{P}_{G_2'A_3, G_2'\Sigma G_2} - \boldsymbol{I})\boldsymbol{G}_2'\boldsymbol{X},$$

which implies that $\boldsymbol{U}_3$ is independent of $\boldsymbol{B}_{3N}$. Thus, $\boldsymbol{U}_3$ can be regarded as an error matrix. Let $\boldsymbol{u}_3 = vec\boldsymbol{U}_3$ and then Theorem 5.3 establishes the following theorem.

Theorem 5.7 *Let $\widehat{\boldsymbol{B}}_3$, $\boldsymbol{B}_{3N}$ and $\boldsymbol{U}_3$ be given by (5.21), (5.22) and (5.23), respectively. Then an Edgeworth-type expansion of the density of $\widehat{\boldsymbol{B}}_3$ equals*

$$f_{\widehat{\boldsymbol{B}}_3}(\boldsymbol{B}_o) = f_{\boldsymbol{B}_{3E}}(\boldsymbol{B}_o) + r_3^\star,$$

where

$$\begin{aligned}f_{\boldsymbol{B}_{3E}}(\boldsymbol{B}_o) &= f_{\boldsymbol{B}_{3N}}(\boldsymbol{B}_o) + \tfrac{1}{2}E[(\boldsymbol{u}_3')^{\otimes 2}]\mathrm{vec}\boldsymbol{f}^2_{\boldsymbol{B}_{3N}}(\boldsymbol{B}_o)\\ &= (1 - \tfrac{1}{2}sk_3m_2 + \tfrac{1}{2}s\,\mathrm{tr}\{\boldsymbol{A}_3'\boldsymbol{G}_2(\boldsymbol{G}_2'\boldsymbol{\Sigma}\boldsymbol{G}_2)^{-1}\boldsymbol{G}_2'\boldsymbol{A}_3(\boldsymbol{B}_o - \boldsymbol{B}_3)\boldsymbol{C}_3\boldsymbol{C}_3'(\boldsymbol{B}_o - \boldsymbol{B}_3)'\})f_{\boldsymbol{B}_{3N}}(\boldsymbol{B}_o),\end{aligned}$$

$$s = \frac{p - m_2}{n - k_3 - p + m_2 - 1}, \qquad n - k_3 - p + m_2 - 1 > 0,$$

m_2 is defined in (4.78) and

$$|r_3^{\star}| \leq \frac{c}{n^2},$$

for some fixed constant c which is a function of the design matrices. The expectation $E[(\boldsymbol{u}_3')^{\otimes 2}]$ equals

$$E[(\boldsymbol{u}_3')^{\otimes 2}] = \tfrac{m_2-q_3}{n-k_3-m_2+q_3-1}\mathrm{vec}'((\boldsymbol{C}_3\boldsymbol{C}_3')^{-1} \otimes (\boldsymbol{A}_3'\boldsymbol{G}_2(\boldsymbol{G}_2'\boldsymbol{\Sigma}\boldsymbol{G}_2)^{-1}\boldsymbol{G}_2'\boldsymbol{A}_3)^{-1}).$$

The density $f_{\boldsymbol{B}_{3E}}(\boldsymbol{B}_o)$ is a real density, i.e. the density of a matrix Kotz-type distribution mixed with a normal density.

In the following $\widehat{\boldsymbol{B}}_2$ will be considered. However, it is convenient first to manipulate

$$\boldsymbol{G}_1'\boldsymbol{A}_2(\widehat{\boldsymbol{B}}_2 - \boldsymbol{B}_2)\boldsymbol{C}_2,$$

which then due to uniqueness assumptions can be transformed into $\widehat{\boldsymbol{B}}_2 - \boldsymbol{B}_2$. From (4.125) it follows that

$$\begin{aligned}\boldsymbol{G}_1'\boldsymbol{A}_2(\widehat{\boldsymbol{B}}_2 - \boldsymbol{B}_2)\boldsymbol{C}_2 &= \boldsymbol{P}_{G_1'A_2,G_1'W_2G_1}\boldsymbol{G}_1'(\boldsymbol{X} - E[\boldsymbol{X}])(\boldsymbol{P}_{C_2'} - \boldsymbol{P}_{C_3'})\\ &+ \boldsymbol{P}_{G_1'A_2,G_1'W_2G_1}\boldsymbol{G}_1'(\boldsymbol{I} - \boldsymbol{P}_{A_3,G_2'W_3G_2,G_2})(\boldsymbol{X} - E[\boldsymbol{X}])\boldsymbol{P}_{C_3'}. \qquad (5.24)\end{aligned}$$

As with $\widehat{\boldsymbol{B}}_3$, the idea is to split this expression into two independent components, one of which is normally distributed, i.e.

$$\boldsymbol{G}_1'\boldsymbol{A}_2(\widehat{\boldsymbol{B}}_2 - \boldsymbol{B}_2)\boldsymbol{C}_2 = \boldsymbol{G}_1'\boldsymbol{A}_2(\boldsymbol{B}_{2N} - \boldsymbol{B}_2)\boldsymbol{C}_2 - \boldsymbol{G}_1'\boldsymbol{A}_2\boldsymbol{U}_2\boldsymbol{C}_2, \qquad (5.25)$$

where it can be shown that

$$\begin{aligned}\boldsymbol{G}_1'\boldsymbol{A}_2(\boldsymbol{B}_{2N} - \boldsymbol{B}_2)\boldsymbol{C}_2 &= \boldsymbol{P}_{G_1'A_2,G_1'\Sigma G_1}\boldsymbol{G}_1'(\boldsymbol{X} - \boldsymbol{A}_2\boldsymbol{B}_2\boldsymbol{C}_2)(\boldsymbol{P}_{C_2'} - \boldsymbol{P}_{C_3'})\\ &+ \boldsymbol{P}_{G_1'A_2,G_1'\Sigma G_1}\boldsymbol{G}_1'(\boldsymbol{I} - \boldsymbol{P}_{A_3,G_2'\Sigma G_2,G_2})\boldsymbol{X}\boldsymbol{P}_{C_3'}, \qquad (5.26)\end{aligned}$$

which is normally distributed, and

$$\begin{aligned}\boldsymbol{G}_1'\boldsymbol{A}_2\boldsymbol{U}_2\boldsymbol{C}_2 = \boldsymbol{P}_{G_1'A_2,G_1'\Sigma G_1}&\boldsymbol{G}_1'\boldsymbol{P}_{A_3,G_2'W_3G_2,G_2}\boldsymbol{P}'_{G_3,\Sigma^{-1}}\boldsymbol{X}\boldsymbol{P}_{C_3'}\\ &- \boldsymbol{P}_{G_1'A_2,G_1'W_2G_1}\boldsymbol{G}_1'\boldsymbol{P}'_{G_2,\Sigma^{-1}}(\boldsymbol{I} - \boldsymbol{P}_{A_3,G_2'W_3G_2,G_2})\boldsymbol{X}\boldsymbol{P}_{C_3'}\\ &- \boldsymbol{P}_{G_1'A_2,G_1'W_2G_1}\boldsymbol{G}_1'\boldsymbol{P}'_{G_2,\Sigma^{-1}}\boldsymbol{X}(\boldsymbol{P}_{C_2'} - \boldsymbol{P}_{C_3'}). \qquad (5.27)\end{aligned}$$

It is now briefly shown how (5.26) and (5.27) arose. First, in (5.24) the trivial identity $\boldsymbol{I} - \boldsymbol{P}_{G_1'A_2,G_1'\Sigma G_1} + \boldsymbol{P}_{G_1'A_2,G_1'\Sigma G_1} = \boldsymbol{I}$ is utilized; i.e. a decomposition of the whole space into $\mathcal{C}(\boldsymbol{G}_1'\boldsymbol{A}_2)$ and its orthogonal complement is applied. Moreover, $\boldsymbol{P}_{G_1'A_2,G_1'W_2G_1}\boldsymbol{G}_1'\boldsymbol{A}_2 = \boldsymbol{G}_1'\boldsymbol{A}_2$. Then (5.24) equals

$$\boldsymbol{P}_{G_1'A_2,G_1'\Sigma G_1}\boldsymbol{G}_1'(\boldsymbol{X} - E[\boldsymbol{X}])(\boldsymbol{P}_{C_2'} - \boldsymbol{P}_{C_3'}) \tag{5.28}$$

$$+\boldsymbol{P}_{G_1'A_2,G_1'W_2G_1}(\boldsymbol{I} - \boldsymbol{P}_{G_1'A_2,G_1'\Sigma G_1})\boldsymbol{G}_1'(\boldsymbol{X} - E[\boldsymbol{X}])(\boldsymbol{P}_{C_2'} - \boldsymbol{P}_{C_3'}) \tag{5.29}$$

$$+\boldsymbol{P}_{G_1'A_2,G_1'\Sigma G_1}\boldsymbol{G}_1'(\boldsymbol{I} - \boldsymbol{P}_{A_3,G_2'W_3G_2,G_2})(\boldsymbol{X} - E[\boldsymbol{X}])\boldsymbol{P}_{C_3'} \tag{5.30}$$

$$+\boldsymbol{P}_{G_1'A_2,G_1'W_2G_1}(\boldsymbol{I} - \boldsymbol{P}_{G_1'A_2,G_1'\Sigma G_1})\boldsymbol{G}_1'(\boldsymbol{I} - \boldsymbol{P}_{A_3,G_2'W_3G_2,G_2}) \times(\boldsymbol{X} - E[\boldsymbol{X}])\boldsymbol{P}_{C_3'}. \tag{5.31}$$

Now, using

$$(\boldsymbol{I} - \boldsymbol{P}_{G_1'A_2,G_1'\Sigma G_1})\boldsymbol{G}_1' = \boldsymbol{G}_1'\boldsymbol{P}'_{G_2,\Sigma^{-1}},$$
$$(\boldsymbol{I} - \boldsymbol{P}_{G_2'A_3,G_2'\Sigma G_2})\boldsymbol{G}_2' = \boldsymbol{G}_2'\boldsymbol{P}'_{G_3,\Sigma^{-1}},$$

splitting (5.30) into the following parts

$$\begin{aligned}
&\boldsymbol{P}_{G_1'A_2,G_1'\Sigma G_1}\boldsymbol{G}_1'(\boldsymbol{I} - \boldsymbol{P}_{A_3,G_2'\Sigma G_2,G_2})(\boldsymbol{X} - E[\boldsymbol{X}])\boldsymbol{P}_{C_3'}\\
&\quad-\boldsymbol{P}_{G_1'A_2,G_1'\Sigma G_1}\boldsymbol{G}_1'\boldsymbol{P}_{A_3,G_2'W_3G_2,G_2}(\boldsymbol{I} - \boldsymbol{P}_{A_3,G_2'\Sigma G_2,G_2})(\boldsymbol{X} - E[\boldsymbol{X}])\boldsymbol{P}_{C_3'}\\
&\quad= \boldsymbol{P}_{G_1'A_2,G_1'\Sigma G_1}\boldsymbol{G}_1'(\boldsymbol{I} - \boldsymbol{P}_{A_3,G_2'\Sigma G_2,G_2})(\boldsymbol{X} - E[\boldsymbol{X}])\boldsymbol{P}_{C_3'}\\
&\quad-\boldsymbol{P}_{G_1'A_2,G_1'\Sigma G_1}\boldsymbol{G}_1'\boldsymbol{P}_{A_3,G_2'W_3G_2,G_2}\boldsymbol{P}'_{G_3,\Sigma^{-1}}(\boldsymbol{X} - E[\boldsymbol{X}])\boldsymbol{P}_{C_3'}
\end{aligned}$$

and observing that (5.31) is identical to

$$\boldsymbol{P}_{G_1'A_2,G_1'W_2G_1}\boldsymbol{G}_1'\boldsymbol{P}'_{G_2,\Sigma^{-1}}(\boldsymbol{I} - \boldsymbol{P}_{A_3,G_2'W_3G_2})(\boldsymbol{X} - E[\boldsymbol{X}])\boldsymbol{P}_{C_3'}$$

yield that (5.28)–(5.31) can be transformed into

$$\boldsymbol{P}_{G_1'A_2,G_1'\Sigma G_1}\boldsymbol{G}_1'(\boldsymbol{X} - E[\boldsymbol{X}])(\boldsymbol{P}_{C_2'} - \boldsymbol{P}_{C_3'}) \tag{5.32}$$

$$+\boldsymbol{P}_{G_1'A_2,G_1'\Sigma G_1}\boldsymbol{G}_1'(\boldsymbol{I} - \boldsymbol{P}_{A_3,G_2'\Sigma G_2,G_2})(\boldsymbol{X} - E[\boldsymbol{X}])\boldsymbol{P}_{C_3'} \tag{5.33}$$

$$+\boldsymbol{P}_{G_1'A_2,G_1'W_2G_1}\boldsymbol{G}_1'\boldsymbol{P}'_{G_2,\Sigma^{-1}}(\boldsymbol{X} - E[\boldsymbol{X}])(\boldsymbol{P}_{C_2'} - \boldsymbol{P}_{C_3'}) \tag{5.34}$$

$$-\boldsymbol{P}_{G_1'A_2,G_1'\Sigma G_1}\boldsymbol{G}_1'\boldsymbol{P}_{A_3,G_2'W_3G_2,G_2}\boldsymbol{P}'_{G_3,\Sigma^{-1}}(\boldsymbol{X} - E[\boldsymbol{X}])\boldsymbol{P}_{C_3'} \tag{5.35}$$

$$+\boldsymbol{P}_{G_1'A_2,G_1'W_2G_1}\boldsymbol{G}_1'\boldsymbol{P}'_{G_2,\Sigma^{-1}}(\boldsymbol{I} - \boldsymbol{P}_{A_3,G_2'W_3G_2,G_2})(\boldsymbol{X} - E[\boldsymbol{X}])\boldsymbol{P}_{C_3'}. \tag{5.36}$$

The sum of the first two equations, i.e. (5.32) and (5.33), is identical to $G_1'A_2(B_{2N}-B_2)C_2$, given in (5.26), and (5.34)–(5.36) imply $G_1'A_2U_2C_2$, presented in (5.27). The reason for presenting slightly more complicated expressions in (5.34)–(5.36) than those in (5.27) is that (5.34)–(5.36) are more suited to showing independence between $G_1'A_2(B_{2N}-B_2)C_2$ and $G_1'A_2U_2C_2$. For $G_1'A_2U_2C_2$ the translation $X-E[X]$ has been replaced by X, since its expectation cancelled out. Note also that $E[G_1'A_2U_2C_2]=\mathbf{0}$ and that W_2 and W_3 in (5.24) have been replaced by Σ, yielding (5.26), where W_2 and W_3 are both consistent estimators of Σ. This motivates the decomposition presented in (5.25).

Now it is shown that $G_1'A_2(B_{2N}-B_2)C_2$ and $G_1'A_2U_2C_2$ are independent so that Corollary 5.2 can be applied. The idea is to show that (5.32) and (5.33) are independent of (5.34)–(5.36). Firstly it is established that (5.32) is independent of (5.34)–(5.36). Note what kinds of projections are used and what space decomposition and inner product estimators are treated. The following facts are applied:

- $X(P_{C_2'}-P_{C_3'})$ is independent of $XP_{C_3'}$ and W_2;
- $G_2'X$ is independent of $P_{G_1'A_2,G_1'\Sigma G_1}G_1'X$.

The second condition implies that $G_2'W_3G_2$ and $P_{G_1'A_2,G_1'\Sigma G_1}G_1'X$ are independent. Thus, (5.32) is independent of (5.34)–(5.36). Furthermore, (5.33) is independent of (5.35)–(5.36), since

- $XP_{C_3'}$ is independent of $X(P_{C_2'}-P_{C_3'})$ and W_i, $i=1,2,3$;
- $G_3'X$ is independent of $P_{G_1'A_2,G_1'\Sigma G_1}G_1'(I-P_{A_3,G_2'\Sigma G_2,G_2})X$.

The last fact above can be verified by calculating the covariance between the expressions.

Since in a forthcoming theorem a few specific results for B_{2N} and U_2 are needed, we note that it follows from the above calculations, provided that inverses exist, that

$$\begin{aligned}
&B_{2N}-B_2\\
&=(A_2'G_1G_1'A_2)^{-1}A_2'G_1P_{G_1'A_2,G_1'\Sigma G_1}G_1'(X-A_2B_2C_2)(P_{C_2'}-P_{C_3'})C_2'(C_2C_2')^{-1}\\
&\quad+(A_2'G_1G_1'A_2)^{-1}A_2'G_1P_{G_1'A_2,G_1'\Sigma G_1}G_1'(I-P_{A_3,G_2'\Sigma G_2,G_2})\\
&\qquad\times(X-A_2B_2C_2)P_{C_3'}C_2'(C_2C_2')^{-1}
\end{aligned}\tag{5.37}$$

and

$$\begin{aligned}
U_2&=(A_2'G_1G_1'A_2)^{-1}A_2'G_1P_{G_1'A_2,G_1'\Sigma G_1}G_1'(I-P_{A_3,G_2'W_3G_2,G_2})XP_{C_3'}C_2'(C_2C_2')^{-1}\\
&-(A_2'G_1G_1'A_2)^{-1}A_2'G_1P_{G_1'A_2,G_1'W_2G_1}G_1'P'_{G_2,\Sigma^{-1}}P_{A_3,G_2'W_3G_2,G_2}XP_{C_3'}C_2'(C_2C_2')^{-1}\\
&-(A_2'G_1G_1'A_2)^{-1}A_2'G_1P_{G_1'A_2,G_1'W_2G_1}G_1'P'_{G_2,\Sigma^{-1}}X(P_{C_2'}-P_{C_3'})C_2'(C_2C_2')^{-1}.
\end{aligned}\tag{5.38}$$

In the Edgeworth-type expansion, $D[\boldsymbol{B}_{2N}]$ is also needed. Since $\boldsymbol{X}(\boldsymbol{P}_{C_2'} - \boldsymbol{P}_{C_3'})$ and $\boldsymbol{X}\boldsymbol{P}_{C_3'}$ are independently distributed,

$$\begin{aligned}
&D[\boldsymbol{B}_{2N}] \\
&= (\boldsymbol{C}_2\boldsymbol{C}_2')^{-1}\boldsymbol{C}_2(\boldsymbol{I} - \boldsymbol{P}_{C_3'})\boldsymbol{C}_2'(\boldsymbol{C}_2\boldsymbol{C}_2')^{-1} \otimes (\boldsymbol{A}_2'\boldsymbol{G}_1(\boldsymbol{G}_1'\boldsymbol{\Sigma}\boldsymbol{G}_1)^{-1}\boldsymbol{G}_1'\boldsymbol{A}_2)^{-1} \\
&\quad +(\boldsymbol{C}_2\boldsymbol{C}_2')^{-1}\boldsymbol{C}_2\boldsymbol{P}_{C_3'}\boldsymbol{C}_2'(\boldsymbol{C}_2\boldsymbol{C}_2')^{-1} \otimes \Big\{(\boldsymbol{A}_2'\boldsymbol{G}_1(\boldsymbol{G}_1'\boldsymbol{\Sigma}\boldsymbol{G}_1)^{-1}\boldsymbol{G}_1'\boldsymbol{A}_2)^{-1} \\
&\quad +(\boldsymbol{A}_2'\boldsymbol{G}_1(\boldsymbol{G}_1'\boldsymbol{\Sigma}\boldsymbol{G}_1)^{-1}\boldsymbol{G}_1'\boldsymbol{A}_2)^{-1} \\
&\quad\quad \times\boldsymbol{A}_2'\boldsymbol{G}_1(\boldsymbol{G}_1'\boldsymbol{\Sigma}\boldsymbol{G}_1)^{-1}\boldsymbol{G}_1'\boldsymbol{A}_3(\boldsymbol{A}_3'\boldsymbol{G}_2(\boldsymbol{G}_2'\boldsymbol{\Sigma}\boldsymbol{G}_2)^{-1}\boldsymbol{G}_2'\boldsymbol{A}_3)^{-}\boldsymbol{A}_3'\boldsymbol{G}_1(\boldsymbol{G}_1'\boldsymbol{\Sigma}\boldsymbol{G}_1)^{-1}\boldsymbol{G}_1'\boldsymbol{A}_2 \\
&\quad\quad \times(\boldsymbol{A}_2'\boldsymbol{G}_1(\boldsymbol{G}_1'\boldsymbol{\Sigma}\boldsymbol{G}_1)^{-1}\boldsymbol{G}_1'\boldsymbol{A}_2)^{-1}\Big\}. \qquad (5.39)
\end{aligned}$$

Although $\boldsymbol{B}_{2N}$ is normally distributed, it does not follow a matrix normal distribution, and as a consequence the inverse of $D[\boldsymbol{B}_{2N}]$ can be difficult to express in a convenient way. However, from a computational point of view it can be shown that $D[\boldsymbol{B}_{2N}]^{-1}$ is not too difficult to obtain and the result is indeed applicable. Using Corollary 5.2 the next theorem can be stated.

Theorem 5.8 *Let* $\widehat{\boldsymbol{B}}_2$, $\boldsymbol{B}_{2N}$ *and* $\boldsymbol{U}_2$ *be defined by (5.25), (5.37) and (5.38), respectively. Then an Edgeworth-type expansion of the density of* $\widehat{\boldsymbol{B}}_2$ *equals*

$$f_{\widehat{\boldsymbol{B}}_2}(\boldsymbol{B}_o) = f_{\boldsymbol{B}_{2E}}(\boldsymbol{B}_o) + r_3^\star,$$

where

$$\begin{aligned}
f_{\boldsymbol{B}_{2E}}(\boldsymbol{B}_o) &= (1 - \tfrac{1}{2}\mathrm{tr}\{D[\widehat{\boldsymbol{B}}_2]D[\boldsymbol{B}_{2N}]^{-1} - \boldsymbol{I}\})f_{\boldsymbol{B}_{2N}}(\boldsymbol{B}_o) \\
&\quad + \tfrac{1}{2}\mathrm{tr}\{(D[\widehat{\boldsymbol{B}}_2]D[\boldsymbol{B}_{2N}]^{-1} - \boldsymbol{I})\mathrm{vec}(\boldsymbol{B}_o - \boldsymbol{B}_2)\mathrm{vec}'(\boldsymbol{B}_o - \boldsymbol{B}_2)D[\boldsymbol{B}_{2N}]^{-1}\}f_{\boldsymbol{B}_{2N}}(\boldsymbol{B}_o);
\end{aligned}$$

$D[\widehat{\boldsymbol{B}}_2]$ *and* $D[\boldsymbol{B}_{2N}]$ *are given in Theorem 4.17 (ii) and (5.39), respectively, and*

$$|r_3^\star| \le \frac{c}{n^2},$$

for some fixed constant c which depends on the design matrices.

It can be noted that the approximating density is not a density where a matrix Kotz-type distribution is included. In fact the density does not even belong to the class of matrix elliptical distributions. From an interpretation point of view, this is slightly unfortunate. To obtain a better and more understandable approximation, the next step is to approximate $D[\widehat{\boldsymbol{B}}_2]$ with an error which is proportional to n^{-2}, so that the overall error of the density approximation will be of the same size as $|r_3^\star|$, given in Theorem 5.8.

The dispersion matrix $D[\widehat{\boldsymbol{B}}_2]$ was presented in Theorem 4.17 (ii), and since $c_2 - 1 = \mathcal{O}(n^{-1})$ and

$$\frac{n - r(\boldsymbol{C}_3) - 1}{n - r(\boldsymbol{C}_3) - m_3 - 1} - (1 + c_2\frac{m_3}{n - r(\boldsymbol{C}_3) - m_3 - 1}) = \mathcal{O}(n^{-2}),$$

an approximative dispersion equals

$$\begin{aligned}\widetilde{D}[\widehat{\boldsymbol{B}}_2] &= s_1(\boldsymbol{C}_2\boldsymbol{C}_2')^{-1}\boldsymbol{C}_2(\boldsymbol{I} - \boldsymbol{P}_{\boldsymbol{C}_3'})\boldsymbol{C}_2'(\boldsymbol{C}_2\boldsymbol{C}_2')^{-1} \otimes \boldsymbol{H}_1\\ &\quad + s_2(\boldsymbol{C}_2\boldsymbol{C}_2')^{-1}\boldsymbol{C}_2\boldsymbol{P}_{\boldsymbol{C}_3'}\boldsymbol{C}_2'(\boldsymbol{C}_2\boldsymbol{C}_2')^{-1} \otimes \boldsymbol{H}_2,\end{aligned}$$

where, if $n - r(\boldsymbol{C}_1) - m_1 + q_2 - 1 > 0$ and $n - r(\boldsymbol{C}_3) - m_3 - 1 > 0$,

$$s_1 = \frac{n - k_2 - 1}{n - r(\boldsymbol{C}_1) - m_1 + q_2 - 1}, \quad s_2 = \frac{n - r(\boldsymbol{C}_3) - 1}{n - r(\boldsymbol{C}_3) - m_3 - 1}, \tag{5.40}$$

$$\boldsymbol{H}_1 = (\boldsymbol{A}_2'\boldsymbol{G}_1(\boldsymbol{G}_1'\boldsymbol{\Sigma}\boldsymbol{G}_1)^{-1}\boldsymbol{G}_1'\boldsymbol{A}_2)^{-1} = (\boldsymbol{A}_2'\boldsymbol{A}_1^o(\boldsymbol{A}_1^{o'}\boldsymbol{\Sigma}\boldsymbol{A}_1^o)^{-1}\boldsymbol{A}_1^{o'}\boldsymbol{A}_2)^{-1}, \tag{5.41}$$

$$\begin{aligned}\boldsymbol{H}_2 &= (\boldsymbol{A}_2'\boldsymbol{G}_1(\boldsymbol{G}_1'\boldsymbol{A}_3)^o((\boldsymbol{G}_1'\boldsymbol{A}_3)^{o'}\boldsymbol{G}_1'\boldsymbol{\Sigma}\boldsymbol{G}_1(\boldsymbol{G}_1'\boldsymbol{A}_3)^o)^-(\boldsymbol{G}_1'\boldsymbol{A}_3)^{o'}\boldsymbol{G}_1'\boldsymbol{A}_2)^{-1}\\ &= (\boldsymbol{A}_2'(\boldsymbol{A}_1 : \boldsymbol{A}_3)^o((\boldsymbol{A}_1 : \boldsymbol{A}_3)^{o'}\boldsymbol{\Sigma}(\boldsymbol{A}_1 : \boldsymbol{A}_3)^o)^-(\boldsymbol{A}_1 : \boldsymbol{A}_3)^{o'}\boldsymbol{A}_2)^{-1}.\end{aligned} \tag{5.42}$$

The matrix $\boldsymbol{H}_2$ is obtained because

$$\begin{aligned}&\boldsymbol{H}_2 = \boldsymbol{H}_1\\ &+\boldsymbol{H}_1\boldsymbol{A}_2'\boldsymbol{G}_1(\boldsymbol{G}_1'\boldsymbol{\Sigma}\boldsymbol{G}_1)^{-1}\boldsymbol{G}_1'\boldsymbol{A}_3(\boldsymbol{A}_3'\boldsymbol{G}_2(\boldsymbol{G}_2'\boldsymbol{\Sigma}\boldsymbol{G}_2)^{-1}\boldsymbol{G}_2'\boldsymbol{A}_3)^-\boldsymbol{A}_3'\boldsymbol{G}_1(\boldsymbol{G}_1'\boldsymbol{\Sigma}\boldsymbol{G}_1)^{-1}\boldsymbol{G}_1'\boldsymbol{A}_2\boldsymbol{H}_1\\ &= (\boldsymbol{I}_{q_2} : \boldsymbol{0})\{(\boldsymbol{A}_2 : \boldsymbol{A}_3)'\boldsymbol{G}_1(\boldsymbol{G}_1'\boldsymbol{\Sigma}\boldsymbol{G}_1)^{-1}\boldsymbol{G}_1'(\boldsymbol{A}_2 : \boldsymbol{A}_3)\}^{-1}(\boldsymbol{I}_{q_2} : \boldsymbol{0})'.\end{aligned}$$

Moreover, $D[\boldsymbol{B}_{2N}]$, given in (5.39), equals

$$\begin{aligned}D[\boldsymbol{B}_{2N}] &= (\boldsymbol{C}_2\boldsymbol{C}_2')^{-1}\boldsymbol{C}_2(\boldsymbol{I} - \boldsymbol{P}_{\boldsymbol{C}_3'})\boldsymbol{C}_2'(\boldsymbol{C}_2\boldsymbol{C}_2')^{-1} \otimes \boldsymbol{H}_1\\ &\quad + (\boldsymbol{C}_2\boldsymbol{C}_2')^{-1}\boldsymbol{C}_2\boldsymbol{P}_{\boldsymbol{C}_3'}\boldsymbol{C}_2'(\boldsymbol{C}_2\boldsymbol{C}_2')^{-1} \otimes \boldsymbol{H}_2.\end{aligned}$$

Hence, $\widetilde{D}[\widehat{\boldsymbol{B}}_N]$ and $D[\boldsymbol{B}_{2N}]$ are of the same form, which helps when exploiting an Edgeworth-type expansion. It follows from Theorem 5.8 that

$$\mathrm{tr}\{\widetilde{D}[\widehat{\boldsymbol{B}}_2]D[\boldsymbol{B}_{2N}]^{-1} - \boldsymbol{I}\} \tag{5.43}$$

and

$$\mathrm{tr}\{(\widetilde{D}[\widehat{\boldsymbol{B}}_2]D[\boldsymbol{B}_{2N}]^{-1} - \boldsymbol{I})\mathrm{vec}(\boldsymbol{B}_o - \boldsymbol{B}_2)\mathrm{vec}'(\boldsymbol{B}_o - \boldsymbol{B}_2)D[\boldsymbol{B}_{2N}]^{-1}\} \tag{5.44}$$

are of interest. To facilitate calculations, based on the decomposition $\mathcal{C}(\boldsymbol{C}_2') = \mathcal{C}(\boldsymbol{C}_3') \boxplus \mathcal{C}(\boldsymbol{C}_2') \cap \mathcal{C}(\boldsymbol{C}_3')^{\perp}$, the following non-singular matrix is used, where, without any loss of generality, it is assumed that the symmetric square roots exist:

$$\boldsymbol{M}_2' = (\boldsymbol{C}_2\boldsymbol{C}_3'(\boldsymbol{C}_3\boldsymbol{C}_3')^{-1/2} : \boldsymbol{C}_2\boldsymbol{C}_2'(\boldsymbol{C}_2\boldsymbol{C}_3')^{o}\{(\boldsymbol{C}_2\boldsymbol{C}_3')^{o'}\boldsymbol{C}_2\boldsymbol{C}_2'(\boldsymbol{C}_2\boldsymbol{C}_3')^{o}\}^{-1/2}). \tag{5.45}$$

To be more explicit about the space decomposition and (5.45), note that (applying Appendix B, Theorem B.3 (v))

$$\mathcal{C}(\boldsymbol{C}_2'(\boldsymbol{C}_2\boldsymbol{C}_3')^{o}\{(\boldsymbol{C}_2\boldsymbol{C}_3')^{o'}\boldsymbol{C}_2\boldsymbol{C}_2'(\boldsymbol{C}_2\boldsymbol{C}_3')^{o}\}^{-}(\boldsymbol{C}_2\boldsymbol{C}_3')^{o'}\boldsymbol{C}_2) = \mathcal{C}(\boldsymbol{C}_2') \cap \mathcal{C}(\boldsymbol{C}_3')^{\perp}.$$

The pre-multiplication by $\boldsymbol{C}_2$ inside $\boldsymbol{M}_2'$ is only needed for technical reasons, which can be seen from the next two equations:

$$\boldsymbol{M}_2(\boldsymbol{C}_2\boldsymbol{C}_2')^{-1}\boldsymbol{C}_2(\boldsymbol{I} - \boldsymbol{P}_{\boldsymbol{C}_3'})\boldsymbol{C}_2'(\boldsymbol{C}_2\boldsymbol{C}_2')^{-1}\boldsymbol{M}_2' = \begin{pmatrix} \boldsymbol{0} & \boldsymbol{0} \\ \boldsymbol{0} & \boldsymbol{I}_{r_1} \end{pmatrix}, \quad r_1 = k_2 - r(\boldsymbol{C}_3), \tag{5.46}$$

$$\boldsymbol{M}_2(\boldsymbol{C}_2\boldsymbol{C}_2')^{-1}\boldsymbol{C}_2\boldsymbol{P}_{\boldsymbol{C}_3'}\boldsymbol{C}_2'(\boldsymbol{C}_2\boldsymbol{C}_2')^{-1}\boldsymbol{M}_2' = \begin{pmatrix} \boldsymbol{I}_{r_2} & \boldsymbol{0} \\ \boldsymbol{0} & \boldsymbol{0} \end{pmatrix}, \quad r_2 = r(\boldsymbol{C}_3). \tag{5.47}$$

Now (5.43) and (5.44) equal

$$\mathrm{tr}\{\widetilde{D}[\widehat{\boldsymbol{B}}_2\boldsymbol{M}_2']D[\boldsymbol{B}_{2N}\boldsymbol{M}_2']^{-1} - \boldsymbol{I}\} = q_2(r_1(s_1-1) + r_2(s_2-1))$$

and

$$\begin{aligned}
&\mathrm{tr}\{(\widetilde{D}[\widehat{\boldsymbol{B}}_2\boldsymbol{M}_2']D[\boldsymbol{B}_{2N}\boldsymbol{M}_2']^{-1} - \boldsymbol{I})\mathrm{vec}((\boldsymbol{B}_o - \boldsymbol{B}_2)\boldsymbol{M}_2')\mathrm{vec}'((\boldsymbol{B}_o - \boldsymbol{B}_2)\boldsymbol{M}_2')D[\boldsymbol{B}_{2N}\boldsymbol{M}_2']^{-1}\} \\
&= (s_2 - 1)\mathrm{tr}\{\boldsymbol{H}_2^{-1}(\boldsymbol{B}_o - \boldsymbol{B}_2)\boldsymbol{C}_2'\boldsymbol{P}_{\boldsymbol{C}_3'}\boldsymbol{C}_2(\boldsymbol{B}_o - \boldsymbol{B}_2)'\} \\
&\quad + (s_1 - 1)\mathrm{tr}\{\boldsymbol{H}_1^{-1}(\boldsymbol{B}_o - \boldsymbol{B}_2)\boldsymbol{C}_2\boldsymbol{C}_2'(\boldsymbol{C}_2\boldsymbol{C}_3')^{o}\{(\boldsymbol{C}_2\boldsymbol{C}_3')^{o'}\boldsymbol{C}_2\boldsymbol{C}_2'(\boldsymbol{C}_2\boldsymbol{C}_3')^{o}\}^{-1} \\
&\qquad \times (\boldsymbol{C}_2\boldsymbol{C}_3')^{o'}\boldsymbol{C}_2\boldsymbol{C}_2'(\boldsymbol{B}_o - \boldsymbol{B}_2)'\},
\end{aligned}$$

where s_1 and s_2 are given in (5.40). Hence, applying Theorem 5.8 and the above calculations then lead to the next theorem which has quite an easily interpretable structure. Furthermore, $s_1 - 1$ and $s_2 - 1$ are both $\mathcal{O}(n^{-1})$.

Theorem 5.9 *Let $\widehat{\boldsymbol{B}}_2$ and $\boldsymbol{B}_{2N}$ be defined by (5.25) and (5.37), respectively. An Edgeworth-type expansion of the density of $\widehat{\boldsymbol{B}}_2$ equals*

$$f_{\widehat{\boldsymbol{B}}_2}(\boldsymbol{B}_o) = f_{\widetilde{\boldsymbol{B}}_{2E}}(\boldsymbol{B}_o) + r_3^{\star},$$

where

$$f_{\widetilde{B}_{2E}}(B_o) = (1 - \tfrac{1}{2}q_2(r_1(s_1-1) + r_2(s_2-1)) f_{B_{2N}}(B_o)$$
$$+\tfrac{1}{2}(s_2-1)\mathrm{tr}\{H_2^{-1}(B_o - B_2)C_2' P_{C_3'} C_2 (B_o - B_2)'\} f_{B_{2N}}(B_o)$$
$$+\tfrac{1}{2}(s_1-1)\mathrm{tr}\{H_1^{-1}(B_o - B_2)C_2(I - P_{C_3'})C_2'(B_o - B_2)'\} f_{B_{2N}}(B_o);$$

r_i, s_i, H_i, $i = 1, 2$, *are given by (5.46), (5.47) and (5.40)–(5.42), and*

$$|r_3^\star| \leq \frac{c}{n^2},$$

for some fixed constant c which depends on the design matrices. The density $f_{B_{2N}}$ *can be factorized as*

$$f_{B_{2N}}(B_o) = |C_2C_2'|^{q_2/2} f_{B_{2N_2}C_2}(B_oC_2) f_{B_{2N_1}C_2}(B_oC_2),$$

where $f_{B_{2N_1}C_2}(B_oC_2)$ *and* $f_{B_{2N_2}C_2}(B_oC_2)$ *are density representations for*

$$B_{2N_1}C_2 = (A_2'G_1(G_1'\Sigma G_1)^{-1}G_1'A_2)^{-1}A_2'G_1(G_1'\Sigma G_1)^{-1}G_1'X(P_{C_2'} - P_{C_3'})$$
$$\sim N_{q_2,n}(B_2C_2(I - P_{C_3'}), H_1, P_{C_2'} - P_{C_3'})$$

within $X(P_{C_2'} - P_{C_3'})$ *and*

$$B_{2N_2}C_2$$
$$= (A_2'G_1(G_1'\Sigma G_1)^{-1}G_1'A_2)^{-1}A_2'G_1(G_1'\Sigma G_1)^{-1}G_1'(I - P_{A_3,G_2'\Sigma G_2,G_2})XP_{C_3'}$$
$$\sim N_{q_2,n}(B_2C_2P_{C_3'}, H_2, P_{C_3'})$$

within $XP_{C_3'}$*, respectively. Moreover,* $B_{2N} = B_{2N_1} + B_{2N_2}$.

Proof From Theorem 5.8 it follows that the only detail which remains to be proven is

$$f_{B_{2N}} = |C_2C_2'|^{q_2/2} f_{B_{2N_2}C_2}(B_oC_2) f_{B_{2N_1}C_2}(B_oC_2).$$

Now, if using M_2, given by (5.45), then

$$f_{B_{2N}}(B_o) \propto |D[B_{2N}]|^{-1/2} e^{-\frac{1}{2}\mathrm{tr}\{D[B_{2N}]^{-1}\mathrm{vec}(B_o - B_2)\mathrm{vec}'(B_o - B_2)\}}$$
$$= |C_2C_2'|^{q_2/2} |D[B_{2N}M_2']|^{-1/2} e^{-\frac{1}{2}\mathrm{tr}\{D[B_{2N}M_2']^{-1}\mathrm{vec}((B_o - B_2)M_2')\mathrm{vec}'((B_o - B_2)M_2')\}}$$
$$= |C_2C_2'|^{q_2/2} f_{B_{2N_2}C_2}(B_oC_2) f_{B_{2N_1}C_2}(B_oC_2).$$

□

The density factorization in Theorem 5.9 was presented in order to give some insight into the structure of the Edgeworth-type expansion. The expression $\boldsymbol{B}_{2N_i}\boldsymbol{C}_2$, $i = 1, 2$, was included in the density functions, but this does not mean that a true variable substitution has taken place, which explains why no Jacobians were included in the expressions. Moreover, the densities $f_{\boldsymbol{B}_{2N_1}\boldsymbol{C}_2}(\boldsymbol{B}_o\boldsymbol{C}_2)$ and $f_{\boldsymbol{B}_{2N_2}\boldsymbol{C}_2}(\boldsymbol{B}_o\boldsymbol{C}_2)$ are representations of densities for normally distributed random variables with singular distributions; i.e. the expressions can only be considered to be real densities on appropriate subspaces.

Finally, $\widehat{\boldsymbol{B}}_1$ is considered, which is more difficult than $\widehat{\boldsymbol{B}}_2$ and $\widehat{\boldsymbol{B}}_3$, because $\widehat{\boldsymbol{B}}_1$ is a function of both $\widehat{\boldsymbol{B}}_2$ and $\widehat{\boldsymbol{B}}_3$. However, the approach to obtaining results concerning a density approximation for $\widehat{\boldsymbol{B}}_1$ will follow the same procedure as that used when obtaining Theorems 5.8 and 5.9. Let us restate $\boldsymbol{A}_1\widehat{\boldsymbol{B}}_1\boldsymbol{C}_1$ as given in (4.137):

$$\begin{aligned}
&\boldsymbol{A}_1(\widehat{\boldsymbol{B}}_1 - \boldsymbol{B}_1)\boldsymbol{C}_1\\
&\quad = \boldsymbol{P}_{A_1,W_1}(\boldsymbol{X} - E[\boldsymbol{X}])(\boldsymbol{P}_{C_1'} - \boldsymbol{P}_{C_2'})\\
&\quad +\boldsymbol{P}_{A_1,W_1}(\boldsymbol{I} - \boldsymbol{P}_{A_2,G_1'W_2G_1,G_1})(\boldsymbol{X} - E[\boldsymbol{X}])(\boldsymbol{P}_{C_2'} - \boldsymbol{P}_{C_3'})\\
&\quad +\boldsymbol{P}_{A_1,W_1}(\boldsymbol{I} - \boldsymbol{P}_{A_2,G_1'W_2G_1,G_1})(\boldsymbol{I} - \boldsymbol{P}_{A_3,G_2'W_3G_2,G_2})(\boldsymbol{X} - E[\boldsymbol{X}])\boldsymbol{P}_{C_3'}.
\end{aligned} \tag{5.48}$$

Similar to the treatment for $\widehat{\boldsymbol{B}}_3$ and $\widehat{\boldsymbol{B}}_2$, the estimator $\boldsymbol{A}_1\widehat{\boldsymbol{B}}_1\boldsymbol{C}_1$ is split into a normally distributed variable and a symmetrically distributed error term $\boldsymbol{A}_1\boldsymbol{U}_1\boldsymbol{C}_1$ with mean $\boldsymbol{0}$, i.e.

$$\boldsymbol{A}_1(\widehat{\boldsymbol{B}}_1 - \boldsymbol{B}_1)\boldsymbol{C}_1 = \boldsymbol{A}_1(\boldsymbol{B}_{1N} - \boldsymbol{B}_1)\boldsymbol{C}_1 - \boldsymbol{A}_1\boldsymbol{U}_1\boldsymbol{C}_1, \tag{5.49}$$

where $\boldsymbol{A}_1\boldsymbol{B}_{1N}\boldsymbol{C}_1$ is a matrix obtained from $\boldsymbol{A}_1\widehat{\boldsymbol{B}}_1\boldsymbol{C}_1$ when $\boldsymbol{W}_i$, $i = 1, 2, 3$, is replaced by $\boldsymbol{\Sigma}$, i.e.

$$\boldsymbol{A}_1(\boldsymbol{B}_{1N} - \boldsymbol{B}_1)\boldsymbol{C}_1 = \boldsymbol{P}_{A_1,\Sigma}(\boldsymbol{X} - E[\boldsymbol{X}])(\boldsymbol{P}_{C_1'} - \boldsymbol{P}_{C_2'}) \tag{5.50}$$

$$+\boldsymbol{P}_{A_1,\Sigma}(\boldsymbol{I} - \boldsymbol{P}_{A_2,G_1'\Sigma G_1,G_1})(\boldsymbol{X} - E[\boldsymbol{X}])(\boldsymbol{P}_{C_2'} - \boldsymbol{P}_{C_3'}) \tag{5.51}$$

$$+\boldsymbol{P}_{A_1,\Sigma}(\boldsymbol{I} - \boldsymbol{P}_{A_2,G_1'\Sigma G_1,G_1})(\boldsymbol{I} - \boldsymbol{P}_{A_3,G_2'\Sigma G_2,G_2})(\boldsymbol{X} - E[\boldsymbol{X}])\boldsymbol{P}_{C_3'}, \tag{5.52}$$

and $\boldsymbol{B}_{1N} - \boldsymbol{B}_1 = (\boldsymbol{A}_1'\boldsymbol{A}_1)^{-1}\boldsymbol{A}_1'\boldsymbol{A}_1(\boldsymbol{B}_{1N} - \boldsymbol{B}_1)\boldsymbol{C}_1\boldsymbol{C}_1'(\boldsymbol{C}_1\boldsymbol{C}_1')^{-1}$. The three terms, (5.50)–(5.52), in $\boldsymbol{A}_1\boldsymbol{B}_{1N}\boldsymbol{C}_1$ are independent since $\boldsymbol{X}(\boldsymbol{P}_{C_1'} - \boldsymbol{P}_{C_2'})$, $\boldsymbol{X}(\boldsymbol{P}_{C_2'} - \boldsymbol{P}_{C_3'})$ and $\boldsymbol{X}\boldsymbol{P}_{C_3'}$ are independently distributed. Therefore,

$$\begin{aligned}
D[\boldsymbol{B}_{1N}] &= (\boldsymbol{C}_1\boldsymbol{C}_1')^{-1}\boldsymbol{C}_1(\boldsymbol{I} - \boldsymbol{P}_{C_2'}) \otimes (\boldsymbol{A}_1'\boldsymbol{\Sigma}^{-1}\boldsymbol{A}_1)^{-1}\\
&\quad +(\boldsymbol{C}_1\boldsymbol{C}_1')^{-1}\boldsymbol{C}_1'(\boldsymbol{P}_{C_2'} - \boldsymbol{P}_{C_3'})\boldsymbol{C}_1'(\boldsymbol{C}_1\boldsymbol{C}_1')^{-1}
\end{aligned}$$

$$\otimes\{(\boldsymbol{A}_1'\boldsymbol{\Sigma}^{-1}\boldsymbol{A}_1)^{-1}+\boldsymbol{F}_2\boldsymbol{A}_2(\boldsymbol{A}_2'\boldsymbol{G}_1(\boldsymbol{G}_1'\boldsymbol{\Sigma}\boldsymbol{G}_1)^{-1}\boldsymbol{G}_1'\boldsymbol{A}_2)^{-}\boldsymbol{A}_2'\boldsymbol{F}_2'\}$$
$$+(\boldsymbol{C}_1\boldsymbol{C}_1')^{-1}\boldsymbol{C}_1'\boldsymbol{P}_{C_3'}\boldsymbol{C}_1'(\boldsymbol{C}_1\boldsymbol{C}_1')^{-1}$$
$$\otimes\{(\boldsymbol{A}_1'\boldsymbol{\Sigma}^{-1}\boldsymbol{A}_1)^{-1}+\boldsymbol{F}_2\boldsymbol{A}_2(\boldsymbol{A}_2'\boldsymbol{G}_1(\boldsymbol{G}_1'\boldsymbol{\Sigma}\boldsymbol{G}_1)^{-1}\boldsymbol{G}_1'\boldsymbol{A}_2)^{-}\boldsymbol{A}_2'\boldsymbol{F}_2$$
$$+\boldsymbol{F}_3\boldsymbol{A}_3(\boldsymbol{A}_3'\boldsymbol{G}_2(\boldsymbol{G}_2'\boldsymbol{\Sigma}\boldsymbol{G}_2)^{-1}\boldsymbol{G}_2'\boldsymbol{A}_3)^{-}\boldsymbol{A}_3'\boldsymbol{F}_3'\},\quad(5.53)$$

where $\boldsymbol{F}_2$ and $\boldsymbol{F}_3$ are given by (4.144) and (4.145), respectively. Moreover, it is obvious that $E[\boldsymbol{A}_1\boldsymbol{B}_{1N}\boldsymbol{C}_1]=\boldsymbol{A}_1\boldsymbol{B}_1\boldsymbol{C}_1$. Now $\boldsymbol{A}_1\boldsymbol{U}_1\boldsymbol{C}_1$ is studied. After some calculations it follows from (5.48) and (5.50)–(5.52) that the "error" term $\boldsymbol{A}_1\boldsymbol{U}_1\boldsymbol{C}_1$ in (5.49) equals

$$\boldsymbol{A}_1\boldsymbol{U}_1\boldsymbol{C}_1=-\boldsymbol{P}_{A_1,W_1}\boldsymbol{P}'_{G_1,\Sigma^{-1}}\boldsymbol{X}(\boldsymbol{P}_{C_1'}-\boldsymbol{P}_{C_2'})\quad(5.54)$$
$$-\boldsymbol{P}_{A_1,W_1}\boldsymbol{P}'_{G_1,\Sigma^{-1}}(\boldsymbol{I}-\boldsymbol{P}_{A_2,G_1'W_2G_1,G_1})\boldsymbol{X}(\boldsymbol{P}_{C_2'}-\boldsymbol{P}_{C_3'})\quad(5.55)$$
$$+\boldsymbol{P}_{A_1,\Sigma}\boldsymbol{P}_{A_2,G_1'W_2G_1,G_1}\boldsymbol{P}'_{G_2,\Sigma^{-1}}\boldsymbol{X}(\boldsymbol{P}_{C_2'}-\boldsymbol{P}_{C_3'})\quad(5.56)$$
$$-\boldsymbol{P}_{A_1,W_1}\boldsymbol{P}'_{G_1,\Sigma^{-1}}(\boldsymbol{I}-\boldsymbol{P}_{A_2,G_1'W_2G_1,G_1})(\boldsymbol{I}-\boldsymbol{P}_{A_3,G_2'W_3G_2,G_2})\boldsymbol{X}\boldsymbol{P}_{C_3'}\quad(5.57)$$
$$+\boldsymbol{P}_{A_1,\Sigma}\boldsymbol{P}_{A_2,G_1'W_2G_1,G_1}\boldsymbol{P}'_{G_2,\Sigma^{-1}}(\boldsymbol{I}-\boldsymbol{P}_{A_3,G_2'W_3G_2,G_2})\boldsymbol{X}\boldsymbol{P}_{C_3'}\quad(5.58)$$
$$+\boldsymbol{P}_{A_1,\Sigma}(\boldsymbol{I}-\boldsymbol{P}_{A_2,G_1'\Sigma G_1,G_1})\boldsymbol{P}_{A_3,G_2'W_3G_2,G_2}\boldsymbol{P}'_{G_3,\Sigma^{-1}}\boldsymbol{X}\boldsymbol{P}_{C_3'},\quad(5.59)$$

and $\boldsymbol{U}_1=(\boldsymbol{A}_1'\boldsymbol{A}_1)^{-1}\boldsymbol{A}_1'\boldsymbol{A}_1\boldsymbol{U}_1\boldsymbol{C}_1\boldsymbol{C}_1'(\boldsymbol{C}_1\boldsymbol{C}_1')^{-1}$. Next the independence between $\boldsymbol{A}_1\boldsymbol{B}_{1N}\boldsymbol{C}_1$ and $\boldsymbol{A}_1\boldsymbol{U}_1\boldsymbol{C}_1$ is established. First it is shown that the right-hand side of (5.50) is independent of (5.54)–(5.59) and thereafter that (5.51) is independent of (5.54)–(5.59), and finally it is established that (5.52) is independent of (5.54)–(5.59).

The expression in (5.50) is independent of (5.54)–(5.59), since

- $\boldsymbol{X}(\boldsymbol{P}_{C_1'}-\boldsymbol{P}_{C_2'})$ is independent of $\boldsymbol{W}_1$ and $\boldsymbol{X}\boldsymbol{P}_{C_3'}$;
- $\boldsymbol{P}_{A_1,\Sigma}\boldsymbol{X}$ is independent of $(\boldsymbol{I}-\boldsymbol{P}_{A_1,\Sigma})\boldsymbol{X}$ and $\boldsymbol{G}_i'\boldsymbol{X}$, $i=1,2,3$, as well as $\boldsymbol{G}_1'\boldsymbol{W}_2\boldsymbol{G}_1$ and $\boldsymbol{G}_2'\boldsymbol{W}_3\boldsymbol{G}_2$.

Moreover, the expression in (5.51) is independent of (5.54)–(5.59), since

- $\boldsymbol{X}(\boldsymbol{P}_{C_2'}-\boldsymbol{P}_{C_3'})$ is independent of $\boldsymbol{W}_1$, $\boldsymbol{W}_2$, $\boldsymbol{X}(\boldsymbol{P}_{C_1'}-\boldsymbol{P}_{C_2'})$ and $\boldsymbol{X}\boldsymbol{P}_{C_3'}$;
- $\boldsymbol{P}_{A_1,\Sigma}(\boldsymbol{I}-\boldsymbol{P}_{A_2,G_1'\Sigma G_1,G_1})\boldsymbol{X}$ is independent of $\boldsymbol{G}_2'\boldsymbol{X}$ and $\boldsymbol{G}_2'\boldsymbol{W}_3\boldsymbol{G}_2$.

Furthermore, the expression in (5.52) is independent of (5.54)–(5.59), since

- $\boldsymbol{X}\boldsymbol{P}_{C_3'}$ is independent of $\boldsymbol{W}_i$, $i=1,2,3$, $\boldsymbol{X}(\boldsymbol{P}_{C_1'}-\boldsymbol{P}_{C_2'})$ and $\boldsymbol{X}(\boldsymbol{P}_{C_2'}-\boldsymbol{P}_{C_3'})$;
- $\boldsymbol{P}_{A_3,G_2'\Sigma G_2,G_2}\boldsymbol{X}$ is independent of $\boldsymbol{G}_3'\boldsymbol{X}$.

Hence, Corollary 5.2 can be applied and the following theorem, corresponding to Theorem 5.9 for $\widehat{\boldsymbol{B}}_2$, has been verified.

Theorem 5.10 *Let $\widehat{B}_1$, B_{1N} and U_1 be defined via (5.48), (5.50)–(5.52) and (5.54)–(5.59), respectively. Then an Edgeworth-type expansion of the density of $\widehat{B}_1$ equals*

$$f_{\widehat{B}_1}(B_o) = f_{B_{1E}}(B_o) + r_3^\star,$$

where

$$\begin{aligned} f_{B_{1E}}(B_o) =& (1 - \tfrac{1}{2}\mathrm{tr}\{D[\widehat{B}_1]D[B_{1N}]^{-1} - I\}) f_{B_{1N}}(B_o) \\ &+ \tfrac{1}{2}\mathrm{tr}\{(D[\widehat{B}_1]D[B_{1N}]^{-1} - I)\mathrm{vec}(B_o - B_1)\mathrm{vec}'(B_o - B_1)D[B_{1N}]^{-1}\} f_{B_{1N}}(B_o); \end{aligned}$$

$D[\widehat{B}_1]$ and $D[B_{1N}]$ are given in Theorem 4.17 (iii) and (5.53), respectively, and

$$|r_3^\star| \le \frac{c}{n^2},$$

for some fixed constant c which depends on the design matrices.

As for $\widehat{B}_2$, in order to obtain a more understandable approximation, the next step is to approximate $D[\widehat{B}_1]$ with an error which is proportional to n^{-2}. From $D[\widehat{B}_1]$ in Theorem 4.17 (iii) it follows, by performing some calculations, that an approximative dispersion equals

$$\begin{aligned} \widetilde{D}[\widehat{B}_1] =& s_3(C_1C_1')^{-1}C_1(I - P_{C_2'})C_1'(C_1C_1')^{-1} \otimes (A_1'\Sigma^{-1}A_1)^{-1} \\ &+ s_4(C_1C_1')^{-1}C_1(P_{C_2'} - P_{C_3'})C_1'(C_1C_1')^{-1} \otimes \{(A_1'\Sigma^{-1}A_1)^{-1} \\ &+ F_2A_2(A_2'G_1(G_1'\Sigma G_1)^{-1}G_1'A_2)^- A_2'F_2'\} \\ &+ (C_1C_1')^{-1}C_1P_{C_3'}C_1'(C_1C_1')^{-1} \otimes \Big\{s_2\{(A_1'\Sigma^{-1}A_1)^{-1} \\ &+ F_3A_3(A_3'G_2(G_2'\Sigma G_2)^{-1}G_2'A_3)^- A_3'F_3'\} \\ &+ F_2A_2(A_2'G_1(G_1'\Sigma G_1)^{-1}G_1'A_2)^- A_2'F_2'\Big\}, \end{aligned}$$

where

$$s_3 = \frac{n - k_1 - 1}{n - r(C_1) - p + q_1 - 1}, \qquad s_4 = \frac{n - r(C_2) - 1}{n - r(C_2) - m_2 - 1} \tag{5.60}$$

and s_2 is given in (5.40). Hence,

$$\begin{aligned} \widetilde{D}[\widehat{B}_1] - D[B_{1N}] =& (s_3 - 1)(C_1C_1')^{-1}C_1(I - P_{C_2'})C_1'(C_1C_1')^{-1} \otimes (A_1'\Sigma^{-1}A_1)^{-1} \\ &+ (s_4 - 1)(C_1C_1')^{-1}C_1(P_{C_2'} - P_{C_3'})C_1'(C_1C_1')^{-1} \otimes \{(A_1'\Sigma^{-1}A_1)^{-1} \\ &+ F_2A_2(A_2'G_1(G_1'\Sigma G_1)^{-1}G_1'A_2)^- A_2'F_2'\} \end{aligned}$$

$$+ (s_2 - 1)(C_1C_1')^{-1}C_1P_{C_3'}C_1'(C_1C_1')^{-1} \otimes \{(A_1'\Sigma^{-1}A_1)^{-1} + F_3A_3(A_3'G_2(G_2'\Sigma G_2)^{-1}G_2'A_3)^{-}A_3'F_3'\}. \quad (5.61)$$

The constants $s_i - 1, i = 2, 3, 4$, are all $\mathcal{O}(n^{-1})$.

When discussing $\widehat{B}_2$, the calculations were simplified by introducing the matrix M_2 in (5.45). Now, when considering $\widehat{B}_1$, the same technique is applied, but instead of M_2, the matrix

$$M_1' = \big(C_1C_3'(C_3C_3')^{-1/2} : C_1C_2'(C_2C_3')^o\{(C_2C_3')^{o'}C_2C_2'(C_2C_3')^o\}^{-1/2} : C_1C_1'(C_1C_2')^o\{(C_1C_2')^{o'}C_1C_1'(C_1C_2')^o\}^{-1/2}\big) \quad (5.62)$$

is used. The matrix is created according to the decomposition

$$\mathcal{C}(C_1') = \mathcal{C}(C_3') \boxplus \mathcal{C}(C_2') \cap \mathcal{C}(C_3')^{\perp} \boxplus \mathcal{C}(C_1') \cap \mathcal{C}(C_2')^{\perp}.$$

Then, (diag($\bullet, \bullet, \bullet$) denotes the block-diagonal operator, see Appendix A, Sect. A.6)

$$M_1(C_1C_1')^{-1}C_1(I - P_{C_2'})C_1'(C_1C_1')^{-1}M_1' = \mathrm{diag}(\mathbf{0}, \mathbf{0}, I_{r_1}), \quad r_1 = k_1 - r(C_2), \quad (5.63)$$

$$M_1(C_1C_1')^{-1}C_1(P_{C_2'} - P_{C_3'})C_1'(C_1C_1')^{-1}M_1' = \mathrm{diag}(\mathbf{0}, I_{r_2}\mathbf{0},), \quad r_2 = r(C_2) - r(C_3), \quad (5.64)$$

$$M_1(C_1C_1')^{-1}C_1P_{C_3'}C_1'(C_1C_1')^{-1}M_1' = \mathrm{diag}(I_{r_3}, \mathbf{0}, \mathbf{0}), \quad r_3 = r(C_3), \quad (5.65)$$

and applying (5.61)

$$\widetilde{D}[\widehat{B}_1M_1'] - D[B_{1N}M_1'] = (s_3 - 1)\mathrm{diag}(\mathbf{0}, \mathbf{0}, I_{r_1}) \otimes (A_1'\Sigma^{-1}A_1)^{-1}$$
$$+ (s_4 - 1)\mathrm{diag}(\mathbf{0}, I_{r_2}, \mathbf{0}) \otimes \{(A_1'\Sigma^{-1}A_1)^{-1} + F_2A_2(A_2'G_1(G_1'\Sigma G_1)^{-1}G_1'A_2)^{-}A_2'F_2'\}$$
$$+ (s_2 - 1)\mathrm{diag}(I_{r_3}, \mathbf{0}, \mathbf{0}) \otimes \{(A_1'\Sigma^{-1}A_1)^{-1} + F_3A_3(A_3'G_2(G_2'\Sigma G_2)^{-1}G_2'A_3)^{-}A_3'F_3'\}. \quad (5.66)$$

Moreover, according to Corollary 5.2 the following two expressions are needed:

$$\mathrm{tr}\{(\widetilde{D}[\widehat{B}_1] - D[B_{1N}])D[B_{1N}]^{-1}\} \quad (5.67)$$

and

$$\mathrm{tr}\{(\widetilde{D}[\widehat{B}_1] - D[B_{1N}])D[B_{1N}]^{-1}\mathrm{vec}(B_o - B_1)\mathrm{vec}'(B_o - B_1)D[B_{1N}]^{-1}\}. \quad (5.68)$$

Explicit calculations of (5.67) and (5.68) are left to the reader. Here it is noted that all calculations become straightforward if one uses the matrix $\boldsymbol{M}_1$, given in (5.62), since

$$\begin{aligned}&\operatorname{tr}\{(\widetilde{D}[\widehat{\boldsymbol{B}}_1]-D[\boldsymbol{B}_{1N}])D[\boldsymbol{B}_{1N}]^{-1}\}\\&\quad=\operatorname{tr}\{(\widetilde{D}[\widehat{\boldsymbol{B}}_1\boldsymbol{M}_1']-D[\boldsymbol{B}_{1N}\boldsymbol{M}_1'])D[\boldsymbol{B}_{1N}\boldsymbol{M}_1']^{-1}\}\end{aligned}$$

and

$$\begin{aligned}&\operatorname{tr}\{(\widetilde{D}[\widehat{\boldsymbol{B}}_1]-D[\boldsymbol{B}_{1N}])D[\boldsymbol{B}_{1N}]^{-1}\operatorname{vec}(\boldsymbol{B}_o-\boldsymbol{B}_1)\operatorname{vec}'(\boldsymbol{B}_o-\boldsymbol{B}_1)D[\boldsymbol{B}_{1N}]^{-1}\}\\&\quad=\operatorname{tr}\Big\{(\widetilde{D}[\widehat{\boldsymbol{B}}_1\boldsymbol{M}_1']-D[\boldsymbol{B}_{1N}\boldsymbol{M}_1'])D[\boldsymbol{B}_{1N}\boldsymbol{M}_1']^{-1}\\&\qquad\qquad\times\operatorname{vec}((\boldsymbol{B}_o-\boldsymbol{B}_1)\boldsymbol{M}_1')\operatorname{vec}'((\boldsymbol{B}_o-\boldsymbol{B}_1)\boldsymbol{M}_1')D[\boldsymbol{B}_{1N}\boldsymbol{M}_1']^{-1}\Big\}.\end{aligned}$$

Among other things, (5.66) presents $\widetilde{D}[\widehat{\boldsymbol{B}}_1\boldsymbol{M}_1']-D[\boldsymbol{B}_{1N}\boldsymbol{M}_1']$, and

$$\begin{aligned}&D[\boldsymbol{B}_{1N}\boldsymbol{M}_1']^{-1}\\&\quad=\operatorname{diag}(\boldsymbol{0},\boldsymbol{0},\boldsymbol{I}_{r_1})\otimes\boldsymbol{A}_1'\boldsymbol{\Sigma}^{-1}\boldsymbol{A}_1+\operatorname{diag}(\boldsymbol{0},\boldsymbol{I}_{r_2},\boldsymbol{0})\otimes\boldsymbol{H}_3^{-1}+\operatorname{diag}(\boldsymbol{I}_{r_3},\boldsymbol{0},\boldsymbol{0})\otimes\boldsymbol{H}_4^{-1},\end{aligned}$$

where

$$\begin{aligned}\boldsymbol{H}_3&=(\boldsymbol{I}:\boldsymbol{0})((\boldsymbol{A}_1:\boldsymbol{A}_2)'\boldsymbol{\Sigma}^{-1}(\boldsymbol{A}_1:\boldsymbol{A}_2))^{-1}(\boldsymbol{I}:\boldsymbol{0})'\\&=(\boldsymbol{A}_1'\boldsymbol{\Sigma}^{-1}\boldsymbol{A}_1)^{-1}+\boldsymbol{F}_2\boldsymbol{A}_2(\boldsymbol{A}_2'\boldsymbol{G}_1(\boldsymbol{G}_1'\boldsymbol{\Sigma}\boldsymbol{G}_1)^{-1}\boldsymbol{G}_1'\boldsymbol{A}_2)^{-}\boldsymbol{A}_2'\boldsymbol{F}_2'\end{aligned}\tag{5.69}$$

and

$$\begin{aligned}\boldsymbol{H}_4&=(\boldsymbol{I}:\boldsymbol{0}:\boldsymbol{0})((\boldsymbol{A}_1:\boldsymbol{A}_2:\boldsymbol{A}_3)'\boldsymbol{\Sigma}^{-1}(\boldsymbol{A}_1:\boldsymbol{A}_2:\boldsymbol{A}_3))^{-1}(\boldsymbol{I}:\boldsymbol{0}:\boldsymbol{0})'\\&=(\boldsymbol{A}_1'\boldsymbol{\Sigma}^{-1}\boldsymbol{A}_1)^{-1}+\sum_{i=1}^{2}\boldsymbol{F}_{i+1}\boldsymbol{A}_{i+1}(\boldsymbol{A}_{i+1}'\boldsymbol{G}_i(\boldsymbol{G}_i'\boldsymbol{\Sigma}\boldsymbol{G}_i)^{-1}\boldsymbol{G}_i'\boldsymbol{A}_{i+1})^{-}\boldsymbol{A}_{i+1}'\boldsymbol{F}_{i+1}'.\end{aligned}\tag{5.70}$$

Moreover, let

$$\boldsymbol{H}_5=(\boldsymbol{A}_1'\boldsymbol{\Sigma}^{-1}\boldsymbol{A}_1)^{-1}+\boldsymbol{F}_3\boldsymbol{A}_3(\boldsymbol{A}_3'\boldsymbol{G}_2(\boldsymbol{G}_2'\boldsymbol{\Sigma}\boldsymbol{G}_2)^{-1}\boldsymbol{G}_2'\boldsymbol{A}_3)^{-}\boldsymbol{A}_3'\boldsymbol{F}_3'.\tag{5.71}$$

Theorem 5.11 *Let $\widehat{\boldsymbol{B}}_1$ and $\boldsymbol{B}_{1N}$ be defined in (5.48) and (5.50)–(5.52). Then an Edgeworth-type expansion of the density of $\widehat{\boldsymbol{B}}_1$, assuming that all the constants given below exist, equals*

$$f_{\widehat{\boldsymbol{B}}_1}(\boldsymbol{B}_o)=f_{\widetilde{\boldsymbol{B}}_{1E}}(\boldsymbol{B}_o)+r_3^{\star},$$

where

$$
\begin{aligned}
f_{\widetilde{B}_{1E}}(B_o) &= (1 - \tfrac{1}{2}(q_1(r_1(s_3-1)+r_2(s_4-1)) + (s_2-1)\mathrm{tr}\{H_5H_4^{-1}\})f_{B_{1N}}(B_o) \\
&+ \tfrac{1}{2}(s_3-1)\mathrm{tr}\{(A_1'\Sigma^{-1}A_1)^{-1}(B_o-B_1)C_1'(I-P_{C_2})C_1(B_o-B_1)'\}f_{B_{1N}}(B_o) \\
&+ \tfrac{1}{2}(s_4-1)\mathrm{tr}\{H_3^{-1}(B_o-B_1)C_1(P_{C_2'}-P_{C_3'})C_1'(B_o-B_1)'\}f_{B_{1N}}(B_o) \\
&+ \tfrac{1}{2}(s_2-1)\mathrm{tr}\{H_4^{-1}H_5H_4^{-1}(B_o-B_1)C_1P_{C_3'}C_1'(B_o-B_1)'\}f_{B_{1N}}(B_o);
\end{aligned}
$$

r_i, $i = 1, 2, 3$, *are defined in (5.63)–(5.65),* s_i, $i = 2, 3, 4$, *in (5.40) and (5.60), and* H_i, $i = 3, 4, 5$, *in (5.69)–(5.71), and*

$$
|r_3^{\star}| \leq \frac{c}{n^2},
$$

for some fixed constant c which depends on the design matrices. The density $f_{B_{1N}}$ *can be factorized as*

$$
f_{B_{1N}}(B_o) = |C_1C_1'|^{q_1/2} f_{B_{1N_3}C_1}(B_oC_1) f_{B_{1N_2}C_1}(B_oC_1) f_{B_{1N_1}C_1}(B_oC_1),
$$

where $f_{B_{1N_i}C_2}(B_oC_2)$, $i = 1, 2, 3$, *are density representations for*

$$
\begin{aligned}
B_{1N_1}C_1 &= (A_1'\Sigma^{-1}A_1)^{-1}A_1'\Sigma^{-1}X(P_{C_1'}-P_{C_2'}) \\
&\sim N_{q_1,n}(B_1C_1(I-P_{C_2'}), (A_1'\Sigma^{-1}A_1)^{-1}, P_{C_1'}-P_{C_2'})
\end{aligned}
$$

within $X(P_{C_1'}-P_{C_2'})$,

$$
\begin{aligned}
B_{1N_2}C_1 &= (A_1'\Sigma^{-1}A_1)^{-1}A_1'\Sigma^{-1}(I-P_{A_2,G_1'\Sigma G_1,G_1})X(P_{C_2'}-P_{C_3'}) \\
&\sim N_{q_1,n}(B_1C_1(P_{C_2'}-P_{C_3'}), H_3, P_{C_2'}-P_{C_3'})
\end{aligned}
$$

within $X(P_{C_2'}-P_{C_3'})$, *and*

$$
\begin{aligned}
B_{1N_3}C_1 &= (A_1'\Sigma^{-1}A_1)^{-1}A_1'\Sigma^{-1}(I-P_{A_2,G_1'\Sigma G_1,G_1})(I-P_{A_3,G_2'\Sigma G_2,G_2})XP_{C_3'} \\
&\sim N_{q_1,n}(B_1C_1P_{C_3'}, H_4, P_{C_3'})
\end{aligned}
$$

within $XP_{C_3'}$, *respectively. Moreover,* $B_{1N} = B_{1N_1} + B_{1N_2} + B_{1N_3}$.

5.5 Density Approximation for the Mean Parameter Estimators in the $EBRM_W^3$

The ideas presented below are the same as those used when working with the $EBRM_B^3$ in the previous Sect. 5.4. In correspondence with Sect. 5.4, it will be shown that the distributions of the estimators $\widehat{B}_i$, $i = 1, 2, 3$, for the $EBRM_W^3$, can all be decomposed into a normally distributed part and an error term which has an expectation equal to $\mathbf{0}$ and is independent of the normal part. Indeed, from a linear model point of view (e.g. see Exercise 1.3, p. 308 in Rao, 1973), the decompositions are both natural and interpretable.

Starting with $\widehat{B}_3$, given in Theorem 3.3, it follows that under full rank conditions

$$\widehat{B}_3 = B_{3N} - U_3,$$

where

$$B_{3N} = (A_3'\Sigma^{-1}A_3)^{-1}A_3'\Sigma^{-1}XQ_2C_3'(C_3Q_2C_3')^{-1}, \tag{5.72}$$

$$U_3 = -(A_3'S_1^{-1}A_3)^{-1}A_3'S_1^{-1}(I - P_{A_3,\Sigma})XQ_2C_3'(C_3Q_2C_3')^{-1}. \tag{5.73}$$

Since S_1 is independent of XQ_2C_3' and $(I - P_{A_3,\Sigma})X$ is independent of $A_3'\Sigma^{-1}X$, the two matrices B_{3N} and U are independently distributed. Moreover,

$$D[B_{3N}] = (C_3Q_2C_3')^{-1} \otimes (A_3'\Sigma^{-1}A_3)^{-1} \tag{5.74}$$

and, if $n - r(C_1' : C_2' : C_3') - p + q_3 - 1 > 0$ (see Theorem 4.25 (i)),

$$D[\widehat{B}_3] = (1 + s_1)(C_3Q_2C_3')^{-1} \otimes (A_3'\Sigma^{-1}A_3)^{-1}, \tag{5.75}$$

where

$$s_1 = \frac{p-q_3}{n-r(C_1':C_2':C_3')-p+q_3-1}. \tag{5.76}$$

Hence, correspondingly to Theorem 5.7, we can present the next theorem, omitting a proof of the statement concerning the error term.

Theorem 5.12 *Let $\widehat{B}_3$, B_{3N} and U_3 ($u_3 = \mathrm{vec}U_3$) be given by Theorem 3.3, (5.72) and (5.73), respectively. Then an Edgeworth-type expansion of the density of $\widehat{B}_3$ equals*

$$f_{\widehat{B}_3}(B_o) = f_{B_{3E}}(B_o) + r_3^\star,$$

where

$$\begin{aligned} f_{B_{3E}}(B_o) &= f_{B_{3N}}(B_o) + \tfrac{1}{2}E[(u_3')^{\otimes 2}]\mathrm{vec} f^2_{B_{3N}}(B_o) \\ &= (1 - \tfrac{1}{2}s_1k_3q_3 + \tfrac{1}{2}s_1\,\mathrm{tr}\{A_3'\Sigma^{-1}A_3(B_o - B_3)C_3Q_2C_3'(B_o - B_3)'\})f_{B_{3N}}(B_o), \end{aligned}$$

with s_1 defined in (5.76) and supposed to exist, and

$$|r_3^\star| \leq \frac{c}{n^2},$$

for some fixed constant c which is a function of the design matrices.

In Theorem 5.12 the density corresponds to a mixture of a Kotz-type distribution (see Appendix A, Sect. A.10) and a normal distribution.

For $\widehat{\boldsymbol{B}}_2$, given in Theorem 3.3, the following decomposition holds under some full rank conditions. Let $\boldsymbol{F}_2 = (\boldsymbol{A}_2'\boldsymbol{A}_2)^{-1}\boldsymbol{A}_2'$, then

$$\widehat{\boldsymbol{B}}_2 = \boldsymbol{F}_2\boldsymbol{P}_{\boldsymbol{A}_2,\widehat{\boldsymbol{S}}_2}\boldsymbol{X}\boldsymbol{Q}_1\boldsymbol{C}_2'(\boldsymbol{C}_2\boldsymbol{Q}_1\boldsymbol{C}_2')^{-1}$$
$$-\boldsymbol{F}_2\boldsymbol{P}_{\boldsymbol{A}_3,\boldsymbol{S}_1}\boldsymbol{X}\boldsymbol{Q}_2\boldsymbol{C}_3'(\boldsymbol{C}_3\boldsymbol{Q}_2\boldsymbol{C}_3')^{-}\boldsymbol{C}_3\boldsymbol{Q}_1\boldsymbol{C}_2'(\boldsymbol{C}_2\boldsymbol{Q}_1\boldsymbol{C}_2')^{-1}, \quad (5.77)$$
$$\boldsymbol{B}_{2N} = \boldsymbol{F}_2\boldsymbol{P}_{\boldsymbol{A}_2,\boldsymbol{\Sigma}}\boldsymbol{X}\boldsymbol{Q}_1\boldsymbol{C}_2'(\boldsymbol{C}_2\boldsymbol{Q}_1\boldsymbol{C}_2')^{-1} \quad (5.78)$$
$$-\boldsymbol{F}_2\boldsymbol{P}_{\boldsymbol{A}_3,\boldsymbol{\Sigma}}\boldsymbol{X}\boldsymbol{Q}_2\boldsymbol{C}_3'(\boldsymbol{C}_3\boldsymbol{Q}_2\boldsymbol{C}_3')^{-}\boldsymbol{C}_3\boldsymbol{Q}_1\boldsymbol{C}_2'(\boldsymbol{C}_2\boldsymbol{Q}_1\boldsymbol{C}_2')^{-1}, \quad (5.79)$$
$$\boldsymbol{U}_2 = -\boldsymbol{F}_2\boldsymbol{P}_{\boldsymbol{A}_2,\widehat{\boldsymbol{S}}_2}(\boldsymbol{I} - \boldsymbol{P}_{\boldsymbol{A}_2,\boldsymbol{\Sigma}})\boldsymbol{X}\boldsymbol{Q}_1\boldsymbol{C}_2'(\boldsymbol{C}_2\boldsymbol{Q}_1\boldsymbol{C}_2')^{-1}$$
$$+\boldsymbol{F}_2\boldsymbol{P}_{\boldsymbol{A}_3,\boldsymbol{S}_1}(\boldsymbol{I} - \boldsymbol{P}_{\boldsymbol{A}_3,\boldsymbol{\Sigma}})\boldsymbol{X}\boldsymbol{Q}_2\boldsymbol{C}_3'(\boldsymbol{C}_3\boldsymbol{Q}_2\boldsymbol{C}_3')^{-}\boldsymbol{C}_3\boldsymbol{Q}_1\boldsymbol{C}_2'(\boldsymbol{C}_2\boldsymbol{Q}_1\boldsymbol{C}_2')^{-1}, \quad (5.80)$$

and

$$\widehat{\boldsymbol{B}}_2 = \boldsymbol{B}_{2N} - \boldsymbol{U}_2.$$

As before, the independence between $\boldsymbol{B}_{2N}$ and $\boldsymbol{U}_2$ has to be proven. Note that $\boldsymbol{X}\boldsymbol{Q}_1\boldsymbol{C}_2'$ is independent of $\boldsymbol{S}_1$, $\widehat{\boldsymbol{S}}_2$ and $\boldsymbol{X}\boldsymbol{Q}_2\boldsymbol{C}_3'$, and $\boldsymbol{P}_{\boldsymbol{A}_2,\boldsymbol{\Sigma}}\boldsymbol{X}$ is independent of $(\boldsymbol{I}-\boldsymbol{P}_{\boldsymbol{A}_2,\boldsymbol{\Sigma}})\boldsymbol{X}$. Hence, the expression on the right-hand side of (5.78) is independent of $\boldsymbol{U}_2$. Moreover, $\boldsymbol{X}\boldsymbol{Q}_2\boldsymbol{C}_3'$ is independent of $\boldsymbol{S}_1$ and $\boldsymbol{P}_{\boldsymbol{A}_3,\boldsymbol{\Sigma}}\boldsymbol{X}\boldsymbol{Q}_2\boldsymbol{C}_3'$ is independent of $\widehat{\boldsymbol{S}}_2$, $(\boldsymbol{I} - \boldsymbol{P}_{\boldsymbol{A}_2,\boldsymbol{\Sigma}})\boldsymbol{X}$ and $(\boldsymbol{I} - \boldsymbol{P}_{\boldsymbol{A}_3,\boldsymbol{\Sigma}})\boldsymbol{X}$. Therefore, (5.79) is independent of $\boldsymbol{U}_2$, implying independence between $\boldsymbol{B}_{2N}$ and $\boldsymbol{U}_2$.

Concerning moments, $E[\boldsymbol{U}_2] = \boldsymbol{0}$,

$$D[\boldsymbol{B}_{2N}] = (\boldsymbol{C}_2\boldsymbol{Q}_1\boldsymbol{C}_2')^{-1} \otimes (\boldsymbol{A}_2'\boldsymbol{\Sigma}^{-1}\boldsymbol{A}_2)^{-1}$$
$$+(\boldsymbol{C}_2\boldsymbol{Q}_1\boldsymbol{C}_2')^{-1}\boldsymbol{C}_2\boldsymbol{Q}_1\boldsymbol{C}_3'(\boldsymbol{C}_3\boldsymbol{Q}_2\boldsymbol{C}_3')^{-}\boldsymbol{C}_3\boldsymbol{Q}_1\boldsymbol{C}_2'(\boldsymbol{C}_2\boldsymbol{Q}_1\boldsymbol{C}_2')^{-1}$$
$$\otimes\boldsymbol{F}_2\boldsymbol{A}_3(\boldsymbol{A}_3'\boldsymbol{\Sigma}^{-1}\boldsymbol{A}_3)^{-}\boldsymbol{A}_3'\boldsymbol{F}_2', \quad (5.81)$$

and according to Theorem 4.25 (ii)

$$D[\widehat{\boldsymbol{B}}_2] = (\boldsymbol{C}_2\boldsymbol{Q}_1\boldsymbol{C}_2')^{-1} \otimes \Big\{(1 + c_1)(\boldsymbol{A}_2'\boldsymbol{\Sigma}^{-1}\boldsymbol{A}_2)^{-1}$$
$$+c_1(c_2 - 1)\boldsymbol{F}_2\boldsymbol{A}_3(\boldsymbol{A}_3'\boldsymbol{\Sigma}^{-1}\boldsymbol{A}_3)^{-}\boldsymbol{A}_3'\boldsymbol{F}_2'\Big\}$$
$$+(1 + c_3)(\boldsymbol{C}_2\boldsymbol{Q}_1\boldsymbol{C}_2')^{-1}\boldsymbol{C}_2\boldsymbol{Q}_1\boldsymbol{C}_3'(\boldsymbol{C}_3\boldsymbol{Q}_2\boldsymbol{C}_3')^{-}\boldsymbol{C}_3\boldsymbol{Q}_1\boldsymbol{C}_2'(\boldsymbol{C}_2\boldsymbol{Q}_1\boldsymbol{C}_2')^{-1}$$
$$\otimes\boldsymbol{F}_2\boldsymbol{A}_3(\boldsymbol{A}_3'\boldsymbol{\Sigma}^{-1}\boldsymbol{A}_3)^{-}\boldsymbol{A}_3'\boldsymbol{F}_2', \quad (5.82)$$

where

$$c_1 = \frac{p-q_2}{n-r(C_1':C_2')-p+q_2-1}, \quad c_2 = \frac{n-r(C_1':C_2')-p+r(A_3)-1}{n-r(C_1':C_2':C_3')-p+r(A_3)-1}, \tag{5.83}$$

$$c_3 = \frac{p-r(A_3)}{n-r(C_1':C_2':C_3')-p+r(A_3)-1}, \tag{5.84}$$

and all three constants are supposed to be positive and finite.

Theorem 5.13 *Let $\widehat{\boldsymbol{B}}_2$, $\boldsymbol{B}_{2N}$ and $\boldsymbol{U}_2$ be defined by (5.77)–(5.80). Then an Edgeworth-type expansion of the density of $\widehat{\boldsymbol{B}}_2$ equals*

$$f_{\widehat{\boldsymbol{B}}_2}(\boldsymbol{B}_o) = f_{\boldsymbol{B}_{2E}}(\boldsymbol{B}_o) + r_3^\star,$$

where

$$\begin{aligned} f_{\boldsymbol{B}_{2E}}(\boldsymbol{B}_o) &= (1 - \tfrac{1}{2}\mathrm{tr}\{D[\widehat{\boldsymbol{B}}_2]D[\boldsymbol{B}_{2N}]^{-1} - \boldsymbol{I}\}) f_{\boldsymbol{B}_{2N}}(\boldsymbol{B}_o) \\ &+ \tfrac{1}{2}\mathrm{tr}\{(D[\widehat{\boldsymbol{B}}_2]D[\boldsymbol{B}_{2N}]^{-1} - \boldsymbol{I})\mathrm{vec}(\boldsymbol{B}_o - \boldsymbol{B}_2)\mathrm{vec}'(\boldsymbol{B}_o - \boldsymbol{B}_2)D[\boldsymbol{B}_{2N}]^{-1}\} f_{\boldsymbol{B}_{2N}}(\boldsymbol{B}_o); \end{aligned}$$

$D[\widehat{\boldsymbol{B}}_2]$ and $D[\boldsymbol{B}_{2N}]$ are supposed to exist and are presented in (5.82) and (5.81), respectively, and

$$|r_3^\star| \le \frac{c}{n^2},$$

for some fixed constant c which depends on the design matrices.

Noting that $c_1(c_2 - 1) = \mathcal{O}(n^{-2})$, it immediately follows that a natural approximation of $D[\widehat{\boldsymbol{B}}_2]$ in (5.82) is given by

$$\begin{aligned} \widetilde{D}[\widehat{\boldsymbol{B}}_2] &= (1 + c_1)(\boldsymbol{C}_2\boldsymbol{Q}_1\boldsymbol{C}_2')^{-1} \otimes (\boldsymbol{A}_2'\boldsymbol{\Sigma}^{-1}\boldsymbol{A}_2)^{-1} \\ &+ (1 + c_3)(\boldsymbol{C}_2\boldsymbol{Q}_1\boldsymbol{C}_2')^{-1}\boldsymbol{C}_2\boldsymbol{Q}_1\boldsymbol{C}_3'(\boldsymbol{C}_3\boldsymbol{Q}_2\boldsymbol{C}_3')^{-}\boldsymbol{C}_3\boldsymbol{Q}_1\boldsymbol{C}_2'(\boldsymbol{C}_2\boldsymbol{Q}_1\boldsymbol{C}_2')^{-1} \\ &\otimes \boldsymbol{F}_2\boldsymbol{A}_3(\boldsymbol{A}_3'\boldsymbol{\Sigma}^{-1}\boldsymbol{A}_3)^{-}\boldsymbol{A}_3'\boldsymbol{F}_2'. \end{aligned} \tag{5.85}$$

Moreover, to simplify calculations, a matrix $\boldsymbol{M}_2$ is introduced which corresponds to the matrix given in (5.45):

$$\begin{aligned} \boldsymbol{M}_2' = \big(&\boldsymbol{A}_2'\boldsymbol{\Sigma}^{-1}\boldsymbol{A}_3(\boldsymbol{A}_3'\boldsymbol{\Sigma}^{-1}\boldsymbol{A}_3)^{-1/2} : \boldsymbol{A}_2'\boldsymbol{\Sigma}^{-1}\boldsymbol{A}_2(\boldsymbol{A}_2'\boldsymbol{\Sigma}^{-1}\boldsymbol{A}_3)^o \\ &\times\{(\boldsymbol{A}_2'\boldsymbol{\Sigma}^{-1}\boldsymbol{A}_3)^{o'}\boldsymbol{A}_2'\boldsymbol{\Sigma}^{-1}\boldsymbol{A}_2(\boldsymbol{A}_2'\boldsymbol{\Sigma}^{-1}\boldsymbol{A}_3)^o\}^{-1/2}\big), \end{aligned}$$

where, without any loss of generality, the square roots are supposed to exist; i.e. it has to be supposed that $\boldsymbol{A}_3$ is of full rank, which we can always assume to hold in (5.82) and (5.85). Then

$$\widetilde{D}[\boldsymbol{M}_2\widehat{\boldsymbol{B}}_2] - D[\boldsymbol{M}_2\boldsymbol{B}_{2N}] = c_1\boldsymbol{H}_1 \otimes \boldsymbol{I}_{q_2} + c_3\boldsymbol{H}_3 \otimes \mathrm{diag}(\boldsymbol{I}_{r(A_3)}, \boldsymbol{0}),$$

where

$$H_1 = (C_2 Q_1 C_2')^{-1}, \tag{5.86}$$

$$H_3 = (C_2 Q_1 C_2')^{-1} C_2 Q_1 C_3' (C_3 Q_2 C_3')^{-} C_3 Q_1 C_2' (C_2 Q_1 C_2')^{-1}. \tag{5.87}$$

Moreover, let

$$H_2 = H_1 + H_3 = (I : 0)((C_2' : C_3')' Q_1 (C_2' : C_3'))^{-1} (I : 0)'. \tag{5.88}$$

Then

$$D[M_2 B_{2N}]^{-1} = H_1^{-1} \otimes \mathrm{diag}(0, I_{q_2 - r(A_3)}) + H_2^{-1} \otimes \mathrm{diag}(I_{r(A_3)}, 0)$$

and

$$\begin{aligned} D[M_2 B_{2N}]^{-1} &\mathrm{vec}(M_2(B_{2N} - B_2)) \\ &= \mathrm{vec}\left\{\{(A_2'\Sigma^{-1}A_3)^{o'} A_2'\Sigma^{-1}A_2(A_2'\Sigma^{-1}A_3)^{o}\}^{-1/2} \right. \\ &\quad \left. \times (A_2'\Sigma^{-1}A_3)^{o'} A_2'\Sigma^{-1}A_2(B_{2N} - B_2)H_1^{-1}\right\} \\ &\quad + \mathrm{vec}\{(A_3'\Sigma^{-1}A_3)^{-1/2} A_3'\Sigma^{-1}A_2(B_{2N} - B_2)H_2^{-1}\}. \end{aligned}$$

Theorem 5.14 *Let $\widehat{B}_2$ and B_{2N} be defined by (5.77)–(5.80). Then an Edgeworth-type expansion of the density of $\widehat{B}_2$ equals*

$$f_{\widehat{B}_2}(B_o) = f_{\widetilde{B}_{2E}}(B_o) + r_3^\star,$$

where

$$\begin{aligned} &f_{\widetilde{B}_{2E}}(B_o) \\ &= (1 - \tfrac{1}{2}(q_2 - r(A_3))k_2 c_1 - \tfrac{1}{2}c_1 r(A_3)\mathrm{tr}\{H_1 H_2^{-1}\} - \tfrac{1}{2}c_3 r(A_3)\mathrm{tr}\{H_3 H_2^{-1}\}) f_{B_{2N}}(B_o) \\ &+ \tfrac{1}{2}c_1 \mathrm{tr}\{H_1^{-1}(B_o - B_2)' A_2' A_3^o (A_3^{o'} \Sigma A_3^o)^{-} A_3^{o'} A_2 (B_o - B_2)\} f_{B_{2N}}(B_o) \\ &+ \tfrac{1}{2}c_1 \mathrm{tr}\{H_2^{-1} H_1 H_2^{-1} (B_o - B_2)' A_2' \Sigma^{-1} P_{A_3,\Sigma} A_2 (B_o - B_2)\} f_{B_{2N}}(B_o) \\ &+ \tfrac{1}{2}c_3 \mathrm{tr}\{H_2^{-1} H_3 H_2^{-1} (B_o - B_2)' A_2' \Sigma^{-1} P_{A_3,\Sigma} A_2 (B_o - B_2)\} f_{B_{2N}}(B_o), \end{aligned}$$

where c_1 and c_3 are supposed to exist and are given by (5.83) and (5.84), respectively, and H_i, $i = 1, 2, 3$, are given by (5.86)–(5.88). Furthermore,

$$|r_3^\star| \le \frac{c}{n^2},$$

for some fixed constant c which depends on the design matrices. The density $f_{\boldsymbol{B}_{2N}}$ can be factorized as

$$f_{\boldsymbol{B}_{2N}}(\boldsymbol{B}_o) = |\boldsymbol{A}_2'\boldsymbol{\Sigma}^{-1}\boldsymbol{A}_2|^{k_2/2} f_{\boldsymbol{A}_2\boldsymbol{B}_{2N_2}}(\boldsymbol{A}_2\boldsymbol{B}_o) f_{\boldsymbol{A}_2\boldsymbol{B}_{2N_1}}(\boldsymbol{A}_2\boldsymbol{B}_o),$$

where $f_{\boldsymbol{A}_2\boldsymbol{B}_{2N_1}}(\boldsymbol{A}_2\boldsymbol{B}_o)$ and $f_{\boldsymbol{A}_2\boldsymbol{B}_{2N_2}}(\boldsymbol{A}_2\boldsymbol{B}_o)$ are density representations for

$$\begin{aligned}\boldsymbol{A}_2\boldsymbol{B}_{2N_1} &= (\boldsymbol{P}_{A_2,\Sigma} - \boldsymbol{P}_{A_3,\Sigma})\boldsymbol{X}\boldsymbol{Q}_1\boldsymbol{C}_2'(\boldsymbol{C}_2\boldsymbol{Q}_1\boldsymbol{C}_2')^{-1}\\ &\sim N_{p,k_2}((\boldsymbol{I} - \boldsymbol{P}_{A_3,\Sigma})\boldsymbol{A}_2\boldsymbol{B}_2, (\boldsymbol{P}_{A_2,\Sigma} - \boldsymbol{P}_{A_3,\Sigma})\boldsymbol{\Sigma}, \boldsymbol{H}_1)\end{aligned}$$

within $(\boldsymbol{P}_{A_2,\Sigma} - \boldsymbol{P}_{A_3,\Sigma})\boldsymbol{X}$ and

$$\begin{aligned}\boldsymbol{A}_2\boldsymbol{B}_{2N_2} &= \boldsymbol{P}_{A_3,\Sigma}\boldsymbol{X}(\boldsymbol{I} - \boldsymbol{Q}_2\boldsymbol{C}_3'(\boldsymbol{C}_3\boldsymbol{Q}_2\boldsymbol{C}_3')^{-}\boldsymbol{C}_3)\boldsymbol{Q}_1\boldsymbol{C}_2'(\boldsymbol{C}_2\boldsymbol{Q}_1\boldsymbol{C}_2')^{-1}\\ &\sim N_{p,q_2}(\boldsymbol{P}_{A_3,\Sigma}\boldsymbol{A}_2\boldsymbol{B}_2, \boldsymbol{P}_{A_3,\Sigma}\boldsymbol{\Sigma}, \boldsymbol{H}_2)\end{aligned}$$

within $\boldsymbol{P}_{A_3,\Sigma}\boldsymbol{X}$, respectively. Moreover, $\boldsymbol{B}_{2N} = \boldsymbol{B}_{2N_1} + \boldsymbol{B}_{2N_2}$.

Finally, $\widehat{\boldsymbol{B}}_1$ is discussed briefly. The results are obtained using a procedure similar to that presented earlier. Now Theorem 3.3, together with a number of calculations, yields

$$\widehat{\boldsymbol{B}}_1 = \boldsymbol{B}_{1N} - \boldsymbol{U}_1,$$

where

$$\boldsymbol{B}_{1N} = \boldsymbol{F}_1\boldsymbol{P}_{A_1,\Sigma}\boldsymbol{X}\boldsymbol{C}_1'(\boldsymbol{C}_1\boldsymbol{C}_1')^{-1} \tag{5.89}$$

$$-\boldsymbol{F}_1\boldsymbol{P}_{A_2,\Sigma}\boldsymbol{X}\boldsymbol{Q}_1\boldsymbol{C}_2'(\boldsymbol{C}_2\boldsymbol{Q}_1\boldsymbol{C}_2')^{-}\boldsymbol{C}_2\boldsymbol{C}_1'(\boldsymbol{C}_1\boldsymbol{C}_1')^{-1} \tag{5.90}$$

$$-\boldsymbol{F}_1\boldsymbol{P}_{A_3,\Sigma}\boldsymbol{X}\boldsymbol{Q}_2\boldsymbol{C}_3'(\boldsymbol{C}_3\boldsymbol{Q}_2\boldsymbol{C}_3')^{-}\boldsymbol{C}_3(\boldsymbol{I} - \boldsymbol{Q}_1\boldsymbol{C}_2'(\boldsymbol{C}_2\boldsymbol{Q}_1\boldsymbol{C}_2')^{-}\boldsymbol{C}_2)\boldsymbol{C}_1'(\boldsymbol{C}_1\boldsymbol{C}_1')^{-1}, \tag{5.91}$$

with $\boldsymbol{F}_1 = (\boldsymbol{A}_1'\boldsymbol{A}_1)^{-1}\boldsymbol{A}_1'$ and

$$\begin{aligned}\boldsymbol{U}_1 = &-\boldsymbol{F}_1\boldsymbol{P}_{A_1,\widehat{S}_3}(\boldsymbol{I} - \boldsymbol{P}_{A_1,\Sigma})\boldsymbol{X}\boldsymbol{C}_1'(\boldsymbol{C}_1\boldsymbol{C}_1')^{-1}\\ &+\boldsymbol{F}_1\boldsymbol{P}_{A_2,\widehat{S}_2}(\boldsymbol{I} - \boldsymbol{P}_{A_2,\Sigma})\boldsymbol{Q}_1\boldsymbol{C}_2'(\boldsymbol{C}_2\boldsymbol{Q}_1\boldsymbol{C}_2')^{-}\boldsymbol{C}_2\boldsymbol{C}_1'(\boldsymbol{C}_1\boldsymbol{C}_1')^{-1} -\\ &+\boldsymbol{F}_1\boldsymbol{P}_{A_3,S_1}(\boldsymbol{I}-\boldsymbol{P}_{A_3,\Sigma})\boldsymbol{X}\boldsymbol{Q}_2\boldsymbol{C}_3'(\boldsymbol{C}_3\boldsymbol{Q}_2\boldsymbol{C}_3')^{-}\boldsymbol{C}_3(\boldsymbol{I}-\boldsymbol{Q}_1\boldsymbol{C}_2'(\boldsymbol{C}_2\boldsymbol{Q}_1\boldsymbol{C}_2')^{-}\boldsymbol{C}_2)\boldsymbol{C}_1'(\boldsymbol{C}_1\boldsymbol{C}_1')^{-1}.\end{aligned} \tag{5.92}$$

The independence between $\boldsymbol{B}_{1N}$ and $\boldsymbol{U}_1$ has to be verified. In the right-hand side of (5.89) the expression is independent of $\boldsymbol{U}_1$, since

- $\boldsymbol{X}\boldsymbol{C}_1'$ is independent of $\widehat{\boldsymbol{S}}_3$, $\widehat{\boldsymbol{S}}_2$, $\boldsymbol{S}_1$, $\boldsymbol{X}\boldsymbol{Q}_1$, $\boldsymbol{X}\boldsymbol{Q}_2$;
- $\boldsymbol{P}_{A_1,\Sigma}\boldsymbol{X}\boldsymbol{C}_1'$ is independent of $(\boldsymbol{I} - \boldsymbol{P}_{A_1,\Sigma})\boldsymbol{X}$.

The second term of $\boldsymbol{B}_{1N}$, given in (5.90), is independent of $\boldsymbol{U}_1$, since

- $\boldsymbol{X}\boldsymbol{Q}_1'\boldsymbol{C}_2'$ is independent of $\widehat{\boldsymbol{S}}_2$, $\boldsymbol{S}_1$, $\boldsymbol{X}\boldsymbol{Q}_2$;
- $\boldsymbol{P}_{A_2,\Sigma}\boldsymbol{X}\boldsymbol{Q}_1\boldsymbol{C}_2'$ is independent of $\widehat{\boldsymbol{S}}_3$, $(\boldsymbol{I}-\boldsymbol{P}_{A_2,\Sigma})\boldsymbol{X}$, $(\boldsymbol{I}-\boldsymbol{P}_{A_1,\Sigma})\boldsymbol{X}$.

The third term, given in (5.91), is independent of $\boldsymbol{U}_1$, since

- $\boldsymbol{X}\boldsymbol{Q}_2'\boldsymbol{C}_3'$ is independent of $\boldsymbol{S}_1$;
- $\boldsymbol{P}_{A_3,\Sigma}\boldsymbol{X}\boldsymbol{Q}_2\boldsymbol{C}_3'$ is independent of $\widehat{\boldsymbol{S}}_3$, $\widehat{\boldsymbol{S}}_2$, $(\boldsymbol{I}-\boldsymbol{P}_{A_1,\Sigma})\boldsymbol{X}$, $(\boldsymbol{I}-\boldsymbol{P}_{A_2,\Sigma})\boldsymbol{X}$, $(\boldsymbol{I}-\boldsymbol{P}_{A_3,\Sigma})\boldsymbol{X}$.

Thus, $\boldsymbol{B}_{1N}$ and $\boldsymbol{U}_1$ are independently distributed. Moreover, in order to perform an Edgeworth-type expansion, dispersion matrices are needed, among others $D[\boldsymbol{B}_{1N}]$, which equals

$$\begin{aligned}
D[\boldsymbol{B}_{1N}] &= (\boldsymbol{C}_1\boldsymbol{C}_1')^{-1}\otimes(\boldsymbol{A}_1'\boldsymbol{\Sigma}^{-1}\boldsymbol{A}_1)^{-1}\\
&+(\boldsymbol{C}_1\boldsymbol{C}_1')^{-1}\boldsymbol{C}_1\boldsymbol{C}_2'(\boldsymbol{C}_2\boldsymbol{Q}_1\boldsymbol{C}_2')^{-}\boldsymbol{C}_2\boldsymbol{C}_1'(\boldsymbol{C}_1\boldsymbol{C}_1')^{-1}\otimes\boldsymbol{F}_1\boldsymbol{A}_2(\boldsymbol{A}_2'\boldsymbol{\Sigma}^{-1}\boldsymbol{A}_2)^{-}\boldsymbol{A}_2'\boldsymbol{F}_1'\\
&+(\boldsymbol{C}_1\boldsymbol{C}_1')^{-1}\boldsymbol{C}_1(\boldsymbol{I}-\boldsymbol{C}_2'(\boldsymbol{C}_2\boldsymbol{Q}_1\boldsymbol{C}_2')^{-}\boldsymbol{C}_2\boldsymbol{Q}_1)\\
&\quad\times\boldsymbol{C}_3'(\boldsymbol{C}_3\boldsymbol{Q}_2\boldsymbol{C}_3')^{-}\boldsymbol{C}_3(\boldsymbol{I}-\boldsymbol{Q}_1\boldsymbol{C}_2'(\boldsymbol{C}_2\boldsymbol{Q}_1\boldsymbol{C}_2')^{-}\boldsymbol{C}_2)\boldsymbol{C}_1'(\boldsymbol{C}_1\boldsymbol{C}_1')^{-1}\\
&\quad\otimes\boldsymbol{F}_1\boldsymbol{A}_3(\boldsymbol{A}_3'\boldsymbol{\Sigma}^{-1}\boldsymbol{A}_3)^{-}\boldsymbol{A}_3'\boldsymbol{F}_1'. \qquad (5.93)
\end{aligned}$$

Theorem 5.15 *Let $\widehat{\boldsymbol{B}}_1$, $\boldsymbol{B}_{1N}$ and $\boldsymbol{U}_1$ be defined by Theorem 3.3, (5.89)–(5.91) and (5.92), respectively. Then an Edgeworth-type expansion of the density of $\widehat{\boldsymbol{B}}_1$ equals*

$$f_{\widehat{\boldsymbol{B}}_1}(\boldsymbol{B}_o) = f_{\boldsymbol{B}_{1E}}(\boldsymbol{B}_o) + r_3^\star,$$

where

$$\begin{aligned}
f_{\boldsymbol{B}_{1E}}(\boldsymbol{B}_o) &= (1-\tfrac{1}{2}\mathrm{tr}\{D[\widehat{\boldsymbol{B}}_1]D[\boldsymbol{B}_{1N}]^{-1}-\boldsymbol{I}\})f_{\boldsymbol{B}_{1N}}(\boldsymbol{B}_o)\\
&+\tfrac{1}{2}\mathrm{tr}\{(D[\widehat{\boldsymbol{B}}_1]D[\boldsymbol{B}_{1N}]^{-1}-\boldsymbol{I})\mathrm{vec}(\boldsymbol{B}_o-\boldsymbol{B}_1)\mathrm{vec}'(\boldsymbol{B}_o-\boldsymbol{B}_1)D[\boldsymbol{B}_{1N}]^{-1}\}f_{\boldsymbol{B}_{1N}}(\boldsymbol{B}_o);
\end{aligned}$$

$D[\widehat{\boldsymbol{B}}_1]$ and $D[\boldsymbol{B}_{1N}]$ are given in Theorem 4.25 (iii) and (5.93), respectively, and

$$|r_3^\star| \le \frac{c}{n^2},$$

for some fixed constant c which depends on the design matrices.

Now $D[\widehat{\boldsymbol{B}}_1]$ is approximated with an error which is proportional to n^{-1}. Using the definition of the constants c_1 and d_1 presented in Lemma 4.6 (see also Theorem 4.25 (iii)), an approximative dispersion equals

$$\begin{aligned}
\widetilde{D}[\widehat{\boldsymbol{B}}_1] &= (1+d_1)(\boldsymbol{C}_1\boldsymbol{C}_1')^{-1}\otimes(\boldsymbol{A}_1'\boldsymbol{\Sigma}^{-1}\boldsymbol{A}_1)^{-1}\\
&+(1+c_1)(\boldsymbol{C}_1\boldsymbol{C}_1')^{-1}\boldsymbol{C}_1\boldsymbol{C}_2'(\boldsymbol{C}_2\boldsymbol{Q}_1\boldsymbol{C}_2')^{-}\boldsymbol{C}_2\boldsymbol{C}_1'(\boldsymbol{C}_1\boldsymbol{C}_1')^{-1}\otimes\boldsymbol{F}_1\boldsymbol{A}_2(\boldsymbol{A}_2'\boldsymbol{\Sigma}^{-1}\boldsymbol{A}_2)^{-}\boldsymbol{A}_2'\boldsymbol{F}_1'
\end{aligned}$$

$$+(1+e)(C_1C_1')^{-1}C_1(I - C_2'(C_2Q_1C_2')^{-}C_2Q_1)C_3'(C_3Q_2C_3')^{-}C_3$$
$$\times(I - Q_1C_2'(C_2Q_1C_2')^{-}C_2)C_1'(C_1C_1')^{-1} \otimes F_1A_3(A_3'\Sigma^{-1}A_3)^{-}A_3'F_1',$$

where

$$e = \frac{p-r(A_3)}{n-r(C_1':C_2':C_3')-p+r(A_3)-1}, \tag{5.94}$$

assuming $n - r(C_1' : C_2' : C_3') - p + r(A_3) - 1 > 0$. Applying the same procedure as was applied to the other parameters for obtaining an Edgeworth-type expansion of the density of the parameter estimators, the next matrix is introduced:

$$M_1' = \Big(A_1'\Sigma^{-1}A_3(A_3'\Sigma^{-1}A_3)^{-1/2}$$
$$: A_1'\Sigma^{-1}A_2(A_2'\Sigma^{-1}A_3)^{o}\{(A_2'\Sigma^{-1}A_3)^{o'}A_2'\Sigma^{-1}A_2(A_2'\Sigma^{-1}A_3)^{o}\}^{-1/2}$$
$$: A_1'\Sigma^{-1}A_1(A_1'\Sigma^{-1}A_2)^{o}\{(A_1'\Sigma^{-1}A_2)^{o'}A_1'\Sigma^{-1}A_1(A_1'\Sigma^{-1}A_2)^{o}\}^{-1/2}\Big),$$

which is inspired by the space decomposition

$$\mathcal{C}_\Sigma(A_1) = \mathcal{C}_\Sigma(A_3) \boxplus \mathcal{C}_\Sigma(A_2) \cap \mathcal{C}_\Sigma(A_3)^{\perp} \boxplus \mathcal{C}_\Sigma(A_1) \cap \mathcal{C}_\Sigma(A_2)^{\perp}$$

with the corresponding dimensions

$$r_1 = r(A_3), \quad r_2 = r(A_2) - r(A_3), \quad r_3 = r(A_1) - r(A_2). \tag{5.95}$$

Hence,

$$\widetilde{D}[M_1\widehat{B}_1] - D[M_1B_{1N}] = d_1H_4 \otimes I + c_1H_5 \otimes \operatorname{diag}(I_{r_1+r_2}, \mathbf{0})$$
$$+eH_6 \otimes \operatorname{diag}(I_{r_1}, \mathbf{0}, \mathbf{0}),$$

where

$$H_4 = (C_1C_1')^{-1}, \tag{5.96}$$
$$H_5 = (C_1C_1')^{-1}C_1C_2'(C_2Q_1C_2')^{-}C_2C_1'(C_1C_1')^{-1}, \tag{5.97}$$
$$H_6 = (C_1C_1')^{-1}C_1(I - C_2'(C_2Q_1C_2')^{-}C_2Q_1)C_3'(C_3Q_2C_3')^{-}C_3$$
$$\times(I - Q_1C_2'(C_2Q_1C_2')^{-}C_2)C_1'(C_1C_1')^{-1}. \tag{5.98}$$

Moreover,

$$D[M_1B_{1N}]^{-1} = H_4^{-1} \otimes \operatorname{diag}(\mathbf{0}, \mathbf{0}, I_{r_3}) + (H_4 + H_5)^{-1} \otimes \operatorname{diag}(\mathbf{0}, I_{r_2}, \mathbf{0})$$
$$+(H_4 + H_5 + H_6)^{-1} \otimes \operatorname{diag}(I_{r_1}, \mathbf{0}, \mathbf{0}).$$

With the above-provided definitions and relations the next theorem can be formulated.

Theorem 5.16 *Let $\widehat{\boldsymbol{B}}_1$ and $\boldsymbol{B}_{1N}$ be defined by Theorem 3.3 and (5.89)–(5.91). Then an Edgeworth-type expansion of the density of $\widehat{\boldsymbol{B}}_1$ equals*

$$f_{\widehat{\boldsymbol{B}}_1}(\boldsymbol{B}_o) = f_{\widetilde{\boldsymbol{B}}_{1E}}(\boldsymbol{B}_o) + r_3^\star,$$

where

$$\begin{aligned}
f_{\widetilde{\boldsymbol{B}}_{1E}}(\boldsymbol{B}_o) &= (1 - \tfrac{1}{2}(d_1k_1r_3 + \mathrm{tr}\{r_2(d_1\boldsymbol{H}_4 + c_1\boldsymbol{H}_5)(\boldsymbol{H}_4 + \boldsymbol{H}_5)^{-1} \\
&\qquad + r_1(d_1\boldsymbol{H}_4 + c_1\boldsymbol{H}_5 + e\boldsymbol{H}_6)(\boldsymbol{H}_4 + \boldsymbol{H}_5 + \boldsymbol{H}_6)^{-1}\}) f_{\boldsymbol{B}_{1N}}(\boldsymbol{B}_o) \\
&+ \tfrac{1}{2}\mathrm{tr}\Big\{d_1\boldsymbol{H}_4^{-1}(\boldsymbol{B}_o - \boldsymbol{B}_1)'\boldsymbol{A}_1'\boldsymbol{\Sigma}^{-1}\boldsymbol{A}_1(\boldsymbol{A}_1'\boldsymbol{\Sigma}^{-1}\boldsymbol{A}_2)^o \\
&\times\{(\boldsymbol{A}_1'\boldsymbol{\Sigma}^{-1}\boldsymbol{A}_2)^{o'}\boldsymbol{A}_1'\boldsymbol{\Sigma}^{-1}\boldsymbol{A}_1(\boldsymbol{A}_1'\boldsymbol{\Sigma}^{-1}\boldsymbol{A}_2)^o\}^{-1}(\boldsymbol{A}_1'\boldsymbol{\Sigma}^{-1}\boldsymbol{A}_2)^{o'}\boldsymbol{A}_1'\boldsymbol{\Sigma}^{-1}\boldsymbol{A}_1(\boldsymbol{B}_o - \boldsymbol{B}_1)\Big\} \\
&\qquad \times f_{\boldsymbol{B}_{1N}}(\boldsymbol{B}_o) \\
&+ \tfrac{1}{2}\mathrm{tr}\Big\{(\boldsymbol{H}_4 + \boldsymbol{H}_5)^{-1}(d_1\boldsymbol{H}_4 + c_1\boldsymbol{H}_5)(\boldsymbol{H}_4 + \boldsymbol{H}_5)^{-1}(\boldsymbol{B}_o - \boldsymbol{B}_1)'\boldsymbol{A}_1'\boldsymbol{\Sigma}^{-1}\boldsymbol{A}_2(\boldsymbol{A}_2'\boldsymbol{\Sigma}^{-1}\boldsymbol{A}_3)^o \\
&\times\{(\boldsymbol{A}_2'\boldsymbol{\Sigma}^{-1}\boldsymbol{A}_3)^{o'}\boldsymbol{A}_2'\boldsymbol{\Sigma}^{-1}\boldsymbol{A}_2(\boldsymbol{A}_2'\boldsymbol{\Sigma}^{-1}\boldsymbol{A}_3)^o\}^{-1}(\boldsymbol{A}_2'\boldsymbol{\Sigma}^{-1}\boldsymbol{A}_3)^{o'}\boldsymbol{A}_2'\boldsymbol{\Sigma}^{-1}\boldsymbol{A}_1(\boldsymbol{B}_o - \boldsymbol{B}_1)\Big\} \\
&\times f_{\boldsymbol{B}_{1N}}(\boldsymbol{B}_o) \\
&+ \tfrac{1}{2}\mathrm{tr}\Big\{(\boldsymbol{H}_4 + \boldsymbol{H}_5 + \boldsymbol{H}_6)^{-1}(d_1\boldsymbol{H}_4 + c_1\boldsymbol{H}_5 + e\boldsymbol{H}_6)(\boldsymbol{H}_4 + \boldsymbol{H}_5 + \boldsymbol{H}_6)^{-1}(\boldsymbol{B}_o - \boldsymbol{B}_1)' \\
&\times\boldsymbol{A}_1'\boldsymbol{\Sigma}^{-1}\boldsymbol{P}_{A_3,\Sigma}\boldsymbol{A}_1(\boldsymbol{B}_o - \boldsymbol{B}_1)\Big\} f_{\boldsymbol{B}_{1N}}(\boldsymbol{B}_o);
\end{aligned}$$

r_i, $i = 1, 2, 3$, are defined in (5.95), c_1, d_1 and e are defined by (5.83), Lemma 4.6 and (5.94), respectively, $\boldsymbol{H}_i$, $i = 3, 4, 5$, are given by (5.96)–(5.98), and

$$|r_3^\star| \leq \frac{c}{n^2},$$

for some fixed constant c which depends on the design matrices. The density $f_{\boldsymbol{B}_{1N}}$ can be factorized as

$$f_{\boldsymbol{B}_{1N}} = |\boldsymbol{A}_1'\boldsymbol{\Sigma}^{-1}\boldsymbol{A}_1|^{k_1/2} f_{\boldsymbol{A}_1\boldsymbol{B}_{1N_3}}(\boldsymbol{A}_1\boldsymbol{B}_o) f_{\boldsymbol{A}_1\boldsymbol{B}_{1N_2}}(\boldsymbol{A}_1\boldsymbol{B}_o) f_{\boldsymbol{A}_1\boldsymbol{B}_{1N_1}}(\boldsymbol{A}_1\boldsymbol{B}_o),$$

where $f_{\boldsymbol{A}_1\boldsymbol{B}_{1N_i}}(\boldsymbol{A}_1\boldsymbol{B}_o)$, $i = 1, 2, 3$, are density representations for

$$\begin{aligned}
\boldsymbol{A}_1\boldsymbol{B}_{1N_1} &= (\boldsymbol{P}_{A_1,\Sigma} - \boldsymbol{P}_{A_2,\Sigma})\boldsymbol{X}\boldsymbol{H}_4^{1/2} \\
&\sim N_{p,k_1}((\boldsymbol{I} - \boldsymbol{P}_{A_2})\boldsymbol{A}_1\boldsymbol{B}_1, (\boldsymbol{P}_{A_1,\Sigma} - \boldsymbol{P}_{A_2,\Sigma})\boldsymbol{\Sigma}, \boldsymbol{H}_4)
\end{aligned}$$

within $(\boldsymbol{P}_{A_1} - \boldsymbol{P}_{A_2})\boldsymbol{X}$,

$$\boldsymbol{A}_1\boldsymbol{B}_{1N_2} = (\boldsymbol{P}_{A_2,\Sigma} - \boldsymbol{P}_{A_3,\Sigma})\boldsymbol{X}(\boldsymbol{H}_4 + \boldsymbol{H}_5)^{1/2}$$
$$\sim N_{p,k_1}((\boldsymbol{P}_{A_2,\Sigma} - \boldsymbol{P}_{A_3,\Sigma})\boldsymbol{A}_1\boldsymbol{B}_1, (\boldsymbol{P}_{A_2,\Sigma} - \boldsymbol{P}_{A_3,\Sigma})\boldsymbol{\Sigma}, \boldsymbol{H}_4 + \boldsymbol{H}_5)$$

within $(\boldsymbol{P}_{A_2} - \boldsymbol{P}_{A_3})\boldsymbol{X}$, *and*

$$\boldsymbol{A}_1\boldsymbol{B}_{1N_3} = \boldsymbol{P}_{A_3,\Sigma}\boldsymbol{X}(\boldsymbol{H}_4 + \boldsymbol{H}_5 + \boldsymbol{H}_6)^{1/2}$$
$$\sim N_{p,k_1}(\boldsymbol{P}_{A_3,\Sigma}\boldsymbol{A}_1\boldsymbol{B}_1, \boldsymbol{P}_{A_3,\Sigma}\boldsymbol{\Sigma}, \boldsymbol{H}_4 + \boldsymbol{H}_5 + \boldsymbol{H}_6)$$

within $\boldsymbol{P}_{A_3}\boldsymbol{X}$. *Moreover,* $\boldsymbol{B}_{1N} = \boldsymbol{B}_{1N_1} + \boldsymbol{B}_{1N_2} + \boldsymbol{B}_{1N_3}$.

Problems

1 Using the matrix derivative given in Definition 5.1, demonstrate the following relations: (a) $\frac{d|\boldsymbol{X}|}{d\boldsymbol{X}} = |\boldsymbol{X}|\text{vec}(\boldsymbol{X}^{-1})'$, (b) $\frac{d\,\text{tr}\{\boldsymbol{A}'\boldsymbol{X}\}}{d\boldsymbol{X}} = \text{vec}\boldsymbol{A}$ and (c) $\frac{d\,\text{tr}\{\boldsymbol{X}'\boldsymbol{X}\}}{d\boldsymbol{X}} = 2\text{vec}\boldsymbol{X}$.

2 Suppose that $\boldsymbol{X}$ is a symmetric matrix. Calculate $\frac{d\,\text{tr}\{\boldsymbol{A}'\boldsymbol{X}\}}{d\boldsymbol{X}}$, $\frac{d|\boldsymbol{X}|}{d\boldsymbol{X}}$ and $\frac{d\,\text{tr}\{\boldsymbol{X}'\boldsymbol{X}\}}{d\boldsymbol{X}}$, using the same matrix derivative as in Problem 1.

3 Prove Lemma 5.1.

4 *GMANOVA + MANOVA* continuation of Problem 2 in Chap. 3 Let

$$\boldsymbol{X} = \boldsymbol{A}\boldsymbol{B}_1\boldsymbol{C}_1 + \boldsymbol{B}_2\boldsymbol{C}_2 + \boldsymbol{E},$$

where all the matrices are given in Problem 2. Consider the MLEs and perform Edgeworth type expansions for $\widehat{\boldsymbol{B}}_1$ and $\widehat{\boldsymbol{B}}_2$, for the case where the estimators are uniquely determined.

5 Prove Corollary 5.1 and determine an upper bound of $|r_3^*|$ as a function of $E[(\text{vec}\boldsymbol{U})^{\otimes 4}]$.

6 Give a complete and detailed proof that $\boldsymbol{B}_{3N}$ in (5.22) and $\boldsymbol{U}_3$ in (5.23) are uncorrelated.

7 Simulate data according to a BRM. For example, use the same design matrices, $\boldsymbol{A}$ and $\boldsymbol{C}$, as in Example 1.7. Apply Theorem 5.2 and try to understand how well the Edgeworth-type expansion works. Consider the centre of the distribution, as well as its tails. What can be said about the upper error bound? Plot the error bound versus the number of independent observations.

8 Let X follow a matrix Kotz-type distribution. Derive $E[X]$ and $D[X]$. Do the marginal distributions of a matrix Kotz-type distribution always follow a Kotz-type distribution? Give a detailed explanation of the reasons for your answer.

9 Calculate (5.67) and (5.68).

10 Approximate the distribution (using an Edgeworth-type expansion) of the maximum likelihood estimators of the mean parameters in the $EBRM_W^2$.

Literature

One tool used in this chapter is the concept of the matrix derivative, which Dwyer and Macphail (1948) were the first to introduce. Since then numerous papers have been written using different versions of matrix derivatives (see MacRae, 1974; Nel, 1980; Polasek, 1985; Wong, 1985; Magnus and Neudecker, 1988; Magnus, 2010). In Kollo and von Rosen (2005), as well as other published works, it has been stressed that a matrix derivative is nothing but a collection of partial derivatives which can be organized in different ways. Moreover, the organization of elements of multivariate moments and cumulants (marginal moments and cumulants) follows the definition of the matrix derivative in use (see Kollo and von Rosen, 2005), which stems from the fact that moments and cumulants can be obtained by differentiation of the characteristic function and the cumulant generating function, respectively.

It is interesting to follow the ideas behind the introduction of cumulants and their relations to moments. In fact these ideas arose from deep studies of the approximation of densities. A survey covering the developments in this field up to the 1940s has been provided by Hald (2002) (see also Hald, 1981, 1998). At the beginning of the nineteenth century, there existed a general idea of approximating a density function with some series where the first term is another density which is easy to use (mostly the normal density), and the other terms may be viewed as correction terms. For details see Hald (2002). One of the main results in this area was presented by Laplace (1811), who used the normal density, derivatives of the normal density (Hermite polynomials) and their expectations. Later Bienaymé (1852) and Chebyshev (1859) improved some of Laplace's work and operated with moments and cumulants, although cumulants at that time had not been explicitly defined. The series which Laplace obtained was called the A-series by Charlier (1905); there are also a B-series and a C-series.

The above-mentioned authors were mainly inspired by the central limit theorem and the average of n independent observations. Around 1870, one started to search for non-normal distributions in order to handle data which obviously could not be normally distributed and instead followed a skewed distribution. Among other discoveries, it was observed that if the normal density function was multiplied by a polynomial the obtained function was not symmetric. It was then that Thiele (1873) rediscovered the A-series and applied it.

Gram (1879, 1883) (see also Hald, 2002), who was a colleague of Thiele at an insurance company in Copenhagen, came up with the idea of using least squares to determine the coefficients of the A-series, i.e. to estimate the coefficients via a specific multiple regression model. Moreover, Gram supposed that in the A-series the approximating functions were orthogonal polynomials and, therefore, one refers to the series as Gram's orthogonal A-series. Thiele (1889) improved Gram's results by assuming a normal density and Hermite polynomials came into the picture. Moreover, Thiele introduced cumulants (half-invariants (semi-invariants) according to Thiele; at that time there existed mathematical results about invariants and semi-invariants which were used in different kinds of linearizations) and used them instead of moments, which Gram had been using. In this way, Thiele reobtained the result of Laplace (1811). Thiele (1899) presented a remarkable non-linear relation between moments and cumulants of an arbitrary order. On the basis of Laplace's results, Edgeworth (1905), among others, presented the A-series in the same fashion as Thiele, but rearranged the terms of the series so that the terms as a function of the number of independent observations decreased. The A-series which Thiele obtained, where normality was used in the approximation, is often called the Gram-Charlier series, but from a historical point of view this name is slightly misleading.

Hald (2002) presents many more contributors to the field of density approximations. In particular he mentions the Danish "school" (Oppermann, Thiele, Gram, Jørgensen), the German "school" (Bruns, Lipps, Hausdorff, von Mises), the British "school" (Edgeworth, among others) and the Swedish "school" (Charlier, among others). Some relations between the different schools can be found, but at the same time it appears from the outside that many scientists (astronomers, mathematicians and statisticians) have been working in parallel without being aware of each other.

Several more results on the A-series were produced from 1920 to 1945, for example by Cramér (1926, 1928) (see also Cramér, 1946, pp. 221–231) and Andersson (1944). Examples of topics focused on during that period are the convergence of the A-series and determination of the coefficients of the series. In articles published during this period one often used the characteristic function, its inverse and the cumulant generating function using techniques similar to those presented in this book.

Although many researchers have been working on the above-mentioned expansions, both the Edgeworth and the Gram-Charlier expansions suffer from the fact that the approximations may not be densities. Moreover, in comparison with the expansion of the centre of the density the expansions of the tails of the density functions may perform poorly. Therefore, research on distribution approximations has continued in various directions. The most commonly applied methods are the tilted Edgeworth expansion, the saddle point approximation and the Cornish-Fisher expansion (see Strawderman, 2000; DasGupta, 2008, which also include many references). For some multivariate distribution expansion, see Kollo and von Rosen (1998), where in particular a q-dimensional density was approximated using a p-dimensional density with $p > q$ (the results comprised Theorem 5.1 in the present book).

When considering the BRM or the $EBRM_{\bullet}^{m}$, the purpose of the density approximations in this book is to approximate the distribution of a given estimator and not, as was the purpose of density approximation for Thiele and others, to find a suitable density for a given data set. A general problem in connection with density approximations is that they are point-wise. For the BRM or the $EBRM_{\bullet}^{m}$, two remarkable results appeared in the presentation. The approximating density happened to be a real density and it was possible to present an upper error bound of the approximation. In Theorem 5.3 the results for the BRM were presented. An early reference to that approximation is Fujikoshi (1985). In Kollo et al. (2007) (see also Kollo and von Rosen, 2005) it was observed that the approximating density was in fact a true density. The upper bound of the density approximation was first obtained by Fujikoshi (1985) (see also Fujikoshi, 1987; Fujikoshi and Shimizu, 1989; Kanda, 1994). The results for the $EBRM_{\bullet}^{3}$ in this chapter, i.e. Theorems 5.7–5.16, are new. However, the derivation of these results is completely based on the technique developed for handling the BRM.

Concerning the exact distribution results for $\widehat{\boldsymbol{B}}$ in the BRM only a few results are available; see, for example, Gleser and Olkin (1972), Kenward (1986) or Bai and Shi (2007). In the paper by Bai and Shi (2007), the GMANOVA+MANOVA model is studied (see also Bai, 2005). The results are, however, difficult to apply.

References

Andersson, W. (1944). Short notes on Charlier's method for expansion of frequency functions in series. *Skandinavisk Aktuarietidskrift, 27*, 16–31.

Bai, P. (2005). Exact distribution of MLE of covariance matrix in a GMANOVA-MANOVA model. *Science in China. Series A, 48*, 1597–1608.

Bai, P., & Shi, L. (2007). Exact distributions of MLEs of regression coefficients in GMANOVA-MANOVA model. *Journal of Multivariate Analysis, 98*, 1840–1852.

Bienaymé, I. J. (1852). Sur la probabilité des erreurs d'après la méthode des moindres carrés. *Journal de Mathématiques Pures et Appliquées, sér. 1, 17*, 33–78; Also: *Mém. Res. Acad. Sci.*. In st. France, sér., 2, t. 15, 1858, 615–663 (in French).

Charlier, C. V. L. (1905). Über das Fehlergesetz. *Arkiv foer Matematik, Astronomi, och Fysik, 2*, 1–9 (in German).

Chebyshev, P. L. (1859). Sur le développement des fonctions à une seule variable. *Bulletin de la Classe physico-mathématique de l'Académie impériale des sciences, Sct. Pétersbourg, 1*, 193–200; Oeuvres 1, 501–508 (in French).

Cramér, H. (1926). On some classes of series used in mathematical statistics. *Den sjette skandinaviska Matematikerkongress, København* (pp. 399–425). Reprinted in Cramér, H. (2013). *Collected works. I.* by A. Martin-Löf, Ed., Reprint of the 1994 edition. *Springer collected works in mathematics*. Heidelberg: Springer.

Cramér, H. (1928). On the composition of elementary errors. *Skandinavisk Aktuarietidskrift, 11*, 13–74, 141–180. Reprinted in Cramér, H. (2013). *Collected works. I.* by A. Martin-Löf, Ed., Reprint of the 1994 edition. *Springer collected works in mathematics*. Heidelberg: Springer.

Cramér, H. (1946). *Mathematical methods of statistics. Vol. 9: Princeton mathematical series*. Princeton: Princeton University Press.

DasGupta, A. (2008). *Asymptotic theory of statistics and probability. Springer texts in statistics*. New York: Springer.

Dwyer, P. S., & Macphail, M. S. (1948). Symbolic matrix derivatives. *Annals of Mathematical Statistics, 19*, 517–534.
Edgeworth, F. Y. (1905). The law of error. *Transactions of the Cambridge Philosophical Society, 20*, Part I, 36–65; Part II, 113–141.
Fujikoshi, Y. (1985). An error bound for an asymptotic expansion of the distribution function of an estimate in a multivariate linear model. *The Annals of Statistics, 13*, 827–831.
Fujikoshi, Y. (1987). Error bounds for asymptotic expansions of the distribution of the MLE in a GMANOVA model. *Annals of the Institute of Statistical Mathematics, 39*, 153–161.
Fujikoshi, Y., & Shimizu, R. (1989). Asymptotic expansions of some mixtures of the multivariate normal distribution and their error bounds. *The Annals of Statistics, 17*, 1124–1132.
Gleser, L. J., & Olkin, I. (1972) Estimation for a regression model with an unknown covariance matrix. In *Proceedings of the Sixth Berkeley Symposium on Mathematical Statistics and Probability (University of California, Berkeley, 1970/1971). Vol. I: Theory of Statistics* (pp. 541–568). Berkeley: University of California Press.
Gram, J. P. (1879). *Om ræckkeudviklinger, bestemte ved hjælp af de mindste kvadraters methode*. Dissertation, Høst og Søn, København (in Danish).
Gram, J. P. (1883). Über die Entwicklung reeller Functionen in Reihen mittelst der Methode der kleinsten Quadrate. *Journal fur die Reine und Angewandte Mathematik, 94*, 41–73 (in German).
Hald, A. (1981). T.N. Thiele's contributions to statistics. *International Statistical Review, 49*, 1–20.
Hald, A. (1998). *A history of mathematical statistics from 1750 to 1930. Wiley series in probability and statistics: Texts and references section*. New York: Wiley.
Hald, A. (2002). On the history of series expansions of frequency functions and sampling distributions. *Matematisk-fysiske meddelelser, 49*, 1873–1944. ISSN: 00233323.
Kanda, T. (1994). Growth curve model with covariance structures. *Hiroshima Mathematical Journal, 24*, 135–176.
Kenward, M. G. (1986). The distribution of a generalized least squares estimator with covariance adjustment. *Journal of Multivariate Analysis, 20*, 244–250.
Kollo, T., Roos, A., & von Rosen, D. (2007). Approximation of the distribution of the location parameter in the growth curve model. *Scandinavian Journal of Statistics, 34*, 499–510.
Kollo, T., & von Rosen, D. (1998). A unified approach to the approximation of multivariate densities. *Scandinavian Journal of Statistics, 25*, 93–109.
Kollo, T., & von Rosen, D. (2005). *Advanced multivariate statistics with matrices. Vol. 579: Mathematics and its applications*. Dordrecht: Springer.
Laplace, P. S. (1811). Mémoire sur les intégrales définies et leur application aux probabilités, et spécialement à la recherche du milieu qu'il faut choisir entre les résultats des observations. *Mémoires de l'Académie Royale des Sciences de Paris, 11*, 279–347. Reprinted in Laplace, 1878–1912, **12**, 357–412 (in French).
MacRae, E. C. (1974). Matrix derivatives with an application to an adaptive linear decision problem. *The Annals of Statistics, 2*, 337–346.
Magnus, J. R. (2010). On the concept of matrix derivative. *Journal of Multivariate Analysis, 101*, 2200–2206.
Magnus, J. R., & Neudecker, H. (1988). *Matrix differential calculus with applications in statistics and econometrics*. New York: Wiley.
Nadarajah, S. (2003). The Kotz-type distribution with applications. *Statistics, 37*, 341–358.
Nel, D. G. (1980). On matrix differentiation in statistics. *South African Statistical Journal, 14*, 137–193.
Polasek, W. (1985). A dual approach for matrix-derivatives. *Metrika, 32*, 275–292.
Rao, C. R. (1973). *Linear statistical inference and its applications. Wiley series in probability and mathematical statistics* (2nd ed). New York: Wiley.
Strawderman, R. L. (2000). Higher-order asymptotic approximation: Laplace, saddlepoint, and related methods. *Journal of the American Statistical Association, 95*, 1358–1364.
Thiele, T. (1873). Om en tilnærmelsesformel. *Tidsskrift for mathematik, Tredie række, 3*, 22–31 (in Danish).

Thiele, T. N. (1889). *Forelæsninger over Almindelig Iagttagelseslære: Sandsynlighedsregning og Mindste Kvadraters Methode*. København: Reitzel (in Danish).
Thiele, T. N. (1899). Om iagttagelseslærens halvinvarianter. *Videnskabernes Selskabs Forhandlinger*, 135–141 (in Danish).
Wong, C. S. (1985). On the use of differentials in statistics. *Linear Algebra and Its Applications, 70*, 285–299.

Chapter 6
Residuals

6.1 Introduction

This chapter is devoted to the study of residuals. Residuals summarize the variation and may be used for estimating parameters connected to the description of uncertainty in a model, identifying outliers (extreme observations) and identifying some of the influential observations (see Chap. 8). Moreover, residuals can be used to construct tests, which is fairly obvious, since statistical hypothesis tests are usually constructed via functions of estimators of parameters describing the variation in the model under consideration.

Generally speaking, residuals can be defined as the difference between the observed and the predicted observations, or as the difference of the random variables corresponding to the observations and the predicted observations. As an introduction to a discussion of residuals and bilinear models, let us consider the general multivariate linear model

$$\boldsymbol{X} = \boldsymbol{BC} + \boldsymbol{E}, \quad \boldsymbol{E} \sim N_{p,n}(\boldsymbol{0}, \boldsymbol{\Sigma}, \boldsymbol{I}), \qquad \boldsymbol{\Sigma} > 0,$$

where $\boldsymbol{B}$ and $\boldsymbol{\Sigma}$ are unknown parameters. The matrix residual $\boldsymbol{R}$, collecting all the residuals, is given by

$$\boldsymbol{R} = \boldsymbol{X} - \widehat{\boldsymbol{B}}\boldsymbol{C} = \boldsymbol{X}(\boldsymbol{I} - \boldsymbol{P}_{C'}),$$

which is illustrated in Fig. 6.1. In the above model, residuals are obtained by projecting $\boldsymbol{X}$ on $\mathcal{C}(\boldsymbol{C}')^{\perp}$. The observed residuals are, of course, given by $\boldsymbol{R}_o = \boldsymbol{X}_o(\boldsymbol{I} - \boldsymbol{P}_{C'})$.

The term "residual", as used in the following, includes the concepts "matrix residual" and "components of the matrix residual". To utilize the residual, since it is a random quantity, it is natural to consider its distribution and then evaluate the observed residual, i.e. $\boldsymbol{R}_o$, with respect to the distribution. In the general

D. von Rosen, *Bilinear Regression Analysis*, Lecture Notes in Statistics 220,
https://doi.org/10.1007/978-3-319-78784-8_6

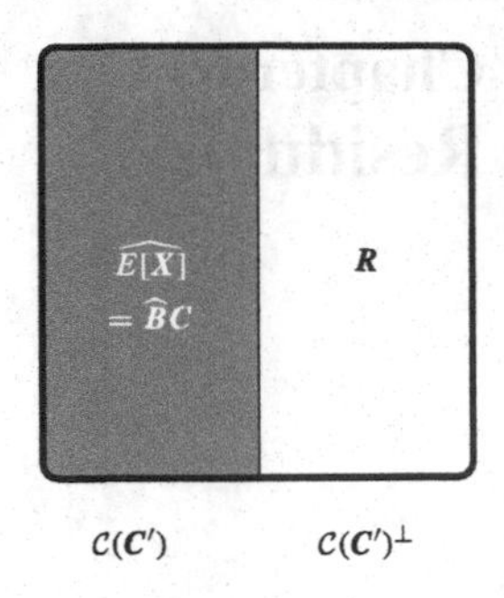

Fig. 6.1 The mean and residual spaces in the general multivariate linear model

multivariate linear case, under the assumption of a normally distributed error, it follows immediately that the distribution equals

$$R \sim N_{p,n}(\mathbf{0}, \boldsymbol{\Sigma}, \boldsymbol{I} - \boldsymbol{P}_{C'}). \tag{6.1}$$

Unfortunately the distribution of $\boldsymbol{R}$ depends on $\boldsymbol{\Sigma}$ and the columns of $\boldsymbol{R}$ are not independent nor identically distributed. Moreover, the dispersion matrix for $\boldsymbol{R}$ is singular. Hence, the relation in (6.1) cannot be used directly. There exist a large number of ways to exploit $\boldsymbol{R}$ and $\boldsymbol{R}_o$, but in this book only a few ideas will be presented. Focus will be set on the basic structures of the residuals in the bilinear models.

A general approach to dealing with residuals, from a distribution point of view, is to study shifts in the mean. One can also adopt approaches based, for example, on the absolute value of each single element of the matrix of residuals, $\boldsymbol{R}_o$. Concerning the mean shift approach, one can study the following five cases, letting $\boldsymbol{R}_{ij}$, $\boldsymbol{R}_j$ and $\boldsymbol{R}_i$ denote $\boldsymbol{R}$ and making some extra model assumption for the ijth element, the jth row or the ith column, respectively.

(i) For $1 \leq i \leq n$, $1 \leq j \leq p$, use

$$\boldsymbol{R}_{ij} \sim N_{p,n}(\boldsymbol{d}_j\theta\boldsymbol{e}_i', \boldsymbol{\Sigma}, \boldsymbol{I} - \boldsymbol{P}_{C'}),$$

where $\boldsymbol{d}_j$: $p \times 1$ and $\boldsymbol{e}_i$: $n \times 1$ are unit basis vectors, e.g. $\boldsymbol{e}_i$ is 1 in the ith position and 0 elsewhere, it is assumed that $\boldsymbol{e}_i \notin \mathcal{C}(\boldsymbol{C}')$ and θ is an unknown parameter (below $\boldsymbol{\theta}$ is an unknown parameter vector).

(ii) For $1 \leq i \leq n$, use

$$\boldsymbol{R}_i \sim N_{p,n}(\mathbf{1}\theta\boldsymbol{e}_i', \boldsymbol{\Sigma}, \boldsymbol{I} - \boldsymbol{P}_{C'})$$

or

(iii)

$$\boldsymbol{R}_i \sim N_{p,n}(\boldsymbol{\theta}\boldsymbol{e}_i', \boldsymbol{\Sigma}, \boldsymbol{I} - \boldsymbol{P}_{C'}).$$

(iv) For $1 \leq j \leq p$, use

$$R_j \sim N_{p,n}(d_j\theta\mathbf{1}', \Sigma, I - P_{C'})$$

or

(v)

$$R_j \sim N_{p,n}(d_j\boldsymbol{\theta}, \Sigma, I - P_{C'}).$$

Note that in cases (i), (ii) and (iv) a bilinear mean structure is imposed, whereas cases (iii) and (v) are described through linear structures. However, without any assumption concerning Σ, the model in case (v) cannot be considered with the usual likelihood-based estimation methods, because there are not enough independent observations (not enough degrees of freedom) for carrying out the estimation. Later the strategy will be first to assume that Σ is known and, when evaluating a test statistic, a plug-in estimator will replace Σ.

Since we plan to make a statistical decision about the residuals, it is natural to set up the problem of identifying large elements of the residual as a statistical decision problem, i.e. a testing problem, which means that we are going to test

$$H_0 : \theta = 0 \qquad \text{against} \qquad H_1 : \theta \text{ differs from } 0$$

in cases (i), (ii) and (iv), or

$$H_0 : \boldsymbol{\theta} = \mathbf{0} \qquad \text{against} \qquad H_1 : \boldsymbol{\theta} \text{ unrestricted}$$

in cases (iii) and (v). However, when evaluating the residual, multiple testing is performed with correlated tests, and one is interested in the large or largest elements of the residual. Based on standard analysis of variance ideas, natural test statistics for testing cases (i), (ii) and (iv) are

$$F_{ij} = \frac{(n - r(C) - 1)d'_j R_{ij} e_i (e'_i(I - P_{C'})e_i)^{-1} e'_i R'_{ij} d_j}{d'_j R_{ij}(I - e_i(e'_i(I - P_{C'})e_i)^{-1}e'_i)R'_{ij} d_j},$$

$$F_i = \frac{(n - r(C) - 1)\mathbf{1}'_p R_i e_i (e'_i(I - P_{C'})e_i)^{-1} e'_i R'_i \mathbf{1}_p}{\mathbf{1}'_p R_i(I - e_i(e'_i(I - P_{C'})e_i)^{-1}e'_i)R'_i \mathbf{1}_p},$$

and

$$F_j = \frac{(n - r(C) - 1)d'_j R_j \mathbf{1}_n (\mathbf{1}'_n(I - P_{C'})\mathbf{1}_n)^{-1} \mathbf{1}'_n R'_j d_j}{d'_j R_j(I - \mathbf{1}_n(\mathbf{1}'_n(I - P_{C'})\mathbf{1}_n)^{-1}\mathbf{1}'_n)R'_j d_j},$$

respectively. The above test statistics are all F-distributed under H_0. For example, let us consider F_{ij}. In case (i), post-multiplying R_{ij} by e_i and pre-multiplying by

$\boldsymbol{d}'_j$ yield, after some further manipulations,

$$(\boldsymbol{d}'_j\boldsymbol{\Sigma}\boldsymbol{d}_j)^{-1/2}(\boldsymbol{d}'_j\boldsymbol{R}_{ij}\boldsymbol{e}_i - \theta)(\boldsymbol{e}'_i(\boldsymbol{I} - \boldsymbol{P}_{C'})\boldsymbol{e}_i)^{-1/2} \sim N(0, 1). \tag{6.2}$$

Furthermore, independently of this expression,

$$(\boldsymbol{d}'_j\boldsymbol{\Sigma}\boldsymbol{d}_j)^{-1}\boldsymbol{d}'_j\boldsymbol{R}_{ij}(\boldsymbol{I} - \boldsymbol{e}_i(\boldsymbol{e}'_i(\boldsymbol{I} - \boldsymbol{P}_{C'})\boldsymbol{e}_i)^{-1}\boldsymbol{e}'_i)\boldsymbol{R}'_{ij}\boldsymbol{d}_j \sim \chi^2(n - r(\boldsymbol{C}) - 1). \tag{6.3}$$

Hence, taking the square in (6.2) and dividing it by (6.3) yield the null distribution, i.e. under H_0 the statistic $F_{ij} \sim F_{1,n-r(C)-1}$. However, we need the distribution of $\max\{F_{ij}\}$ or the second largest observation of $\{F_{ij}\}$, the third largest, etc. These distribution problems can be studied in depth, but here it is suggested that one should apply a straightforward parametric bootstrap approach as a tool for finding an approximate solution, i.e. to simulate the distributions.

Alternatively the mean shift could also have been introduced in the original model, i.e.

$$\boldsymbol{X} \sim N_{p,n}(\boldsymbol{B}\boldsymbol{C} + \boldsymbol{d}_j\theta\boldsymbol{e}'_i, \boldsymbol{\Sigma}, \boldsymbol{I}). \tag{6.4}$$

If $\boldsymbol{e}_i \notin \mathcal{C}(\boldsymbol{C}')$, which usually is true, the F-test statistic presented for testing case (i) is not the same as the likelihood ratio test for testing H_0 in model (6.4). Choosing between the two approaches is an interesting philosophical question. Since our intention is to evaluate a given model, the residuals are the main objects to exploit. However, if our intention had been to find deviating observations among the set of all the observations, (6.4) would have been the model to discuss. To some extent the approach used in this book is a marginal inferential procedure and hence also simpler than the approach based on (6.4).

Returning to the bootstrap simulations for the MANOVA case, which are needed in order to determine the distribution of the large F_{ij} values, we need to generate observations from $N_{p,n}(\boldsymbol{0}, \boldsymbol{\Sigma}, \boldsymbol{I} - \boldsymbol{P}_{C'})$ which is impossible since $\boldsymbol{\Sigma}$ is unknown. However, if we replace $\boldsymbol{\Sigma}$ by an unbiased estimate, e.g.

$$\widehat{\boldsymbol{\Sigma}}_o = \frac{1}{n - r(\boldsymbol{C}')}\boldsymbol{X}_o(\boldsymbol{I} - \boldsymbol{P}_{C'})\boldsymbol{X}'_o$$

or the maximum likelihood estimate, and then generate observations from $N_{p,n}(\boldsymbol{0}, \widehat{\boldsymbol{\Sigma}}_o, \boldsymbol{I} - \boldsymbol{P}_{C'})$, this gives the possibility of finding an approximative distribution for $\max\{F_{ij}\}$, $\max\{F_i\}$ and $\max\{F_j\}$, as well as finding the distributions of the second largest elements, and so on; i.e. for each generated $\boldsymbol{X}_o$ we calculate $\max\{F_{ij}\}$, for example, and then the procedure of generating $\boldsymbol{X}_o$ is repeated many times which leads to an estimate of the distribution for $\max\{F_{ij}\}$.

6.2 Residuals for the BRM

In this subsection quite a large number of results and ideas are presented which do not follow general practise and are open to discussion. In general, for each residual we first derive an approximate density which will later be used in a "mean shift" testing approach. The ideas are backed up via some data analysis.

In Fig. 3.1 a decomposition of the overall residual was shown which was based on the following space decomposition:

$$
\begin{aligned}
(\mathcal{C}(\boldsymbol{C}')\otimes\mathcal{C}_{\boldsymbol{\Sigma}}(\boldsymbol{A}))^{\perp} &= \mathcal{C}(\boldsymbol{C}')^{\perp}\otimes\mathcal{C}_{\boldsymbol{\Sigma}}(\mathcal{R}^{p})\boxplus\mathcal{C}(\boldsymbol{C}')\otimes\mathcal{C}_{\boldsymbol{\Sigma}}(\boldsymbol{A})^{\perp}\\
&= \mathcal{C}(\boldsymbol{C}')^{\perp}\otimes\mathcal{C}_{\boldsymbol{\Sigma}}(\boldsymbol{A})\boxplus\mathcal{C}(\boldsymbol{C}')^{\perp}\otimes\mathcal{C}_{\boldsymbol{\Sigma}}(\boldsymbol{A})^{\perp}\boxplus\mathcal{C}(\boldsymbol{C}')\otimes\mathcal{C}_{\boldsymbol{\Sigma}}(\boldsymbol{A})^{\perp}.
\end{aligned}
$$

Moreover, it was shown in Chap. 3 how the defining inner product quantity, i.e. $\boldsymbol{\Sigma}$, should be estimated and then, instead of the decomposition given above,

$$
\begin{aligned}
(\mathcal{C}(\boldsymbol{C}')\otimes\mathcal{C}_{\widehat{\boldsymbol{\Sigma}}}(\boldsymbol{A}))^{\perp} &= \mathcal{C}(\boldsymbol{C}')^{\perp}\otimes\mathcal{C}_{\widehat{\boldsymbol{\Sigma}}}(\mathcal{R}^{p})\boxplus\mathcal{C}(\boldsymbol{C}')\otimes\mathcal{C}_{\widehat{\boldsymbol{\Sigma}}}(\boldsymbol{A})^{\perp}\\
&= \mathcal{C}(\boldsymbol{C}')^{\perp}\otimes\mathcal{C}_{\widehat{\boldsymbol{\Sigma}}}(\boldsymbol{A})\boxplus\mathcal{C}(\boldsymbol{C}')^{\perp}\otimes\mathcal{C}_{\widehat{\boldsymbol{\Sigma}}}(\boldsymbol{A})^{\perp}\boxplus\mathcal{C}(\boldsymbol{C}')\otimes\mathcal{C}_{\widehat{\boldsymbol{\Sigma}}}(\boldsymbol{A})^{\perp}
\end{aligned}
\tag{6.5}
$$

was suggested as a basis for inference. Concerning the estimator of the inner product, the sums of squares matrix $\boldsymbol{S}$ (omitting $1/(n-r(\boldsymbol{C}))$, which could have been used when estimating $\boldsymbol{\Sigma}$) was used, which, as before, equals $\boldsymbol{S}=\boldsymbol{X}(\boldsymbol{I}-\boldsymbol{P}_{\boldsymbol{C}'})\boldsymbol{X}'$. It has been mentioned that residuals can be defined through $\boldsymbol{X}-\widehat{E[\boldsymbol{X}]}$, which means that for the BRM

$$
\begin{aligned}
\boldsymbol{X}-\widehat{E[\boldsymbol{X}]} &= \boldsymbol{X}-\boldsymbol{A}\widehat{\boldsymbol{B}}\boldsymbol{C}=\boldsymbol{X}-\boldsymbol{P}_{A,S}\boldsymbol{X}\boldsymbol{P}_{C'}\\
&= \boldsymbol{X}(\boldsymbol{I}-\boldsymbol{P}_{C'})+(\boldsymbol{I}-\boldsymbol{P}_{A,S})\boldsymbol{X}\boldsymbol{P}_{C'}\\
&= \boldsymbol{P}_{A,S}\boldsymbol{X}(\boldsymbol{I}-\boldsymbol{P}_{C'})+(\boldsymbol{I}-\boldsymbol{P}_{A,S})\boldsymbol{X}(\boldsymbol{I}-\boldsymbol{P}_{C'})+(\boldsymbol{I}-\boldsymbol{P}_{A,S})\boldsymbol{X}\boldsymbol{P}_{C'}
\end{aligned}
$$

gives three natural residuals obtained by projecting $\boldsymbol{X}$ on appropriate subspaces. The residuals are in complete agreement with the subspace decomposition given in (6.5).

Definition 6.1 For the BRM presented in Definition 2.1 the following residuals are considered:

(i) $\boldsymbol{R}_1=\boldsymbol{X}(\boldsymbol{I}-\boldsymbol{P}_{C'})$,
(ii) $\boldsymbol{R}_2=(\boldsymbol{I}-\boldsymbol{P}_{A,S})\boldsymbol{X}\boldsymbol{P}_{C'}$;
moreover, $\boldsymbol{R}_1=\boldsymbol{R}_{11}+\boldsymbol{R}_{12}$, where
(iii) $\boldsymbol{R}_{11}=\boldsymbol{P}_{A,S}\boldsymbol{X}(\boldsymbol{I}-\boldsymbol{P}_{C'})$,
(iv) $\boldsymbol{R}_{12}=(\boldsymbol{I}-\boldsymbol{P}_{A,S})\boldsymbol{X}(\boldsymbol{I}-\boldsymbol{P}_{C'})$.

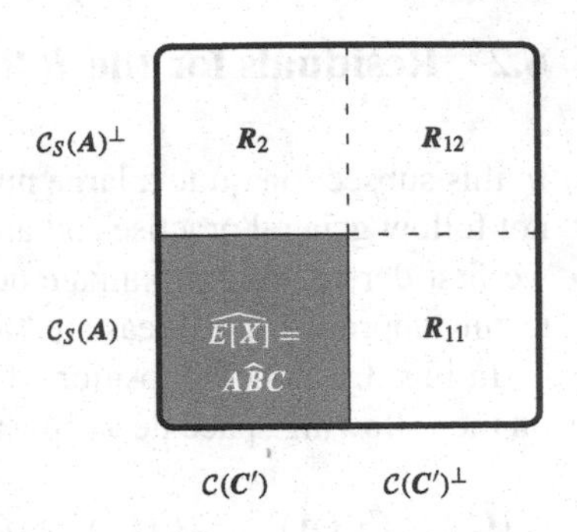

Fig. 6.2 For the BRM the three different residuals, $\boldsymbol{R}_{11}$, $\boldsymbol{R}_{12}$ and $\boldsymbol{R}_2$, are presented. Moreover, the residual $\boldsymbol{R}_1 = \boldsymbol{R}_{11} + \boldsymbol{R}_{12}$ can be understood

These residuals are illustrated in Fig. 6.2. Note that in Chap. 3, instead of $\boldsymbol{R}_{11}$, $\boldsymbol{R}_{12}$ and $\boldsymbol{R}_2$, the following notations were used, $\widehat{\boldsymbol{R}}_{11}$, $\widehat{\boldsymbol{R}}_{12}$ and $\widehat{\boldsymbol{R}}_2$, because there the aim was to highlight the fact that the inner product had been estimated.

In principle one would like to find the distribution of the residuals, but, as for the MLEs of the parameters in the BRM, useful expressions for the distributions (densities) do not exist for $\boldsymbol{R}_{11}$, $\boldsymbol{R}_{12}$ and $\boldsymbol{R}_2$. Therefore, density approximations will also take place for the residuals and these approximations will serve as a basis for an evaluation via a likelihood based test procedure. However, note that, in particular, the residual $\boldsymbol{R}_1 = \boldsymbol{R}_{11} + \boldsymbol{R}_{12} = \boldsymbol{X}(\boldsymbol{I} - \boldsymbol{P}_{C'})$ is normally distributed.

Moreover, although the decomposition of the tensor space seems to be natural, it is even more important that the objects, i.e. the residuals, should be interpretable. Therefore, it is of interest to note that the quantities in Definition 6.1 have a clear meaning, explained below.

- $\boldsymbol{R}_1$ gathers the differences between the "observations", $\boldsymbol{X}$, and the "mean", $\boldsymbol{X}\boldsymbol{P}_{C'}$. The residual can be used to detect observations which deviate from the others without taking into account any model assumption.
- $\boldsymbol{R}_2$ gathers the differences between the "mean", $\boldsymbol{X}\boldsymbol{P}_{C'}$, and the estimated model, $\boldsymbol{A}\widehat{\boldsymbol{B}}\boldsymbol{C} = \boldsymbol{P}_{A,S}\boldsymbol{X}\boldsymbol{P}_{C'}$. The residual gives a hint of the appropriateness of the model assumptions about the mean structure.
- $\boldsymbol{R}_{11}$ gathers the differences between the "observations", $\boldsymbol{X}$, and the "mean", $\boldsymbol{X}\boldsymbol{P}_{C'}$, relative to the within-individuals model. The residual is useful for detecting if observations do not follow the "within-individuals" model.
- $\boldsymbol{R}_{12}$ is the overall residual and gathers the differences between the "observations", $\boldsymbol{X}$, and the "mean", $\boldsymbol{X}\boldsymbol{P}_{C'}$, relative to the case where the within-individuals model does not hold.

In Fig. 6.3 the four different residuals are presented for the Potthoff and Roy (1964) data set previously considered in Example 1.7. In Fig. 6.3d the model is evaluated via $\boldsymbol{R}_2$. One can observe that there is a better fit for the girls than for the boys, and it is clearly indicated that it is worthwhile investigating whether different models can be used for the girls and for the boys. For example, it can be of interest to apply an $EBRM_B^2$. Moreover, in Fig. 6.3a–c there are interesting observations which will be highlighted in the following presentation. However, the main problem which we are

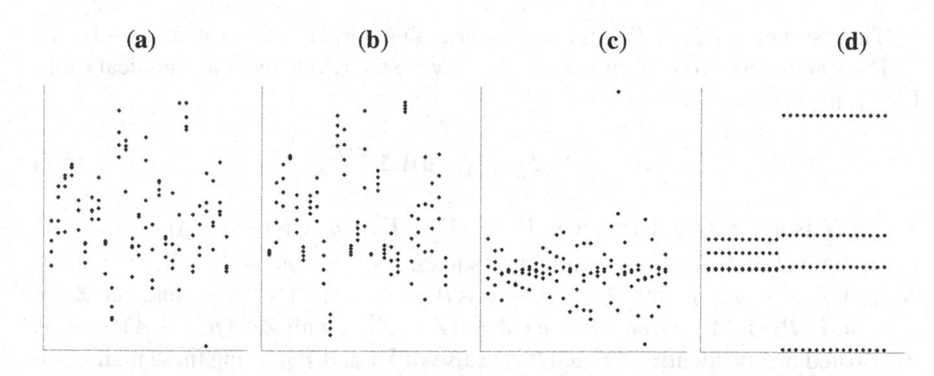

Fig. 6.3 The residuals $\boldsymbol{R}_{1o}$, $\boldsymbol{R}_{2o}$, $\boldsymbol{R}_{11o}$ and $\boldsymbol{R}_{12o}$ (see Definition 6.1) for the Potthoff and Roy (1964) data presented in Table 1.2. On the x-axis the 27 observations are listed. The first 11 observations concern the girls and the others concern the boys. On the y-axis the values of the residuals are presented. A linear model over time has been applied and the estimators are given in Example 3.1. Under **(a)**, $\boldsymbol{R}_{1o}$ is presented and then in **(b)** and **(c)** the split into $\boldsymbol{R}_{11o}$ and $\boldsymbol{R}_{12o}$ is given. The plot in **(d)** shows $\boldsymbol{R}_{2o}$, with the four lines per gender corresponding to the four ages and the four estimated mean values

going to address is to obtain the distribution of the largest residual and, as mentioned above, this will be dealt with using probabilistic arguments.

Next we prepare for density approximations of the residuals, i.e. we derive the mean and dispersion for the different residuals. Additionally, the moments give a basic understanding of the residuals.

Theorem 6.1 *Let* $\boldsymbol{R}_1$, $\boldsymbol{R}_2$, $\boldsymbol{R}_{11}$ *and* $\boldsymbol{R}_{12}$ *be given in Definition 6.1, and*

$$c_1 = \frac{n - r(\boldsymbol{C}) - p + r(\boldsymbol{A})}{n - r(\boldsymbol{C})}, \qquad c_2 = \frac{p - r(\boldsymbol{A})}{n - r(\boldsymbol{C}) - p + r(\boldsymbol{A}) - 1}, \tag{6.6}$$

where it is assumed that $n - r(\boldsymbol{C}) - p + r(\boldsymbol{A}) - 1 > 0$. *Then*

(i) $E[\boldsymbol{R}_1] = \boldsymbol{0}$, $E[\boldsymbol{R}_2] = \boldsymbol{0}$, $E[\boldsymbol{R}_{11}] = \boldsymbol{0}$, $E[\boldsymbol{R}_{12}] = \boldsymbol{0}$;
(ii) $D[\boldsymbol{R}_1] = (\boldsymbol{I} - \boldsymbol{P}_{C'}) \otimes \boldsymbol{\Sigma}$;
(iii) $C[\boldsymbol{R}_1, \boldsymbol{R}_2] = \boldsymbol{0}$, $C[\boldsymbol{R}_2, \boldsymbol{R}_{12}] = \boldsymbol{0}$, $C[\boldsymbol{R}_2, \boldsymbol{R}_{11}] = \boldsymbol{0}$, $C[\boldsymbol{R}_{11}, \boldsymbol{R}_{12}] = \boldsymbol{0}$;
(iv) $D[\boldsymbol{R}_2] = \boldsymbol{P}_{C'} \otimes \boldsymbol{\Sigma} \boldsymbol{P}_{A^o, \Sigma^{-1}} + c_2 \boldsymbol{P}_{C'} \otimes \boldsymbol{P}_{A,\Sigma} \boldsymbol{\Sigma}$;
(v) $D[\boldsymbol{R}_{11}] = c_1 (\boldsymbol{I} - \boldsymbol{P}_{C'}) \otimes \boldsymbol{P}_{A,\Sigma} \boldsymbol{\Sigma}$;
(vi) $D[\boldsymbol{R}_{12}] = (\boldsymbol{I} - \boldsymbol{P}_{C'}) \otimes \boldsymbol{\Sigma} \boldsymbol{P}_{A^o, \Sigma^{-1}} + (1 - c_1)(\boldsymbol{I} - \boldsymbol{P}_{C'}) \otimes \boldsymbol{P}_{A,\Sigma} \boldsymbol{\Sigma}$.

Proof Since $\boldsymbol{A}^{o'} \boldsymbol{X}$ and $\boldsymbol{X}(\boldsymbol{I} - \boldsymbol{P}_{C'})$ both have an expectation equal to $\boldsymbol{0}$ and the residuals are odd functions in $\boldsymbol{X}$, the expectation of any residual in statement (i) equals $\boldsymbol{0}$.

The result in statement (ii) follows because $X(I-P_{C'}) \sim N_{p,n}(0, \Sigma, (I-P_{C'}))$.

For statements (iii)–(vi), it is useful to rewrite the residuals in a canonical form. Let, as in (4.32),

$$A^{o'} = H(I_{p-r(A)} : 0)\Gamma\Sigma^{-1/2}, \tag{6.7}$$

where H is a non-singular matrix, $\Gamma' = (\Gamma_1' : \Gamma_2')$: $p \times (p - r(A)) : p \times r(A)$ is orthogonal and $\Sigma^{1/2}$ is a symmetric square root. Define $Y = (Y_1' : Y_2')' \sim N_{p,n}(0, I, I - P_{C'})$ with Y_1: $(p - r(A)) \times n$, Y_2: $r(A) \times n$, and let $Z \sim N_{p,n}(0, I, P_{C'})$. Moreover, note that $Z = (Z_1' : Z_2')'$, with Z_1: $(p - r(A)) \times n$, is distributed independently of Y and hence also of Y_1 and Y_2. Using these matrices it follows that the distribution of the residuals given in Definition 6.1 can be described as follows:

$$\begin{aligned}
&\bullet\ R_2 = (I - P_{A,S})XP_{C'} \text{ is distributed as } \Sigma^{1/2}\Gamma_1'Z_1 + \Sigma^{1/2}\Gamma_2'Y_2Y_1'(Y_1Y_1')^{-1}Z_1;\\
&\bullet\ R_1 = X(I - P_{C'}) \text{ is distributed as } \Sigma^{1/2}\Gamma'Y, \text{ i.e. is normally distributed};\\
&\bullet\ R_{11} = P_{A,S}X(I - P_{C'}) \text{ is distributed as } \Sigma^{1/2}\Gamma_2'Y_2(I - Y_1'(Y_1Y_1')^{-1}Y_1);
\end{aligned} \tag{6.8}$$

- $R_{12} = (I - P_{A,S})X(I - P_{C'})$ is distributed as

$$\Sigma^{1/2}\Gamma_1'Y_1 + \Sigma^{1/2}\Gamma_2'Y_2Y_1'(Y_1Y_1')^{-1}Y_1.$$

Moreover,

$$\Sigma^{1/2}\Gamma_1'\Gamma_1\Sigma^{1/2} = \Sigma - A(A'\Sigma^{-1}A)^{-}A', \quad \Sigma^{1/2}\Gamma_2'\Gamma_2\Sigma^{1/2} = A(A'\Sigma^{-1}A)^{-}A'. \tag{6.9}$$

In statement (iii) it is affirmed that the residuals R_{11}, R_{12} and R_2 are uncorrelated. Because Y_1 and Y_2 are independent,

$$\begin{aligned}
C[R_{11}, R_{12}] &= E[\mathrm{vec}\{\Sigma^{1/2}\Gamma_2'Y_2(I - P_{Y_1'})\}\mathrm{vec}'\{\Sigma^{1/2}\Gamma_1'Y_1\}]\\
&\quad + E[\mathrm{vec}\{\Sigma^{1/2}\Gamma_2'Y_2(I - P_{Y_1'})\}\mathrm{vec}'\{\Sigma^{1/2}\Gamma_1'Y_2P_{Y_1'}\}]\\
&= E[(I - Y_1'(Y_1Y_1')^{-1}Y_1)Y_1'(Y_1Y_1')^{-1}Y_1] \otimes \Sigma^{1/2}\Gamma_2'\Gamma_2\Sigma^{1/2} = 0.
\end{aligned}$$

Furthermore, because Z_1 is independent of Y, $C[R_2, R_{12}] = 0$ and $C[R_2, R_{11}] = 0$. Hence, statement (iii) has been established.

Now it is shown concisely that statements (iv)–(vi) are true. Concerning statement (iv), it follows, since $\boldsymbol{Y}_2$ is independent of $\boldsymbol{Y}_1$ and $\boldsymbol{Z}_1$, that

$$D[\boldsymbol{R}_2] = \boldsymbol{P}_{C'} \otimes \Big(\boldsymbol{\Sigma}^{1/2}\boldsymbol{\Gamma}_1'\boldsymbol{\Gamma}_1\boldsymbol{\Sigma}^{1/2} + \boldsymbol{\Sigma}^{1/2}\boldsymbol{\Gamma}_2'E[\boldsymbol{Y}_2\boldsymbol{Y}_1'(\boldsymbol{Y}_1\boldsymbol{Y}_1')^{-1}(\boldsymbol{Y}_1\boldsymbol{Y}_1')^{-1}\boldsymbol{Y}_1\boldsymbol{Y}_2']\boldsymbol{\Gamma}_2\boldsymbol{\Sigma}^{1/2}\Big)$$

and the expectation in this expression is given in Appendix B, Theorem B.21 (vii). Next, when studying $D[\boldsymbol{R}_{12}]$ in statement (vi), since $\boldsymbol{Y}_2$ is independent of $\boldsymbol{Y}_1$,

$$D[\boldsymbol{R}_{12}] = (\boldsymbol{I} - \boldsymbol{P}_{C'}) \otimes (\boldsymbol{\Sigma}^{1/2}\boldsymbol{\Gamma}_1'\boldsymbol{\Gamma}_1\boldsymbol{\Sigma}^{1/2} + E[\boldsymbol{P}_{Y_1'}] \otimes \boldsymbol{\Sigma}^{1/2}\boldsymbol{\Gamma}_2'\boldsymbol{\Gamma}_2\boldsymbol{\Sigma}^{1/2}).$$

Theorem B.23 (ii) in Appendix B implies

$$E[\boldsymbol{P}_{Y_1'}] = \frac{p - r(\boldsymbol{A})}{n - r(\boldsymbol{C})}(\boldsymbol{I} - \boldsymbol{P}_{C'})$$

and thus statement (vi) is verified. Finally, for statement (v), one can note that $\boldsymbol{R}_{11}$ and $\boldsymbol{R}_{12}$ are uncorrelated and sum to $\boldsymbol{R}_1$, from which the expression in statement (v) can be obtained. □

In Theorem 6.1 (iii) it was given that the three different residuals are pairwise uncorrelated. A natural question arises as to whether the residuals are indeed independent. Unfortunately the answer is negative, i.e. the residuals are not independent. One way of showing this is to study higher-order mixed moments of the residuals; e.g. one can show that

$$E[\boldsymbol{R}_{11}\boldsymbol{R}_{11}' \otimes \boldsymbol{R}_2\boldsymbol{R}_2'] \neq E[\boldsymbol{R}_{11}\boldsymbol{R}_{11}'] \otimes E[\boldsymbol{R}_2\boldsymbol{R}_2'].$$

In univariate linear models or the MANOVA model the residuals and the estimated mean are independent. If this were true for the BRM, this fact could be exploited, but once again a negative answer appears. Concerning the correlation between the residuals and the mean estimator, the following theorem holds.

Theorem 6.2 *Let* $\boldsymbol{R}_2$, $\boldsymbol{R}_{11}$ *and* $\boldsymbol{R}_{12}$ *be given in Definition 6.1, and* $\widehat{\boldsymbol{ABC}} = \boldsymbol{P}_{A,S}\boldsymbol{X}\boldsymbol{P}_{C'}$. *Then*

(i) $C[\boldsymbol{R}_{11}, \widehat{\boldsymbol{ABC}}] = \boldsymbol{0}$;
(ii) $C[\boldsymbol{R}_{12}, \widehat{\boldsymbol{ABC}}] = \boldsymbol{0}$;
(iii) $C[\boldsymbol{R}_2, \widehat{\boldsymbol{ABC}}] = -\frac{p-r(\boldsymbol{A})}{n-r(\boldsymbol{C})-p+r(\boldsymbol{A})-1}\boldsymbol{P}_{C'}\otimes\boldsymbol{P}_{A,\Sigma}\boldsymbol{\Sigma}$, *if* $n-r(\boldsymbol{C})-p+r(\boldsymbol{A})-1>0$.

Proof Since $\boldsymbol{X}\boldsymbol{P}_{C'}$ is independent of $\boldsymbol{R}_{11}$ and $\boldsymbol{R}_{12}$ both statements (i) and (ii) follow immediately. Concerning statement (iii),

$$C[\boldsymbol{R}_2, \widehat{\boldsymbol{ABC}}] = C[\boldsymbol{X}\boldsymbol{P}_{C'}, \widehat{\boldsymbol{ABC}}] - D[\widehat{\boldsymbol{ABC}}] = \boldsymbol{P}_{C'} \otimes \boldsymbol{P}_{a,\Sigma}\boldsymbol{\Sigma} - D[\widehat{\boldsymbol{ABC}}],$$

and $D[\widehat{\boldsymbol{ABC}}]$ was presented in Theorem 4.3 (ii). Hence, statement (iii) is verified. □

Since $\boldsymbol{R}_2$ measures the deviation from the model, but according to statement (iii) of the theorem is also correlated with $\boldsymbol{A}\widehat{\boldsymbol{B}}\boldsymbol{C}$, any conclusion based on $\boldsymbol{R}_2$ should also take this fact into account; i.e. marginal inference based on $\boldsymbol{R}_2$ should not be performed uncritically. Moreover, note that the covariance is negative and that it "diminishes" when n increases.

The next theorem includes unbiased estimators of the dispersion of the residuals which can be used when quickly evaluating them, i.e. to decide about the tails of the distribution of the residuals. However, it is questionable to suppose unbiasedness for functions of quadratic expressions, since in general quadratic forms are not symmetrically distributed. On the other hand, there are no obvious alternative estimators which are easily calculated.

Theorem 6.3 *Let* $D[\boldsymbol{R}_2]$, $D[\boldsymbol{R}_{11}]$ *and* $D[\boldsymbol{R}_{12}]$ *be given in Theorem 6.1 and* $\widehat{\boldsymbol{\Sigma}}$ *in Theorem 3.1. Then, the following estimators are unbiased estimators of the dispersion of the residuals (the constants* c_1 *and* c_2 *are presented in Theorem 6.1):*

(i) *if* $n - r(\boldsymbol{C}) - p + r(\boldsymbol{A}) > 0$,

$$\widehat{D[\boldsymbol{R}_{11}]} = \frac{n}{n-r(\boldsymbol{C})}(\boldsymbol{I} - \boldsymbol{P}_{C'}) \otimes \boldsymbol{P}_{A,\widehat{\Sigma}}\widehat{\boldsymbol{\Sigma}};$$

(ii) *if* $n - r(\boldsymbol{C}) - p + r(\boldsymbol{A}) - 1 > 0$,

$$\widehat{D[\boldsymbol{R}_{12}]} = (\boldsymbol{I} - \boldsymbol{P}_{C'}) \otimes (\widehat{\boldsymbol{\Sigma}} + (\tfrac{r(\boldsymbol{C})}{n}(1 - c_2) - c_1)\frac{n}{n-r(\boldsymbol{C})-p+r(\boldsymbol{A})}\boldsymbol{P}_{A,\widehat{\Sigma}}\widehat{\boldsymbol{\Sigma}});$$

(iii) *if* $n - r(\boldsymbol{C}) - p + r(\boldsymbol{A}) - 1 > 0$,

$$\widehat{D[\boldsymbol{R}_2]} = \boldsymbol{P}_{C'} \otimes (\widehat{\boldsymbol{\Sigma}} + (c_2 - 1 + \tfrac{r(\boldsymbol{C})}{n}(1 - c_2))\frac{n}{n-r(\boldsymbol{C})-p+r(\boldsymbol{A})}\boldsymbol{P}_{A,\widehat{\Sigma}}\widehat{\boldsymbol{\Sigma}}).$$

Proof The proof of the three statements is based on a combination of $E[\widehat{\boldsymbol{\Sigma}}]$, given in Theorem 4.6 (ii), and (see Theorem B.20 (v) in Appendix B)

$$n\boldsymbol{A}(\boldsymbol{A}'\widehat{\boldsymbol{\Sigma}}^{-1}\boldsymbol{A})^{-}\boldsymbol{A}' = \boldsymbol{A}(\boldsymbol{A}'\boldsymbol{S}^{-1}\boldsymbol{A})^{-}\boldsymbol{A}'$$
$$\sim W_p(\boldsymbol{A}(\boldsymbol{A}'\boldsymbol{\Sigma}^{-1}\boldsymbol{A})^{-}\boldsymbol{A}', n - r(\boldsymbol{C}) - p + r(\boldsymbol{A})).$$

□

The condition $n-r(\boldsymbol{C})-p+r(\boldsymbol{A}) > 0$ in statement (i) and $n-r(\boldsymbol{C})-p+r(\boldsymbol{A})-1 > 0$ in statements (ii) and (iii) are needed to secure existence of c_1 and c_2.

6.3 Distribution Approximations of the Residuals in the BRM

In the previous section the most basic properties for the three residuals $\boldsymbol{R}_{11}$, $\boldsymbol{R}_{12}$ and $\boldsymbol{R}_2$ were presented. Next the distribution of the residuals is studied, but this can only be performed approximately. As for the MLEs, an Edgeworth-type density approximation will be derived.

Since $n^{-1}\boldsymbol{S}$ converges to $\boldsymbol{\Sigma}$ in probability, as $n \to \infty$ (see Appendix B, Theorem B.18 (ii)), the residuals $\boldsymbol{R}_{11}$, $\boldsymbol{R}_{12}$ and $\boldsymbol{R}_2$ can respectively be approximated as follows by

$$\boldsymbol{R}_{11N} = \boldsymbol{P}_{A,\Sigma}\boldsymbol{X}(\boldsymbol{I} - \boldsymbol{P}_{C'}) \sim N_{p,n}(\boldsymbol{0}, \boldsymbol{A}(\boldsymbol{A}'\boldsymbol{\Sigma}^{-1}\boldsymbol{A})^{-}\boldsymbol{A}', \boldsymbol{I} - \boldsymbol{P}_{C'}), \quad (6.10)$$

$$\boldsymbol{R}_{12N} = (\boldsymbol{I} - \boldsymbol{P}_{A,\Sigma})\boldsymbol{X}(\boldsymbol{I} - \boldsymbol{P}_{C'}) \sim N_{p,n}(\boldsymbol{0}, \boldsymbol{\Sigma}\boldsymbol{A}^o(\boldsymbol{A}^{o\prime}\boldsymbol{\Sigma}\boldsymbol{A}^o)^{-}\boldsymbol{A}^{o\prime}\boldsymbol{\Sigma}, \boldsymbol{I} - \boldsymbol{P}_{C'}), \quad (6.11)$$

and

$$\boldsymbol{R}_{2N} = (\boldsymbol{I} - \boldsymbol{P}_{A,\Sigma})\boldsymbol{X}\boldsymbol{P}_{C'} \sim N_{p,n}(\boldsymbol{0}, \boldsymbol{\Sigma}\boldsymbol{A}^o(\boldsymbol{A}^{o\prime}\boldsymbol{\Sigma}\boldsymbol{A}^o)^{-}\boldsymbol{A}^{o\prime}\boldsymbol{\Sigma}, \boldsymbol{P}_{C'}), \quad (6.12)$$

respectively. Moreover, $\boldsymbol{R}_{11} = \boldsymbol{R}_{11N} - \boldsymbol{U}_{11}$, $\boldsymbol{R}_{12} = \boldsymbol{R}_{12N} - \boldsymbol{U}_{12}$, $\boldsymbol{R}_2 = \boldsymbol{R}_{2N} - \boldsymbol{U}_2$, where

$$\boldsymbol{U}_{11} = (\boldsymbol{P}_{A,\Sigma} - \boldsymbol{P}_{A,S})\boldsymbol{X}(\boldsymbol{I} - \boldsymbol{P}_{C'}), \qquad \boldsymbol{U}_{12} = -\boldsymbol{U}_{11} \quad (6.13)$$

and

$$\boldsymbol{U}_2 = (\boldsymbol{P}_{A,\Sigma} - \boldsymbol{P}_{A,S})\boldsymbol{X}\boldsymbol{P}_{C'}. \quad (6.14)$$

In Sect. 5.3 the density approximation of the mean estimator in the BRM was considered and a $\boldsymbol{U}$-matrix ("error matrix") was obtained, which in turn was independent of the normally distributed approximating quantity. This is not true for the above-suggested $\boldsymbol{U}_{11}$, $\boldsymbol{U}_{12}$ and $\boldsymbol{U}_2$. These quantities only satisfy $C[\boldsymbol{R}_{\bullet N}, \boldsymbol{U}_{\bullet}] = \boldsymbol{0}$, i.e. the $\boldsymbol{U}$-matrices are uncorrelated with the quantities which approximate the residuals. Under some mild conditions, according to Corollary 5.3, we can approximate the density of the residual with another density, although this time no error bound for the approximation can be presented. Concerning $\boldsymbol{U}_{11}$ and $\boldsymbol{U}_{12}$, the main difference compared with the mean estimator in the BRM is that $\boldsymbol{X}(\boldsymbol{I} - \boldsymbol{P}_{C'})$ is not independent of $\boldsymbol{S}$, unlike $\boldsymbol{X}\boldsymbol{P}_{C'}$ which is part of the mean. The independence between $\boldsymbol{S}$ and $\boldsymbol{X}\boldsymbol{P}_{C'}$ was important when considering the mean estimator. To find an error bound of the approximation is, of course, of interest. However, this is more crucial for the density approximation of the mean estimators than that of the residuals. One reason is that in this case one intends to compare the residuals from all the different subjects and, since one is carrying out the same procedure for each subject, it is often not very essential to find an upper error bound, because it will not increase the discrimination power among the subjects. The matter of importance is the distribution of the multiple comparison procedure which is applied for each residual, which will be treated in detail in Sect. 6.4.

Now some basic moment relations are presented which will be used in the theorems presented below where Edgeworth-type approximations are presented. The results follow from Theorem 6.1, where c_2 (used below) is also defined and supposed to exist. From (6.10) to (6.12) the said moment relations are as follows:

$$E[\boldsymbol{R}_{11}] = E[\boldsymbol{R}_{11N}] = \boldsymbol{0}, \quad E[\boldsymbol{R}_{12}] = E[\boldsymbol{R}_{12N}] = \boldsymbol{0}, \quad E[\boldsymbol{R}_2] = E[\boldsymbol{R}_{2N}] = \boldsymbol{0}, \tag{6.15}$$

$$D[\boldsymbol{R}_{11}] - D[\boldsymbol{R}_{11N}] = -\frac{p - r(\boldsymbol{A})}{n - r(\boldsymbol{C})}(\boldsymbol{I} - \boldsymbol{P}_{C'}) \otimes \boldsymbol{P}_{A,\Sigma}\boldsymbol{\Sigma}, \tag{6.16}$$

$$D[\boldsymbol{R}_{12}] - D[\boldsymbol{R}_{12N}] = \frac{p - r(\boldsymbol{A})}{n - r(\boldsymbol{C})}(\boldsymbol{I} - \boldsymbol{P}_{C'}) \otimes \boldsymbol{P}_{A,\Sigma}\boldsymbol{\Sigma}, \tag{6.17}$$

$$D[\boldsymbol{R}_2] - D[\boldsymbol{R}_{2N}] = c_2\boldsymbol{P}_{C'} \otimes \boldsymbol{P}_{A,\Sigma}\boldsymbol{\Sigma}. \tag{6.18}$$

Note that (6.16) shows that the approximation suggested by (6.10) has a larger variation than the quantity which is to be approximated and this is not desirable. The result in (6.16) indicates that something is not optimal, which follows from the fact that $\boldsymbol{S}$ and $\boldsymbol{X}(\boldsymbol{I} - \boldsymbol{P}_{C'})$ are dependent.

However, the approximation can be sharpened, somewhat, and an approximation will indeed be derived whose error has a mean which equals $\boldsymbol{0}$ and is independent of the approximating variable. The idea is to manipulate $\boldsymbol{R}_{11N}$ in $\boldsymbol{R}_{11} = \boldsymbol{R}_{11N} - \boldsymbol{U}_{11}$. Instead of $\boldsymbol{R}_{11N}$,

$$\begin{aligned}\boldsymbol{P}_{A,\Sigma}\boldsymbol{X}\boldsymbol{M}(\boldsymbol{I} - \boldsymbol{P}_{C'}) &= \boldsymbol{P}_{A,\Sigma}\boldsymbol{X}\boldsymbol{M}\begin{pmatrix} \boldsymbol{0} & \boldsymbol{0} \\ \boldsymbol{0} & \boldsymbol{I}_{n-p+r(A)} \end{pmatrix}(\boldsymbol{I} - \boldsymbol{P}_{C'}) \\ &\quad + \boldsymbol{P}_{A,\Sigma}\boldsymbol{X}\boldsymbol{M}\begin{pmatrix} \boldsymbol{I}_{p-r(A)} & \boldsymbol{0} \\ \boldsymbol{0} & \boldsymbol{0} \end{pmatrix}(\boldsymbol{I} - \boldsymbol{P}_{C'})\end{aligned}$$

will be used, where $\boldsymbol{M}$ is an orthogonal matrix which satisfies

$$\boldsymbol{P}'_{A^o,S^{-1}}\boldsymbol{X}(\boldsymbol{I} - \boldsymbol{P}_{C'}) = \boldsymbol{X}\boldsymbol{M}\begin{pmatrix} \boldsymbol{I}_{p-r(A)} & \boldsymbol{0} \\ \boldsymbol{0} & \boldsymbol{0} \end{pmatrix}\boldsymbol{M}';$$

i.e. an eigenvalue decomposition of the idempotent matrix $(I-P_{C'})X'A^o(A^{o'}X(I-P_{C'})(I-P_{C'})X'A^o)^-A^{o'}X(I-P_{C'})$ has taken place. Thus,

$$R_{11} = P_{A,\Sigma}XM\begin{pmatrix} 0 & 0 \\ 0 & I_{n-p+r(A)} \end{pmatrix}(I-P_{C'})$$
$$+ P_{A,\Sigma}XM\begin{pmatrix} I_{p-r(A)} & 0 \\ 0 & 0 \end{pmatrix}(I-P_{C'}) - U_{11}.$$

The explanation for our next result is that $P_{A,\Sigma}X$ and $P_{A,\Sigma}XM$ have marginally the same normal distribution, since $M'M = I$ and M is independent of $P_{A,\Sigma}X$, but $P_{A,\Sigma}XM$ has some advantages in comparison with $P_{A,\Sigma}X$, i.e. it is possible to have an approximating quantity which is independent of the error.

Theorem 6.4 *The distribution of the residual R_{11} given in Definition 6.1 can be approximated through the difference*

$$R_{11} = \widetilde{R}_{11N} - U_{11x},$$

where

$$\widetilde{R}_{11N} = P_{A,\Sigma}XM\begin{pmatrix} 0 & 0 \\ 0 & I_{n-p+r(A)} \end{pmatrix}(I-P_{C'})$$

is normally distributed and

$$U_{11x} = -P_{A,\Sigma}XM\begin{pmatrix} I_{p-r(A)} & 0 \\ 0 & 0 \end{pmatrix}(I-P_{C'}) + (P_{A,\Sigma}-P_{A,S})X(I-P_{C'}),$$

with $\widetilde{R}_{11N}$ and U_{11x} being independently distributed and M satisfying

$$M\begin{pmatrix} I_{p-r(A)} & 0 \\ 0 & 0 \end{pmatrix}M'$$
$$= (I-P_{C'})X'A^o(A^{o'}X(I-P_{C'})(I-P_{C'})X'A^o)^-A^{o'}X(I-P_{C'}).$$

Proof First note that

$$(P_{A,\Sigma}-P_{A,S})X(I-P_{C'}) = P_{A,\Sigma}(I-P_{A,S})X(I-P_{C'})$$
$$= P_{A,\Sigma}P'_{A^o,S^{-1}}X(I-P_{C'}) = P_{A,\Sigma}XM\begin{pmatrix} I_{p-r(A)} & 0 \\ 0 & 0 \end{pmatrix}M'.$$

It will be proved that $\widetilde{\boldsymbol{R}}_{11N}$ and $\boldsymbol{U}_{11x}$ are independently distributed. Note that $\boldsymbol{A}'\boldsymbol{\Sigma}^{-1}\boldsymbol{X}$ and $\boldsymbol{A}^{o'}\boldsymbol{X}$ are independent, which implies that $\boldsymbol{P}_{A,\Sigma}\boldsymbol{X}\boldsymbol{M}$ and $\boldsymbol{M}$ are independent, since $\boldsymbol{M}$ is a function of $\boldsymbol{A}^{o'}\boldsymbol{X}$ and the distribution of $\boldsymbol{X}\boldsymbol{M}$ is independent of $\boldsymbol{M}$. Moreover, $\boldsymbol{P}_{A,\Sigma}\boldsymbol{X}\boldsymbol{M}\begin{pmatrix}\boldsymbol{0} & \boldsymbol{0}\\ \boldsymbol{0} & \boldsymbol{I}_{n-p+r(A)}\end{pmatrix}$ is independent of $\boldsymbol{P}_{A,\Sigma}\boldsymbol{X}\boldsymbol{M}\begin{pmatrix}\boldsymbol{I}_{p-r(A)} & \boldsymbol{0}\\ \boldsymbol{0} & \boldsymbol{0}\end{pmatrix}$, since the expressions comprise different independent observations. Thus, the theorem has been established. □

Note that the sizes of $\boldsymbol{I}_\bullet$ in the decomposition, i.e. $\boldsymbol{I}_{p-r(A)}$ and $\boldsymbol{I}_{n-p+r(A)}$, follow from

$$r((\boldsymbol{I}-\boldsymbol{P}_{C'})\boldsymbol{X}'\boldsymbol{A}^o) = r(\boldsymbol{S}\boldsymbol{A}^o) = r(\boldsymbol{A}^o) = p - r(\boldsymbol{A}).$$

Hence, the distribution of $\boldsymbol{R}_{11}$ is approximated with a subset of $\boldsymbol{X}\boldsymbol{M}$. It is somewhat unsatisfactory that the decomposition is not unique and there are in fact $\binom{n}{p-r(A)}$ possibilities to approximate.

For the Edgeworth-type approximations of the density for $\boldsymbol{R}_{11}$ in the following, moments of order 1 and 2 are needed and for their error terms moments of the fourth order have to be obtained. Therefore, it is noted that

$$\begin{aligned}
&E[\boldsymbol{R}_{11}] = E[\widetilde{\boldsymbol{R}}_{11N}] = \boldsymbol{0},\\
&D[\boldsymbol{R}_{11}] - D[\widetilde{\boldsymbol{R}}_{11N}]\\
&= (c_1(\boldsymbol{I}-\boldsymbol{P}_{C'}) - (\boldsymbol{I}-\boldsymbol{P}_{C'})\begin{pmatrix}\boldsymbol{0} & \boldsymbol{0}\\ \boldsymbol{0} & \boldsymbol{I}_{n-p+r(A)}\end{pmatrix}(\boldsymbol{I}-\boldsymbol{P}_{C'}))\otimes \boldsymbol{P}_{A,\Sigma}\boldsymbol{\Sigma}, \qquad (6.19)
\end{aligned}$$

with c_1 defined in Theorem 6.1. Unfortunately, the difference in (6.19) is not positive definite. The derivation of the fourth-order moments will be omitted, since this needs relatively lengthy calculations, but these calculations follow those performed when obtaining higher-order moments for the estimators in the BRM. Moreover, since the densities for $\boldsymbol{R}_{11}$ and $\widetilde{\boldsymbol{R}}_{11N}$ do not exist, linear combinations of the residuals with dispersion matrices which are of full rank will be considered. Indeed, residuals are commonly evaluated via $\boldsymbol{K}\boldsymbol{R}_\bullet\boldsymbol{L}$, where $\boldsymbol{K}$ and $\boldsymbol{L}$ may be vectors and, in particular, unit basis vectors which select one element of $\boldsymbol{R}_\bullet$ ($\bullet$ means that it can be $\boldsymbol{R}_{11}$, $\boldsymbol{R}_{12}$, $\boldsymbol{R}_1$ or $\boldsymbol{R}_2$). The proof of the next theorem follows from Theorem 5.2 and (6.19).

Theorem 6.5 *For the BRM, let the residual $\boldsymbol{R}_{11}$ be as given in Definition 6.1, let $\boldsymbol{K}$: $p_1\times p$ and $\boldsymbol{L}$: $n\times n_1$, both of which are known, and let*

$$\begin{aligned}
\boldsymbol{K}\widetilde{\boldsymbol{R}}_{11N}\boldsymbol{L} &\sim N_{p_1,n_1}(\boldsymbol{0}, \boldsymbol{K}\boldsymbol{A}(\boldsymbol{A}'\boldsymbol{\Sigma}^{-1}\boldsymbol{A})^-\boldsymbol{A}'\boldsymbol{K}', \boldsymbol{D}),\\
\boldsymbol{D} &= \boldsymbol{L}'(\boldsymbol{I}-\boldsymbol{P}_{C'})\begin{pmatrix}\boldsymbol{0} & \boldsymbol{0}\\ \boldsymbol{0} & \boldsymbol{I}_{n-p+r(A)}\end{pmatrix}(\boldsymbol{I}-\boldsymbol{P}_{C'})\boldsymbol{L}.
\end{aligned}$$

Then an Edgeworth-type expansion of the density of $\boldsymbol{K}\boldsymbol{R}_{11}\boldsymbol{L}$, *via the density of* $\boldsymbol{K}\widetilde{\boldsymbol{R}}_{11N}\boldsymbol{L}$ *and under the assumption that* $D[\boldsymbol{K}\widetilde{\boldsymbol{R}}_{11N}\boldsymbol{L}]$ *is p.d., equals*

$$f_{\boldsymbol{K}\boldsymbol{R}_{11E}\boldsymbol{L}}(\boldsymbol{K}\boldsymbol{R}_o\boldsymbol{L}) + r^\star,$$

where

$$\begin{aligned}f_{\boldsymbol{K}\boldsymbol{R}_{11E}\boldsymbol{L}}(\boldsymbol{K}\boldsymbol{R}_o\boldsymbol{L}) = \big\{&1 - \tfrac{1}{2}c_1 p_1 \mathrm{tr}\{\boldsymbol{L}'(\boldsymbol{I} - \boldsymbol{P}_{\boldsymbol{C}'})\boldsymbol{L}\boldsymbol{D}^{-1}\} + \tfrac{1}{2}p_1 n_1\\ &+ \tfrac{1}{2}\mathrm{tr}\{(\boldsymbol{K}\boldsymbol{A}(\boldsymbol{A}'\boldsymbol{\Sigma}^{-1}\boldsymbol{A})^{-}\boldsymbol{A}'\boldsymbol{K}')^{-1}\boldsymbol{K}\boldsymbol{R}_o\boldsymbol{L}\boldsymbol{D}^{-1}\\ &\times(c_1\boldsymbol{L}'(\boldsymbol{I} - \boldsymbol{P}_{\boldsymbol{C}'})\boldsymbol{L} - \boldsymbol{D})\boldsymbol{D}^{-1}\boldsymbol{L}'\boldsymbol{R}_o'\boldsymbol{K}'\}\big\}\\ &\times f_{\boldsymbol{K}\widetilde{\boldsymbol{R}}_{11N}\boldsymbol{L}}(\boldsymbol{K}\boldsymbol{R}_o\boldsymbol{L});\end{aligned}$$

c_1 *is supposed to exist and is defined in Theorem 6.1, and the leading term of* $|r^\star|$ *is proportional to* $E[vec(\boldsymbol{K}(\boldsymbol{R}_{11} - \widetilde{\boldsymbol{R}}_{11N})\boldsymbol{L})^{\otimes 4}]$ *which is a function of* $\boldsymbol{A}$, $\boldsymbol{C}$, $\boldsymbol{K}$ *and* $\boldsymbol{L}$.

The two most basic moment properties of $\boldsymbol{K}\boldsymbol{R}_{11E}\boldsymbol{L}$ are now given. Statement (ii) in particular will be used later.

Corollary 6.1 *Let* $\boldsymbol{K}\boldsymbol{R}_{11E}\boldsymbol{L}$ *be defined via* $f_{\boldsymbol{K}\boldsymbol{R}_{11E}\boldsymbol{L}}(\boldsymbol{K}\boldsymbol{R}_o\boldsymbol{L})$, *presented in Theorem 6.5, where it is assumed that* $f_{\boldsymbol{K}\boldsymbol{R}_{11E}\boldsymbol{L}}(\boldsymbol{K}\boldsymbol{R}_o\boldsymbol{L}) \geq 0$. *Then*

(i) $E[\boldsymbol{K}\boldsymbol{R}_{11E}\boldsymbol{L}] = \boldsymbol{0}$;
(ii) $D[\boldsymbol{K}\boldsymbol{R}_{11E}\boldsymbol{L}] = c_1\boldsymbol{L}'(\boldsymbol{I} - \boldsymbol{P}_{\boldsymbol{C}'})\boldsymbol{L} \otimes \boldsymbol{K}\boldsymbol{A}(\boldsymbol{A}'\boldsymbol{\Sigma}^{-1}\boldsymbol{A})^{-}\boldsymbol{A}'\boldsymbol{K}'$.

Proof The derivation of statement (ii) follows from Appendix B, Theorem B.23 (i), because according to the theorem

$$\begin{aligned}D[\boldsymbol{K}\boldsymbol{R}_{11E}\boldsymbol{L}] = &\big(1 - \tfrac{1}{2}c_1 p_1 \mathrm{tr}\{\boldsymbol{L}'(\boldsymbol{I} - \boldsymbol{P}_{\boldsymbol{C}'})\boldsymbol{L}\boldsymbol{D}^{-1}\} + \tfrac{1}{2}p_1 n_1\big)\boldsymbol{D} \otimes \boldsymbol{K}\boldsymbol{A}(\boldsymbol{A}'\boldsymbol{\Sigma}^{-1}\boldsymbol{A})^{-}\boldsymbol{A}'\boldsymbol{K}'\\ &+ \tfrac{1}{2}p_1 \mathrm{tr}\{\boldsymbol{D}^{-1}(c_1\boldsymbol{L}'(\boldsymbol{I} - \boldsymbol{P}_{\boldsymbol{C}'})\boldsymbol{L} - \boldsymbol{D})\}\boldsymbol{D} \otimes \boldsymbol{K}\boldsymbol{A}(\boldsymbol{A}'\boldsymbol{\Sigma}^{-1}\boldsymbol{A})^{-}\boldsymbol{A}'\boldsymbol{K}'\\ &+ (c_1\boldsymbol{L}'(\boldsymbol{I} - \boldsymbol{P}_{\boldsymbol{C}'})\boldsymbol{L} - \boldsymbol{D}) \otimes \boldsymbol{K}\boldsymbol{A}(\boldsymbol{A}'\boldsymbol{\Sigma}^{-1}\boldsymbol{A})^{-}\boldsymbol{A}'\boldsymbol{K}'\end{aligned}$$

which is identical to statement (ii). □

Now we switch from a discussion of $\boldsymbol{R}_{11}$ to a discussion of the other two residuals, $\boldsymbol{R}_{12}$ and $\boldsymbol{R}_2$, presented in Definition 6.1. However, for these residuals no results will be presented which correspond to Theorem 6.4, i.e. no modification like the one which led to $\widetilde{\boldsymbol{R}}_{11N}$ will take place. The next two theorems are based on Corollary 5.3, and density approximations for $\boldsymbol{R}_{12}$ and $\boldsymbol{R}_2$ are presented.

Theorem 6.6 *The distribution of the residual* $\boldsymbol{R}_{12}$ *given in Definition 6.1, can be approximated through the difference*

$$\boldsymbol{R}_{12} = \boldsymbol{R}_{12N} - \boldsymbol{U}_{12},$$

where $\boldsymbol{R}_{12N}$ *and* $\boldsymbol{U}_{12}$ *are defined by (6.11) and (6.13), respectively. Let* $\boldsymbol{K}$*:* $p_1 \times p$ *and* $\boldsymbol{L}$*:* $n \times n_1$*, both of which are known, and*

$$\boldsymbol{K}\boldsymbol{R}_{12N}\boldsymbol{L} \sim N_{p_1,n_1}(\boldsymbol{0}, \boldsymbol{K}\boldsymbol{\Sigma}\boldsymbol{P}_{A^o,\Sigma^{-1}}\boldsymbol{K}', \boldsymbol{L}'(\boldsymbol{I}-\boldsymbol{P}_{C'})\boldsymbol{L}).$$

Then an Edgeworth-type expansion $f_{\boldsymbol{K}\boldsymbol{R}_{12E}\boldsymbol{L}}(\boldsymbol{K}\boldsymbol{R}_o\boldsymbol{L})$ *of the density of* $\boldsymbol{K}\boldsymbol{R}_{12}\boldsymbol{L}$*, via the density of* $\boldsymbol{K}\boldsymbol{R}_{12N}\boldsymbol{L}$*, under the assumption that* $D[\boldsymbol{K}\boldsymbol{R}_{12N}\boldsymbol{L}]$ *is p.d., is given by*

$$\begin{aligned} f_{\boldsymbol{K}\boldsymbol{R}_{12E}\boldsymbol{L}}(\boldsymbol{K}\boldsymbol{R}_o\boldsymbol{L}) = \big\{1 &- \tfrac{1}{2}\tfrac{p-r(A)}{n-r(C)}n_1\mathrm{tr}\{\boldsymbol{K}\boldsymbol{P}_{A,\Sigma}\boldsymbol{\Sigma}\boldsymbol{K}'(\boldsymbol{K}\boldsymbol{\Sigma}\boldsymbol{P}_{A^o,\Sigma^{-1}}\boldsymbol{K}')^{-1}\} \\ &+ \tfrac{1}{2}c_1\mathrm{tr}\{(\boldsymbol{K}\boldsymbol{\Sigma}\boldsymbol{P}_{A^o,\Sigma^{-1}}\boldsymbol{K}')^{-1}\boldsymbol{K}\boldsymbol{P}_{A,\Sigma}\boldsymbol{\Sigma}\boldsymbol{K}'(\boldsymbol{K}\boldsymbol{\Sigma}\boldsymbol{P}_{A^o,\Sigma^{-1}}\boldsymbol{K}')^{-1} \\ &\times \boldsymbol{K}\boldsymbol{R}_o\boldsymbol{L}(\boldsymbol{L}'(\boldsymbol{I}-\boldsymbol{P}_{C'})\boldsymbol{L})^{-1}\boldsymbol{L}'\boldsymbol{R}_o'\boldsymbol{K}'\}\big\} f_{\boldsymbol{K}\boldsymbol{R}_{12N}\boldsymbol{L}}(\boldsymbol{K}\boldsymbol{R}_o\boldsymbol{L}), \end{aligned}$$

where c_1*, supposed to exist, is defined in Theorem 6.1.*

Corollary 6.2 *Let* $\boldsymbol{K}\boldsymbol{R}_{12E}\boldsymbol{L}$ *be defined via* $f_{\boldsymbol{K}\boldsymbol{R}_{12E}\boldsymbol{L}}(\boldsymbol{K}\boldsymbol{R}_o\boldsymbol{L})$*, given in Theorem 6.6, where it is assumed that* $f_{\boldsymbol{K}\boldsymbol{R}_{12E}\boldsymbol{L}}(\boldsymbol{K}\boldsymbol{R}_o\boldsymbol{L}) \geq 0$*. Then*

(i) $E[\boldsymbol{K}\boldsymbol{R}_{12E}\boldsymbol{L}] = \boldsymbol{0}$;
(ii) $D[\boldsymbol{K}\boldsymbol{R}_{12E}\boldsymbol{L}] = \boldsymbol{L}'(\boldsymbol{I}-\boldsymbol{P}_{C'})\boldsymbol{L} \otimes (f_1\boldsymbol{K}\boldsymbol{\Sigma}\boldsymbol{P}_{A^o,\Sigma^{-1}}\boldsymbol{K}' + c_1\boldsymbol{K}\boldsymbol{P}_{A,\Sigma}\boldsymbol{\Sigma}\boldsymbol{K}')$,
where

$$\begin{aligned} f_1 = 1 &- \tfrac{1}{2}\tfrac{p-r(A)}{n-r(C)}n_1\mathrm{tr}\{\boldsymbol{K}\boldsymbol{P}_{A,\Sigma}\boldsymbol{\Sigma}\boldsymbol{K}'(\boldsymbol{K}\boldsymbol{\Sigma}\boldsymbol{P}_{A^o,\Sigma^{-1}}\boldsymbol{K}')^{-1}\} \\ &+ \tfrac{1}{2}c_1n_1\mathrm{tr}\{(\boldsymbol{K}\boldsymbol{\Sigma}\boldsymbol{P}_{A^o,\Sigma^{-1}}\boldsymbol{K}')^{-1}\boldsymbol{K}\boldsymbol{P}_{A,\Sigma}\boldsymbol{\Sigma}\boldsymbol{K}'\}. \end{aligned}$$

Theorem 6.7 *The distribution of the residual* $\boldsymbol{R}_2$*, given in Definition 6.1, can be approximated through the difference*

$$\boldsymbol{R}_2 = \boldsymbol{R}_{2N} - \boldsymbol{U}_2,$$

where $\boldsymbol{R}_{2N}$ *and* $\boldsymbol{U}_2$ *are defined by (6.12) and (6.14), respectively. Let* $\boldsymbol{K}$*:* $p_1 \times p$ *and* $\boldsymbol{L}$*:* $n \times n_1$*, both of which are known, and*

$$\boldsymbol{K}\boldsymbol{R}_{2N}\boldsymbol{L} \sim N_{p_1,n_1}(\boldsymbol{0}, \boldsymbol{K}\boldsymbol{\Sigma}\boldsymbol{P}_{A^o,\Sigma^{-1}}\boldsymbol{K}', \boldsymbol{L}'\boldsymbol{P}_{C'}\boldsymbol{L}).$$

Then an Edgeworth-type expansion $f_{\boldsymbol{K}\boldsymbol{R}_{2E}\boldsymbol{L}}(\boldsymbol{K}\boldsymbol{R}_o\boldsymbol{L})$ *of the density of* $\boldsymbol{K}\boldsymbol{R}_2\boldsymbol{L}$*, via the density of* $\boldsymbol{K}\boldsymbol{R}_{2N}\boldsymbol{L}$*, under the assumption that* $D[\boldsymbol{K}\boldsymbol{R}_{2N}\boldsymbol{L}]$ *is p.d., is given by*

$$\begin{aligned} f_{\boldsymbol{K}\boldsymbol{R}_{2E}\boldsymbol{L}}(\boldsymbol{K}\boldsymbol{R}_o\boldsymbol{L}) = \big\{1 &- \tfrac{1}{2}c_2p_1n_1 \\ &+\mathrm{tr}\{(\boldsymbol{K}\boldsymbol{P}_{A,\Sigma}\boldsymbol{\Sigma}\boldsymbol{K}')^{-1}\boldsymbol{K}\boldsymbol{R}_o\boldsymbol{L}(\boldsymbol{L}'\boldsymbol{P}_{C'}\boldsymbol{L})^{-1}\boldsymbol{L}'\boldsymbol{R}_o'\boldsymbol{K}'\}\big\} f_{\boldsymbol{K}\boldsymbol{R}_{2N}\boldsymbol{L}}(\boldsymbol{K}\boldsymbol{R}_o\boldsymbol{L}), \end{aligned}$$

where c_2*, supposed to exist, is defined in Theorem 6.1.*

Corollary 6.3 *Let $KR_{2E}L$ be defined via $f_{KR_{2E}L}(KR_oL)$, given in Theorem 6.7, where it is assumed that $f_{KR_{2E}L}(KR_oL) \geq 0$, and suppose that $c_2p_1n_1 \leq 2$. Then*

(i) $E[KR_{2E}L] = \mathbf{0}$;

(ii) $$D[KR_{2E}L] = \big(1-\tfrac{1}{2}c_2p_1n_1+n_1\mathrm{tr}\{(KP_{A,\Sigma}\Sigma K')^{-1}K\Sigma P_{A^o,\Sigma^{-1}}K'\}\big)L'P_{C'}L \otimes K\Sigma P_{A^o,\Sigma^{-1}}K' + 2L'P_{C'}L\otimes K\Sigma P_{A^o,\Sigma^{-1}}K'(KP_{A,\Sigma}\Sigma K')^{-1}K\Sigma P_{A^o,\Sigma^{-1}}K'.$$

6.4 Mean Shift Evaluations of the Residuals in the BRM

In the presentation of Sect. 6.3, approximate densities of the residual matrices R_{11}, R_{12} and R_2 have been obtained. The expressions depend on unknown dispersion parameters and if one uses the densities directly, the parameters have to be replaced by estimates. This can be carried out and then it is possible to look for extreme values in the data set i.e., one tries to understand if the extreme observations are in the tail of the distribution.

However, one should remember that a weak point of Edgeworth-type expansions is that the tails of the distributions may be poorly estimated.

Another approach, already demonstrated in Sect. 6.1, where it was shown how it can work for the MANOVA model, is based on statistical testing for extreme observations. This can be achieved by studying the so-called mean shift assumptions. In this case a model is assumed for the residuals. Let $R_\bullet$ represent any of the residuals R_{11}, R_{12}, R_1 and R_2. Then the model which will be studied can, in principle, be written as follows:

$$R_\bullet = F\Theta G + E_\bullet, \tag{6.20}$$

where the density for $E_\bullet$ is one of the densities presented in Theorem 6.5, Theorems 6.6 and 6.7 or the matrix normal density.

The F and G matrices in (6.20) can correspond to the five cases mentioned in Sect. 6.1, i.e. $F = \mathbf{1}$, $F = d_j$ or $F = I$, and $G = \mathbf{1}'$, $G = e_i'$ or $G = I$, where d_j and e_i stand as usual for the unit basis vectors.

A test can be constructed for testing $H_0 : \Theta = \mathbf{0}$ via the previous theorems where density approximations were derived. The idea is to construct, for any given Σ, a test which is similar to the likelihood ratio test. Many tests will be performed, e.g. for each i and j in $\{d_i, e_j\}$, and the maximum value or some of the largest values of the test statistics are of interest. Even if we were to estimate Σ, the distribution of the test statistic would still be a function of Σ. Therefore, no energy will be spent on obtaining special estimators of Σ so that pivot quantities will appear which are completely independent of all the parameters. Instead, when interpreting the distribution of the mean shift test, only the MLE of Σ from the BRM will be utilized as a consistent plug-in estimator. An obvious alternative estimator which might be used is the unbiased estimator presented in Theorem 4.7.

In the following a number of test statistics will be presented which will later be evaluated through a parametric bootstrap approach. Let us start with $\boldsymbol{R}_{12}$ and some preparations. The density approximation given by Theorem 6.6 cannot be directly applied if $D[\boldsymbol{K}\boldsymbol{R}_{12E}\boldsymbol{L}]$ is singular, and therefore an appropriate working density has to be found. For example, when applying a likelihood-based approach, densities have to exist. Under H_0, i.e. with no mean shift, the information about the residuals is solely available on the space connected to the eigenvalues of $D[\boldsymbol{R}_{12N}]$ which are larger than 0, where the dispersion is given in Theorem 6.6. Therefore, $D[\boldsymbol{R}_{12N}]$ is spectrally decomposed as

$$D[\boldsymbol{R}_{12N}] = \boldsymbol{V}\boldsymbol{V}' \otimes \boldsymbol{W}\boldsymbol{W}', \quad \boldsymbol{V} : n \times (n - r(\boldsymbol{C})), \quad \boldsymbol{W} : p \times (p - r(\boldsymbol{A}));$$

i.e. $\boldsymbol{\Sigma}\boldsymbol{P}_{A^o,\Sigma^{-1}} = \boldsymbol{W}\boldsymbol{W}'$ and $\boldsymbol{I} - \boldsymbol{P}_{C'} = \boldsymbol{V}\boldsymbol{V}'$. Note that $\boldsymbol{W}$ is a function of $\boldsymbol{\Sigma}$, and later, when analysing data, $\boldsymbol{W}$ is obtained by factorizing $\widehat{\boldsymbol{\Sigma}}\boldsymbol{P}_{A^o,\widehat{\Sigma}^{-1}}$, i.e. $\widehat{\boldsymbol{\Sigma}}\boldsymbol{P}_{A^o,\widehat{\Sigma}^{-1}} = \boldsymbol{W}\boldsymbol{W}'$. A modified non-singular residual can be obtained by pre- and post-multiplying $\boldsymbol{R}_{12}$ in the following suitable way:

$$\boldsymbol{R}_{12}^N = (\boldsymbol{W}'\boldsymbol{W})^{-1}\boldsymbol{W}'\boldsymbol{R}_{12}\boldsymbol{V}(\boldsymbol{V}'\boldsymbol{V})^{-1};$$

this density approximation leads to a non-singular distribution. By choosing $\boldsymbol{K} = (\boldsymbol{W}'\boldsymbol{W})^{-1}\boldsymbol{W}'$ and $\boldsymbol{L} = \boldsymbol{V}(\boldsymbol{V}'\boldsymbol{V})^{-1}$ Theorem 6.6 can be applied directly and an appropriate density has been obtained. Hence, the following formal model will be "tested":

$$\boldsymbol{R}_{12;ij}^N = \boldsymbol{K}\boldsymbol{d}_j\theta\boldsymbol{e}_i'\boldsymbol{L} + \boldsymbol{E}_{12}, \tag{6.21}$$

where $\boldsymbol{E}_{12}$ has the density presented in Theorem 6.6 with the particular choices of $\boldsymbol{K}$ and $\boldsymbol{L}$ provided above. Moreover, note that $\boldsymbol{R}_{12;ij}^N$ is the same matrix as $\boldsymbol{R}_{12}^N$ but in order to indicate which residual is to be tested, $\boldsymbol{R}_{12;ij}^N$ is used. It follows that $D[\boldsymbol{K}\boldsymbol{R}_{12}^N\boldsymbol{L}] = \boldsymbol{I}_{p_1n_1}$, where $p_1 = p - r(\boldsymbol{A})$, $n_1 = n - r(\boldsymbol{C})$ and it is supposed that $\boldsymbol{K}$ is a function of $\boldsymbol{\Sigma}$, not $\widehat{\boldsymbol{\Sigma}}$. Note that $\boldsymbol{R}_{12}^N$ bears the same amount of information as $\boldsymbol{R}_{12}$.

Let $L_{12;ij}^N(\widehat{\theta})$ and $L_{12;ij}^N$ denote the likelihood for $\boldsymbol{R}_{12;ij}^N$ under $H_1\colon \theta \neq 0$ and H_0: $\theta = 0$, respectively, where under H_1 an estimator of θ is needed. If a strict likelihood ratio test were to be constructed, $\widehat{\theta}$ would have to be the MLE for θ. However, this estimator can only be obtained via an iterative algorithm due to the expression for the density of $\boldsymbol{E}_{12}$ given in Theorem 6.6. Instead a least squares approach can be used, e.g.

$$\min_{\theta} \operatorname{tr}\{\boldsymbol{T}^{-1}(\boldsymbol{R}_{12;ijo}^N - \boldsymbol{K}\boldsymbol{d}_j\theta\boldsymbol{e}_i'\boldsymbol{L})()'\},$$

where

$$\boldsymbol{T} = f_1\boldsymbol{I} + c_1\boldsymbol{K}\boldsymbol{P}_{A,\Sigma}\boldsymbol{\Sigma}\boldsymbol{K}'; \tag{6.22}$$

f_1 and c_1 are presented in Corollary 6.2 and Theorem 6.1, respectively, and $\boldsymbol{R}^N_{12;ijo}$ is the observation of $\boldsymbol{R}^N_{12;ij}$ which equals

$$\boldsymbol{R}^N_{12;ijo} = (\boldsymbol{W}'\boldsymbol{W})^{-1}\boldsymbol{W}'\boldsymbol{R}_{12o}\boldsymbol{V}(\boldsymbol{V}'\boldsymbol{V})^{-1}.$$

A unique least squares solution under the assumption of a known $\boldsymbol{\Sigma}$ is given by

$$\widehat{\theta}_o = (\boldsymbol{d}'_j\boldsymbol{K}'\boldsymbol{T}^{-1}\boldsymbol{K}\boldsymbol{d}_j)^{-1}\boldsymbol{d}'_j\boldsymbol{K}'\boldsymbol{T}^{-1}\boldsymbol{R}^N_{12;ijo}\boldsymbol{L}'\boldsymbol{e}_i(\boldsymbol{e}'_i\boldsymbol{L}\boldsymbol{L}'\boldsymbol{e}_i)^{-1}. \tag{6.23}$$

If one replaces $\boldsymbol{\Sigma}$ by its MLE presented in Theorem 3.1, there is enough information for forming a test statistic for testing H_0: $\theta = 0$, which is then given by

$$T_{ijo} = \frac{L^N_{12;ij}(\widehat{\theta}_o)}{L^N_{12;ij}}. \tag{6.24}$$

However, one may question this approach, because it depends on the approximating density and its singularity; i.e. one may question whether an estimator should be based on the matrices $\boldsymbol{K}$ and $\boldsymbol{L}$, which appear because of the choice of the approximating distribution.

An alternative approach is to use the observation $(\boldsymbol{R}_{12o})_{ij}$ as an estimate of θ when considering $\boldsymbol{d}_j\theta\boldsymbol{e}'_i$. This implies that the likelihood ratio in (6.24) is in fact a ratio between a density without the ijth observation (with an improper standardizing constant) and a density for all the observations. In the following examples this latter choice of $\widehat{\theta}_o$ will be applied.

Let ij^1 denote the pair of indices which corresponds to $\max_{ij} T_{ijo}$, ij^2 is the pair of indices which corresponds to the second largest value in $\{T_{ijo}\}$ and ij^3 is the pair of indices which identifies the third largest value in $\{T_{ijo}\}$. Now the remaining task is to determine the distribution of the corresponding T_{ij^1}, T_{ij^2} and T_{ij^3}.

The statistic in (6.24) has been constructed via density approximations and a "semi-likelihood ratio test" approach. If the observations are replaced by their corresponding random variables, we can write as follows:

$$T_{ij} = \frac{L^N_{12;ij}(\widehat{\theta})}{L^N_{12;ij}}, \qquad \widehat{\theta} = \boldsymbol{d}'_j\boldsymbol{R}_{12}\boldsymbol{e}_i, \tag{6.25}$$

and our interest is, for example, T_{ij^1} and its distribution. One way of handling this distribution is via simulations. However, it is less clear how these simulations should be performed. The density presented in Theorem 6.6 can be used and via a random number generating algorithm, suited to handling a known multivariate density, one can obtain observations so that the distribution for T_{ij^1} can be described.

In this book a somewhat easier approach is applied. The proposed strategy is to generate observations, $\boldsymbol{X}_o$, according to

$$\boldsymbol{X} \sim N_{p,n}(\boldsymbol{0}, \widehat{\boldsymbol{\Sigma}}_o, \boldsymbol{I}),$$

where $\widehat{\boldsymbol{\Sigma}}$ is presented in Theorem 3.1. In other words the parametric bootstrap philosophy is applied. Note that other relevant estimators of $\boldsymbol{\Sigma}$ could also have been used. The observations $\boldsymbol{X}_o$ are then used to calculate $\boldsymbol{R}_{12o} = (\boldsymbol{I} - \boldsymbol{P}_{A,\widehat{\Sigma}_o})\boldsymbol{X}_o(\boldsymbol{I} - \boldsymbol{P}_{C'})$. Thereafter $L^N_{12;ij}(\widehat{\theta}_o)$ and $L^N_{12;ij}$ are calculated, as well as $\{T_{ijo}\}$. Thus, T_{ij^k}, $k = 1, 2, 3$, is obtained. This process can be repeated a large number of times, and a density can thereby be estimated, which can be used to determine how far out in the tails of the distributions the original deviating residuals appear.

When working with vector-valued residuals, instead of single elements of the residual matrix, as above, there is one immediate advantage of using a test statistic instead of directly working with the density. The advantage is that it is easier to draw conclusions from a one-dimensional test statistic than to draw conclusions based on an evaluation of a multivariate density function.

In the next example the above ideas are illustrated.

Example 6.1 (The Classical Potthoff and Roy (1964) Data Set) The data have already been used for illustration, see Examples 1.7 and 3.1. The residual $\boldsymbol{R}_{12o} = (\boldsymbol{I} - \boldsymbol{P}_{A,S_o^{-1}})\boldsymbol{X}_o(\boldsymbol{I} - \boldsymbol{P}_{C'})$ is presented in Table 6.1 together with the test statistic presented in (6.25).

It is seen from Table 6.1 that the test statistic reflects the size of the components in $\boldsymbol{R}_{12o}$, which supports the presented approach. Hence, the remaining task is to find the distribution of the large residuals, taking into account the fact that one has to investigate 108 correlated observations from 27 independently distributed individuals. In Table 6.2, simulated quantiles for T_{ij^1}, T_{ij^2} and T_{ij^3} are presented. It is only $T_{203o} = 1367.0$ which is significant, since it is larger than T_{ij^1o} at a 95% level. Moreover, note the small value $T_{201o} = 0.5$. Since maximum likelihood estimators are not used, the test statistic can become smaller than 1, but this value is clearly much smaller than the other values. Since both the smallest and the largest value appeared for the same individual, i.e. #20, and we know beforehand that observations within individuals are correlated, we can only conclude that individual #20 deviates from the others. Table 6.2 also gives simulated quantiles for the residuals corresponding to the three largest (by absolute value) residuals, $R_{12;ij^1o}$, $R_{12;ij^2o}$ and $R_{12;ij^3o}$. The results are in agreement with those based on the test statistic given by (6.25); i.e. individual #20 deviates. It is interesting to determine how large the residuals need to be in order to become significant; i.e. even if the residuals are asymptotically normally distributed with mean 0 and a variance which, according to Table 6.1, does not seem to imply great variability, large values are still not very unlikely to appear. □

Table 6.1 The residuals $\boldsymbol{R}_{12o} = (\boldsymbol{I} - \boldsymbol{P}_{A,S_o^{-1}})\boldsymbol{X}_o(\boldsymbol{I} - \boldsymbol{P}_{C'}) = (R_{12;ijo})$ and the test statistic given in (6.25) applied to the Potthoff and Roy (1964) data presented in Table 1.2

		Residuals				Test statistics			
id	Gender	$R_{12;i1o}$	$R_{12;i2o}$	$R_{12;i3o}$	$R_{12;i4o}$	T_{i1o}	T_{i2o}	T_{i3o}	T_{i4o}
1	F	1.22	−0.87	−0.29	0.16	2.0	1.5	1.1	1.0
2	F	0.77	−0.54	0.33	0.07	1.2	1.1	1.0	1.0
3	F	−1.12	0.80	−0.10	−0.13	1.7	1.4	1.0	1.0
4	F	0.05	−0.04	−0.44	0.03	1.0	1.0	1.1	1.0
5	F	−0.54	0.38	−0.51	0.04	1.1	1.1	1.0	1.0
6	F	−0.08	0.05	−0.64	0.03	1.0	1.0	1.1	1.0
7	F	0.16	−0.12	−0.71	0.06	1.0	1.0	1.2	1.0
8	F	0.29	−0.21	−0.02	0.03	1.0	1.0	1.0	1.0
9	F	−0.28	0.21	0.88	−0.08	1.1	1.0	1.3	1.0
10	F	−1.00	0.71	0.11	−0.12	1.6	1.3	1.0	1.0
11	F	0.55	−0.38	1.37	−0.01	1.0	1.0	1.3	1.0
12	M	1.47	−1.04	0.47	0.15	2.2	1.6	0.9	1.0
13	M	0.02	−0.03	−1.55	0.09	1.0	1.0	1.8	1.0
14	M	0.97	−0.70	−1.34	0.19	1.8	1.4	2.2	1.0
15	M	−1.49	1.05	−0.38	−0.15	2.3	1.7	0.9	1.0
16	M	−1.51	1.06	−1.84	−0.08	1.6	1.4	1.1	1.0
17	M	−0.18	0.13	−0.02	−0.02	1.0	1.0	1.0	1.0
18	M	0.64	−0.45	−0.02	0.02	1.2	1.1	1.0	1.0
19	M	1.71	−1.21	0.41	0.18	3.0	2.0	0.9	1.0
20	M	2.18	−1.49	6.87	−0.12	0.5	0.9	1367.0	1.0
21	M	0.10	0.13	1.09	−0.04	1.0	1.0	1.3	1.0
22	M	0.04	−0.03	−0.58	0.04	1.0	1.0	1.1	1.0
23	M	−0.33	0.22	−1.69	0.05	0.9	1.0	1.7	1.0
24	M	−2.78	1.97	−0.25	−0.31	22.2	6.9	0.8	1.1
25	M	−1.71	1.22	0.18	−0.21	3.6	2.2	1.1	1.0
26	M	0.14	−0.11	−1.34	0.09	1.0	1.0	1.6	1.0
27	M	0.64	−0.45	−0.02	0.08	1.2	1.1	1.0	1.0

Up to now only single observations, i.e. $\boldsymbol{d}'_j\boldsymbol{R}_{12}\boldsymbol{e}_i$, have been studied. If instead individuals are of interest, $\boldsymbol{R}_{12}\boldsymbol{e}_i$ will be exploited and there are two different models which one should, "naturally", investigate. The first model equals

$$\boldsymbol{R}^N_{12;i} = \boldsymbol{K}\boldsymbol{\theta}\boldsymbol{e}'_i\boldsymbol{L} + \boldsymbol{E}_{12}, \tag{6.26}$$

where $\boldsymbol{K}$, $\boldsymbol{L}$ and $\boldsymbol{E}_{12}$ are as in (6.21) and $\boldsymbol{R}^N_{12;i} = \boldsymbol{R}^N_{12}$, where i is only used to indicate the mean shift for the ith observation; the notation also applies to the likelihood functions $L^N_{12;i}(\widehat{\boldsymbol{\theta}}_o)$ and $L^N_{12;i}$ given below. Now $\boldsymbol{\theta}$ is a vector of size p, meaning that there is a shift for each component of the residual connected to the ith observation vector. If, however, the mean shift is the same for each component, then

Table 6.2 Estimated quantiles for T_{ij^1}, T_{ij^2} and T_{ij^3} connected to the test statistics T_{ij^1o}, T_{ij^2o} and T_{ij^3o}, with T_{ij} defined in (6.25), and applied to the Potthoff and Roy data set presented in Table 1.2

Quantile	T_{ij^1o}	T_{ij^2o}	T_{ij^3o}	$R_{12;ij^1o}$	$R_{12;ij^2o}$	$R_{12;ij^3o}$
100% max	1.7×10^6	1.3×10^4	1.9×10^3	8.6	7.5	6.0
99%	3.9×10^3	2.2×10^2	66.3	6.4	5.2	4.6
95%	4.2×10^2	64.2	27.4	5.5	4.5	4.0
90%	1.7×10^2	37.7	18.1	5.0	4.2	3.7
75%	51.3	17.5	10.2	4.3	3.7	3.3
50%	18.5	9.1	6.3	3.7	3.1	2.8
25%	8.9	5.5	4.2	3.1	2.7	2.5
10%	5.3	3.8	3.1	2.7	2.4	2.2
5%	4.1	3.1	2.6	2.5	2.2	2.0
1%	2.7	2.3	2.1	2.1	1.9	1.8
0% min	1.6	1.5	1.5	1.6	1.5	1.5

Estimated quantiles are given for the three largest (by absolute value) residuals, $R_{12;ij^ko}$, $k = 1, 2, 3$, obtained from the same data set. The estimated quantiles are based on 10,000 simulations

instead of (6.26) the following second model can be used:

$$\boldsymbol{R}_{12;i}^N = \boldsymbol{K}\boldsymbol{1}_p\theta\boldsymbol{e}_i'\boldsymbol{L} + \boldsymbol{E}_{12}, \tag{6.27}$$

where $\boldsymbol{E}_{12}$ follows the distribution (density) presented in Theorem 6.6.

Let us start by constructing a test for H_0: $\boldsymbol{\theta} = \boldsymbol{0}$ in (6.26). Via a least squares approach, an estimate of $\boldsymbol{\theta}$ is given by

$$\widehat{\boldsymbol{\theta}}_o = (\boldsymbol{K}'\boldsymbol{T}^{-1}\boldsymbol{K})^{-1}\boldsymbol{K}'\boldsymbol{T}^{-1}\boldsymbol{R}_{12;io}^N\boldsymbol{L}'\boldsymbol{e}_i(\boldsymbol{e}_i'\boldsymbol{L}\boldsymbol{L}'\boldsymbol{e}_i)^{-1},$$

where $\boldsymbol{T}$ is given in (6.22), and in $\boldsymbol{T}$ as well as $\boldsymbol{R}_{12;i}^N$ the unknown $\boldsymbol{\Sigma}$ is replaced by an appropriate estimate. Alternatively, similar to the treatment of $\boldsymbol{R}_{12;ij}$, an unweighted estimator,

$$\widehat{\boldsymbol{\theta}} = \boldsymbol{R}_{12}\boldsymbol{e}_i, \tag{6.28}$$

can be utilized. In this case, a test statistic corresponding to (6.24), when, for example, (6.28) is used, equals

$$T_{io} = \frac{L_{12;i}^N(\widehat{\boldsymbol{\theta}}_o)}{L_{12;i}^N}, \tag{6.29}$$

where $L_{12;i}^N$ equals $L_{12;ij}^N$, given above, i.e. the likelihood under the H_0 of no mean shift. Moreover, $L_{12;i}^N(\widehat{\boldsymbol{\theta}}_o)$ is the likelihood under the alternative hypothesis where $\boldsymbol{\theta}$

Table 6.3 The same data as in Table 6.1 are analysed, but in this table the test statistic for column-wise mean shift, T_{io}, based on (6.28) and (6.29), is presented

	Individual													
	1	2	3	4	5	6	7	8	9	10	11	12	13	14
T_{io}	2.4	1.3	1.8	1.1	1.1	1.1	1.2	1.0	1.4	1.7	1.5	2.5	1.8	3.5
$\overline{T}_{io}$	1.0	1.0	1.0	1.0	1.1	1.1	1.1	1.0	1.2	1.0	1.5	1.0	1.6	1.5
	Individual													
	15	16	17	18	19	20	21	22	23	24	25	26	27	
T_{io}	2.6	3.2	1.0	1.2	3.5	9379.2	1.3	1.1	1.8	36.0	4.6	1.7	1.2	
$\overline{T}_{io}$	1.0	2.0	1.0	1.0	1.0	9486.7	1.3	1.1	1.8	1.0	1.0	1.4	1.0	

The test statistic for column-wise mean shift, $\overline{T}_{io}$, based on (6.30) and (6.31), is also shown

has been estimated by the ith column of $\boldsymbol{R}_{12o}$, and hence the likelihood $L^N_{12;i}(\widehat{\boldsymbol{\theta}}_o)$, besides including a correct standardization constant, is the likelihood of all the observations except the ith one. Based on T_{io} in (6.29), the distribution of the test statistic T_{ik}, $k = 1, 2, 3$, can be simulated, i.e. the distribution of the largest, second largest and third largest value of the statistic can be simulated. The procedure is illustrated in the next example.

Example 6.2 (The Classical Potthoff and Roy (1964) Data Set, Given in Table 1.2.) The residual $\boldsymbol{R}_{12o} = (\boldsymbol{I} - \boldsymbol{P}_{A,S^{-1}})\boldsymbol{X}_o(\boldsymbol{I} - \boldsymbol{P}_{C'})$ was presented in Table 6.1, and in Table 6.3 the test statistic of no mean shift in columns according to (6.29) is shown for the case where (6.28) is used as an estimate of $\boldsymbol{\theta}$. Moreover, the quantiles of the three largest values of the test statistic are presented in Table 6.4.

From Tables 6.3 and 6.4 it follows that only individual #20 has an extreme residual, since $T_{20o} = 9379.2$ is larger than T_{i1_o} at a 95% level, which is in complete agreement with the results of the mean shift analysis presented in Tables 6.1 and 6.2. Furthermore, in Tables 6.1 and 6.3, one can observe that the behaviour of individual #24 is peculiar too, but it is not significantly peculiar. □

Now the alternative test procedure based on H_0: $\theta = 0$ in (6.27) is discussed in some detail. It is assumed that there is a mean shift which is equal for all the components in a column of $\boldsymbol{R}_{12}$, for example the ith column. The least squares approach yields an estimate of θ which equals

$$\widehat{\theta}_o = (\boldsymbol{1}'\boldsymbol{K}'\boldsymbol{T}^{-1}\boldsymbol{K}\boldsymbol{1})^{-1}\boldsymbol{1}'\boldsymbol{K}'\boldsymbol{T}^{-1}\boldsymbol{R}^N_{12io}\boldsymbol{L}'\boldsymbol{e}_i(\boldsymbol{e}_i'\boldsymbol{L}\boldsymbol{L}'\boldsymbol{e}_i)^{-1}, \qquad (6.30)$$

where $\boldsymbol{T}$ is given in (6.22) with $\boldsymbol{\Sigma}$ in $\boldsymbol{T}$ replaced by an estimator, for example the unbiased one presented in Theorem 4.7. The replacement of $\boldsymbol{\Sigma}$ by $\widehat{\boldsymbol{\Sigma}}$ also applies to $\boldsymbol{R}^N_{12io}$. Moreover, the hypothesis concerning H_0, together with the least squares approach, implies a somewhat different interpretation of the residual evaluation than that given above, i.e. the interpretation of the test statistic in (6.29). A test statistic

Table 6.4 Estimated quantiles connected to the test statistics T_{ik_o} and $\overline{T}_{ik_o}$, $k = 1, 2, 3$, respectively, defined in (6.29) and (6.31), are presented

Quantile	T_{i1_o}	T_{i2_o}	T_{i3_o}	$\overline{T}_{i1_o}$	$\overline{T}_{i2_o}$	$\overline{T}_{i3_o}$
100% max	7.6×10^6	4.1×10^4	2.5×10^3	3.0×10^6	4.0×10^4	1.9×10^3
99%	1.7×10^4	6.3×10^2	1.7×10^2	4.4×10^3	2.3×10^2	59.5
95%	1.6×10^3	1.6×10^2	59.9	4.2×10^2	57.0	22.5
90%	5.6×10^2	91.4	37.7	1.5×10^2	29.5	13.8
75%	1.5×10^2	37.2	19.3	37.8	12.2	7.1
50%	44.8	17.3	10.5	11.0	5.5	3.8
25%	18.3	9.1	6.2	4.6	2.9	2.3
10%	9.6	5.7	4.2	2.5	2.0	1.7
5%	7.0	4.4	3.4	2.0	1.6	1.5
1%	4.0	3.1	2.5	1.3	1.2	1.2
0% min	1.7	1.6	1.6	1.0	1.0	1.0

The estimated quantiles are based on 10,000 simulations

corresponding to (6.29) equals

$$\overline{T}_{io} = \frac{L_{12;i}^N(\widehat{\theta}_o)}{L_{12;i}^N}, \tag{6.31}$$

where $\widehat{\theta}_o$ is presented in (6.30). Indeed a test based on (6.31) is close to a traditional likelihood ratio test based on a normally distributed sample with known dispersion, although instead of the normal density, the density in Theorem 6.6 is used. The test statistic is illustrated in the next example. However, any significant results only reflect that the equal mean shift hypothesis is not true and do not automatically imply that the residuals are extreme.

Example 6.3 (The Classical Potthoff and Roy (1964) Data Set Given in Table 1.2) The residual $\boldsymbol{R}_{12o} = (\boldsymbol{I} - \boldsymbol{P}_{A,S_o^{-1}})\boldsymbol{X}_o(\boldsymbol{I} - \boldsymbol{P}_{C'})$ was presented in Table 6.1, and in Table 6.3 the test statistic for no equal mean shift in columns according to (6.31) is shown. Moreover, in Table 6.4 the distribution for the three largest values of the test statistic is presented. Once again it follows that individual #20 deviates from the others. □

Finally, concerning the residual $\boldsymbol{R}_{12}$, the mean shift tests within the rows of $\boldsymbol{R}_{12}$ are presented. A test statistic corresponding to (6.29) for testing $H_0 : \boldsymbol{\theta} = \boldsymbol{0}$ in

$$\boldsymbol{R}_{12;j} = \boldsymbol{K}\boldsymbol{d}_j\boldsymbol{\theta}\boldsymbol{L} + \boldsymbol{E}_{12},$$

where $\boldsymbol{\theta}$ is a row vector of proper size and the density for $\boldsymbol{E}_{12}$ is presented in Theorem 6.6, equals

$$T_{jo} = \frac{L^N_{12;j}(\widehat{\boldsymbol{\theta}}_o)}{L^N_{12;j}}, \tag{6.32}$$

where $\widehat{\boldsymbol{\theta}}_o = \boldsymbol{d}'_j \boldsymbol{R}_{12o}$. The notation follows the same ideas as those used when constructing (6.25) or (6.29). Concerning (6.32), the reader should be warned that there are too many parameters involved and the test statistic is rather heuristic. Moreover, a test statistic corresponding to (6.31) for testing $H_0 : \theta = 0$ in

$$\boldsymbol{R}^N_{12;j} = \boldsymbol{K}\boldsymbol{d}_j\theta\boldsymbol{1}'\boldsymbol{L} + \boldsymbol{E}_{12}$$

equals

$$\overline{T}_{jo} = \frac{L^N_{12;j}(\widehat{\theta}_o)}{L^N_{12;j}}, \tag{6.33}$$

where (with an estimated $\boldsymbol{\Sigma}$)

$$\widehat{\theta}_o = (\boldsymbol{d}'_j\boldsymbol{K}'\boldsymbol{T}^{-1}\boldsymbol{K}\boldsymbol{d}_j)^{-1}\boldsymbol{d}'_j\boldsymbol{K}'\boldsymbol{T}^{-1}\boldsymbol{R}^N_{12;jo}\boldsymbol{L}'\boldsymbol{1}(\boldsymbol{1}'\boldsymbol{L}\boldsymbol{L}'\boldsymbol{1})^{-1},$$

and $\boldsymbol{T}$ is given in (6.22). Example 6.4 presents some explicit data analysis.

Example 6.4 (The Classical Potthoff and Roy (1964) Data Set Given in Table 1.2) The residual $\boldsymbol{R}_{12o} = (\boldsymbol{I} - \boldsymbol{P}_{A,S_o^{-1}})\boldsymbol{X}_o(\boldsymbol{I} - \boldsymbol{P}_{C'})$ was presented in Table 6.1, and in Table 6.5 the test statistic for no mean shift in rows according to (6.32) or (6.33) is shown. Simulations did not reveal any significant values. Because the tests are across individuals, a significant difference in this example would have been somewhat difficult to explain. □

Above, $\boldsymbol{R}_{12}$ has been exploited and next $\boldsymbol{R}_{11}$ will come into focus. However, all the expressions concerning testing for mean shifts in $\boldsymbol{R}_{11}$ are similar to the corresponding expressions for $\boldsymbol{R}_{12}$. Therefore, a theorem will be presented which covers both residuals, but first a number of preparatory notations will be introduced. As before, the problem of singularity of the distribution has to be taken care of

Table 6.5 The data in Table 6.1 are analysed and the test statistics for row-wise mean shift, T_{jo} and $\overline{T}_{jo}$, given in (6.32) and (6.33), respectively, are presented

	Time			
	8	12	14	16
T_{jo}	1.4×10^4	6.1×10^2	6.8×10^3	1.3
$\overline{T}_{jo}$	0.7	2.0	0.8	0.7

via bilinear transformations. Let $\widetilde{\boldsymbol{R}}_{11N}$ and $\boldsymbol{R}_{12}$ be defined in Theorem 6.4 and Definition 6.1, respectively. From the above discussion concerning $\boldsymbol{R}_{12}$, it follows that one can use

$$\boldsymbol{K}_{12} = (\boldsymbol{W}_2'\boldsymbol{W}_2)^{-1}\boldsymbol{W}_2', \quad \boldsymbol{L}_{12} = \boldsymbol{V}_2(\boldsymbol{V}_2'\boldsymbol{V}_2)^{-1}, \tag{6.34}$$

where it is assumed that $D[\boldsymbol{R}_{12N}] = \boldsymbol{V}_2\boldsymbol{V}_2' \otimes \boldsymbol{W}_2\boldsymbol{W}_2'$ and

$$\boldsymbol{K}_{11} = (\boldsymbol{W}_1'\boldsymbol{W}_1)^{-1}\boldsymbol{W}_1', \quad \boldsymbol{L}_{11} = \boldsymbol{V}_1(\boldsymbol{V}_1'\boldsymbol{V}_1)^{-1}, \tag{6.35}$$

since

$$\begin{aligned} D[\widetilde{\boldsymbol{R}}_{11N}] &= \boldsymbol{V}_1\boldsymbol{V}_1' \otimes \boldsymbol{W}_1\boldsymbol{W}_1' \\ &= (\boldsymbol{I} - \boldsymbol{P}_{C'})\begin{pmatrix} \boldsymbol{0} & \boldsymbol{0} \\ \boldsymbol{0} & \boldsymbol{I}_{n-p+r(A)} \end{pmatrix}(\boldsymbol{I} - \boldsymbol{P}_{C'}) \otimes \boldsymbol{A}(\boldsymbol{A}'\boldsymbol{\Sigma}^{-1}\boldsymbol{A})^{-}\boldsymbol{A}' \end{aligned}$$

for some $\boldsymbol{V}_i$, $\boldsymbol{W}_i$, $i = 1, 2$, obtained via a spectral decomposition. Note that $\boldsymbol{V}_i$ and $\boldsymbol{W}_i$ are not unique and we always assume that $\boldsymbol{\Sigma}$ in $\boldsymbol{K}_{1i}$, $i = 1, 2$, has been estimated. Five types of mean shift hypothesis will be considered, i.e.

$$\text{(a) } \boldsymbol{d}_j\theta\boldsymbol{e}_i', \qquad \text{(b) } \boldsymbol{\theta}\boldsymbol{e}_i', \qquad \text{(c) } \boldsymbol{1}\theta\boldsymbol{e}_i', \qquad \text{(d) } \boldsymbol{d}_j\theta\boldsymbol{1}', \qquad \text{(e) } \boldsymbol{d}_j\boldsymbol{\theta}, \tag{6.36}$$

with the tests $H_0\colon \theta = 0$ against $H_1\colon \theta \neq 0$ and $H_0\colon \boldsymbol{\theta} = \boldsymbol{0}$ against $H_1\colon \boldsymbol{\theta}$ unrestricted. In the following definition, models with the above types of mean shift hypothesis are presented, as well as the notation for the likelihood under H_0 and its alternative.

Definition 6.2 Models and notation are presented for the likelihood functions related to $\boldsymbol{R}_{11}$ and $\boldsymbol{R}_{12}$, given in Definition 6.1; these models and notation are used when testing for mean shifts under the conditions stated in (6.36).

$$\begin{aligned} \text{(a)}\quad & \boldsymbol{R}^N_{11;ij} = \boldsymbol{K}_{11}\boldsymbol{d}_j\theta\boldsymbol{e}_i'\boldsymbol{L}_{11} + \boldsymbol{E}_{11}, \quad \boldsymbol{R}^N_{11;ijo} = \boldsymbol{K}_{11}\boldsymbol{R}_{11o}\boldsymbol{L}_{11}, L^N_{11;ij}(\widehat{\theta}_o), \quad L^N_{11;ij}, \\ & \boldsymbol{R}^N_{12;ij} = \boldsymbol{K}_{12}\boldsymbol{d}_j\theta\boldsymbol{e}_i'\boldsymbol{L}_{12} + \boldsymbol{E}_{12}, \quad \boldsymbol{R}^N_{12;ijo} = \boldsymbol{K}_{12}\boldsymbol{R}_{12o}\boldsymbol{L}_{12}, L^N_{12;ij}(\widehat{\theta}_o), \quad L^N_{12;ij}; \end{aligned}$$

$$\begin{aligned} \text{(b)}\quad & \boldsymbol{R}^N_{11;i} = \boldsymbol{K}_{11}\boldsymbol{\theta}\boldsymbol{e}_i'\boldsymbol{L}_{11} + \boldsymbol{E}_{11}, \quad \boldsymbol{R}^N_{11;io} = \boldsymbol{K}_{11}\boldsymbol{R}_{11o}\boldsymbol{L}_{11}, L^N_{11;i}(\widehat{\boldsymbol{\theta}}_o), \quad L^N_{11;i}, \\ & \boldsymbol{R}^N_{12;i} = \boldsymbol{K}_{12}\boldsymbol{\theta}\boldsymbol{e}_i'\boldsymbol{L}_{12} + \boldsymbol{E}_{12}, \quad \boldsymbol{R}^N_{12;io} = \boldsymbol{K}_{12}\boldsymbol{R}_{12o}\boldsymbol{L}_{12}, L^N_{12;i}(\widehat{\boldsymbol{\theta}}_o), \quad L^N_{12;i}; \end{aligned}$$

$$\begin{aligned} \text{(c)}\quad & \boldsymbol{R}^N_{11;i} = \boldsymbol{K}_{11}\boldsymbol{1}\theta\boldsymbol{e}_i'\boldsymbol{L}_{11} + \boldsymbol{E}_{11}, \quad \boldsymbol{R}^N_{11;io} = \boldsymbol{K}_{11}\boldsymbol{R}_{11o}\boldsymbol{L}_{11}, L^N_{11;i}(\widehat{\theta}_o), \quad L^N_{11;i}, \\ & \boldsymbol{R}^N_{12;i} = \boldsymbol{K}_{12}\boldsymbol{1}\theta\boldsymbol{e}_i'\boldsymbol{L}_{12} + \boldsymbol{E}_{12}, \quad \boldsymbol{R}^N_{12;io} = \boldsymbol{K}_{120}\boldsymbol{R}_{12o}\boldsymbol{L}_{12}, L^N_{12;i}(\widehat{\theta}_o), \quad L^N_{12;i}; \end{aligned}$$

(d) $R_{11;j}^N = K_{11}d_j\theta 1'L_{11} + E_{11}, \quad R_{11;jo}^N = K_{11}R_{11o}L_{11}, L_{11;j}^N(\widehat{\theta}_o), \quad L_{11;j}^N,$

$R_{12;j}^N = K_{12}d_j\theta 1'L_{12} + E_{12}, \quad R_{12;jo}^N = K_{12}R_{12o}L_{12}, L_{12;j}^N(\widehat{\theta}_o), \quad L_{12;j}^N;$

(e) $R_{11;j}^N = K_{11}d_j\boldsymbol{\theta} L_{11} + E_{11}, \quad R_{11;jo}^N = K_{11}R_{11o}L_{11}, L_{11;j}^N(\widehat{\boldsymbol{\theta}}_o), \quad L_{11j}^N,$

$R_{12;j}^N = K_{12}d_j\boldsymbol{\theta} L_{12} + E_{12}, \quad R_{12;jo}^N = K_{12}R_{12o}L_{12}, L_{12;j}^N(\widehat{\boldsymbol{\theta}}_o), \quad L_{12;j}^N;$

E_{11} and E_{12} follow the densities given in Theorems 6.5 and 6.6, respectively, and K_{11}, K_{12}, L_{11} and L_{12} are given in (6.34) and (6.35). The estimates of θ and $\boldsymbol{\theta}$ are presented in Theorem 6.8. Moreover, $L_{1k;\bullet}^N(\widehat{\theta}_o)$ and $L_{1k;\bullet}^N$, $k = 1, 2$, denote the likelihood under H_0 and the alternative hypothesis, respectively, which are based on $E_{1k}, k = 1, 2$.

Enough preparations have now been completed for the presentation of the next theorem; the results concerning R_{12} have already been given in detail above.

Theorem 6.8 *In Definition 6.2 notation and models with five types of mean shift were presented for testing for no shift in the residuals R_{11} and R_{12}. The test statistics for each type are presented below.*

(i) *Let the models and mean shift be as in Definition 6.2 (a). Then the test statistics $T_{11;ijo}$ and $T_{12;ijo}$ for R_{11} and R_{12}, respectively, equal*

$$T_{1k;ijo} = \frac{L_{1k;ij}^N(\widehat{\theta}_o)}{L_{1k;ij}^N}, \qquad \widehat{\theta}_o = d_j' R_{1ko}e_i, \quad k = 1, 2.$$

(ii) *Let the models and mean shift be as in Definition 6.2 (b). Then the test statistics $T_{11;io}$ and $T_{12;io}$ for R_{11} and R_{12}, respectively, equal*

$$T_{1k;io} = \frac{L_{1k;i}^N(\widehat{\boldsymbol{\theta}}_o)}{L_{1k;i}^N}, \qquad \widehat{\boldsymbol{\theta}}_o = R_{1ko}e_i, \quad k = 1, 2.$$

(iii) *Let the models and mean shift be as in Definition 6.2 (c). Then the test statistics $T_{11;io}$ and $T_{12;io}$ for R_{11} and R_{12}, respectively, equal*

$$\overline{T}_{1k;io} = \frac{L_{1k;i}^N(\widehat{\theta}_o)}{L_{1k;i}^N}, \qquad k = 1, 2;$$

if $k = 1$

$$\widehat{\theta}_o = (\mathbf{1}'\boldsymbol{K}'_{11}\boldsymbol{K}_{11}\mathbf{1})^{-1}\mathbf{1}'\boldsymbol{K}'_{11}\boldsymbol{R}^N_{11;io}(\boldsymbol{L}'_{11}(\boldsymbol{I} - \boldsymbol{P}_{C'})\boldsymbol{L}_{11})^{-1}\boldsymbol{L}'_{11}\boldsymbol{e}_i \times(\boldsymbol{e}'_i\boldsymbol{L}_{11}(\boldsymbol{L}'_{11}(\boldsymbol{I} - \boldsymbol{P}_{C'})\boldsymbol{L}_{11})^{-1}\boldsymbol{L}'_{11}\boldsymbol{e}_i)^{-1},$$

and if $k = 2$

$$\widehat{\theta}_o = (\mathbf{1}'\boldsymbol{K}'_{12}\boldsymbol{T}^{-1}_{12}\boldsymbol{K}_{12}\mathbf{1})^{-1}\mathbf{1}'\boldsymbol{K}'_{12}\boldsymbol{T}^{-1}_{12}\boldsymbol{R}^N_{12;io}\boldsymbol{L}'_{11}\boldsymbol{e}_i(\boldsymbol{e}'_i\boldsymbol{L}_{11}\boldsymbol{L}'_{11}\boldsymbol{e}_i)^{-1},$$

where $\boldsymbol{T}_{12}$ *equals* $\boldsymbol{T}$*, given by (6.22), where an estimate of* $\boldsymbol{\Sigma}$ *has been plugged-in.*

(iv) *Let the models and mean shift be as in Definition 6.2 (d). Then the test statistics* $T_{11;jo}$ *and* $T_{12;jo}$ *for* $\boldsymbol{R}_{11}$ *and* $\boldsymbol{R}_{12}$*, respectively, equal*

$$\overline{T}_{1k;jo} = \frac{L^N_{1k;j}(\widehat{\theta}_o)}{L^N_{1k;j}}, \quad k = 1, 2;$$

if $k = 1$

$$\widehat{\theta}_o = (\boldsymbol{d}'_j\boldsymbol{K}'_{11}\boldsymbol{K}_{11}\boldsymbol{d}_j)^{-1}\boldsymbol{d}'_j\boldsymbol{K}'_{11}\boldsymbol{R}^N_{11;jo}(\boldsymbol{L}'_{11}(\boldsymbol{I} - \boldsymbol{P}_{C'})\boldsymbol{L}_{11})^{-1}\boldsymbol{L}'_{11}\mathbf{1} \times(\mathbf{1}'\boldsymbol{L}_{11}(\boldsymbol{L}'_{11}(\boldsymbol{I} - \boldsymbol{P}_{C'})\boldsymbol{L}_{11})^{-1}\boldsymbol{L}'_{11}\mathbf{1})^{-1},$$

and if $k = 2$

$$\widehat{\theta}_o = (\boldsymbol{d}'_j\boldsymbol{K}'_{12}\boldsymbol{T}^{-1}_{12}\boldsymbol{K}_{12}\boldsymbol{d}_j)^{-1}\boldsymbol{d}'_j\boldsymbol{K}'_{12}\boldsymbol{T}^{-1}_{12}\boldsymbol{R}^N_{12;jo}\boldsymbol{L}'_{11}\mathbf{1}(\mathbf{1}'\boldsymbol{L}_{11}\boldsymbol{L}'_{11}\mathbf{1})^{-1},$$

where $\boldsymbol{T}_{12}$ *equals* $\boldsymbol{T}$ *given by (6.22).*

(v) *Let the models and mean shift be as in Definition 6.2 (e). Then the test statistics* $T_{11;jo}$ *and* $T_{12;jo}$ *for* $\boldsymbol{R}_{11}$ *and* $\boldsymbol{R}_{12}$*, respectively, equal*

$$T_{1k;jo} = \frac{L^N_{1k;j}(\widehat{\boldsymbol{\theta}}_o)}{L^N_{1k;j}}, \qquad \widehat{\boldsymbol{\theta}}_o = \boldsymbol{d}'_j\boldsymbol{R}_{1ko}, \quad k = 1, 2.$$

Proof Almost all the statements of the theorem were explained when considering $\boldsymbol{R}_{12}$ above. It should be added here that a weighted least squares estimator is used for $k = 1$ in statements (iii) and (iv), based on Corollary 6.1 (ii). □

All the five types of mean shifts can now be investigated. The ideas will once again be illustrated by analysing the Potthoff and Roy data, and this time $\boldsymbol{R}_{11}$ is considered. However, our focus will be fixed on individuals, i.e. cases (a)–(c) in Definition 6.2, and therefore Theorem 6.8 (i)–(iii) are applied.

Table 6.6 The residual $\boldsymbol{R}_{11o} = \boldsymbol{P}_{A,S_o^{-1}}\boldsymbol{X}_o(\boldsymbol{I} - \boldsymbol{P}_{C'}) = (R_{11;ijo})$ and the test statistic given in Theorem 6.8 (i) applied to the Potthoff and Roy (1964) data given in Table 1.2

		Residuals				Test statistics			
id	Gender	$R_{11;i1o}$	$R_{11;i2o}$	$R_{11;i3o}$	$R_{11;i4o}$	$T_{11;i1o}$	$T_{11;i2o}$	$T_{11;i3o}$	$T_{11;i4o}$
1	F	−1.41	−01.35	−1.30	−1.25	2.8	2.0	0.7	0.2
2	F	−0.95	−0.19	0.58	1.34	2.6	1.1	1.1	2.4
3	F	0.44	0.97	1.50	2.03	1.0	1.0	1.2	1.1
4	F	2.27	2.31	2.34	2.38	1.4	1.7	1.2	1.1
5	F	0.86	0.39	−0.08	−0.56	1.5	1.1	1.0	1.3
6	F	−1.11	−1.28	−1.45	−1.62	0.7	0.9	1.2	1.3
7	F	0.16	0.39	0.62	0.85	1.0	1.0	1.0	0.9
8	F	1.53	0.98	0.43	−0.13	2.3	1.3	0.9	1.1
9	F	−0.90	−1.44	−1.97	−2.51	0.6	0.8	1.6	2.4
10	F	−3.68	−3.94	−4.20	−4.47	0.2	1.4	3.3	1.1
11	F	2.77	3.15	3.54	3.92	0.5	1.0	2.1	0.5
12	M	1.65	2.23	2.81	3.39	0.5	1.0	2.0	1.8
13	M	−1.40	−1.29	−1.17	−1.06	1.1	1.1	1.0	0.9
14	M	−0.84	−0.61	−0.38	−0.15	1.1	1.1	1.0	1.0
15	M	4.11	2.63	1.16	−0.32	34.1	3.9	0.8	1.4
16	M	−1.36	−1.37	−1.38	−1.39	1.0	1.1	1.1	0.9
17	M	1.81	1.56	1.30	1.05	1.3	1.3	1.0	0.8
18	M	−1.5	−1.4	−1.2	−1.0	1.1	1.2	1.0	0.9
19	M	−0.58	−1.1	−1.6	−2.1	0.8	0.9	1.3	1.6
20	M	−2.06	−1.82	−1.59	−1.35	1.3	1.4	1.0	0.7
21	M	4.43	4.31	1.19	4.07	1.0	3.7	2.1	0.3
22	M	0.08	−0.78	−1.64	−2.51	1.0	0.9	1.5	2.9
23	M	−1.04	−0.53	−0.03	0.48	1.4	1.1	1.0	2.9
24	M	−3.10	−1.28	0.53	2.34	29.0	1.9	1.2	12.1
25	M	1.33	0.47	−0.39	−1.26	2.0	1.1	1.1	1.9
26	M	−0.02	0.80	1.62	2.44	1.0	0.9	1.5	2.6
27	M	−1.51	−1.86	−2.20	−2.54	0.7	1.1	1.5	1.2

Example 6.5 (The Classical Potthoff and Roy (1964) Data Set Given in Table 1.2) The residual $\boldsymbol{R}_{11o} = \boldsymbol{P}_{A,S_o^{-1}}\boldsymbol{X}_o(\boldsymbol{I} - \boldsymbol{P}_{C'})$ is presented in Table 6.6 and will first be analysed via the test statistic given in Theorem 6.8 (i). It is seen from Table 6.6 that individuals #15 and #24 may deviate from the other individuals. It is remarkable that individuals #10, #11 and #21 do not show up in the test, although they have relatively large residuals. One possible explanation is that within individuals there is a strong interdependence, so that, when testing for no mean shift, single elements will not influence the likelihood much; i.e. some kind of masking effect exists. Moreover, note that once there is a program for calculating the residuals, it is possible to generate knowledge about the data and model by perturbing observations and then studying the effects of the perturbations. The situation is rather complex, although the model is simple; i.e. there are two groups of individuals of different group sizes

and for each group a separate model is assumed to hold. In addition to this, repeated correlated observations are gathered. If we want to validate the model via a multiple testing procedure, it follows from Table 6.7 and the parametric bootstrap approach that none of the residuals presented in Table 6.6 have a significant mean shift. One can artificially perturb the data to understand how large residuals should be in order to have significant mean shifts.

In Table 6.8 the statements of Theorem 6.8 (ii) and (iii) have been applied for testing all the observations from an individual for a mean shift. Theorem 6.8 (ii) concerns simultaneously testing for a mean shift within an individual and Theorem 6.8 (iii) assumes that the same mean shift appears within an individual. In the analysis, individuals #15, #21 and #24 are highlighted. However, according to Table 6.7 the mean shifts for these observations are not significant. □

Table 6.7 Estimated quantiles for $T_{11;ij^1}$, $T_{11;ij^2}$ and $T_{11;ij^3}$ corresponding to the test statistics $T_{11;ij^1o}$, $T_{11;ij^2o}$ and $T_{11;ij^3o}$ ($T_{11;ijo}$ was presented in Theorem 6.8 (i)) as well as for $T_{11;i^ko}$ and $\overline{T}_{11;i^ko}$, $k = 1, 2$ ($T_{11;io}$ and $\overline{T}_{11;io}$ were given in Theorem 6.8 (ii), and (iii), respectively)

Quantile	$T_{11;ij^1o}$	$T_{11;ij^2o}$	$T_{11;ij^3o}$	$T_{11;i^1o}$	$T_{11;i^2o}$	$\overline{T}_{11;i^1o}$	$\overline{T}_{11;i^2o}$
100% max	5.8×10^{11}	8.9×10^{7}	1.2×10^{7}	1.5×10^{16}	1.3×10^{10}	1.7×10^{15}	1.7×10^{15}
99%	1.8×10^{5}	5.2×10^{3}	5.3×10^{2}	1.1×10^{7}	8.7×10^{4}	1.2×10^{6}	1.2×10^{6}
95%	1.9×10^{3}	2.5×10^{2}	65.4	2.1×10^{4}	9.0×10^{2}	1.0×10^{3}	5.1×10^{2}
90%	3.4×10^{2}	77.2	29.9	1.9×10^{3}	1.7×10^{3}	1.7×10^{2}	54.6
75%	55.5	20.3	11.6	1.8×10^{2}	42.2	35.5	12.4
50%	17.4	9.0	6.3	44.9	17.3	12.7	6.1
25%	8.5	5.5	4.2	18.8	9.6	6.5	3.8
10%	5.5	3.9	3.2	10.8	6.4	4.1	2.8
5%	4.4	3.3	2.8	8.1	5.2	3.3	2.4
1%	3.1	2.6	2.3	5.1	3.7	2.4	1.9
0% min	2.0	2.0	1.8	2.5	2.1	1.1	1.1

The estimated quantiles are based on 10,000 simulations

Table 6.8 The data in Table 6.1 are analysed and the test statistic for column-wise mean shift, $T_{11;io}$, based on Theorem 6.8 (ii), is presented

	Individual													
	1	2	3	4	5	6	7	8	9	10	11	12	13	14
$T_{11;io}$	2.1	2.4	1.4	3.1	1.9	1.3	1.0	2.6	2.4	9.2	7.6	3.8	1.3	1.1
$\overline{T}_{11;io}$	1.9	1.9	1.4	3.2	1.1	1.1	1.1	1.3	1.1	6.4	8.1	2.4	1.3	1.1
	Individual													
	15	16	17	18	19	20	21	22	23	24	25	26	27	
$T_{11;io}$	45.9	1.4	1.6	1.4	1.8	1.8	20.7	3.1	1.5	93.5	2.8	2.8	2.1	
$\overline{T}_{11;io}$	2.5	1.4	1.5	1.3	1.3	1.7	20.5	1.2	1.0	1.2	1.0	1.2	1.8	

The test statistic for column-wise mean shift, $\overline{T}_{11;io}$, based on Theorem 6.8 (iii), is also shown

6.5 Residual Analysis for R_1 in the BRM

So far R_{11} and R_{12} have been exploited. However, since these residuals are not independently distributed, it can be worthwhile performing a residual analysis of

$$R_1 = X(I - P_{C'}) = R_{11} + R_{12}.$$

Because $R_1 \sim N_{p,n}(0, \Sigma, I - P_{C'})$, i.e. the distribution is known, this case should be both simpler and more reliable than considering R_{11} and R_{12} separately, although R_1 cannot completely contain the same amount of information as R_{11} and R_{12}. Moreover, since R_1 is also the residual in the MANOVA model, R_1 has in fact already been considered in Sect. 6.1. Next some of the statements of Sect. 6.1 are repeated, but the idea now is to carry out the presentation, although very briefly, relatively systematically in line with the treatments of R_{11} and R_{12}. Let

$$I - P_{C'} = VV', \quad V : n \times n_1, \quad n_1 = n - r(C)),$$

and by post-multiplying R_1 one eliminates the singularity, i.e.

$$R_1^N = R_1 L_1, \quad L_1 = V(V'V)^{-1}. \tag{6.37}$$

Now Definition 6.2 and Theorem 6.8 are adjusted so that the presentation fits R_1^N. The results of the theorem will, however, not be proved, since all the results are obtained by simply copying the results presented in earlier sections.

Definition 6.3 Models and notation are presented for the likelihood functions related to $R_1 = X(I - P_{C'})$; these models and this notation are used when testing for mean shifts under the conditions given in (6.36):

(a) $\quad R_{1;ij}^N = d_j \theta e_i' L_1 + E_1, \qquad R_{1;ijo}^N = R_{1o} L_1;$

(b) $\quad R_{1;i}^N = \theta e_i' L_1 + E_1, \qquad R_{1;io}^N = R_{1o} L_1;$

(c) $\quad R_{1;i}^N = 1\theta e_i' L_1 + E_1, \qquad R_{1;io}^N = R_{1o} L_1;$

(d) $\quad R_{1;j}^N = d_j \theta 1' L_1 + E_1, \qquad R_{1;jo}^N = R_{1o} L_1;$

$E_1 \sim N_{p,n_1}(0, \Sigma, I)$, $n_1 = n - r(C)$, L_1 is defined by (6.37), and d_j and e_i are unit basis vectors.

Denote the observed value of $\boldsymbol{R}_1$ by $\boldsymbol{R}_{1o}$. Moreover, $\boldsymbol{R}_{1;ijo}$, $\boldsymbol{R}_{1;io}$ and $\boldsymbol{R}_{1;jo}$ are all equal to $\boldsymbol{R}_{1o}$, given in Definition 6.1, and as before the subscripts ij, i and j only indicate which type of mean shift and which element is being studied.

Theorem 6.9 *In Definition 6.3, in order to test for no mean shift in the residual $\boldsymbol{R}_1$, models with four types of mean shift were presented. The test statistics for the four types are presented below.*

(i) *Let the model and mean shift be as in Definition 6.3 (a). The test statistic for $\boldsymbol{R}^N_{1;ij}$, testing for no mean shift, is given by*

$$T_{1;ijo} = \frac{(n - r(\boldsymbol{C}) - 1)\boldsymbol{d}'_j\boldsymbol{R}_{1o}(\boldsymbol{I} - \boldsymbol{P}_{C'})\boldsymbol{e}_i(\boldsymbol{e}'_i(\boldsymbol{I} - \boldsymbol{P}_{C'})\boldsymbol{e}_i)^{-1}\boldsymbol{e}'_i(\boldsymbol{I} - \boldsymbol{P}_{C'})\boldsymbol{R}'_{1o}\boldsymbol{d}_j}{\boldsymbol{d}'_j\boldsymbol{R}_{1o}(\boldsymbol{I} - \boldsymbol{P}_{C'})(\boldsymbol{I} - \boldsymbol{e}_i(\boldsymbol{e}'_i(\boldsymbol{I} - \boldsymbol{P}_{C'})\boldsymbol{e}_i)^{-1}\boldsymbol{e}'_i)(\boldsymbol{I} - \boldsymbol{P}_{C'})\boldsymbol{R}'_{1o}\boldsymbol{d}_j}.$$

(ii) *Let the model and mean shift be as in Definition 6.3 (b). Then the test statistic for $\boldsymbol{R}^N_{1;i}$, testing for no mean shift, is given by*

$$T_{1;io} = \frac{|\boldsymbol{R}_{1o}(\boldsymbol{I} - \boldsymbol{P}_{C'})\boldsymbol{R}'_{1o}|}{|\boldsymbol{R}_{1o}(\boldsymbol{I} - \boldsymbol{P}_{C'})(\boldsymbol{I} - \boldsymbol{e}_i(\boldsymbol{e}'_i(\boldsymbol{I} - \boldsymbol{P}_{C'})\boldsymbol{e}_i)^{-1}\boldsymbol{e}'_i)(\boldsymbol{I} - \boldsymbol{P}_{C'})\boldsymbol{R}'_{1o}|}.$$

(iii) *Let the model and mean shift be as in Definition 6.3 (c). Then the test statistic for $\boldsymbol{R}_1$, testing for no mean shift, is given by*

$$\overline{T}_{1;io} = \frac{(n - r(\boldsymbol{C}) - 1)\boldsymbol{1}'\boldsymbol{R}_{1o}(\boldsymbol{I} - \boldsymbol{P}_{C'})\boldsymbol{e}_i(\boldsymbol{e}'_i(\boldsymbol{I} - \boldsymbol{P}_{C'})\boldsymbol{e}_i)^{-1}\boldsymbol{e}'_i(\boldsymbol{I} - \boldsymbol{P}_{C'})\boldsymbol{R}'_{1o}\boldsymbol{1}}{\boldsymbol{1}'\boldsymbol{R}_{1o}(\boldsymbol{I} - \boldsymbol{P}_{C'})(\boldsymbol{I} - \boldsymbol{e}_i(\boldsymbol{e}'_i(\boldsymbol{I} - \boldsymbol{P}_{C'})\boldsymbol{e}_i)^{-1}\boldsymbol{e}'_i)(\boldsymbol{I} - \boldsymbol{P}_{C'})\boldsymbol{R}'_{1o}\boldsymbol{1}}.$$

(iv) *Let the model and mean shift be as in Definition 6.3 (d). Then the test statistic for $\boldsymbol{R}_1$, testing for no mean shift, is given by*

$$\overline{T}_{1;jo} = \frac{(n - r(\boldsymbol{C}) - 1)\boldsymbol{d}'_j\boldsymbol{R}_{1o}(\boldsymbol{I} - \boldsymbol{P}_{C'})\boldsymbol{1}_n(\boldsymbol{1}'_n(\boldsymbol{I} - \boldsymbol{P}_{C'})\boldsymbol{1}_n)^{-1}\boldsymbol{1}'_n(\boldsymbol{I} - \boldsymbol{P}_{C'})\boldsymbol{R}'_{1o}\boldsymbol{d}_j}{\boldsymbol{d}'_j\boldsymbol{R}_{1o}(\boldsymbol{I} - \boldsymbol{P}_{C'})(\boldsymbol{I} - \boldsymbol{1}_n(\boldsymbol{1}'_n(\boldsymbol{I} - \boldsymbol{P}_{C'})\boldsymbol{1}_n)^{-1}\boldsymbol{1}'_n)(\boldsymbol{I} - \boldsymbol{P}_{C'})\boldsymbol{R}'_{1o}\boldsymbol{d}_j}.$$

Proof Since $\boldsymbol{I} - \boldsymbol{P}_{C'}$ is idempotent, $\boldsymbol{L}_1$ in (6.37) equals $\boldsymbol{V}$ because $\boldsymbol{V}$ is a semi-orthogonal matrix, i.e. $\boldsymbol{V}'\boldsymbol{V} = \boldsymbol{I}_{n_1}$. Moreover, note that all the models of the theorem are of the form

$$\boldsymbol{X}\boldsymbol{V} = \boldsymbol{\mu}\boldsymbol{V} + \boldsymbol{E}_1, \qquad \boldsymbol{E}_1 \sim N_{p,n_1}(\boldsymbol{0}, \boldsymbol{\Sigma}, \boldsymbol{I}),$$

where $\boldsymbol{\mu}$ equals $\boldsymbol{d}_j\theta\boldsymbol{e}'_i$, $\boldsymbol{\theta}\boldsymbol{e}'_i$, $\boldsymbol{1}\theta\boldsymbol{e}'_i$ or $\boldsymbol{d}_j\theta\boldsymbol{1}'$. This is a standard MANOVA model with bilinear restrictions on the mean and the results will be verified in detail in the next section under more general assumptions. □

To understand best what may occur when performing data analysis, once again the Potthoff and Roy (1964) data set is used. It is also of particular interest to

Table 6.9 Estimated quantiles for $T_{1;ij^1}$, $T_{1;ij^2}$ and $T_{1;ij^3}$ connected to the test statistics $T_{1;ij^1o}$, $T_{1;ij^2o}$ and $T_{1;ij^3o}$ (with $T_{1;ijo}$ defined in Theorem 6.9 (i)) are given, and applied to the Potthoff and Roy data set presented in Table 1.2

Quantile	$T_{1;ij^1o}$	$T_{1;ij^2o}$	$T_{1;ij^3o}$	$R_{12;ij^1o}$	$R_{12;ij^2o}$	$R_{12;ij^3o}$
100%max	45.6	25.2	17.5	11.1	9.2	8.8
99%	21.7	14.2	10.8	8.6	7.3	6.6
95%	16.2	11.1	8.6	7.6	6.6	6.0
90%	13.9	9.7	7.8	7.1	6.2	5.7
75%	11.1	8.1	6.7	6.4	5.6	5.2
50%	8.8	6.9	5.8	5.7	5.1	4.8
25%	7.3	5.9	5.1	5.2	4.6	4.4
10%	6.3	5.2	4.6	4.7	4.3	4.0
5%	5.8	4.9	4.4	4.5	4.1	3.8
1%	5.0	4.3	3.9	4.1	3.7	3.5
0% min	4.0	3.4	3.1	3.4	3.2	3.1

Estimated quantiles are given for the three largest (by absolute value) residuals, $R_{1ij^ko}, k = 1, 2, 3$, obtained from the same data set. The estimated quantiles are based on 10,000 simulations

compare the results for $\boldsymbol{R}_1$ with those for $\boldsymbol{R}_{11}$ and $\boldsymbol{R}_{12}$ to determine whether there is any significant advantage in decomposing $\boldsymbol{R}_1$ (Table 6.9).

Example 6.6 (The Classical Potthoff and Roy (1964) Data Set Given in Table 1.2) The residual $\boldsymbol{R}_{1o} = \boldsymbol{X}_o(\boldsymbol{I} - \boldsymbol{P}_{C'})$ is presented in Table 6.10. Also shown in this table are the values of the test statistic of Theorem 6.9 (i). It can be observed that individuals #10, #11, #21 and #24 differ from the other individuals, with the largest value for individual #24 when $j = 1$, i.e. at age 8. However, from Table 6.9 it follows that no residuals have a significant mean shift, i.e. even the value $T_{1;241o} = 9.0$ is not significant.

Since there seem to be some individuals which deviate from the rest, we now test for a mean shift for a whole individual or for an equal mean shift for a whole individual. The results are presented in Table 6.11. For $T_{1;io}$ only individual #20 seems to stand out, whereas according to $\overline{T}_{1;io}$, individuals #10, #11 and #21 should be investigated. The appropriate distributions for decision making are presented in Table 6.12 and it is $T_{1;201_o} = 5.2$ which exhibits a mean shift which is significant, as well as $\overline{T}_{1;113_o} = 4.6$. The last result is interesting, but difficult to interpret, since neither $\overline{T}_{1;111_o}$ nor $\overline{T}_{1;112_o}$ are significant. Therefore, the final conclusion from the residual analysis for the residual $\boldsymbol{R}_1$ and the split $\boldsymbol{R}_1 = \boldsymbol{R}_{11} + \boldsymbol{R}_{12}$ is that only the residual from individual #20 is too far away from 0 to be deemed non-significant.

Now all the significant findings concerning $\boldsymbol{R}_1$ are hereby summarized. In Table 6.1 the observation $T_{12;2031_o}$ was significant, as well as $R_{12;2031_o}$. Moreover, in Table 6.3 the statistics $T_{12;201_o} = 9379.2$ and $\overline{T}_{12;201_o} = 9486.7$ were significant. Tables 6.6 and 6.8 give indications that observations or individuals deviate, but the overall conclusion is that no elements in $\boldsymbol{R}_{11}$, with its mean shift, deviate

Table 6.10 The residual $R_{1o} = X_o(I - P_{C'}) = (R_{1;ijo})$ and the test statistic given in Theorem 6.9 (i) applied to the Potthoff and Roy (1964) data presented in Table 1.2

		Residuals				Test statistics			
id	Gender	$R_{1;i1o}$	$R_{1;i2o}$	$R_{1;i3o}$	$R_{1;i4o}$	$T_{1;i1o}$	$T_{1;i2o}$	$T_{1;i3o}$	$T_{1;i4o}$
1	F	−0.18	−2.23	−1.59	−1.09	0.0	1.3	0.4	0.3
2	F	−0.18	−0.73	0.91	1.41	0.0	0.1	0.1	0.4
3	F	−0.68	1.77	1.41	1.91	0.1	0.8	0.3	0.8
4	F	2.32	2.27	1.91	2.41	1.1	1.4	0.6	1.3
5	F	0.32	0.77	−0.59	−0.59	0.0	0.2	0.1	0.1
6	F	−1.18	−1.23	−2.09	−1.59	0.3	0.4	0.7	0.5
7	F	0.32	0.27	−0.09	0.91	0.0	0.0	0.0	0.2
8	F	1.82	0.77	0.41	−0.09	0.7	0.2	0.0	0.0
9	F	−1.18	−1.23	−1.09	−2.59	0.3	0.4	0.2	1.5
10	F	−4.68	−3.23	−4.09	−4.59	5.2	3.0	3.1	5.5
11	F	3.32	2.77	4.91	3.91	2.4	2.1	4.7	3.7
12	M	3.12	1.19	3.28	3.53	2.0	0.4	1.8	2.9
13	M	−1.38	−1.31	−2.72	−0.97	0.3	0.4	1.2	0.2
14	M	0.12	−1.31	−1.72	0.03	0.0	0.4	0.5	0.0
15	M	2.62	3.69	0.78	−0.47	1.4	3.9	0.1	0.0
16	M	−2.88	−0.31	−3.22	−1.47	1.7	0.0	1.8	0.5
17	M	1.62	1.69	1.28	1.03	0.5	0.7	0.3	0.2
18	M	−0.88	−1.81	−1.22	−0.97	0.1	0.8	0.2	0.2
19	M	1.12	−2.31	−1.22	−1.97	0.2	1.4	0.2	0.8
20	M	0.12	−3.31	5.28	−1.47	0.0	3.0	5.4	0.5
21	M	4.62	4.19	5.28	4.03	4.9	5.2	5.4	3.9
22	M	0.12	−0.81	−2.22	−2.47	0.0	0.2	0.8	1.3
23	M	−1.38	−0.31	−1.72	0.53	0.4	0.0	0.5	0.1
24	M	−5.88	0.69	0.28	2.03	9.0	0.1	0.0	0.9
25	M	−0.38	1.69	−0.22	−1.47	0.0	0.7	0.0	0.5
26	M	0.12	0.69	0.28	2.53	0.0	0.1	0.0	1.4
27	M	−0.88	−2.31	−2.22	−2.47	0.1	1.4	0.8	1.3

significantly from 0. For $\boldsymbol{R}_1 = \boldsymbol{R}_{11} + \boldsymbol{R}_{12}$, the results were presented in Tables 6.10 and 6.11, and it was concluded that only individual #20 had a significant mean shift. Thus, it can be stated that only individual #20 had a large residual, which to some extent can also be seen in an ocular data inspection. Finally we claim that the residual analysis has shown that if one just observes data without referring to distributions and probability statements, it is difficult to determine how large deviating values should be to be deemed as outlying (extreme) observations. □

In the residual analysis so far, the residual $\boldsymbol{R}_1$ has been scrutinized; i.e. the residual has been decomposed and various mean shift tests have been performed. Now $\boldsymbol{R}_{2o} = (\boldsymbol{I} - \boldsymbol{P}_{A,S_o})\boldsymbol{X}_o\boldsymbol{P}_{C'}$ is considered. As noted before, $\boldsymbol{R}_2$ is suitable for validating the model, but is not connected to single observations or columns in $\boldsymbol{X}$. In Theorem 6.7 it was noted that $\boldsymbol{R}_2$ has the same distribution as $\boldsymbol{R}_{2N} - \boldsymbol{U}_2$.

Table 6.11 The data in Table 6.10 are analysed and the test statistic for column-wise mean shift, $T_{1;io}$, based on Theorem 6.9 (ii), is presented

	Individual													
	1	2	3	4	5	6	7	8	9	10	11	12	13	14
$T_{1;io}$	1.1	1.1	1.1	1.1	1.0	1.0	1.0	1.0	1.1	1.3	1.2	1.2	1.1	1.1
$\overline{T}_{1;io}$	0.5	0.0	0.3	1.5	0.0	0.7	0.0	0.1	0.7	6.0	4.6	2.3	0.7	0.1
	Individual													
	15	16	17	18	19	20	21	22	23	24	25	26	27	
$T_{1;io}$	1.6	1.1	1.0	1.0	1.2	5.2	1.3	1.1	1.1	2.7	1.3	1.1	1.1	
$\overline{T}_{1;io}$	0.8	1.1	0.5	0.4	0.3	0.0	7.2	0.5	0.1	0.1	0.0	0.2	1.1	

The test statistic for column-wise mean shift, $\overline{T}_{1;io}$, based on Theorem 6.9 (iii), is also shown

Table 6.12 Estimated quantiles connected to the test statistics $T_{1;i^k o}$ and $\overline{T}_{1;i^k o}$, respectively, defined in Theorem 6.9 (ii) and (iii), are presented for the Potthoff and Roy (1964) data given in Table 1.2

Quantile	$T_{1;i^1 o}$	$T_{1;i^2 o}$	$T_{1;i^3 o}$	$\overline{T}_{1;i^1 o}$	$\overline{T}_{1;i^2 o}$	$\overline{T}_{1;i^3 o}$
100% max	3.7	2.4	2.0	34.4	10.6	6.9
99%	2.5	1.9	1.7	17.4	7.6	5.1
95%	2.2	1.8	1.6	12.3	6.3	4.4
90%	2.0	1.7	1.5	10.4	5.6	4.0
75%	1.8	1.6	1.5	8.0	4.8	3.5
50%	1.7	1.5	1.4	6.1	4.0	3.0
25%	1.6	1.5	1.4	4.9	3.4	2.6
10%	1.5	1.4	1.4	4.1	3.0	2.3
5%	1.5	1.4	1.3	3.7	2.8	2.2
1%	1.4	1.4	1.3	3.2	2.4	1.8
0% min	1.3	1.3	1.3	2.2	1.8	1.1

The estimated quantiles are based on 10,000 simulations

The approximating density $f_{\boldsymbol{K}\boldsymbol{R}_{2N}\boldsymbol{L}}(\boldsymbol{K}\boldsymbol{R}_0\boldsymbol{L})$ is utilized for specific $\boldsymbol{K}$ and $\boldsymbol{L}$, and $D[\boldsymbol{R}_{2N}]$ is decomposed spectrally, i.e.

$$D[\boldsymbol{R}_{2N}] = \boldsymbol{V}\boldsymbol{V}' \otimes \boldsymbol{W}\boldsymbol{W}', \quad \boldsymbol{V} : n \times r(\boldsymbol{C}), \ \boldsymbol{W} : p \times (p - r(\boldsymbol{A})),$$

which follows from $\boldsymbol{\Sigma}\boldsymbol{P}_{A^o,\Sigma^{-1}} = \boldsymbol{W}\boldsymbol{W}'$ and $\boldsymbol{P}_{C'} = \boldsymbol{V}\boldsymbol{V}'$. In the same way as $\boldsymbol{R}_{12}^N$ was introduced, let

$$\boldsymbol{R}_{2;ij}^N = \boldsymbol{K}\boldsymbol{R}_2\boldsymbol{L}, \quad \boldsymbol{K} = (\boldsymbol{W}'\boldsymbol{W})^{-1}\boldsymbol{W}', \ \boldsymbol{L} = \boldsymbol{V}(\boldsymbol{V}'\boldsymbol{V})^{-1},$$

and then with these choices of $\boldsymbol{K}$ and $\boldsymbol{L}$ in Theorem 6.7, a non-singular density approximation exists. The model for testing for a mean shift, e.g. following (6.21), is written as

$$\boldsymbol{R}_{2;ij}^N = \boldsymbol{K}\boldsymbol{d}_j\theta\boldsymbol{e}_i'\boldsymbol{L} + \boldsymbol{E}_2, \quad \boldsymbol{d}_j : p \times 1, \ \boldsymbol{e}_i : r(\boldsymbol{C}) \times 1, \tag{6.38}$$

where $\boldsymbol{E}_2$ has the approximating density given in Theorem 6.7. The density depends on $\boldsymbol{\Sigma}$, but if one replaces it by $\widehat{\boldsymbol{\Sigma}}$, given in Theorem 3.1, or by $\widehat{\boldsymbol{\Sigma}}_U$, given in Theorem 4.7, we have a complete specification of the likelihood and can formulate the following test quantity for $H_0 : \theta = 0$ versus $H_1 : \theta \neq 0$:

$$T_{2;ijo} = \frac{L^N_{2;qij}(\widehat{\theta_o})}{L^N_{2;ij}}, \tag{6.39}$$

where $L^N_{2;ij}$ is the likelihood for $\boldsymbol{R}^N_2$ under H_0 and $\boldsymbol{R}^N_2(\widehat{\theta_o})$ under H_1 with $\widehat{\theta_o} = \boldsymbol{d}'_j\boldsymbol{R}_{2o}\boldsymbol{e}_i$. Moreover, a parallel discussion of testing for mean shifts via

$$\begin{aligned}
\boldsymbol{R}^N_{2;i} &= \boldsymbol{K}\boldsymbol{\theta}\boldsymbol{e}'_i\boldsymbol{L} + \boldsymbol{E}_2,\\
\boldsymbol{R}^N_{2;i} &= \boldsymbol{K}\boldsymbol{1}\theta\boldsymbol{e}'_i\boldsymbol{L} + \boldsymbol{E}_2,\\
\boldsymbol{R}^N_{2;j} &= \boldsymbol{K}\boldsymbol{d}_j\theta\boldsymbol{1}'\boldsymbol{L} + \boldsymbol{E}_2
\end{aligned}$$

follows the same ideas as before; $\boldsymbol{R}^N_{2;i}$ and $\boldsymbol{R}^N_{2;j}$ are identical to $\boldsymbol{R}^N_2$. However, one should remember that $r(\boldsymbol{C})$ is often a small value, meaning that there are only a few independent observations available, and therefore formal tests usually have low power.

6.6 Residuals for the $EBRM^3_B$

In this section the basis for studying residuals for the $EBRM^3_B$ is given. Figure 2.7 presented a decomposition of the whole tensor space showing the characteristic "stairs structure". The next figure (Fig. 6.4) once again shows the spaces, but now the focus is directed on the residuals.

In Fig. 6.4, for any given $\boldsymbol{\Sigma}$, ten different residuals are presented. All these residuals can be studied, as well as linear combinations of them. In a textbook this is impossible and only the following four residuals will be highlighted:

(i) $\boldsymbol{R}_{1N} = \boldsymbol{R}_{11} + \boldsymbol{R}_{12} + \boldsymbol{R}_{13} + \boldsymbol{R}_{14}$;
(ii) $\boldsymbol{R}_{2N} = \boldsymbol{R}_{21} + \boldsymbol{R}_{22} + \boldsymbol{R}_{23}$;
(iii) $\boldsymbol{R}_{3N} = \boldsymbol{R}_{31} + \boldsymbol{R}_{32}$;
(iv) $\boldsymbol{R}_{4N} = \boldsymbol{R}_{4N}$.

Explicit expressions for any given $\boldsymbol{\Sigma}$ can be obtained by projecting $\boldsymbol{X}$ on $\mathcal{W}_i \otimes \mathcal{V}_j$, $i \leq j$, i.e. $\mathrm{vec}\boldsymbol{R}_{5-i,j} = (\boldsymbol{P}_{\mathcal{W}_i} \otimes \boldsymbol{P}_{\mathcal{V}_j,\Sigma})\mathrm{vec}\boldsymbol{X}$, where $\mathcal{W}_i$ and $\mathcal{V}_j$ are defined in Fig. 6.4. However, $\boldsymbol{\Sigma}$ is unknown and then the inner product has to be estimated. Therefore, the residual analysis will rest on Corollary 3.3, i.e. $\boldsymbol{X} - \widehat{E[\boldsymbol{X}]}$ will be

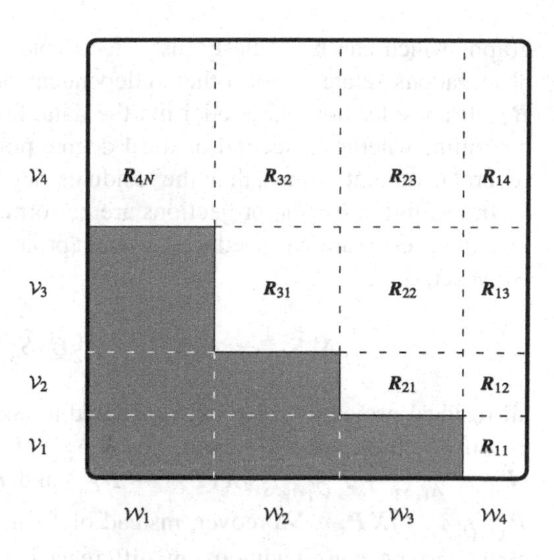

Fig. 6.4 Decomposition of the whole space according to the within-individuals and the between-individuals designs, illustrating the mean and residual spaces in $EBRM_B^3$: $\mathcal{V}_1 = \mathcal{C}_\Sigma(A_1)$, $\mathcal{V}_2 = \mathcal{C}_\Sigma(A_1 : A_2) \cap \mathcal{C}_\Sigma(A_1)^\perp$, $\mathcal{V}_3 = \mathcal{C}_\Sigma(A_1 : A_2 : A_3) \cap \mathcal{C}_\Sigma(A_1 : A_2)^\perp$, $\mathcal{V}_4 = \mathcal{C}_\Sigma(A_1 : A_2 : A_3)^\perp$, $\mathcal{W}_1 = \mathcal{C}(C_3')$, $\mathcal{W}_2 = \mathcal{C}(C_2') \cap \mathcal{C}(C_3')^\perp$, $\mathcal{W}_3 = \mathcal{C}(C_1') \cap \mathcal{C}(C_2')^\perp$, $\mathcal{W}_4 = \mathcal{C}(C_1')^\perp$

considered. The fact will be utilized that (using the notations of Theorem 3.2)

$$\begin{aligned}
X - \widehat{E[X]} &= X - P_{A_1,S_1} X P_{C_1'} - P_{\widehat{Q}_1' A_2, \widehat{S}_2} X P_{C_2'} - P_{\widehat{Q}_2' \widehat{Q}_1' A_3, \widehat{S}_3} X P_{C_3'} \\
&= X(I - P_{C_1'}) + (I - P_{A_1,S_1}) X (P_{C_1'} - P_{C_2'}) \\
&\quad + (I - P_{A_1,S_1} - P_{\widehat{Q}_1' A_2, \widehat{S}_2}) X (P_{C_2'} - P_{C_3'}) \\
&\quad + (I - P_{A_1,S_1} - P_{\widehat{Q}_1' A_2, \widehat{S}_2} - P_{\widehat{Q}_2' \widehat{Q}_1' A_3, \widehat{S}_3}) X P_{C_3'}.
\end{aligned}$$

Thus, since $\mathcal{C}(I - P_{C_1'}) = \mathcal{W}_4$, $\mathcal{C}(P_{C_1'} - P_{C_2'}) = \mathcal{W}_3$, $\mathcal{C}(P_{C_2'} - P_{C_3'}) = \mathcal{W}_2$ and $\mathcal{C}(P_{C_3'}) = \mathcal{W}_1$, the next definitions make sense.

Definition 6.4 Let $\widehat{Q}_i$, S_1 and $\widehat{S}_i$, $i = 2, 3$, be as in Theorem 3.2. For the $EBRM_B^3$ the following residuals will be considered:

(i) $R_1 = X(I - P_{C_1'})$;
(ii) $R_2 = (I - P_{A_1,S_1}) X (P_{C_1'} - P_{C_2'})$;
(iii) $R_3 = (I - P_{A_1,S_1} - P_{\widehat{Q}_1' A_2, \widehat{S}_2}) X (P_{C_2'} - P_{C_3'})$;
(iv) $R_4 = (I - P_{A_1,S_1} - P_{\widehat{Q}_1' A_2, \widehat{S}_2} - P_{\widehat{Q}_2' \widehat{Q}_1' A_3, \widehat{S}_3}) X P_{C_3'}$.

Note that the residual R_1 is identical to $R_1 \sim N_{p,n}(\mathbf{0}, \Sigma, I - P_{C_1'})$ for the BRM and, therefore, for R_1 only the mean shift test of the residual analysis will be provided. Missing details can be found in Sect. 6.2. However, it should be remembered that in many applications only the residual in Definition 6.4 (i) bears enough information to be analysed in detail, for example via statistical tests. This does not mean that R_2, R_3 and R_4 should be discarded, but it may happen that for these residuals there is only enough information available for presenting some graphs which can be ocularly inspected. Note that $\boldsymbol{R}_1$ concerns how independent observations relate to the other independent observations, whereas $\boldsymbol{R}_2$, $\boldsymbol{R}_3$ and $\boldsymbol{R}_4$ all consider how the model fits the data. For example, if one's intention is to determine whether a second or third degree polynomial growth model fits one of several treatment groups, then the residuals can be supportive.

In Definition 6.4 the projections are performed with the help of inner products. Due to the estimation procedure, different projections have different inner products. However, since

$$\boldsymbol{A}_1'\widehat{\boldsymbol{S}}_3^{-1} = \boldsymbol{A}_1'\boldsymbol{S}_1^{-1}, \quad \boldsymbol{A}_2'\widehat{\boldsymbol{Q}}_1\widehat{\boldsymbol{S}}_3^{-1} = \boldsymbol{A}_2'\widehat{\boldsymbol{Q}}_1\widehat{\boldsymbol{S}}_2^{-1},$$

all residual projections can be considered to take place on spaces where the inner product defined via $\widehat{\boldsymbol{S}}_3$ is used, i.e. $\boldsymbol{R}_2 = (\boldsymbol{I} - \boldsymbol{P}_{A_1,\widehat{S}_3})\boldsymbol{X}(\boldsymbol{P}_{C_1'} - \boldsymbol{P}_{C_2'})$, $\boldsymbol{R}_3 = (\boldsymbol{I} - \boldsymbol{P}_{A_1,\widehat{S}_3} - \boldsymbol{P}_{\widehat{Q}_1'A_2,\widehat{S}_3})\boldsymbol{X}(\boldsymbol{P}_{C_2'} - \boldsymbol{P}_{C_3'})$ and $\boldsymbol{R}_4 = (\boldsymbol{I} - \boldsymbol{P}_{A_1,\widehat{S}_3} - \boldsymbol{P}_{\widehat{Q}_1'A_2,\widehat{S}_3} - \boldsymbol{P}_{\widehat{Q}_2'\widehat{Q}_1'A_3,\widehat{S}_3})\boldsymbol{X}\boldsymbol{P}_{C_3'}$. Moreover, instead of $\widehat{\boldsymbol{S}}_3$ the MLE $\widehat{\boldsymbol{\Sigma}}$, given by Theorem 3.2, could have been used without any difference in the performed projections.

Concerning the stochastic properties of the residuals the basic relations which will be utilized are the following:

- $\boldsymbol{S}_1$ is independent of $\boldsymbol{X}(\boldsymbol{P}_{C_1'} - \boldsymbol{P}_{C_2'})$, $\boldsymbol{X}(\boldsymbol{P}_{C_2'} - \boldsymbol{P}_{C_3'})$ and $\boldsymbol{X}\boldsymbol{P}_{C_3'}$;
- $\widehat{\boldsymbol{S}}_2$ is independent of $\boldsymbol{X}(\boldsymbol{P}_{C_2'} - \boldsymbol{P}_{C_3'})$ and $\boldsymbol{X}\boldsymbol{P}_{C_3'}$;
- $\widehat{\boldsymbol{S}}_3$ is independent of $\boldsymbol{X}\boldsymbol{P}_{C_3'}$.

Applying these properties it can be shown that

$$E[\boldsymbol{R}_2] = E[\boldsymbol{R}_3] = E[\boldsymbol{R}_4] = \boldsymbol{0}.$$

The result follows from the fact that

$$(\boldsymbol{I} - \boldsymbol{P}_{A_1,S_1} - \boldsymbol{P}_{\widehat{Q}_1'A_2,\widehat{S}_2})\boldsymbol{A}_2 = \boldsymbol{0},$$
$$(\boldsymbol{I} - \boldsymbol{P}_{A_1,S_1} - \boldsymbol{P}_{\widehat{Q}_1'A_2,\widehat{S}_2} - \boldsymbol{P}_{\widehat{Q}_2'\widehat{Q}_1'A_3,\widehat{S}_3})\boldsymbol{A}_3 = \boldsymbol{0}.$$

The next theorem is a direct consequence of the above-mentioned independence relations and the detailed moment calculations performed in Chap. 4. It is based on the fact that the following alternative expressions for the residuals can be obtained ($\boldsymbol{G}_i$, $\boldsymbol{W}_i$ and $\boldsymbol{Z}_{1,s}$ are defined in Table 4.1):

$$\begin{aligned}\boldsymbol{R}_2 &= \boldsymbol{P}'_{G_1,W_1^{-1}}\boldsymbol{X}(\boldsymbol{P}_{C_1'} - \boldsymbol{P}_{C_2'}) = \widehat{\boldsymbol{Q}}_1'\boldsymbol{X}(\boldsymbol{P}_{C_1'} - \boldsymbol{P}_{C_2'}) \\ &= \boldsymbol{Z}_{1,1}\boldsymbol{X}(\boldsymbol{P}_{C_1'} - \boldsymbol{P}_{C_2'}),\end{aligned} \tag{6.40}$$

$$\begin{aligned}\boldsymbol{R}_3 &= \boldsymbol{P}'_{G_1,W_1^{-1}}\boldsymbol{P}'_{G_2,W_2^{-1}}\boldsymbol{X}(\boldsymbol{P}_{C_2'} - \boldsymbol{P}_{C_3'}) = \widehat{\boldsymbol{Q}}_2'\widehat{\boldsymbol{Q}}_1'\boldsymbol{X}(\boldsymbol{P}_{C_2'} - \boldsymbol{P}_{C_3'}) \\ &= \boldsymbol{Z}_{1,2}\boldsymbol{X}(\boldsymbol{P}_{C_2'} - \boldsymbol{P}_{C_3'}),\end{aligned} \tag{6.41}$$

$$R_4 = P'_{G_1,W_1^{-1}} P'_{G_2,W_2^{-1}} P'_{G_3,W_3^{-1}} X P_{C_3'} = \widehat{Q}_3' \widehat{Q}_2' \widehat{Q}_1' X P_{C_3'}$$
$$= Z_{1,3} X P_{C_3'}. \tag{6.42}$$

Theorem 6.10 *Let R_2, R_3 and R_4 be as in Definition 6.4. Then*

(i) $D[R_2] = (P_{C_1'} - P_{C_2'}) \otimes E[\widehat{Q}_1' \Sigma \widehat{Q}_1]$, *where* $E[\widehat{Q}_1' \Sigma \widehat{Q}_1]$ *is given by (4.120);*
(ii) $D[R_3] = (P_{C_2'} - P_{C_3'}) \otimes E[\widehat{Q}_2' \widehat{Q}_1' \Sigma \widehat{Q}_1 \widehat{Q}_2]$, *where* $E[\widehat{Q}_2' \widehat{Q}_1' \Sigma \widehat{Q}_1 \widehat{Q}_2]$ *is given by (4.121);*
(iii) $D[R_4] = P_{C_3'} \otimes E[\widehat{Q}_3' \widehat{Q}_2' \widehat{Q}_1' \Sigma \widehat{Q}_1 \widehat{Q}_2 \widehat{Q}_3]$, *where* $E[\widehat{Q}_3' \widehat{Q}_2' \widehat{Q}_1' \Sigma \widehat{Q}_1 \widehat{Q}_2 \widehat{Q}_3]$ *is given by (4.122);*
(iv) $C[R_1, R_2] = C[R_1, R_3] = C[R_1, R_4] = 0$; $C[R_2, R_3] = C[R_2, R_4] = 0$; $C[R_3, R_4] = 0$.

It is noted that the unbiased estimators of the dispersion matrices in Theorem 6.10 can be obtained via the unbiased estimators of the K-matrices in Theorem 4.16.

Since the residuals R_2, R_3 and R_4 follow complicated distributions which are not available in any practical form, Edgeworth-type approximations will be used. The approximations will be based on the following decompositions:

$$R_2 = R_{2N} - U_2, \quad R_3 = R_{3N} - U_3, \quad R_4 = R_{4N} - U_4, \tag{6.43}$$

where

$$R_{2N} = (I - P_{A_1,\Sigma}) X (P_{C_1'} - P_{C_2'}) = P'_{G_1,\Sigma^{-1}} X (P_{C_1'} - P_{C_2'}), \tag{6.44}$$

$$U_2 = (P'_{G_1,\Sigma^{-1}} - P'_{G_1,W_1^{-1}}) X (P_{C_1'} - P_{C_2'}), \tag{6.45}$$

$$R_{3N} = (I - P_{A_1,\Sigma} - P_{Q_1'A_2,\Sigma}) X (P_{C_2'} - P_{C_3'})$$
$$= P'_{G_2,\Sigma^{-1}} X (P_{C_2'} - P_{C_3'}), \tag{6.46}$$

$$U_3 = \big(P'_{G_1,\Sigma^{-1}} (P'_{G_2,\Sigma^{-1}} - P'_{G_2,W_2^{-1}})$$
$$+ (P'_{G_1,\Sigma^{-1}} - P'_{G_1,W_1^{-1}}) P'_{G_2,W_2^{-1}}\big) X (P_{C_2'} - P_{C_3'}), \tag{6.47}$$

$$R_{4N} = (I - P_{A_1,\Sigma} - P_{Q_1'A_2,\Sigma} - P_{Q_2'Q_1'A_3,\Sigma}) = P'_{G_3,\Sigma^{-1}} X P_{C_3'}, \tag{6.48}$$

$$U_4 = \big(P'_{G_1,\Sigma^{-1}} P'_{G_2,\Sigma^{-1}} (P'_{G_3,\Sigma^{-1}} - P'_{G_3,W_3^{-1}})$$
$$+ P'_{G_1,\Sigma^{-1}} (P'_{G_2,\Sigma^{-1}} - P'_{G_2,W_2^{-1}}) P'_{G_3,W_3^{-1}}$$
$$+ (P'_{G_1,\Sigma^{-1}} - P'_{G_1,W_1^{-1}}) P'_{G_2,W_2^{-1}} P'_{G_3,W_3^{-1}})\big) X P_{C_3'}. \tag{6.49}$$

The residuals R_{2N}, R_{3N} and R_{4N} are all normally distributed. Moreover, demonstrating (6.43) for R_3 and R_4 is a rather straightforward task. The idea is to replace by Σ the matrices in the projections which define the inner product. The decomposition of $\boldsymbol{R}_2$ is trivial. For $\boldsymbol{R}_3$ it is noted that

$$\boldsymbol{P}'_{G_1,W_1^{-1}}\boldsymbol{P}'_{G_2,W_2^{-1}} = \boldsymbol{P}'_{G_1,\Sigma^{-1}}\boldsymbol{P}'_{G_2,\Sigma^{-1}} \\ -\boldsymbol{P}'_{G_1,\Sigma^{-1}}(\boldsymbol{P}'_{G_2,\Sigma^{-1}} - \boldsymbol{P}'_{G_2,W_2^{-1}}) - (\boldsymbol{P}'_{G_1,\Sigma^{-1}} - \boldsymbol{P}'_{G_1,W_1^{-1}})\boldsymbol{P}'_{G_2,W_2^{-1}}$$

and $\boldsymbol{P}'_{G_1,\Sigma^{-1}}\boldsymbol{P}'_{G_2,\Sigma^{-1}} = \boldsymbol{P}'_{G_2,\Sigma^{-1}}$. Moreover, concerning $\boldsymbol{R}_4$, calculations applied to $\boldsymbol{R}_3$ yield

$$\begin{aligned}\boldsymbol{P}'_{G_1,W_1^{-1}}\boldsymbol{P}'_{G_2,W_2^{-1}}\boldsymbol{P}'_{G_3,W_3^{-1}} &= \boldsymbol{P}'_{G_1,\Sigma^{-1}}\boldsymbol{P}'_{G_2,\Sigma^{-1}}\boldsymbol{P}'_{G_3,\Sigma^{-1}} \\ &\quad -\boldsymbol{P}'_{G_1,\Sigma^{-1}}\boldsymbol{P}'_{G_2,\Sigma^{-1}}(\boldsymbol{P}'_{G_3,\Sigma^{-1}} - \boldsymbol{P}'_{G_3,W_3^{-1}}) \\ &\quad -\boldsymbol{P}'_{G_1,\Sigma^{-1}}(\boldsymbol{P}'_{G_2,\Sigma^{-1}} - \boldsymbol{P}'_{G_2,W_2^{-1}})\boldsymbol{P}'_{G_3,W_3^{-1}} \\ &\quad -(\boldsymbol{P}'_{G_1,\Sigma^{-1}} - \boldsymbol{P}'_{G_1,W_1^{-1}})\boldsymbol{P}'_{G_2,W_2^{-1}}\boldsymbol{P}'_{G_3,W_3^{-1}}\end{aligned}$$

and $\boldsymbol{P}'_{G_1,\Sigma^{-1}}\boldsymbol{P}'_{G_2,\Sigma^{-1}}\boldsymbol{P}'_{G_3,\Sigma^{-1}} = \boldsymbol{P}'_{G_3,\Sigma^{-1}}$.

Hence, the approximating quantities $\boldsymbol{R}_{2N}$, $\boldsymbol{R}_{3N}$ and $\boldsymbol{R}_{4N}$ have been established. To validate if they make sense, it will be shown that $E[\boldsymbol{U}_i] = \boldsymbol{0}$ and $C[\boldsymbol{R}_{iN}, \boldsymbol{U}_i] = \boldsymbol{0}$, $i = 2, 3, 4$. Concerning the expectation, $E[\boldsymbol{U}_i] = E[\boldsymbol{R}_{iN}] + E[\boldsymbol{R}_i] = \boldsymbol{0}$. For the covariance it is noted that (see also Theorem B.21 (viii) in Appendix B and its proof)

$$\begin{aligned}&E[\boldsymbol{P}_{G_1,W_1^{-1}}] = \boldsymbol{P}_{G_1,\Sigma^{-1}}, && E[\boldsymbol{P}_{G_2,W_2^{-1}}] = \boldsymbol{P}_{G_2,\Sigma^{-1}},\ E[\boldsymbol{P}_{G_3,W_3^{-1}}] = \boldsymbol{P}_{G_3,\Sigma^{-1}}, \\ &E[\boldsymbol{P}_{G_3,W_3^{-1}}\boldsymbol{P}_{G_2,W_2^{-1}}] = \boldsymbol{P}_{G_3,\Sigma^{-1}}, && E[\boldsymbol{Z}'_{1,s}] = \boldsymbol{P}_{G_s,\Sigma^{-1}},\end{aligned}$$

which, if one applies one or more of these results directly to $C[\boldsymbol{R}_{iN}, \boldsymbol{U}_i]$, $i = 1, 2, 3$, will show that the covariance equals $\boldsymbol{0}$. For example,

$$\begin{aligned}C[\boldsymbol{R}_{3N}, \boldsymbol{U}_3] = (\boldsymbol{P}_{C'_2} - \boldsymbol{P}_{C'_3}) \otimes \Big\{&E[\boldsymbol{P}'_{G_2,\Sigma^{-1}}\boldsymbol{\Sigma}(\boldsymbol{P}_{G_2,\Sigma^{-1}} - \boldsymbol{P}_{G_2,W_2^{-1}})\boldsymbol{P}_{G_1,\Sigma^{-1}}] \\ &+ E[\boldsymbol{P}'_{G_2,\Sigma^{-1}}\boldsymbol{\Sigma}\boldsymbol{P}_{G_2,W_2^{-1}}(\boldsymbol{P}_{G_1,\Sigma^{-1}} - \boldsymbol{P}_{G_1,W_1^{-1}})]\Big\} = \boldsymbol{0},\end{aligned}$$

since

$$\begin{aligned}&E[(\boldsymbol{P}_{G_2,\Sigma^{-1}} - \boldsymbol{P}_{G_2,W_2^{-1}})] = \boldsymbol{0}, \\ &E[\boldsymbol{P}_{G_2,W_2^{-1}}(\boldsymbol{P}_{G_1,\Sigma^{-1}} - \boldsymbol{P}_{G_1,W_1^{-1}})] = \boldsymbol{P}_{G_2,\Sigma^{-1}} - \boldsymbol{P}_{G_2,\Sigma^{-1}} = \boldsymbol{0}.\end{aligned}$$

With these calculations, the preparations for presenting Edgeworth-type approximations are now completed. The first result concerns $\boldsymbol{R}_2$ and it is given in the next theorem.

Theorem 6.11 *The distribution of the residual* $\boldsymbol{R}_2$*, given in (6.40), can be approximated through the difference*

$$\boldsymbol{R}_2 = \boldsymbol{R}_{2N} - \boldsymbol{U}_2,$$

where $\boldsymbol{R}_{2N}$ *and* $\boldsymbol{U}_2$ *are defined by (6.44) and (6.45), respectively. Let* $\boldsymbol{K}$*:* $p_1 \times p$ *and* $\boldsymbol{L}$*:* $n \times n_1$*, both of which are known, and*

$$\boldsymbol{K}\boldsymbol{R}_{2N}\boldsymbol{L} \sim N_{p_1,n_1}(\boldsymbol{0}, \boldsymbol{K}\boldsymbol{\Sigma}\boldsymbol{P}_{A_1^o,\Sigma^{-1}}\boldsymbol{K}', \boldsymbol{L}'(\boldsymbol{P}_{C_1'} - \boldsymbol{P}_{C_2'})\boldsymbol{L}).$$

Then an Edgeworth-type expansion $f_{\boldsymbol{K}\boldsymbol{R}_{2E}\boldsymbol{L}}(\boldsymbol{K}\boldsymbol{R}_o\boldsymbol{L})$ *of the density of* $\boldsymbol{K}\boldsymbol{R}_2\boldsymbol{L}$*, via the density of* $\boldsymbol{K}\boldsymbol{R}_{2N}\boldsymbol{L}$*, assuming* $D[\boldsymbol{K}\boldsymbol{R}_{2N}\boldsymbol{L}]$ *is p.d., is given by*

$$f_{\boldsymbol{K}\boldsymbol{R}_{2E}\boldsymbol{L}}(\boldsymbol{K}\boldsymbol{R}_o\boldsymbol{L}) = \{1 - \tfrac{1}{2}\tfrac{p-r(A_1)}{n-r(C_1)-p+r(A_1)-1}n_1\mathrm{tr}\{\boldsymbol{K}\boldsymbol{P}_{A_1,\Sigma}\boldsymbol{\Sigma}\boldsymbol{K}'(\boldsymbol{K}\boldsymbol{\Sigma}\boldsymbol{P}_{A_1^o,\Sigma^{-1}}\boldsymbol{K}')^{-1}\}$$
$$+ \tfrac{1}{2}\tfrac{p-r(A_1)}{n-r(C_1)-p+r(A_1)-1}\mathrm{tr}\{(\boldsymbol{K}\boldsymbol{\Sigma}\boldsymbol{P}_{A_1^o,\Sigma^{-1}}\boldsymbol{K}')^{-1}\boldsymbol{K}\boldsymbol{P}_{A_1,\Sigma}\boldsymbol{\Sigma}\boldsymbol{K}'(\boldsymbol{K}\boldsymbol{\Sigma}\boldsymbol{P}_{A_1^o,\Sigma^{-1}}\boldsymbol{K}')^{-1}$$
$$\times \boldsymbol{K}\boldsymbol{R}_o\boldsymbol{L}(\boldsymbol{L}'(\boldsymbol{I} - \boldsymbol{P}_{C'})\boldsymbol{L})^{-1}\boldsymbol{L}'\boldsymbol{R}_o'\boldsymbol{K}'\}\}f_{\boldsymbol{K}\boldsymbol{R}_{2N}\boldsymbol{L}}(\boldsymbol{K}\boldsymbol{R}_o\boldsymbol{L}).$$

Proof The proof follows by applying Corollary 5.3, Theorem 6.10 and (4.120). □

Using Appendix B, Theorem B.23 (i) gives the dispersion of the approximating distribution.

Corollary 6.4 *Let* $\boldsymbol{K}\boldsymbol{R}_{2E}\boldsymbol{L}$ *be defined via* $f_{\boldsymbol{K}\boldsymbol{R}_{2E}\boldsymbol{L}}(\boldsymbol{K}\boldsymbol{R}_o\boldsymbol{L})$*, given in Theorem 6.11, where it is assumed that* $f_{\boldsymbol{K}\boldsymbol{R}_{2E}\boldsymbol{L}}(\boldsymbol{K}\boldsymbol{R}_o\boldsymbol{L}) \geq 0$*. Then*

(i) $E[\boldsymbol{K}\boldsymbol{R}_{2E}\boldsymbol{L}] = \boldsymbol{0}$;
(ii) $D[\boldsymbol{K}\boldsymbol{R}_{2E}\boldsymbol{L}] = \boldsymbol{L}'(\boldsymbol{I} - \boldsymbol{P}_{C'})\boldsymbol{L} \otimes \boldsymbol{K}(\boldsymbol{\Sigma}\boldsymbol{P}_{A_1^o,\Sigma^{-1}} + g_{1,1}\boldsymbol{P}_{A_1,\Sigma}\boldsymbol{\Sigma})\boldsymbol{K}'$,
where $g_{1,1}$ *is given in Theorem 4.15.*

Similar results to those presented above for $\boldsymbol{R}_2$ are now given for $\boldsymbol{R}_3$.

Theorem 6.12 *The distribution of the residual* $\boldsymbol{R}_3$*, given in (6.41), can be approximated through the difference*

$$\boldsymbol{R}_3 = \boldsymbol{R}_{3N} - \boldsymbol{U}_3,$$

where $\boldsymbol{R}_{3N}$ *and* $\boldsymbol{U}_3$ *are defined by (6.46) and (6.47), respectively. Let* $\boldsymbol{K}$*:* $p_1 \times p$ *and* $\boldsymbol{L}$*:* $n \times n_1$*, both of which are known, and*

$$\boldsymbol{K}\boldsymbol{R}_{3N}\boldsymbol{L} \sim N_{p_1,n_1}(\boldsymbol{0}, \boldsymbol{K}\boldsymbol{\Sigma}\boldsymbol{P}_{G_2',\Sigma^{-1}}\boldsymbol{K}', \boldsymbol{L}'(\boldsymbol{P}_{C_2'} - \boldsymbol{P}_{C_3'})\boldsymbol{L}).$$

Then an Edgeworth-type expansion $f_{\boldsymbol{KR}_{3E}\boldsymbol{L}}(\boldsymbol{KR}_o\boldsymbol{L})$ *of the density of* $\boldsymbol{KR}_3\boldsymbol{L}$*, via the density of* $\boldsymbol{KR}_{3N}\boldsymbol{L}$*, under the assumption that* $D[\boldsymbol{KR}_{3N}\boldsymbol{L}]$ *is p.d., is given by*

$$\begin{aligned} f_{\boldsymbol{KR}_{3E}\boldsymbol{L}}(\boldsymbol{KR}_o\boldsymbol{L}) &= \big\{1 - \tfrac{1}{2}n_1\mathrm{tr}\{\boldsymbol{K}(g_{1,2}\boldsymbol{K}_1 + g_{2,2}\boldsymbol{K}_2)\boldsymbol{K}'(\boldsymbol{K\Sigma P}_{G_2,\Sigma^{-1}}\boldsymbol{K}')^{-1}\} \\ &+ \tfrac{1}{2}\mathrm{tr}\big\{(\boldsymbol{K\Sigma P}_{G_2,\Sigma^{-1}}\boldsymbol{K}')^{-1}\boldsymbol{K}(g_{1,2}\boldsymbol{K}_1 + g_{2,2}\boldsymbol{K}_2)\boldsymbol{K}'(\boldsymbol{K\Sigma P}_{G_2,\Sigma^{-1}}\boldsymbol{K}')^{-1} \\ &\times \boldsymbol{KR}_o\boldsymbol{L}(\boldsymbol{L}'(\boldsymbol{P}_{C_2'} - \boldsymbol{P}_{C_3'})\boldsymbol{L})^{-1}\boldsymbol{L}'\boldsymbol{R}_o'\boldsymbol{K}'\big\}\big\} f_{\boldsymbol{KR}_{3N}\boldsymbol{L}}(\boldsymbol{KR}_o\boldsymbol{L}), \end{aligned}$$

where $g_{i,2}$ *is defined in Theorem 4.15 and* $\boldsymbol{K}_i$*,* $i = 1, 2$*, in Theorem 4.12.*

Corollary 6.5 *Let* $\boldsymbol{KR}_{3E}\boldsymbol{L}$ *be defined via* $f_{\boldsymbol{KR}_{3E}\boldsymbol{L}}(\boldsymbol{KR}_o\boldsymbol{L})$*, given in Theorem 6.12, where it is assumed that* $f_{\boldsymbol{KR}_{3E}\boldsymbol{L}}(\boldsymbol{KR}_o\boldsymbol{L}) \geq 0$*. Then*

(i) $E[\boldsymbol{KR}_{3E}\boldsymbol{L}] = \boldsymbol{0}$;
(ii) $D[\boldsymbol{KR}_{3E}\boldsymbol{L}] = \boldsymbol{L}'(\boldsymbol{P}_{C_2'} - \boldsymbol{P}_{C_3'})\boldsymbol{L} \otimes \boldsymbol{K}(\boldsymbol{\Sigma P}_{G_2,\Sigma^{-1}} + g_{1,2}\boldsymbol{K}_1 + g_{2,2}\boldsymbol{K}_2)\boldsymbol{K}'$.

Finally, $\boldsymbol{R}_4$ is considered.

Theorem 6.13 *The distribution of the residual* $\boldsymbol{R}_4$*, given in (6.42), can be approximated through the difference*

$$\boldsymbol{R}_4 = \boldsymbol{R}_{4N} - \boldsymbol{U}_4,$$

where $\boldsymbol{R}_{4N}$ *and* $\boldsymbol{U}_4$ *are defined by (6.48) and (6.49), respectively. Let* $\boldsymbol{K}$*:* $p_1 \times p$ *and* $\boldsymbol{L}$*:* $n \times n_1$*, both of which are known, and*

$$\boldsymbol{KR}_{4N}\boldsymbol{L} \sim N_{p_1,n_1}(\boldsymbol{0}, \boldsymbol{K\Sigma P}_{G_3',\Sigma^{-1}}\boldsymbol{K}', \boldsymbol{L}'\boldsymbol{P}_{C_3'}\boldsymbol{L}).$$

Then an Edgeworth-type expansion $f_{\boldsymbol{KR}_{4E}\boldsymbol{L}}(\boldsymbol{KR}_o\boldsymbol{L})$ *of the density of* $\boldsymbol{KR}_4\boldsymbol{L}$*, via the density of* $\boldsymbol{KR}_{4N}\boldsymbol{L}$*, under the assumption that* $D[\boldsymbol{KR}_{4N}\boldsymbol{L}]$ *is p.d., is given by*

$$\begin{aligned} f_{\boldsymbol{KR}_{4E}\boldsymbol{L}}(\boldsymbol{KR}_o\boldsymbol{L}) &= \big\{1 - \tfrac{1}{2}n_1\mathrm{tr}\{\boldsymbol{K}(g_{1,3}\boldsymbol{K}_1 + g_{2,3}\boldsymbol{K}_2 + g_{3,3}\boldsymbol{K}_3)\boldsymbol{K}'(\boldsymbol{K\Sigma P}_{G_3,\Sigma^{-1}}\boldsymbol{K}')^{-1}\} \\ &+ \tfrac{1}{2}\mathrm{tr}\big\{(\boldsymbol{K\Sigma P}_{A^o,\Sigma^{-1}}\boldsymbol{K}')^{-1}\boldsymbol{K}(g_{1,3}\boldsymbol{K}_1 + g_{2,3}\boldsymbol{K}_2 + g_{3,3}\boldsymbol{K}_3)\boldsymbol{K}'(\boldsymbol{K\Sigma P}_{A^o,\Sigma^{-1}}\boldsymbol{K}')^{-1} \\ &\times \boldsymbol{KR}_o\boldsymbol{L}(\boldsymbol{L}'\boldsymbol{P}_{C_3'}\boldsymbol{L})^{-1}\boldsymbol{L}'\boldsymbol{R}_o'\boldsymbol{K}'\big\}\big\} f_{\boldsymbol{KR}_{4N}\boldsymbol{L}}(\boldsymbol{KR}_o\boldsymbol{L}), \end{aligned}$$

where $g_{i,3}$ *is defined in Theorem 4.15 and* $\boldsymbol{K}_i$*,* $i = 1, 2, 3$*, in Theorem 4.12.*

Corollary 6.6 *Let* $\boldsymbol{KR}_{4E}\boldsymbol{L}$ *be defined via* $f_{\boldsymbol{KR}_{4E}\boldsymbol{L}}(\boldsymbol{KR}_o\boldsymbol{L})$*, given in Theorem 6.13, where it is assumed that* $f_{\boldsymbol{KR}_{4E}\boldsymbol{L}}(\boldsymbol{KR}_o\boldsymbol{L}) \geq 0$*. Then*

(i) $E[\boldsymbol{KR}_{4E}\boldsymbol{L}] = \boldsymbol{0}$;
(ii) $D[\boldsymbol{KR}_{4E}\boldsymbol{L}] = \boldsymbol{L}'\boldsymbol{P}_{C_3'}\boldsymbol{L} \otimes \boldsymbol{K}(\boldsymbol{\Sigma P}_{G_3,\Sigma^{-1}} + g_{1,3}\boldsymbol{K}_1 + g_{2,3}\boldsymbol{K}_2 + g_{3,3}\boldsymbol{K}_3)\boldsymbol{K}'$.

Hence, a basis for validating the residuals in the $EBRM_B^3$ has been established. As for the BRM, it is suggested that the validation should be carried out via mean shift tests. For the BRM five different tests have been suggested, see Sect. 6.1, although details have not been given for all of them. Here we have four different residuals and the task of constructing most of the possible alternative tests is left to the reader. The case which will be treated here is that where the mean shift is of the form $\boldsymbol{d}_j\theta\boldsymbol{e}_i'$.

Consider $\boldsymbol{R}_1 = \boldsymbol{X}(\boldsymbol{I} - \boldsymbol{P}_{\boldsymbol{C}_1'})$, which bears information on how columns (individuals) deviate from the average of the columns (individuals). The residual $\boldsymbol{R}_1$ is identical to $\boldsymbol{R}_1$ for the BRM, and all BRM-results connected to $\boldsymbol{R}_1$ can be copied. First we have to eliminate the singularity (see (6.37)), and thereafter the test statistic is presented which corresponds to the mean shift hypothesis in Theorem 6.9. As before, the parametric bootstrap is suggested for evaluating which elements in $\boldsymbol{R}_1$ are truly large.

Turning to $\boldsymbol{R}_2$, we also have a very similar quantity to $\boldsymbol{R}_2$, obtained from a BRM and presented in Definition 6.1 (ii). Thus, with minor modifications, i.e. changing $\boldsymbol{P}_{\boldsymbol{C}'}$ to $\boldsymbol{P}_{\boldsymbol{C}_1'} - \boldsymbol{P}_{\boldsymbol{C}_2'} = \boldsymbol{P}_{\boldsymbol{Q}\boldsymbol{C}_2'}$, $\boldsymbol{Q} = \boldsymbol{I} - \boldsymbol{P}_{\boldsymbol{C}_1'}$, one can use the same ideas as those used for the BRM and the same results as those obtained for the BRM. When further considering $\boldsymbol{R}_3$ and $\boldsymbol{R}_4$, one can use the same statistic as was used for $\boldsymbol{R}_2$, since the approximate likelihood in all cases will be of the same form. For example, see Theorems 6.11–6.13 and note that nothing unexpected happens when moving from $\boldsymbol{R}_2$ to $\boldsymbol{R}_3$ or $\boldsymbol{R}_4$. Thus, in the next theorem we can immediately summarize the appropriate test statistics for a relatively detailed residual analysis of the $EBRM_B^3$.

The same notation will be adopted as that used when working with the BRM, i.e.

$$\boldsymbol{R}_{k;ij}^N = \boldsymbol{K}\boldsymbol{d}_j\theta\boldsymbol{e}_i'\boldsymbol{L} + \boldsymbol{E}_k, \quad k = 1, 2, 3, 4.$$

The residual $\boldsymbol{R}_{k;ij}^N$ is the same as $\boldsymbol{R}_k^N = \boldsymbol{K}\boldsymbol{R}_k\boldsymbol{L}$, $k = 1, 2, 3, 4$, and, as before, ij only indicates which element is supposed to have a mean shift, while $\boldsymbol{R}_k^N$ is presented in (6.37) and (6.38) for $k = 1$ and $k = 2$, respectively, and for $k = 3, 4$ it will be defined in the following. The vectors $\boldsymbol{d}_j$ and $\boldsymbol{e}_i$ are unit basis vectors, θ is an unknown parameter, $\boldsymbol{E}_1 \sim N_{p,n_1}(\boldsymbol{0}, \boldsymbol{\Sigma}, \boldsymbol{I})$, and $\boldsymbol{E}_i$, $i = 2, 3, 4$, are defined through the densities in Theorems 6.11, 6.12 and 6.13, respectively. The matrices $\boldsymbol{K}$ and $\boldsymbol{L}$ depend also on k, $k = 1, 2, 3, 4$, and are chosen so that non-singular distributions are obtained. Finally, it is noted that $T_{k;ijo}$, $k = 1, 2, 3, 4$, represents the observed test statistic, $L_{k;ij}^N(\widehat{\theta})$ is the likelihood based on $\boldsymbol{E}_k$, and as $\widehat{\theta}$ the estimator $\widehat{\theta} = \boldsymbol{d}_j'\boldsymbol{R}_k\boldsymbol{e}_i$ is used, $L_{k;ij}$ is the likelihood under H_0, i.e. with no mean shift, and $\boldsymbol{R}_{ko}$ is the observed version of $\boldsymbol{R}_k$. In the likelihood, both under H_0 and H_1, the dispersion matrix has been replaced by $\widehat{\boldsymbol{\Sigma}}_o$, the maximum likelihood estimate, given in Theorem 3.2.

Theorem 6.14 *Consider $\boldsymbol{R}_i$, $i = 1, 2, 3, 4$, given in Definition 6.4.*

(i) *For $\boldsymbol{R}_1$ let*

$$\boldsymbol{R}_{1;ij}^N = \boldsymbol{d}_j\theta\boldsymbol{e}_i'\boldsymbol{L} + \boldsymbol{E}_1, \quad \boldsymbol{R}_{1;ij}^N = \boldsymbol{R}_1\boldsymbol{L}, \quad \boldsymbol{L} = \boldsymbol{V}(\boldsymbol{V}'\boldsymbol{V})^{-1}, \quad (\boldsymbol{I} - \boldsymbol{P}_{\boldsymbol{C}_1'}) = \boldsymbol{V}\boldsymbol{V}';$$

($\boldsymbol{V}$ is of full rank), $\quad \boldsymbol{E}_1 \sim N_{p,n_1}(\boldsymbol{0}, \boldsymbol{\Sigma}, \boldsymbol{I}_{n_1})$.

Then a test statistic for testing $H_0 : \theta = 0$ against $H_1 : \theta \neq 0$ is given by

$$T_{1;ijo} = \frac{(n - r(\boldsymbol{C}_1) - 1)\boldsymbol{d}'_j \boldsymbol{R}_{1o}(\boldsymbol{I} - \boldsymbol{P}_{C'_1})\boldsymbol{e}_i(\boldsymbol{e}'_i(\boldsymbol{I} - \boldsymbol{P}_{C'_1})\boldsymbol{e}_i)^{-1}\boldsymbol{e}'_i(\boldsymbol{I} - \boldsymbol{P}_{C'_1})\boldsymbol{R}'_{1o}\boldsymbol{d}_j}{\boldsymbol{d}'_j \boldsymbol{R}_{1o}(\boldsymbol{I} - \boldsymbol{P}_{C'_1})(\boldsymbol{I} - \boldsymbol{e}_i(\boldsymbol{e}'_i(\boldsymbol{I} - \boldsymbol{P}_{C'_1})\boldsymbol{e}_i)^{-1}\boldsymbol{e}'_i)(\boldsymbol{I} - \boldsymbol{P}_{C'_1})\boldsymbol{R}'_{1o}\boldsymbol{d}_j}.$$

(ii) *For $\boldsymbol{R}_2$ let*

$$\boldsymbol{R}^N_{2;ij} = \boldsymbol{K}\boldsymbol{d}_j\theta\boldsymbol{e}'_i\boldsymbol{L} + \boldsymbol{E}_2, \quad \boldsymbol{R}^N_{2;ij} = \boldsymbol{K}\boldsymbol{R}_2\boldsymbol{L}, \quad \boldsymbol{K} = (\boldsymbol{W}'\boldsymbol{W})^{-1}\boldsymbol{W}' \quad \boldsymbol{L} = \boldsymbol{V}(\boldsymbol{V}'\boldsymbol{V})^{-1},$$

$$(\boldsymbol{W} \text{ and } \boldsymbol{V} \text{ are of full rank}), \quad \widehat{\boldsymbol{\Sigma}}\boldsymbol{P}_{A_1^o,\widehat{\Sigma}^{-1}} = \boldsymbol{W}\boldsymbol{W}', \quad \boldsymbol{P}_{C'_1} - \boldsymbol{P}_{C'_2} = \boldsymbol{V}\boldsymbol{V}';$$

$\boldsymbol{E}_2$ has the approximating density given in Theorem 6.11. Then a test statistic for testing $H_0 : \theta = 0$ against $H_1 : \theta \neq 0$ is given by

$$T_{2;ijo} = \frac{L^N_{2;ij}(\widehat{\theta}_o)}{L^N_{2;ij}},$$

where $L^N_{2;ij}$ is the likelihood for $\boldsymbol{R}^N_2$ (obtained via $\boldsymbol{E}_2$) under H_0 and $L^N_{2;ij}(\widehat{\theta}_o)$ is obtained under H_1, with $\widehat{\theta}_o = \boldsymbol{d}'_j\boldsymbol{R}_{2o}\boldsymbol{e}_i$.

(iii) *For $\boldsymbol{R}_3$ let*

$$\boldsymbol{R}^N_{3;ij} = \boldsymbol{K}\boldsymbol{d}_j\theta\boldsymbol{e}'_i\boldsymbol{L} + \boldsymbol{E}_3, \quad \boldsymbol{R}^N_{3;ij} = \boldsymbol{K}\boldsymbol{R}_3\boldsymbol{L}, \quad \boldsymbol{K} = (\boldsymbol{W}'\boldsymbol{W})^{-1}\boldsymbol{W}', \quad \boldsymbol{L} = \boldsymbol{V}(\boldsymbol{V}'\boldsymbol{V})^{-1},$$

$$(\boldsymbol{W} \text{ and } \boldsymbol{V} \text{ are of full rank}), \quad \widehat{\boldsymbol{\Sigma}}\boldsymbol{P}_{G_2^o,\widehat{\Sigma}^{-1}} = \boldsymbol{W}\boldsymbol{W}', \quad \boldsymbol{P}_{C'_2} - \boldsymbol{P}_{C'_3} = \boldsymbol{V}\boldsymbol{V}';$$

$\boldsymbol{E}_3$ has the approximating density given in Theorem 6.12. Then a test statistic for testing $H_0 : \theta = 0$ against $H_1 : \theta \neq 0$ is given by

$$T_{3;ijo} = \frac{L^N_{3;ij}(\widehat{\theta}_o)}{L^N_{3;ij}},$$

where $L^N_{3;ij}$ is the likelihood for $\boldsymbol{R}^N_3$ (obtained via $\boldsymbol{E}_3$) under H_0 and $L^N_{3;ij}(\widehat{\theta}_o)$ is the likelihood under H_1 with $\widehat{\theta}_o = \boldsymbol{d}'_j\boldsymbol{R}_{3o}\boldsymbol{e}_i$.

(iv) *For $\boldsymbol{R}_4$ let*

$$\boldsymbol{R}^N_{4;ij} = \boldsymbol{K}\boldsymbol{d}_j\theta\boldsymbol{e}'_i\boldsymbol{L} + \boldsymbol{E}_4, \quad \boldsymbol{R}^N_{4;ij} = \boldsymbol{K}\boldsymbol{R}_4\boldsymbol{L}, \quad \boldsymbol{K} = (\boldsymbol{W}'\boldsymbol{W})^{-1}\boldsymbol{W}' \quad \boldsymbol{L} = \boldsymbol{V}(\boldsymbol{V}'\boldsymbol{V})^{-1},$$

$$(\boldsymbol{W} \text{ and } \boldsymbol{V} \text{ are of full rank}), \quad \widehat{\boldsymbol{\Sigma}}\boldsymbol{P}_{G_3^o,\widehat{\Sigma}^{-1}} = \boldsymbol{W}\boldsymbol{W}', \quad \boldsymbol{P}_{C'_3} = \boldsymbol{V}\boldsymbol{V}';$$

$\boldsymbol{E}_4$ has the approximating density given in Theorem 6.13. Then a test statistic for testing $H_0 : \theta = 0$ against $H_1 : \theta \neq 0$ is given by

$$T_{4;ijo} = \frac{L^N_{4;ij}(\widehat{\theta}_o)}{L^N_{4;ij}},$$

where $L_{4;ij}^N$ is the likelihood for $L_{4;ij}^N$ (obtained via $\boldsymbol{E}_4$) under H_0 and $\boldsymbol{R}_4^N(\widehat{\theta_o})$ is obtained under H_1, with $\widehat{\theta_o} = \boldsymbol{d}'_j \boldsymbol{R}_{4o} \boldsymbol{e}_i$.

To finalize the residual analysis, one has to take care of the large residuals, i.e. those residuals which significantly deviate from the other residuals, for example when testing hypotheses. A pure data analysis approach is suggested for determining the distribution of these large/largest residuals; i.e. $\boldsymbol{X}_o$ is simulated from $N_{p,n_1}(\boldsymbol{0}, \widehat{\boldsymbol{\Sigma}}_o, \boldsymbol{I})$, which can then be used to generate the residuals and thereby the largest values of the residuals, as well as the distributions of the large/largest residuals. The estimate $\widehat{\boldsymbol{\Sigma}}_o$ is for example the observed maximum likelihood estimator, presented in Theorem 3.2.

This section is concluded by an example which shows how the residuals $\boldsymbol{R}_i$, $i = 1, 2, 3, 4$, can be utilized when evaluating an $EBRM_B^3$.

Example 6.7 In this example the aim is to demonstrate how outlying observations will show up in the residuals $\boldsymbol{R}_i$, $i = 1, 2, 3, 4$, presented in Definition 6.4, and not to present a residual analysis where the distribution of the largest residuals is investigated. The approach is completely in line with what was performed with the BRM. Consider the model presented in Example 1.9. Based on the given design and parameter matrices, a data matrix $\boldsymbol{X}: 10 \times 45$ can be generated. Here in Example 6.7 some values are replaced by outlying observations. The effect of the contamination is studied with the help of the absolute difference $m_{k;ij}$, defined as

$$m_{k;ij} = |\boldsymbol{d}'_j(\widetilde{\boldsymbol{R}}_{ko} - \boldsymbol{R}_{ko})\boldsymbol{e}_i|, k = 1, 2, 3, 4, j = 1, 2, \ldots p_k, i = 1, 2, \ldots n_k, \tag{6.50}$$

where $\boldsymbol{d}_j$ and $\boldsymbol{e}_i$ are unit basis vectors of proper size, i.e. depend on p_k and n_k, which in turn are given by the size of $\boldsymbol{R}_{ko}$, $\widetilde{\boldsymbol{R}}_{ko}$ is the observed residual based on the manipulated data and $\boldsymbol{R}_{ko}$ is the observed residual for the original data. To summarize the difference $\widetilde{\boldsymbol{R}}_{ko} - \boldsymbol{R}_{ko}$, for example, the following three measures can be used: m_k^1, the absolute largest difference, i.e. $m_k^1 = \max_{ij}\{m_{k;ij}\}$, m_k^2, the second largest difference and m_k^3, the third largest difference.

Before calculating (6.50), in this example it is relatively easy to interpret the four residuals and it is suggested that this is carried out before doing explicit calculations. The main issue is to understand $\mathcal{C}(\boldsymbol{P}_{C'_1} - \boldsymbol{P}_{C'_2})$, $\mathcal{C}(\boldsymbol{P}_{C'_2} - \boldsymbol{P}_{C'_3})$ and $\mathcal{C}(\boldsymbol{P}_{C'_3})$, and then relate, in this example, these spaces to the different groups of individuals. Note that

$$\boldsymbol{C}_1 = \begin{pmatrix} \boldsymbol{1}'_{10} & \boldsymbol{0} & \boldsymbol{0} \\ \boldsymbol{0} & \boldsymbol{1}'_{15} & \boldsymbol{0} \\ \boldsymbol{0} & \boldsymbol{0} & \boldsymbol{1}'_{20} \end{pmatrix}, \quad \boldsymbol{C}_2 = \begin{pmatrix} \boldsymbol{1}'_{10} & \boldsymbol{0} & \boldsymbol{0} \\ \boldsymbol{0} & \boldsymbol{1}'_{15} & \boldsymbol{0} \end{pmatrix}, \quad \boldsymbol{C}_3 = \begin{pmatrix} \boldsymbol{1}'_{10} & \boldsymbol{0} & \boldsymbol{0} \end{pmatrix}.$$

Then

$$\mathcal{C}(\boldsymbol{P}_{C_1'} - \boldsymbol{P}_{C_2'}) = \mathcal{C}(\boldsymbol{C}_1') \cap \mathcal{C}(\boldsymbol{C}_2')^{\perp} = \mathcal{C}((\boldsymbol{0} : \boldsymbol{0} : \boldsymbol{1}_{20}')'),$$
$$\mathcal{C}(\boldsymbol{P}_{C_2'} - \boldsymbol{P}_{C_3'}) = \mathcal{C}(\boldsymbol{C}_2') \cap \mathcal{C}(\boldsymbol{C}_3')^{\perp} = \mathcal{C}((\boldsymbol{0} : \boldsymbol{1}_{15}' : \boldsymbol{0})'),$$
$$\mathcal{C}(\boldsymbol{P}_{C_3'}) = \mathcal{C}((\boldsymbol{1}_{10}' : \boldsymbol{0} : \boldsymbol{0})').$$

Hence, $\boldsymbol{P}_{C_1'} - \boldsymbol{P}_{C_2'}$ is connected to the third group, $\boldsymbol{P}_{C_2'} - \boldsymbol{P}_{C_3'}$ is connected to the second group and $\boldsymbol{P}_{C_3'}$ is connected to the first group, and these three facts can constitute the basis in any residual analysis.

As before, $\boldsymbol{R}_1$ shows the difference between individuals and the "group means". The residual $\boldsymbol{R}_2$ indicates if the third group can be described by the parameters in $\boldsymbol{B}_1$, since $\boldsymbol{P}_{C_1'} - \boldsymbol{P}_{C_2'}$ is a projection of the individuals in the third group, with $\boldsymbol{X}(\boldsymbol{P}_{C_1'} - \boldsymbol{P}_{C_2'})$ being the "mean" which is then compared to the model $\boldsymbol{P}_{A_1,S_1}\boldsymbol{X}(\boldsymbol{P}_{C_1'} - \boldsymbol{P}_{C_2'})$. The residual $\boldsymbol{R}_3$ indicates if the second group is described by the parameters in $\boldsymbol{B}_1$ and $\boldsymbol{B}_2$, and $\boldsymbol{R}_4$ can be used to determine whether the first group follows the proposed model, i.e. whether the complete set of parameters, $\boldsymbol{B}_1$, $\boldsymbol{B}_2$ and $\boldsymbol{B}_3$, describes the data. Indeed, it is interesting to note that by studying the different residuals, quite a large amount of information on the model fit can be obtained.

Let us first perturb one single observation in $\boldsymbol{X}_o$. In order to highlight the consequences, the choices are all extreme:

$$\mathrm{P}_{(\mathrm{i})}: \text{ add 60 to } (X_{5,30}); \quad \mathrm{P}_{(\mathrm{ii})}: \text{ add60 to } (X_{5,15}); \quad \mathrm{P}_{(\mathrm{iii})}: \text{ add 60 to } (X_{5,5}).$$

Note that the above perturbed observations in $\mathrm{P}_{(\mathrm{i})}$, $\mathrm{P}_{(\mathrm{ii})}$ and $\mathrm{P}_{(\mathrm{iii})}$ belong to different groups. According to Table 6.13, all three perturbations show up very clearly in $\widetilde{\boldsymbol{R}}_{1o}$. Moreover, $\mathrm{P}_{(\mathrm{i})}$, which is a modification of an observation in group 3, is also visible in $\widetilde{\boldsymbol{R}}_{2o}$, i.e. the residuals connected to group 3 are affected. Concerning $\mathrm{P}_{(\mathrm{ii})}$, the effect of the perturbation, besides showing up in $\widetilde{\boldsymbol{R}}_{1o}$, appears in $\widetilde{\boldsymbol{R}}_{3o}$ (i.e. residuals connected to group 2 are affected), and for $\mathrm{P}_{(\mathrm{iii})}$ the residual $\widetilde{\boldsymbol{R}}_{4o}$ is highlighted, which means that group 1 is influenced. Thus the residuals behave as expected and it seems that a residual analysis based on single observations has the possibility of strengthening the statistical analysis.

Another type of perturbation occurs when the mean for an individual is shifted, i.e. all the observations of an individual are altered with the same value:

$$\mathrm{P}_{(\mathrm{iv})}: \text{ add 60 to the elements in } \boldsymbol{x}_{30} \ (\boldsymbol{x}_{30} \text{ stands for the } 30th \text{ column of } \boldsymbol{X}_o);$$
$$\mathrm{P}_{(\mathrm{v})}: \text{ add 60 to the elements in } \boldsymbol{x}_{15}; \quad \mathrm{P}_{(\mathrm{vi})}: \text{ add 60 to the elements in } \boldsymbol{x}_5.$$

The different perturbed individuals given in $\mathrm{P}_{(\mathrm{iv})}$, $\mathrm{P}_{(\mathrm{v})}$ and $\mathrm{P}_{(\mathrm{vi})}$ belong, as do those in $\mathrm{P}_{(\mathrm{i})}$, $\mathrm{P}_{(\mathrm{ii})}$ and $\mathrm{P}_{(\mathrm{iii})}$, to different groups. From Table 6.13 it follows that the outlying observations are visible only in $\widetilde{\boldsymbol{R}}_{1o}$ and it does not seem that there is any information in $\widetilde{\boldsymbol{R}}_{2o}$, $\widetilde{\boldsymbol{R}}_{3o}$ and $\widetilde{\boldsymbol{R}}_{4o}$. This is, however, expected, because in $\boldsymbol{A}_1$

Table 6.13 The largest value m_k^1, and the second largest value m_k^2, defined via (6.50), are calculated for the perturbations $P_{(i)}$–$P_{(vi)}$ in the model considered in Example 6.7

	$\widetilde{R}_{1o}$		$\widetilde{R}_{2o}$		$\widetilde{R}_{3o}$		$\widetilde{R}_{4o}$	
	Value	Obs	Value	Obs	Value	Obs	Value	Obs
	The largest value, m_k^1							
$P_{(i)}$	57	$X_{5,30}$	3	$X_{5,26-45}$	$*$	$**$	$*$	$**$
$P_{(ii)}$	56	$X_{5,15}$	$*$	$**$	4	$X_{5,11-25}$	$*$	$**$
$P_{(iii)}$	54	$X_{5,5}$	$*$	$**$	$*$	$**$	6	$X_{5,1-10}$
$P_{(iv)}$	57	$X_{1-10,30}$	$*$	$**$	$*$	$**$	$*$	$**$
$P_{(v)}$	56	$X_{1-10,15}$	$*$	$**$	$*$	$**$	$*$	$**$
$P_{(vi)}$	54	$X_{1-10,5}$	$*$	$**$	$*$	$**$	$*$	$**$
	The second largest value, m_k^2							
$P_{(i)}$	3	$X_{5;26-29,31-45}$	$*$	$**$	$*$	$**$	$*$	$**$
$P_{(ii)}$	4	$X_{5;11-14,16-25}$	$*$	$**$	$*$	$**$	$*$	$**$
$P_{(iii)}$	6	$X_{5;1-4,6-10}$	$*$	$**$	$*$	$**$	$*$	$**$
$P_{(iv)}$	3	$X_{1-10;25-29,31-45}$	$*$	$**$	$*$	$**$	$*$	$**$
$P_{(v)}$	4	$X_{1-10;11-14,16-25}$	$*$	$**$	$*$	$**$	$*$	$**$
$P_{(vi)}$	6	$X_{1-10;1-4,6-10}$	$*$	$**$	$*$	$**$	$*$	$**$

In the table "Value" stands for the value of m_k^i and "Obs" for the observation which it concerns. If there is only one observation, $X_{i,j}$ is used, and if all the rows between k and l for the jth observation are included, then $X_{k-l,j}$ is used. If a given row and a sequence of observations are included, then $X_{i,k-l}$ is used, and if two sequences of columns have to be indicated, then $X_{i;k_1-l_1,k_2-l_2}$ is used. Moreover, "$*$" means that the value < 1.5, and in this case "$**$" indicates that no specific observation is highlighted

(see Example 1.9) the first column equals $\mathbf{1}_{10}$ and thus, when all the observations of an individual are shifted with the same amount, this will take place within the regression space which is orthogonal to the residual space, i.e. the basis for the residuals. Moreover, in Table 6.13 there is a threshold of 1.5. The reason for introducing it is that there are some small effects on several observations, but these effects appear due to the estimated weights used in the projections and are not really related to the mean shift of the residual. However, if the weights play a key role in the analysis, then thresholding may not be appropriate. □

6.7 Residuals for the $EBRM_W^3$

This section consists of a suggested residual analysis for the $EBRM_W^3$ which follows very closely the residual analysis for the $EBRM_B^3$, considered in Sect. 6.6. The procedure for the proposed residual analysis for the $EBRM_W^3$ is the same as that for the $EBRM_B^3$ (see Fig. 6.4), but includes some changes of the spaces defining the tensor products.

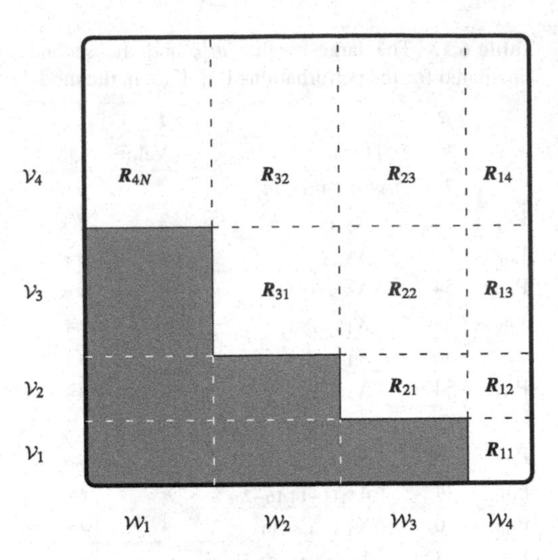

Fig. 6.5 Decomposition of the whole space according to the within-individuals and the between-individuals designs, illustrating the mean and residual spaces in the $EBRM_W^3$: $\mathcal{V}_1 = \mathcal{C}_\Sigma(A_3)$, $\mathcal{V}_2 = \mathcal{C}_\Sigma(A_2) \cap \mathcal{C}_\Sigma(A_3)^\perp$, $\mathcal{V}_3 = \mathcal{C}_\Sigma(A_1) \cap \mathcal{C}_\Sigma(A_2)^\perp$, $\mathcal{V}_4 = \mathcal{C}_\Sigma(A_1)^\perp$, $\mathcal{W}_1 = \mathcal{C}(C_1')$, $\mathcal{W}_2 = \mathcal{C}(C_1' : C_2') \cap \mathcal{C}(C_1')^\perp$, $\mathcal{W}_3 = \mathcal{C}(C_1' : C_2' : C_3') \cap \mathcal{C}(C_1' : C_2')^\perp$, $\mathcal{W}_4 = \mathcal{C}(C_1' : C_2' : C_3')^\perp$

As was suggested for the $EBRM_B^3$, the proposed residuals in Fig. 6.5, i.e. R_{ij}, will be merged:

(i) $R_{1N} = R_{11} + R_{12} + R_{13} + R_{14}$;
(ii) $R_{2N} = R_{21} + R_{22} + R_{23}$;
(iii) $R_{3N} = R_{31} + R_{32}$;
(iv) $R_{4N} = R_{4N}$.

Moreover, explicit expressions for any given Σ can be obtained by projecting X on $\mathcal{W}_i \otimes \mathcal{V}_j$, $i \leq j$, i.e. $R_{5-i,j} = (P_{\mathcal{W}_i} \otimes P_{\mathcal{V}_j,\Sigma})\text{vec}X$. To handle the case of an unknown Σ, Theorem 3.3 is applied, where, in particular, several of the matrices utilized below are identified, i.e.

$$\begin{aligned}
X - \widehat{E[X]} &= X - P_{A_1,\widehat{S}_3} X P_{C_1'} - P_{A_2,\widehat{S}_2} X P_{Q_1 C_2'} - P_{A_3,S_1} X P_{Q_2 C_3'} \\
&= X(I - P_{C_1'} - P_{Q_1 C_2'} - P_{Q_2 C_3'}) + (I - P_{A_1,\widehat{S}_3}) \\
&\quad + X P_{C_1'} + (I - P_{A_2,\widehat{S}_2}) X P_{Q_1 C_2'} + (I - P_{A_3,S_1}) X P_{Q_2 C_3'},
\end{aligned}$$

where, according to the projection theorem (see Appendix B, Theorem B.11 (iv))

$$\begin{aligned}
&\mathcal{C}(C_1' : C_2' : C_3') = \mathcal{C}(C_1') + \mathcal{C}(Q_1 C_2') + \mathcal{C}(Q_2 C_3'), \\
&\mathcal{C}(Q_1 C_2') = \mathcal{C}(C_1')^\perp \cap \mathcal{C}(C_1' : C_2'), \\
&\mathcal{C}(Q_2 C_3') = \mathcal{C}(C_1' : C_2')^\perp \cap \mathcal{C}(C_1' : C_2' : C_3').
\end{aligned}$$

These spaces are illustrated in Fig. 6.5 and it makes sense to define the four residuals given in the next definition.

Definition 6.5 Let S_1, $\widehat{S}_i$, $i = 2, 3$, and Q_i, $i = 1, 2, 3$, be as in Theorem 3.3. For the $EBRM_W^3$ the following residuals will be considered:

(i) $R_1 = X(I - P_{C_1':C_2':C_3'})$;
(ii) $R_2 = (I - P_{A_3,S_1})XP_{Q_2C_3'}$;
(iii) $R_3 = (I - P_{A_2,\widehat{S}_2})XP_{Q_1C_2'}$;
(iv) $R_4 = (I - P_{A_1,\widehat{S}_3})XP_{C_1'}$.

The residuals presented in Definitions 6.4 and 6.5 are identical in the following sense: if starting with an $EBRM_B^3$ and applying the transformation in Sect. 3.5, which yielded an $EBRM_W^3$, then inserting the transformed matrices in Definition 6.5 will give the same residuals as when the original matrices are inserted in Definition 6.4. Thus, in principle, it is enough to study either the $EBRM_B^3$ or the $EBRM_W^3$, although it is mostly beneficial to investigate the "original" model in the "original" matrices.

A common inner product for all the projectors presented in Definition 6.5 can be based on either $\widehat{S}_3$ or $\widehat{\Sigma}$, since, for example,

$$A_3'S_1^{-1} = A_3'\widehat{S}_2^{-1} = A_3'\widehat{S}_3^{-1}, \quad A_2'\widehat{S}_2^{-1} = A_2'\widehat{S}_3^{-1}.$$

Moreover, R_1 is normally distributed, similar to R_1 in the $EBRM_B^3$, which in turn was similarly distributed to R_1 in the BRM. Hence, most attention will be focused on R_2, R_3 and R_4. Now,

(i) S_1 is independent of XQ_2C_3', XQ_1C_2' and XC_1';
(ii) $\widehat{S}_2$ is independent of XQ_1C_2' and XC_1';
(iii) $\widehat{S}_3$ is independent of XC_1'.

Hence, because $\mathcal{C}(A_3) \subseteq \mathcal{C}(A_2) \subseteq \mathcal{C}(A_1)$, $E[R_i] = \mathbf{0}$, $i = 2, 3, 4$. The dispersion matrices of the different residuals follow from the next theorem.

Theorem 6.15 *Let R_2, R_3 and R_4 be as in Definition 6.5. Then*

(i) $D[R_2] = P_{Q_2C_3'} \otimes E[P'_{A_3^o,S_1^{-1}}\Sigma P_{A_3^o,S_1^{-1}}]$, *where* $E[P'_{A_3^o,S_1^{-1}}\Sigma P_{A_3^o,S_1^{-1}}]$ *is given in Theorem 4.23;*
(ii) $D[R_3] = P_{Q_1C_2'} \otimes E[P'_{A_2^o,\widehat{S}_2^{-1}}\Sigma P_{A_2^o,\widehat{S}_2^{-1}}]$, *where* $E[P'_{A_2^o,\widehat{S}_2^{-1}}\Sigma P_{A_2^o,\widehat{S}_2^{-1}}]$ *is given in Theorem 4.23;*
(iii) $D[R_4] = P_{C_1'} \otimes E[P'_{A_1^o,\widehat{S}_3^{-1}}\Sigma P_{A_1^o,\widehat{S}_3^{-1}}]$, *where* $E[P'_{A_1^o,\widehat{S}_3^{-1}}\Sigma P_{A_1^o,\widehat{S}_3^{-1}}]$ *is given in Theorem 4.23;*
(iv) $C[R_1, R_2] = C[R_1, R_3] = C[R_1, R_4] = \mathbf{0}$; $C[R_2, R_3] = C[R_2, R_4] = \mathbf{0}$; $C[R_3, R_4] = \mathbf{0}$.

Following the presentation for the $EBRM_B^3$, the next issue will be to prepare for Edgeworth-type approximations; i.e. it is noted that

$$R_2 = R_{2N} - U_2, \quad R_3 = R_{3N} - U_3, \quad R_4 = R_{4N} - U_4, \tag{6.51}$$

where

$$R_{2N} = (I - P_{A_3,\Sigma})XP_{Q_2C_3'}, \quad U_2 = (P_{A_3,S_1} - P_{A_3,\Sigma})XP_{Q_2C_3'}, \tag{6.52}$$

$$R_{3N} = (I - P_{A_2,\Sigma})XP_{Q_1C_2'}, \quad U_3 = (P_{A_2,\widehat{S}_2} - P_{A_2,\Sigma})XP_{Q_1C_2'}, \tag{6.53}$$

$$R_{4N} = (I - P_{A_1,\Sigma})XP_{C_1'}, \quad U_4 = (P_{A_1,\widehat{S}_3} - P_{A_1,\Sigma})XP_{C_1'}. \tag{6.54}$$

The residuals R_{2N}, R_{3N} and R_{4N} are all normally distributed. Furthermore, $E[U_2] = E[U_3] = E[U_4] = \mathbf{0}$ and $C[R_{iN}, U_i] = \mathbf{0}$, $i = 1, 2, 3, 4$, hold and are established by direct calculations. Hence, by referring to Corollary 5.3, several results can be proven when combining it with Theorem 6.15 (i)–(iii). In the results given below we assume that the sample size is large enough for the included constants to exist.

Theorem 6.16 *The distribution of the residual R_2, given in Definition 6.5 (ii), can be approximated through the difference*

$$R_2 = R_{2N} - U_2,$$

where R_{2N} and U_2 are defined by (6.52). Let K: $p_1 \times p$ and L: $n \times n_1$, both of which are known, and

$$KR_{2N}L \sim N_{p_1,n_1}(\mathbf{0}, K\Sigma P_{A_3^o,\Sigma^{-1}}K', L'P_{Q_2C_3'}L).$$

Then an Edgeworth-type expansion $f_{KR_{2E}L}(KR_oL)$ of the density of KR_2L, via the density of $KR_{2N}L$, under the assumption that $D[KR_{2N}L]$ is p.d., is given by

$$\begin{aligned} f_{KR_{2E}L}(KR_oL) = \big\{1 + \tfrac{1}{2}n_1p_1 - \tfrac{1}{2}\mathrm{tr}\{D[KR_2L](D[KR_{2N}L])^{-1}\} \\ -\tfrac{1}{2}\mathrm{tr}\big\{(D[KR_{2N}L])^{-1}(D[KR_2L] - D[KR_{2N}L])(D[KR_{2N}L])^{-1} \\ \times\mathrm{vec}(KR_oL)\mathrm{vec}'(KR_oL)\big\}\big\} f_{KR_{2N}L}(KR_oL), \end{aligned}$$

where

$$\begin{aligned} D[KR_2L] &= L'P_{Q_2C_3'}L \otimes \big(\tfrac{p-r(A_3)}{n-r(C_1':C_2':C_3')-p+r(A_3)-1}KA_3(A_3'\Sigma^{-1}A_3)^-A_3'K \\ &\quad +KA_3^o(A_3^{o'}\Sigma A_3^o)^-A_3^{o'}K'\big), \\ D[KR_{2N}L] &= L'P_{Q_2C_3'}L \otimes K\Sigma A_3^o(A_3^{o'}\Sigma A_3^o)^-A_3^{o'}\Sigma K'. \end{aligned}$$

Using Theorem B.23 (i) in Appendix B gives the dispersion of the approximating distribution.

Corollary 6.7 *Let $\boldsymbol{K}\boldsymbol{R}_{2E}\boldsymbol{L}$ be defined via $f_{\boldsymbol{K}\boldsymbol{R}_{2E}\boldsymbol{L}}(\boldsymbol{K}\boldsymbol{R}_o\boldsymbol{L})$, given in Theorem 6.16, where it is assumed that $f_{\boldsymbol{K}\boldsymbol{R}_{2E}\boldsymbol{L}}(\boldsymbol{K}\boldsymbol{R}_o\boldsymbol{L}) \geq 0$. Then*

(i) $E[\boldsymbol{K}\boldsymbol{R}_{2E}\boldsymbol{L}] = \boldsymbol{0}$;
(ii) $D[\boldsymbol{K}\boldsymbol{R}_{2E}\boldsymbol{L}] = t\boldsymbol{N} \otimes \boldsymbol{M} - \frac{1}{2}n_1\mathrm{tr}\{\boldsymbol{M}^{-1}(\boldsymbol{M}_1 - \boldsymbol{M})\}\boldsymbol{N} \otimes \boldsymbol{M} - \boldsymbol{N} \otimes (\boldsymbol{M}_1 - \boldsymbol{M})$, *where*

$$
\begin{aligned}
t &= 1 + \tfrac{1}{2}n_1p_1 - \tfrac{1}{2}\mathrm{tr}\{D[\boldsymbol{K}\boldsymbol{R}_2\boldsymbol{L}](D[\boldsymbol{K}\boldsymbol{R}_{2N}\boldsymbol{L}])^{-1}\},\\
\boldsymbol{M} &= \boldsymbol{K}\boldsymbol{\Sigma}\boldsymbol{A}_3^o(\boldsymbol{A}_3^{o\prime}\boldsymbol{\Sigma}\boldsymbol{A}_3^o)^-\boldsymbol{A}_3^{o\prime}\boldsymbol{\Sigma}\boldsymbol{K}',\\
\boldsymbol{M}_1 &= \tfrac{p-r(\boldsymbol{A}_3)}{n-r(\boldsymbol{C}_1':\boldsymbol{C}_2':\boldsymbol{C}_3')-p+r(\boldsymbol{A}_3)-1}\boldsymbol{K}\boldsymbol{A}_3(\boldsymbol{A}_3'\boldsymbol{\Sigma}^{-1}\boldsymbol{A}_3)^-\boldsymbol{A}_3'\boldsymbol{K}\\
&\quad +\boldsymbol{K}\boldsymbol{A}_3^o(\boldsymbol{A}_3^{o\prime}\boldsymbol{\Sigma}\boldsymbol{A}_3^o)^-\boldsymbol{A}_3^{o\prime}\boldsymbol{K}',\\
\boldsymbol{N} &= \boldsymbol{L}'\boldsymbol{P}_{\boldsymbol{Q}_2\boldsymbol{C}_3'}\boldsymbol{L};
\end{aligned}
$$

$D[\boldsymbol{K}\boldsymbol{R}_2\boldsymbol{L}]$ and $D[\boldsymbol{K}\boldsymbol{R}_{2N}\boldsymbol{L}]$ are presented in Theorem 6.16.

Now the Edgeworth-type expansion for $\boldsymbol{R}_3$ is stated.

Theorem 6.17 *The distribution of the residual $\boldsymbol{R}_3$, given in Definition 6.5 (iii), can be approximated through the difference*

$$
\boldsymbol{R}_3 = \boldsymbol{R}_{3N} - \boldsymbol{U}_3,
$$

where $\boldsymbol{R}_{3N}$ and $\boldsymbol{U}_3$ are defined by (6.53). Let $\boldsymbol{K}$: $p_1 \times p$ and $\boldsymbol{L}$: $n \times n_1$, both of which are known, and

$$
\boldsymbol{K}\boldsymbol{R}_{3N}\boldsymbol{L} \sim N_{p_1,n_1}(\boldsymbol{0}, \boldsymbol{K}\boldsymbol{\Sigma}\boldsymbol{P}_{\boldsymbol{A}_2^o,\boldsymbol{\Sigma}^{-1}}\boldsymbol{K}', \boldsymbol{L}'\boldsymbol{P}_{\boldsymbol{Q}_1\boldsymbol{C}_2'}\boldsymbol{L}).
$$

Then an Edgeworth-type expansion $f_{\boldsymbol{K}\boldsymbol{R}_{3E}\boldsymbol{L}}(\boldsymbol{K}\boldsymbol{R}_o\boldsymbol{L})$ of the density of $\boldsymbol{K}\boldsymbol{R}_3\boldsymbol{L}$, via the density of $\boldsymbol{K}\boldsymbol{R}_{3N}\boldsymbol{L}$, under the assumption that $D[\boldsymbol{K}\boldsymbol{R}_{3N}\boldsymbol{L}]$ is p.d., is given by

$$
\begin{aligned}
f_{\boldsymbol{K}\boldsymbol{R}_{3E}\boldsymbol{L}}(\boldsymbol{K}\boldsymbol{R}_o\boldsymbol{L}) &= \big\{1 + \tfrac{1}{2}n_1p_1 - \tfrac{1}{2}\mathrm{tr}\{D[\boldsymbol{K}\boldsymbol{R}_3\boldsymbol{L}](D[\boldsymbol{K}\boldsymbol{R}_{3N}\boldsymbol{L}])^{-1}\}\\
&\quad -\tfrac{1}{2}\mathrm{tr}\big\{(D[\boldsymbol{K}\boldsymbol{R}_{3N}\boldsymbol{L}])^{-1}(D[\boldsymbol{K}\boldsymbol{R}_3\boldsymbol{L}] - D[\boldsymbol{K}\boldsymbol{R}_{3N}\boldsymbol{L}])(D[\boldsymbol{K}\boldsymbol{R}_{3N}\boldsymbol{L}])^{-1}\\
&\qquad \times\mathrm{vec}(\boldsymbol{K}\boldsymbol{R}_o\boldsymbol{L})\mathrm{vec}'(\boldsymbol{K}\boldsymbol{R}_o\boldsymbol{L})\big\}\big\}f_{\boldsymbol{K}\boldsymbol{R}_{3N}\boldsymbol{L}}(\boldsymbol{K}\boldsymbol{R}_o\boldsymbol{L}),
\end{aligned}
$$

where

$$
\begin{aligned}
D[\boldsymbol{K}\boldsymbol{R}_3\boldsymbol{L}] &= \boldsymbol{L}'\boldsymbol{P}_{\boldsymbol{Q}_1\boldsymbol{C}_2'}\boldsymbol{L}\otimes\big(\boldsymbol{K}\boldsymbol{A}_2^o(\boldsymbol{A}_2^{o\prime}\boldsymbol{\Sigma}\boldsymbol{A}_2^o)^{-1}\boldsymbol{A}_2^{o\prime}\boldsymbol{K}' + \boldsymbol{K}\boldsymbol{A}_3(\boldsymbol{A}_3'\boldsymbol{\Sigma}^{-1}\boldsymbol{A}_3)^-\boldsymbol{A}_3'\boldsymbol{K}'\\
&\quad +c_1\boldsymbol{K}\boldsymbol{P}'_{\boldsymbol{A}_3^o,\boldsymbol{\Sigma}^{-1}}\boldsymbol{A}_2(\boldsymbol{A}_2'\boldsymbol{\Sigma}^{-1}\boldsymbol{A}_2)^{-1}\boldsymbol{A}_2'\boldsymbol{P}_{\boldsymbol{A}_3^o,\boldsymbol{\Sigma}^{-1}}\boldsymbol{K}'\\
&\quad +c_1c_2\boldsymbol{K}\boldsymbol{A}_3(\boldsymbol{A}_3'\boldsymbol{\Sigma}^{-1}\boldsymbol{A}_3)^-\boldsymbol{A}_3'\boldsymbol{K}'\big),\\
D[\boldsymbol{K}\boldsymbol{R}_{3N}\boldsymbol{L}] &= \boldsymbol{L}'\boldsymbol{P}_{\boldsymbol{Q}_1\boldsymbol{C}_2'}\boldsymbol{L}\otimes\boldsymbol{K}\boldsymbol{\Sigma}\boldsymbol{A}_2^o(\boldsymbol{A}_2^{o\prime}\boldsymbol{\Sigma}\boldsymbol{A}_2^o)^-\boldsymbol{A}_2^{o\prime}\boldsymbol{\Sigma}\boldsymbol{K}',
\end{aligned}
$$

with c_1 and c_2 defined in Lemma 4.6 (ii).

Corollary 6.8 *Let $\boldsymbol{K R}_{3E}\boldsymbol{L}$ be defined via $f_{\boldsymbol{K R}_{3E}\boldsymbol{L}}(\boldsymbol{K R}_o\boldsymbol{L})$, given in Theorem 6.12, where it is assumed that $f_{\boldsymbol{K R}_{3E}\boldsymbol{L}}(\boldsymbol{K R}_o\boldsymbol{L}) \geq 0$. Then*

(i) $E[\boldsymbol{K R}_{3E}\boldsymbol{L}] = \boldsymbol{0}$;
(ii) $D[\boldsymbol{K R}_{3E}\boldsymbol{L}] = t\boldsymbol{N} \otimes \boldsymbol{M} - \frac{1}{2}n_1\mathrm{tr}\{\boldsymbol{M}^{-1}(\boldsymbol{M}_1 - \boldsymbol{M})\}\boldsymbol{N} \otimes \boldsymbol{M} - \boldsymbol{N} \otimes (\boldsymbol{M}_1 - \boldsymbol{M})$, *where*

$$\begin{aligned} t &= 1 + \tfrac{1}{2}n_1p_1 - \tfrac{1}{2}\mathrm{tr}\{D[\boldsymbol{K R}_3\boldsymbol{L}](D[\boldsymbol{K R}_{3N}\boldsymbol{L}])^{-1}\}, \\ \boldsymbol{M} &= \boldsymbol{K\Sigma A}_2^o(\boldsymbol{A}_2^{o\prime}\boldsymbol{\Sigma A}_2^o)^-\boldsymbol{A}_2^{o\prime}\boldsymbol{\Sigma K}', \\ \boldsymbol{M}_1 &= \boldsymbol{K A}_2^o(\boldsymbol{A}_2^{o\prime}\boldsymbol{\Sigma A}_2^o)^{-1}\boldsymbol{A}_2^{o\prime}\boldsymbol{K}' + \boldsymbol{K A}_3(\boldsymbol{A}_3'\boldsymbol{\Sigma}^{-1}\boldsymbol{A}_3)^-\boldsymbol{A}_3'\boldsymbol{K}' \\ &\quad +c_1\boldsymbol{K P}'_{\boldsymbol{A}_3^o,\boldsymbol{\Sigma}^{-1}}\boldsymbol{A}_2(\boldsymbol{A}_2'\boldsymbol{\Sigma}^{-1}\boldsymbol{A}_2)^{-1}\boldsymbol{A}_2'\boldsymbol{P}_{\boldsymbol{A}_3^o,\boldsymbol{\Sigma}^{-1}}\boldsymbol{K}' \\ &\quad +c_1c_2\boldsymbol{K A}_3(\boldsymbol{A}_3'\boldsymbol{\Sigma}^{-1}\boldsymbol{A}_3)^-\boldsymbol{A}_3'\boldsymbol{K}', \\ \boldsymbol{N} &= \boldsymbol{L}'\boldsymbol{P}_{\boldsymbol{Q}_1\boldsymbol{C}_2'}\boldsymbol{L}; \end{aligned}$$

$D[\boldsymbol{K R}_3\boldsymbol{L}]$ and $D[\boldsymbol{K R}_{3N}\boldsymbol{L}]$ are presented in Theorem 6.17. Moreover, c_1 and c_2 are defined in Lemma 4.6 (ii).

Finally, results for $\boldsymbol{R}_4$ are presented.

Theorem 6.18 *The distribution of the residual $\boldsymbol{R}_4$, given in Definition 6.5 (iv), can be approximated through the difference*

$$\boldsymbol{R}_4 = \boldsymbol{R}_{4N} - \boldsymbol{U}_4,$$

where $\boldsymbol{R}_{4N}$ and $\boldsymbol{U}_4$ are defined by (6.54). Let $\boldsymbol{K}$: $p_1 \times p$ and $\boldsymbol{L}$: $n \times n_1$, both of which are known, and

$$\boldsymbol{K R}_{4N}\boldsymbol{L} \sim N_{p_1,n_1}(\boldsymbol{0}, \boldsymbol{K\Sigma P}_{\boldsymbol{A}_1^o,\boldsymbol{\Sigma}^{-1}}\boldsymbol{K}', \boldsymbol{L}'\boldsymbol{P}_{\boldsymbol{C}_1'}\boldsymbol{L}).$$

Then an Edgeworth-type expansion $f_{\boldsymbol{K R}_{4E}\boldsymbol{L}}(\boldsymbol{K R}_o\boldsymbol{L})$ of the density of $\boldsymbol{K R}_4\boldsymbol{L}$, via the density of $\boldsymbol{K R}_{4N}\boldsymbol{L}$, under the assumption that $D[\boldsymbol{K R}_{4N}\boldsymbol{L}]$ is p.d., is given by

$$\begin{aligned} f_{\boldsymbol{K R}_{4E}\boldsymbol{L}}(\boldsymbol{K R}_o\boldsymbol{L}) &= \big\{1 + \tfrac{1}{2}n_1p_1 - \tfrac{1}{2}\mathrm{tr}\{D[\boldsymbol{K R}_4\boldsymbol{L}](D[\boldsymbol{K R}_{4N}\boldsymbol{L}])^{-1}\} \\ &\quad -\tfrac{1}{2}\mathrm{tr}\big\{(D[\boldsymbol{K R}_{4N}\boldsymbol{L}])^{-1}(D[\boldsymbol{K R}_4\boldsymbol{L}] - D[\boldsymbol{K R}_{4N}\boldsymbol{L}])(D[\boldsymbol{K R}_{4N}\boldsymbol{L}])^{-1} \\ &\quad \times\mathrm{vec}(\boldsymbol{K R}_o\boldsymbol{L})\mathrm{vec}'(\boldsymbol{K R}_o\boldsymbol{L})\big\}\big\} f_{\boldsymbol{K R}_{4N}\boldsymbol{L}}(\boldsymbol{K R}_o\boldsymbol{L}), \end{aligned}$$

where

$$
\begin{aligned}
D[\boldsymbol{K}\boldsymbol{R}_4\boldsymbol{L}] = {} & \boldsymbol{K}\boldsymbol{A}_1^o(\boldsymbol{A}_1^{o'}\boldsymbol{\Sigma}\boldsymbol{A}_1^o)^{-1}\boldsymbol{A}_1^{o'}\boldsymbol{K}' \\
& + d_1\boldsymbol{K}\boldsymbol{P}'_{A_2^o,\Sigma^{-1}}\boldsymbol{A}_1(\boldsymbol{A}_1'\boldsymbol{\Sigma}^{-1}\boldsymbol{A}_1)^-\boldsymbol{A}_1'\boldsymbol{P}_{A_2^o,\Sigma^{-1}}\boldsymbol{K}' \\
& + d_1d_2\boldsymbol{K}\boldsymbol{A}_{23}(\boldsymbol{A}_{23}'\boldsymbol{\Sigma}^{-1}\boldsymbol{A}_{23})^-\boldsymbol{A}_{23}'\boldsymbol{K}' \\
& + c_2d_1d_2\boldsymbol{K}\boldsymbol{A}_3(\boldsymbol{A}_3'\boldsymbol{\Sigma}^{-1}\boldsymbol{A}_3)^-\boldsymbol{A}_3'\boldsymbol{K}', \\
D[\boldsymbol{K}\boldsymbol{R}_{4N}\boldsymbol{L}] = {} & \boldsymbol{L}'\boldsymbol{P}_{C_1'}\boldsymbol{L} \otimes \boldsymbol{K}\boldsymbol{\Sigma}\boldsymbol{A}_1^o(\boldsymbol{A}_1^{o'}\boldsymbol{\Sigma}\boldsymbol{A}_1^o)^-\boldsymbol{A}_1^{o'}\boldsymbol{\Sigma}\boldsymbol{K}',
\end{aligned}
$$

with c_2, d_1 and d_2 defined in Lemma 4.6 (ii) and (iii), and

$$\boldsymbol{A}_{23}(\boldsymbol{A}_{23}'\boldsymbol{\Sigma}^{-1}\boldsymbol{A}_{23})^-\boldsymbol{A}_{23}' = \boldsymbol{A}_2(\boldsymbol{A}_2'\boldsymbol{\Sigma}^{-1}\boldsymbol{A}_2)^-\boldsymbol{A}_2' - \boldsymbol{A}_3(\boldsymbol{A}_3'\boldsymbol{\Sigma}^{-1}\boldsymbol{A}_3)^-\boldsymbol{A}_3'.$$

Corollary 6.9 *Let $\boldsymbol{K}\boldsymbol{R}_{4E}\boldsymbol{L}$ be defined via $f_{\boldsymbol{K}\boldsymbol{R}_{4E}\boldsymbol{L}}(\boldsymbol{K}\boldsymbol{R}_o\boldsymbol{L})$, given in Theorem 6.13, where it is assumed that $f_{\boldsymbol{K}\boldsymbol{R}_{4E}\boldsymbol{L}}(\boldsymbol{K}\boldsymbol{R}_o\boldsymbol{L}) \geq 0$. Then*

(i) $E[\boldsymbol{K}\boldsymbol{R}_{4E}\boldsymbol{L}] = \boldsymbol{0}$;
(ii) $D[\boldsymbol{K}\boldsymbol{R}_{4E}\boldsymbol{L}] = t\boldsymbol{N} \otimes \boldsymbol{M} - \frac{1}{2}n_1\mathrm{tr}\{\boldsymbol{M}^{-1}(\boldsymbol{M}_1 - \boldsymbol{M})\}\boldsymbol{N} \otimes \boldsymbol{M} - \boldsymbol{N} \otimes (\boldsymbol{M}_1 - \boldsymbol{M})$,
where

$$
\begin{aligned}
t &= 1 + \tfrac{1}{2}n_1p_1 - \tfrac{1}{2}\mathrm{tr}\{D[\boldsymbol{K}\boldsymbol{R}_4\boldsymbol{L}](D[\boldsymbol{K}\boldsymbol{R}_{4N}\boldsymbol{L}])^{-1}\}, \\
\boldsymbol{M} &= \boldsymbol{K}\boldsymbol{\Sigma}\boldsymbol{A}_1^o(\boldsymbol{A}_1^{o'}\boldsymbol{\Sigma}\boldsymbol{A}_1^o)^-\boldsymbol{A}_1^{o'}\boldsymbol{\Sigma}\boldsymbol{K}', \\
\boldsymbol{M}_1 &= \boldsymbol{K}\boldsymbol{A}_1^o(\boldsymbol{A}_1^{o'}\boldsymbol{\Sigma}\boldsymbol{A}_1^o)^{-1}\boldsymbol{A}_1^{o'}\boldsymbol{K}' + d_1\boldsymbol{K}\boldsymbol{P}'_{A_2^o,\Sigma^{-1}}\boldsymbol{A}_1(\boldsymbol{A}_1'\boldsymbol{\Sigma}^{-1}\boldsymbol{A}_1)^-\boldsymbol{A}_1'\boldsymbol{P}_{A_2^o,\Sigma^{-1}}\boldsymbol{K}' \\
&\quad + d_1d_2\boldsymbol{K}\boldsymbol{A}_{23}(\boldsymbol{A}_{23}'\boldsymbol{\Sigma}^{-1}\boldsymbol{A}_{23})^-\boldsymbol{A}_{23}'\boldsymbol{K}' + c_2d_1d_2\boldsymbol{K}\boldsymbol{A}_3(\boldsymbol{A}_3'\boldsymbol{\Sigma}^{-1}\boldsymbol{A}_3)^-\boldsymbol{A}_3'\boldsymbol{K}', \\
\boldsymbol{N} &= \boldsymbol{L}'\boldsymbol{P}_{C_1'}\boldsymbol{L};
\end{aligned}
$$

$D[\boldsymbol{K}\boldsymbol{R}_4\boldsymbol{L}]$, $D[\boldsymbol{K}\boldsymbol{R}_{4N}\boldsymbol{L}]$ and $\boldsymbol{A}_{23}(\boldsymbol{A}_{23}'\boldsymbol{\Sigma}^{-1}\boldsymbol{A}_{23})^-\boldsymbol{A}_{23}'$ are presented in Theorem 6.18. Moreover, d_1, d_2 and c_2 are defined in Lemma 4.6 (ii) and (iii).

Using the above results concerning the residuals $\boldsymbol{R}_i$, $i = 1, 2, 3, 4$, model validation can take place for the $EBRM_W^3$. As for the BRM and $EBRM_B^3$, it is suggested that mean shift tests should be carried out. Now the case is briefly treated where the mean shift is of the form $\boldsymbol{d}_j\theta\boldsymbol{e}_i'$.

Consider, among other things, $\boldsymbol{R}_1 = \boldsymbol{X}(\boldsymbol{I} - \boldsymbol{P}_{C_1':C_2':C_3'})$, which includes information on how columns (individuals) deviate from the average of the columns (individuals). As usual when performing the residual analysis, we have to eliminate the singularity, e.g. see (6.37), and thereafter the test statistic corresponding to the mean shift hypothesis can be presented as in Theorem 6.19, given below. Moreover, as previously, a parametric bootstrap is suggested for evaluating which elements in $\boldsymbol{R}_1$ are really large.

The same notation will be adopted as that used when working with the BRM or $EBRM_B^3$, i.e.

$$\boldsymbol{R}_{k;ij}^N = \boldsymbol{K}\boldsymbol{d}_j\theta\boldsymbol{e}_i'\boldsymbol{L} + \boldsymbol{E}_k, \quad k = 1,2,3,4; \tag{6.55}$$

$\boldsymbol{R}_{k;ij}^N$ is the same as $\boldsymbol{R}_k^N$ and, as before, ij only indicates which element is supposed to have a mean shift. The residual $\boldsymbol{R}_k^N$, $k = 1,2,3,4$, is obtained from $\boldsymbol{R}_k^N$ by removing the deterministic part (remember that the dispersion matrix is singular) in order to utilize the existence of a density. The vectors $\boldsymbol{d}_j$ and $\boldsymbol{e}_i$ are unit basis vectors, $\boldsymbol{E}_1 \sim N_{p,n_1}(\boldsymbol{0}, \boldsymbol{\Sigma}, \boldsymbol{I})$, $n_1 = n - r(\boldsymbol{C}_1' : \boldsymbol{C}_2' : \boldsymbol{C}_3')$, and $\boldsymbol{E}_i$, $i = 2,3,4$, are defined through the densities in Theorems 6.16, 6.17 and 6.18, respectively. Moreover, as before, it is noted that $T_{k;ijo}$, $k = 1,2,3,4$, represents the observed test statistic, $L_{k;ij}^N(\widehat{\theta})$ is the likelihood based on $\boldsymbol{E}_k$, and as $\widehat{\theta}$ the estimator $\widehat{\theta} = \boldsymbol{d}_j'\boldsymbol{R}_k\boldsymbol{e}_i$ is used, $L_{k;ij}$ is the likelihood under H_0, i.e. with no mean shift in the model in (6.55), and $\boldsymbol{R}_{1o}$ is the observed version of $\boldsymbol{R}_1$. In the likelihood, the dispersion matrix has been replaced by $\widehat{\boldsymbol{\Sigma}}_o$, the maximum likelihood estimate, given in Theorem 3.3.

Theorem 6.19 *Consider $\boldsymbol{R}_i$, $i = 1,2,3,4$, given in Definition 6.5.*

(i) *For $\boldsymbol{R}_1$ let*

$$\boldsymbol{R}_{1;ij}^N = \boldsymbol{d}_j\theta\boldsymbol{e}_i'\boldsymbol{L}_1 + \boldsymbol{E}_1, \quad \boldsymbol{R}_{1;ij}^N = \boldsymbol{R}_1\boldsymbol{L}, \quad \boldsymbol{L}{=}\boldsymbol{V}(\boldsymbol{V}'\boldsymbol{V})^{-1}, \quad (\boldsymbol{V} \textit{ is of full rank}),$$
$$(\boldsymbol{I} - \boldsymbol{P}_{\boldsymbol{C}_1':\boldsymbol{C}_2':\boldsymbol{C}_3'}) = \boldsymbol{V}\boldsymbol{V}', \quad \boldsymbol{E}_1 \sim N_{p,n_1}(\boldsymbol{0}, \boldsymbol{\Sigma}, \boldsymbol{I}_{n_1}), \quad n_1 = n - r(\boldsymbol{C}_1' : \boldsymbol{C}_2' : \boldsymbol{C}_3').$$

Then a test statistic for testing $H_0 : \theta = 0$ against $H_1 : \theta \neq 0$ (with $\boldsymbol{P}_1 = \boldsymbol{P}_{\boldsymbol{C}_1':\boldsymbol{C}_2':\boldsymbol{C}_3'}$) is given by

$$T_{1;ijo} = \frac{(n - r(\boldsymbol{P}_1) - 1)\boldsymbol{d}_j'\boldsymbol{R}_{1o}(\boldsymbol{I} - \boldsymbol{P}_1)\boldsymbol{e}_i(\boldsymbol{e}_i'(\boldsymbol{I} - \boldsymbol{P}_1)\boldsymbol{e}_i)^{-1}\boldsymbol{e}_i'(\boldsymbol{I} - \boldsymbol{P}_1)\boldsymbol{R}_{1o}'\boldsymbol{d}_j}{\boldsymbol{d}_j'\boldsymbol{R}_{1o}(\boldsymbol{I} - \boldsymbol{P}_1)(\boldsymbol{I} - \boldsymbol{e}_i(\boldsymbol{e}_i'(\boldsymbol{I} - \boldsymbol{P}_1)\boldsymbol{e}_i)^{-1}\boldsymbol{e}_i')(\boldsymbol{I} - \boldsymbol{P}_1)\boldsymbol{R}_{1o}'\boldsymbol{d}_j}.$$

(ii) *For $\boldsymbol{R}_2$ let*

$$\boldsymbol{R}_{2;ij}^N = \boldsymbol{K}\boldsymbol{d}_j\theta\boldsymbol{e}_i'\boldsymbol{L} + \boldsymbol{E}_2, \boldsymbol{R}_{2;ij}^N = \boldsymbol{K}\boldsymbol{R}_2\boldsymbol{L}, \boldsymbol{K} = (\boldsymbol{W}'\boldsymbol{W})^{-1}\boldsymbol{W}', \boldsymbol{L} = \boldsymbol{V}(\boldsymbol{V}'\boldsymbol{V})^{-1},$$
$$(\boldsymbol{W} \textit{ and } \boldsymbol{V} \textit{ are of full rank}), \widehat{\boldsymbol{\Sigma}}\boldsymbol{P}_{\boldsymbol{A}_3^o,\widehat{\boldsymbol{\Sigma}}^{-1}} = \boldsymbol{W}\boldsymbol{W}', \boldsymbol{P}_{\boldsymbol{Q}_2\boldsymbol{C}_3'} = \boldsymbol{V}\boldsymbol{V}',$$

where $\boldsymbol{E}_2$ has the approximating density given in Theorem 6.16. Then a test statistic for testing $H_0 : \theta = 0$ against $H_1 : \theta \neq 0$ is given by

$$T_{2;ijo} = \frac{L_{2;ij}^N(\widehat{\theta}_o)}{L_{2;ij}^N},$$

where $L_{2;ij}^N$ is the likelihood for R_2^N (obtained via E_2) under H_0 and $R_2^N(\widehat{\theta}_o)$ under H_1 with $\widehat{\theta}_o = d'_j R_{2o} e_i$.

(iii) *For R_3 let*

$$R_{3;ij}^N = K d_j \theta e_i' L + E_3, \; R_{3;ij}^N = K R_3 L, \; K = (W'W)^{-1}W', \; L = V(V'V)^{-1},$$

$$(W \text{ and } V \text{ are of full rank}), \; \widehat{\Sigma} P_{A_2^o, \widehat{\Sigma}^{-1}} = WW', \; P_{Q_1 C_2'} = VV',$$

where E_3 has the approximating density given in Theorem 6.17. Then a test statistic for testing $H_0 : \theta = 0$ against $H_1 : \theta \neq 0$ is given by

$$T_{3;ijo} = \frac{L_{3;ij}^N(\widehat{\theta}_o)}{L_{3;ij}^N},$$

where $L_{3;ij}^N$ is the likelihood for R_3^N (obtained via E_3) under H_0 and $R_3^N(\widehat{\theta}_o)$ under H_1 with $\widehat{\theta}_o = d'_j R_{3o} e_i$.

(iv) *For R_4 let*

$$R_{4;ij}^N = K d_j \theta e_i' L + E_4, \; R_{4;ij}^N = K R_4 L, \; K = (W'W)^{-1}W', \; L = V(V'V)^{-1},$$

$$(W \text{ and } V \text{ are of full rank}), \; \widehat{\Sigma} P_{A_1^o, \widehat{\Sigma}^{-1}} = WW', \; P_{C_3'} = VV',$$

where E_4 has the approximating density given in Theorem 6.18. Then a test statistic for testing $H_0 : \theta = 0$ against $H_1 : \theta \neq 0$ is given by

$$T_{4;ijo} = \frac{L_{4;ij}^N(\widehat{\theta}_o)}{L_{4;ij}^N},$$

where $L_{4;ij}^N$ is the likelihood for R_4^N (obtained via E_4) under H_0 and $R_4^N(\widehat{\theta}_o)$ under H_1 with $\widehat{\theta}_o = d'_j R_{4o} e_i$.

Finally, as before, to complete the analysis of residuals, X is simulated from $N_{p,n_1}(\mathbf{0}, \widehat{\Sigma}_o, I)$ to obtain the distribution of the large/largest residuals.

This chapter is ended by copying Example 6.7 and then reparameterizing the model so that it becomes an $EBRM_W^3$.

Example 6.8 Consider the model presented in Example 1.9 and let it be reformulated as an $EBRM_W^3$. Put

$$\widetilde{A}_1 = (A_1 : A_2 : A_3), \quad \widetilde{A}_2 = (A_1 : A_2), \quad \widetilde{A}_3 = A_1,$$

where A_i, $i = 1, 2, 3$, is defined in Example 1.9,

$$\widetilde{C}_1 = (\mathbf{1}_{10}' : \mathbf{1}_{35}' \otimes 0), \quad \widetilde{C}_2 = (\mathbf{1}_{10}' \otimes 0 : \mathbf{1}_{15}' : \mathbf{1}_{25}' \otimes 0), \quad \widetilde{C}_3 = (\mathbf{1}_{25}' \otimes 0 : \mathbf{1}_{20}')$$

and then instead of the model in Example 1.9, the following $EBRM_W^3$ has emerged:

$$
\begin{aligned}
\boldsymbol{X} &= \widetilde{\boldsymbol{A}}_1\boldsymbol{\Theta}_1\widetilde{\boldsymbol{C}}_1 + \widetilde{\boldsymbol{A}}_2\boldsymbol{\Theta}_2\widetilde{\boldsymbol{C}}_2 + \widetilde{\boldsymbol{A}}_3\boldsymbol{\Theta}_3\widetilde{\boldsymbol{C}}_3 + \boldsymbol{E},\\
\boldsymbol{E} &\sim N_{p,n}(\boldsymbol{0}, \boldsymbol{\Sigma}, \boldsymbol{I}), \quad \mathcal{C}(\widetilde{\boldsymbol{A}}_3) \subseteq \mathcal{C}(\widetilde{\boldsymbol{A}}_2) \subseteq \mathcal{C}(\widetilde{\boldsymbol{A}}_1),
\end{aligned}
$$

and $\boldsymbol{\Theta}_i$, $i = 1, 2, 3$, are new parameters.

Now $\widetilde{\boldsymbol{C}}_i$, $i = 1, 2, 3$, correspond to the different groups, which leads to an excellent direct interpretation of the model. However, since the residuals in Definition 6.4 "equal" the residuals in Definition 6.5; i.e. in this case the proposed residuals for the $EBRM_W^3$ and $EBRM_B^3$ are identical and no more calculations have to take place. □

Problems

1 (*GMANOVA + MANOVA*, continuation of Problem 2 in Chap. 3) Let

$$\boldsymbol{X} = \boldsymbol{A}\boldsymbol{B}_1\boldsymbol{C}_1 + \boldsymbol{B}_2\boldsymbol{C}_2 + \boldsymbol{E},$$

where all the matrices are given in Problem 2 in Chap. 3. Define residuals. Estimate the dispersion of the residuals and calculate the covariances among them.

2 Is the proposed density approximation in Theorem 6.5 a true density?

3 Give a detailed derivation of the test statistic in (6.31).

4 Derive appropriate residuals for the $EBRM_B^2$.

5 Derive appropriate residuals for the $EBRM_W^2$.

6 Find appropriate density approximations for some of the residuals in Problem 4 or 5

7 Perform a residual analysis of the data in Table 1.1.

8 In Table 1.1, strongly contaminate three observations and perform a residual analysis.

9 Try to challenge some of the results in this chapter by constructing a data set with "extreme observations" which cannot be identified by the given theorems.

10 In this chapter a parametric bootstrap approach was suggested. If instead a standard bootstrap approach (with resampling from the residuals) was to be applied, identify what would be problematic with this approach and suggest how to proceed in order to apply a standard bootstrap approach.

Literature

It may be worthwhile thinking of a residual as something which is left over. The study of residuals and outlying observations has followed the theory of least squares for a long time. Wright (1884) frequently used the term "residual". Farebrother (1978) discusses Pizzetti (1891) in relation to the so-called recursive residuals. The Danish scientist Thiele and colleagues of his used residuals at the end of the 19th century (e.g. see Lauritzen, 2002). Anscombe and Guttman (1960) also gave several earlier references where the problem of outlying observations was discussed. Indeed, there is a huge body of literature on outliers, which often by definition can be linked to residuals. Some of the literature on outliers falls within the subject areas of robust statistics, explorative data analysis and regression analysis, among others, but this literature will not be considered in this brief survey of literature on residuals.

Broadly speaking, residuals were from the beginning used for model evaluation and this is still the case. Checking the linearity of the mean, checking the homoscedasticity of variances and checking distributions for normality can all be performed via residuals. Today in many standard books which include regression/variance analysis some kind of residual analysis is also performed.

Below a concise survey of the topics that have been discussed over the years and a few of the authors who have treated these topics are now presented. In the well-known book by Fisher (1925), the terms "residual", "mean square residue" and "residual variance" were used. Later Fisher (1935) used the terms "residual sums of squares", "residual error" and "residual deviations". In particular "residual sums of squares" is frequently used today. Bartlett (1934) used the term "residual" when showing how matrices and vectors can be used in least squares analysis. Yates (1937) used the term "residual effect", which nowadays is a common term in experimental design, for example when carry-over effects occur in cross-over studies (see also Anscombe, 1948; Tocher, 1952; Box and Hunter, 1957; Yates et al., 1957). Dwyer (1941) investigated skewness, i.e. normality, with the help of residuals and Durbin and Watson (1950) used residuals for testing for serial covariance. Rushton (1951) utilized residuals when presenting a specific computational algorithm for polynomial regression models.

Around 1960 many interesting articles appeared where residuals and outliers were discussed. In particular, the work by Anscombe and colleagues of his is worth mentioning. Anscombe and Guttman (1960) defined outliers as observations of abnormally large residuals, presented approaches to the rejection of outliers and provided a brief history of this topic (see also Srivastava and von Rosen, 1998, where several references are given). Anscombe (1961) discusses the distribution of residuals, including skewness and kurtosis. In Anscombe and Tukey (1963) residuals are exploited in detail and some graphical plots are provided to assist in the joint understanding of data and model assumptions. Anscombe (1967) discussed residual analysis from the perspective of making computations easier to carry out. Moreover, Zyskind (1963) considered what may be termed "variable selection" with the help of residuals. An old problem, and one which is also mentioned by Anscombe and Tukey (1963), is deciding if an observation which corresponds to a large residual is an outlier and should perhaps be removed (see also Kruskal, 1960, who gives general comments and a number of references). Grubbs (1950) published a well-written article focusing on the testing of large residuals. In Grubbs (1950) one can find several older interesting references.

In the 1970s, residual analysis for linear models became more sophisticated and researchers studied what types of deviance from the models could be found via residuals. An interesting article, which in a way summarizes the results of the 1970s, is that written by Draper and John (1981) (see also Cook, 1977, 1979; Andrews and Pregibon, 1978; Draper and Smith, 1981; Cook and Weisberg, 1982; Jørgensen, 1993). In the 1980s, mixed linear models started to become popular, and therefore one started to develop residual analysis for mixed linear models, including longitudinal models and random coefficient regression models (e.g. see Verbeke and Molenberghs, 2009). In particular, Longford (2001) can be mentioned, where a parametric bootstrap approach is applied and where several references on handling outliers in mixed linear models are given. An excellent overview of residual analysis in mixed linear models is presented by Schützenmeister and Piepho (2012).

In Chap. 6 we have used parametric bootstrap simulations (Efron and Tibshirani, 1993) to find an approximation of the distribution of extreme residuals. For references on bootstrap methods see, for example, Davison and Hinkley (1997) or Chernick (2008); many more references exist which treat various aspects of bootstrapping. In particular, bootstrapping theory has been developed for performing residual analysis within the context of regression analysis (Wakefield, 2013; Weisberg, 2014) or within time series analysis (e.g. see Krampe et al., 2015). Moreover, there are interesting connections between the bootstrap method and Edgeworth expansions (Hall, 1992).

Residuals are often exploited through graphical methods using different types of plots. Examples can be found in many books, for example those by Atkinson (1987), Cook (1998) and Atkinson and Riani (2000).

In this chapter, via simulations, test have been performed for a mean shift in the residuals. For some analytical results on mean shift testing in multivariate regression models, including the BRM, see Srivastava and von Rosen (1998). Moreover, through a decomposition of linear spaces residuals for bilinear models have been presented by von Rosen (1995) and Hamid and von Rosen (2006). However, many of the results presented in this chapter have not been presented earlier, for example the density approximations presented in various places and all the results connected to the $EBRM_W^3$.

References

Andrews, D. F., & Pregibon, D. (1978). Finding the outliers that matter. *Journal of the Royal Statistical Society, Series B, 40*, 85–93.

Anscombe, F. J. (1948). The validity of comparative experiments. *Journal of the Royal Statistical Society Series A, 111*, 181–211.

Anscombe, F. J. (1961). Examination of residuals. In *Proceedings of the 4th Berkeley Symposium on Mathematical Statistics and Probability* (Vol. I, pp. 1–36). Berkeley: University of California Press.

Anscombe, F. J. (1967). Topics in the investigation of linear relations fitted by the method of least squares (with discussion). *Journal of the Royal Statistical Society, Series B, 29*, 1–52.

Anscombe, F. J., & Guttman, I. (1960). Rejection of outliers. *Technometrics, 2*, 123–147.

Anscombe, F. J., & Tukey, J. W. (1963). The examination and analysis of residuals. *Technometrics, 5*, 141–160.

Atkinson, A. C. (1987). *Plots, transformations, and regression: An introduction to graphical methods of diagnostic regression analysis. Oxford statistical science series* (Vol. 1). Oxford: Oxford University Press.

Atkinson, A. C., & Riani, M. (2000). *Robust diagnostic regression analysis*. Springer series in statistics. New York: Springer.

Bartlett, M. S. (1934). The vector representation of a sample. *Mathematical Proceedings of the Cambridge Philosophical Society, 30*, 327–340.

Box, G. E. P., & Hunter, J. S. (1957). Multi-factor experimental designs for exploring response surfaces. *Annals of Mathematical Statistics, 28*, 195–241.

Chernick, M. R. (2008). *Bootstrap methods: A guide for practitioners and researchers. Wiley series in probability and statistics* (2nd ed.). Hoboken: Wiley-Interscience.

Cook, R. D. (1977). Detection of influential observations in linear regression. *Technometrics, 19*, 15–18. Additional correspondence, 348–350.

Cook, R. D. (1979). Influential observations in linear regression. *Journal of the American Statistical Association, 74*, 169–174.

Cook, R. D. (1998). *Regression graphics. Ideas for studying regressions through graphics. Wiley series in probability and statistics: Probability and statistics*. A Wiley-Interscience Publication. New York: Wiley.

Cook, R. D., & Weisberg, S. (1982). *Residuals and influence in regression*. London: Chapman and Hall.

Davison, A. C., & Hinkley, D. V. (1997). *Bootstrap methods and their application. Cambridge series in statistical and probabilistic mathematics* (Vol. 1). Cambridge: Cambridge University Press.

Draper, N. R., & John, J. A. (1981). Influential observations and outliers in regression. *Technometrics, 23*, 21–26.

Draper, N. R., & Smith, H. (1981). *Applied regression analysis. Wiley series in probability and mathematical statistics* (2nd ed.). New York: Wiley.

Durbin, J., & Watson, G. S. (1950). Testing for serial correlation in least squares regression. I. *Biometrika, 37*, 409–428.

Dwyer, P. S. (1941). The skewness of the residuals in linear regression theory. *Annals of Mathematical Statistics, 12*, 104–110.

Efron, B., & Tibshirani, R. J. (1993). *An introduction to the bootstrap*. New York: Chapman and Hall.

Farebrother, R. W. (1978). An historical note on recursive residuals. *Journal of the Royal Statistical Society, Series B, 40*, 373–375.

Fisher, R. A. (1925). *Statistical methods for research workers*. Edinburgh: Oliver and Boyd.

Fisher, R. A. (1935). *The design of experiments*. Edinburgh: Oliver and Boyd.

Grubbs, F. E. (1950). Sample criteria for testing outlying observations. *Annals of Mathematical Statistics, 21*, 27–58.

Hall, P. (1992). *The bootstrap and Edgeworth expansion. Springer series in statistics*. New York: Springer.
Hamid, J., & von Rosen, D. (2006). Residuals in the extended growth curve model. *Scandinavian Journal of Statistics, 33*, 121–138.
Jørgensen, B. (1993). *The theory of linear models*. New York: Chapman and Hall.
Krampe, J., Kreiss, J.-P., & Paparoditis, E. (2015). Hybrid wild bootstrap for nonparametric trend estimation in locally stationary time series. *Statistics & Probability Letters, 101*, 54–63.
Kruskal, W. H. (1960). Some remarks on wild observations. *Technometrics, 2*, 1–3.
Lauritzen, S. L. (2002). *Thiele: Pioneer in statistics*. Oxford: Oxford University Press.
Longford, N. T. (2001). Simulation-based diagnostics in random-coefficient models. *Journal of the Royal Statistical Society, Series A, 164*, 259–273.
Pizzetti, P. (1891). I Fondamenti Matematici per la Critica dei Risultati Sperimentali. Genoa. Reprinted in Atti della Universita di Genova, 1892 (reference taken from Farebrother, 1978)
Potthoff, R. F., & Roy, S. N. (1964). A generalized multivariate analysis of variance model useful especially for growth curve problems. *Biometrika, 51*, 313–326.
Rushton, S. (1951). On least squares fitting by orthonormal polynomials using the Choleski method. *Journal of the Royal Statistical Society, Series B, 13*, 92–99.
Schützenmeister, A., & Piepho, H. P. (2012). Residual analysis of linear mixed models using a simulation approach. *Computational Statistics and Data Analysis, 56*, 1405–1416.
Srivastava, M. S., & von Rosen, D. (1998). Outliers in multivariate regression models. *Journal of Multivariate Analysis, 65*, 195–208.
Tocher, K. D. (1952). The design and analysis of block experiments. *Journal of the Royal Statistical Society, Series B, 14*, 45–100.
Verbeke, G., & Molenberghs, G. (2009). *Linear mixed models for longitudinal data*. Reprint of the 2000 original. *Springer series in statistics*. New York: Springer.
von Rosen, D. (1995). Residuals in the growth curve model. *Annals of the Institute of Statistical Mathematics, 47*, 129–136.
Wakefield, J. (2013). *Bayesian and Frequentist regression methods*. Springer series in statistics. New York: Springer.
Weisberg, S. (2014). *Applied linear regression* (4th ed.). Wiley series in probability and statistics. Hoboken: Wiley.
Wright, T. W. (1884). *A treatise on the adjustment of observations with applications to geodetic work and other measures of precision*. New York: van Nostrand.
Yates, F. (1937). *The design and analysis of factorial experiments*. Technical Communication, no. 35. Harpenden: Imperail Bureau of Soil Science.
Yates, F., Healy, M. J. R., & Lipton, S. (1957). Routine analysis of replicated experiments on an electronic computer. *Journal of the Royal Statistical Society, Series B, 19*, 234–254.
Zyskind, G. (1963). A note on residual analysis. *Journal of the American Statistical Association, 58*, 1125–1132.

Chapter 7
Testing Hypotheses

7.1 Introduction

Up to now the focus has been on point estimation, interpretation of estimators and model validation. In this chapter, the important concept of hypothesis testing is considered and various tests for the BRM are derived. It is interesting to note that in order to achieve some of the results for the BRM, knowledge about the $EBRM_B^2$ and the $EBRM_W^2$ is useful. Concerning the $EBRM_B^m$ or $EBRM_W^m$, there exist a large number of possibilities of testing various hypotheses, but only a few will be considered. On the other hand, readers who understand how to construct tests for the BRM will also be able to obtain many results for the $EBRM_B^m$ or $EBRM_W^m$.

This chapter will only present work on tests under the null distribution. There are still several open problems concerning, for example, the power of tests and approximations of non-null distributions. Some results exist for the BRM and several of them are connected to the theory about invariant tests. In particular, invariance together with sufficiency has been used to find tests with good properties. In this chapter, tests based on the likelihood ratio are presented, as well as some alternatives. In particular, the interpretations of the tests are highlighted.

7.2 Background

The general multivariate linear model, as formulated in Sect. 1.4, equals

$$\boldsymbol{X} = \boldsymbol{B}\boldsymbol{C} + \boldsymbol{E}, \qquad \boldsymbol{E} \sim N_{p,n}(\boldsymbol{0}, \boldsymbol{\Sigma}, \boldsymbol{I}), \quad \boldsymbol{\Sigma} > 0, \tag{7.1}$$

where $\boldsymbol{C}$ is a given design matrix and $\boldsymbol{B}$ and $\boldsymbol{\Sigma}$ are unknown parameter matrices. Moreover, suppose that there are the linear restrictions $\boldsymbol{B}\boldsymbol{G} = \boldsymbol{0}$ on the parameter

D. von Rosen, *Bilinear Regression Analysis*, Lecture Notes in Statistics 220,
https://doi.org/10.1007/978-3-319-78784-8_7

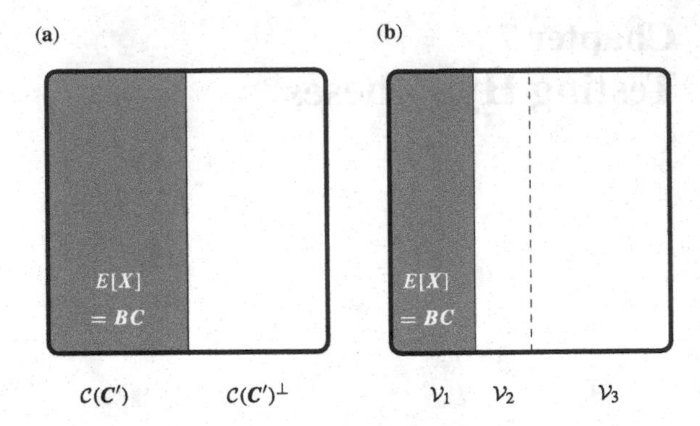

Fig. 7.1 Consider the model in (7.1). A decomposition is presented of the whole space according to the design and restrictions. In (**a**), there are no restrictions and the decomposition consists of the subspaces $\mathcal{C}(\boldsymbol{C}')$ and $\mathcal{C}(\boldsymbol{C}')^{\perp}$. In (**b**), with the restrictions $\boldsymbol{BG} = \boldsymbol{0}$, $\mathcal{V}_1 = \mathcal{C}(\boldsymbol{C}'\boldsymbol{G}^o)$, $\mathcal{V}_2 = \mathcal{C}(\boldsymbol{C}'\boldsymbol{G}^o)^{\perp} \cap \mathcal{C}(\boldsymbol{C}')$ and $\mathcal{V}_3 = \mathcal{C}(\boldsymbol{C}')^{\perp}$

space, where $\boldsymbol{G}$ is known, corresponding, for example, to a hypothesis testing problem. The model with and without restrictions is illustrated in Fig. 7.1.

Note that $\boldsymbol{BG} = \boldsymbol{0}$ is equivalent to $\boldsymbol{B} = \boldsymbol{\Theta}\boldsymbol{G}^{o'}$, where $\boldsymbol{\Theta}$ is an unknown new parameter matrix. Thus, a reparametrization may take place and under the restrictions the model can equivalently be written as follows:

$$\boldsymbol{X} = \boldsymbol{\Theta}\boldsymbol{G}^{o'}\boldsymbol{C} + \boldsymbol{E}, \qquad \boldsymbol{E} \sim N_{p,n}(\boldsymbol{0}, \boldsymbol{\Sigma}, \boldsymbol{I}). \tag{7.2}$$

This means, among other things, that the model with restrictions belongs to the same class of models as the unrestricted one. Estimating $\boldsymbol{\Theta}$ yields a maximum likelihood estimator of $\boldsymbol{B}$, i.e. $\widehat{\boldsymbol{B}} = \widehat{\boldsymbol{\Theta}}\boldsymbol{G}^{o'}$, which satisfies $\widehat{\boldsymbol{B}}\boldsymbol{G} = \boldsymbol{0}$.

In Fig. 7.1b, the decomposition

$$\mathcal{C}(\boldsymbol{C}') = \mathcal{C}(\boldsymbol{C}'\boldsymbol{G}^o) \boxplus \mathcal{C}(\boldsymbol{C}'\boldsymbol{G}^o)^{\perp} \cap \mathcal{C}(\boldsymbol{C}')$$

is illustrated. It is natural to believe that if the variation is large for observations which have been projected on $\mathcal{C}(\boldsymbol{C}'\boldsymbol{G}^o)^{\perp} \cap \mathcal{C}(\boldsymbol{C}')$, then the null hypothesis H_0 : $\boldsymbol{BG} = \boldsymbol{0}$ should be rejected. In statistics, this is then formally verified using distribution theory. Let us follow this decision process in some detail. The estimated likelihood without restrictions is proportional to $|\boldsymbol{X}(\boldsymbol{I} - \boldsymbol{P}_{C'})\boldsymbol{X}'|^{-n/2}$ and that with restrictions is proportional to $|\boldsymbol{X}(\boldsymbol{I} - \boldsymbol{P}_{C'G^o})\boldsymbol{X}'|^{-n/2}$, both of which results follow from the estimation of $\boldsymbol{\Sigma}$. Let $\widehat{\boldsymbol{\Sigma}}_{H_0}$ denote the MLE of $\boldsymbol{\Sigma}$ under the null hypothesis, and $\widehat{\boldsymbol{\Sigma}}_{H_1}$ the MLE of $\boldsymbol{\Sigma}$ under the alternative hypothesis, i.e. the unrestricted case. The likelihood ratio statistic is equivalent to (see Theorem 3.1 with $\boldsymbol{A} = \boldsymbol{I}$)

$$\begin{aligned}\lambda^{\frac{2}{n}} &= \frac{|n\widehat{\boldsymbol{\Sigma}}_{H_0}|}{|n\widehat{\boldsymbol{\Sigma}}_{H_1}|} = \frac{|\boldsymbol{X}(\boldsymbol{I} - \boldsymbol{P}_{C'G^o})\boldsymbol{X}'|}{|\boldsymbol{X}(\boldsymbol{I} - \boldsymbol{P}_{C'})\boldsymbol{X}'|} \\ &= \frac{|\boldsymbol{X}(\boldsymbol{I} - \boldsymbol{P}_{C'})\boldsymbol{X}' + \boldsymbol{X}\boldsymbol{C}'(\boldsymbol{C}\boldsymbol{C}')^{-}\boldsymbol{N}(\boldsymbol{N}'(\boldsymbol{C}\boldsymbol{C}')^{-}\boldsymbol{N})^{-}\boldsymbol{N}'(\boldsymbol{C}\boldsymbol{C}')^{-}\boldsymbol{C}\boldsymbol{X}'|}{|\boldsymbol{X}(\boldsymbol{I} - \boldsymbol{P}_{C'})\boldsymbol{X}'|},\end{aligned} \tag{7.3}$$

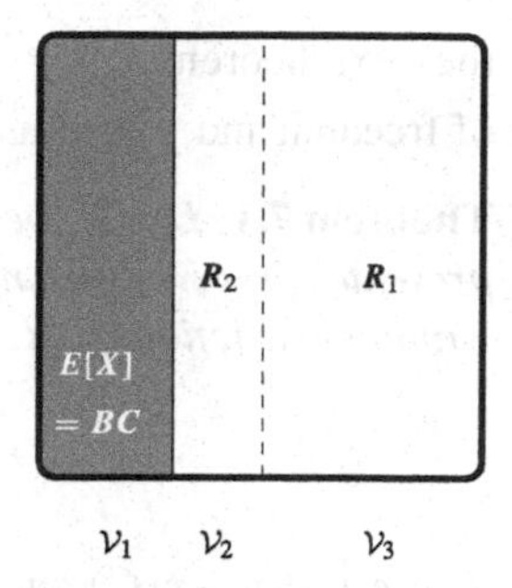

Fig. 7.2 Consider the model in (7.1). A decomposition is presented of the whole space according to the design and the restrictions $\boldsymbol{BG} = \boldsymbol{0}$, and the residuals $\boldsymbol{R}_1$ and $\boldsymbol{R}_2$, given in (7.5) and (7.6), are illustrated. $\mathcal{V}_1 = \mathcal{C}(\boldsymbol{C}'\boldsymbol{G}^o)$, $\mathcal{V}_2 = \mathcal{C}(\boldsymbol{C}'\boldsymbol{G}^o)^{\perp} \cap \mathcal{C}(\boldsymbol{C}')$ and $\mathcal{V}_3 = \mathcal{C}(\boldsymbol{C}')^{\perp}$

where $\boldsymbol{N}$ is any matrix satisfying $\mathcal{C}(\boldsymbol{N}) = \mathcal{C}(\boldsymbol{C}) \cap \mathcal{C}(\boldsymbol{G})$. The numerator in (7.3) is obtained from Appendix B, Theorem B.12. Moreover,

$$\mathcal{C}(\boldsymbol{C}'(\boldsymbol{CC}')^{-}\boldsymbol{N}) = \mathcal{C}(\boldsymbol{C}'\boldsymbol{G}^o)^{\perp} \cap \mathcal{C}(\boldsymbol{C}'). \tag{7.4}$$

Now, the observed λ, i.e. λ_o, is large when

$$\boldsymbol{X}_o\boldsymbol{C}'(\boldsymbol{CC}')^{-}\boldsymbol{N}(\boldsymbol{N}'(\boldsymbol{CC}')^{-}\boldsymbol{N})^{-}\boldsymbol{N}'(\boldsymbol{CC}')^{-}\boldsymbol{C}\boldsymbol{X}_o'$$

is "large", which is what we would like to see, for example, when testing a hypothesis and desiring a clear interpretation of the test. The remaining task is to find out if λ_o, the observed λ is "extreme", and to verify such a property, the distribution for λ is needed, which we will return to in detail later in Sect. 7.3. An interesting fact is that a similar ratio to the one in (7.3) will be obtained when testing general hypotheses in the BRM, which indeed is quite remarkable.

In Chap. 6, residuals were considered. We know that quadratic forms of residuals summarize information and thus can be used as a basis for constructing tests. In Fig. 7.2, corresponding to Fig. 7.1b, the residuals

$$\boldsymbol{R}_1 = \boldsymbol{X}(\boldsymbol{I} - \boldsymbol{P}_{C'}), \tag{7.5}$$

$$\boldsymbol{R}_2 = \boldsymbol{X}\boldsymbol{P}_{C'(CC')^{-}N} \tag{7.6}$$

are presented.

It is of interest to note that the test statistic $\lambda^{\frac{2}{n}}$, given in (7.3), is identical to

$$\lambda^{\frac{2}{n}} = \frac{|\boldsymbol{R}_1\boldsymbol{R}_1' + \boldsymbol{R}_2\boldsymbol{R}_2'|}{|\boldsymbol{R}_1\boldsymbol{R}_1'|}, \tag{7.7}$$

meaning that the likelihood ratio test is based on a decision as to whether $\boldsymbol{R}_2\boldsymbol{R}_2'$ is "large". Moreover, it follows immediately that $\boldsymbol{R}_1\boldsymbol{R}_1' \sim W_p(\boldsymbol{\Sigma}, n - r(\boldsymbol{C}))$ and $\boldsymbol{R}_2\boldsymbol{R}_2' \sim W_p(\boldsymbol{\Sigma}, r(\boldsymbol{N}))$ are independently distributed (see Appendix B, Theorem B.19 (ix)). Hence, Theorem C.3 in Appendix C can be used, which verifies the next theorem. Let χ_f^2 denote a chi-squared distributed variable with f degrees of freedom and $\chi_\beta^2(f)$ its β-percentile (see Appendix A, Sect. A.9).

Theorem 7.1 *Let λ_o be the observed value of λ, given in (7.7). For the model presented in (7.1), the null hypothesis $\boldsymbol{BG} = \boldsymbol{0}$ is tested against an alternative without restrictions. Let*

$$t_o = \tfrac{2}{n}(f - \tfrac{1}{2}(p - m + 1)) \ln \lambda_o,$$

where $f = n - r(\boldsymbol{C})$ and $m = \dim\{\mathcal{C}(\boldsymbol{G}) \cap \mathcal{C}(\boldsymbol{C})\} = \dim\{\mathcal{C}(\boldsymbol{C}'\boldsymbol{G}^{o'})^\perp \cap \mathcal{C}(\boldsymbol{C}')\}$. The likelihood ratio test, approximately at significance level α, rejects the hypothesis if t_o satisfies

$$P\{\chi_{pm}^2 \geq t_o\} + c_1(1 - c_1)(P\{\chi_{pm+4}^2 \geq t_o\} - P\{\chi_{pm}^2 \geq t_o\})$$
$$+ c_2(P\{\chi_{pm+8}^2 \geq t_o\} - P\{\chi_{pm}^2 \geq t_o\}) \leq \alpha,$$

where c_1 and c_2 are defined in Appendix C, Theorem C.3. □

Suppose that for the model in (7.1), there are bilinear restrictions on the parameter space which equal $\boldsymbol{FBG} = \boldsymbol{0}$, where $\boldsymbol{F}$ and $\boldsymbol{G}$ are known matrices. By using Theorem B.10 (i) in Appendix B, it follows that the MANOVA model with the bilinear restrictions can be written as follows:

$$\boldsymbol{X} = (\boldsymbol{F}')^o \boldsymbol{\Theta}_1 \boldsymbol{C} + \boldsymbol{F}'\boldsymbol{\Theta}_2 \boldsymbol{G}^{o'} \boldsymbol{C} + \boldsymbol{E}, \qquad \boldsymbol{E} \sim N_{p,n}(\boldsymbol{0}, \boldsymbol{\Sigma}, \boldsymbol{I}), \tag{7.8}$$

which belongs to the class of $EBRM_B^2$, since $\mathcal{C}(\boldsymbol{C}'\boldsymbol{G}^o) \subseteq \mathcal{C}(\boldsymbol{C}')$. Thus, by introducing bilinear restrictions, without further assumptions, the MANOVA model turns into an $EBRM_B^2$. Figure 7.3 shows what happens when a bilinear restriction is imposed.

The illustration in Fig. 7.3b is based on the decompositions $\mathcal{C}_\Sigma(\boldsymbol{F}') \boxplus \mathcal{C}_\Sigma(\boldsymbol{F}')^\perp$ and

$$\mathcal{C}(\boldsymbol{C}') = \mathcal{C}(\boldsymbol{C}'\boldsymbol{G}^o) \boxplus \mathcal{C}(\boldsymbol{C}'\boldsymbol{G}^o)^\perp \cap \mathcal{C}(\boldsymbol{C}').$$

Suppose that the aim is to test

$$H_0: \boldsymbol{FBG} = \boldsymbol{0} \quad versus \;\; H_1: \boldsymbol{B} \text{ unrestricted}.$$

It follows from Fig. 7.3 that this case can be handled in a fairly straightforward manner. Under the alternative H_1, i.e. with no restrictions,

$$n\widehat{\boldsymbol{\Sigma}}_{H_1} = \boldsymbol{S}_1 = \boldsymbol{X}(\boldsymbol{I} - \boldsymbol{P}_{C'})\boldsymbol{X}',$$

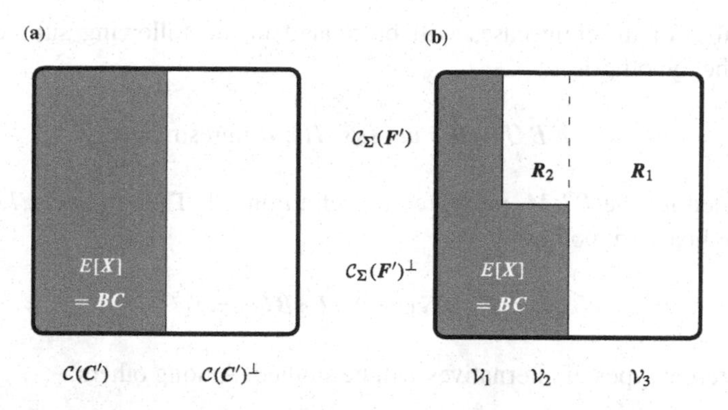

Fig. 7.3 Consider the model in (7.1). A decomposition is presented of the whole space according to the design and restrictions. In (**a**), there are no restrictions and the decomposition consists of the subspaces $\mathcal{C}(\boldsymbol{C}')$ and $\mathcal{C}(\boldsymbol{C}')^\perp$. In (**b**), with the restrictions $\boldsymbol{FBG} = \boldsymbol{0}$, $\mathcal{V}_1 = \mathcal{C}(\boldsymbol{C}'\boldsymbol{G}^o)$, $\mathcal{V}_2 = \mathcal{C}(\boldsymbol{C}'\boldsymbol{G}^o)^\perp \cap \mathcal{C}(\boldsymbol{C}')$ and $\mathcal{V}_3 = \mathcal{C}(\boldsymbol{C}')^\perp$. The residuals equal $\boldsymbol{R}_1 = \boldsymbol{X}(\boldsymbol{I} - \boldsymbol{P}_{C'})$ and $\boldsymbol{R}_2 = \boldsymbol{P}'_{F',S_1^{-1}}\boldsymbol{X}\boldsymbol{P}_{C'(CC')^-N}$

and under H_0 (see Theorem 3.2)

$$n\widehat{\boldsymbol{\Sigma}}_{H_0} = \boldsymbol{S}_1 + \boldsymbol{P}'_{F',S_1^{-1}}\boldsymbol{X}\boldsymbol{P}_{C'(CC')^-N}\boldsymbol{X}'\boldsymbol{P}_{F',S_1^{-1}},$$

where $\boldsymbol{C}'(\boldsymbol{C}\boldsymbol{C}')^-\boldsymbol{N}$ is justified by (7.4). Suppose that, without any loss of generality, $\boldsymbol{H} = (\boldsymbol{F}', \boldsymbol{S}_1^{-1}(\boldsymbol{F}')^o)$ is of full rank. The likelihood ratio criterion is equivalent to

$$\lambda_o^{\frac{2}{n}} = \frac{|\widehat{\boldsymbol{\Sigma}}_{H_0}|}{|\widehat{\boldsymbol{\Sigma}}_{H_1}|} = \frac{|\boldsymbol{H}'\widehat{\boldsymbol{\Sigma}}_{H_0}\boldsymbol{H}|}{|\boldsymbol{H}'\widehat{\boldsymbol{\Sigma}}_{H_1}\boldsymbol{H}|} = \frac{|\boldsymbol{F}\boldsymbol{S}_1\boldsymbol{F}' + \boldsymbol{F}\boldsymbol{X}_o\boldsymbol{P}_{C'(CC')^-N}\boldsymbol{X}_o'\boldsymbol{F}'|}{|\boldsymbol{F}\boldsymbol{S}_1\boldsymbol{F}'|}$$
$$= \frac{|\boldsymbol{F}\boldsymbol{R}_{1o}\boldsymbol{R}_{1o}'\boldsymbol{F}' + \boldsymbol{F}\boldsymbol{R}_{2o}\boldsymbol{R}_{2o}'\boldsymbol{F}'|}{|\boldsymbol{F}\boldsymbol{R}_{1o}\boldsymbol{R}_{1o}'\boldsymbol{F}'|}, \tag{7.9}$$

where $\boldsymbol{R}_{1o}$ and $\boldsymbol{R}_{2o}$ are observed versions of $\boldsymbol{R}_1$ and $\boldsymbol{R}_2$ which are defined in Fig. 7.3 and $\boldsymbol{S}_1 = \boldsymbol{X}_o(\boldsymbol{I} - \boldsymbol{P}_{C'})\boldsymbol{X}_o'$. In the forthcoming presentation, for notational convenience, $\boldsymbol{S}_1$ will represent either $\boldsymbol{S}_1 = \boldsymbol{X}(\boldsymbol{I} - \boldsymbol{P}_{C'})\boldsymbol{X}'$ or $\boldsymbol{S}_1 = \boldsymbol{X}_o(\boldsymbol{I} - \boldsymbol{P}_{C'})\boldsymbol{X}_o'$. The same understanding also applies to $\boldsymbol{S}$, $\boldsymbol{S}_2$ and $\boldsymbol{S}_3$. For a detailed explanation of how to obtain the relations in (7.9), see the more general BRM case presented in the next section. It is important to note that since $\boldsymbol{F}\boldsymbol{P}'_{F',S_1^{-1}} = \boldsymbol{F}$, $\boldsymbol{F}\boldsymbol{R}_1\boldsymbol{R}_1'\boldsymbol{F}' \sim W_{r(\boldsymbol{F})}(\boldsymbol{F}\boldsymbol{\Sigma}\boldsymbol{F}', n - r(\boldsymbol{C}))$, which then under H_0 is distributed independently of $\boldsymbol{F}\boldsymbol{R}_2\boldsymbol{R}_2'\boldsymbol{F}' \sim W_{r(\boldsymbol{F})}(\boldsymbol{F}\boldsymbol{\Sigma}\boldsymbol{F}', r(\boldsymbol{N}))$. Hence, even if the bilinear restrictions give non-linear MLEs, the test statistic has the same form as that used when linear restrictions $\boldsymbol{BG} = \boldsymbol{0}$ are imposed.

A number of different cases will be treated in the following subsections. In Sect. 7.3 the hypothesis

$$H_0: \boldsymbol{FBG} = \mathbf{0} \quad versus \ H_1\colon \boldsymbol{B} \text{ unrestricted}$$

will be tested for the BRM, presented in Definition 2.1. Then in Sects. 7.4–7.7 the more complicated hypothesis

$$H_0: \boldsymbol{F}_1\boldsymbol{B}\boldsymbol{G}_1 = \mathbf{0},\ \boldsymbol{F}_2\boldsymbol{B}\boldsymbol{G}_2 = \mathbf{0}$$

versus different types of alternatives will be studied. Among others,

$$H_0: \boldsymbol{F}_1\boldsymbol{B}\boldsymbol{G}_1 = \mathbf{0},\ \boldsymbol{F}_2\boldsymbol{B}\boldsymbol{G}_2 = \mathbf{0} \quad versus \ H_1\colon \boldsymbol{B} \text{ unrestricted}$$

will be discussed, which turns out to be rather difficult. Moreover, in Sect. 7.11, an $EBRM_B^3$ versus a BRM will be tested and in Sect. 7.12

$$H_0: \boldsymbol{F}_1\boldsymbol{B}\boldsymbol{G}_1 = \boldsymbol{F}_2\boldsymbol{\Theta}\boldsymbol{G}_2 \quad versus \ H_1\colon \boldsymbol{B} \text{ unrestricted}$$

will be tested for the BRM; in this hypothesis, $\boldsymbol{\Theta}$ is also an unknown parameter. All the above-mentioned hypotheses will be tested via the likelihood ratio statistic, but in Sects. 7.8–7.10, alternative test statistics will be considered.

7.3 Likelihood Ratio Testing, $H_0: FBG = 0$, in the BRM

A likelihood ratio test statistic for testing bilinear restrictions in the BRM is now derived. This can be achieved in many ways. In this presentation the concept of dispersion in particular is utilized. Tests for general linear or multivariate models utilize functions of residuals measuring deviances from the model. The residuals are obtained by projections of $\boldsymbol{X}$ on certain between-individuals subspaces. For the BRM, it follows from Sect. 6.2 that natural residuals are obtained via projections of $\boldsymbol{X}$ on between-individuals spaces and within-individuals spaces. Because projections are idempotent matrices and not of full rank, it appears that the concept of "residual" has to be modified somewhat when performing likelihood ratio testing in the BRM. The projection on the within-individuals space causes the problem. However, all the spaces which were of interest when constructing residuals for model validation are also of interest when constructing likelihood ratio tests.

Definition 7.1 The dispersion $\boldsymbol{D}$ on the tensor space $\mathcal{V} \otimes \mathcal{W}$ is given by

$$\boldsymbol{D} = \boldsymbol{H}'\boldsymbol{Y}\boldsymbol{P}\boldsymbol{Y}'\boldsymbol{H},$$

where $\boldsymbol{H}$ is a basis matrix of full rank on $\mathcal{W}$, $\boldsymbol{P}$ is a projector on $\mathcal{V}$ and $E[\boldsymbol{Y}] = \mathbf{0}$.

Note that in Definition 7.1, the projector $\boldsymbol{P}$ can very well include random variables which, however, in this book have to be independent of $\boldsymbol{H}'\boldsymbol{Y}$. Moreover, if $\boldsymbol{Y} \sim N_{p,n}(\mathbf{0}, \boldsymbol{\Sigma}, \boldsymbol{I})$, then $\boldsymbol{D}$ is Wishart-distributed. We remark that the parameter $\boldsymbol{\Sigma}$ in the BRM also often is called dispersion matrix, but $\boldsymbol{\Sigma}$ is obviously not related to Definition 7.1. In (7.9), $\boldsymbol{FR}_1\boldsymbol{R}_1'\boldsymbol{F}'$ and $\boldsymbol{FR}_2\boldsymbol{R}_2'\boldsymbol{F}'$ can be thought of as two independently distributed dispersions.

In the following presentation, the results concerning the MLEs obtained in Chap. 3 will be applied. Let

$$\boldsymbol{X} = \boldsymbol{ABC} + \boldsymbol{E}, \qquad \boldsymbol{E} \sim N_{p,n}(\mathbf{0}, \boldsymbol{\Sigma}, \boldsymbol{I}), \quad \boldsymbol{\Sigma} > 0,$$

where all the matrices are defined in Definition 2.1. Moreover, the testing problem is identified by

$$H_0 : \boldsymbol{FBG} = \mathbf{0} \quad versus \quad H_1 : \boldsymbol{B} \text{ unrestricted},$$

where $\boldsymbol{F}$ and $\boldsymbol{G}$ are known matrices. It is noted that all the matrices represent a specific quantity of interest.

Example 7.1 For the BRM, let $\boldsymbol{X} = \boldsymbol{ABC} + \boldsymbol{E}$ and suppose that

$$\boldsymbol{A} = \begin{pmatrix} 1 & t_1 & t_1^2 \\ 1 & t_2 & t_2^2 \\ \vdots & \vdots & \vdots \\ 1 & t_p & t_p^2 \end{pmatrix}, \qquad \boldsymbol{C} = (\mathbf{1}_{n_1}' \otimes (1:0)' : \mathbf{1}_{n_2}' \otimes (0:1)'),$$

indicating that there is a quadratic within-individuals model and two treatment groups. If one is testing for a linear within-individuals structure, then

$$H_0 : \boldsymbol{FB} = \mathbf{0} \quad versus \quad H_1 : \boldsymbol{B} \text{ unrestricted},$$

where $\boldsymbol{F} = (0:0:1)$ can be an appropriate specification. Furthermore, if only one of the treatment groups follows a quadratic structure, this can be tested by

$$H_0 : \boldsymbol{FBG} = \mathbf{0} \quad versus \quad H_1 : \boldsymbol{B} \text{ unrestricted},$$

where $\boldsymbol{F} = (0:0:1)$ and $\boldsymbol{G} = (0:1)'$. □

A common strategy for obtaining tests based on the likelihood ratio is to obtain estimators under the hypothesis H_0 and under the alternative hypothesis H_1, which are inserted in the likelihoods corresponding to H_0 and H_1. Moreover, as seen above, the models under H_0 and H_1 generate the following two models:

$$H_1 : \qquad \boldsymbol{X} = \boldsymbol{ABC} + \boldsymbol{E}, \tag{7.10}$$

$$H_0 : \qquad \boldsymbol{X} = \boldsymbol{A}(\boldsymbol{F}')^o\boldsymbol{\Theta}_1\boldsymbol{C} + \boldsymbol{AF}'\boldsymbol{\Theta}_2\boldsymbol{G}^{o'}\boldsymbol{C} + \boldsymbol{E}, \tag{7.11}$$

where $\boldsymbol{\Theta}_1$ and $\boldsymbol{\Theta}_2$ are unknown parameters. Under the alternative H_1, according to Theorem 3.1,

$$\boldsymbol{A}\widehat{\boldsymbol{B}}\boldsymbol{C} = \boldsymbol{P}_{A,S_1}\boldsymbol{X}\boldsymbol{P}_{C'},$$
$$n\widehat{\boldsymbol{\Sigma}} = (\boldsymbol{X} - \boldsymbol{A}\widehat{\boldsymbol{B}}\boldsymbol{C})()' = \boldsymbol{S}_1 + \boldsymbol{P}'_{A^o,S_1^{-1}}\boldsymbol{X}\boldsymbol{P}_{C'}\boldsymbol{X}'\boldsymbol{P}_{A^o,S_1^{-1}},$$

where $\boldsymbol{S}_1 = \boldsymbol{X}(\boldsymbol{I} - \boldsymbol{P}_{C'})\boldsymbol{X}'$, which yields that the maximum of the likelihood is proportional to

$$|\boldsymbol{S}_1 + \boldsymbol{P}'_{A^o,S_1^{-1}}\boldsymbol{X}_o\boldsymbol{P}_{C'}\boldsymbol{X}'_o\boldsymbol{P}_{A^o,S_1^{-1}}|^{-n/2}, \tag{7.12}$$

and now $\boldsymbol{S}_1 = \boldsymbol{X}_o(\boldsymbol{I} - \boldsymbol{P}_{C'})\boldsymbol{X}'_o$, where it has been indicated that observed values are used. Under H_0 the corresponding quantities equal, according to Theorem 3.2 (taking $\boldsymbol{C}_3$=$\boldsymbol{0}$),

$$\boldsymbol{A}\widehat{\boldsymbol{B}}\boldsymbol{C} = \boldsymbol{A}(\boldsymbol{F}')^o\widehat{\boldsymbol{\Theta}}_1\boldsymbol{C} + \boldsymbol{A}\boldsymbol{F}'\widehat{\boldsymbol{\Theta}}_2\boldsymbol{G}^{o'}\boldsymbol{C} = \boldsymbol{P}_{A_1,S_1}\boldsymbol{X}\boldsymbol{P}_{C'_1} + \boldsymbol{P}_{\widehat{Q}'_1A_2,\widehat{S}_2}\boldsymbol{X}\boldsymbol{P}_{C'_2},$$
$$n\widehat{\boldsymbol{\Sigma}} = (\boldsymbol{X} - \boldsymbol{A}\widehat{\boldsymbol{B}}\boldsymbol{C})()' = \widehat{\boldsymbol{S}}_2 + \widehat{\boldsymbol{Q}}'_2\widehat{\boldsymbol{Q}}'_1\boldsymbol{X}\boldsymbol{P}_{C'_2}\boldsymbol{X}'\widehat{\boldsymbol{Q}}_1\widehat{\boldsymbol{Q}}_2,$$

where

$$\boldsymbol{S}_1 = \boldsymbol{X}(\boldsymbol{I} - \boldsymbol{P}_{C'})\boldsymbol{X}', \quad \boldsymbol{C}_1 = \boldsymbol{C}, \quad \boldsymbol{C}_2 = \boldsymbol{G}^{o'}\boldsymbol{C},$$
$$\boldsymbol{A}_1 = \boldsymbol{A}(\boldsymbol{F}')^o, \quad \boldsymbol{A}_2 = \boldsymbol{A}\boldsymbol{F}', \quad \widehat{\boldsymbol{Q}}_1 = \boldsymbol{I} - \boldsymbol{P}'_{A_1,S_1}, \quad \widehat{\boldsymbol{Q}}_2 = \boldsymbol{I} - \boldsymbol{P}'_{\widehat{Q}'_1A_2,\widehat{S}_2},$$
$$\widehat{\boldsymbol{Q}}'_2\widehat{\boldsymbol{Q}}'_1 = \boldsymbol{I} - \boldsymbol{P}_{A_1,S_1} - \boldsymbol{P}_{\widehat{Q}'_1A_2,\widehat{S}_2}, \quad \widehat{\boldsymbol{S}}_2 = \boldsymbol{S}_1 + \widehat{\boldsymbol{Q}}'_1\boldsymbol{X}(\boldsymbol{P}_{C'_1} - \boldsymbol{P}_{C'_2})\boldsymbol{X}'\widehat{\boldsymbol{Q}}_1.$$

At this stage the parameters will not be put into focus. Here, in Sect. 7.3, the purpose is to present the general mathematics for performing likelihood ratio testing. When deriving the distribution of the likelihood ratio statistic, it will be apparent that we relatively freely will switch between observed random variables and random variables. This is legitimate if experiments and calculations are repeated, but there is no real mathematical justification for the approach. For notational convenience, in the following, we will not normally distinguish between random and observed random variables when a hat, "$\widehat{\ }$", is used and it will be clear from the presentations what is meant.

The maximum of the likelihood under H_0 can be shown, as with (7.12), to be proportional to

$$|\widehat{\boldsymbol{S}}_2 + \widehat{\boldsymbol{Q}}'_2\widehat{\boldsymbol{Q}}'_1\boldsymbol{X}_o\boldsymbol{P}_{C'_2}\boldsymbol{X}'_o\widehat{\boldsymbol{Q}}_1\widehat{\boldsymbol{Q}}_2|^{-n/2}.$$

Thus, the likelihood ratio for testing H_0 in (7.11) versus H_1 in (7.10) is equivalent to

$$\lambda_o^{\frac{2}{n}} = \frac{|\widehat{\boldsymbol{\Sigma}}_{H_0}|}{|\widehat{\boldsymbol{\Sigma}}_{H_1}|} = \frac{|\widehat{\boldsymbol{S}}_2 + \widehat{\boldsymbol{Q}}_2'\widehat{\boldsymbol{Q}}_1'\boldsymbol{X}_o\boldsymbol{P}_{\boldsymbol{C}_2'}\boldsymbol{X}_o'\widehat{\boldsymbol{Q}}_1\widehat{\boldsymbol{Q}}_2|}{|\boldsymbol{S}_1 + \boldsymbol{P}'_{\boldsymbol{A}^o,\boldsymbol{S}_1^{-1}}\boldsymbol{X}_o\boldsymbol{P}_{\boldsymbol{C}_1'}\boldsymbol{X}_o'\boldsymbol{P}_{\boldsymbol{A}^o,\boldsymbol{S}_1^{-1}}|}, \tag{7.13}$$

which seems to be a difficult expression to handle. However, $\lambda_o^{\frac{2}{n}}$ can be manipulated so that a satisfactory and interpretable test statistic appears. First, it is noted that $\widehat{\boldsymbol{Q}}_1\widehat{\boldsymbol{Q}}_2$ is a projection on a space where the inner product is defined through $\widehat{\boldsymbol{S}}_2^{-1}$ and (see Appendix B, Theorem B.3 (v))

$$\mathcal{C}(\widehat{\boldsymbol{Q}}_1\widehat{\boldsymbol{Q}}_2) = \mathcal{C}(\widehat{\boldsymbol{Q}}_1(\widehat{\boldsymbol{Q}}_1'\boldsymbol{A}_2^o)^o) = \mathcal{C}(\widehat{\boldsymbol{Q}}_1) \cap \mathcal{C}(\boldsymbol{A}_2)^{\perp} = \mathcal{C}(\boldsymbol{A}_1)^{\perp} \cap \mathcal{C}(\boldsymbol{A}_2)^{\perp} = \mathcal{C}(\boldsymbol{A})^{\perp}.$$

Hence,

$$\begin{aligned}
\lambda_o^{\frac{2}{n}} &= \frac{|\widehat{\boldsymbol{S}}_2 + \boldsymbol{P}'_{\boldsymbol{A}^o,\widehat{\boldsymbol{S}}_2^{-1}}\boldsymbol{X}_o\boldsymbol{P}_{\boldsymbol{C}'\boldsymbol{G}^o}\boldsymbol{X}_o'\boldsymbol{P}_{\boldsymbol{A}^o,\widehat{\boldsymbol{S}}_2^{-1}}|}{|\boldsymbol{S}_1 + \boldsymbol{P}'_{\boldsymbol{A}^o,\boldsymbol{S}_1^{-1}}\boldsymbol{X}_o\boldsymbol{P}_{\boldsymbol{C}'}\boldsymbol{X}_o'\boldsymbol{P}_{\boldsymbol{A}^o,\boldsymbol{S}_1^{-1}}|} \\
&= \frac{|\widehat{\boldsymbol{S}}_2||\boldsymbol{A}^{o\prime}\widehat{\boldsymbol{S}}_2\boldsymbol{A}^o|^{-1}|\boldsymbol{A}^{o\prime}\widehat{\boldsymbol{S}}_2\boldsymbol{A}^o + \boldsymbol{A}^{o\prime}\boldsymbol{X}_o\boldsymbol{P}_{\boldsymbol{C}'\boldsymbol{G}^o}\boldsymbol{X}_o'\boldsymbol{A}^o|}{|\boldsymbol{S}_1||\boldsymbol{A}^{o\prime}\boldsymbol{S}_1\boldsymbol{A}^o|^{-1}|\boldsymbol{A}^{o\prime}\boldsymbol{X}_o\boldsymbol{X}_o'\boldsymbol{A}^o|} \\
&= \frac{|\widehat{\boldsymbol{S}}_2||\boldsymbol{A}^{o\prime}\widehat{\boldsymbol{S}}_2\boldsymbol{A}^o|^{-1}|\boldsymbol{A}^{o\prime}\boldsymbol{X}_o\boldsymbol{X}_o'\boldsymbol{A}^o|}{|\boldsymbol{S}_1||\boldsymbol{A}^{o\prime}\boldsymbol{S}_1\boldsymbol{A}^o|^{-1}|\boldsymbol{A}^{o\prime}\boldsymbol{X}_o\boldsymbol{X}_o'\boldsymbol{A}^o|} = \frac{|\widehat{\boldsymbol{S}}_2||\boldsymbol{A}^{o\prime}\widehat{\boldsymbol{S}}_2\boldsymbol{A}^o|^{-1}}{|\boldsymbol{S}_1||\boldsymbol{A}^{o\prime}\boldsymbol{S}_1\boldsymbol{A}^o|^{-1}}.
\end{aligned} \tag{7.14}$$

Put $\boldsymbol{H} = (\boldsymbol{A}^o : \boldsymbol{S}_1^{-1}\underline{\boldsymbol{A}})$, where $\boldsymbol{A}^o$ is supposed to be of full rank and $\underline{\boldsymbol{A}}$ is any matrix of full rank satisfying $\mathcal{C}(\underline{\boldsymbol{A}}) = \mathcal{C}(\boldsymbol{A})$, and note that $\boldsymbol{H}$ is of full rank. Then

$$|\boldsymbol{H}'\boldsymbol{S}_1\boldsymbol{H}| = |\boldsymbol{A}^{o\prime}\boldsymbol{S}_1\boldsymbol{A}^o||\underline{\boldsymbol{A}}'\boldsymbol{S}_1^{-1}\underline{\boldsymbol{A}}|$$

and since $\underline{\boldsymbol{A}}(\underline{\boldsymbol{A}}'\widehat{\boldsymbol{S}}_2^{-1}\underline{\boldsymbol{A}})^{-1}\underline{\boldsymbol{A}}' = \widehat{\boldsymbol{S}}_2 - \widehat{\boldsymbol{S}}_2\boldsymbol{A}^o(\boldsymbol{A}^{o\prime}\widehat{\boldsymbol{S}}_2\boldsymbol{A}^o)^{-1}\boldsymbol{A}^{o\prime}\widehat{\boldsymbol{S}}_2$,

$$|\boldsymbol{H}'\widehat{\boldsymbol{S}}_2\boldsymbol{H}| = |\boldsymbol{A}^{o\prime}\widehat{\boldsymbol{S}}_2\boldsymbol{A}^o||\underline{\boldsymbol{A}}'\boldsymbol{S}_1^{-1}\underline{\boldsymbol{A}}(\underline{\boldsymbol{A}}'\widehat{\boldsymbol{S}}_2^{-1}\underline{\boldsymbol{A}})^{-1}\underline{\boldsymbol{A}}'\boldsymbol{S}_1^{-1}\underline{\boldsymbol{A}}|.$$

Thus, because $\boldsymbol{H}$ is non-singular, it follows from (7.14) that

$$\lambda_o^{\frac{2}{n}} = \frac{|\underline{\boldsymbol{A}}'\boldsymbol{S}_1^{-1}\underline{\boldsymbol{A}}|}{|\underline{\boldsymbol{A}}'\widehat{\boldsymbol{S}}_2^{-1}\underline{\boldsymbol{A}}|}. \tag{7.15}$$

Next $|\underline{\boldsymbol{A}}'\widehat{\boldsymbol{S}}_2^{-1}\underline{\boldsymbol{A}}|$ is manipulated. Let $\boldsymbol{N}$ be any matrix of full rank such that $\mathcal{C}(\boldsymbol{N}) = \mathcal{C}(\boldsymbol{C}) \cap \mathcal{C}(\boldsymbol{G})$ and define (see also Theorem B.12 in Appendix B)

$$\boldsymbol{P}_{\mathcal{B}} = \boldsymbol{P}_{\boldsymbol{C}'} - \boldsymbol{P}_{\boldsymbol{C}'\boldsymbol{G}^o} = \boldsymbol{P}_{\boldsymbol{C}'(\boldsymbol{C}\boldsymbol{C}')^{-}\boldsymbol{N}}.$$

Note that $\mathcal{B}$ indicates that this is a projection on a between-individuals subspace. Then, by calculating $\widehat{\boldsymbol{S}}_2^{-1}$ via Appendix B, Theorem B.6 (i) and using the fact that $\boldsymbol{P}_{C_1'} - \boldsymbol{P}_{C_2'} = \boldsymbol{P}_{\mathcal{B}}$,

$$
\begin{aligned}
|\underline{\boldsymbol{A}}'\widehat{\boldsymbol{S}}_2^{-1}\underline{\boldsymbol{A}}| &= |\underline{\boldsymbol{A}}'\boldsymbol{S}_1^{-1}\underline{\boldsymbol{A}}||\boldsymbol{I} - \boldsymbol{P}_{A,S_1}\widehat{\boldsymbol{Q}}_1'\boldsymbol{X}_o\boldsymbol{P}_{\mathcal{B}} \\
&\quad (\boldsymbol{P}_{\mathcal{B}}\boldsymbol{X}_o'\widehat{\boldsymbol{Q}}_1\boldsymbol{S}_1^{-1}\widehat{\boldsymbol{Q}}_1'\boldsymbol{X}_o\boldsymbol{P}_{\mathcal{B}} + \boldsymbol{I})^{-1}\boldsymbol{P}_{\mathcal{B}}\boldsymbol{X}_o'\widehat{\boldsymbol{Q}}_1\boldsymbol{S}_1^{-1}| \\
&= |\underline{\boldsymbol{A}}'\boldsymbol{S}_1^{-1}\underline{\boldsymbol{A}}||\boldsymbol{I} + \boldsymbol{P}_{\mathcal{B}}\boldsymbol{X}_o'\boldsymbol{P}_{A_1^o,S_1^{-1}}\boldsymbol{S}_1^{-1}\boldsymbol{X}_o\boldsymbol{P}_{\mathcal{B}}|^{-1}|\boldsymbol{I} \\
&\quad + \boldsymbol{P}_{\mathcal{B}}\boldsymbol{X}_o'\boldsymbol{P}_{A^o,S_1^{-1}}\boldsymbol{S}_1^{-1}\boldsymbol{X}_o\boldsymbol{P}_{\mathcal{B}}|
\end{aligned}
$$

and

$$
\lambda_o^{\frac{2}{n}} = \frac{|\boldsymbol{I} + \boldsymbol{P}_{\mathcal{B}}\boldsymbol{X}_o'\boldsymbol{P}_{A_1^o,S_1^{-1}}\boldsymbol{S}_1^{-1}\boldsymbol{X}_o\boldsymbol{P}_{\mathcal{B}}|}{|\boldsymbol{I} + \boldsymbol{P}_{\mathcal{B}}\boldsymbol{X}_o'\boldsymbol{P}_{A^o,S_1^{-1}}\boldsymbol{S}_1^{-1}\boldsymbol{X}_o\boldsymbol{P}_{\mathcal{B}}|}. \tag{7.16}
$$

Using the definition of $\boldsymbol{P}_{\mathcal{B}}$ and taking out $(\boldsymbol{N}'(\boldsymbol{C}\boldsymbol{C}')^-\boldsymbol{N})^{-1}$ yield

$$
\lambda_o^{\frac{2}{n}} = \frac{|\boldsymbol{N}'(\boldsymbol{C}\boldsymbol{C}')^-\boldsymbol{C}(\boldsymbol{I} + \boldsymbol{X}_o'\boldsymbol{P}_{A_1^o,S_1^{-1}}\boldsymbol{S}_1^{-1}\boldsymbol{X}_o)\boldsymbol{C}'(\boldsymbol{C}\boldsymbol{C}')^-\boldsymbol{N}|}{|\boldsymbol{N}'(\boldsymbol{C}\boldsymbol{C}')^-\boldsymbol{C}(\boldsymbol{I} + \boldsymbol{X}_o'\boldsymbol{P}_{A^o,S_1^{-1}}\boldsymbol{S}_1^{-1}\boldsymbol{X}_o)\boldsymbol{C}'(\boldsymbol{C}\boldsymbol{C}')^-\boldsymbol{N}|}.
$$

Moreover, from Appendix B, Theorem B.12, the following relation between projectors appears to be useful for the presentation (remember that $\boldsymbol{A}_1^o = (\boldsymbol{A}(\boldsymbol{F}')^o)^o$):

$$
\boldsymbol{P}_{A_1^o,S_1^{-1}} = \boldsymbol{P}_{A^o,S_1^{-1}} + \boldsymbol{P}_{\mathcal{W}},
$$

where

$$
\boldsymbol{P}_{\mathcal{W}} = \boldsymbol{P}_{S_1^{-1}A(A'S_1^{-1}A)^-M,S_1^{-1}}, \tag{7.17}
$$

$\boldsymbol{M}$ is any matrix of full rank satisfying $\mathcal{C}(\boldsymbol{M}) = \mathcal{C}(\boldsymbol{A}') \cap \mathcal{C}(\boldsymbol{F}')$, and $\mathcal{W}$ denotes that the projection takes place on a within-individual subspace. The application of this relation between projectors is crucial for deriving a good approximation of the distribution for λ. The next issue is to understand the following chain of equalities, where in particular (7.17) has been applied:

$$
\begin{aligned}
\lambda_o^{\frac{2}{n}} &= \frac{|\boldsymbol{N}'(\boldsymbol{C}\boldsymbol{C}')^-\boldsymbol{C}(\boldsymbol{I} + \boldsymbol{X}_o'(\boldsymbol{P}_{A^o,S_1^{-1}} + \boldsymbol{P}_{\mathcal{W}})\boldsymbol{S}_1^{-1}\boldsymbol{X}_o)\boldsymbol{C}'(\boldsymbol{C}\boldsymbol{C}')^-\boldsymbol{N}|}{|\boldsymbol{N}'(\boldsymbol{C}\boldsymbol{C}')^-\boldsymbol{C}(\boldsymbol{I} + \boldsymbol{X}_o'\boldsymbol{P}_{A^o,S_1^{-1}}\boldsymbol{S}_1^{-1}\boldsymbol{X}_o)\boldsymbol{C}'(\boldsymbol{C}\boldsymbol{C}')^-\boldsymbol{N}|} \\
&= |\boldsymbol{I} + \boldsymbol{P}_{\mathcal{W}}\boldsymbol{S}_1^{-1}\boldsymbol{X}_o\boldsymbol{C}'(\boldsymbol{C}\boldsymbol{C}')^-\boldsymbol{N} \\
&\qquad \times\{\boldsymbol{N}'(\boldsymbol{C}\boldsymbol{C}')^-\boldsymbol{C}(\boldsymbol{I} + \boldsymbol{X}_o'\boldsymbol{P}_{A^o,S_1^{-1}}\boldsymbol{S}_1^{-1}\boldsymbol{X}_o)\boldsymbol{C}'(\boldsymbol{C}\boldsymbol{C}')^-\boldsymbol{N}\}^{-1}\boldsymbol{N}'(\boldsymbol{C}\boldsymbol{C}')^-\boldsymbol{C}\boldsymbol{X}_o'|
\end{aligned}
$$

$$= |M'(A'S_1^{-1}A)^- M + M'(A'S_1^{-1}A)^- A'S_1^{-1}X_o C'(CC')^- N \\ \times \{N'(CC')^- C(I + X_o' P_{A^o, S_1^{-1}} S_1^{-1} X_o) C'(CC')^- N\}^{-1} \\ \times N'(CC')^- C X_o' S_1^{-1} A(A'S_1^{-1}A)^- M||M'(A'S_1^{-1}A)^- M|^{-1}. \quad (7.18)$$

From a distributional point of view, the expression in (7.18) seems rather awkward. However, it will be shown that $\lambda_o^{\frac{2}{n}}$ has the same form as the test statistic presented in (7.9); details are presented below after Theorem 7.3. Now we replace the observed variables in (7.18) by the corresponding random variables. From Appendix B, Theorem B.20 (v), it follows that

$$M'(A'S_1^{-1}A)^- M \sim W_{r(M)}(M'(A'\Sigma^{-1}A)^- M, n - r(C) - p + r(A))$$

and $A^{o'}X$ is independent of $A'\Sigma^{-1}X$, see Appendix B, Theorem B.19 (xiii). Moreover,

$$M'(A'S_1^{-1}A)^- A'S_1^{-1}X \\ = M'(A'\Sigma^{-1}A)^- A'\Sigma^{-1}X(I - (I - P_{C'})X'A^o(A^{o'}S_1A^o)^- A^{o'}X),$$

which, given $A^{o'}X$, is normally distributed. Thus, conditionally on $A^{o'}X$, for

$$M'(A'S_1^{-1}A)^- A'S_1^{-1}X \\ \times C'(CC')^- N(N'(CC')^- C(I + X'P_{A^o, S_1^{-1}} S_1^{-1} X)C'(CC')^- N)^{-1/2}, \quad (7.19)$$

under H_0, i.e. $FBG = 0$, the mean and dispersion equal 0 and $I \otimes M'(A'\Sigma^{-1}A)^- M$, respectively, with the remarkable conclusion that the distribution of (7.19) is indeed independent of $A^{o'}X$, and thus (7.19) is normally distributed and its "square" Wishart distributed. If, inside the determinants of $\lambda_o^{\frac{2}{n}}$ in (7.18), one pre- and post-multiplies by the matrix $(M'(A'\Sigma^{-1}A)^- M)^{-1/2}$, the result of the multiplication establishes that $\lambda^{\frac{2}{n}}$ follows the same distribution as

$$\frac{|V + U|}{|V|}, \quad (7.20)$$

where V and U are independent, with $V \sim W_{r(M)}(I, n - r(C) - p + r(A))$ and under H_0, $U \sim W_{r(M)}(I, r(N))$. Hence, the likelihood ratio (7.13) has been turned into a well-known form of a ratio of determinants of Wishart-distributed variables and then the results given in Appendix C.3 can be utilized. Note that in the above derivation, it has implicitly been assumed that both M and N differ from 0. If one of the matrices equals $\mathbf{0}$, then it can be shown that $\lambda_o = 1$, i.e. the hypothesis does not put any restrictions on the parameter space and thus the hypothesis is not meaningful to test. However, it is worth noting that the usual testability conditions $\mathcal{C}(\boldsymbol{F}') \subseteq \mathcal{C}(\boldsymbol{A}')$ and $\mathcal{C}(\boldsymbol{G}) \subseteq \mathcal{C}(\boldsymbol{C})$ are not needed. On the other hand, it is much easier to interpret a test under these nested subspace conditions than without them.

Theorem 7.2 *For the BRM presented in Definition 2.1, the null hypothesis* H_0: $\boldsymbol{FBG} = \mathbf{0}$ *is tested against an alternative without restrictions on* $\boldsymbol{B}$. *Let* λ_o *be the observed value of* λ, *given in (7.13), and let*

$$t_o = \tfrac{2}{n}(f - \tfrac{1}{2}(p_o - m + 1)) \ln \lambda_o,$$

where $f = n - r(\boldsymbol{C}) - p + r(\boldsymbol{A})$, $p_o = \dim\{\mathcal{C}(\boldsymbol{F}') \cap \mathcal{C}(\boldsymbol{A}')\}$ *and* $m = \dim\{\mathcal{C}(\boldsymbol{G}) \cap \mathcal{C}(\boldsymbol{C})\}$. *The likelihood ratio test, approximately at significance level* α, *rejects the hypothesis if* t_o *satisfies*

$$P\{\chi^2_{p_o m} \geq t_o\} + c_1(1 - c_1)(P\{\chi^2_{p_o m+4} \geq t_o\} - P\{\chi^2_{p_o m} \geq t_o\})$$
$$+ c_2(P\{\chi^2_{p_o m+8} \geq t_o\} - P\{\chi^2_{p_o m} \geq t_o\}) \leq \alpha,$$

where

$$c_1 = \frac{p_o m(p_o^2 + m^2 - 5)}{48(f - \frac{1}{2}(p_o - m + 1))^2},$$

$$c_2 = \frac{1}{2}c_1^2 + \frac{p_o m(3p_o^4 + 3m^4 + 10p_o^2 m^2 - 50(p_o^2 + m^2) + 159)}{1920(f - \frac{1}{2}(p_o - m + 1))^4}.$$

□

Corollary 7.1 *If* $\boldsymbol{F} = \boldsymbol{I}$, *for the BRM, presented in Definition 2.1, the test of the null hypothesis* $\boldsymbol{BG} = \mathbf{0}$ *against an alternative without restriction is obtained from Theorem 7.2 if one uses* $p_o = r(\boldsymbol{A})$. □

Corollary 7.2 *If* $\boldsymbol{G} = \boldsymbol{I}$, *for the BRM, presented in Definition 2.1, the test of the null hypothesis* $\boldsymbol{FB} = \mathbf{0}$ *against an alternative without a restriction is obtained from Theorem 7.2 if one uses* $m = r(\boldsymbol{C})$. □

Note that if $p_o = 1$ or $p_o = 2$, instead of Theorem C.3 in Appendix C, the reader is referred to Theorem C.2 (ii) or (iii) in Appendix C, leading to a simplified version of Theorem 7.2. Let $F_{m,f}$ and $F_\beta(m, f)$ denote the F-distribution and its β-percentile (see Appendix A, Sect. A.9).

Theorem 7.3 *The model and hypothesis are the same as those in Theorem 7.2. Let* λ *be given in (7.13) and put* $U_{p_o,m,f} = \lambda^{-\frac{2}{n}}$, *where* $p_o = \dim\{\mathcal{C}(\boldsymbol{F}') \cap \mathcal{C}(\boldsymbol{A}')\}$, $f = n - r(\boldsymbol{C}) - p + r(\boldsymbol{A})$ *and* $m = \dim\{\mathcal{C}(\boldsymbol{G}) \cap \mathcal{C}(\boldsymbol{C})\}$. *Then*

(i) *if* $p_o = 2$, $\quad T_{11} = \frac{(f-1)}{m}(1 - U_{2,m,f}^{1/2})/U_{2,m,f}^{1/2} \sim F_{2m,2(f-1)}$;

(ii) *if* $p_o = 1$, $T_{12} = \frac{f}{m}(1 - U_{1,m,f})/U_{1,m,f} \sim F_{m,f}$.

□

Note that for notational convenience we do not distinguish between an observed $U_{p_o,m,f}$ and a random $U_{p_o,m,f}$. The appropriate interpretation is obvious from the context. Above were presented a number of complicated relations leading to quite a good result, stated in Theorem 7.2. However, it is possible to extract more insight into the construction of the test statistic, as well as increase our understanding of the test, if one exploits some details. First, consider the proof of (see also Appendix B, Theorem B.20 (v))

$$M'(A'S_1^{-1}A)^-M \sim W_{r(M)}(M'(A'\Sigma^{-1}A)^-M, n - r(C) - p + r(A)), \quad (7.21)$$

where M satisfies $\mathcal{C}(M) \subseteq \mathcal{C}(A')$. This proof can run as follows:

$$\begin{aligned} M'(A'S_1^{-1}A)^-M &= M'(A'\Sigma^{-1}A)^-A'\Sigma^{-1}A(A'S_1^{-1}A)^-A'\Sigma^{-1}A(A'\Sigma^{-1}A)^-M \\ &= M'(A'\Sigma^{-1}A)^-A'\Sigma^{-1}(S_1 - S_1A^o(A^{o'}S_1A^o)^-A^{o'}S_1)\Sigma^{-1}A(A'\Sigma^{-1}A)^-M \\ &= M'(A'\Sigma^{-1}A)^-A'\Sigma^{-1}XPX'\Sigma^{-1}A(A'\Sigma^{-1}A)^-M, \end{aligned}$$

where

$$P = I - P_{C'} - (I - P_{C'})X'A^o(A^{o'}S_1A^o)^-A^{o'}X(I - P_{C'}). \quad (7.22)$$

Now $A'\Sigma^{-1}X$ is independent of $A^{o'}X$ and $P^2 = P$, i.e. P is idempotent of rank $n - r(C) - r(A^o)$. Thus, it is possible to establish (7.21) by using a conditional argument, i.e. condition with respect to $A^{o'}X$, and then conditionally (7.21) is true, which, however, due to the idempotency of P, with probability 1, does not depend on $A^{o'}X$ and hence holds unconditionally. This also means that according to Definition 7.1, we may consider $M'(A'S_1^{-1}A)^-M$ to be interpreted as a dispersion quantity. Furthermore, it is interesting to note that when conditioning with respect to $A^{o'}X$, information is moved from the within-individuals subspace to the between-individuals subspace.

Next $M'(A'S_1^{-1}A)^-A'S_1^{-1}XC'(CC')^-N$ in (7.18) is exploited. It follows that

$$\begin{aligned} &M'(A'S_1^{-1}A)^-A'S_1^{-1}XC'(CC')^-N \\ &\quad = M'(A'\Sigma^{-1}A)^-A'\Sigma^{-1}A(A'S_1^{-1}A)^-A'S_1^{-1}XC'(CC')^-N \\ &\quad = M'(A'\Sigma^{-1}A)^-A'\Sigma^{-1}(I - S_1A^o(A^{o'}S_1A^o)^-A^{o'})XC'(CC')^-N \\ &\quad = M'(A'\Sigma^{-1}A)^-A'\Sigma^{-1}XP_1C'(CC')^-N, \end{aligned}$$

where

$$P_1 = I - (I - P_{C'})X'A^o(A^{o'}S_1A^o)^-A^{o'}X. \quad (7.23)$$

It can be shown that $\boldsymbol{P}_1$ is idempotent, $\mathcal{C}(\boldsymbol{P}_1) = \mathcal{C}(\boldsymbol{X}'\boldsymbol{A}^o)^\perp$ and $\mathcal{N}(\boldsymbol{P}_1) = \mathcal{C}((\boldsymbol{I} - \boldsymbol{P}_{C'})\boldsymbol{X}'\boldsymbol{A}^o)$. Therefore, according to Appendix B, Theorem B.11 (iv)

$$\mathcal{C}(\boldsymbol{P}_1\boldsymbol{C}'(\boldsymbol{C}\boldsymbol{C}')^-\boldsymbol{N}) = \mathcal{C}(\boldsymbol{X}'\boldsymbol{A}^o)^\perp \cap \{\mathcal{C}((\boldsymbol{I} - \boldsymbol{P}_{C'})\boldsymbol{X}'\boldsymbol{A}^o) \boxplus \mathcal{C}(\boldsymbol{C}'(\boldsymbol{C}\boldsymbol{C}')^-\boldsymbol{N})\} \quad (7.24)$$

and $\boldsymbol{P}\boldsymbol{P}_1\boldsymbol{C}'(\boldsymbol{C}\boldsymbol{C}')^-\boldsymbol{N} = \boldsymbol{0}$. Thus, with probability 1, (7.18) is identical to

$$\lambda^{\frac{2}{n}} = \frac{|\widetilde{\boldsymbol{V}} + \widetilde{\boldsymbol{U}}|}{|\widetilde{\boldsymbol{V}}|},$$

where

$$\begin{aligned}
\widetilde{\boldsymbol{V}} &= (\boldsymbol{M}'(\boldsymbol{A}'\boldsymbol{\Sigma}^{-1}\boldsymbol{A})^-\boldsymbol{M})^{-1/2}\boldsymbol{M}'(\boldsymbol{A}'\boldsymbol{\Sigma}^{-1}\boldsymbol{A})^-\boldsymbol{A}'\boldsymbol{\Sigma}^{-1}\boldsymbol{X}\boldsymbol{P}\boldsymbol{X}' \\
&\quad \times\boldsymbol{\Sigma}^{-1}\boldsymbol{A}(\boldsymbol{A}'\boldsymbol{\Sigma}^{-1}\boldsymbol{A})^-\boldsymbol{M}(\boldsymbol{M}'(\boldsymbol{A}'\boldsymbol{\Sigma}^{-1}\boldsymbol{A})^-\boldsymbol{M})^{-1/2}, \\
\widetilde{\boldsymbol{U}} &= (\boldsymbol{M}'(\boldsymbol{A}'\boldsymbol{\Sigma}^{-1}\boldsymbol{A})^-\boldsymbol{M})^{-1/2}\boldsymbol{M}'(\boldsymbol{A}'\boldsymbol{\Sigma}^{-1}\boldsymbol{A})^-\boldsymbol{A}'\boldsymbol{\Sigma}^{-1}\boldsymbol{X} \\
&\quad \times\boldsymbol{P}_1\boldsymbol{C}'(\boldsymbol{C}\boldsymbol{C}')^-\boldsymbol{N}(\boldsymbol{N}'(\boldsymbol{C}\boldsymbol{C}')^-\boldsymbol{C}\boldsymbol{P}_1'\boldsymbol{P}_1\boldsymbol{C}'(\boldsymbol{C}\boldsymbol{C}')^-\boldsymbol{N})^-\boldsymbol{N}'(\boldsymbol{C}\boldsymbol{C}')^-\boldsymbol{C}\boldsymbol{P}_1' \\
&\quad \times\boldsymbol{X}'\boldsymbol{\Sigma}^{-1}\boldsymbol{A}(\boldsymbol{A}'\boldsymbol{\Sigma}^{-1}\boldsymbol{A})^-\boldsymbol{M}(\boldsymbol{M}'(\boldsymbol{A}'\boldsymbol{\Sigma}^{-1}\boldsymbol{A})^-\boldsymbol{M})^{-1/2},
\end{aligned}$$

and $\widetilde{\boldsymbol{V}}$ and $\widetilde{\boldsymbol{U}}$ are, conditionally on $\boldsymbol{A}^{o'}\boldsymbol{X}$, independently distributed. Moreover, conditionally on $\boldsymbol{A}^{o'}\boldsymbol{X}$, $\widetilde{\boldsymbol{V}} \sim W_{r(M)}(\boldsymbol{I}, r(\boldsymbol{P}))$ and, under H_0, $\widetilde{\boldsymbol{U}} \sim W_{r(M)}(\boldsymbol{I}, r(\boldsymbol{P}_1\boldsymbol{C}'(\boldsymbol{C}\boldsymbol{C}')^-\boldsymbol{N}))$, which then also hold unconditionally, where

$$\begin{aligned}
r(\boldsymbol{P}) &= n - r(\boldsymbol{C}) - p + r(\boldsymbol{A}), \quad (7.25)\\
r(\boldsymbol{P}_1\boldsymbol{C}'(\boldsymbol{C}\boldsymbol{C}')^-\boldsymbol{N}) &= r(\boldsymbol{N}),
\end{aligned}$$

and it also follows that $\widetilde{\boldsymbol{V}}$ and $\widetilde{\boldsymbol{U}}$ are independently distributed. Furthermore, it is possible to interpret λ via dispersion quantities; i.e. it has in fact been shown above that in (7.18)

$$\boldsymbol{D}_{12} = \boldsymbol{M}'(\boldsymbol{A}'\boldsymbol{S}_1^{-1}\boldsymbol{A})^-\boldsymbol{M}, \quad (7.26)$$

$$\begin{aligned}
\boldsymbol{D}_{21} &= \boldsymbol{M}'(\boldsymbol{A}'\boldsymbol{S}_1^{-1}\boldsymbol{A})^-\boldsymbol{A}'\boldsymbol{S}_1^{-1}\boldsymbol{X}\boldsymbol{C}'(\boldsymbol{C}\boldsymbol{C}')^-\boldsymbol{N}(\boldsymbol{N}'(\boldsymbol{C}\boldsymbol{C}')^-\boldsymbol{C}\boldsymbol{P}_1'\boldsymbol{P}_1\boldsymbol{C}'(\boldsymbol{C}\boldsymbol{C}')^-\boldsymbol{N})^- \\
&\quad \times\boldsymbol{N}'(\boldsymbol{C}\boldsymbol{C}')^-\boldsymbol{C}\boldsymbol{X}'\boldsymbol{S}_1^{-1}\boldsymbol{A}(\boldsymbol{A}'\boldsymbol{S}_1^{-1}\boldsymbol{A})^-\boldsymbol{M}, \quad (7.27)
\end{aligned}$$

both of which, according to Definition 7.1, are dispersion quantities which are independent and Wishart-distributed. Therefore, the test criterion λ_o has the same distribution as

$$\lambda^{\frac{2}{n}} = \frac{|\boldsymbol{D}_{12} + \boldsymbol{D}_{21}|}{|\boldsymbol{D}_{12}|}. \quad (7.28)$$

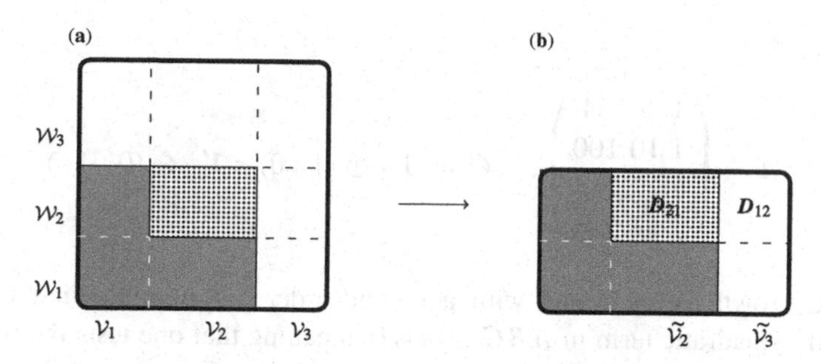

Fig. 7.4 In (**a**), the dotted area corresponds to H_0: $\boldsymbol{FBG} = \boldsymbol{0}$. In (**b**), those areas are given which are of interest for the likelihood ratio test. Furthermore, $\mathcal{W}_1 = \mathcal{C}_{\bullet}(\boldsymbol{A}(\boldsymbol{F}')^o)$, $\mathcal{W}_2 = \mathcal{C}_{\bullet}(\boldsymbol{A}) \cap \mathcal{C}_{\bullet}(\boldsymbol{A}(\boldsymbol{F}')^o)^{\perp}$, $\mathcal{W}_3 = \mathcal{C}_{\bullet}(\boldsymbol{A})^{\perp}$, $\mathcal{V}_1 = \mathcal{C}(\boldsymbol{C}'\boldsymbol{G}^o)$, $\mathcal{V}_2 = \mathcal{C}(\boldsymbol{C}') \cap \mathcal{C}(\boldsymbol{C}'\boldsymbol{G}^o)^{\perp}$, $\mathcal{V}_3 = \mathcal{C}(\boldsymbol{C}')^{\perp}$, $\widetilde{\mathcal{V}}_2 = \mathcal{C}(\boldsymbol{P}_1\boldsymbol{C}'(\boldsymbol{C}\boldsymbol{C}')^{-}\boldsymbol{N})$ and $\widetilde{\mathcal{V}}_3 = \mathcal{C}(\boldsymbol{P}_1(\boldsymbol{C}')^o)$, where $\boldsymbol{P}_1$ is defined in (7.23). The dispersion matrices $\boldsymbol{D}_{12}$ and $\boldsymbol{D}_{21}$ are defined in (7.26) and (7.27), respectively

Before leaving the likelihood ratio test statistic $\lambda_o^{\frac{2}{n}}$, given in (7.18), the following reflections seem to be appropriate. The distribution of $\lambda^{\frac{2}{n}}$ is described through a ratio of determinants of Wishart-distributed dispersion matrices. Moreover, it was shown that the distribution does not depend on $\boldsymbol{A}^{o'}\boldsymbol{X}$. Unfortunately, this does not mean that when replacing $\boldsymbol{X}$ by the data $\boldsymbol{X}_o$, in order to calculate $\lambda_o^{\frac{2}{n}}$, the observed likelihood ratio statistic will be functionally independent of $\boldsymbol{A}^{o'}\boldsymbol{X}_o$. Hence, when evaluating this fact, the projectors $\boldsymbol{P}$ and $\boldsymbol{P}_1$ or $(\boldsymbol{I} - \boldsymbol{P}_{C'})\boldsymbol{X}_o'\boldsymbol{A}^o(\boldsymbol{A}^{o'}\boldsymbol{S}_1\boldsymbol{A}^o)^{-}\boldsymbol{A}^{o'}\boldsymbol{X}_o(\boldsymbol{I} - \boldsymbol{P}_{C'})$ have to be investigated. If, for example, $\boldsymbol{P}$ is "small", the observed likelihood ratio, $\lambda_o^{\frac{2}{n}}$, may be "large". This occurs if $r(\boldsymbol{X}_o'\boldsymbol{A}^o)$ is close to $n - r(\boldsymbol{C})$, which may take place in high-dimensional problems when p and n are close to each other (see also (7.25)), although it is still important to assume that $p \leq n - r(\boldsymbol{C})$, which means that "real" high-dimensional problems are not covered by the present approach. The effect of $\boldsymbol{A}^{o'}\boldsymbol{X}_o$ is usually not serious. However, performing some simulations may help us to understand if a particular choice of $\boldsymbol{A}$ in a particular situation may have the potential to harm conclusions.

In Fig. 7.4, those spaces are presented which are involved in building the test statistic. The conditioning by $\boldsymbol{A}^{o'}\boldsymbol{X}$ has an influence on the result via the projection $\boldsymbol{P}_1$. In particular, $\widetilde{\mathcal{V}}_2 = \mathcal{C}(\boldsymbol{P}_1\boldsymbol{C}'(\boldsymbol{C}\boldsymbol{C}')^{-}\boldsymbol{N})$ and $\widetilde{\mathcal{V}}_3 = \mathcal{C}(\boldsymbol{P}) = \mathcal{C}(\boldsymbol{P}_1(\boldsymbol{C}')^o)$ should be understood, since the dispersions on these spaces build up the likelihood ratio test. This means that we have spaces which depend on $\boldsymbol{A}^{o'}\boldsymbol{X}_o$, i.e. depend on data when the test concerns the mean parameters. However, this is not very satisfactory, because it is more difficult to interpret the outcome of this test than, for example, to interpret the outcome of the most commonly applied test in MANOVA (see e.g. Fig. 7.2). On the other hand, it can be shown via (7.24) that $\widetilde{\mathcal{W}_2}$ equals $\{\boldsymbol{0}\}$ if $\mathcal{C}(\boldsymbol{N}) = \{\boldsymbol{0}\}$, which is exactly what we want to test.

Example 7.2 Consider the Potthoff and Roy data presented in Table 1.2 and analysed in Example 3.1. Let, as in Model IIa of Example 3.1, $\boldsymbol{X} = \boldsymbol{ABC} + \boldsymbol{E}$,

where

$$A = \begin{pmatrix} 1 & 8 & 64 \\ 1 & 10 & 100 \\ 1 & 12 & 144 \\ 1 & 14 & 196 \end{pmatrix}, \qquad C = (\mathbf{1}'_{11} \otimes (1:0)' : \mathbf{1}'_{16} \otimes (0:1)').$$

Thus, the growth is modelled with a second-order polynomial. First one tests whether the quadratic term in ABC equals $\mathbf{0}$, meaning that one tests the following hypothesis:

$$H_0 : FB = \mathbf{0}, \quad versus \ H_1 : B \text{ unrestricted},$$

where $F = (0 : 0 : 1)$. In Theorem 7.2 it follows that $f = 24$, $p_o = 1$ and $m = 2$. Since $p_o = 1$, instead of Theorem 7.2, Theorem 7.3 (ii) is utilized. Moreover, the calculations show that $\lambda_o^{2/27} = 1.0976$. Thus, $U_{1,2,24} = \lambda_o^{-2/27} = 0.911$ and

$$T_{12o} = \frac{24}{2}(1 - U_{1,2,24})/U_{1,2,24} = 1.2 < F_{0.05}(2, 24) = 3.4.$$

Hence H_0 cannot be rejected at significance level 0.05.

Next it is supposed that only the girls follow a quadratic growth, which is reflected in the following test:

$$H_0 : FBG = \mathbf{0}, \quad versus \ H_1 : B \text{ unrestricted},$$

where $F = (0 : 0 : 1)$ and $G = (0 : 1)'$. Theorem 7.3 (ii) informs us that the hypothesis should not be rejected, since

$$T_{12o} = 24(1 - U_{1,1,24})/U_{1,1,24} = 2.3 < F_{0.05}(1, 24) = 4.3.$$

Finally, it is tested whether there is no growth between age 8 and age 14 for both the boys and the girls, i.e. H_0: $FB = \mathbf{0}$, where

$$F = \begin{pmatrix} 0 & 1 & 0 \\ 0 & 0 & 1 \end{pmatrix}.$$

In this case, according to Theorem 7.2, $f = 24$, $p_o = 2$ and $m = 2$. Since $p_o = 2$, Theorem 7.3 (i) can be applied. The calculations yield $\lambda_o^{2/27} = 6.123$. Thus, $U_{2,2,24} = \lambda_o^{-2/27} = 0.16$ and

$$T_{11o} = \frac{23}{2}(1 - U_{2,2,24}^{\frac{1}{2}})/U_{2,2,24}^{\frac{1}{2}} = 17.0 > F_{0.05}(4, 46) = 2.6.$$

Hence, H_0 can be rejected at significance level 0.05. Of course, if there is any power in the test, this hypothesis should be rejected, which was fortunately also what took place. □

Example 7.3 Below, a couple of tests are performed which are based on the melatonin data described in Example 1.6. The data were generated with the help of the following design and parameter matrices. Let $\omega = \pi/24$,

$$
\boldsymbol{A}_1 = \begin{pmatrix} 1 & \sin(\omega) & \cos(\omega) \\ 1 & \sin(4\omega) & \cos(4\omega) \\ 1 & \sin(8\omega) & \cos(8\omega) \\ 1 & \sin(12\omega) & \cos(12\omega) \\ 1 & \sin(14\omega) & \cos(14\omega) \\ 1 & \sin(16\omega) & \cos(16\omega) \\ 1 & \sin(18\omega) & \cos(18\omega) \\ 1 & \sin(20\omega) & \cos(20\omega) \\ 1 & \sin(22\omega) & \cos(22\omega) \\ 1 & \sin(24\omega) & \cos(24\omega) \end{pmatrix}, \quad \boldsymbol{A}_2 = \begin{pmatrix} \sin(2\omega) \\ \sin(4*2\omega) \\ \sin(8*2\omega) \\ \sin(12*2\omega) \\ \sin(14*2\omega) \\ \sin(16*2\omega) \\ \sin(18*2\omega) \\ \sin(20*2\omega) \\ \sin(22*2\omega) \\ \sin(24*2\omega) \end{pmatrix}, \quad \boldsymbol{A}_3 = \begin{pmatrix} \cos(2\omega) \\ \cos(4*2\omega) \\ \cos(8*2\omega) \\ \cos(12*2\omega) \\ \cos(14*2\omega) \\ \cos(16*2\omega) \\ \cos(18*2\omega) \\ \cos(20*2\omega) \\ \cos(22*2\omega) \\ \cos(24*2\omega) \end{pmatrix},
$$

$$
\boldsymbol{C}_1 = (\mathbf{1}'_{10} \otimes \begin{pmatrix} 1 \\ 0 \\ 0 \end{pmatrix} : \mathbf{1}'_{15} \otimes \begin{pmatrix} 0 \\ 1 \\ 0 \end{pmatrix} : \mathbf{1}'_{20} \otimes \begin{pmatrix} 0 \\ 0 \\ 1 \end{pmatrix}),
$$

$$
\boldsymbol{C}_2 = (\mathbf{1}'_{10} \otimes \begin{pmatrix} 1 \\ 0 \end{pmatrix} : \mathbf{1}'_{15} \otimes \begin{pmatrix} 0 \\ 1 \end{pmatrix} : \mathbf{1}'_{20} \otimes \begin{pmatrix} 0 \\ 0 \end{pmatrix}), \quad \boldsymbol{C}_3 = (\mathbf{1}'_{10} : \mathbf{1}'_{35} \otimes 0),
$$

$$
\boldsymbol{B}_1 = \begin{pmatrix} 0.01 & 0.14 & 0.20 \\ 0.21 & -0.01 & -0.004 \\ 0.02 & 0.03 & -0.01 \end{pmatrix}, \quad \boldsymbol{B}_2 = (-0.04 : -0.06), \quad \boldsymbol{B}_3 = (0.10);
$$

$\boldsymbol{\Sigma}$ is given in Example 1.9. Then data according to

$$
\boldsymbol{X} = \boldsymbol{A}_1\boldsymbol{B}_1\boldsymbol{C}_1 + \boldsymbol{A}_2\boldsymbol{B}_2\boldsymbol{C}_2 + \boldsymbol{A}_3\boldsymbol{B}_3\boldsymbol{C}_3 + \boldsymbol{E}, \quad \boldsymbol{E} \sim N_{10,45}(\mathbf{0}, \boldsymbol{\Sigma}, \boldsymbol{I})
$$

are simulated. Note that the data set consists of three different groups of independent observations, each of which has a somewhat different within-individuals means structure. Moreover, no explicit data values are presented, since it is expected that the readers can generate their own data with the help of the matrices given above. Thus, it is not possible to copy the calculations in this example exactly, but the sizes of the estimates and the tests should be the same. (This will also be the case in several of the following examples.)

Now the BRM is studied and, therefore, we put $\boldsymbol{A} = (\boldsymbol{A}_1 : \boldsymbol{A}_2 : \boldsymbol{A}_3)$, i.e.

$$\boldsymbol{A} = \begin{pmatrix} 1 & \sin(\omega) & \cos(\omega) & \sin(2\omega) & \cos(2\omega) \\ 1 & \sin(4\omega) & \cos(4\omega) & \sin(4 * 2\omega) & \cos(4 * 2\omega) \\ 1 & \sin(8\omega) & \cos(8\omega) & \sin(8 * 2\omega) & \cos(8 * 2\omega) \\ 1 & \sin(12\omega) & \cos(12\omega) & \sin(12 * 2\omega) & \cos(12 * 2\omega) \\ 1 & \sin(14\omega) & \cos(14\omega) & \sin(14 * 2\omega) & \cos(14 * 2\omega) \\ 1 & \sin(16\omega) & \cos(16\omega) & \sin(16 * 2\omega) & \cos(16 * 2\omega) \\ 1 & \sin(18\omega) & \cos(18\omega) & \sin(18 * 2\omega) & \cos(18 * 2\omega) \\ 1 & \sin(20\omega) & \cos(20\omega) & \sin(20 * 2\omega) & \cos(20 * 2\omega) \\ 1 & \sin(22\omega) & \cos(22\omega) & \sin(22 * 2\omega) & \cos(22 * 2\omega) \\ 1 & \sin(24\omega) & \cos(24\omega) & \sin(24 * 2\omega) & \cos(24 * 2\omega) \end{pmatrix},$$

$$\boldsymbol{C} = (\boldsymbol{1}'_{10} \otimes \begin{pmatrix} 1 \\ 0 \\ 0 \end{pmatrix} : \boldsymbol{1}'_{15} \otimes \begin{pmatrix} 0 \\ 1 \\ 0 \end{pmatrix} : \boldsymbol{1}'_{20} \otimes \begin{pmatrix} 0 \\ 0 \\ 1 \end{pmatrix}).$$

On the basis of how the data were generated, it is known that they do not follow the BRM model. In fact, the true model is a BRM with $\boldsymbol{F}_i \boldsymbol{B} \boldsymbol{G}_i = \boldsymbol{0}$, $i = 1, 2$, where

$$\boldsymbol{F}_1 = (0 : 0 : 0 : 0 : 1), \;\; \boldsymbol{G}_1 = (0 : 1 : 0)', \;\; \boldsymbol{F}_2 = \begin{pmatrix} 0\,0\,0\,1\,0 \\ 0\,0\,0\,0\,1 \end{pmatrix}, \;\; \boldsymbol{G}_2 = (0 : 0 : 1)', \tag{7.29}$$

which equivalently can be stated as: for $\boldsymbol{B} = (b_{ij})$, $b_{52} = b_{43} = b_{53} = 0$.

If there is a reasonable power of the likelihood ratio test, which is not obvious since $p = 10$ is relatively large, the observed test statistic should lead to rejection. First H_0: $\boldsymbol{F}\boldsymbol{B} = \boldsymbol{0}$ against H_1: $\boldsymbol{B}$ unrestricted is tested, where

$$\boldsymbol{F} = \begin{pmatrix} 0\,0\,0\,1\,0 \\ 0\,0\,0\,0\,1 \end{pmatrix},$$

which is identical to $\boldsymbol{F}_2$ in (7.29). Here it is tested if H_0 is "true", with the knowledge that since the data consist of three groups with different mean structures, as assumed above, this cannot be correct; i.e. $\boldsymbol{G}_2$ indicates that only one group out of the three is restricted by $\boldsymbol{F}$. Additionally, $\boldsymbol{F}_1 \boldsymbol{B} \boldsymbol{G}_1 = \boldsymbol{0}$ should be valid. Hence, whether or not the difference is uncovered is only a matter of power. The test statistic equals $\lambda_o^{2/45} = 2.49$. In order to choose an appropriate transformation of λ, for example T_{11} or T_{12} of Theorem 7.3 (i) or (ii), one needs to determine p_o. It can be shown that $p_o = \dim\{\mathcal{C}(\boldsymbol{F}') \cap \mathcal{C}(\boldsymbol{A}')\} = 2$. Moreover, $m = \dim\{\mathcal{C}(\boldsymbol{I}_3) \cap \mathcal{C}(\boldsymbol{C})\} = 3$ and $f = n - r(\boldsymbol{C}) - p + r(\boldsymbol{A}) = 37$. Thus, Theorem 7.3 (i) can be used and $U_{2,3,37} = \lambda_o^{-2/45} = 0.40$, leading to

$$T_{11o} = \frac{36}{3}(1 - U_{2,3,37}^{\frac{1}{2}})/U_{2,3,37}^{\frac{1}{2}} = 6.9 > F_{0.05}(6, 74) = 2.2.$$

Hence, H_0 is rejected at significance level 0.05.

Furthermore, H_0: $\boldsymbol{FBG} = \boldsymbol{0}$ versus H_1: $\boldsymbol{B}$ unrestricted can be tested with an $\boldsymbol{F}$ which is identical to the $\boldsymbol{F}$ of the previous test and $\boldsymbol{G} = (1 : 0 : 0)'$. In this case $\lambda_o^{2/45} = 1.31$, $p_o = 2$ and $m = 1$. Then, according to Theorem 7.3 (i), $U_{2,1,37} = \lambda_o^{-2/45} = 0.76$ and, since

$$T_{11o} = 36(1 - U_{2,1,37}^{\frac{1}{2}})/U_{2,1,37}^{\frac{1}{2}} = 5.2 > F_{0.05}(2, 74) = 3.1,$$

the hypothesis H_0 is rejected at significance level 0.05. If instead of via $\boldsymbol{G} = (1 : 0 : 0)'$, the restrictions in H_0 are defined via $\boldsymbol{G} = (0 : 0 : 1)'$, the test statistic $T_{11o} = 1.4$ implies that the hypothesis should not be rejected, which is in complete agreement with the data-generating assumptions in (7.29).

Finally, the hypothesis H_0: $\boldsymbol{FBG} = \boldsymbol{0}$ is tested against an unrestricted $\boldsymbol{B}$, where $\boldsymbol{G} = (1 : 0 : 0)'$ and $\boldsymbol{F} = (\boldsymbol{0} : \boldsymbol{I}_4)$, i.e. the first group has a constant mean. As before, in order to choose an appropriate test statistic, p_o has to be determined and in this case equals $p_o = 4$. Thus, there is no test statistic with an exact F-distribution and the result will rely on Theorem 7.2. Now $m = 1$, $f = 37$ and the value of t_o of the theorem is 10.2. Therefore,

$$\begin{aligned} &P\{\chi_4^2 \geq t_o\} + c_1(1 - c_1)(P\{\chi_8^2 \geq t_o\} - P\{\chi_4^2 \geq t_o\}) \\ &\quad + c_2(P\{\chi_{12}^2 \geq t_o\} - P\{\chi_4^2 \geq t_o\}) \approx P\{\chi_4^2 \geq t_o\} = 0.04, \end{aligned}$$

since c_1 and c_2 are small, and therefore H_0 is rejected at the significance level $\alpha = 0.05$. □

7.4 Likelihood Ratio Testing $H_0 : \boldsymbol{F}_1\boldsymbol{B}\boldsymbol{G}_1 = \boldsymbol{0}$ in the BRM with the Restrictions $\boldsymbol{F}_2\boldsymbol{B}\boldsymbol{G}_2 = \boldsymbol{0}$, $\mathcal{C}(\boldsymbol{F}_1') \subseteq \mathcal{C}(\boldsymbol{F}_2')$

In this section, the BRM is treated, together with two bilinear restrictions on $\boldsymbol{B}$, i.e. $\boldsymbol{F}_i\boldsymbol{B}\boldsymbol{G}_i = \boldsymbol{0}$, $i = 1, 2$, where $\boldsymbol{F}_i$ and $\boldsymbol{G}_i$ are known matrices. The presentation closely follows the one given in the previous section. Theorem B.10 (iii) in Appendix B implies that

$$\boldsymbol{F}_i\boldsymbol{B}\boldsymbol{G}_i = \boldsymbol{0}, \qquad i = 1, 2,$$

is equivalent to

$$\begin{aligned} \boldsymbol{B} &= (\boldsymbol{F}_1' : \boldsymbol{F}_2')^o\boldsymbol{\Theta}_1 + (\boldsymbol{F}_2' : (\boldsymbol{F}_1' : \boldsymbol{F}_2')^o)^o\boldsymbol{\Theta}_2\boldsymbol{G}_1^{o'} \\ &\quad +(\boldsymbol{F}_1' : (\boldsymbol{F}_1' : \boldsymbol{F}_2')^o)^o\boldsymbol{\Theta}_3\boldsymbol{G}_2^{o'} + ((\boldsymbol{F}_1')^o : (\boldsymbol{F}_2')^o)^o\boldsymbol{\Theta}_4(\boldsymbol{G}_1 : \boldsymbol{G}_2)^{o'}, \end{aligned}$$

where $\boldsymbol{\Theta}_1 - \boldsymbol{\Theta}_4$ are new parameters, which, however, are not considered in this section. Then, multiplying by $\boldsymbol{A}$ and $\boldsymbol{C}$, the mean structure for the BRM with double bilinear restrictions is obtained:

$$E[\boldsymbol{X}] = \boldsymbol{ABC} = \boldsymbol{A}(\boldsymbol{F}_1' : \boldsymbol{F}_2')^o\boldsymbol{\Theta}_1\boldsymbol{C} + \boldsymbol{A}(\boldsymbol{F}_2' : (\boldsymbol{F}_1' : \boldsymbol{F}_2')^o)^o\boldsymbol{\Theta}_2\boldsymbol{G}_1^{o'}\boldsymbol{C}$$
$$+ \boldsymbol{A}(\boldsymbol{F}_1' : (\boldsymbol{F}_1' : \boldsymbol{F}_2')^o)^o\boldsymbol{\Theta}_3\boldsymbol{G}_2^{o'}\boldsymbol{C} + \boldsymbol{A}((\boldsymbol{F}_1')^o : (\boldsymbol{F}_2')^o)^o\boldsymbol{\Theta}_4(\boldsymbol{G}_1 : \boldsymbol{G}_2)^{o'}\boldsymbol{C}. \tag{7.30}$$

Because (7.30) does not expose a hierarchical subspace structure (stairs structure), it follows that in order to utilize results for either the $EBRM_B^\bullet$ or $EBRM_W^\bullet$, an additional assumption has to be introduced. For example, any of the following assumption can be chosen:

$$\mathcal{C}(\boldsymbol{F}_1') \subseteq \mathcal{C}(\boldsymbol{F}_2'), \quad \boldsymbol{A}(\boldsymbol{F}_2' : (\boldsymbol{F}_1' : \boldsymbol{F}_2')^o)^o = \boldsymbol{0}, \quad \mathcal{C}(\boldsymbol{G}_2^o) \subseteq \mathcal{C}(\boldsymbol{G}_1^o),$$
$$\mathcal{C}(\boldsymbol{C}'\boldsymbol{G}_2^o) \subseteq \mathcal{C}(\boldsymbol{C}'\boldsymbol{G}_1^o).$$

In this section, $\mathcal{C}(\boldsymbol{F}_1') \subseteq \mathcal{C}(\boldsymbol{F}_2')$ is discussed, but the other cases which are listed can be handled in a similar fashion. Under the assumption $\mathcal{C}(\boldsymbol{F}_1') \subseteq \mathcal{C}(\boldsymbol{F}_2')$, an $EBRM_B^3$ emerges with a mean structure given by

$$E[\boldsymbol{X}] = \boldsymbol{ABC} = \boldsymbol{A}(\boldsymbol{F}_2')^o\boldsymbol{\Theta}_1\boldsymbol{C} + \boldsymbol{A}(\boldsymbol{F}_1' : (\boldsymbol{F}_2')^o)^o\boldsymbol{\Theta}_3\boldsymbol{G}_2^{o'}\boldsymbol{C} + \boldsymbol{A}\boldsymbol{F}_1'\boldsymbol{\Theta}_4(\boldsymbol{G}_1 : \boldsymbol{G}_2)^{o'}\boldsymbol{C}. \tag{7.31}$$

Note that the nested subspace condition $\mathcal{C}(\boldsymbol{C}'(\boldsymbol{G}_1 : \boldsymbol{G}_2)^o) \subseteq \mathcal{C}(\boldsymbol{C}'\boldsymbol{G}_2^o) \subseteq \mathcal{C}(\boldsymbol{C}')$ holds. Before starting the mathematical derivation of the test, a simple example is presented illustrating the model assumptions.

Example 7.4 (Similar to the Potthoff and Roy Data Presented in Example 1.7) To illustrate the test presented and the assumptions made in this section, the following BRM is supposed to be valid: $E[\boldsymbol{X}] = \boldsymbol{ABC}$ with $\boldsymbol{F}_2\boldsymbol{B}\boldsymbol{G}_2 = \boldsymbol{0}$, where

$$\boldsymbol{A} = \begin{pmatrix} 1 & t_1 & t_1^2 \\ 1 & t_2 & t_2^2 \\ \vdots & \vdots & \vdots \\ 1 & t_p & t_p^2 \end{pmatrix}, \quad \boldsymbol{C} = (\mathbf{1}_{n_1}' \otimes (1 : 0 : 0)' : \mathbf{1}_{n_2}' \otimes (0 : 1 : 0)' : \mathbf{1}_{n_3}' \otimes (0 : 0 : 1)'),$$

$$\boldsymbol{F}_2 = \begin{pmatrix} 0 & 0 & 1 \\ 0 & 1 & 0 \end{pmatrix}, \quad \boldsymbol{G}_2 = (0 : 1 : 0)'.$$

The hypothesis is specified as $H_0 : \boldsymbol{F}_1\boldsymbol{B}\boldsymbol{G}_1 = \boldsymbol{0}$, where

$$\boldsymbol{F}_1 = (0 : 0 : 1), \qquad \boldsymbol{G}_1 = (0 : 0 : 1)'.$$

Hence, $\mathcal{C}(F_1') \subseteq \mathcal{C}(F_2')$ and we have an example reflecting (7.31), similar to the Potthoff and Roy data set. However, instead of two groups (girls and boys), as in the data set of Potthoff and Roy, there are three groups of individuals whose members have a constant mean, or follow a linear or a quadratic mean structure over time. The restriction $F_2BG_2 = 0$ states that for the second group, the mean over time is constant. The hypothesis $F_1BG_1 = 0$ is supposed to test whether the mean over time for the third group is linear. □

For the model of this section, the likelihood ratio for testing $H_0 : F_iBG_i = 0$, $i = 1, 2$, against $H_1 : F_2BG_2 = 0$, i.e. testing $H_0 : F_1BG_1 = 0$ within the BRM with the restriction $F_2BG_2 = 0$, according to Theorem 3.2, is equivalent to

$$\lambda_o^{\frac{2}{n}} = \frac{|\widehat{\Sigma}_{H_0}|}{|\widehat{\Sigma}_{H_1}|} = \frac{|\widehat{S}_3 + \widehat{Q}_3'\widehat{Q}_2'\widehat{Q}_1' X_o P_{C_3'} X_o' \widehat{Q}_1\widehat{Q}_2\widehat{Q}_3|}{|\widehat{S}_2 + P'_{A^o,\widehat{S}_2^{-1}} X_o P_{C_2'} X_o' P_{A^o,\widehat{S}_2^{-1}}|},$$

where

$$A_1 = A(F_2')^o, \quad C_1 = C, \quad A_2 = A(F_1' : (F_2')^o)^o, \quad C_2 = G_2^{o'}C,$$

$$A_3 = AF_1', \quad C_3 = (G_1 : G_2)^{o'}C,$$

$$n\widehat{\Sigma}_{H_0} = \widehat{S}_3 + P'_{A^o,\widehat{S}_3^{-1}} X_o P_{C_3} X_o' P_{A^o,\widehat{S}_3^{-1}},$$

$$\widehat{S}_3 = \widehat{S}_2 + P'_{(A_1:A_2)^o,\widehat{S}_2^{-1}} X_o(P_{C_2'} - P_{C_3'})X_o' P_{(A_1:A_2)^o,\widehat{S}_2^{-1}},$$

$$\widehat{S}_2 = S_1 + P'_{A_1^o,S_1^{-1}} X_o(P_{C_1'} - P_{C_2'})X_o' P_{A_1^o,S_1^{-1}}, \quad S_1 = X_o(I - P_{C_1'})X_o',$$

$$\widehat{Q}_1 = I - P'_{A_1,S_1}, \quad \widehat{Q}_2 = I - P'_{\widehat{Q}_1'A_2,\widehat{S}_2},$$

$$\widehat{Q}_3 = I - P'_{\widehat{Q}_2'\widehat{Q}_1'A_3,\widehat{S}_3}, \quad \widehat{Q}_1\widehat{Q}_2\widehat{Q}_3 = P_{A^o,\widehat{S}_3^{-1}}.$$

In order to determine the distribution of the test statistic, a somewhat technical treatment takes place. It is suggested that those who are only interested in the results should jump directly to Theorem 7.4.

Taking out $\widehat{S}_2$ and $\widehat{S}_3$ from the determinants of the numerator and the denominator yields after a few calculations

$$\lambda_o^{\frac{2}{n}} = \frac{|\widehat{S}_3 + P'_{A^o,\widehat{S}_3^{-1}} X_o P_{C_3} X_o' P_{A^o,\widehat{S}_3^{-1}}|}{|\widehat{S}_2 + P'_{A^o,\widehat{S}_2^{-1}} X_o P_{C_2'} X_o' P_{A^o,\widehat{S}_2^{-1}}|} = \frac{|\widehat{S}_3||A^{o'}\widehat{S}_3A^o|^{-1}}{|\widehat{S}_2||A^{o'}\widehat{S}_2A^o|^{-1}}.$$

Put $H = (A^o : \widehat{S}_2^{-1}\underline{A})$, where, as previously, $\underline{A}$ is any matrix of full rank satisfying $\mathcal{C}(\underline{A}) = \mathcal{C}(A)$ and A^o is of full rank. Thus, H is of full rank and

$$|H'\widehat{S}_2H| = |A^{o'}\widehat{S}_2A^o||\underline{A}'\widehat{S}_2^{-1}\underline{A}|.$$

Since $\underline{A}(\underline{A}'\widehat{S}_3^{-1}\underline{A})^{-1}\underline{A}' = \widehat{S}_3 - \widehat{S}_3A^o(A^{o'}\widehat{S}_3A^o)^{-1}A^{o'}\widehat{S}_3$ (see Appendix B, Theorem B.13),

$$|H'\widehat{S}_3H| = |A^{o'}\widehat{S}_3A^o||\underline{A}'\widehat{S}_2^{-1}\underline{A}(\underline{A}'\widehat{S}_3^{-1}\underline{A})^{-1}\underline{A}'\widehat{S}_2^{-1}\underline{A}|.$$

These calculations show, because H is non-singular, that

$$\lambda_o^{\frac{2}{n}} = \frac{|\underline{A}'\widehat{S}_2^{-1}\underline{A}|}{|\underline{A}'\widehat{S}_3^{-1}\underline{A}|}. \tag{7.32}$$

Neither $\widehat{S}_2$ nor $\widehat{S}_3$ are Wishart-distributed and, therefore, this ratio is slightly more complicated to handle than (7.15). Let N be any matrix of full rank satisfying $\mathcal{C}(N) = \mathcal{C}(G_2^{o'}C) \cap \mathcal{C}(G_2^{o'}G_1)$ and define

$$P_{\mathcal{B}} = P_{C'G_2^o(G_2^{o'}CC'G_2^o)^-N},$$

implying that $P_{C_2'} - P_{C_3'} = P_{\mathcal{B}}$, since

$$\begin{aligned}\mathcal{C}(C'G_2^o(G_2^{o'}CC'G_2^o)^-N) &= \mathcal{C}(C'G_2^o(G_2^{o'}CC'G_2^o)^-G_2^{o'}C(C'G_2^o(G_2^{o'}G_1)^o)^o)\\ &= \mathcal{C}(C'G_2^o(G_2^{o'}CC'G_2^o)^-G_2^{o'}C(C'(G_1 : G_2)^o)^o) = \mathcal{C}(C'G_2^o) \cap \mathcal{C}(C'(G_1 : G_2)^o)^{\perp},\end{aligned}$$

where in the last equality the projection theorem, Appendix B, Theorem B.11 (iv), has been utilized. Then, by calculating $\widehat{S}_3^{-1}$ as a function of $\widehat{S}_2^{-1}$, according to Appendix B, Theorem B.6 (i),

$$\begin{aligned}|\underline{A}'\widehat{S}_3^{-1}\underline{A}| &= |\underline{A}'\widehat{S}_2^{-1}\underline{A}|\\ &\quad\times|I - P_{A,\widehat{S}_2}\widehat{Q}_2'\widehat{Q}_1'X_oP_{\mathcal{B}}(P_{\mathcal{B}}X_o'\widehat{Q}_1\widehat{Q}_2\widehat{S}_2^{-1}\widehat{Q}_2'\widehat{Q}_1'X_oP_{\mathcal{B}} + I)^{-1}\\ &\quad\times P_{\mathcal{B}}X_o'\widehat{Q}_1\widehat{Q}_2\widehat{S}_2^{-1}|\\ &= |\underline{A}'\widehat{S}_2^{-1}\underline{A}||I + P_{\mathcal{B}}X_o'P_{(A_1:A_2)^o,\widehat{S}_2^{-1}}\widehat{S}_2^{-1}X_oP_{\mathcal{B}}|^{-1}\\ &\quad\times|I + P_{\mathcal{B}}X_o'P_{A^o,\widehat{S}_2^{-1}}\widehat{S}_2^{-1}X_oP_{\mathcal{B}}|.\end{aligned}$$

Hence,

$$\begin{aligned}\lambda_o^{\frac{2}{n}} &= \frac{|I + P_{\mathcal{B}}X_o'P_{(A_1:A_2)^o,\widehat{S}_2^{-1}}\widehat{S}_2^{-1}X_oP_{\mathcal{B}}|}{|I + P_{\mathcal{B}}X_o'P_{A^o,\widehat{S}_2^{-1}}\widehat{S}_2^{-1}X_oP_{\mathcal{B}}|}\\ &= \frac{|N'(G_2^{o'}CC'G_2^o)^-G_2^{o'}C(I + X_o'P_{(A_1:A_2)^o,\widehat{S}_2^{-1}}\widehat{S}_2^{-1}X_o)C'G_2^o(G_2^{o'}CC'G_2^o)^-N|}{|N'(G_2^{o'}CC'G_2^o)^-G_2^{o'}C(I + X_o'P_{A^o,\widehat{S}_2^{-1}}\widehat{S}_2^{-1}X_o)C'G_2^o(G_2^{o'}CC'G_2^o)^-N|}.\end{aligned}$$

Moreover, once again applying Appendix B, Theorem B.12,

$$P_{(A_1:A_2)^o,\widehat{S}_2^{-1}} = P_{A^o,\widehat{S}_2^{-1}} + P_{\mathcal{W}},$$

where, since $\mathcal{C}(A_1 : A_2) = \mathcal{C}(A(F_1')^o)$,

$$P_{\mathcal{W}} = P_{\widehat{S}_2^{-1}A(A'\widehat{S}_2^{-1}A)^-M,\widehat{S}_2^{-1}},$$

and M is any matrix of full rank satisfying $\mathcal{C}(M) = \mathcal{C}(F_1') \cap \mathcal{C}(A')$. Thus, by copying the calculations presented when deriving (7.18),

$$\begin{aligned}\lambda_o^{\frac{2}{n}} &= |M'(A'\widehat{S}_2^{-1}A)^-M + M'(A'\widehat{S}_2^{-1}A)^-A'\widehat{S}_2^{-1}X_oC'G_2^o(G_2^{o'}CC'G_2^o)^-N\\ &\quad\times\{N'(G_2^{o'}CC'G_2^o)^-G_2^{o'}C(I + X_o'P_{A^o,\widehat{S}_2^{-1}}\widehat{S}_2^{-1}X_o)C'G_2^o(G_2^{o'}CC'G_2^o)^-N\}^{-1}\\ &\quad\times N'(G_2^{o'}CC'G_2^o)^-G_2^{o'}CX_o'\widehat{S}_2^{-1}A(A'\widehat{S}_2^{-1}A)^-M||M'(A'\widehat{S}_2^{-1}A)^-M|^{-1}.\end{aligned} \tag{7.33}$$

The remaining task is to study the distributional properties of the corresponding statistic $\lambda^{\frac{2}{n}}$. Let

$$W = X(I - P_{C_2'})X' \sim W_p(\Sigma, n - r(C_2)).$$

Noting that (7.33) does not depend on the choice of M as long as it satisfies $\mathcal{C}(M) = \mathcal{C}(A') \cap \mathcal{C}(F_1')$, the representation $M = A'(A(F_1')^o)^o$ can be used and

$$\begin{aligned}M'(A'\widehat{S}_2^{-1}A)^-M &= (A(F_1')^o)^{o'}A(A'\widehat{S}_2^{-1}A)^-A'(A(F_1')^o)^o\\ &= (A(F_1')^o)^{o'}\widehat{S}_2(A(F_1')^o)^o - (A(F_1')^o)^{o'}\widehat{S}_2A^o(A^{o'}\widehat{S}_2A^o)^-A^{o'}\widehat{S}_2(A(F_1')^o)^o\\ &= (A(F_1')^o)^{o'}W(A(F_1')^o)^o - (A(F_1')^o)^{o'}WA^o(A^{o'}WA^o)^-A^{o'}W(A(F_1')^o)^o\\ &= M'(A'W^{-1}A)^-M \sim W_{r(M)}(M'(A'\Sigma^{-1}A)^-M, n - r(C_2) - p + r(A)),\end{aligned}$$

where Theorem B.13 in Appendix B has been applied. Moreover,

$$M'(A'\widehat{S}_2^{-1}A)^-A'\widehat{S}_2^{-1} = M'(A'W^{-1}A)^-A'W^{-1}.$$

Thus, using (7.33),

$$\begin{aligned}\lambda^{\frac{2}{n}} &= |M'(A'W^{-1}A)^-M + M'(A'W^{-1}A)^-A'W^{-1}XC'G_2^o(G_2^{o'}CC'G_2^o)^-N\\ &\quad\times\{N'(G_2^{o'}CC'G_2^o)^-G_2^{o'}C(I + X'P_{A^o,W^{-1}}W^{-1}X)C'G_2^o(G_2^{o'}CC'G_2^o)^-N\}^{-1}\\ &\quad\times N'(G_2^{o'}CC'G_2^o)^-G_2^{o'}CX'W^{-1}A(A'W^{-1}A)^-M||M'(A'W^{-1}A)^-M|^{-1}.\end{aligned} \tag{7.34}$$

Since $XC'G_2^o$ is independent of W, the expression in (7.34) has the same form as (7.18) and it can immediately be stated that $\lambda^{2/n}$ follows the distribution of

$$\frac{|V+U|}{|V|}, \tag{7.35}$$

where V and U are independent, $V \sim W_{r(M)}(I, n-r(C_2)-p+r(A))$ and under H_0, $U \sim W_{r(M)}(I, r(N))$. Hence, the next two theorems can be stated and they are similar to Theorems 7.2 and 7.3.

Theorem 7.4 *For the BRM presented in Definition 2.1 with the restrictions $F_2BG_2 = 0$, the null hypothesis H_0: $F_1BG_1 = 0$, $F_2BG_2 = 0$, where $\mathcal{C}(F_1') \subseteq \mathcal{C}(F_2')$, is tested against H_1: $F_2BG_2 = 0$. Let λ_o be the observed value of λ, given in (7.32), and let*

$$t_o = \tfrac{2}{n}(f - \tfrac{1}{2}(p_o - m + 1)) \ln \lambda_o,$$

where $f = n - r(G_2^{o'}C) - p + r(A)$, $p_o = \dim\{\mathcal{C}(F_1') \cap \mathcal{C}(A')\}$ and $m = \dim\{\mathcal{C}(G_2^{o'}C) \cap \mathcal{C}(G_2^{o'}G_1)\}$. The likelihood ratio test, approximately at significance level α, rejects the hypothesis if t_o satisfies

$$\begin{aligned} P\{\chi^2_{p_om} \geq t_o\} &+ c_1(1-c_1)(P\{\chi^2_{p_om+4} \geq t_o\} - P\{\chi^2_{p_om} \geq t_o\}) \\ &+ c_2(P\{\chi^2_{p_om+8} \geq t_o\} - P\{\chi^2_{p_om} \geq t_o\}) \leq \alpha, \end{aligned}$$

where c_1 and c_2 are defined in Theorem 7.2. □

Theorem 7.5 *The model and hypothesis are the same as those in Theorem 7.4. Let λ_o be given in (7.32) with a corresponding λ and put $U_{p_o,m,f} = \lambda^{-\frac{2}{n}}$, where $p_o = \dim\{\mathcal{C}(F_1') \cap \mathcal{C}(A')\}$, $f = n - r(G_2^{o'}C) - p + r(A)$ and $m = \dim\{\mathcal{C}(G_2^{o'}C) \cap \mathcal{C}(G_2^{o'}G_1)\}$. Then*

(i) *if $p_o = 2$,* $T_{21} = \frac{(f-1)}{m}(1 - U_{2,m,f}^{1/2})/U_{2,m,f}^{1/2} \sim F_{2m,2(f-1)}$;
(ii) *if $p_o = 1$,* $T_{22} = \frac{f}{m}(1 - U_{1,m,f})/U_{1,m,f} \sim F_{m,f}$.

□

Moreover, as with (7.20), the final result presented in (7.35) was obtained by conditioning on $A^{o'}X$. Correspondingly to (7.22) and (7.23), which were used in (7.26) and (7.27), the following projections were utilized:

$$P = P_1(I - P_{C_2'}) = I - P_{C_2'} - (I - P_{C_2'})X'A^o(A^{o'}WA^o)^- A^{o'}X(I - P_{C_2'}),$$

$$P_1 = I - (I - P_{C_2'})X'A^o(A^{o'}WA^o)^- A^{o'}X.$$

Via these projections, dispersion matrices can be defined and random properties of the presented test statistic stem from the obtained dispersion matrices. The

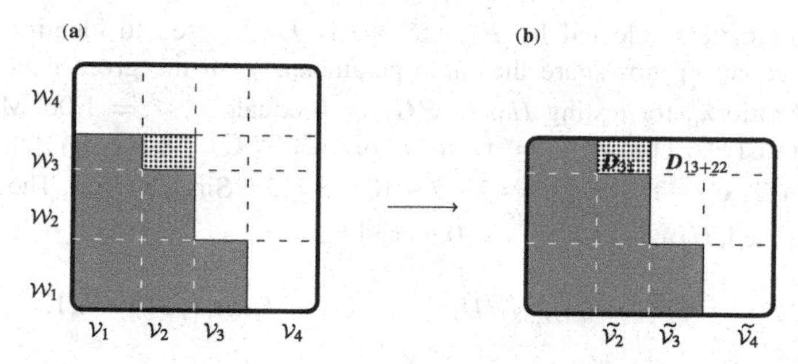

Fig. 7.5 In (**a**), the dotted area corresponds to H_0: $F_1BG_1 = 0$ in the BRM with the restrictions $F_2BG_2 = 0$, where $\mathcal{C}(F_1') \subseteq \mathcal{C}(F_2')$. In (**b**), those areas are given which, after conditioning with respect to $A^{o'}X$, contribute to the likelihood ratio test. Furthermore, $\mathcal{W}_1 = \mathcal{C}_\bullet(A(F_2')^o)$, $\mathcal{W}_2 = \mathcal{C}_\bullet(A(F_1')^o) \cap \mathcal{C}_\bullet(A(F_2')^o)^\perp$, $\mathcal{W}_3 = \mathcal{C}_\bullet(A) \cap \mathcal{C}_\bullet(A(F_1')^o)^\perp$, $\mathcal{W}_4 = \mathcal{C}_\bullet(A)^\perp$, $\mathcal{V}_1 = \mathcal{C}(C'(G_1 : G_2)^o)$, $\mathcal{V}_2 = \mathcal{C}(C'G_2^o) \cap \mathcal{C}(C'(G_1 : G_2)^o)^\perp$, $\mathcal{V}_3 = \mathcal{C}(C') \cap \mathcal{C}(C'G_2^o)^\perp$, $\mathcal{V}_4 = \mathcal{C}(C')^\perp$, $\widetilde{\mathcal{V}}_2 = \mathcal{C}(P_{P_1C'G_2^o(G_2^{o'}CC'G_2^o)^-N})$, $\mathcal{C}(N) = \mathcal{C}(G_2^{o'}C) \cap \mathcal{C}(G_2^{o'}G_1)$ and $\widetilde{\mathcal{V}}_3 + \widetilde{\mathcal{V}}_4 = \mathcal{C}(P_{C_2'})^\perp$. The dispersion matrices D_{31} and D_{13+22} are defined in (7.37) and (7.36), respectively

dispersion matrices of interest are

$$D_{13+22} = M'(A'W^{-1}A)^-M = M'(A'\Sigma^{-1}A)^-A'\Sigma^{-1}XPX'\Sigma^{-1}A(A'\Sigma^{-1}A)^-M, \tag{7.36}$$

$$D_{31} = M'(A'\Sigma^{-1}A)^-A'\Sigma^{-1}XP_{P_1C'G_2^o(G_2^{o'}CC'G_2^o)^-N}X'\Sigma^{-1}A(A'\Sigma^{-1}A)^-M. \tag{7.37}$$

Therefore,

$$\lambda^{\frac{2}{n}} = \frac{|D_{13+22} + D_{31}|}{|D_{13+22}|}. \tag{7.38}$$

The likelihood ratio test, the dispersion matrices and the spaces which are involved in building up the test are illustrated in Fig. 7.5. It is recommended that one should compare Fig. 7.5 with Fig. 7.4 in order to understand the similarities and differences between deriving the tests in Sect. 7.3 and deriving those in Sect. 7.4.

In the above derivation, the likelihood ratio test for testing $H_0 : F_1BG_1 = 0$ was derived when $F_2BG_2 = 0$ and $\mathcal{C}(F_1') \subseteq \mathcal{C}(F_2')$ held. However, it follows from the derivation of the test that the same test statistic is obtained when $\mathcal{C}(F_1') = \mathcal{C}(F_2')$, which in fact leads to a case where the result of the test is often easier to interpret than when $\mathcal{C}(F_1') \subseteq \mathcal{C}(F_2')$ occurs.

Example 7.5 In this example the same data as those in Example 7.3 are used. The matrices which are considered are the following:

$$F_1 = (0:0:0:0:1),\quad G_1 = (1:-1:0)',\quad F_2 = \begin{pmatrix} 0\,0\,0\,1\,0 \\ 0\,0\,0\,0\,1 \end{pmatrix},\quad G_2 = (0:0:1)'.$$

For the parameters selected by $\boldsymbol{F}_1$, the matrix $\boldsymbol{G}_1$ is used to identify that the first and second groups share the same parameter. With the given matrices, the likelihood ratio λ_o for testing H_0: $\boldsymbol{F}_1\boldsymbol{B}\boldsymbol{G}_1 = \boldsymbol{0}$ equals $\lambda_o^{2/45} = 1.06$. Moreover, $p_o = \dim\{\mathcal{C}(\boldsymbol{F}_1') \cap \mathcal{C}(\boldsymbol{A}')\} = 1$, $m = \dim\{\mathcal{C}(\boldsymbol{G}_2^{o'}\boldsymbol{C}) \cap \mathcal{C}(\boldsymbol{G}_2^{o'}\boldsymbol{G}_1)\} = 1$ and $f = n - r(\boldsymbol{G}_2^{o'}\boldsymbol{C}) - p + r(\boldsymbol{A}) = 45 - 2 - 10 + 5 = 38$. Since $p_o = 1$, Theorem 7.5 (ii) can be used, $U_{1,1,38} = \lambda_o^{-2/45} = 0.94$ and

$$T_{22o} = 38(1 - U_{1,1,38})/U_{1,1,38} = 2.4 < F_{0.05}(1, 38) = 4.1.$$

Hence, H_0 cannot be rejected at significance level 0.05. □

7.5 Likelihood Ratio Testing $H_0: \boldsymbol{F}_2\boldsymbol{B}\boldsymbol{G}_2 = \boldsymbol{0}$ in the BRM with the Restrictions $\boldsymbol{F}_1\boldsymbol{B}\boldsymbol{G}_1 = \boldsymbol{0}$, $\mathcal{C}(\boldsymbol{F}_1') \subseteq \mathcal{C}(\boldsymbol{F}_2')$ and $\mathcal{C}(\boldsymbol{G}_2) \subseteq \mathcal{C}(\boldsymbol{G}_1)$

In the previous section, when testing $H_0 : \boldsymbol{F}_1\boldsymbol{B}\boldsymbol{G}_1 = \boldsymbol{0}$ in the BRM with the restrictions $\boldsymbol{F}_2\boldsymbol{B}\boldsymbol{G}_2 = \boldsymbol{0}$ and $\mathcal{C}(\boldsymbol{F}_1') \subseteq \mathcal{C}(\boldsymbol{F}_2')$, the $EBRM_B^3$ was utilized. Now the following testing problem in the BRM with the restrictions $\boldsymbol{F}_1\boldsymbol{B}\boldsymbol{G}_1 = \boldsymbol{0}$ is considered:

$$H_0 : \boldsymbol{F}_2\boldsymbol{B}\boldsymbol{G}_2 = \boldsymbol{0},\ \boldsymbol{F}_1\boldsymbol{B}\boldsymbol{G}_1 = \boldsymbol{0}, \quad \text{versus } H_1 : \boldsymbol{F}_1\boldsymbol{B}\boldsymbol{G}_1 = \boldsymbol{0}, \tag{7.39}$$

where $\mathcal{C}(\boldsymbol{F}_1') \subseteq \mathcal{C}(\boldsymbol{F}_2')$ and $\mathcal{C}(\boldsymbol{G}_2) \subseteq \mathcal{C}(\boldsymbol{G}_1)$. One reason for discussing this testing problem is to present an alternative approach to the one given in the previous section. Without any loss of generality, it can be shown that it is appropriate to assume $\mathcal{C}(\boldsymbol{G}_2) = \mathcal{C}(\boldsymbol{G}_1)$ instead of $\mathcal{C}(\boldsymbol{G}_2) \subseteq \mathcal{C}(\boldsymbol{G}_1)$, which, however, will not take place. Moreover, assume that $\mathcal{C}(\boldsymbol{G}_2) \subseteq \mathcal{C}(\boldsymbol{G}_1)$ does not hold, i.e. the same assumptions as in Sect. 7.4 hold. If one only focuses on H_0, it follows from the assumption $\boldsymbol{F}_2\boldsymbol{B}\boldsymbol{G}_2 = \boldsymbol{0}$ that $\boldsymbol{F}_1\boldsymbol{B}\boldsymbol{G}_2 = \boldsymbol{0}$ also holds. Hence, under H_0, $\boldsymbol{F}_1\boldsymbol{B}\boldsymbol{G}_1 = \boldsymbol{0}$ is identical to $\boldsymbol{F}_1\boldsymbol{B}(\boldsymbol{G}_1 : \boldsymbol{G}_2) = \boldsymbol{0}$ and, of course, $\mathcal{C}(\boldsymbol{G}_1) \subseteq \mathcal{C}(\boldsymbol{G}_1 : \boldsymbol{G}_2)$. Thus, the restrictions on the parameter space of $\boldsymbol{B}$ under H_0 are the same in Sects. 7.4 and 7.5.

Example 7.6 To illustrate the test and model assumptions of this section, we use three groups of individuals with different mean structures. Let $E[\boldsymbol{X}] = \boldsymbol{A}\boldsymbol{B}\boldsymbol{C}$ with $\boldsymbol{F}_1\boldsymbol{B}\boldsymbol{G}_1 = \boldsymbol{0}$ and under H_0: $\boldsymbol{F}_2\boldsymbol{B}\boldsymbol{G}_2 = \boldsymbol{0}$, where

$$\boldsymbol{A} = \begin{pmatrix} 1 & t_1 & t_1^2 \\ 1 & t_2 & t_2^2 \\ \vdots & \vdots & \vdots \\ 1 & t_p & t_p^2 \end{pmatrix}, \qquad \boldsymbol{C} = (\mathbf{1}_{n_1}' \otimes (1:0:0)' : \mathbf{1}_{n_2}' \otimes (0:1:0)' : \mathbf{1}_{n_3}' \otimes (0:0:1)'),$$

$$\boldsymbol{F}_1 = (0:0:1), \quad \boldsymbol{G}_1 = \begin{pmatrix} 0\,0 \\ 0\,1 \\ 1\,0 \end{pmatrix}, \quad \boldsymbol{F}_2 = \begin{pmatrix} 0\,0\,1 \\ 0\,1\,0 \end{pmatrix}, \quad \boldsymbol{G}_2 = (0:1:0)'.$$

Hence, $\mathcal{C}(\boldsymbol{F}_1') \subseteq \mathcal{C}(\boldsymbol{F}_2')$ and $\mathcal{C}(\boldsymbol{G}_2) \subseteq \mathcal{C}(\boldsymbol{G}_1)$. The "growth" for one of the groups is modelled with a second-order polynomial; i.e. one of the groups has a quadratic growth and the two other groups follow a linear growth. Moreover, it is tested whether one of the two groups with a linear growth has a constant mean. Thus, under H_0, one group has a constant mean, one group follows a linear mean model and one group follows a quadratic mean model.

It is clear that under H_0, the mean has a nested structure in the same way as it has with the $EBRM_B^3$ or $EBRM_W^3$. Under the alternative hypothesis, the treatment groups follow either a linear or a quadratic mean model. Let $\boldsymbol{B} = (b_{ij})$, and then alternatively to the matrix formulation of the restrictions $\boldsymbol{F}_i\boldsymbol{B}\boldsymbol{G}_i = \boldsymbol{0}$, $i = 1, 2$, the hypothesis can be written as H_0: $b_{32} = b_{33} = b_{22} = 0$. □

The general solution to the system of equations $\boldsymbol{F}_1\boldsymbol{B}\boldsymbol{G}_1 = \boldsymbol{0}$, $\boldsymbol{F}_2\boldsymbol{B}\boldsymbol{G}_2 = \boldsymbol{0}$ is presented in Appendix B, Theorem B.10 (iii). With the additional subspace conditions, the results imply the following mean structure:

$$E[\boldsymbol{X}] = \boldsymbol{A}\boldsymbol{\Theta}_1\boldsymbol{G}_1^{o'}\boldsymbol{C} + \boldsymbol{A}(\boldsymbol{F}_1')^o\boldsymbol{\Theta}_2(\boldsymbol{G}_2 : \boldsymbol{G}_1^o)^{o'}\boldsymbol{C} + \boldsymbol{A}(\boldsymbol{F}_2')^o\boldsymbol{\Theta}_3\boldsymbol{G}_2'\boldsymbol{C}.$$

This means that under $\boldsymbol{H}_0$, since $\mathcal{C}(\boldsymbol{A}(\boldsymbol{F}_2')^o) \subseteq \mathcal{C}(\boldsymbol{A}(\boldsymbol{F}_1')^o) \subseteq \mathcal{C}(\boldsymbol{A})$, the mean model yields an $EBRM_W^3$. Hence, Theorem 3.3 provides the MLE for $\boldsymbol{\Sigma}$, i.e.

$$\begin{aligned} n\widehat{\boldsymbol{\Sigma}}_{H_0} &= \widehat{\boldsymbol{S}}_3 + \boldsymbol{P}'_{A_1^o,\widehat{S}_3^{-1}}\boldsymbol{X}\boldsymbol{P}_{C_1'}\boldsymbol{X}'\boldsymbol{P}_{A_1^o,\widehat{S}_3^{-1}}, \\ \widehat{\boldsymbol{S}}_3 &= \widehat{\boldsymbol{S}}_2 + \boldsymbol{P}'_{A_2^o,\widehat{S}_2^{-1}}\boldsymbol{X}\boldsymbol{P}_2\boldsymbol{X}'\boldsymbol{P}_{A_2^o,\widehat{S}_2^{-1}}, \\ \widehat{\boldsymbol{S}}_2 &= \boldsymbol{S}_1 + \boldsymbol{P}'_{A_3^o,S_1^{-1}}\boldsymbol{X}\boldsymbol{P}_3\boldsymbol{X}'\boldsymbol{P}_{A_3^o,S_1^{-1}}, \end{aligned}$$

where $\boldsymbol{P}_2$ and $\boldsymbol{P}_3$ are orthogonal projectors on $\mathcal{C}(\boldsymbol{C}_1')^\perp \cap \mathcal{C}(\boldsymbol{C}_1' : \boldsymbol{C}_2')$ and $\mathcal{C}(\boldsymbol{C}_1' : \boldsymbol{C}_2')^\perp \cap \mathcal{C}(\boldsymbol{C}')$, respectively, $\boldsymbol{A}_1 = \boldsymbol{A}$, $\boldsymbol{A}_2 = \boldsymbol{A}(\boldsymbol{F}_1')^o$, $\boldsymbol{A}_3 = \boldsymbol{A}(\boldsymbol{F}_2')^o$, $\boldsymbol{S}_1 = \boldsymbol{X}(\boldsymbol{I} - \boldsymbol{P}_{C'})\boldsymbol{X}'$, $\boldsymbol{C}_1 = \boldsymbol{G}_1^{o'}\boldsymbol{C}$, $\boldsymbol{C}_2 = (\boldsymbol{G}_2 : \boldsymbol{G}_1^o)^{o'}\boldsymbol{C}$ and $\boldsymbol{C}_3 = \boldsymbol{G}_2'\boldsymbol{C}$.

For the alternative hypothesis there is only the restriction $\boldsymbol{F}_1\boldsymbol{B}\boldsymbol{G}_1 = \boldsymbol{0}$ on the mean parameter space and in this case the mean of the model may be written as follows:

$$E[\boldsymbol{X}] = \boldsymbol{A}\boldsymbol{\Theta}_1\boldsymbol{G}_1^{o'}\boldsymbol{C} + \boldsymbol{A}(\boldsymbol{F}_1')^o\boldsymbol{\Theta}_2\boldsymbol{G}_1'\boldsymbol{C}. \tag{7.40}$$

Since $\mathcal{C}(\boldsymbol{A}(\boldsymbol{F}_1')^o) \subseteq \mathcal{C}(\boldsymbol{A})$, it follows that in this case there is an $EBRM_W^2$ which has to be considered. Thus, from Theorem 3.3,

$$\begin{aligned} n\widehat{\boldsymbol{\Sigma}}_{H_1} &= \widehat{\boldsymbol{S}}_2 + \boldsymbol{P}'_{\boldsymbol{A}_1^o,\widehat{\boldsymbol{S}}_2^{-1}}\boldsymbol{X}\boldsymbol{P}_{\boldsymbol{C}_1'}\boldsymbol{X}'\boldsymbol{P}_{\boldsymbol{A}_1^o,\widehat{\boldsymbol{S}}_2^{-1}}, \\ \widehat{\boldsymbol{S}}_2 &= \boldsymbol{S}_1 + \boldsymbol{P}'_{\boldsymbol{A}_2^o,\boldsymbol{S}_1^{-1}}\boldsymbol{X}\boldsymbol{P}_4\boldsymbol{X}'\boldsymbol{P}_{\boldsymbol{A}_2^o,\boldsymbol{S}_1^{-1}}, \end{aligned} \tag{7.41}$$

where $\boldsymbol{P}_4$ is the orthogonal projector on $\mathcal{C}(\boldsymbol{C}') \cap \mathcal{C}(\boldsymbol{C}_1')^\perp$, $\boldsymbol{A}_1 = \boldsymbol{A}$, $\boldsymbol{A}_2 = \boldsymbol{A}(\boldsymbol{F}_1')^o$, $\boldsymbol{C}_1 = \boldsymbol{G}_1^{o'}\boldsymbol{C}$, $\boldsymbol{C}_2 = \boldsymbol{G}_1'\boldsymbol{C}$ and $\boldsymbol{S}_1 = \boldsymbol{X}(\boldsymbol{I} - \boldsymbol{P}_{\boldsymbol{C}'})\boldsymbol{X}'$. This implies that under H_0 and H_1, the matrices $\boldsymbol{A}_1$, $\boldsymbol{A}_2$, $\boldsymbol{C}_1$ and $\boldsymbol{S}_1$ are the same. Note also that the parameter $\boldsymbol{\Theta}_1$ in (7.40) is not affected by the hypothesis.

Using the same type of calculations as in the previous sections, it can be shown that the likelihood ratio statistic is equivalent to

$$\lambda_o^{\frac{2}{n}} = \frac{|\widehat{\boldsymbol{\Sigma}}_{H_0}|}{|\widehat{\boldsymbol{\Sigma}}_{H_1}|} = \frac{|\widehat{\boldsymbol{S}}_3||\boldsymbol{A}^{o'}\widehat{\boldsymbol{S}}_3\boldsymbol{A}^o|^{-1}|\boldsymbol{A}^{o'}\boldsymbol{X}_o\boldsymbol{X}_o'\boldsymbol{A}^o|}{|\widehat{\boldsymbol{S}}_2||\boldsymbol{A}^{o'}\widehat{\boldsymbol{S}}_2\boldsymbol{A}^o|^{-1}|\boldsymbol{A}^{o'}\boldsymbol{X}_o\boldsymbol{X}_o'\boldsymbol{A}^o|}. \tag{7.42}$$

Since $\boldsymbol{P}_4 = \boldsymbol{P}_2 + \boldsymbol{P}_3$ it follows that $\boldsymbol{A}^{o'}\widehat{\boldsymbol{S}}_3\boldsymbol{A}^o = \boldsymbol{A}^{o'}\widehat{\boldsymbol{S}}_2\boldsymbol{A}^o$ and $\boldsymbol{A}_2^{o'}\widehat{\boldsymbol{S}}_3\boldsymbol{A}_2^o = \boldsymbol{A}_2^{o'}\widehat{\boldsymbol{S}}_2\boldsymbol{A}_2^o$. Moreover, expanding $|\widehat{\boldsymbol{S}}_3|$ and $|\widehat{\boldsymbol{S}}_2|$ yields

$$\begin{aligned} \lambda_o^{\frac{2}{n}} &= \frac{|\widehat{\boldsymbol{S}}_2||\boldsymbol{A}_2^{o'}\widehat{\boldsymbol{S}}_2\boldsymbol{A}_2^o|^{-1}|\boldsymbol{A}_2^{o'}(\boldsymbol{S}_1 + \boldsymbol{X}_o\boldsymbol{P}_3\boldsymbol{X}_o' + \boldsymbol{X}_o\boldsymbol{P}_2\boldsymbol{X}_o')\boldsymbol{A}_2^o|}{|\boldsymbol{S}_1||\boldsymbol{A}_2^{o'}\boldsymbol{S}_1\boldsymbol{A}_2^o|^{-1}|\boldsymbol{A}_2^{o'}(\boldsymbol{S}_1 + \boldsymbol{X}_o\boldsymbol{P}_4\boldsymbol{X}_o')\boldsymbol{A}_2^o|} \\ &= \frac{|\widehat{\boldsymbol{S}}_2||\boldsymbol{A}_2^{o'}\widehat{\boldsymbol{S}}_2\boldsymbol{A}_2^o|^{-1}}{|\boldsymbol{S}_1||\boldsymbol{A}_2^{o'}\boldsymbol{S}_1\boldsymbol{A}_2^o|^{-1}}, \end{aligned} \tag{7.43}$$

which has the same form as (7.14); i.e. replacing $\boldsymbol{A}$ in (7.14) by $\boldsymbol{A}_2 = \boldsymbol{A}(\boldsymbol{F}_1')^o$ and replacing $\boldsymbol{A}_1 = \boldsymbol{A}(\boldsymbol{F}')^o$ in (7.14) by $\boldsymbol{A}_3 = \boldsymbol{A}(\boldsymbol{F}_2')^o$ lead to (7.14) being identical to (7.43), where in particular

$$\widehat{\boldsymbol{S}}_2 = \boldsymbol{S}_1 + \boldsymbol{P}'_{\boldsymbol{A}_3^o,\boldsymbol{S}_1^{-1}}\boldsymbol{X}(\boldsymbol{P}_{\boldsymbol{C}_1'} - \boldsymbol{P}_{\boldsymbol{C}_2'})\boldsymbol{X}'\boldsymbol{P}_{\boldsymbol{A}_3^o,\boldsymbol{S}_1^{-1}}.$$

Thus, if one replaces observations by random variables,

$$\lambda^{\frac{2}{n}} = \frac{|\boldsymbol{A}_2'\boldsymbol{S}_1^{-1}\boldsymbol{A}_2|}{|\boldsymbol{A}_2'\widehat{\boldsymbol{S}}_2^{-1}\boldsymbol{A}_2|}. \tag{7.44}$$

Indeed, the above observations immediately show the possibility of using (7.18) (see also (7.15)), which implies that the likelihood ratio test statistic is given by

$$\lambda^{\frac{2}{n}} = |\boldsymbol{M}'(\boldsymbol{A}_2'\boldsymbol{S}_1^{-1}\boldsymbol{A}_2)^-\boldsymbol{M} + \boldsymbol{M}'(\boldsymbol{A}_2'\boldsymbol{S}_1^{-1}\boldsymbol{A}_2)^-\boldsymbol{A}_2'\boldsymbol{S}_1^{-1}\boldsymbol{X}\boldsymbol{C}'(\boldsymbol{C}\boldsymbol{C}')^-\boldsymbol{N}$$
$$\times\{\boldsymbol{N}'(\boldsymbol{C}\boldsymbol{C}')^-\boldsymbol{C}(\boldsymbol{I} + \boldsymbol{X}'\boldsymbol{P}_{\boldsymbol{A}_2^o,\boldsymbol{S}_1^{-1}}\boldsymbol{S}_1^{-1}\boldsymbol{X})\boldsymbol{C}'(\boldsymbol{C}\boldsymbol{C}')^-\boldsymbol{N}\}^{-1}$$
$$\times\boldsymbol{N}'(\boldsymbol{C}\boldsymbol{C}')^-\boldsymbol{C}\boldsymbol{X}'\boldsymbol{S}_1^{-1}\boldsymbol{A}_2(\boldsymbol{A}_2'\boldsymbol{S}_1^{-1}\boldsymbol{A}_2)^-\boldsymbol{M}||\boldsymbol{M}'(\boldsymbol{A}_2'\boldsymbol{S}_1^{-1}\boldsymbol{A}_2)^-\boldsymbol{M}|^{-1}, \quad (7.45)$$

where $\boldsymbol{S}_1 = \boldsymbol{X}(\boldsymbol{I} - \boldsymbol{P}_{\boldsymbol{C}'})\boldsymbol{X}'$, and $\boldsymbol{M}$ and $\boldsymbol{N}$ are any matrices of full rank satisfying

$$\mathcal{C}(\boldsymbol{M}) = \mathcal{C}((\boldsymbol{F}_1')^{o'}\boldsymbol{A}'(\boldsymbol{A}(\boldsymbol{F}_2')^o)^o),$$
$$\mathcal{C}(\boldsymbol{N}) = \mathcal{C}(\boldsymbol{C}) \cap \mathcal{C}(\boldsymbol{G}_2).$$

Put

$$\boldsymbol{P}_1 = \boldsymbol{I} - (\boldsymbol{I} - \boldsymbol{P}_{\boldsymbol{C}'})\boldsymbol{X}'\boldsymbol{A}_2^o(\boldsymbol{A}_2^{o'}\boldsymbol{S}_1\boldsymbol{A}_2^o)^-\boldsymbol{A}_2^{o'}\boldsymbol{X}, \quad (7.46)$$
$$\boldsymbol{P} = \boldsymbol{P}_1(\boldsymbol{I} - \boldsymbol{P}_{\boldsymbol{C}'}) = \boldsymbol{I} - \boldsymbol{P}_{\boldsymbol{C}'} - (\boldsymbol{I} - \boldsymbol{P}_{\boldsymbol{C}'})\boldsymbol{X}'\boldsymbol{A}_2^o(\boldsymbol{A}_2^{o'}\boldsymbol{S}_1\boldsymbol{A}_2^o)^-\boldsymbol{A}_2^{o'}\boldsymbol{X}(\boldsymbol{I} - \boldsymbol{P}_{\boldsymbol{C}'}). \quad (7.47)$$

Then it can be shown that $\lambda^{\frac{2}{n}}$ has the same distribution as (see also Theorem 7.4 and (7.28))

$$\frac{|\boldsymbol{V} + \boldsymbol{U}|}{|\boldsymbol{V}|}, \quad (7.48)$$

where $\boldsymbol{V} \sim W_{r(\boldsymbol{M})}(\boldsymbol{I}, r(\boldsymbol{P}))$ and $\boldsymbol{U} \sim W_{r(\boldsymbol{M})}(\boldsymbol{I}, r(\boldsymbol{P}_1\boldsymbol{C}'(\boldsymbol{C}\boldsymbol{C}')^-\boldsymbol{N}))$ with $r(\boldsymbol{P}) = n - r(\boldsymbol{C}) - p + r(\boldsymbol{A}' : \boldsymbol{F}_1') - r(\boldsymbol{F}_1)$ and $r(\boldsymbol{P}_1\boldsymbol{C}'(\boldsymbol{C}\boldsymbol{C}')^-\boldsymbol{N}) = r(\boldsymbol{N})$. Hence, the next two theorems have been verified.

Theorem 7.6 *For the BRM presented in Definition 2.1 with the restrictions $\boldsymbol{F}_2\boldsymbol{B}\boldsymbol{G}_2 = \boldsymbol{0}$, the null hypothesis H_0: $\boldsymbol{F}_1\boldsymbol{B}\boldsymbol{G}_1 = \boldsymbol{0}$, $\boldsymbol{F}_2\boldsymbol{B}\boldsymbol{G}_2 = \boldsymbol{0}$ is tested against H_1: $\boldsymbol{F}_1\boldsymbol{B}\boldsymbol{G}_1 = \boldsymbol{0}$; i.e. all elements in $\boldsymbol{F}_2\boldsymbol{B}\boldsymbol{G}_2$ differ from $\boldsymbol{0}$, with $\mathcal{C}(\boldsymbol{F}_1') \subseteq \mathcal{C}(\boldsymbol{F}_2')$ and $\mathcal{C}(\boldsymbol{G}_2) \subseteq \mathcal{C}(\boldsymbol{G}_1)$. Let λ_o be the observed value of λ, given in (7.44), and let*

$$t_o = \tfrac{2}{n}(f - \tfrac{1}{2}(p_o - m + 1))\ln\lambda_o,$$

where $f = n - r(\boldsymbol{C}) - p + r(\boldsymbol{A}' : \boldsymbol{F}_1') - r(\boldsymbol{F}_1)$, $p_o = \dim\{\mathcal{C}((\boldsymbol{F}_1')^{o'}\boldsymbol{A}'(\boldsymbol{A}(\boldsymbol{F}_2')^o)^o)\}$ and $m = \dim\{\mathcal{C}(\boldsymbol{G}_2) \cap \mathcal{C}(\boldsymbol{C})\}$. The likelihood ratio test, approximately at significance level α, rejects the hypothesis if t_o satisfies

$$P\{\chi^2_{p_om} \geq t_o\} + c_1(1 - c_1)(P\{\chi^2_{p_om+4} \geq t_o\} - P\{\chi^2_{p_om} \geq t_o\})$$
$$+ c_2(P\{\chi^2_{p_om+8} \geq t_o\} - P\{\chi^2_{p_om} \geq t_o\}) \leq \alpha,$$

where c_1 and c_2 are defined in Theorem 7.2. □

Theorem 7.7 *The model and hypothesis given below are the same as those in Theorem 7.6. Let* λ *be given in (7.44) and put* $U_{p_o,m,f} = \lambda^{-\frac{2}{n}}$, *where* $p_o = \dim\{\mathcal{C}((\boldsymbol{F}_1')^{o'}\boldsymbol{A}'(\boldsymbol{A}(\boldsymbol{F}_2')^o)^o)\}$, $f = n - r(\boldsymbol{C}) - p + r(\boldsymbol{A}' : \boldsymbol{F}_1') - r(\boldsymbol{F}_1)$ *and* $m = \dim\{\mathcal{C}(\boldsymbol{G}_2) \cap \mathcal{C}(\boldsymbol{C})\}$. *Then*

(i) *if* $p_o = 2$, $T_{23} = \frac{(f-1)}{m}(1 - U_{2,m,f}^{1/2})/U_{2,m,f}^{1/2} \sim F_{2m,2(f-1)}$;
(ii) *if* $p_o = 1$, $T_{24} = \frac{f}{m}(1 - U_{1,m,f})/U_{1,m,f} \sim F_{m,f}$.

□

As in the previous sections, we can try to understand what we are testing and how we are testing the hypothesis H_0: $\boldsymbol{F}_2\boldsymbol{B}\boldsymbol{G}_2 = \boldsymbol{0}$ when applying the likelihood ratio statistic, i.e. try to find some expressions which correspond to (7.36) and (7.37). Define the dispersion matrices

$$\boldsymbol{D}_{12} = \boldsymbol{M}'(\boldsymbol{A}_2'\boldsymbol{S}_1^{-1}\boldsymbol{A}_2)^-\boldsymbol{M} = \boldsymbol{M}'(\boldsymbol{A}_2'\boldsymbol{\Sigma}^{-1}\boldsymbol{A}_2)^-\boldsymbol{A}_2'\boldsymbol{\Sigma}^{-1}\boldsymbol{X}\boldsymbol{P}\boldsymbol{X}'\boldsymbol{\Sigma}^{-1}\boldsymbol{A}_2(\boldsymbol{A}_2'\boldsymbol{\Sigma}^{-1}\boldsymbol{A}_2)^-\boldsymbol{M}, \quad (7.49)$$

$$\boldsymbol{D}_{22} = \boldsymbol{M}'(\boldsymbol{A}_2'\boldsymbol{\Sigma}^{-1}\boldsymbol{A}_2)^-\boldsymbol{A}_2'\boldsymbol{\Sigma}^{-1}\boldsymbol{X}\boldsymbol{P}_{\boldsymbol{P}_1\boldsymbol{C}'(\boldsymbol{C}\boldsymbol{C}')^-\boldsymbol{N}}\boldsymbol{X}'\boldsymbol{\Sigma}^{-1}\boldsymbol{A}_2(\boldsymbol{A}_2'\boldsymbol{\Sigma}^{-1}\boldsymbol{A}_2)^-\boldsymbol{M}, \quad (7.50)$$

where $\boldsymbol{P}$ and $\boldsymbol{P}_1$ are defined in (7.47) and (7.46). Then applying these definitions to (7.45) yields after some calculations, similar to those used for handling (7.34) and (7.18),

$$\lambda^{\frac{2}{n}} = \frac{|\boldsymbol{D}_{12} + \boldsymbol{D}_{22}|}{|\boldsymbol{D}_{12}|},$$

which in fact also explains (7.48). The dispersion matrices are illustrated in Fig. 7.6. The figure should be compared to Fig. 7.5, and the difference between the figures shows how the different hypotheses (restrictions) act on the mean space.

Moreover, it is interesting to note, concerning the way in which the test is derived, that one could consider the calculations as using a conditional approach, i.e. conditioning with respect to $\boldsymbol{A}_2^{o'}\boldsymbol{X}$. Note that at the end of the derivation, the distribution of the test statistic is indeed independent of $\boldsymbol{A}_2^{o'}\boldsymbol{X}$. This idea will also be utilized later in Sect. 7.7.

Example 7.7 In this example, the data which were generated in Example 7.3 are considered again. However, now the additional condition $\mathcal{C}(\boldsymbol{G}_2) \subseteq \mathcal{C}(\boldsymbol{G}_1)$ is imposed. The matrices which define the restrictions on the parameter space are

$$\boldsymbol{F}_1 = (0:0:0:0:1),\ \boldsymbol{G}_1 = \begin{pmatrix} 0\,0 \\ 0\,1 \\ 1\,0 \end{pmatrix},\ \boldsymbol{F}_2 = \begin{pmatrix} 0\,0\,0\,0\,1 \\ 0\,0\,0\,1\,0 \end{pmatrix},\ \boldsymbol{G}_2 = (0:1:0)',$$

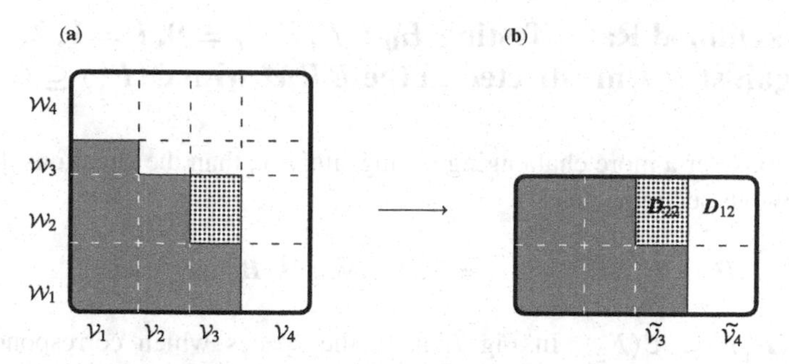

Fig. 7.6 In (**a**), the dotted area corresponds to H_0: $F_2BG_2 = 0$ in the BRM with the restrictions $F_1BG_1 = 0$, where $\mathcal{C}(F_1') \subseteq \mathcal{C}(F_2')$ and $\mathcal{C}(G_2') \subseteq \mathcal{C}(G_1')$. In (**b**), those areas are given, which after conditioning with respect to $A_2^{o'}X$, contribute to the likelihood ratio test. Furthermore, $\mathcal{W}_1 = \mathcal{C}_{\bullet}(A(F_2')^o)$, $\mathcal{W}_2 = \mathcal{C}_{\bullet}(A(F_1')^o) \cap \mathcal{C}_{\bullet}(A(F_2')^o)^{\perp}$, $\mathcal{W}_3 = \mathcal{C}_{\bullet}(A) \cap \mathcal{C}_{\bullet}(A(F_1')^o)^{\perp}$, $\mathcal{W}_4 = \mathcal{C}_{\bullet}(A)^{\perp}$, $\mathcal{V}_1 = \mathcal{C}(C'G_1^o)$, $\mathcal{V}_2 = \mathcal{C}(C'G_2^o) \cap \mathcal{C}(C'G_1^o)^{\perp}$, $\mathcal{V}_3 = \mathcal{C}(C') \cap \mathcal{C}(C'G_2^o)^{\perp}$, $\mathcal{V}_4 = \mathcal{C}(C')^{\perp}$, $\widetilde{\mathcal{V}}_3 = \mathcal{C}(P_{P_1C'(CC')^-N})$, $\mathcal{C}(N) = \mathcal{C}(G_2^{o'}C) \cap \mathcal{C}(G_2^{o'}G_1)$ and $\widetilde{\mathcal{V}}_4 = \mathcal{C}(P)$, where P_1 and P are defined in (7.46) and (7.47), respectively. Moreover, the dispersion matrices D_{22} and D_{12} are defined in (7.50) and (7.49), respectively

which satisfy $\mathcal{C}(F_1') \subseteq \mathcal{C}(F_2)$ and $\mathcal{C}(G_2) \subseteq \mathcal{C}(G_1)$. The restrictions under H_0: $F_1BG_1 = 0$, $F_2BG_2 = 0$, if $B = (b_{ij})$, yield $b_{42} = 0$, $b_{52} = 0$ and $b_{53} = 0$. In this case, the test statistic given by (7.42) takes the value $\lambda_o^{2/45} = 1.9$ and, hence, $U_{p_o,m,f} = 0.51$. Moreover, $p_o = 1$, $m = 1$ and $f = 36$. Thus, from Theorem 7.7 (ii),

$$T_{24o} = 36(1 - U_{1,1,36})/U_{1,1,36} = 34.1 > F_{0.05}(1, 36) = 4.1$$

and the hypothesis H_0: $F_2BG_2 = 0$ is rejected.

Instead of G_1, the subvector $\widetilde{G}_1 = (0 : 0 : 1)'$ can be used in order to avoid any overlap between $F_1BG_1 = 0$ and $F_2BG_2 = 0$; for instance in the present example $F_1BG_2 = 0$ appears in both $F_1BG_1 = 0$ and $F_2BG_2 = 0$. In this case, of course, we are back in Sect. 7.4.

If instead of $G_2 = (0 : 1 : 0)'$, the between-individuals matrix $G_2 = (0 : 0 : 1)'$ is used, we are closer to the model which generated the data in Example 7.3 and obtain

$$T_{24o} = 36(1 - U_{1,1,36})/U_{1,1,36} = 1.6 < F_{0.05}(1, 36) = 4.1,$$

and this time H_0 is not rejected. □

7.6 Likelihood Ratio Testing $H_0: F_iBG_i = 0, i = 1, 2,$ Against B Unrestricted in the BRM with $\mathcal{C}(F_1') \subseteq \mathcal{C}(F_2')$

Now we consider a more challenging testing situation than the situations discussed in the previous sections, i.e.

$$H_0: \ \boldsymbol{F}_i\boldsymbol{B}\boldsymbol{G}_i = \boldsymbol{0}, \ i = 1, 2, \quad \text{versus } \boldsymbol{B} \text{ unrestricted}, \tag{7.51}$$

where $\mathcal{C}(\boldsymbol{F}_1') \subseteq \mathcal{C}(\boldsymbol{F}_2')$. In Fig. 7.7a, b, the spaces which correspond to the hypotheses tested in Sects. 7.3 and 7.4 are illustrated. In this section the structure presented in Fig. 7.7c is discussed. It is immediately seen that the hypothesis generates a restriction on the parameter space which has a different form compared with the restrictions in the previous sections, and therefore it also appears that the testing problem differs from the problems in the previous sections. Unfortunately, the spaces connected to the indicated area of Fig. 7.7c will generate a likelihood ratio which is more difficult to handle as precisely as the ratios in the earlier sections were handled. On the other hand, the hypothesis treated in this section, i.e. (7.51), is in a sense the most natural extension of $H_0: \ \boldsymbol{FBG} = \boldsymbol{0}$, which was discussed, in Sect. 7.3 in particular.

From Theorems 3.1 and 3.2 (see also (7.31)), it follows that the likelihood ratio for testing (7.51) is equivalent to

$$\lambda_o^{\frac{2}{n}} = \frac{|\widehat{\boldsymbol{\Sigma}}_{H_0}|}{|\widehat{\boldsymbol{\Sigma}}_{H_1}|} = \frac{|\widehat{\boldsymbol{S}}_3 + \widehat{\boldsymbol{Q}}_3'\widehat{\boldsymbol{Q}}_2'\widehat{\boldsymbol{Q}}_1'\boldsymbol{X}_o\boldsymbol{P}_{\boldsymbol{C}_3'}\boldsymbol{X}_o'\widehat{\boldsymbol{Q}}_1\widehat{\boldsymbol{Q}}_2\widehat{\boldsymbol{Q}}_3|}{|\boldsymbol{S}_1 + \boldsymbol{P}'_{\boldsymbol{A}^o,\boldsymbol{S}_1^{-1}}\boldsymbol{X}_o\boldsymbol{P}_{\boldsymbol{C}'}\boldsymbol{X}_o'\boldsymbol{P}_{\boldsymbol{A}^o,\boldsymbol{S}_1^{-1}}|}, \tag{7.52}$$

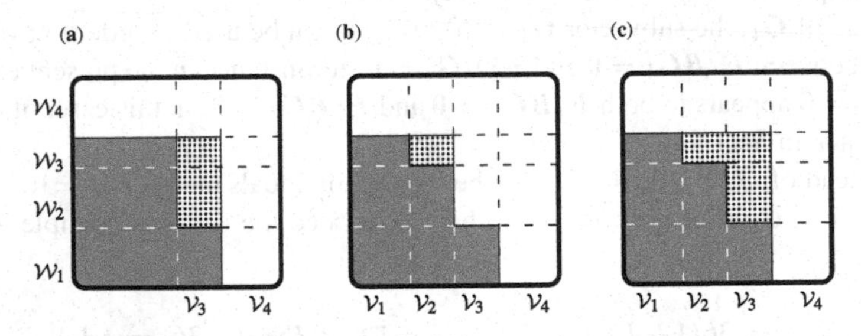

Fig. 7.7 In (**a**), the dotted area corresponds to H_0: $\boldsymbol{F}_2\boldsymbol{B}\boldsymbol{G}_2 = \boldsymbol{0}$ in the BRM. In (**b**), the area is shown for testing H_0: $\boldsymbol{F}_1\boldsymbol{B}\boldsymbol{G}_1 = \boldsymbol{0}$ in the BRM, given $\boldsymbol{F}_2\boldsymbol{B}\boldsymbol{G}_2 = \boldsymbol{0}$, where $\mathcal{C}(\boldsymbol{F}_1') \subseteq \mathcal{C}(\boldsymbol{F}_2')$, and in (**c**), the area is shown for testing H_0: $\boldsymbol{F}_i\boldsymbol{B}\boldsymbol{G}_i = \boldsymbol{0}, i = 1, 2$, in the BRM, where $\mathcal{C}(\boldsymbol{F}_1') \subseteq \mathcal{C}(\boldsymbol{F}_2')$ holds. Furthermore, $\mathcal{W}_1 = \mathcal{C}_\bullet(\boldsymbol{A}(\boldsymbol{F}_2')^o)$, $\mathcal{W}_2 = \mathcal{C}_\bullet(\boldsymbol{A}(\boldsymbol{F}_1')^o) \cap \mathcal{C}_\bullet(\boldsymbol{A}(\boldsymbol{F}_2')^o)^\perp$, $\mathcal{W}_3 = \mathcal{C}_\bullet(\boldsymbol{A}) \cap \mathcal{C}_\bullet(\boldsymbol{A}(\boldsymbol{F}_1')^o)^\perp$, $\mathcal{W}_4 = \mathcal{C}_\bullet(\boldsymbol{A})^\perp$, $\mathcal{V}_1 = \mathcal{C}(\boldsymbol{C}'(\boldsymbol{G}_1 : \boldsymbol{G}_2)^o)$, $\mathcal{V}_2 = \mathcal{C}(\boldsymbol{C}'\boldsymbol{G}_2^o) \cap \mathcal{C}(\boldsymbol{C}'(\boldsymbol{G}_1 : \boldsymbol{G}_2)^o)^\perp$, $\mathcal{V}_3 = \mathcal{C}(\boldsymbol{C}') \cap \mathcal{C}(\boldsymbol{C}'\boldsymbol{G}_2^o)^\perp$ and $\mathcal{V}_4 = \mathcal{C}(\boldsymbol{C}')^\perp$

where the notation follows that of Sect. 7.4. However, an interesting factorization of λ_o can take place, namely

$$\lambda_o = \lambda_{1o}\lambda_{2o},$$

where

$$\lambda_{1o}^{\frac{2}{n}} = \frac{|\widehat{\boldsymbol{S}}_2 + \boldsymbol{P}'_{A^o,\widehat{S}_2^{-1}}\boldsymbol{X}_o\boldsymbol{P}_{C_2'}\boldsymbol{X}_o'\boldsymbol{P}_{A^o,\widehat{S}_2^{-1}}|}{|\boldsymbol{S}_1 + \boldsymbol{P}'_{A^o,S_1^{-1}}\boldsymbol{X}_o\boldsymbol{P}_{C'}\boldsymbol{X}_o'\boldsymbol{P}_{A^o,S_1^{-1}}|}, \tag{7.53}$$

$$\lambda_{2o}^{\frac{2}{n}} = \frac{|\widehat{\boldsymbol{S}}_3 + \boldsymbol{P}'_{A^o,\widehat{S}_3^{-1}}\boldsymbol{X}_o\boldsymbol{P}_{C_3'}\boldsymbol{X}_o'\boldsymbol{P}_{A^o,\widehat{S}_3^{-1}}|}{|\widehat{\boldsymbol{S}}_2 + \boldsymbol{P}'_{A^o,\widehat{S}_2^{-1}}\boldsymbol{X}_o\boldsymbol{P}_{C_2'}\boldsymbol{X}_o'\boldsymbol{P}_{A^o,\widehat{S}_2^{-1}}|}. \tag{7.54}$$

Then it is noted that, correspondingly to λ_{1o}, given in (7.53), λ_1 is the test statistic for testing a BRM with respect to H_0: $\boldsymbol{F}_2\boldsymbol{B}\boldsymbol{G}_2 = \boldsymbol{0}$ against $\boldsymbol{B}$ unrestricted, which was presented in Sect. 7.3, i.e. Theorems 7.2 and 7.3. Moreover, correspondingly to λ_{2o}, given in (7.54), λ_2 is the statistic used for testing, within a BRM framework, H_0: $\boldsymbol{F}_1\boldsymbol{B}\boldsymbol{G}_1 = \boldsymbol{0}$, given that $\boldsymbol{F}_2\boldsymbol{B}\boldsymbol{G}_2 = \boldsymbol{0}$ holds, which was treated in Sect. 7.4, i.e. Theorems 7.4 and 7.5.

Expressing the statistics with the help of dispersion matrices, it follows from Sect. 7.3 and (7.28) that

$$\lambda_1^{\frac{2}{n}} = \frac{|\underline{\boldsymbol{A}}'\boldsymbol{S}_1^{-1}\underline{\boldsymbol{A}}|}{|\underline{\boldsymbol{A}}'\widehat{\boldsymbol{S}}_2^{-1}\underline{\boldsymbol{A}}|} = \frac{|\boldsymbol{D}_{12} + \boldsymbol{D}_{21}|}{|\boldsymbol{D}_{12}|}, \tag{7.55}$$

where

$$\begin{aligned}\boldsymbol{D}_{12} &\sim W_{r(\boldsymbol{M}_1)}(\boldsymbol{M}_1'(\boldsymbol{A}'\boldsymbol{\Sigma}^{-1}\boldsymbol{A})^-\boldsymbol{M}_1, r(\boldsymbol{P})),\\ &\quad r(\boldsymbol{P}) = n - r(\boldsymbol{C}) - p + r(\boldsymbol{A}),\\ \boldsymbol{D}_{21} &\sim W_{r(\boldsymbol{M}_1)}(\boldsymbol{M}_1'(\boldsymbol{A}'\boldsymbol{\Sigma}^{-1}\boldsymbol{A})^-\boldsymbol{M}_1, r(\boldsymbol{N}_1)),\end{aligned}$$

with $\boldsymbol{M}_1$ and $\boldsymbol{N}_1$ satisfying

$$\mathcal{C}(\boldsymbol{M}_1) = \mathcal{C}(\boldsymbol{F}_2') \cap \mathcal{C}(\boldsymbol{A}'), \qquad \mathcal{C}(\boldsymbol{N}_1) = \mathcal{C}(\boldsymbol{G}_2) \cap \mathcal{C}(\boldsymbol{C}).$$

Section 7.4 and (7.38) yield that λ_2 can be expressed as follows:

$$\lambda_2^{\frac{2}{n}} = \frac{|\underline{\boldsymbol{A}}'\boldsymbol{S}_2^{-1}\underline{\boldsymbol{A}}|}{|\underline{\boldsymbol{A}}'\widehat{\boldsymbol{S}}_3^{-1}\underline{\boldsymbol{A}}|} = \frac{|\boldsymbol{D}_{13+22} + \boldsymbol{D}_{31}|}{|\boldsymbol{D}_{13+22}|}, \tag{7.56}$$

where

$$D_{13+22} \sim W_{r(M_2)}(M_2'(A'\Sigma^{-1}A)^- M_2, r(P)),$$
$$r(P) = n - r(C_2) - p + r(A),$$
$$D_{31} \sim W_{r(M_2)}(M_2'(A'\Sigma^{-1}A)^- M_2, r(N_2)),$$

with M_2 and N_2 satisfying

$$\mathcal{C}(M_2) = \mathcal{C}(F_1') \cap \mathcal{C}(A'), \qquad \mathcal{C}(N_2) = \mathcal{C}(G_2^{o'}C) \cap \mathcal{C}(G_2^{o'}G_1).$$

However, it can be shown that λ_1 and λ_2 are not independently distributed, which means that the interpretation of the statistics becomes complicated. Unfortunately, the joint distribution of λ_1 and λ_2 is not easy to obtain. In order to find an approximate upper bound of the p-value for testing (7.51) via (7.52), a Bonferroni correction may take place. In general, the Bonferroni approach also overcomes the difficulty associated with any dependence among the tests and is definitely suitable when only a few tests are to be considered. For example, in our case this approach can be used since there are only two tests to be performed. Moreover, it is interesting to discover that the factorization of the likelihood ratio test statistic has a natural hierarchy; i.e. one should first apply λ_1 and thereafter λ_2, given that H_0: $F_2BG_2 = 0$ has not been rejected. If the test is rejected in the first step, then the test described in (7.51) should, of course, also be rejected. Hence, a testing strategy has been derived which is similar, for example, to classical profile analysis in multivariate analysis. Since the tests based on λ_1 and λ_2 are not independent, it is quite natural to use equal rejection probabilities, although it is not necessary to carry out the overall test in this way.

Theorem 7.8 *For the BRM presented in Definition 2.1, let, as in (7.51), the null hypothesis H_0: $F_iBG_i = 0, i = 1, 2$, where $\mathcal{C}(F_1') \subseteq \mathcal{C}(F_2')$ holds, be tested against the alternative hypothesis H_1: B is unrestricted. Let λ_{1o} and λ_{2o} be the observed values of λ_1 and λ_2, defined by (7.53) and (7.54), respectively. Moreover, let*

$$t_{1o} = \tfrac{2}{n}(f_1 - \tfrac{1}{2}(p_{1o} - m_1 + 1)) \ln \lambda_{1o},$$
$$t_{2o} = \tfrac{2}{n}(f_2 - \tfrac{1}{2}(p_{2o} - m_2 + 1)) \ln \lambda_{2o},$$

where

$$f_1 = n - r(C) - p + r(A), \qquad f_2 = n - r(C_2) - p + r(A),$$
$$p_{1o} = \dim\{\mathcal{C}(F_2') \cap \mathcal{C}(A')\}, \qquad p_{2o} = \dim\{\mathcal{C}(F_1') \cap \mathcal{C}(A')\},$$
$$m_1 = \dim\{\mathcal{C}(G_2) \cap \mathcal{C}(C)\}, \qquad m_2 = \dim\{\mathcal{C}(G_2^{o'}C) \cap \mathcal{C}(G_2^{o'}G_1)\}.$$

The likelihood ratio test for this hypothesis, approximately on level α, rejects the hypothesis if

$$P\{\chi^2_{p_{1o}m_1} \geq t_{1o}\} + c_{11}(1-c_{11})(P\{\chi^2_{p_{1o}m_1+4} \geq t_{1o}\} - P\{\chi^2_{p_{1o}m_1} \geq t_{1o}\})$$
$$+ c_{12}(P\{\chi^2_{p_{1o}m_1+8} \geq t_{1o}\} - P\{\chi^2_{p_{1o}m_1} \geq t_{1o}\}) \leq \alpha_1,$$

or

$$P\{\chi^2_{p_{2o}m_2} \geq t_{2o}\} + c_{21}(1-c_{21})(P\{\chi^2_{p_{2o}m_2+4} \geq t_{2o}\} - P\{\chi^2_{p_{2o}m_2} \geq t_{2o}\})$$
$$+ c_{22}(P\{\chi^2_{p_{2o}m_2+8} \geq t_{2o}\} - P\{\chi^2_{p_{2o}m_2} \geq t_{2o}\}) \leq \alpha_2,$$

where c_{11} and c_{12} correspond to c_1 and c_2 in Theorem 7.2, with p_{1o}, m_1 and f_1 inserted, c_{21} and c_{22} correspond to c_1 and c_2 in the same theorem, with p_{2o}, m_2 and f_2 inserted, and $\alpha_1 + \alpha_2 = \alpha$. □

In Theorem 7.8 it was suggested to use $\alpha_1 + \alpha_2 = \alpha$, where α is the prespecified significance level. Since λ_1 and λ_2 are not independently distributed it is difficult to find α_1 and α_2 so that the Type I error equals exactly α. Therefore it is reasonable to apply the Bonferroni approach when choosing α_1 and α_2. However, note that under independence of the two hypotheses we can use the relation

$$(1-\alpha) = (1-\alpha_1)(1-\alpha_2) = 1 - \alpha_1 - \alpha_2 + \alpha_1\alpha_2,$$

i.e. the overall hypothesis is not rejected if the hypothesis connected to λ_1 and the hypothesis connected to λ_2 are not rejected. Since $\alpha_1\alpha_2$ will be small it makes sense to also under independence use $\alpha_1 + \alpha_2 = \alpha$. An exception would be if the distribution of $\lambda_1\lambda_2$ could be found.

Example 7.8 Here, once again, the melatonin data generated in Example 7.3 are considered. Now, for the BRM, H_0: $\boldsymbol{F}_i\boldsymbol{B}\boldsymbol{G}_i = \boldsymbol{0}$, $i = 1, 2$, against $\boldsymbol{B}$ unrestricted is tested with the following matrices:

$$\boldsymbol{F}_1 = (0:0:0:0:1), \quad \boldsymbol{G}_1 = (0:0:1)', \quad \boldsymbol{F}_2 = \begin{pmatrix} 0&0&0&0&1 \\ 0&0&0&1&0 \end{pmatrix}, \quad \boldsymbol{G}_2 = (0:1:0)',$$

and in comparison with Example 7.3, $\boldsymbol{G}_1$ and $\boldsymbol{G}_2$ are interchanged, which means that the hypothesis which is tested in this example differs from the true model from which data have been generated. Moreover, alternatively, it can be stated that for $\boldsymbol{B} = (b_{ij})$, the restrictions equal $b_{53} = b_{52} = b_{42} = 0$. From the derivation, it follows that λ_1 is a test statistic for testing $b_{52} = b_{42} = 0$, and λ_2 tests $b_{53} = 0$ given that $b_{52} = b_{42} = 0$.

To calculate λ_{1o}, the matrices $\boldsymbol{S}_1$ and $\widehat{\boldsymbol{S}}_2$ are needed, which equal $\boldsymbol{S}_1 = \boldsymbol{X}_o(\boldsymbol{I} - \boldsymbol{P}_{C'})\boldsymbol{X}'_o$ and

$$\widehat{\boldsymbol{S}}_2 = \boldsymbol{S}_1 + \boldsymbol{P}'_{A_1^o,S_1^{-1}}\boldsymbol{X}_o(\boldsymbol{P}_{C_1'} - \boldsymbol{P}_{C_2'})\boldsymbol{X}'_o\boldsymbol{P}_{A_1^o,S_1^{-1}},$$

where $\boldsymbol{A}_1 = \boldsymbol{A}(\boldsymbol{F}'_2)^o$, $\boldsymbol{C}_1 = \boldsymbol{C}$ and $\boldsymbol{C}_2 = \boldsymbol{G}_2^{o'}\boldsymbol{C}$. Moreover, $(\boldsymbol{F}'_2)^o = (\boldsymbol{I}_3 : \boldsymbol{0})$ and

$$\boldsymbol{G}_2^{o'} = \begin{pmatrix} 1\,0\,0 \\ 0\,0\,1 \end{pmatrix}.$$

Concerning the second test, to calculate λ_{2o}, additionally the following definition is needed:

$$\widehat{\boldsymbol{S}}_3 = \widehat{\boldsymbol{S}}_2 + \boldsymbol{P}'_{(A_1:A_2)^o,\widehat{S}_2^{-1}}\boldsymbol{X}_o(\boldsymbol{P}_{C_2'} - \boldsymbol{P}_{C_3'})\boldsymbol{X}'_o\boldsymbol{P}_{(A_1:A_2)^o,\widehat{S}_2^{-1}},$$

where $\boldsymbol{A}_2 = \boldsymbol{A}(\boldsymbol{F}'_1 : (\boldsymbol{F}'_2)^o)^o = \boldsymbol{A}(0 : 0 : 0 : 1 : 0)'$, $\boldsymbol{C}_1 = \boldsymbol{C}$, and $\boldsymbol{C}_3 = (\boldsymbol{G}_1 : \boldsymbol{G}_2)^{o'}\boldsymbol{C} = (1 : 0 : 0)\boldsymbol{C}$.

The test connected with λ_1, H_0: $\boldsymbol{F}_2\boldsymbol{B}\boldsymbol{G}_2 = \boldsymbol{0}$ versus $\boldsymbol{B}$ unrestricted, is rejected since $U_{2,1,37} = \lambda_{2o}^{-2/45} = 1.95^{-1} = 0.51$, and from Theorem 7.3 (i)

$$T_{11o} = 36(1 - U_{2,1,37}^{1/2})/U_{2,1,37}^{1/2} = 14.3 > F_{0.05}(2, 72) = 4.1.$$

Thus, the overall hypothesis H_0: $\boldsymbol{F}_i\boldsymbol{B}\boldsymbol{G}_i = \boldsymbol{0}$, $i = 1, 2$, is rejected.

Parenthetically it is noted that the test connected with λ_2, H_0: $\boldsymbol{F}_1\boldsymbol{B}\boldsymbol{G}_1 = \boldsymbol{0}$ given $\boldsymbol{F}_2\boldsymbol{B}\boldsymbol{G}_2 = \boldsymbol{0}$, is not rejected since $U_{1,1,38} = \lambda_{2o}^{-2/45} = 1.03^{-1} = 0.97$, and from Theorem 7.5 (ii)

$$T_{22o} = 38(1 - U_{1,1,38})/U_{1,1,38} = 1.2 < F_{0.05}(1, 38) = 3.1.$$

Next we investigate what happens if

$$\boldsymbol{F}_1 = (0 : 0 : 0 : 0 : 1),\ \ \boldsymbol{G}_1 = (0 : 0 : 1)',\ \ \boldsymbol{F}_2 = \begin{pmatrix} 0\,0\,0\,0\,1 \\ 0\,0\,0\,1\,0 \\ 0\,0\,1\,0\,0 \\ 0\,1\,0\,0\,0 \end{pmatrix},\ \ \boldsymbol{G}_2 = (1 : 0 : 0)'$$

are used, which is a rather extreme suggestion in relation to how the data have been generated. Thus, $\boldsymbol{C}_1 = \boldsymbol{C}, \boldsymbol{C}_2 = \boldsymbol{G}_2^{o'}\boldsymbol{C} = (\boldsymbol{0} : \boldsymbol{I}_2)\boldsymbol{C}, \boldsymbol{C}_3 = (\boldsymbol{G}_1 : \boldsymbol{G}_2)^{o'}\boldsymbol{C} = (0 : 1 : 0)\boldsymbol{C}$,

$$\boldsymbol{A}_1 = \boldsymbol{A}(\boldsymbol{F}_2')^o = \boldsymbol{A}\begin{pmatrix}1\\0\\0\\0\\0\end{pmatrix}, \quad \boldsymbol{A}_2 = \boldsymbol{A}(\boldsymbol{F}_1' : (\boldsymbol{F}_2')^o)^o = \boldsymbol{A}\begin{pmatrix}0&0&0\\1&0&0\\0&1&0\\0&0&1\\0&0&0\end{pmatrix},$$

and $\boldsymbol{A}_3 = \boldsymbol{A}\boldsymbol{F}_1'$. When testing $\boldsymbol{F}_2\boldsymbol{B}\boldsymbol{G}_2 = \boldsymbol{0}$, since $p_{1o} = 4$, Theorem 7.8 is suggested to be used. In this case, $\lambda_{1o}^{2/45} = 1.34$, $t_{1o} = 10.2$ and applying the theorem yields $P\{\chi_4^2 \geq t_{1o}\} = 0.04 < 0.05$ and thus H_0 is rejected. Note that the same test was performed in Sect. 7.3, in Example 7.3. Moreover, $\lambda_{2o}^{2/45} = 1.0$ and then the corresponding H_0 is not rejected, which, however, is extraneous to the conclusions concerning the rejection of the hypothesis about the double bilinear restrictions. It is worth noting that as long as $\mathcal{C}(\boldsymbol{F}_1') \subseteq \mathcal{C}(\boldsymbol{F}_2')$, the value λ_{1o} will not depend on the choice of $\boldsymbol{F}_1'$ and λ_{2o} will not depend on the choice of $\boldsymbol{F}_2'$. This observation helps us to evaluate and break down the overall test defined through the double bilinear restrictions; i.e. we can, for example, marginally interpret $\boldsymbol{F}_1\boldsymbol{B}\boldsymbol{G}_1 = \boldsymbol{0}$. □

7.7 Likelihood Ratio Testing $H_0 : \boldsymbol{F}_i\boldsymbol{B}\boldsymbol{G}_i = \boldsymbol{0}, i = 1, 2$, Against $\boldsymbol{B}$ Unrestricted in the $\boldsymbol{BRM}$ with $\mathcal{C}(\boldsymbol{F}_1') \subseteq \mathcal{C}(\boldsymbol{F}_2')$ and $\mathcal{C}(\boldsymbol{G}_2) \subseteq \mathcal{C}(\boldsymbol{G}_1)$

It was seen in the previous section that a test statistic appeared which was somewhat different from the test statistics of the other sections, since it "naturally" presented a product of two test statistics instead of being only one statistic. The tests in the previous section were, however, not independently distributed, which should be taken into account when interpreting them. The fact is, however, that the dependence of these tests is difficult to handle in a precise manner. Now we exploit what happens if, additionally, the condition $\mathcal{C}(\boldsymbol{G}_2) \subseteq \mathcal{C}(\boldsymbol{G}_1)$ is imposed on the testing problem of the previous section, i.e. what happens in the BRM when $\mathcal{C}(\boldsymbol{F}_1') \subseteq \mathcal{C}(\boldsymbol{F}_2')$ and $\mathcal{C}(\boldsymbol{G}_2) \subseteq \mathcal{C}(\boldsymbol{G}_1)$ hold. The hypothesis of interest is given by

$$H_0 : \boldsymbol{F}_i\boldsymbol{B}\boldsymbol{G}_i = \boldsymbol{0}, \; i = 1, 2, \quad \text{versus } \boldsymbol{B} \text{ unrestricted.} \tag{7.57}$$

From Sect. 7.5, recall the following matrices:

$$\begin{aligned} A_1 = A, \quad A_2 = A(F_1')^o, \quad A_3 = A(F_2')^o, \\ C_1 = G_1^{o'}C, \quad C_2 = (G_2 : G_1^o)^{o'}C, \quad C_3 = G_2'C, \end{aligned} \tag{7.58}$$

which can be used to express $\widehat{\Sigma}_{H_0}$. Then, as in Sect. 7.5,

$$\begin{aligned} \widehat{S}_3 &= \widehat{S}_2 + P'_{A_2^o, \widehat{S}_2^{-1}} X P_2 X' P_{A_2^o, \widehat{S}_2^{-1}}, \\ \widehat{S}_2 &= S_1 + P'_{A_3^o, S_1^{-1}} X P_3 X' P_{A_3^o, S_1^{-1}}, \\ S_1 &= X(I - P_{C'})X', \\ \widehat{\mathcal{S}}_2 &= S_1 + P'_{A_2^o, S_1^{-1}} X P_4 X' P_{A_2^o, S_1^{-1}}, \end{aligned}$$

where P_2, P_3 and P_4 are orthogonal projectors on $\mathcal{C}(C_1')^\perp \cap \mathcal{C}(C_1' : C_2')$, $\mathcal{C}(C_1' : C_2')^\perp \cap \mathcal{C}(C')$ and $\mathcal{C}(C') \cap \mathcal{C}(C_1')^\perp$, respectively.

Utilizing the maximum likelihood estimator of Σ in the BRM, i.e. the unrestricted case, and $\widehat{\Sigma}_{H_0}$ of Sect. 7.5, it follows that the likelihood ratio test for testing H_0 in (7.57) is based on

$$\lambda_o^{\frac{2}{n}} = \frac{|\widehat{\Sigma}_{H_0}|}{|\widehat{\Sigma}_{H_1}|} = \frac{|\widehat{S}_3 + P'_{A_1^o, \widehat{S}_3^{-1}} X_o P_{C_1'} X_o' P_{A_1^o, \widehat{S}_3^{-1}}|}{|S_1 + P'_{A_1^o, S_1^{-1}} X_o P_{C'} X_o' P_{A_1^o, S_1^{-1}}|}.$$

In Sect. 7.6, as already mentioned, it was shown that the ratio λ_o could be factorized. Since, in the present section, only the condition $\mathcal{C}(G_2') \subseteq \mathcal{C}(G_1')$ has been added, this may of course also take place here. It follows that

$$\lambda_o = \lambda_{1o}\lambda_{2o},$$

where

$$\lambda_{1o}^{\frac{2}{n}} = \frac{|\widehat{\mathcal{S}}_2 + P'_{A_1^o, \widehat{\mathcal{S}}_2^{-1}} X_o P_{C_1'} X_o' P_{A_1^o, \widehat{\mathcal{S}}_2^{-1}}|}{|S_1 + P'_{A_1^o, S_1^{-1}} X_o P_{C'} X_o' P_{A_1^o, S_1^{-1}}|}, \tag{7.59}$$

$$\lambda_{2o}^{\frac{2}{n}} = \frac{|\widehat{S}_3 + P'_{A_1^o, \widehat{S}_3^{-1}} X_o P_{C_1'} X_o' P_{A_1^o, \widehat{S}_3^{-1}}|}{|\widehat{\mathcal{S}}_2 + P'_{A_1^o, \widehat{\mathcal{S}}_2^{-1}} X_o P_{C_1'} X_o' P_{A_1^o, \widehat{\mathcal{S}}_2^{-1}}|}, \tag{7.60}$$

with the important observation that within the BRM frame, correspondingly to (7.59) and (7.60), λ_1 is a statistic for testing H_0: $F_1BG_1 = 0$ against no restrictions on B (which was presented in Sect. 7.3, Theorems 7.2 and 7.3), and λ_2

is a statistic for testing H_0: $F_2BG_2 = 0$, $\mathcal{C}(F_1') \subseteq \mathcal{C}(F_2')$, $\mathcal{C}(G_2) \subseteq \mathcal{C}(G_1)$, given that $F_1BG_1 = 0$ (which was considered in Theorems 7.6 and 7.7 of Sect. 7.5).

Now we investigate the role which the condition $\mathcal{C}(G_2) \subseteq \mathcal{C}(G_1)$ can play when obtaining the distribution of the test statistic $\lambda^{\frac{2}{n}}$. Note that $\widehat{S}_2$, given by (7.41), equals $\widehat{S}_2$ of Sect. 7.3 if one replaces F by F_1 and since P_4 is identical to $P_{C_1'} - P_{C_2'}$ of Sect. 7.3. Moreover, from Sect. 7.3, it follows that λ_1 can be written as follows:

$$\lambda_1^{\frac{2}{n}} = \frac{|V_1 + U_1|}{|V_1|},$$

with

$$\begin{aligned} V_1 &= (M_1'(A'\Sigma^{-1}A)^- M_1)^{-1/2} M_1'(A'\Sigma^{-1}A)^- A'\Sigma^{-1} XPX'\Sigma^{-1}A(A'\Sigma^{-1}A)^- \\ &\quad \times M_1(M_1'(A'\Sigma^{-1}A)^- M_1)^{-1/2} \sim W_{r(M_1)}(I, n - r(C) - p + r(A)), \end{aligned} \tag{7.61}$$

$$\begin{aligned} U_1 &= (M_1'(A'\Sigma^{-1}A)^- M_1)^{-1/2} M_1'(A'\Sigma^{-1}A)^- A'\Sigma^{-1} X \\ &\quad \times P_1 C'(CC')^- N_1 (N_1'(CC')^- C P_1' P_1 C'(CC')^- N_1)^- N_1'(CC')^- C P_1' \\ &\quad \times X'\Sigma^{-1}A(A'\Sigma^{-1}A)^- M_1 (M_1'(A'\Sigma^{-1}A)^- M_1)^{-1/2} \sim W_{r(M_1)}(I, r(N_1)), \end{aligned} \tag{7.62}$$

where M_1 satisfies $\mathcal{C}(M_1) = \mathcal{C}(A') \cap \mathcal{C}(F_1')$, $\mathcal{C}(N_1) = \mathcal{C}(C) \cap \mathcal{C}(G_1)$, P and P_1 are defined in (7.22) and (7.23), respectively; V_1 and U_1 are independently distributed.

Turning to λ_2 and applying the results of Sect. 7.5 yield

$$\lambda_2^{\frac{2}{n}} = \frac{|V_2 + U_2|}{|V_2|},$$

with

$$\begin{aligned} V_2 &= (M_2'(A_2'\Sigma^{-1}A_2)^- M_2)^{-1/2} M_2'(A_2'\Sigma^{-1}A_2)^- A_2'\Sigma^{-1} X P_{22} X' \\ &\quad \times \Sigma^{-1}A_2(A_2'\Sigma^{-1}A_2)^- M_2 (M_2'(A_2'\Sigma^{-1}A_2)^- M_2)^{-1/2} \sim W_{r(M_2)}(I, r(P_{22})), \\ U_2 &= (M_2'(A_2'\Sigma^{-1}A_2)^- M_2)^{-1/2} M_2'(A_2'\Sigma^{-1}A_2)^- A_2'\Sigma^{-1} X \\ &\quad \times P_{12} C'(CC')^- N_2 (N_2'(CC')^- C P_{12}' P_{12} C'(CC')^- N_2)^- N_2'(CC')^- C P_{12}' \\ &\quad \times X'\Sigma^{-1}A_2(A_2'\Sigma^{-1}A_2)^- M_2 (M_2'(A_2'\Sigma^{-1}A_2)^- M_2)^{-1/2} \sim W_{r(M_2)}(I, r(N_2)), \end{aligned}$$

where M_2 satisfies $\mathcal{C}(M_2) = \mathcal{C}((F_1')^{o'} A'(A(F_2')^o)^o)$, $\mathcal{C}(N_2) = \mathcal{C}(C) \cap \mathcal{C}(G_2)$, and P_{22} and P_{12} correspond to P and P_1, defined in (7.47) and (7.46), respectively; V_2 and U_2 are independently distributed.

Both λ_1 and λ_2 are functions of Wishart-distributed random variables. In Sect. 7.6, λ_i, $i = 1, 2$, were not functions of independently distributed variables. However, with regard to λ_1 and λ_2 of this section is now shown that they are independently distributed test statistics. Let

$$\begin{aligned}
\boldsymbol{Y}_1 &= \boldsymbol{M}_1'(\boldsymbol{A}'\boldsymbol{\Sigma}^{-1}\boldsymbol{A})^{-}\boldsymbol{A}'\boldsymbol{\Sigma}^{-1}\boldsymbol{X},\\
\boldsymbol{Y}_2 &= \boldsymbol{M}_2'(\boldsymbol{A}_2'\boldsymbol{\Sigma}^{-1}\boldsymbol{A}_2)^{-}\boldsymbol{A}_2'\boldsymbol{\Sigma}^{-1}\boldsymbol{X}
\end{aligned}$$

and note that

$$C[\boldsymbol{Y}_1, \boldsymbol{Y}_2] = \boldsymbol{I} \otimes \boldsymbol{M}_1'(\boldsymbol{A}'\boldsymbol{\Sigma}^{-1}\boldsymbol{A})^{-}\boldsymbol{A}'\boldsymbol{\Sigma}^{-1}\boldsymbol{A}_2(\boldsymbol{A}_2'\boldsymbol{\Sigma}^{-1}\boldsymbol{A}_2)^{-}\boldsymbol{M}_2.$$

Since $\mathcal{C}(\boldsymbol{M}_1) = \mathcal{C}(\boldsymbol{A}') \cap \mathcal{C}(\boldsymbol{F}_1')$, one can, without any loss of generality, choose $\boldsymbol{M}_1$ to equal

$$\boldsymbol{M}_1 = \boldsymbol{A}'(\boldsymbol{A}(\boldsymbol{F}_1')^o)^o.$$

Thus,

$$\begin{aligned}
&\boldsymbol{M}_1'(\boldsymbol{A}'\boldsymbol{\Sigma}^{-1}\boldsymbol{A})^{-}\boldsymbol{A}'\boldsymbol{\Sigma}^{-1}\boldsymbol{A}_2(\boldsymbol{A}_2'\boldsymbol{\Sigma}^{-1}\boldsymbol{A}_2)^{-}\boldsymbol{M}_2\\
&= (\boldsymbol{A}(\boldsymbol{F}_1')^o)^{o'}\boldsymbol{A}_2(\boldsymbol{A}_2'\boldsymbol{\Sigma}^{-1}\boldsymbol{A}_2)^{-}\boldsymbol{M}_2 = \boldsymbol{0},
\end{aligned}$$

since by the definition of $\boldsymbol{A}_2$ in (7.58), it is trivially obtained that $(\boldsymbol{A}(\boldsymbol{F}_1')^o)^{o'}\boldsymbol{A}_2 = \boldsymbol{0}$. Hence, $\boldsymbol{Y}_1$ and $\boldsymbol{Y}_2$ are independently distributed. Now $\boldsymbol{U}_1$ and $\boldsymbol{V}_1$ are functions of $\boldsymbol{Y}_1$ and at the same time independent of $\boldsymbol{A}^{o'}\boldsymbol{X}$. Moreover, $\boldsymbol{U}_2$ and $\boldsymbol{V}_2$ are functions of $\boldsymbol{Y}_2$, as well as being independent of $\boldsymbol{A}_2^{o'}\boldsymbol{X}$. Therefore, based on these observations, λ_1 and λ_2 are independently distributed.

In Fig. 7.8 the spaces which are involved in testing (7.57) are presented. A comparison of Fig. 7.7 with Fig. 7.8 yields that the figures are very similar. The only difference is that the space $\mathcal{V}_2 = \mathcal{C}(\boldsymbol{C}'\boldsymbol{G}_2^o) \cap \mathcal{C}(\boldsymbol{C}'(\boldsymbol{G}_1 : \boldsymbol{G}_2)^o)^{\perp}$ in Fig. 7.7

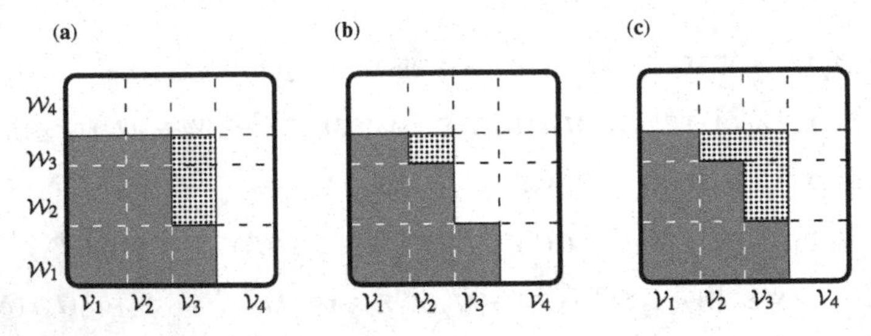

Fig. 7.8 In (**a**), the dotted area corresponds to H_0: $\boldsymbol{F}_2\boldsymbol{B}\boldsymbol{G}_2 = \boldsymbol{0}$ in the BRM. In (**b**), the area is shown for testing H_0: $\boldsymbol{F}_1\boldsymbol{B}\boldsymbol{G}_1 = \boldsymbol{0}$ in the BRM, given $\boldsymbol{F}_2\boldsymbol{B}\boldsymbol{G}_2 = \boldsymbol{0}$, where $\mathcal{C}(\boldsymbol{F}_1') \subseteq \mathcal{C}(\boldsymbol{F}_2')$, and in (**c**), the area is shown for testing H_0: $\boldsymbol{F}_i\boldsymbol{B}\boldsymbol{G}_i = \boldsymbol{0}, i = 1, 2$, in the BRM, where $\mathcal{C}(\boldsymbol{F}_1') \subseteq \mathcal{C}(\boldsymbol{F}_2')$ and $\mathcal{C}(\boldsymbol{G}_2) \subseteq \mathcal{C}(\boldsymbol{G}_1)$ hold. Furthermore, $\mathcal{W}_1 = \mathcal{C}_\bullet(\boldsymbol{A}(\boldsymbol{F}_2')^o)$, $\mathcal{W}_2 = \mathcal{C}_\bullet(\boldsymbol{A}(\boldsymbol{F}_1')^o) \cap \mathcal{C}_\bullet(\boldsymbol{A}(\boldsymbol{F}_2')^o)^{\perp}$, $\mathcal{W}_3 = \mathcal{C}_\bullet(\boldsymbol{A}) \cap \mathcal{C}_\bullet(\boldsymbol{A}(\boldsymbol{F}_1')^o)^{\perp}$, $\mathcal{W}_4 = \mathcal{C}_\bullet(\boldsymbol{A})^{\perp}$, $\mathcal{V}_1 = \mathcal{C}(\boldsymbol{C}'\boldsymbol{G}_1^o)$, $\mathcal{V}_2 = \mathcal{C}(\boldsymbol{C}'\boldsymbol{G}_2^o) \cap \mathcal{C}(\boldsymbol{C}'\boldsymbol{G}_1^o)^{\perp}$, $\mathcal{V}_3 = \mathcal{C}(\boldsymbol{C}') \cap \mathcal{C}(\boldsymbol{C}'\boldsymbol{G}_2^o)^{\perp}$ and $\mathcal{V}_4 = \mathcal{C}(\boldsymbol{C}')^{\perp}$

differs from $\mathcal{V}_2 = \mathcal{C}(\boldsymbol{C}'\boldsymbol{G}_2^o) \cap \mathcal{C}(\boldsymbol{C}'\boldsymbol{G}_1^o)^\perp$ in Fig. 7.8. The question arises, of course, of whether the difference is crucial, and the answer is that this difference may be important, but that it will not matter in many cases. However, one approach to adopt is that if there is a risk of a problem arising, then, if possible, one should try to design the experiment so that $\mathcal{C}(\boldsymbol{G}_2) \subseteq \mathcal{C}(\boldsymbol{G}_1)$ holds.

Theorem 7.9 *For the BRM presented in Definition 2.1 let the null hypothesis H_0: $\boldsymbol{F}_i\boldsymbol{B}\boldsymbol{G}_i = \boldsymbol{0}$, $i = 1, 2$, where $\mathcal{C}(\boldsymbol{F}_1') \subseteq \mathcal{C}(\boldsymbol{F}_2')$ and $\mathcal{C}(\boldsymbol{G}_2) \subseteq \mathcal{C}(\boldsymbol{G}_1)$ hold, be tested against the alternative hypothesis H_1: $\boldsymbol{B}$ is unrestricted. Let λ_{1o} and λ_{2o} be defined by (7.59) and (7.60), respectively. Moreover, let*

$$t_{1o} = \tfrac{2}{n}(f_1 - \tfrac{1}{2}(p_{1o} - m_1 + 1)) \ln \lambda_{1o},$$
$$t_{2o} = \tfrac{2}{n}(f_2 - \tfrac{1}{2}(p_{2o} - m_2 + 1)) \ln \lambda_{2o},$$

where

$$f_1 = n - r(\boldsymbol{C}) - p + r(\boldsymbol{A}), \qquad f_2 = n - r(\boldsymbol{C}'(\boldsymbol{G}_2 : \boldsymbol{G}_1^o)^o) - p + r(\boldsymbol{A}),$$
$$p_{1o} = \dim\{\mathcal{C}(\boldsymbol{F}_1') \cap \mathcal{C}(\boldsymbol{A}')\}, \qquad p_{2o} = \dim\{\mathcal{C}((\boldsymbol{F}_1')^{o'}\boldsymbol{A}'(\boldsymbol{A}(\boldsymbol{F}_2')^o)^o)\},$$
$$m_1 = \dim\{\mathcal{C}(\boldsymbol{G}_1) \cap \mathcal{C}(\boldsymbol{C})\}, \qquad m_2 = \dim\{\mathcal{C}(\boldsymbol{G}_2) \cap \mathcal{C}(\boldsymbol{C})\}.$$

Then the likelihood ratio test for testing H_0, approximately at significance level α, rejects the hypothesis if

$$P\{\chi^2_{p_{1o}m_1} \geq t_{1o}\} + c_{11}(1 - c_{11})(P\{\chi^2_{p_{1o}m_1+4} \geq t_{1o}\} - P\{\chi^2_{p_{1o}m_1} \geq t_{1o}\})$$
$$+ c_{12}(P\{\chi^2_{p_{1o}m_1+8} \geq t_{1o}\} - P\{\chi^2_{p_{1o}m_1} \geq t_{1o}\}) \leq \alpha_1,$$

or

$$P\{\chi^2_{p_{2o}m_2} \geq t_{2o}\} + c_{21}(1 - c_{21})(P\{\chi^2_{p_{2o}m_2+4} \geq t_{2o}\} - P\{\chi^2_{p_{2o}m_2} \geq t_{2o}\})$$
$$+ c_{22}(P\{\chi^2_{p_{2o}m_2+8} \geq t_{2o}\} - P\{\chi^2_{p_{2o}m_2} \geq t_{2o}\}) \leq \alpha_2,$$

where c_{11} and c_{12} correspond to c_1 and c_2 in Theorem 7.2, with p_{1o}, m_1 and f_1 inserted, c_{21} and c_{22} correspond to c_1 and c_2 in the same theorem, with p_{2o}, m_2 and f_2 inserted, and $\alpha_1 + \alpha_2 = \alpha$. □

Note that if $p_{io} = 1$ or $p_{io} = 2$, $i = 1, 2$, one can use Theorems 7.3 and 7.7.

Example 7.9 Reconsider the melatonin data given in Example 7.3. All the design matrices are the same as those in Example 7.3. For the BRM, this time the null hypothesis H_0: $\boldsymbol{F}_i\boldsymbol{B}\boldsymbol{G}_i = \boldsymbol{0}$, $i = 1, 2$, is tested against the alternative hypothesis

H_1: $\boldsymbol{B}$ unrestricted, with

$$\boldsymbol{F}_1 = (0:0:0:0:1),\ \boldsymbol{G}_1' = \begin{pmatrix} 0\,0\,1 \\ 0\,1\,0 \end{pmatrix},\ \boldsymbol{F}_2 = \begin{pmatrix} 0\,0\,0\,0\,1 \\ 0\,0\,0\,1\,0 \end{pmatrix},\ \boldsymbol{G}_2' = (0:1:0).$$

These matrices generate in $\boldsymbol{B} = (b_{ij})$ the restrictions $b_{52} = b_{53} = b_{42} = 0$, and λ_1 is the test statistic for testing $b_{52} = b_{53} = 0$ versus $\boldsymbol{B}$ unrestricted, while λ_2 is the test statistic for testing $b_{42} = 0$, given $b_{52} = b_{53} = 0$. Hence, the intention is to test H_0 as in Example 7.8, but the test is carried out differently. Moreover,

$$(\boldsymbol{F}_1')^o = \begin{pmatrix} 1\,0\,0\,0 \\ 0\,1\,0\,0 \\ 0\,0\,1\,0 \\ 0\,0\,0\,1 \\ 0\,0\,0\,0 \end{pmatrix}, \qquad (\boldsymbol{F}_2')^o = \begin{pmatrix} 1\,0\,0 \\ 0\,1\,0 \\ 0\,0\,1 \\ 0\,0\,0 \\ 0\,0\,0 \end{pmatrix},$$

$\boldsymbol{G}_1^{o'} = (1:0:0)$ and $(\boldsymbol{G}_2 : \boldsymbol{G}_1^o)^{o'} = (0:0:1)$. Then,

$$\begin{aligned} &\boldsymbol{A}_1 = \boldsymbol{A}, \quad \boldsymbol{A}_2 = \boldsymbol{A}(\boldsymbol{F}_1')^o, \quad \boldsymbol{A}_3 = \boldsymbol{A}(\boldsymbol{F}_2')^o, \\ &\boldsymbol{C}_1 = \boldsymbol{G}_1^{o'}\boldsymbol{C} = (1:0:0)\boldsymbol{C}, \quad \boldsymbol{C}_2 = (\boldsymbol{G}_2 : \boldsymbol{G}_1^o)^{o'}\boldsymbol{C} = (0:0:1)\boldsymbol{C}, \quad \boldsymbol{C}_3 = \boldsymbol{G}_2'\boldsymbol{C}. \end{aligned}$$

According to Theorem 7.9, the test based on λ_1, given in (7.59), is not rejected since $\lambda_{1o}^{2/45} = 1.1$. However, the second test, based on λ_2 which is presented in (7.60), is rejected since $\lambda_{2o}^{2/45} = 1.9$, which corresponds to $U_{1,1,39} = 0.52$, and Theorem 7.7 implies that

$$T_{24o} = 39(1 - U_{1,1,39})/U_{1,1,39} = 35.7 > F_{0.05}(1, 39) = 4.1.$$

Thus the overall test is rejected. Now, because of the results of Example 7.8, it is reasonable to test H_0: $b_{42} = 0$, since in Example 7.8, λ_{1o} was large and in the present example λ_{2o} was large. When testing H_0: $b_{42} = 0$, this hypothesis can be stated in matrix form as $\boldsymbol{FBG} = \boldsymbol{0}$, where $\boldsymbol{F} = (0:0:0:1:0)$ and $\boldsymbol{G}' = (0:1:0)$. Theorem 7.3 (ii) yields that H_0: $b_{42} = 0$ is rejected since $\lambda_o^{2/45} = 1.94$ and

$$T_{12o} = 37(1 - U_{1,1,37})/U_{1,1,3} = 34.7 > F_{1,39;0.05} = 4.1.$$

Thus, it can be concluded that $b_{42} = 0$ is not in agreement with the observations, as was expected based on how the data were generated in Example 7.3. □

7.8 A "Trace Test" for the BRM, $H_0 : \boldsymbol{FBG} = \boldsymbol{0}$ Against Unrestricted $\boldsymbol{B}$

Previously, for the BRM, likelihood ratio tests for the hypotheses $H_0 : \boldsymbol{FBG} = \boldsymbol{0}$ and $H_0 : \boldsymbol{F}_i\boldsymbol{BG}_i = \boldsymbol{0}$, $i = 1, 2$, were considered, and the latter case was treated under various types of additional conditions. In this section, an alternative procedure to the likelihood ratio testing procedure is presented. The hypothesis $H_0 : \boldsymbol{FBG} = \boldsymbol{0}$ is treated in this section, while $H_0 : \boldsymbol{F}_i\boldsymbol{BG}_i = \boldsymbol{0}$, $i = 1, 2$, will be in focus in the next section. In addition to a presentation of the explicit derivation of the tests, a number of differences from the likelihood ratio tests will be pointed out. Moreover, the differences will be summarized in Sect. 7.10.

Before starting with $H_0 : \boldsymbol{FBG} = \boldsymbol{0}$, an introduction to the construction of the "trace test" statistic is presented where the hypothesis $H_0 : \boldsymbol{BG} = \boldsymbol{0}$ is discussed and several reflections on the approach are made. Consider the BRM

$$\boldsymbol{X} = \boldsymbol{ABC} + \boldsymbol{E}, \qquad \boldsymbol{E} \sim N_{p,n}(\boldsymbol{0}, \boldsymbol{\Sigma}, \boldsymbol{I}), \tag{7.63}$$

and temporarily $\boldsymbol{\Sigma}$ is supposed to be known. In Sect. 2.4, based on linear models theory, the use of the estimator

$$\boldsymbol{A}\widehat{\boldsymbol{B}}\boldsymbol{C} = \boldsymbol{P}_{A,\Sigma}\boldsymbol{X}\boldsymbol{P}_{C'}$$

was justified, and using that, $D[\boldsymbol{X}] = \boldsymbol{I} \otimes \boldsymbol{\Sigma}$ yields

$$D[\boldsymbol{A}\widehat{\boldsymbol{B}}\boldsymbol{C}] = \boldsymbol{P}_{C'} \otimes \boldsymbol{A}(\boldsymbol{A}'\boldsymbol{\Sigma}^{-1}\boldsymbol{A})^{-}\boldsymbol{A}'. \tag{7.64}$$

It could be asserted that if one's purpose was to make inference concerning $\boldsymbol{B}$, it would be of interest to consider $\boldsymbol{\Sigma}$ to be a nuisance parameter. However, it has already been established in the special case $\boldsymbol{A} = \boldsymbol{I}$ that, although $\widehat{\boldsymbol{B}}\boldsymbol{C}$ does not depend functionally on $\boldsymbol{\Sigma}$, the distribution for $\widehat{\boldsymbol{B}}\boldsymbol{C}$ does, and in particular $D[\widehat{\boldsymbol{B}}\boldsymbol{C}] = \boldsymbol{P}_{C'} \otimes \boldsymbol{\Sigma}$. Thus, strictly speaking, $\boldsymbol{\Sigma}$ cannot be considered as a nuisance parameter. Moreover, for the interpretation of $\boldsymbol{A}\widehat{\boldsymbol{B}}\boldsymbol{C}$, it may be fruitful to recall that the parameter matrix $\boldsymbol{\Sigma}$ plays two roles; i.e. it is used to mimic the variation in the data and also is used to define the inner product. Hence, from a nuisance parameter point of view, the inclusion of $\boldsymbol{\Sigma}$ in $\boldsymbol{P}_{A,\Sigma}$ when estimating $\boldsymbol{ABC}$ is conceptually not very problematic and is to some extent independent of the variation in the data. However, one cannot circumvent the fact that the distribution connected with $\widehat{\boldsymbol{B}}$ depends on $\boldsymbol{\Sigma}$.

Now, consider

$$\boldsymbol{S} = \boldsymbol{X}(\boldsymbol{I} - \boldsymbol{P}_{C'})\boldsymbol{X}'.$$

It is known that $\boldsymbol{S}$ is independent of $\boldsymbol{X}\boldsymbol{P}_{C'}$, and $\boldsymbol{S}$ and $\boldsymbol{X}\boldsymbol{P}_{C'}$, are statistics which are jointly sufficient, with $\boldsymbol{S}$ not bearing any information about $\boldsymbol{B}$. Thus, it is natural to replace $\boldsymbol{\Sigma}$ by $\frac{1}{n}\boldsymbol{S}$ (or $\frac{1}{n-r(C)}\boldsymbol{S}$) in (7.64), leading to the maximum likelihood estimator

$$\boldsymbol{A}\widehat{\boldsymbol{B}}\boldsymbol{C} = \boldsymbol{P}_{A,S}\boldsymbol{X}\boldsymbol{P}_{C'}. \tag{7.65}$$

Moreover, similar to the conditional principle and the use of ancillarity, it is reasonable to evaluate $\boldsymbol{A}\widehat{\boldsymbol{B}}\boldsymbol{C}$ conditionally on $\boldsymbol{S}$, i.e.

$$\boldsymbol{A}\widehat{\boldsymbol{B}}\boldsymbol{C}|\boldsymbol{S} \sim N_{p,n}(\boldsymbol{ABC}, \boldsymbol{P}_{A,S}\boldsymbol{\Sigma}\boldsymbol{P}'_{A,S}, \boldsymbol{P}_{C'}),$$

or by performing an estimation of the variation

$$\boldsymbol{A}\widehat{\boldsymbol{B}}\boldsymbol{C}|\boldsymbol{S} \sim N_{p,n}(\boldsymbol{ABC}, \tfrac{1}{n}\boldsymbol{A}(\boldsymbol{A}'\boldsymbol{S}\boldsymbol{A})^{-}\boldsymbol{A}', \boldsymbol{P}_{C'}),$$

where the distribution, given $\boldsymbol{S} = \boldsymbol{S}_o$ and $\boldsymbol{B}$, is now completely known.

A competitive estimator to the maximum likelihood estimator in (7.65) is

$$\boldsymbol{A}\widetilde{\boldsymbol{B}}\boldsymbol{C} = \boldsymbol{P}_A\boldsymbol{X}\boldsymbol{P}_{C'} \sim N_{p,n}(\boldsymbol{ABC}, \boldsymbol{P}_A\boldsymbol{\Sigma}\boldsymbol{P}_A, \boldsymbol{P}_{C'}),$$

and in this case too, a conditional argument can be used to replace $\boldsymbol{\Sigma}$, i.e.

$$\boldsymbol{A}\widetilde{\boldsymbol{B}}\boldsymbol{C}|\boldsymbol{S} \sim N_{p,n}(\boldsymbol{ABC}, \tfrac{1}{n}\boldsymbol{P}_A\boldsymbol{S}\boldsymbol{P}_A, \boldsymbol{P}_{C'}).$$

However, it is interesting to note that

$$\boldsymbol{P}_A\boldsymbol{S}\boldsymbol{P}_A - \boldsymbol{A}(\boldsymbol{A}'\boldsymbol{S}\boldsymbol{A})^{-}\boldsymbol{A}' = \boldsymbol{P}_A(\boldsymbol{S} - \boldsymbol{A}(\boldsymbol{A}'\boldsymbol{S}\boldsymbol{A})^{-}\boldsymbol{A}')\boldsymbol{P}_A$$

is positive semi-definite (see Appendix B, Theorem B.13). Thus, when carrying out the conditional inference, the use of $\boldsymbol{A}\widehat{\boldsymbol{B}}\boldsymbol{C}$ has some advantages in comparison with $\boldsymbol{A}\widetilde{\boldsymbol{B}}\boldsymbol{C}$.

Next, as promised at the beginning of this section, the basic ideas are illustrated with the help of a simple testing problem. For the BRM in (7.63), the hypothesis and its alternative equal

$$H_0: \ \boldsymbol{BG} = \boldsymbol{0}, \quad versus \ H_1\text{: } \boldsymbol{B} \text{ unrestricted.} \tag{7.66}$$

Thus, since $\boldsymbol{BG} = \boldsymbol{0}$ is equivalent to $\boldsymbol{B} = \boldsymbol{\Theta}\boldsymbol{G}^{o'}$, where $\boldsymbol{\Theta}$ is an arbitrary matrix, under H_0 the BRM is defined as

$$\boldsymbol{X} = \boldsymbol{A}\boldsymbol{\Theta}\boldsymbol{G}^{o'}\boldsymbol{C} + \boldsymbol{E}, \quad \boldsymbol{E} \sim N_{p,n}(\boldsymbol{0}, \boldsymbol{\Sigma}, \boldsymbol{I}).$$

For any given $\boldsymbol{\Sigma}$, it follows that the likelihood ratio test for H_0 versus $\boldsymbol{B}$ unrestricted is proportional to

$$e^{-\frac{1}{2}\mathrm{tr}\{\boldsymbol{\Sigma}^{-1}(\boldsymbol{X}_o - \boldsymbol{A}\widehat{\boldsymbol{B}}\boldsymbol{C})()'\}}e^{\frac{1}{2}\mathrm{tr}\{\boldsymbol{\Sigma}^{-1}(\boldsymbol{X}_o - \boldsymbol{A}\widehat{\boldsymbol{\Theta}}\boldsymbol{G}^{o'}\boldsymbol{C})()'\}}, \tag{7.67}$$

where

$$\boldsymbol{A}\widehat{\boldsymbol{B}}\boldsymbol{C} = \boldsymbol{P}_{A,\Sigma}\boldsymbol{X}_o\boldsymbol{P}_{C'}, \quad \boldsymbol{A}\widehat{\boldsymbol{\Theta}}\boldsymbol{G}^{o'}\boldsymbol{C} = \boldsymbol{P}_{A,\Sigma}\boldsymbol{X}_o\boldsymbol{P}_{C'G^o}.$$

The relation in (7.67) can be written as follows:

$$e^{-\frac{1}{2}\mathrm{tr}\{\boldsymbol{\Sigma}^{-1}(\boldsymbol{S}_1+(\boldsymbol{I}-\boldsymbol{P}_{\mathrm{A},\Sigma})\boldsymbol{X}_{\mathrm{o}}\boldsymbol{P}_{\mathrm{C}'}\boldsymbol{X}_{\mathrm{o}}'(\boldsymbol{I}-\boldsymbol{P}_{\mathrm{A},\Sigma})')\}+\frac{1}{2}\mathrm{tr}\{\boldsymbol{\Sigma}^{-1}(\boldsymbol{S}_2+(\boldsymbol{I}-\boldsymbol{P}_{\mathrm{A},\Sigma})\boldsymbol{X}_{\mathrm{o}}\boldsymbol{P}_{\mathrm{C}'\mathrm{G}^{\mathrm{o}}}\boldsymbol{X}_{\mathrm{o}}'(\boldsymbol{I}-\boldsymbol{P}_{\mathrm{A},\Sigma})')\}}, \qquad (7.68)$$

where

$$\boldsymbol{S}_1 = \boldsymbol{X}_o(\boldsymbol{I} - \boldsymbol{P}_{C'})\boldsymbol{X}_o', \qquad \boldsymbol{S}_2 = \boldsymbol{X}_o(\boldsymbol{I} - \boldsymbol{P}_{C'G^o})\boldsymbol{X}_o',$$
$$\boldsymbol{S}_2 - \boldsymbol{S}_1 = \boldsymbol{X}_o(\boldsymbol{P}_{C'} - \boldsymbol{P}_{C'G^o})\boldsymbol{X}_o' = \boldsymbol{X}_o\boldsymbol{P}_{C'(CC')^-N}\boldsymbol{X}_o',$$

remembering that (see Appendix B, Theorem B.12)

$$\boldsymbol{P}_{C'} - \boldsymbol{P}_{C'G^o} = \boldsymbol{P}_{C'(CC')^-N},$$

where $\boldsymbol{N}$ is any matrix satisfying $\mathcal{C}(\boldsymbol{N}) = \mathcal{C}(\boldsymbol{G}) \cap \mathcal{C}(\boldsymbol{C})$. The expression $\boldsymbol{S}_2 - \boldsymbol{S}_1$ can be viewed as the square of the difference of two residuals.

A few manipulations in (7.68) yield that the likelihood ratio test is proportional to

$$e^{\frac{1}{2}\mathrm{tr}\{\boldsymbol{\Sigma}^{-1}\boldsymbol{P}_{\mathrm{A},\Sigma}\boldsymbol{X}_{\mathrm{o}}\boldsymbol{P}_{\mathrm{C}'(\mathrm{CC}')^-\mathrm{N}}\boldsymbol{X}_{\mathrm{o}}'\boldsymbol{P}_{\mathrm{A},\Sigma}'\}}.$$

Thus, a natural test statistic for testing (7.66) is

$$\mathrm{tr}\{\boldsymbol{\Sigma}^{-1}\boldsymbol{P}_{\mathrm{A},\Sigma}\boldsymbol{X}\boldsymbol{P}_{\mathrm{C}'(\mathrm{CC}')^-\mathrm{N}}\boldsymbol{X}'\boldsymbol{P}_{\mathrm{A},\Sigma}'\}. \qquad (7.69)$$

In order to acquire a deeper understanding of the test statistic in (7.69), one should note that $\boldsymbol{X}\boldsymbol{P}_{C'(CC')^-N}$ is a projection on the between-individual subspace, and the statistic is built up by a projection of $\boldsymbol{X}\boldsymbol{P}_{C'(CC')^-N}$ on the within-individuals space $\mathcal{C}_\Sigma(\boldsymbol{A})$, i.e.

$$\boldsymbol{P}_{A,\Sigma}\boldsymbol{X}\boldsymbol{P}_{C'(CC')^-N},$$

and then the projection is squared. Since this takes place on the within-individual space, the inner product has to be taken into account, meaning that

$$\boldsymbol{P}_{C'(CC')^-N}\boldsymbol{X}'\boldsymbol{P}_{A,\Sigma}'\boldsymbol{\Sigma}^{-1}\boldsymbol{P}_{A,\Sigma}\boldsymbol{X}\boldsymbol{P}_{C'(CC')^-N} \qquad (7.70)$$

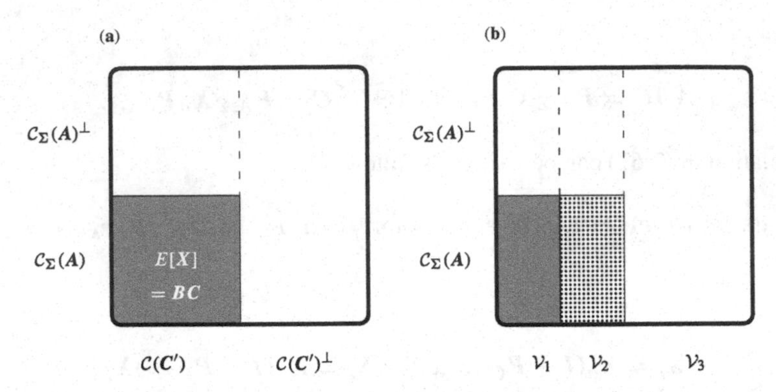

Fig. 7.9 Consider the BRM model in (7.63). A decomposition is presented of the whole space according to the design and the restrictions $BF = 0$. In **(a)**, where there are no restrictions the decomposition consists of the subspaces $\mathcal{C}(C')$ and $\mathcal{C}(C')^\perp$, as well as $\mathcal{C}_\Sigma(A)$ and $\mathcal{C}_\Sigma(A)^\perp$. In **(b)**, with the restrictions $BG = 0$, $\mathcal{V}_1 = \mathcal{C}(C'G^o)$, $\mathcal{V}_2 = \mathcal{C}(C'G^o)^\perp \cap \mathcal{C}(C')$ and $\mathcal{V}_3 = \mathcal{C}(C')^\perp$

should be calculated. Finally, in order to summarize the information in this expression, the trace is taken in (7.70), which leads to an expression which is identical to (7.69).

For (7.69) to become applicable, Σ has to be replaced by an estimator. Consider Fig. 7.9, which illustrates the fact that the hypothesis (7.66) concerns the testing of

$$\mathcal{C}(C'G^o)^\perp \cap \mathcal{C}(C') \otimes \mathcal{C}_\Sigma(A) = \mathcal{C}(C'(CC')^- N) \otimes \mathcal{C}_\Sigma(A),$$

i.e. testing whether the dimension of this space equals 0. This space is highlighted in Fig. 7.9b. However, the inner product in $\mathcal{C}_\Sigma(A)$ has to be estimated, which means that a suitable estimator of Σ has to be found. The variation in the BRM is uncovered via projections of the observations on $\mathcal{C}(C')^\perp \otimes \mathcal{W}$ and $\mathcal{C}(C') \cap \mathcal{C}_\Sigma(A)^\perp$, with $\mathcal{W}$ representing the whole within-individuals space. However, it is natural only to use $\mathcal{C}(C')^\perp \otimes \mathcal{W}$, since $\mathcal{C}(C') \cap \mathcal{C}_\Sigma(A)^\perp$ depends on Σ; i.e. it is proposed that $(I - P_{C'})X$ should be the basis of the space where an estimator of Σ is obtained. Hence, as an estimator of Σ, when using the dispersion matrix to define the inner product, the quantity to use is

$$\widehat{\Sigma} = \frac{1}{n} S = \frac{1}{n} X(I - P_{C'})X'. \tag{7.71}$$

Remember that when obtaining the maximum likelihood estimators of the mean parameters in the BRM, the data were projected on the space $\mathcal{C}(C') \cap \mathcal{C}_S(A)^\perp$; i.e. the inner product was estimated using S, which is in agreement with the above discussion concerning the estimation of Σ.

Now, since $P_{C'(CC')^- N}$ is a projection on $\mathcal{C}(C'G^o)^\perp \cap \mathcal{C}(C')$, $P_{A,\Sigma}$ is a projection on $\mathcal{C}_\Sigma(A)$ and $n^{-1}S$ can be used to estimate the inner product, instead of (7.69), a test statistic which is functionally independent of the parameters under

H_0 is given by

$$T_3 = \mathrm{tr}\{\boldsymbol{S}^{-1}\boldsymbol{P}_{\mathrm{A,S}}\boldsymbol{X}\boldsymbol{P}_{\mathrm{C'(CC')^-N}}\boldsymbol{X}'\boldsymbol{P}'_{\mathrm{A,S}}\}.$$

This statistic is called the "trace test" statistic. More precisely, it is a statistic which belongs to a class of "trace tests".

Proposition 7.1 *For the BRM presented in Definition 2.1, let the null hypothesis H_0 : $\boldsymbol{BG} = \boldsymbol{0}$ be tested against H_1: $\boldsymbol{B}$ unrestricted. Let $\boldsymbol{S}$ be defined in (7.71) and let $\boldsymbol{N}$ be any matrix satisfying $\mathcal{C}(\boldsymbol{N}) = \mathcal{C}(\boldsymbol{G}) \cap \mathcal{C}(\boldsymbol{C})$. A test statistic is given by*

$$T_3 = \mathrm{tr}\{\boldsymbol{S}^{-1}\boldsymbol{P}_{\mathrm{A,S}}\boldsymbol{X}\boldsymbol{P}_{\mathrm{C'(CC')^-N}}\boldsymbol{X}'\boldsymbol{P}'_{\mathrm{A,S}}\}.$$

The hypothesis is rejected when the observed value of T_3 is large.

Moreover, it has been observed several times that $\boldsymbol{S}$ is independent of $\boldsymbol{X}\boldsymbol{P}_{C'(CC')^-N}\boldsymbol{X}'$, and in the next theorem the fundamental property is stated that the distribution of T_3, under H_0, is independent of the parameters. Hence, replacing $\boldsymbol{\Sigma}$ in (7.69) by $\boldsymbol{S}$ makes sense.

Theorem 7.10 *For the BRM presented in Definition 2.1, let the null hypothesis H_0 : $\boldsymbol{BG} = \boldsymbol{0}$ be tested against H_1: $\boldsymbol{B}$ unrestricted. Under H_0 the distribution of the test statistic T_3, presented in Proposition 7.1, is independent of $\boldsymbol{\Sigma}$ and $\boldsymbol{B}$.*

Proof Rewrite T_3 as

$$\begin{aligned}T_3 = &\ \mathrm{tr}\{\boldsymbol{S}^{-1}\boldsymbol{X}\boldsymbol{P}_{\mathrm{C'(CC')^-N}}\boldsymbol{X}'\}\\ &-\mathrm{tr}\{\boldsymbol{A}^{\mathrm{o}}(\boldsymbol{A}^{\mathrm{o}'}\boldsymbol{S}\boldsymbol{A}^{\mathrm{o}})^{-1}\boldsymbol{A}^{\mathrm{o}'}\boldsymbol{X}\boldsymbol{P}_{\mathrm{C'(CC')^-N}}\boldsymbol{X}'\boldsymbol{A}^{\mathrm{o}}(\boldsymbol{A}^{\mathrm{o}'}\boldsymbol{S}\boldsymbol{A}^{\mathrm{o}})^{-1}\boldsymbol{A}^{\mathrm{o}'}\},\end{aligned}$$

for an appropriately chosen $\boldsymbol{A}^{o}$. It is noted that the first term in T_3 equals

$$\begin{aligned}\mathrm{tr}\{\boldsymbol{S}^{-1}\boldsymbol{X}\boldsymbol{P}_{\mathrm{C'(CC')^-N}}\boldsymbol{X}'\} = &\ \mathrm{tr}\{(\boldsymbol{\Sigma}^{-1/2}\boldsymbol{S}\boldsymbol{\Sigma}^{-1/2})^{-1}\boldsymbol{\Sigma}^{-1/2}(\boldsymbol{X} - \boldsymbol{A}\boldsymbol{\Theta}\boldsymbol{G}^{\mathrm{o}'}\boldsymbol{C})\boldsymbol{P}_{\mathrm{C'(CC')^-N}}\\ &\times(\boldsymbol{X} - \boldsymbol{A}\boldsymbol{\Theta}\boldsymbol{G}^{o'}\boldsymbol{C})'\boldsymbol{\Sigma}^{-1/2}\},\end{aligned}$$

since for any $\boldsymbol{\Theta}$, $\boldsymbol{A}\boldsymbol{\Theta}\boldsymbol{G}^{o'}\boldsymbol{C}\boldsymbol{C}'(\boldsymbol{C}\boldsymbol{C}')^{-}\boldsymbol{N} = \boldsymbol{0}$. Then under H_0 the distribution is independent of $\boldsymbol{\Sigma}$ and $\boldsymbol{B}$. Moreover, the second term can be rewritten in the following way:

$$\begin{aligned}&\mathrm{tr}\{\boldsymbol{A}^{\mathrm{o}}(\boldsymbol{A}^{\mathrm{o}'}\boldsymbol{S}\boldsymbol{A}^{\mathrm{o}})^{-1}\boldsymbol{A}^{\mathrm{o}'}\boldsymbol{X}\boldsymbol{P}_{\mathrm{C'(CC')^-N}}\boldsymbol{X}'\boldsymbol{A}^{\mathrm{o}}(\boldsymbol{A}^{\mathrm{o}'}\boldsymbol{S}\boldsymbol{A}^{\mathrm{o}})^{-1}\boldsymbol{A}^{\mathrm{o}'}\}\\ &= \mathrm{tr}\{\boldsymbol{A}^{\mathrm{o}}(\boldsymbol{A}^{\mathrm{o}'}\boldsymbol{\Sigma}\boldsymbol{A}^{\mathrm{o}})^{-1/2}((\boldsymbol{A}^{\mathrm{o}'}\boldsymbol{\Sigma}\boldsymbol{A}^{\mathrm{o}})^{-1/2}\boldsymbol{A}^{\mathrm{o}'}\boldsymbol{S}\boldsymbol{A}^{\mathrm{o}}(\boldsymbol{A}^{\mathrm{o}'}\boldsymbol{\Sigma}\boldsymbol{A}^{\mathrm{o}})^{-1/2})^{-1}\\ &\quad\times(\boldsymbol{A}^{o'}\boldsymbol{\Sigma}\boldsymbol{A}^{o})^{-1/2}\boldsymbol{A}^{o'}\boldsymbol{X}\boldsymbol{P}_{C'(CC')^-N}\boldsymbol{X}'\}.\end{aligned}$$

Since the distribution of $(A^{o'}\Sigma A^{o})^{-1/2}A^{o'}X$ is independent of Σ and B, the distribution of

$$(A^{o'}\Sigma A^{o})^{-1/2}A^{o'}SA^{o}(A^{o'}\Sigma A^{o})^{-1/2}$$

is also independent of the unknown parameters, which establishes the theorem. □

Theorem 7.11 *Let T_3 be defined in Proposition 7.1, and let the constants $c_{0;n,s}$ and $c_{i;n,s,t}$, $i = 1, 2, 3$, be given in Definition B.1 (i)–(iv), of Appendix B, Sect. B.15. Moreover, let $r_N = r(N)$, $r_A = r(A)$ and $r_C = r(C)$. Then*

(i)

$$E[T_3] = c_0 + \frac{1}{n - r_C - p - 1}\mathrm{tr}\{\Sigma^{-1}ABN(N'(CC')^{-}N)^{-}N'B'A'\},$$

where

$$c_0 = \frac{r_N r_A(n-r_C-1)}{(n-r_C-p-1)(n-r_C-p+r_A-1)};$$

(ii) *under H_0*

$$D[T_3] = c_1 + c_2 + c_3 + c_4 - E[T_3]^2,$$

where $E[T_3] = c_0$, with c_0 defined in statement (i), and

$$c_1 = r_N^2 p^2 c_{1;n-r_C,p} + 2r_N p c_{2;n-r_C,p},$$
$$c_2 = r_N^2(p - r_A)^2 c_{1;n-r_C,p-r_A} + 2r_N(p - r_A)c_{2;n-r_C,p-r_A},$$
$$c_3 = -2r_N^2(p - r_A)^2 c_{1;n-r_C,p-r_A} - 4r_N^2(p - r_A)c_{2;n-r_C,p-r_A}$$
$$-\frac{2r_N^2 r_A(p-r_A)}{(n-r_C-p-1)(n-r_C-(p-r_A))},$$
$$c_4 = 2r_N r_A(n - r_C - 1)c_{0;n-r_C,p-r_A}.$$

Proof According to Appendix B, Theorem B.19 (iv)

$$E[XP_{C'(CC')^{-}N}X'] = r_N\Sigma + ABN(N'(CC')^{-}N)^{-}N'B'A',$$

and using the independence between $XP_{C'(CC')^{-}N}X'$ and S, together with Theorem B.26 (ii) in Appendix B, establishes statement (i).

Concerning statement (ii), since $D[T_3] = E[T_3^2] - E[T_3]^2$, the expectation $E[T_3^2]$ has to be determined. First it is noted that

$$E[T_3^2] = \mathrm{tr}\{\mathrm{E}[(S^{-1}P_{\mathrm{A,S}})^{\otimes 2}(XP_{\mathrm{C'(CC')^{-}N}}X')^{\otimes 2}]\}$$
$$= \mathrm{tr}\{\mathrm{E}[(S^{-1}P_{\mathrm{A,S}})^{\otimes 2}]\mathrm{E}[(XP_{\mathrm{C'(CC')^{-}N}}X')^{\otimes 2}]\},$$

and according to Appendix B, Theorem B.19 (vii)

$$E[(\boldsymbol{X}\boldsymbol{P}_{C'(CC')^-N}\boldsymbol{X}')^{\otimes 2}] = r_N^2 \boldsymbol{\Sigma} \otimes \boldsymbol{\Sigma} + r_N(\text{vec}\boldsymbol{\Sigma}\text{vec}'\boldsymbol{\Sigma} + \boldsymbol{K}_{p,p}\boldsymbol{\Sigma} \otimes \boldsymbol{\Sigma}).$$

Now

$$\begin{aligned}
&\text{tr}\{\text{E}[(\boldsymbol{S}^{-1}\boldsymbol{P}_{\text{A,S}})^{\otimes 2}\text{r}_\text{N}(\text{vec}\boldsymbol{\Sigma}\text{vec}'\boldsymbol{\Sigma} + \boldsymbol{K}_{\text{p,p}}\boldsymbol{\Sigma} \otimes \boldsymbol{\Sigma})]\} \\
&\quad = 2r_N\text{tr}\{\text{E}[\boldsymbol{\Sigma}^{1/2}\boldsymbol{S}^{-1}\boldsymbol{A}(\boldsymbol{A}'\boldsymbol{S}^{-1}\boldsymbol{A})^-\boldsymbol{A}'\boldsymbol{S}^{-1}\boldsymbol{\Sigma}\boldsymbol{S}^{-1}\boldsymbol{A}(\boldsymbol{A}'\boldsymbol{S}^{-1}\boldsymbol{A})^-\boldsymbol{A}'\boldsymbol{S}^{-1}\boldsymbol{\Sigma}^{1/2}]\},
\end{aligned}$$

which, according to Appendix B, Theorem B.26 (iii) equals c_4. The remaining task is to derive the quantity $r_N^2\text{tr}\{\text{E}[(\boldsymbol{S}^{-1}\boldsymbol{P}_{\text{A,S}})^{\otimes 2}\boldsymbol{\Sigma} \otimes \boldsymbol{\Sigma}]\}$, which can be written as

$$r_N^2\text{tr}\{\text{E}[(\boldsymbol{\Sigma}^{1/2}\boldsymbol{S}^{-1}\boldsymbol{\Sigma}^{1/2} - \boldsymbol{\Sigma}^{1/2}\boldsymbol{A}^o(\boldsymbol{A}^{o'}\boldsymbol{S}^{-1}\boldsymbol{A}^o)^-\boldsymbol{A}^{o'}\boldsymbol{\Sigma}^{1/2})^{\otimes 2}]\}$$

and is obtained via

$$\begin{aligned}
c_1 &= r_N^2\text{tr}\{\text{E}[(\boldsymbol{\Sigma}^{1/2} \otimes \boldsymbol{\Sigma}^{1/2})(\boldsymbol{S}^{-1} \otimes \boldsymbol{S}^{-1})(\boldsymbol{\Sigma}^{1/2} \otimes \boldsymbol{\Sigma}^{1/2})]\}, \\
c_2 &= r_N^2\text{tr}\{\text{E}[(\boldsymbol{\Sigma}^{1/2}\boldsymbol{A}^o(\boldsymbol{A}^{o'}\boldsymbol{S}\boldsymbol{A}^o)^{-1}\boldsymbol{A}^{o'}\boldsymbol{\Sigma}^{1/2})^{\otimes 2}]\},
\end{aligned}$$

where Theorem B.21 (iii) in Appendix B has been used. Finally, Theorem B.24 in Appendix B determines that

$$\begin{aligned}
c_3 = &-r_N^2\text{tr}\{\text{E}[\boldsymbol{\Sigma}^{1/2}\boldsymbol{S}^{-1}\boldsymbol{\Sigma}^{1/2} \otimes \boldsymbol{\Sigma}^{1/2}\boldsymbol{A}^o(\boldsymbol{A}^{o'}\boldsymbol{S}\boldsymbol{A}^o)^{-1}\boldsymbol{A}^{o'}\boldsymbol{\Sigma}^{1/2}]\} \\
&-r_N^2\text{tr}\{\text{E}[\boldsymbol{\Sigma}^{1/2}\boldsymbol{A}^o(\boldsymbol{A}^{o'}\boldsymbol{S}\boldsymbol{A}^o)^{-1}\boldsymbol{A}^{o'}\boldsymbol{\Sigma}^{1/2} \otimes \boldsymbol{\Sigma}^{1/2}\boldsymbol{S}^{-1}\boldsymbol{\Sigma}^{1/2}]\},
\end{aligned}$$

and thus the proof of the theorem is complete. □

From Theorem 7.11 (i), it follows that when $\boldsymbol{B} \neq \mathbf{0}$, the expected value of T_3 is larger than c_0. Moreover, if

$$\boldsymbol{B}_1\boldsymbol{N}(\boldsymbol{N}'(\boldsymbol{C}\boldsymbol{C}')^-\boldsymbol{N})^-\boldsymbol{N}'\boldsymbol{B}_1' - \boldsymbol{B}_2\boldsymbol{N}(\boldsymbol{N}'(\boldsymbol{C}\boldsymbol{C}')^-\boldsymbol{N})^-\boldsymbol{N}'\boldsymbol{B}_2'$$

is positive semi-definite, then (see Appendix B, Theorem B.9 (ii))

$$\text{tr}\{\boldsymbol{\Sigma}^{-1}\boldsymbol{A}\boldsymbol{B}_1\boldsymbol{N}(\boldsymbol{N}'(\boldsymbol{C}\boldsymbol{C}')^-\boldsymbol{N})^-\boldsymbol{N}'\boldsymbol{B}_1'\boldsymbol{A}'\} \geq \text{tr}\{\boldsymbol{\Sigma}^{-1}\boldsymbol{A}\boldsymbol{B}_2\boldsymbol{N}(\boldsymbol{N}'(\boldsymbol{C}\boldsymbol{C}')^-\boldsymbol{N})^-\boldsymbol{N}'\boldsymbol{B}_2'\boldsymbol{A}'\}.$$

Hence, it makes sense to use T_3 as a test statistic, because deviances from H_0 are reflected in the test statistic.

Unfortunately, the exact distribution for T_3, given by Proposition 7.1, is not available. There are several ways to solve this problem approximately and it is worthwhile examining T_3 more closely. First it can be noted that $\boldsymbol{S}^{-1/2}\boldsymbol{X}\boldsymbol{P}_{C'(CC')^-N}\boldsymbol{X}'\boldsymbol{S}^{-1/2}$ is multivariate β-distributed of type II (see Appendix

A, Sect. A.9), and $\boldsymbol{H} = (\boldsymbol{A}'\boldsymbol{S}^{-1}\boldsymbol{A})^{-1/2}\boldsymbol{A}'\boldsymbol{S}^{-1/2}$ is semi-orthogonal, i.e. $\boldsymbol{H}\boldsymbol{H}' = \boldsymbol{I}$. Thus,

$$T_3 = \mathrm{tr}\{\boldsymbol{H}\boldsymbol{S}^{-1/2}\boldsymbol{X}\boldsymbol{P}_{\mathrm{C}'(\mathrm{CC}')^{-}\mathrm{N}}\boldsymbol{X}'\boldsymbol{S}^{-1/2}\boldsymbol{H}'\}.$$

Exploiting this expression is somewhat difficult, since $\boldsymbol{H}$ and

$$\boldsymbol{S}^{-1/2}\boldsymbol{X}\boldsymbol{P}_{C'(CC')^{-}N}\boldsymbol{X}'\boldsymbol{S}^{-1/2}$$

are not independently distributed. Therefore, to gain a better understanding of the statistic, a canonical version of T_3 can be derived. As has been done many times before, let $\boldsymbol{A}' = \boldsymbol{T}(\boldsymbol{I}_{r(A)} : \boldsymbol{0})\boldsymbol{\Gamma}\boldsymbol{\Sigma}^{1/2}$, where $\boldsymbol{T}$ is a non-singular matrix and $\boldsymbol{\Gamma}$ is an orthogonal matrix (see Appendix B, Theorem B.1 (i)). Moreover, let $\boldsymbol{Y} = \boldsymbol{\Gamma}\boldsymbol{\Sigma}^{-1/2}\boldsymbol{X}$ and $\boldsymbol{V} = \boldsymbol{\Gamma}\boldsymbol{\Sigma}^{-1/2}\boldsymbol{S}\boldsymbol{\Sigma}^{-1/2}\boldsymbol{\Gamma}'$. Then

$$T_3 = \mathrm{tr}\{\boldsymbol{V}^{-1}(\boldsymbol{I} : \boldsymbol{0})'((\boldsymbol{I} : \boldsymbol{0})\boldsymbol{V}^{-1}(\boldsymbol{I} : \boldsymbol{0})')^{-1}(\boldsymbol{I} : \boldsymbol{0})\boldsymbol{V}^{-1}\boldsymbol{Y}\boldsymbol{P}_{\mathrm{C}'(\mathrm{CC}')^{-}\mathrm{N}}\boldsymbol{Y}'\}.$$

Through a spectral decomposition, it follows that

$$T_3 = \sum_{i=1}^{r(A)} \lambda_i \chi^2_{r(N);i}, \tag{7.72}$$

where λ_i are eigenvalues of

$$\boldsymbol{V}^{-1}(\boldsymbol{I} : \boldsymbol{0})'((\boldsymbol{I} : \boldsymbol{0})\boldsymbol{V}^{-1}(\boldsymbol{I} : \boldsymbol{0})')^{-1}(\boldsymbol{I} : \boldsymbol{0})\boldsymbol{V}^{-1} = \begin{pmatrix} \boldsymbol{V}^{11} & \boldsymbol{V}^{12} \\ \boldsymbol{V}^{21} & \boldsymbol{V}^{21}(\boldsymbol{V}^{11})^{-1}\boldsymbol{V}^{12} \end{pmatrix},$$

which contains already known notation. Note that in (7.72) the index i is used to indicate that we have different chi-square variables. The distribution for T_3 is relatively easy to simulate, i.e. only $\boldsymbol{V}$ needs to be simulated. Then λ_i are obtained and, given λ_i, the test statistic T_3 has a weighted chi-square distribution. Approximating a weighted chi-square distribution with a chi-square distribution is a classical problem which has been studied by many authors. In the next proposition, a well-known idea is presented. However, note that λ_i is random, which usually is not the case.

Proposition 7.2 *For the BRM presented in Definition 2.1, let the null hypothesis* H_0 : $\boldsymbol{B}\boldsymbol{G} = \boldsymbol{0}$ *be tested against* H_1: $\boldsymbol{B}$ *unrestricted. The corresponding test statistic* T_3 *is given by Proposition 7.1. Then the hypothesis connected to* T_3 *is rejected at approximate significance level* α *if* $P(T_{3o} \geq a\chi^2_{[f]}) \leq \alpha$, *where* T_{3o} *is the observed value of* T_3, $[f]$ *denotes the integer part of either* f *or* $f+1$ *and the integer part* *which is closest to f is chosen;*

$$a = \frac{c_1 + c_2 + c_3 + c_4 - c_0^2}{2c_0}, \qquad f = \frac{2c_0^2}{c_1 + c_2 + c_3 + c_4 - c_0^2},$$

where $c_0 - c_4$ are defined in Theorem 7.11.

Proof Below are presented a few hints explaining the choices of a and f. In (7.72) it was seen that the test statistic is a weighted sum of χ^2-distributed variables. This type of distribution appears frequently and is often approximated by an adjustment of a chi-square distribution where one uses a scaling parameter, a, and a degrees-of-freedom parameter, f. These parameters will be determined by identification of the mean and dispersion, i.e.

$$E[T_3] = af, \qquad D[T_3] = 2a^2 f.$$

Solving these equations, where the results of Theorem 7.11 are utilized, establishes the theorem. □

Note that it is possible to have non-integer degrees of freedom in a chi-square distribution and in Proposition 7.2 it is not necessary to use $|f|$ instead of f, in particular since the distribution is only used to approximate another distribution.

Now a trace test for $\boldsymbol{B}$ in the BRM, i.e. H_0: $\boldsymbol{FBG} = \mathbf{0}$ against H_1: $\boldsymbol{B}$ arbitrary, is derived. First $\boldsymbol{\Sigma}$ is assumed to be known. Following the ideas previously presented in this section, a reparametrization takes place and it is noted that $\boldsymbol{FBG} = \mathbf{0}$ is equivalent to

$$\boldsymbol{B} = (\boldsymbol{F}')^o \boldsymbol{\Theta}_1 + \boldsymbol{F}' \boldsymbol{\Theta}_2 \boldsymbol{G}^{o'},$$

where $\boldsymbol{\Theta}_1$ and $\boldsymbol{\Theta}_2$ are new parameters. Thus, the following models under H_1 and H_0, respectively, are considered:

$$\begin{aligned} H_1 &: \ E[\boldsymbol{X}] = \boldsymbol{ABC}, \\ H_0 &: \ E[\boldsymbol{X}] = \boldsymbol{A}(\boldsymbol{F}')^o \boldsymbol{\Theta}_1 \boldsymbol{C} + \boldsymbol{AF}' \boldsymbol{\Theta}_2 \boldsymbol{G}^{o'} \boldsymbol{C}. \end{aligned}$$

Since $\boldsymbol{\Sigma}$ is supposed to be known, the likelihood ratio statistic can be shown to be equivalent to

$$\mathrm{tr}\{\boldsymbol{\Sigma}^{-1}(\boldsymbol{X} - \boldsymbol{A}\widehat{\boldsymbol{B}}_{\mathrm{H}_0}\boldsymbol{C})()'\} - \mathrm{tr}\{\boldsymbol{\Sigma}^{-1}(\boldsymbol{X} - \boldsymbol{A}\widehat{\boldsymbol{B}}_{\mathrm{H}_1}\boldsymbol{C})()'\}, \qquad (7.73)$$

where $\widehat{\boldsymbol{B}}_{H_1}$ and $\widehat{\boldsymbol{B}}_{H_0}$ denote the maximum likelihood estimators of $\boldsymbol{B}$ under H_1 and H_0, respectively.

Let

$$\begin{aligned}
&\boldsymbol{A}_1 = \boldsymbol{A}(\boldsymbol{F}')^o, \quad \boldsymbol{C}_1 = \boldsymbol{C}, \quad \boldsymbol{A}_2 = \boldsymbol{A}\boldsymbol{F}', \quad \boldsymbol{C}_2 = \boldsymbol{G}^{o'}\boldsymbol{C},\\
&\boldsymbol{Q}_0' = \boldsymbol{I} - \boldsymbol{P}_{A,\Sigma}, \quad \boldsymbol{Q}_1' = \boldsymbol{I} - \boldsymbol{P}_{A_1,\Sigma}, \quad \boldsymbol{Q}_2' = \boldsymbol{I} - \boldsymbol{P}_{Q_1'A_2,\Sigma},\\
&\boldsymbol{S}_1 = \boldsymbol{S} = \boldsymbol{X}(\boldsymbol{I} - \boldsymbol{P}_{C'})\boldsymbol{X}', \quad \boldsymbol{S}_2 = \boldsymbol{S}_1 + \boldsymbol{Q}_1'\boldsymbol{X}(\boldsymbol{P}_{C_1'} - \boldsymbol{P}_{C_2'})\boldsymbol{X}'\boldsymbol{Q}_1.
\end{aligned}$$

Then (7.73) can be rewritten as

$$\mathrm{tr}\{\boldsymbol{\Sigma}^{-1}(\boldsymbol{S}_2 + \boldsymbol{Q}_2'\boldsymbol{Q}_1'\boldsymbol{X}\boldsymbol{P}_{C_2'}\boldsymbol{X}'\boldsymbol{Q}_1\boldsymbol{Q}_2)\} - \mathrm{tr}\{\boldsymbol{\Sigma}^{-1}(\boldsymbol{S}_1 + \boldsymbol{Q}_0'\boldsymbol{X}\boldsymbol{P}_{C_1'}\boldsymbol{X}'\boldsymbol{Q}_0)\}, \tag{7.74}$$

which, since $\boldsymbol{Q}_1\boldsymbol{Q}_2 = \boldsymbol{Q}_0$, equals

$$\begin{aligned}
&\mathrm{tr}\{\boldsymbol{\Sigma}^{-1}(\boldsymbol{S}_2 + \boldsymbol{Q}_0'\boldsymbol{X}\boldsymbol{P}_{C_2'}\boldsymbol{X}'\boldsymbol{Q}_0 - \boldsymbol{S}_1 - \boldsymbol{Q}_0'\boldsymbol{X}\boldsymbol{P}_{C_1'}\boldsymbol{X}'\boldsymbol{Q}_0)\}\\
&= \mathrm{tr}\{\boldsymbol{\Sigma}^{-1}(\boldsymbol{Q}_1'\boldsymbol{X}(\boldsymbol{P}_{C_1'} - \boldsymbol{P}_{C_2'})\boldsymbol{X}'\boldsymbol{Q}_1 - \boldsymbol{Q}_0'\boldsymbol{X}(\boldsymbol{P}_{C_1'} - \boldsymbol{P}_{C_2'})\boldsymbol{X}'\boldsymbol{Q}_0)\}.
\end{aligned}$$

From Theorem B.12 in Appendix B, it follows that the differences between the projections equal

$$\boldsymbol{P}_{C_1'} - \boldsymbol{P}_{C_2'} = \boldsymbol{P}_{C'(CC')^-N}, \quad \boldsymbol{Q}_1 - \boldsymbol{Q}_0 = \boldsymbol{P}_{A(A'\Sigma^{-1}A)^-M,\Sigma},$$

where $\boldsymbol{N}$ and $\boldsymbol{M}$ are arbitrary matrices satisfying $\mathcal{C}(\boldsymbol{N}) = \mathcal{C}(\boldsymbol{C}) \cap \mathcal{C}(\boldsymbol{G})$ and $\mathcal{C}(\boldsymbol{M}) = \mathcal{C}(\boldsymbol{A}') \cap \mathcal{C}(\boldsymbol{F}')$, respectively. Thus, with a known $\boldsymbol{\Sigma}$ (since $\boldsymbol{Q}_0\boldsymbol{Q}_1 = \boldsymbol{Q}_1\boldsymbol{Q}_0 = \boldsymbol{Q}_0$),

$$\mathrm{tr}\{\boldsymbol{\Sigma}^{-1}\boldsymbol{P}_{A(A'\Sigma^{-1}A)^-M,\Sigma}\boldsymbol{X}\boldsymbol{P}_{C'(CC')^-N}\boldsymbol{X}'\boldsymbol{P}'_{A(A'\Sigma^{-1}A)^-M,\Sigma}\} \tag{7.75}$$

is a natural test statistic. However, if $\boldsymbol{\Sigma}$ is unknown, the inner product which is behind the expression in (7.75) has to be estimated.

It is of interest to note that

$$\begin{aligned}
\mathcal{C}(\boldsymbol{C}'(\boldsymbol{C}\boldsymbol{C}')^-\boldsymbol{N}) &= \mathcal{C}(\boldsymbol{C}') \cap \mathcal{C}(\boldsymbol{C}'\boldsymbol{G}^o)^\perp,\\
\mathcal{C}_\Sigma(\boldsymbol{A}(\boldsymbol{A}'\boldsymbol{\Sigma}^{-1}\boldsymbol{A})^-\boldsymbol{M}) &= \mathcal{C}_\Sigma(\boldsymbol{A}(\boldsymbol{A}'\boldsymbol{\Sigma}^{-1}\boldsymbol{A})^-\boldsymbol{A}'\boldsymbol{\Sigma}^{-1}(\boldsymbol{\Sigma}^{-1}\boldsymbol{A}\boldsymbol{F}')^o)\\
&= \mathcal{C}_\Sigma(\boldsymbol{A}) \cap \mathcal{C}_\Sigma(\boldsymbol{A}(\boldsymbol{F}')^o)^\perp.
\end{aligned}$$

These expressions give clear interpretations of the spaces involved in (7.75). Consider Fig. 7.10, where it can be seen that the tensor space

$$\mathcal{V}_2 \otimes \mathcal{W}_2 = \mathcal{C}(\boldsymbol{C}'(\boldsymbol{C}\boldsymbol{C}')^-\boldsymbol{N}) \otimes \mathcal{C}_\Sigma(\boldsymbol{A}(\boldsymbol{A}'\boldsymbol{\Sigma}^{-1}\boldsymbol{A})^-\boldsymbol{M})$$

should be studied, and the test statistic, given in (7.75), is used for deciding if $\mathcal{V}_2 \otimes \mathcal{W}_2$ equals $\{\boldsymbol{0}\}$. Since $\boldsymbol{\Sigma}$ is involved in the expression, $\boldsymbol{\Sigma}$ has to be estimated and, in order to avoid the estimator exerting too much influence on the test, a natural quantity to use, as before, is $n^{-1}\boldsymbol{S}$, since, both under H_0 and H_1, the distribution

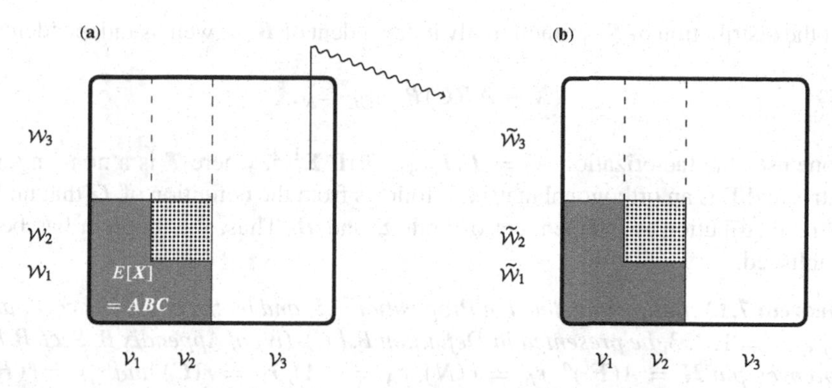

Fig. 7.10 Consider the BRM model in (7.63). A decomposition is presented of the whole space according to the design and the restrictions $\boldsymbol{FBG} = \boldsymbol{0}$. In **(a)**, $\boldsymbol{\Sigma}$ is known, whereas in **(b)**, $\boldsymbol{\Sigma}$ has been replaced by $\frac{1}{n}\boldsymbol{S}$. The decomposition in **(a)** is based on the subspaces $\mathcal{V}_1 = \mathcal{C}(\boldsymbol{C}'\boldsymbol{G}^o)$, $\mathcal{V}_2 = \mathcal{C}(\boldsymbol{C}'\boldsymbol{G}^o)^{\perp} \cap \mathcal{C}(\boldsymbol{C}')$, $\mathcal{V}_3 = \mathcal{C}(\boldsymbol{C}')^{\perp}$, $\mathcal{W}_1 = \mathcal{C}_{\Sigma}(\boldsymbol{A}(\boldsymbol{F}')^o)$, $\mathcal{W}_2 = \mathcal{C}_{\Sigma}(\boldsymbol{A}(\boldsymbol{F}')^o)^{\perp} \cap \mathcal{C}_{\Sigma}(\boldsymbol{A})$ and $\mathcal{W}_3 = \mathcal{C}_{\Sigma}(\boldsymbol{A})^{\perp}$. In **(b)**, the subspaces $\mathcal{V}_1$, $\mathcal{V}_2$ and $\mathcal{V}_3$ are the same as in **(a)**, whereas the within-individuals decomposition is based on $\widetilde{\mathcal{W}}_1 = \mathcal{C}_S(\boldsymbol{A}(\boldsymbol{F}')^o)$, $\widetilde{\mathcal{W}}_2 = \mathcal{C}_S(\boldsymbol{A}(\boldsymbol{F}')^o)^{\perp} \cap \mathcal{C}_S(\boldsymbol{A})$ and $\widetilde{\mathcal{W}}_3 = \mathcal{C}_S(\boldsymbol{A})^{\perp}$

of $\boldsymbol{S}$ is independent of $\boldsymbol{B}$. Note that when constructing the likelihood ratio test in Sect. 7.3, different estimators of the inner product were obtained under H_0 and H_1, i.e. $\boldsymbol{S}_1$ and $\widehat{\boldsymbol{S}}_2$, defined in Sect. 7.3, were utilized. In the present situation, the statistic was derived by first assuming $\boldsymbol{\Sigma}$ to be known and then replacing the dispersion with $n^{-1}\boldsymbol{S}$; i.e. the same estimator was chosen irrespective of the hypothesis, which in a way makes sense since we are interested only in $\boldsymbol{B}$ and not in $\boldsymbol{\Sigma}$. Hence, the next proposition has been motivated.

Proposition 7.3 *For the BRM presented in Definition 2.1, let the null hypothesis $H_0: \boldsymbol{FBG} = \boldsymbol{0}$ be tested against H_1: $\boldsymbol{B}$ unrestricted. Let $\boldsymbol{S}$ be defined in (7.71), and $\boldsymbol{N}$ and $\boldsymbol{M}$ be matrices satisfying $\mathcal{C}(\boldsymbol{N}) = \mathcal{C}(\boldsymbol{G}) \cap \mathcal{C}(\boldsymbol{C})$ and $\mathcal{C}(\boldsymbol{M}) = \mathcal{C}(\boldsymbol{A}') \cap \mathcal{C}(\boldsymbol{F}')$, respectively. A test statistic is given by*

$$T_4 = \mathrm{tr}\{\boldsymbol{S}^{-1}\boldsymbol{P}_{\mathrm{A(A'S^{-1}A)^{-}M,S}}\boldsymbol{X}\boldsymbol{P}_{\mathrm{C'(CC')^{-}N}}\boldsymbol{X}'\boldsymbol{P}'_{\mathrm{A(A'S^{-1}A)^{-}M,S}}\}.$$

The hypothesis is rejected when the observed value of T_4 is large.

Theorem 7.12 *For the BRM presented in Definition 2.1, let the null hypothesis $H_0: \boldsymbol{FBG} = \boldsymbol{0}$ be tested against H_1: $\boldsymbol{B}$ unrestricted. Under H_0 the distribution for the test statistic T_4, presented in Proposition 7.3, is independent of $\boldsymbol{\Sigma}$ and $\boldsymbol{B}$.*

Proof Under H_0 the statistic T_4 equals

$$T_4 = \mathrm{tr}\{\boldsymbol{S}^{-1}\boldsymbol{P}_{\mathrm{A(A'S^{-1}A)^{-}M,S}}(\boldsymbol{X} - \boldsymbol{ABC})\boldsymbol{P}_{\mathrm{C'(CC')^{-}N}}(\boldsymbol{X} - \boldsymbol{ABC})'\boldsymbol{P}'_{\mathrm{A(A'S^{-1}A)^{-}M,S}}\}$$

and the distribution of $\boldsymbol{S}$ is functionally independent of $\boldsymbol{B}$, as well as independent of

$$(\boldsymbol{X}-\boldsymbol{ABC})\boldsymbol{P}_{C'(CC')^{-}N}.$$

If one uses the factorization $\boldsymbol{A}' = \boldsymbol{T}(\boldsymbol{I}_{r(A)} : \boldsymbol{0})\boldsymbol{\Gamma}'\boldsymbol{\Sigma}^{1/2}$, where $\boldsymbol{T}$ is a non-singular matrix and $\boldsymbol{\Gamma}$ is an orthogonal matrix, it follows from the definition of T_4 that under H_0 its distribution is independent of both $\boldsymbol{\Sigma}$ and $\boldsymbol{B}$. Thus, the theorem has been established. □

Theorem 7.13 *Let T_4 be defined in Proposition 7.3, and let the constants $c_{0;n,s}$ and $c_{i;n,s,t}$, $i=1,2,3$, be presented in Definition B.1 (i)–(iv) of Appendix B, Sect. B.15. Moreover, put $\boldsymbol{H} = \boldsymbol{A}(\boldsymbol{F}')^{o}$, $r_N = r(\boldsymbol{N})$, $r_A = r(\boldsymbol{A})$, $r_C = r(\boldsymbol{C})$ and $r_H = r(\boldsymbol{H})$. Then*

(i) $E[T_4] = r(\boldsymbol{N})((p-r_H)c_{0;n-r(C),p-r_H} - (p-r_A)c_{0;n-r_C,p-r_A})$
$\qquad + c_{0;n-r_C,p-r_H}\mathrm{tr}\{(\boldsymbol{H}^{o'}\boldsymbol{\Sigma}\boldsymbol{H}^{o})^{-}\boldsymbol{H}^{o'}\boldsymbol{ABN}(\boldsymbol{N}'(\boldsymbol{CC}')^{-}\boldsymbol{N})^{-}\boldsymbol{N}'\boldsymbol{B}'\boldsymbol{A}'\boldsymbol{H}^{o}\}$;

(ii) *under H_0*

$$D[T_4] = c_1 + c_2 - 2c_3 - E[T_4]^2,$$

where

$$\begin{aligned}
E[T_4] &= r(\boldsymbol{N})((p-r_H)c_{0;n-r(C),p-r_H} - (p-r_A)c_{0;n-r_C,p-r_A}),\\
c_1 &= r_N^2(p-r_A)^2c_{1;n-r_C,p-r_A} + r_N^2((p-r_A)+(p-r_A)^2)c_{2;n-r_C,p-r_A}\\
&\quad +2r_N(p-r_A)c_{1;n-r_C,p-r_A} + 2r_N((p-r_A)+(p-r_A)^2)c_{2;n-r_C,p-r_A},\\
c_2 &= r_N^2(p-r_H)^2c_{1;n-r_C,p-r_H} + r_N^2((p-r_H)+(p-r_H)^2)c_{2;n-r_C,p-r_H}\\
&\quad +2r_N(p-r_H)c_{1;n-r_C,p-r_H} + 2r_N((p-r_H)+(p-r_H)^2)c_{2;n-r_C,p-r_H},\\
c_3 &= r_N^2(p-r_A)^2c_{1;n-r_C,p-r_A,p-r_H} + 2r_N^2(p-r_A)c_{2;n-r_C,p-r_A,p-r_H}\\
&\quad +r_N^2(p-r_A)(r_A-r_H)c_{3;n-r_C,p-r_A,p-r_H}\\
&\quad +2r_N(p-r_A)c_{1;n-r_C,p-r_A,p-r_H}\\
&\quad +2r_N((p-r_A)+(p-r_A)^2)c_{2;n-r_C,p-r_A,p-r_H}.
\end{aligned}$$

Proof Since (see Appendix B, Theorem B.13)

$$\boldsymbol{P}_{A(A'S^{-1}A)^{-}M,S} = \boldsymbol{P}_{A,S} - \boldsymbol{P}_{A(F')^{o},S} = \boldsymbol{P}'_{(A(F')^{o})^{o},S^{-1}} - \boldsymbol{P}'_{A^{o},S^{-1}},$$

it follows, by assuming the generators of the orthogonal complements to be of full rank, that

$$\begin{aligned}
T_4 &= \mathrm{tr}\{(\boldsymbol{H}^{o'}\boldsymbol{S}\boldsymbol{H}^{o})^{-1}\boldsymbol{H}^{o'}\boldsymbol{X}\boldsymbol{P}_{C'(CC')^{-}N}\boldsymbol{X}'\boldsymbol{H}^{o}\}\\
&\quad -\mathrm{tr}\{(\boldsymbol{A}^{o'}\boldsymbol{S}\boldsymbol{A}^{o})^{-1}\boldsymbol{A}^{o'}\boldsymbol{X}\boldsymbol{P}_{C'(CC')^{-}N}\boldsymbol{X}'\boldsymbol{A}^{o}\}.
\end{aligned}$$

Thus, since $\boldsymbol{S}$ and $\boldsymbol{XP}_{C'(CC')^- N}$ are independent, statement (i) follows by application of Theorems B.20 (ii) and B.21 (i) in Appendix B.

Turning to statement (ii), since $D[T_4] = E[T_4^2] - E[T_4]^2$, the expectation $E[T_4^2]$ has to be determined. Let $T_4 = v - u$, where

$$u = \mathrm{tr}\{(\boldsymbol{A}^{o'}\boldsymbol{S}\boldsymbol{A}^{o})^{-1}\boldsymbol{A}^{o'}\boldsymbol{X}\boldsymbol{P}_{\mathrm{C'(CC')^- N}}\boldsymbol{X}'\boldsymbol{A}^{o}\},$$

$$v = \mathrm{tr}\{(\boldsymbol{H}^{o'}\boldsymbol{S}\boldsymbol{H}^{o})^{-1}\boldsymbol{H}^{o'}\boldsymbol{X}\boldsymbol{P}_{\mathrm{C'(CC')^- N}}\boldsymbol{X}'\boldsymbol{H}^{o}\}.$$

Then $E[T_4^2] = E[u^2] + E[v^2] - 2E[uv]$ and each of these terms has to be determined. Since $\boldsymbol{XP}_{C'(CC')^- N}\boldsymbol{X}'$ is independent of $\boldsymbol{S}$ it is noted, as when discussing T_3 (see Appendix B, Theorem B.19 (vii)), that

$$E[(\boldsymbol{XP}_{C'(CC')^- N}\boldsymbol{X}')^{\otimes 2}] = r_N^2\boldsymbol{\Sigma}\otimes\boldsymbol{\Sigma} + r_N(\boldsymbol{K}_{p,p}(\boldsymbol{\Sigma}\otimes\boldsymbol{\Sigma}) + \mathrm{vec}\boldsymbol{\Sigma}\mathrm{vec}'\boldsymbol{\Sigma}).$$

This relation leads to

$$E[u^2] = r_N^2\mathrm{tr}\{\mathrm{E}[(\boldsymbol{A}^{o'}\boldsymbol{S}\boldsymbol{A}^{o})^{-1}\otimes(\boldsymbol{A}^{o'}\boldsymbol{S}\boldsymbol{A}^{o})^{-1}]\boldsymbol{A}^{o'}\boldsymbol{\Sigma}\boldsymbol{A}^{o}\otimes\boldsymbol{A}^{o'}\boldsymbol{\Sigma}\boldsymbol{A}^{o}\}$$
$$+2r_N\mathrm{tr}\{\mathrm{E}[(\boldsymbol{A}^{o'}\boldsymbol{S}\boldsymbol{A}^{o})^{-1}\boldsymbol{A}^{o'}\boldsymbol{\Sigma}\boldsymbol{A}^{o}(\boldsymbol{A}^{o'}\boldsymbol{S}\boldsymbol{A}^{o})^{-1}\boldsymbol{A}^{o'}\boldsymbol{\Sigma}\boldsymbol{A}^{o}]\}.$$

Hence, using Appendix B, Theorem B.21 (iii) and (v) it can be shown that $c_1 = E[u^2]$. Similarly, the expectation for v^2 can be obtained and $c_2 = E[v^2]$. Finally, $E[uv]$ is to be determined. However, using Theorems B.19 (vii) and B.25 in Appendix B, as well as copying the calculations for obtaining $E[u^2]$, yields $c_3 = E[uv]$, which establishes the theorem. □

Proposition 7.4 *For the BRM presented in Definition 2.1, let the null hypothesis H_0 : $\boldsymbol{FBG} = \boldsymbol{0}$ be tested against H_1: $\boldsymbol{B}$ unrestricted. The corresponding test statistic T_4 is given by Proposition 7.3. Then the hypothesis connected to T_4 is rejected at approximate significance level α if $P(T_{4o} \geq a\chi^2_{[f]}) \leq \alpha$, where T_{4o} is the observed value of T_4, $[f]$ denotes the integer part of either f or $f+1$ and the integer part which is closest to f is chosen;*

$$a = \frac{c_1 + c_2 - 2c_3 - c_0^2}{2c_0}, \qquad f = \frac{2c_0^2}{c_1 + c_2 - 2c_3 - c_0^2},$$

where $c_0 = E[T_4]$ and $c_1 - c_3$ are presented in Theorem 7.13.

Proof As in Proposition 7.2, the coefficients a and f are obtained by solving

$$E[T_4] = af, \qquad D[T_4] = 2a^2 f,$$

which via Theorem 7.13 then suggests the statement. □

Now the proposition is illustrated via one of our data sets which has been used several times before.

Example 7.10 Our main interest is to compare the "trace test" with the likelihood ratio test. Therefore, consider the Potthoff and Roy data presented in Table 1.2, which have been analysed in Example 7.2, among other places in the book. Let $\boldsymbol{X} = \boldsymbol{ABC} + \boldsymbol{E}$, whose matrices have previously been defined. In particular, note that

$$\boldsymbol{A} = \begin{pmatrix} 1 & 8 & 64 \\ 1 & 10 & 100 \\ 1 & 12 & 144 \\ 1 & 14 & 196 \end{pmatrix}, \qquad \boldsymbol{C} = (\mathbf{1}'_{11} \otimes (1:0)' : \mathbf{1}'_{16} \otimes (0:1)'),$$

meaning that the growth for both the girls and the boys is modelled with a second-order polynomial.

In Example 7.2, three tests were carried out using the following hypotheses:

(i) no quadratic term in $\boldsymbol{ABC}$;
(ii) only girls follow a quadratic growth model;
(iii) no growth exists for both the boys and the girls between age 8 and age 14.

Both the hypotheses related to statement (i) and statement (ii) were deemed to be non-significant when performing a likelihood ratio test, while the hypothesis linked to statement (iii) was rejected, which was in accordance with our expectations.

Concerning the "trace-test", the results are in agreement. For statement (i) it is obtained that $T_{4o} = 0.1$ and $T_{4o}/a = 1.4$, which are non-significant since the values of the test statistics are below $\chi^2_{0.05}(3) = 7.8$. However, the exact probabilities for rejection differ somewhat between the likelihood ratio test ($p = 0.32$) and the "trace test" ($p = 0.67$). This discrepancy may be due to the ad hoc procedure implemented when deriving the "trace test" statistic or the relatively crude method used for technically determining the probability for the "trace test".

For statement (ii) the corresponding numbers are $T_{4o} = 0.1$, $T_{4o}/a = 1.5$ and $\chi^2_{0.05}(2) = 6.0$, and thus this test is not rejected. The rejection probabilities for the likelihood ratio test and the "trace test" are given by $p = 0.14$ and $p = 0.34$, respectively.

For the third hypothesis, presented in statement (iii), i.e. the most extreme hypothesis, the following were obtained: $T_{4o} = 5.1$, $T_{4o}/a = 82.4$ and $\chi^2_{0.05}(2) = 6.0$. Both the "trace test" and the likelihood ratio test provide very small rejection probabilities. □

7.9 A "Trace Test" for the BRM, $H_0: F_iBG_i = 0, i = 1, 2$, $\mathcal{C}(F_1') \subseteq \mathcal{C}(F_2')$, Against Unrestricted B

As when performing tests with the help of the likelihood ratio criterion in Sect. 7.4 and other places in the book, the condition $\mathcal{C}(F_1') \subseteq \mathcal{C}(F_2')$ is supposed to hold. The reason for assuming such an condition is that, as before, the theory developed for the class of $EBRM_B^3$ is going to be utilized. Note that $F_iBG_i = 0$, $i = 1, 2$, with $\mathcal{C}(F_1') \subseteq \mathcal{C}(F_2')$, is equivalent to

$$B = (F_2')^o\Theta_1 + (F_1' : (F_2')^o)^o\Theta_3 G_2^{o'} + F_1'\Theta_4(G_1 : G_2)^{o'},$$

where Θ_i are new unknown parameters which have to be estimated and, of course, $\mathcal{C}((G_1 : G_2)^o) \subset \mathcal{C}(G_2^o)$. Thus the reparametrization implies that the mean structure of the BRM under H_0 becomes

$$E[X] = ABC = A(F_2')^o\Theta_1 C + A(F_1' : (F_2')^o)^o\Theta_3 G_2^{o'} C + AF_1'\Theta_4(G_1 : G_2)^{o'} C,$$

i.e. an $EBRM_B^3$. For the time being, suppose that the dispersion matrix Σ is known. The following notations, also used in Sect. 7.4, will be applied, but now the projections are solely functions of Σ:

$$A_1 = A(F_2')^o, \quad C_1 = C, \quad A_2 = A(F_1' : (F_2')^o)^o, \quad C_2 = G_2^{o'}C,$$
$$A_3 = AF_1', \quad C_3 = (G_1 : G_2)^{o'}C,$$
$$S_3 = S_2 + P'_{(A_1:A_2)^o,\Sigma^{-1}}X(P_{C_2'} - P_{C_3'})X'P_{(A_1:A_2)^o,\Sigma^{-1}},$$
$$S_2 = S_1 + P'_{A_1^o,\Sigma^{-1}}X(P_{C_1'} - P_{C_2'})X'P_{A_1^o,\Sigma^{-1}}, \quad S_1 = S = X(I - P_{C_1'})X',$$
$$Q_1 = I - P'_{A_1,\Sigma}, \quad Q_2 = I - P'_{Q_1'A_2,\Sigma},$$
$$Q_3 = I - P'_{Q_2'Q_1'A_3,\Sigma}, \quad Q_1Q_2Q_3 = P_{A^o,\Sigma^{-1}}.$$

Under the alternative hypothesis, i.e. with an unrestricted mean assumed to hold, the estimated mean equals (e.g. see Sect. 2.4)

$$\widehat{E_{H_1}[X]} = P_{A,\Sigma}XP_{C'},$$

whereas from (2.39)

$$\widehat{E_{H_0}[X]} = (I - Q_1')XP_{C_1'} + (I - Q_2')XP_{C_2'} + (I - Q_3')XP_{C_3'}. \tag{7.76}$$

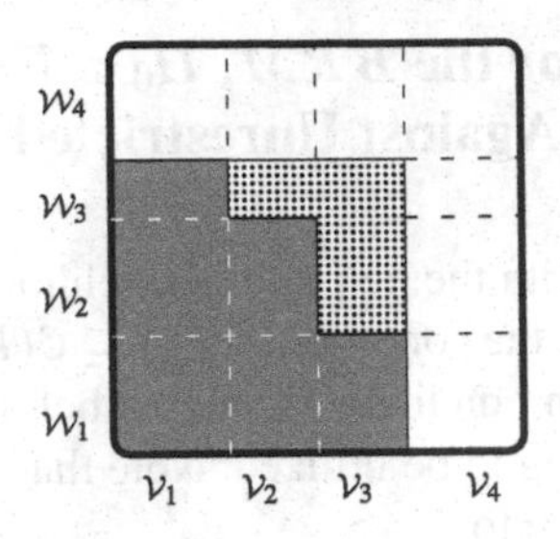

Fig. 7.11 The dotted area corresponds to H_0: $\boldsymbol{F}_i\boldsymbol{B}\boldsymbol{G}_i = \boldsymbol{0}, i = 1, 2$, in the BRM, where $\mathcal{C}(\boldsymbol{F}_1') \subseteq \mathcal{C}(\boldsymbol{F}_2')$. Furthermore, $\mathcal{W}_1 = \mathcal{C}_\bullet(\boldsymbol{A}(\boldsymbol{F}_2')^o)$, $\mathcal{W}_2 = \mathcal{C}_\bullet(\boldsymbol{A}(\boldsymbol{F}_1')^o) \cap \mathcal{C}_\bullet(\boldsymbol{A}(\boldsymbol{F}_2')^o)^\perp$, $\mathcal{W}_3 = \mathcal{C}_\bullet(\boldsymbol{A}) \cap \mathcal{C}_\bullet(\boldsymbol{A}(\boldsymbol{F}_1')^o)^\perp$, $\mathcal{W}_4 = \mathcal{C}_\bullet(\boldsymbol{A})^\perp$, $\mathcal{V}_1 = \mathcal{C}(\boldsymbol{C}'(\boldsymbol{G}_1 : \boldsymbol{G}_2)^o)$, $\mathcal{V}_2 = \mathcal{C}(\boldsymbol{C}'\boldsymbol{G}_2^o) \cap \mathcal{C}(\boldsymbol{C}'(\boldsymbol{G}_1 : \boldsymbol{G}_2)^o)^\perp$, $\mathcal{V}_3 = \mathcal{C}(\boldsymbol{C}') \cap \mathcal{C}(\boldsymbol{C}'\boldsymbol{G}_2^o)^\perp$ and $\mathcal{V}_4 = \mathcal{C}(\boldsymbol{C}')^\perp$

Hence, similar to when tests were performed within the BRM, in Sect. 7.8, a trace test statistic can be constructed via

$$\mathrm{tr}\{\boldsymbol{\Sigma}^{-1}(\boldsymbol{X} - \widehat{\mathrm{E}_{\mathrm{H}_0}[\boldsymbol{X}]})()'\} - \mathrm{tr}\{\boldsymbol{\Sigma}^{-1}(\boldsymbol{X} - \widehat{\mathrm{E}_{\mathrm{H}_1}[\boldsymbol{X}]})()'\}. \tag{7.77}$$

In Sect. 7.8, it was relatively easy to simplify the test statistic. Because $E_{H_0}[\boldsymbol{X}]$ and $E_{H_1}[\boldsymbol{X}]$ are built up with the help of projections of observations on certain spaces, it makes sense to consider the corresponding spaces and their decompositions. In fact, what are needed are the projections of spaces indicated in Fig. 7.11 (the dotted area), which are in agreement with the construction of Fig. 7.7.

Now, instead of performing a large number of calculations, the idea is to rely on one's intuition. Based on Fig. 7.11, the spaces which are involved in the test are given by

$$\mathcal{V}_2 \otimes \mathcal{W}_3 + \mathcal{V}_3 \otimes (\mathcal{W}_2 + \mathcal{W}_3), \tag{7.78}$$

where $\mathcal{V}_i$ and $\mathcal{W}_i$, $i = 2, 3$, are defined in Fig. 7.11. The test which will be constructed is to some extent a goodness-of-fit test which will help us to decide if the space given in (7.78) differs from $\{\boldsymbol{0}\}$. What is needed to construct the test is the construction of projections on the spaces in (7.78). Firstly, note that $\boldsymbol{Q}_1'$, $\boldsymbol{Q}_2'\boldsymbol{Q}_1'$ and $\boldsymbol{Q}_3'\boldsymbol{Q}_2'\boldsymbol{Q}_1'$ in (7.77) and (7.76) are all projectors and

$$\mathcal{C}_\Sigma(\boldsymbol{Q}_1') = \mathcal{C}_\Sigma(\boldsymbol{A}_1)^\perp, \quad \mathcal{C}_\Sigma(\boldsymbol{Q}_2'\boldsymbol{Q}_1') = \mathcal{C}_\Sigma(\boldsymbol{A}_1 : \boldsymbol{A}_2)^\perp,$$
$$\mathcal{C}_\Sigma(\boldsymbol{Q}_3'\boldsymbol{Q}_2'\boldsymbol{Q}_1') = \mathcal{C}_\Sigma(\boldsymbol{A}_1 : \boldsymbol{A}_2 : \boldsymbol{A}_3)^\perp = \mathcal{C}_\Sigma(\boldsymbol{A})^\perp.$$

Moreover,

$$\mathcal{C}_\Sigma(\boldsymbol{A}_1)^\perp = \mathcal{C}_\Sigma(\boldsymbol{A}_1)^\perp \cap \mathcal{C}_\Sigma(\boldsymbol{A}) + \mathcal{C}_\Sigma(\boldsymbol{A})^\perp,$$
$$\mathcal{C}_\Sigma(\boldsymbol{A}_1 : \boldsymbol{A}_2)^\perp = \mathcal{C}_\Sigma(\boldsymbol{A}_1 : \boldsymbol{A}_2)^\perp \cap \mathcal{C}_\Sigma(\boldsymbol{A}) + \mathcal{C}_\Sigma(\boldsymbol{A})^\perp,$$
$$\mathcal{C}_\Sigma(\boldsymbol{A}_1 : \boldsymbol{A}_2 : \boldsymbol{A}_3)^\perp = \mathcal{C}_\Sigma(\boldsymbol{A})^\perp,$$

and let

$$\begin{aligned}
\mathcal{V}_2 &= \mathcal{C}(\boldsymbol{N}_1) = \mathcal{C}(\boldsymbol{C}'\boldsymbol{G}_2^o) \cap \mathcal{C}(\boldsymbol{C}'(\boldsymbol{G}_1 : \boldsymbol{G}_2)^o)^\perp,\\
\mathcal{V}_3 &= \mathcal{C}(\boldsymbol{N}_2) = \mathcal{C}(\boldsymbol{C}') \cap \mathcal{C}(\boldsymbol{C}'\boldsymbol{G}_2^o)^\perp,\\
\mathcal{C}_\Sigma(\boldsymbol{M}_1) &= \mathcal{C}_\Sigma(\boldsymbol{A}) \cap \mathcal{C}_\Sigma(\boldsymbol{A}(\boldsymbol{F}_1')^o)^\perp,\\
\mathcal{C}_\Sigma(\boldsymbol{M}_2) &= \mathcal{C}_\Sigma(\boldsymbol{A}) \cap \mathcal{C}_\Sigma(\boldsymbol{A}(\boldsymbol{F}_2')^o)^\perp,
\end{aligned}$$

with the corresponding projections

$$\begin{aligned}
&\boldsymbol{P}_{N_1} = \boldsymbol{P}_{C'G_2^o} - \boldsymbol{P}_{C'(G_1:G_2)^o}, \quad \boldsymbol{P}_{N_2} = \boldsymbol{P}_{C'} - \boldsymbol{P}_{C'G_2^o},\\
&\boldsymbol{P}_{M_1,\Sigma} = \boldsymbol{P}_{A,\Sigma} - \boldsymbol{P}_{A_1(F_1')^o,\Sigma}, \quad \boldsymbol{P}_{M_2,\Sigma} = \boldsymbol{P}_{A,\Sigma} - \boldsymbol{P}_{A_1(F_2')^o,\Sigma}.
\end{aligned}$$

Therefore, the test statistic presented in (7.77), where $\boldsymbol{\Sigma}$ is known, equals

$$\begin{aligned}
\operatorname{tr}\{\boldsymbol{\Sigma}^{-1}((&\boldsymbol{P}_{A,\Sigma} - \boldsymbol{P}_{A_1(F_1')^o,\Sigma})\boldsymbol{X}(\boldsymbol{P}_{C'G_2^o} - \boldsymbol{P}_{C'(G_1:G_2)^o})\boldsymbol{X}'\\
&+(\boldsymbol{P}_{A,\Sigma} - \boldsymbol{P}_{A_1(F_2')^o,\Sigma})\boldsymbol{X}(\boldsymbol{P}_{C'} - \boldsymbol{P}_{C'G_2^o})\boldsymbol{X}')\}.
\end{aligned}$$

Since the distribution of $\boldsymbol{S}$ does not depend on $\boldsymbol{B}$, either under H_0 or under H_1, the same argument as that applied when obtaining T_3 in Proposition 7.1 can be used; i.e. replacing $\boldsymbol{\Sigma}$ by $n^{-1}\boldsymbol{S}$, in order to present a test statistic for the hypothesis involving the bilinear restrictions $\boldsymbol{F}_i\boldsymbol{B}\boldsymbol{G}_i = \boldsymbol{0}$, $i = 1, 2$, and $\mathcal{C}(\boldsymbol{F}_1') \subseteq \mathcal{C}(\boldsymbol{F}_2')$ is a natural procedure.

Proposition 7.5 *For the BRM presented in Definition 2.1, let the null hypothesis $H_0 : \boldsymbol{F}_i\boldsymbol{B}\boldsymbol{G}_i = \boldsymbol{0}$, $i = 1, 2$, $\mathcal{C}(\boldsymbol{F}_1') \subseteq \mathcal{C}(\boldsymbol{F}_2')$, be tested against H_1: $\boldsymbol{B}$ unrestricted. Let $\boldsymbol{S}$ be defined in (7.71). A test statistic is given by*

$$T_5 = T_{51} + T_{52},$$

where

$$T_{51} = \operatorname{tr}\{\boldsymbol{S}^{-1}(\boldsymbol{P}_{A,S} - \boldsymbol{P}_{A(F_1')^o,S})\boldsymbol{X}(\boldsymbol{P}_{C'G_2^o} - \boldsymbol{P}_{C'(G_1:G_2)^o})\boldsymbol{X}'\},$$

$$T_{52} = \operatorname{tr}\{\boldsymbol{S}^{-1}(\boldsymbol{P}_{A,S} - \boldsymbol{P}_{A(F_2')^o,S})\boldsymbol{X}(\boldsymbol{P}_{C'} - \boldsymbol{P}_{C'G_2^o})\boldsymbol{X}'\}.$$

The hypothesis may be rejected if any of the observed values of T_{51}, T_{52} or T_5 is large.

The statistics T_{51} and T_{52} are also test statistics. In particular, they are both positive and, therefore, it is possible to consider them separately. From Proposition 7.5, since

$$\boldsymbol{P}_{A,S} - \boldsymbol{P}_{A(F_2')^o,S} = \boldsymbol{P}_{A(A'S^{-1}A)^-M}, \qquad \boldsymbol{P}_{C'} - \boldsymbol{P}_{C'G_2^o} = \boldsymbol{P}_{C'(CC')^-N},$$

where $\mathcal{C}(\boldsymbol{M}) = \mathcal{C}(\boldsymbol{A}') \cap \mathcal{C}(\boldsymbol{F}_2')$ and $\mathcal{C}(\boldsymbol{N}) = \mathcal{C}(\boldsymbol{C}) \cap \mathcal{C}(\boldsymbol{G}_2)$, it follows that T_{52} tests H_0: $\boldsymbol{F}_2\boldsymbol{B}\boldsymbol{G}_2 = \boldsymbol{0}$ in the BRM against $\boldsymbol{B}$ being arbitrary. Moreover, T_{51} is a test statistic for testing H_0: $\boldsymbol{F}_1\boldsymbol{B}\boldsymbol{G}_1 = \boldsymbol{0}$ in the BRM given $\boldsymbol{B}\boldsymbol{G}_2 = \boldsymbol{0}$. The latter statement follows from the fact that $E[\boldsymbol{X}] = \boldsymbol{A}\boldsymbol{B}\boldsymbol{C} = \boldsymbol{A}\boldsymbol{\Theta}\boldsymbol{G}_2^{o'}\boldsymbol{C}$ for some $\boldsymbol{\Theta}$, and $\boldsymbol{F}_1\boldsymbol{B}\boldsymbol{G}_1 = \boldsymbol{0}$ is equivalent to $\boldsymbol{F}_1\boldsymbol{\Theta}\boldsymbol{G}_2^{o'}\boldsymbol{G}_1 = \boldsymbol{0}$. Furthermore, $\mathcal{C}(\boldsymbol{G}_2^o(\boldsymbol{G}_2^{o'}\boldsymbol{G}_1)^o) = \mathcal{C}(\boldsymbol{G}_1 : \boldsymbol{G}_2)^\perp$, which altogether implies the expression for T_{51}. It is also worth noting that $\boldsymbol{X}(\boldsymbol{P}_{\boldsymbol{C}'\boldsymbol{G}_2^o} - \boldsymbol{P}_{\boldsymbol{C}'(\boldsymbol{G}_1:\boldsymbol{G}_2)^o})\boldsymbol{X}'$ and $\boldsymbol{X}(\boldsymbol{P}_{\boldsymbol{C}'} - \boldsymbol{P}_{\boldsymbol{C}'\boldsymbol{G}_2^o})\boldsymbol{X}'$ are independently distributed. This implies that T_{51} and T_{52} are uncorrelated, and given $\boldsymbol{S}$, also independent.

Now a few results will be presented without proofs, since the statements can be verified using the same procedure as was applied in Sect. 7.8.

Theorem 7.14 *For the BRM presented in Definition 2.1, let the null hypothesis H_0 : $\boldsymbol{F}_i\boldsymbol{B}\boldsymbol{G}_i = \boldsymbol{0}$, $i = 1, 2$, $\mathcal{C}(\boldsymbol{F}_1') \subseteq \mathcal{C}(\boldsymbol{F}_2')$, be tested against H_1: $\boldsymbol{B}$ unrestricted. Under H_0 the test statistics T_{51} and T_{52}, presented in Proposition 7.5, are functionally independent of $\boldsymbol{B}$ and $\boldsymbol{\Sigma}$.*

Theorem 7.15 *Let T_{51} and T_{52} be defined in Proposition 7.5, and let the constants $c_{0;n,s}$ and $c_{i;n,s,t}$, $i = 1, 2, 3$, be given in Definition B.1 (i)–(iv) of Appendix B, Sect. B.15. Moreover, let $\boldsymbol{N}_1$ and $\boldsymbol{N}_2$ be any matrices satisfying $\mathcal{C}(\boldsymbol{N}_1) = \mathcal{C}(\boldsymbol{G}_2^{o'}\boldsymbol{C}) \cap \mathcal{C}(\boldsymbol{G}_2^{o'}\boldsymbol{G}_1)$ and $\mathcal{C}(\boldsymbol{N}_2) = \mathcal{C}(\boldsymbol{C}) \cap \mathcal{C}(\boldsymbol{G}_2)$, respectively, and let $\boldsymbol{H}_1 = \boldsymbol{A}(\boldsymbol{F}_1')^o$, $\boldsymbol{H}_2 = \boldsymbol{A}(\boldsymbol{F}_2')^o$, $r_{H_1} = r(\boldsymbol{H}_1)$, $r_{H_2} = r(\boldsymbol{H}_2)$, $r_A = r(\boldsymbol{A})$ and $r_C = r(\boldsymbol{C})$. Then*

(i)

$$E[T_{52}] = r_{N_2}((p - r_{H_2})c_{0;n-r(\boldsymbol{C}),p-r_{H_2}} - (p - r_A)c_{0;n-r_C,p-r_A})$$
$$+c_{0;n-r_C,p-r_{H_2}}\mathrm{tr}\{(\boldsymbol{H}_2^{o'}\boldsymbol{\Sigma}\boldsymbol{H}_2^o)^-\boldsymbol{H}_2^{o'}\boldsymbol{A}\boldsymbol{B}\boldsymbol{N}_2(\boldsymbol{N}_2'(\boldsymbol{C}\boldsymbol{C}')^-\boldsymbol{N}_2)^-\boldsymbol{N}_2'\boldsymbol{B}'\boldsymbol{A}'\boldsymbol{H}_2^o\};$$

(ii) *under H_0*

$$D[T_{52}] = c_1 + c_2 - 2c_3 - E[T_{52}]^2,$$

where

$$E[T_{52}] = r_{N_2}((p - r_{H_2})c_{0;n-r(\boldsymbol{C}),p-r_{H_2}} - (p - r_A)c_{0;n-r_C,p-r_A}),$$
$$c_1 = r_{N_2}^2(p - r_A)^2c_{1;n-r_C,p-r_A} + r_{N_2}^2((p - r_A) + (p - r_A)^2)$$
$$\times c_{2;n-r(\boldsymbol{C}),p-r(\boldsymbol{A})} + 2r_{N_2}(p - r_A)c_{1;n-r_C,p-r_A}$$
$$+2r_{N_2}((p - r_A) + (p - r_A)^2)$$
$$\times c_{2;n-r_C,p-r_A},$$

$$
\begin{aligned}
c_2 &= r_{N_2}^2(p - r_{H_2})^2 c_{1;n-r_C,p-r_{H_2}} + r_{N_2}^2((p - r_{H_2}) + (p - r_{H_2})^2) \\
&\quad \times c_{2;n-r_C,p-r_{H_2}} + 2r_{N_2}(p - r_{H_2})c_{1,n-r_C,p-r_{H_2}} \\
&\quad + 2r_{N_2}((p - r_{H_2}) + (p - r_{H_2})^2)c_{2;n-r_C,p-r_{H_2}}, \\
c_3 &= r_{N_2}^2(p - r_A)^2 c_{1;n-r_C,p-r_A,p-r_{H_2}} + 2r_{N_2}^2(p - r_A)c_{2;n-r_C,p-r_A,p-r_{H_2}} \\
&\quad + r_{N_2}^2(p - r_A)(r_A - r_{H_2})c_{3;n-r(C),p-r_A,p-r_{H_2}} \\
&\quad + 2r_{N_2}(p - r_A)c_{1;n-r_C,p-r_A,p-r_{H_2}} \\
&\quad + 2r_{N_2}((p - r_A) + (p - r_A)^2)c_{2;n-r_C,p-r_A,p-r_{H_2}};
\end{aligned}
$$

(iii)

$$
\begin{aligned}
E[T_{51}] &= r_{N_1}((p - r_{H_1})c_{0;n-r(C),p-r_{H_1}} - (p - r_A))c_{0;n-r_C,p-r_A} \\
&\quad + c_{0;n-r_C,p-r_{H_1}} \mathrm{tr}\{\boldsymbol{H}_1^{o'}\boldsymbol{\Sigma}\boldsymbol{H}_1^o)^- \boldsymbol{H}_1^{o'}\boldsymbol{A}\boldsymbol{B}\boldsymbol{N}_1(\boldsymbol{N}_1'(\boldsymbol{C}\boldsymbol{C}')^-\boldsymbol{N}_1)^-\boldsymbol{N}_1'\boldsymbol{B}'\boldsymbol{A}'\boldsymbol{H}_1^o\};
\end{aligned}
$$

(iv) *under* H_0

$$
D[T_{51}] = c_1 + c_2 - 2c_3 - E[T_{51}]^2,
$$

where

$$
\begin{aligned}
E[T_{51}] &= r_{N_1}((p - r_{H_1})c_{0;n-r(C),p-r_{H_1}} - (p - r_A))c_{0;n-r_C,p-r_A}, \\
c_1 &= r_{N_1}^2(p - r_A)^2 c_{1;n-r_C,p-r_A} + r_{N_1}^2((p - r_A) + (p - r_A)^2)c_{2;n-r(C),p-r(A)} \\
&\quad + 2r_{N_1}(p - r_A)c_{1;n-r_C,p-r_A} + 2r_{N_1}((p - r_A) + (p - r_A)^2)c_{2;n-r_C,p-r_A}, \\
c_2 &= r_{N_1}^2(p - r_{H_1})^2 c_{1;n-r_C,p-r_{H_1}} + r_{N_1}^2((p - r_{H_1}) + (p - r_{H_1})^2)c_{2;n-r_C,p-r_{H_1}} \\
&\quad + 2r_{N_1}(p - r_{H_1})c_{1;n-r_C,p-r_{H_1}} + 2r_{N_1}((p - r_{H_1}) + (p - r_{H_1})^2)c_{2;n-r_C,p-r_{H_1}}, \\
c_3 &= r_{N_1}^2(p - r_A)^2 c_{1;n-r_C,p-r_A,p-r_{H_1}} + 2r_{N_1}^2(p - r_A)c_{2;n-r_C,p-r_A,p-r_{H_1}} \\
&\quad + r_{N_1}^2(p - r_A)(r_A - r_{H_1})c_{3;n-r(C),p-r_A,p-r_{H_1}} + 2r_{N_1}(p - r_A)c_{1;n-r_C,p-r_A,p-r_{H_1}} \\
&\quad + 2r_{N_1}((p - r_A) + (p - r_A)^2)c_{2;n-r_C,p-r_A,p-r_{H_1}}.
\end{aligned}
$$

Proposition 7.6 *Let the test statistic T_{52} be given by Proposition 7.5. Then the hypothesis connected to T_{52} is rejected at approximate significance level α if $P(T_{52o} \geq a\chi^2_{[f]}) \leq \alpha$, where T_{52o} is the observed value of T_{52}, $[f]$ denotes the integer part of either f or $f+1$ and the integer part which is closest to f is chosen;*

$$
a = \frac{c_1 + c_2 - 2c_3 - c_0^2}{2c_0}, \qquad f = \frac{2c_0^2}{c_1 + c_2 - 2c_3 - c_0^2},
$$

where $c_0 = E[T_{52}]$ and $c_1 - c_3$ are presented in Theorem 7.15 (i) and (ii).

Proposition 7.7 *Let the test statistic T_{51} be given by Proposition 7.5. Then the hypothesis connected to T_{51} is rejected at approximate significance level α if $P(T_{51o} \geq a\chi^2_{[f]}) \leq \alpha$, where T_{51o} is the observed value of T_{51}, $[f]$ denotes the integer part of either f or $f+1$ and the the integer part which is closest to f is chosen;*

$$a = \frac{c_1 + c_2 - 2c_3 - c_0^2}{2c_0}, \quad f = \frac{2c_0^2}{c_1 + c_2 - 2c_3 - c_0^2},$$

where $c_0 = E[T_{51}]$ and $c_1 - c_3$ are presented in Theorem 7.15 (iii) and (iv).

Example 7.11 The melatonin data generated in Example 7.3 are considered one final time. In Example 7.8 the likelihood ratio test was carried out for these data. More precisely, for the BRM, H_0: $\boldsymbol{F}_i\boldsymbol{B}\boldsymbol{G}_i = \boldsymbol{0}$, $i = 1, 2$, was tested against $\boldsymbol{B}$ unrestricted. The likelihood ratio statistic equals a product, $\lambda_1\lambda_2$, of two test statistics. For these tests, λ_1 tests $H_0 : \boldsymbol{F}_2\boldsymbol{B}\boldsymbol{G}_2 = \boldsymbol{0}$ versus $\boldsymbol{B}$ unrestricted, which turned out to be far below the critical value, while λ_2, which tests $H_0 : \boldsymbol{F}_1\boldsymbol{B}\boldsymbol{G}_1 = \boldsymbol{0}$ given that $\boldsymbol{F}_2\boldsymbol{B}\boldsymbol{G}_2 = \boldsymbol{0}$, was not significant.

Concerning the "trace-test" for the hypothesis H_0: $\boldsymbol{F}_i\boldsymbol{B}\boldsymbol{G}_i = \boldsymbol{0}$, $i = 1, 2$, versus $\boldsymbol{B}$ unrestricted, it follows from Propositions 7.6 and 7.7 that the test statistics T_{52}, for testing H_0: $\boldsymbol{F}_2\boldsymbol{B}\boldsymbol{G}_2 = \boldsymbol{0}$ versus $\boldsymbol{B}$ unrestricted, and T_{51}, for testing H_0: $\boldsymbol{F}_1\boldsymbol{B}\boldsymbol{G}_1 = \boldsymbol{0}$ versus $\boldsymbol{B}\boldsymbol{G}_2 = \boldsymbol{0}$, are of interest. Note that T_{52} corresponds to λ_1, mentioned above.

The results of the "trace-test" are as follows: $T_{52o} = 1.1$, $T_{52o}/a = 22.0 > \chi^2_{0.05}(1) = 3.84$, $T_{51o} = 0.03$ and $T_{51o}/a = 0.6 < \chi^2_{0.05}(1) = 3.84$. Thus, there is a very strong agreement between the likelihood ratio test and the "trace-test". Note that three parameters are put to zero under the null hypothesis and that this hypothesis is tested via two chi-square distributions which both have one degree of freedom. From an asymptotic point of view this is somewhat unnatural and should be exploited further. □

7.10 The Likelihood Ratio Test Versus the "Trace Test"

Firstly, it is noted that if the dispersion matrix $\boldsymbol{\Sigma}$ is known, the likelihood ratio test and the "trace test" for a given hypothesis connected to the BRM, with restrictions on the mean, will yield identical test statistics. However, a known $\boldsymbol{\Sigma}$ will never occur and when $\boldsymbol{\Sigma}$ is unknown, the construction of the two types of tests culminates in different tests.

The likelihood ratio procedure considers the whole space, i.e. a tensor space which consists of the within-individuals subspace and the between-individuals subspace. Moreover, the likelihood ratio procedure is a precise mathematical formulation of the testing problem and has for a couple of centuries been known to be the best test from an asymptotic point of view. However, with many parameters being included in a model, there are situations where the likelihood ratio test is not useful, since, for example, the test may reject the null hypothesis too often. There can also be a problem understanding what is really being tested when many parameters appear in the model, in particular when there are several nuisance parameters in the model.

In Sects. 7.3–7.7, likelihood ratio tests of hypotheses concerning $\boldsymbol{B}$ in the BRM were mainly of interest, whereas $\boldsymbol{\Sigma}$ played a secondary role; i.e. knowledge about $\boldsymbol{\Sigma}$ was only applied when evaluating the distribution of $\widehat{\boldsymbol{B}}$. In the likelihood ratio test the maximum likelihood estimator of $\boldsymbol{\Sigma}$ was used whereas for the "trace test" it was decided to use $n^{-1}\boldsymbol{S}$. Since $n^{-1}\boldsymbol{S}$ and the maximum likelihood estimator of $\boldsymbol{\Sigma}$ both converge to $\boldsymbol{\Sigma}$ with the same "speed", the two different testing approaches are asymptotically equivalent. However, small sample comparisons between the approaches have yet to be performed. One advantage of the "trace test", when $n^{-1}\boldsymbol{S}$ is used, is that the spaces which are involved in the construction of the test statistic are easier to interpret than the projections used in the construction of the likelihood ratio statistic, where some kind of conditional approach is applied; for example see Sect. 7.3. Moreover, when considering H_0: $\boldsymbol{F}_i\boldsymbol{B}\boldsymbol{G}_i = \boldsymbol{0}$, $i = 1, 2$, $\mathcal{C}(\boldsymbol{F}_1') \subseteq \mathcal{C}(\boldsymbol{F}_2')$, in the BRM, the derivation and the construction of the test statistic are more straightforward for the "trace test" than for the likelihood ratio test.

It can be mentioned that the "trace test" is a goodness-of-fit test in the sense that it compares the fit under H_0 with the fit under H_1, i.e. it highlights the difference of fit under H_0 and H_1. The drawback of "trace tests" is that their distributions and power for various alternatives have not yet been studied in detail, whereas the likelihood ratio test has been scrutinized with respect to different statistical properties. In the previous sections, we have been relying on some ad hoc approximations, which seems to work, but no real proofs are given. On the other hand, although likelihood ratio statistics are associated with certain errors no sharp upper error bounds are available for the tests of the hypotheses in Sects. 7.3–7.7.

7.11 Testing an $EBRM_B^3$ Against a BRM

Now we return to exploiting likelihood ratio tests, and the results of Sects. 7.6 and 7.7 will be slightly extended. The reason is that in the next section, restrictions of a different type than $\boldsymbol{F}_i\boldsymbol{B}\boldsymbol{G}_i = \boldsymbol{0}$, $i = 1, 2$, are considered and the results will rely on the present section. In the previous sections, restrictions were put on $\boldsymbol{B}$ in the BRM, $\boldsymbol{X} = \boldsymbol{A}\boldsymbol{B}\boldsymbol{C} + \boldsymbol{E}$, through $\boldsymbol{F}_i\boldsymbol{B}\boldsymbol{G}_i = \boldsymbol{0}$, $i = 1, 2$, $\mathcal{C}(\boldsymbol{F}_2) \subseteq \mathcal{C}(\boldsymbol{F}_1)$. In this section it is assumed that under H_0

$$E[\boldsymbol{X}] = \boldsymbol{A}_1\boldsymbol{B}_1\boldsymbol{C}_1 + \boldsymbol{A}_2\boldsymbol{B}_2\boldsymbol{C}_2 + \boldsymbol{A}_3\boldsymbol{B}_3\boldsymbol{C}_3, \quad \mathcal{C}(\boldsymbol{C}_3') \subseteq \mathcal{C}(\boldsymbol{C}_2') \subseteq \mathcal{C}(\boldsymbol{C}_1'), \tag{7.79}$$

where $\boldsymbol{B}_i$, $i = 1, 2, 3$, are the parameters of interest. Under the alternative hypothesis we have

$$E[\boldsymbol{X}] = \boldsymbol{A}\boldsymbol{B}\boldsymbol{C},$$

where in particular $\mathcal{C}(\boldsymbol{A}_1 : \boldsymbol{A}_2 : \boldsymbol{A}_3) \subseteq \mathcal{C}(\boldsymbol{A})$, $\mathcal{C}(\boldsymbol{C}_1) \subseteq \mathcal{C}(\boldsymbol{C})$ and $\boldsymbol{B}$ is completely unknown, i.e. no restrictions apply to $\boldsymbol{B}$. Thus, an $EBRM_B^3$ is tested against a BRM. From Theorems 3.1 and 3.2, it follows that the likelihood ratio test statistic for testing (7.79) is equivalent to

$$\lambda^{\frac{2}{n}} = \frac{|\widehat{\boldsymbol{\Sigma}}_{H_0}|}{|\widehat{\boldsymbol{\Sigma}}_{H_1}|} = \frac{|\widehat{\boldsymbol{S}}_3 + \widehat{\boldsymbol{Q}}_3'\widehat{\boldsymbol{Q}}_2'\widehat{\boldsymbol{Q}}_1'\boldsymbol{X}\boldsymbol{P}_{C_3'}\boldsymbol{X}'\widehat{\boldsymbol{Q}}_1\widehat{\boldsymbol{Q}}_2\widehat{\boldsymbol{Q}}_3|}{|\boldsymbol{S} + \boldsymbol{P}'_{A^o,S^{-1}}\boldsymbol{X}\boldsymbol{P}_{C'}\boldsymbol{X}'\boldsymbol{P}_{A^o,S^{-1}}|}, \tag{7.80}$$

where the notation follows that of Sect. 7.4, except that $\boldsymbol{A}_i$, $i = 1, 2, 3$, and $\boldsymbol{C}_i$, $i = 1, 2, 3$, are arbitrary known matrices following the conditions

$$\begin{aligned}&\mathcal{C}(\boldsymbol{C}_3') \subseteq \mathcal{C}(\boldsymbol{C}_2') \subseteq \mathcal{C}(\boldsymbol{C}_1') \subseteq \mathcal{C}(\boldsymbol{C}'),\\ &\mathcal{C}(\boldsymbol{A}_1 : \boldsymbol{A}_2 : \boldsymbol{A}_3) \subseteq \mathcal{C}(\boldsymbol{A}).\end{aligned} \tag{7.81}$$

Let $\widetilde{\boldsymbol{A}}$ be any matrix such that

$$\mathcal{C}(\widetilde{\boldsymbol{A}}) = \mathcal{C}(\boldsymbol{A}_1 : \boldsymbol{A}_2 : \boldsymbol{A}_3).$$

As in Sects. 7.6 and 7.7, the test statistic in (7.80) can be factorized, but this time it is natural to work with three factors (see Fig. 7.12):

$$\lambda = \lambda_1\lambda_2\lambda_3,$$

where

$$\lambda_1^{\frac{2}{n}} = \frac{|\boldsymbol{S}_1 + \boldsymbol{P}'_{\widetilde{A}^o,S_1^{-1}}\boldsymbol{X}\boldsymbol{P}_{C_1'}\boldsymbol{X}'\boldsymbol{P}_{\widetilde{A}^o,S_1^{-1}}|}{|\boldsymbol{S} + \boldsymbol{P}'_{A^o,S^{-1}}\boldsymbol{X}\boldsymbol{P}_{C'}\boldsymbol{X}'\boldsymbol{P}_{A^o,S^{-1}}|}, \tag{7.82}$$

$$\lambda_2^{\frac{2}{n}} = \frac{|\widehat{\boldsymbol{S}}_2 + \boldsymbol{P}'_{\widetilde{A}^o,\widehat{S}_2^{-1}}\boldsymbol{X}\boldsymbol{P}_{C_2'}\boldsymbol{X}'\boldsymbol{P}_{\widetilde{A}^o,\widehat{S}_2^{-1}}|}{|\boldsymbol{S}_1 + \boldsymbol{P}'_{\widetilde{A}^o,S_1^{-1}}\boldsymbol{X}\boldsymbol{P}_{C_1'}\boldsymbol{X}'\boldsymbol{P}_{\widetilde{A}^o,S_1^{-1}}|}, \tag{7.83}$$

$$\lambda_3^{\frac{2}{n}} = \frac{|\widehat{\boldsymbol{S}}_3 + \boldsymbol{P}_{\widetilde{A}^o,\widehat{S}_3^{-1}}\boldsymbol{X}\boldsymbol{P}_{C_3'}\boldsymbol{X}'\boldsymbol{P}_{\widetilde{A}^o,\widehat{S}_3^{-1}}|}{|\widehat{\boldsymbol{S}}_2 + \boldsymbol{P}'_{\widetilde{A}^o,\widehat{S}_2^{-1}}\boldsymbol{X}\boldsymbol{P}_{C_2'}\boldsymbol{X}'\boldsymbol{P}_{\widetilde{A}^o,\widehat{S}_2^{-1}}|}, \tag{7.84}$$

and for clarity $\boldsymbol{S}_1$, $\widehat{\boldsymbol{S}}_2$ and $\widehat{\boldsymbol{S}}_3$ are also given:

$$\begin{aligned}\boldsymbol{S}_1 &= \boldsymbol{X}(\boldsymbol{I} - \boldsymbol{P}_{C_1'})\boldsymbol{X}',\\ \widehat{\boldsymbol{S}}_2 &= \boldsymbol{S}_1 + \boldsymbol{P}'_{A_1^o,S_1^{-1}}\boldsymbol{X}(\boldsymbol{P}_{C_1'} - \boldsymbol{P}_{C_2'})\boldsymbol{X}'\boldsymbol{P}_{A_1^o,S_1^{-1}},\\ \widehat{\boldsymbol{S}}_3 &= \boldsymbol{S}_2 + \boldsymbol{P}'_{(A_1:A_2)^o,\widehat{S}_2^{-1}}\boldsymbol{X}(\boldsymbol{P}_{C_2'} - \boldsymbol{P}_{C_3'})\boldsymbol{X}'\boldsymbol{P}_{(A_1:A_2)^o,\widehat{S}_2^{-1}}.\end{aligned}$$

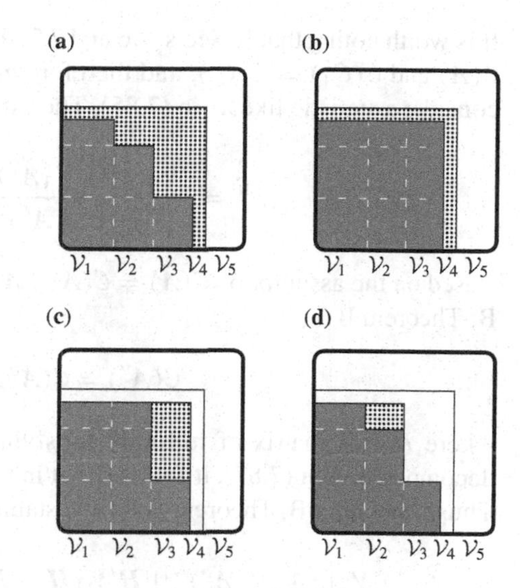

Fig. 7.12 In **(a)**, the dotted area corresponds to the likelihood ratio test H_0: $E[\boldsymbol{X}] = \boldsymbol{A}_1\boldsymbol{B}_1\boldsymbol{C}_1 + \boldsymbol{A}_2\boldsymbol{B}_2\boldsymbol{C}_2 + \boldsymbol{A}_3\boldsymbol{B}_3\boldsymbol{C}_3$ against H_1: $E[\boldsymbol{X}] = \boldsymbol{A}\boldsymbol{B}\boldsymbol{C}$, where $\mathcal{C}(\boldsymbol{A}_1 : \boldsymbol{A}_2 : \boldsymbol{A}_3) \subseteq \mathcal{C}(\boldsymbol{A})$ and $\mathcal{C}(\boldsymbol{C}_3') \subseteq \mathcal{C}(\boldsymbol{C}_2') \subseteq \mathcal{C}(\boldsymbol{C}_1') \subseteq \mathcal{C}(\boldsymbol{C})$. The test statistic λ is presented in (7.80). In **(b)**, the test statistic λ_1 in (7.82) is illustrated, and **(c)** and **(d)** show what is tested with λ_2 and λ_3, respectively. Furthermore, $\mathcal{V}_1 = \mathcal{C}(\boldsymbol{C}_3')$, $\mathcal{V}_2 = \mathcal{C}(\boldsymbol{C}_2') \cap \mathcal{C}(\boldsymbol{C}_3')^\perp$, $\mathcal{V}_3 = \mathcal{C}(\boldsymbol{C}_1') \cap \mathcal{C}(\boldsymbol{C}_2)^\perp$, $\mathcal{V}_4 = \mathcal{C}(\boldsymbol{C}_1) \cap \mathcal{C}(\boldsymbol{C}')^\perp$ and $\mathcal{V}_5 = \mathcal{C}(\boldsymbol{C}')^\perp$

Note that λ_2 and λ_3 correspond to (7.53) and (7.54), respectively, and Theorem 7.8 describes how the tests based on λ_2 and λ_3 should be performed. In Fig. 7.12 the three different test statistics are illustrated. Here it can be seen that λ_1 tests if the space $(\mathcal{C}(\boldsymbol{C}_1')^\perp \otimes \mathcal{C}(\widetilde{\boldsymbol{A}})^\perp) \cap (\mathcal{C}(\boldsymbol{C}) \otimes \mathcal{C}(\boldsymbol{A}))$ equals $\{\boldsymbol{0}\}$. If this test is rejected, then the overall hypothesis about the $EBRM_B^3$ against the BRM is also rejected. However, if it is not rejected, then it makes sense to investigate λ_2, which tests if the space $(\mathcal{C}(\boldsymbol{C}_2')^\perp \cap \mathcal{C}(\boldsymbol{C}_1')) \otimes (\mathcal{C}(\boldsymbol{A}_1)^\perp \cap \mathcal{C}(\widetilde{\boldsymbol{A}}))$ equals $\{\boldsymbol{0}\}$. Moreover, if λ_2 is not rejected either, then the test statistic λ_3 should be considered, and in this case it will be tested whether the space $(\mathcal{C}(\boldsymbol{C}_3')^\perp \cap \mathcal{C}(\boldsymbol{C}_2')) \otimes (\mathcal{C}(\boldsymbol{A}_1 : \boldsymbol{A}_2)^\perp \cap \mathcal{C}(\widetilde{\boldsymbol{A}}))$ equals $\{\boldsymbol{0}\}$, given that $(\mathcal{C}(\boldsymbol{C}_2')^\perp \cap \mathcal{C}(\boldsymbol{C}_1')) \otimes (\mathcal{C}(\boldsymbol{A}_1)^\perp \cap \mathcal{C}(\widetilde{\boldsymbol{A}})) = \{\boldsymbol{0}\}$.

Before deriving the approximating distributions of the three test statistics mentioned above, it can be noted that if one wants to simplify the technical treatment, which, however, is not necessary, $\boldsymbol{\Sigma}$ can be replaced by $\boldsymbol{I}$ without any loss of generality; i.e. the distribution of the test statistic does not depend on $\boldsymbol{\Sigma}$. Therefore, in order to indicate that $\boldsymbol{\Sigma} = \boldsymbol{I}$ is assumed to hold, $\boldsymbol{X}$ is replaced by $\boldsymbol{Y} \sim N_{p,n}(\boldsymbol{0}, \boldsymbol{I}_p, \boldsymbol{I}_n)$, $\boldsymbol{S}_i$ by $\boldsymbol{V}_i$ (defined as the matrix where in $\boldsymbol{S}_i$ the matrix $\boldsymbol{X}$ has been replaced by $\boldsymbol{Y}$), and $\boldsymbol{S}$ is replaced by $\boldsymbol{V} \sim W_p(\boldsymbol{I}, n - r(\boldsymbol{C}))$. Moreover, instead of $\boldsymbol{A}_i$, $i = 1, 2, 3$, and $\boldsymbol{A}$ one should now have $\boldsymbol{\Sigma}^{1/2}\boldsymbol{A}_i$ and $\boldsymbol{\Sigma}^{1/2}\boldsymbol{A}$, but it is not necessary to emphasize this. The obtained distributions will not depend on $\boldsymbol{A}_i$ or $\boldsymbol{A}$, and only the ranks of these matrices are important; these do not change with pre-multiplication by $\boldsymbol{\Sigma}^{1/2}$. Now we start to derive an approximation of the distribution of the likelihood ratio test and to consider

$$\lambda_1^{\frac{2}{n}} = \frac{|\boldsymbol{V}_1 + \boldsymbol{P}'_{\widetilde{A}^o, V_1^{-1}} \boldsymbol{Y} \boldsymbol{P}_{C_1'} \boldsymbol{Y}' \boldsymbol{P}_{\widetilde{A}^o, V_1^{-1}}|}{|\boldsymbol{V} + \boldsymbol{P}'_{A^o; V^{-1}} \boldsymbol{Y} \boldsymbol{P}_{C'} \boldsymbol{Y}' \boldsymbol{P}_{A^o; V^{-1}}|}. \tag{7.85}$$

It is worth noting that in Sects. 7.6 and 7.7, the matrices satisfied $\mathcal{C}(\boldsymbol{A}_1 : \boldsymbol{A}_2 : \boldsymbol{A}_3) = \mathcal{C}(\boldsymbol{A})$ and $\mathcal{C}(\boldsymbol{C}_1') = \mathcal{C}(\boldsymbol{C}')$, and therefore in these sections it was not necessary to consider a statistic like λ_1 in (7.85). The expression in (7.85) can be rewritten as

$$\lambda_1^{\frac{2}{n}} = \frac{|\boldsymbol{V}_1||(\widetilde{\boldsymbol{A}}^{o'}\boldsymbol{V}_1\widetilde{\boldsymbol{A}}^{o})^{-1}||(\widetilde{\boldsymbol{A}}^{o'}\boldsymbol{Y}\boldsymbol{Y}'\widetilde{\boldsymbol{A}}^{o})|}{|\boldsymbol{V}||(\boldsymbol{A}^{o'}\boldsymbol{V}\boldsymbol{A}^{o})^{-1}||(\boldsymbol{A}^{o'}\boldsymbol{Y}\boldsymbol{Y}'\boldsymbol{A}^{o})|}. \tag{7.86}$$

Based on the assumption $\mathcal{C}(\widetilde{\boldsymbol{A}}) = \mathcal{C}(\boldsymbol{A}_1 : \boldsymbol{A}_2 : \boldsymbol{A}_3) \subseteq \mathcal{C}(\boldsymbol{A})$ and utilizing Appendix B, Theorem B.3 (ii)

$$\mathcal{C}(\widetilde{\boldsymbol{A}}^{o}) = \mathcal{C}(\boldsymbol{A}^{o}) \boxplus \mathcal{C}(\boldsymbol{H}), \tag{7.87}$$

where $\boldsymbol{H}$ is a matrix of full rank satisfying $\mathcal{C}(\boldsymbol{H}) = \mathcal{C}(\boldsymbol{A}) \cap \mathcal{C}(\widetilde{\boldsymbol{A}})^{\perp}$. Using the decomposition in (7.87), it follows that in (7.86), $\widetilde{\boldsymbol{A}}^{o}$ can be replaced by $(\boldsymbol{A}^{o} : \boldsymbol{H})$. Thus, Appendix B, Theorem B.8 (iv) establishes that

$$\lambda_1^{\frac{2}{n}} = \frac{|\boldsymbol{V}_1||(\boldsymbol{A}^{o'}\boldsymbol{V}_1\boldsymbol{A}^{o})^{-1}||\boldsymbol{H}'\boldsymbol{V}_1\boldsymbol{H} - \boldsymbol{H}'\boldsymbol{V}_1\boldsymbol{A}^{o}(\boldsymbol{A}^{o'}\boldsymbol{V}_1\boldsymbol{A}^{o})^{-1}\boldsymbol{A}^{o'}\boldsymbol{V}_1\boldsymbol{H}|^{-1}}{|\boldsymbol{V}||(\boldsymbol{A}^{o'}\boldsymbol{V}\boldsymbol{A}^{o})^{-1}|}$$
$$\times \frac{|(\boldsymbol{A}^{o'}\boldsymbol{Y}\boldsymbol{Y}'\boldsymbol{A}^{o})||\boldsymbol{H}'\boldsymbol{Y}\boldsymbol{Y}'\boldsymbol{H} - \boldsymbol{H}'\boldsymbol{Y}\boldsymbol{Y}'\boldsymbol{A}^{o}(\boldsymbol{A}^{o'}\boldsymbol{Y}\boldsymbol{Y}'\boldsymbol{A}^{o})^{-1}\boldsymbol{A}^{o'}\boldsymbol{Y}\boldsymbol{Y}'\boldsymbol{H}|}{|(\boldsymbol{A}^{o'}\boldsymbol{Y}\boldsymbol{Y}'\boldsymbol{A}^{o})|}.$$

Hence, the test statistic can be factored into

$$\lambda_1 = \lambda_{11}\lambda_{12},$$

where

$$\lambda_{11}^{\frac{2}{n}} = \frac{|\boldsymbol{V}_1||(\boldsymbol{A}^{o'}\boldsymbol{V}_1\boldsymbol{A}^{o})^{-1}|}{|\boldsymbol{V}||(\boldsymbol{A}^{o'}\boldsymbol{V}\boldsymbol{A}^{o})^{-1}|}, \tag{7.88}$$

$$\lambda_{12}^{\frac{2}{n}} = \frac{|\boldsymbol{H}'\boldsymbol{Y}\boldsymbol{Y}'\boldsymbol{H} - \boldsymbol{H}'\boldsymbol{Y}\boldsymbol{Y}'\boldsymbol{A}^{o}(\boldsymbol{A}^{o'}\boldsymbol{Y}\boldsymbol{Y}'\boldsymbol{A}^{o})^{-1}\boldsymbol{A}^{o'}\boldsymbol{Y}\boldsymbol{Y}'\boldsymbol{H}|}{|\boldsymbol{H}'\boldsymbol{V}_1\boldsymbol{H} - \boldsymbol{H}'\boldsymbol{V}_1\boldsymbol{A}^{o}(\boldsymbol{A}^{o'}\boldsymbol{V}_1'\boldsymbol{A}^{o})^{-1}\boldsymbol{A}^{o'}\boldsymbol{V}_1'\boldsymbol{H}|}$$
$$= \frac{|\boldsymbol{H}'\underline{\boldsymbol{A}}(\underline{\boldsymbol{A}}'(\boldsymbol{Y}\boldsymbol{Y}')^{-1}\underline{\boldsymbol{A}})^{-1}\underline{\boldsymbol{A}}'\boldsymbol{H}|}{|\boldsymbol{H}'\underline{\boldsymbol{A}}(\underline{\boldsymbol{A}}'\boldsymbol{V}_1^{-1}\underline{\boldsymbol{A}})^{-1}\underline{\boldsymbol{A}}'\boldsymbol{H}|}, \tag{7.89}$$

and $\underline{\boldsymbol{A}}$ is any matrix of full rank satisfying $\mathcal{C}(\underline{\boldsymbol{A}}) = \mathcal{C}(\boldsymbol{A})$. The appearance of two test statistics instead of λ_1 is in agreement with Fig. 7.12b.

Concerning $\lambda_{11}^{\frac{2}{n}}$ this expression is similar to (7.14). Therefore, it is possible to copy all the calculations from (7.14) into the final expression in (7.20). The only issue that has to be addressed is the definition of the corresponding $\boldsymbol{M}$ and $\boldsymbol{N}$ matrices, which are similar to those used in (7.18). It follows that $\boldsymbol{N}$ has to satisfy

$$\boldsymbol{P}_{C'} - \boldsymbol{P}_{C_1'} = \boldsymbol{P}_{C'(CC')^{-}N},$$

i.e. $\boldsymbol{N} = \mathcal{C}(\boldsymbol{C}_1')^o$. Moreover, $\boldsymbol{M}$ must satisfy

$$\mathcal{C}(\boldsymbol{M}) = \mathcal{C}(\boldsymbol{A}')$$

and $\boldsymbol{M}$ should be of full rank. Then the result of Theorem 7.2 can be utilized. Another way of obtaining the result is to suppose that $\boldsymbol{F} = \boldsymbol{I}$ in Sect. 7.3 and apply Corollary 7.1.

In the following, (7.89) is exploited. First it is noted (putting $\boldsymbol{P}_{\mathcal{B}} = \boldsymbol{P}_{C'(CC')^- N}$, $\boldsymbol{N} = \mathcal{C}(\boldsymbol{C}_1')^o$), that

$$\boldsymbol{YY}' = \boldsymbol{V}_1 + \boldsymbol{Y}\boldsymbol{P}_{\mathcal{B}}\boldsymbol{Y}',$$

and applying Theorem B.6 (i) in Appendix B yields (since $\boldsymbol{P}_{\mathcal{B}}$ is idempotent)

$$(\boldsymbol{YY}')^{-1} = \boldsymbol{V}_1^{-1} - \boldsymbol{V}_1^{-1}\boldsymbol{Y}\boldsymbol{P}_{\mathcal{B}}(\boldsymbol{P}_{\mathcal{B}}\boldsymbol{Y}'\boldsymbol{V}_1^{-1}\boldsymbol{Y}\boldsymbol{P}_{\mathcal{B}} + \boldsymbol{I})^{-1}\boldsymbol{P}_{\mathcal{B}}\boldsymbol{Y}'\boldsymbol{V}_1^{-1}.$$

Thus, using Appendix B, Theorem B.6 (i) once again,

$$\begin{aligned}
(\underline{\boldsymbol{A}}'(\boldsymbol{YY}')^{-1}\underline{\boldsymbol{A}})^{-1} &= (\underline{\boldsymbol{A}}'\boldsymbol{V}_1^{-1}\underline{\boldsymbol{A}})^{-1} + (\underline{\boldsymbol{A}}'\boldsymbol{V}_1^{-1}\underline{\boldsymbol{A}})^{-1}\underline{\boldsymbol{A}}'\boldsymbol{V}_1^{-1}\boldsymbol{Y}\boldsymbol{P}_{\mathcal{B}}(\boldsymbol{I} + \boldsymbol{P}_{\mathcal{B}}\boldsymbol{Y}'\boldsymbol{V}_1^{-1}\boldsymbol{Y}\boldsymbol{P}_{\mathcal{B}} \\
&\quad - \boldsymbol{P}_{\mathcal{B}}\boldsymbol{Y}'\boldsymbol{V}_1^{-1}\underline{\boldsymbol{A}}(\underline{\boldsymbol{A}}'\boldsymbol{V}_1^{-1}\underline{\boldsymbol{A}})^{-1}\underline{\boldsymbol{A}}'\boldsymbol{V}_1^{-1}\boldsymbol{Y}\boldsymbol{P}_{\mathcal{B}})^{-1}\boldsymbol{P}_{\mathcal{B}}\boldsymbol{Y}'\boldsymbol{V}_1^{-1}\underline{\boldsymbol{A}}(\underline{\boldsymbol{A}}'\boldsymbol{V}_1^{-1}\underline{\boldsymbol{A}})^{-1} \\
&= (\underline{\boldsymbol{A}}'\boldsymbol{V}_1^{-1}\underline{\boldsymbol{A}})^{-1} + (\underline{\boldsymbol{A}}'\boldsymbol{V}_1^{-1}\underline{\boldsymbol{A}})^{-1}\underline{\boldsymbol{A}}'\boldsymbol{V}_1^{-1}\boldsymbol{Y}\boldsymbol{P}_{\mathcal{B}}(\boldsymbol{I} + \boldsymbol{P}_{\mathcal{B}}\boldsymbol{Y}'\boldsymbol{A}^o(\boldsymbol{A}^{o'}\boldsymbol{V}_1\boldsymbol{A}^o)^{-1}\boldsymbol{A}^{o'}\boldsymbol{Y}\boldsymbol{P}_{\mathcal{B}})^{-1} \\
&\quad \times \boldsymbol{P}_{\mathcal{B}}\boldsymbol{Y}'\boldsymbol{V}_1^{-1}\underline{\boldsymbol{A}}(\underline{\boldsymbol{A}}'\boldsymbol{V}_1^{-1}\underline{\boldsymbol{A}})^{-1}.
\end{aligned}$$

Utilizing the above derivation, λ_{12} in (7.89) can be shown to equal

$$\begin{aligned}
\lambda_{12}^{\frac{2}{n}} &= |\boldsymbol{I} + \boldsymbol{P}_{\mathcal{B}}\boldsymbol{Y}'\boldsymbol{A}^o(\boldsymbol{A}^{o'}\boldsymbol{V}_1\boldsymbol{A}^o)^{-1}\boldsymbol{A}^{o'}\boldsymbol{Y}\boldsymbol{P}_{\mathcal{B}}|^{-1}|\boldsymbol{I} + \boldsymbol{P}_{\mathcal{B}}\boldsymbol{Y}'\boldsymbol{A}^o(\boldsymbol{A}^{o'}\boldsymbol{V}_1\boldsymbol{A}^o)^{-1}\boldsymbol{A}^{o'}\boldsymbol{Y}\boldsymbol{P}_{\mathcal{B}} \\
&\quad + \boldsymbol{P}_{\mathcal{B}}\boldsymbol{Y}'\underline{\boldsymbol{A}}(\underline{\boldsymbol{A}}'\boldsymbol{V}_1^{-1}\boldsymbol{A})^{-1} \\
&\qquad \times \underline{\boldsymbol{A}}'\boldsymbol{H}(\boldsymbol{H}'\underline{\boldsymbol{A}}(\underline{\boldsymbol{A}}'\boldsymbol{V}_1^{-1}\underline{\boldsymbol{A}})^{-1}\underline{\boldsymbol{A}}'\boldsymbol{H})^{-1}\boldsymbol{H}'\underline{\boldsymbol{A}}(\boldsymbol{A}'\boldsymbol{V}_1^{-1}\underline{\boldsymbol{A}})^{-1}\underline{\boldsymbol{A}}'\boldsymbol{Y}\boldsymbol{P}_{\mathcal{B}}| \\
&= |\boldsymbol{I} + \boldsymbol{P}_{\mathcal{B}}\boldsymbol{Y}'\boldsymbol{A}^o(\boldsymbol{A}^{o'}\boldsymbol{V}_1\boldsymbol{A}^o)^{-1}\boldsymbol{A}^{o'}\boldsymbol{Y}\boldsymbol{P}_{\mathcal{B}}|^{-1}|\boldsymbol{I} + \boldsymbol{P}_{\mathcal{B}}\boldsymbol{Y}'\boldsymbol{V}_1^{-1}\boldsymbol{Y}\boldsymbol{P}_{\mathcal{B}} \\
&\quad - \boldsymbol{P}_{\mathcal{B}}\boldsymbol{Y}'\boldsymbol{A}(\boldsymbol{A}'\boldsymbol{H})^o((\boldsymbol{A}'\boldsymbol{H})^{o'}\boldsymbol{A}'\boldsymbol{V}_1\boldsymbol{A}(\boldsymbol{A}'\boldsymbol{H})^o)^{-1}(\boldsymbol{A}'\boldsymbol{H})^{o'}\boldsymbol{A}'\boldsymbol{Y}\boldsymbol{P}_{\mathcal{B}}| \\
&= |\boldsymbol{I} + \boldsymbol{P}_{\mathcal{B}}\boldsymbol{Y}'\boldsymbol{A}^o(\boldsymbol{A}^{o'}\boldsymbol{V}_1\boldsymbol{A}^o)^{-1}\boldsymbol{A}^{o'}\boldsymbol{Y}\boldsymbol{P}_{\mathcal{B}}|^{-1} \\
&\quad \times |\boldsymbol{I} + \boldsymbol{P}_{\mathcal{B}}\boldsymbol{Y}'(\boldsymbol{A}(\boldsymbol{A}'\boldsymbol{H})^o)^o((\boldsymbol{A}(\boldsymbol{A}'\boldsymbol{H})^o)^{o'}\boldsymbol{V}_1(\boldsymbol{A}(\boldsymbol{A}'\boldsymbol{H})^o)^o)^{-1}(\boldsymbol{A}(\boldsymbol{A}'\boldsymbol{H})^o)^{o'}\boldsymbol{Y}\boldsymbol{P}_{\mathcal{B}}|.
\end{aligned}$$

However, $\lambda_{12}^{\frac{2}{n}}$ has the same form as the expression in (7.16). Thus, the remaining task is to determine an $\boldsymbol{M}$ such that

$$\boldsymbol{P}_{(A(A'H)^o)^o, V_1^{-1}} - \boldsymbol{P}_{A^o, V_1^{-1}} = \boldsymbol{P}_{V_1^{-1}A(A'V_1^{-1}A)^- M, V_1^{-1}},$$

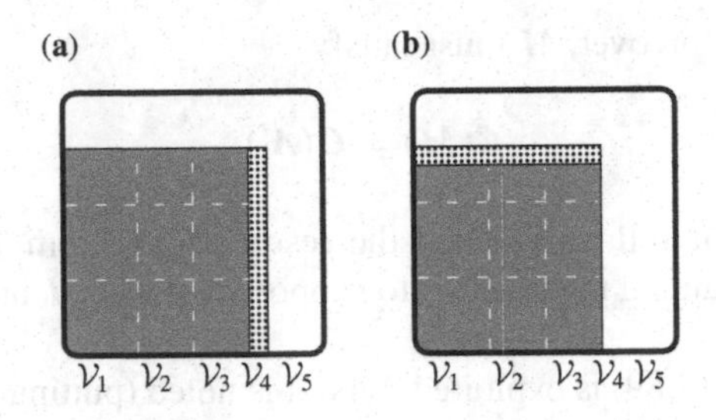

Fig. 7.13 In (**a**), the dotted area corresponds to the likelihood ratio test statistic λ_{11}, given in (7.88). In (**b**), the test statistic λ_{12} in (7.89) is illustrated. Furthermore, $\mathcal{V}_1 = \mathcal{C}(\boldsymbol{C}_3')$, $\mathcal{V}_2 = \mathcal{C}(\boldsymbol{C}_2') \cap \mathcal{C}(\boldsymbol{C}_3')^{\perp}$, $\mathcal{V}_3 = \mathcal{C}(\boldsymbol{C}_1') \cap \mathcal{C}(\boldsymbol{C}_2)^{\perp}$, $\mathcal{V}_4 = \mathcal{C}(\boldsymbol{C}_1) \cap \mathcal{C}(\boldsymbol{C}')^{\perp}$ and $\mathcal{V}_5 = \mathcal{C}(\boldsymbol{C}')^{\perp}$

implying that $\boldsymbol{M}$ can be chosen as $\boldsymbol{M} = \boldsymbol{A}'\widetilde{\boldsymbol{A}}^o$ (see Appendix B, Theorem B.12). Hence, with $\boldsymbol{N} = \boldsymbol{C}'\boldsymbol{C}_1^o$ and $\boldsymbol{M} = \boldsymbol{A}'\widetilde{\boldsymbol{A}}^o$, the relation in (7.20) can be utilized.

The test statistics λ_{11} and λ_{12} given in (7.88) and (7.89), respectively, are illustrated in Fig. 7.13.

Theorem 7.16 *Testing an $EBRM_B^3$ presented in Definition 2.2 against a BRM presented in Definition 2.1. Under H_0 the data are assumed to follow an $EBRM_B^3$ with the mean*

$$E[\boldsymbol{X}] = \boldsymbol{A}_1\boldsymbol{B}_1\boldsymbol{C}_1 + \boldsymbol{A}_2\boldsymbol{B}_2\boldsymbol{C}_2 + \boldsymbol{A}_3\boldsymbol{B}_3\boldsymbol{C}_3, \quad \mathcal{C}(\boldsymbol{C}_3') \subseteq \mathcal{C}(\boldsymbol{C}_2') \subseteq \mathcal{C}(\boldsymbol{C}_1').$$

Moreover, under H_1 the data are modelled by a standard BRM with the mean

$$E[\boldsymbol{X}] = \boldsymbol{ABC}, \qquad \mathcal{C}(\boldsymbol{C}_1') \subseteq \mathcal{C}(\boldsymbol{C}'), \quad \mathcal{C}(\widetilde{\boldsymbol{A}}) = \mathcal{C}(\boldsymbol{A}_1 : \boldsymbol{A}_2 : \boldsymbol{A}_3) \subseteq \mathcal{C}(\boldsymbol{A}).$$

Then the likelihood ratio test statistic λ for testing H_0 against H_1 can be factored into four components:

$$\lambda = \lambda_{11}\lambda_{12}\lambda_2\lambda_3,$$

where λ_{11}, λ_{12}, λ_2 and λ_3 are identified via (7.88), (7.89), (7.83) and (7.84), respectively.

Each component can be considered to be a test statistic and H_0 is rejected if one or several of the observed test statistics are in the tails of their corresponding distributions.

The next proposition utilizes Theorem C.3 in Appendix C. Note that the results concerning λ_2 and λ_3 stem from Theorem 7.9.

Proposition 7.8 *Let*

$$c_1(p_o, f, m) = \frac{p_o m(p_o^2 + m^2 - 5)}{48(f - \frac{1}{2}(p_o - m + 1))^2},$$

$$c_2(p_o, f, m) = \tfrac{1}{4608} p_o^2 m^2 (p_o^2 + m^2 - 5)^2 + \frac{p_o m(3p_o^4 + 3m^4 + 10p_o^2 m^2 - 50(p_o^2 + m^2) + 159)}{1920(f - \frac{1}{2}(p_o - m + 1))^4}.$$

(i) *Let λ_{11o} be the observed value of λ_{11}, given by (7.88) and used in the expression of the likelihood ratio test, presented in Theorem 7.16. Put*

$$t_o = -\tfrac{2}{n}(f - \tfrac{1}{2}(p_o - m + 1)) \ln \lambda_{11o},$$

where $f = n - r(\mathbf{C}) - p + r(\mathbf{A})$, $p_o = r(\mathbf{A})$ and $m = r(\mathbf{C}) - r(\mathbf{C}_1)$. Moreover, let $c_1 = c_1(p_o, f, m)$ and $c_2 = c_2(p_o, f, m)$. The hypothesis corresponding to the statistic λ_{11} in Theorem 7.16 is rejected, approximately at significance level α, if t_o satisfies

$$P\{\chi^2_{p_o m} \geq t_o\} + c_1(1 - c_1)(P\{\chi^2_{p_o m+4} \geq t_o\} - P\{\chi^2_{p_o m} \geq t_o\}) + c_2(P\{\chi^2_{p_o m+8} \geq t_o\} - P\{\chi^2_{p_o m} \geq t_o\}) \leq \alpha.$$

(ii) *Let λ_{12o} be the observed value of λ_{12}, given by (7.89) and used in the expression of the likelihood ratio test in Theorem 7.16. Put*

$$t_o = \tfrac{2}{n}(f - \tfrac{1}{2}(p_o - m + 1)) \ln \lambda_{12o},$$

where $f = n - r(\mathbf{C}) - p + r(\mathbf{A})$, $p_o = r(\mathbf{A}) - r(\widetilde{\mathbf{A}})$ and $m = r(\mathbf{C}) - r(\mathbf{C}_1)$. Moreover, let $c_1 = c_1(p_o, f, m)$ and $c_2 = c_2(p_o, f, m)$. The hypothesis corresponding to the statistic λ_{12} in Theorem 7.16 is rejected, approximately at significance level α, if t_o satisfies

$$P\{\chi^2_{p_o m} \geq t_o\} + c_1(1 - c_1)(P\{\chi^2_{p_o m+4} \geq t_o\} - P\{\chi^2_{p_o m} \geq t_o\}) + c_2(P\{\chi^2_{p_o m+8} \geq t_o\} - P\{\chi^2_{p_o m} \geq t_o\}) \leq \alpha.$$

(iii) *Let λ_{2o} be the observed value of λ_2, given by (7.83) and used in the expression of the likelihood ratio test in Theorem 7.16. Put*

$$t_o = \tfrac{2}{n}(f - \tfrac{1}{2}(p_o - m + 1)) \ln \lambda_{2o},$$

where $f = n - r(\boldsymbol{C}) - p + r(\boldsymbol{A})$, $p_o = r(\widetilde{\boldsymbol{A}}) - r(\boldsymbol{A}_1)$ *and* $m = r(\boldsymbol{C}_1) - r(\boldsymbol{C}_2)$. *Moreover, let* $c_1 = c_1(p_o, f, m)$ *and* $c_2 = c_2(p_o, f, m)$. *The hypothesis corresponding to the statistic* λ_1 *in Theorem 7.8 is rejected, approximately at significance level* α, *if* t_o *satisfies*

$$P\{\chi^2_{p_om} \geq t_o\} + c_1(1-c_1)(P\{\chi^2_{p_om+4} \geq t_o\} - P\{\chi^2_{p_om} \geq t_o\})$$
$$+ c_2(P\{\chi^2_{p_om+8} \geq t_o\} - P\{\chi^2_{p_om} \geq t_o\}) \leq \alpha.$$

(iv) *Let* λ_{3o} *be the observed value of* λ_3, *given by (7.84) and used in the expression of the likelihood ratio test in Theorem 7.16. Put*

$$t_o = \tfrac{2}{n}(f - \tfrac{1}{2}(p_o - m + 1)) \ln \lambda_{3o},$$

where $f = n - r(\boldsymbol{C}) - p + r(\boldsymbol{A})$, $p_o = r(\widetilde{\boldsymbol{A}}) - r(\boldsymbol{A}_1 : \boldsymbol{A}_2)$ *and* $m = r(\boldsymbol{C}_2) - r(\boldsymbol{C}_3)$. *Moreover, let* $c_1 = c_1(p_o, f, m)$ *and* $c_2 = c_2(p_o, f, m)$. *The hypothesis corresponding to the statistic* λ_2 *in Theorem 7.8 is rejected, approximately at significance level* α, *if* t_o *satisfies*

$$P\{\chi^2_{p_om} \geq t_o\} + c_1(1-c_1)(P\{\chi^2_{p_om+4} \geq t_o\} - P\{\chi^2_{p_om} \geq t_o\})$$
$$+ c_2(P\{\chi^2_{p_om+8} \geq t_o\} - P\{\chi^2_{p_om} \geq t_o\}) \leq \alpha.$$

7.12 Estimating and Testing in the BRM with $\boldsymbol{F}_1\boldsymbol{B}\boldsymbol{G}_1 = \boldsymbol{F}_2\boldsymbol{\Theta}\boldsymbol{G}_2$

In this section, a new way of formulating restrictions is presented. However, it can be worth noting that most of the mathematical treatment is not presented. The reader who has understood the previous sections is supposed to be able to fill in the gaps, and one may regard this section as a kind of follow-up section. The restrictions for the BRM with the mean $E[\boldsymbol{X}] = \boldsymbol{ABC}$ are in this section assumed to satisfy

$$\boldsymbol{F}_1\boldsymbol{B}\boldsymbol{G}_1 = \boldsymbol{F}_2\boldsymbol{\Theta}\boldsymbol{G}_2, \tag{7.90}$$

where $\boldsymbol{F}_i$ and $\boldsymbol{G}_i$, $i = 1, 2$, are known matrices, and $\boldsymbol{\Theta}$ and $\boldsymbol{B}$ unknown parameters. The purpose is to estimate the parameters in (7.90) and test (7.90) against $\boldsymbol{B}$ unstructured. It is natural to consider (7.90) as a system of linear equations whose solution is generated by free parameters (i.e. a reparametrization will take place), and then use knowledge about the $EBRM^3_B$. However, before a detailed presentation and discussion are provided, an explanatory and illustrative example is given.

Example 7.12 Suppose that there are two samples of different types of plants where a linear growth over time is observed by following each plant at the same time points, i.e.

$$E[X_{ijk}] = \alpha_i + \beta_i t_j, \quad k = 1, 2, \ldots, n_i.$$

However, if α_i is proportional to another factor (let us say the temperature), then

$$\alpha_i = \theta \,\text{temp}_i, \quad i = 1, 2,$$

for some unknown θ. Thus, the following mean structure emerges:

$$E[X_{ijk}] = \theta \,\text{temp}_i + \beta_i t_j, \quad i = 1, 2; \quad j = 1, 2, \ldots, p; \quad k = 1, 2, \ldots, n_i.$$

In matrix notation the model can be written as follows:

$$\begin{aligned}
E[\boldsymbol{X}] &= \boldsymbol{A}\boldsymbol{B}\boldsymbol{C} + \boldsymbol{E}, \quad \boldsymbol{E} \sim N_{p,n}(\boldsymbol{0}, \boldsymbol{\Sigma}, \boldsymbol{I}),\\
\boldsymbol{B} &= \begin{pmatrix} \alpha_1 & \alpha_2 \\ \beta_1 & \beta_2 \end{pmatrix},\\
\boldsymbol{A}' &= \begin{pmatrix} 1 & 1 & \ldots & 1 \\ t_1 & t_2 & \ldots & t_p \end{pmatrix}, \quad \boldsymbol{C} = \begin{pmatrix} 1\,1 \ldots 1\,0\,0 \ldots 0 \\ 0\,0 \ldots 0\,1\,1 \ldots 1 \end{pmatrix},\\
\boldsymbol{F}_1 &= (1 : 0), \quad \boldsymbol{G}_2 = (\text{temp}_1 : \text{temp}_2),
\end{aligned}$$

where $\boldsymbol{F}_1\boldsymbol{B} = \theta\boldsymbol{G}_2$.

If instead of two groups, there are three groups, two of which only are affected, then

$$\boldsymbol{B} = \begin{pmatrix} \alpha_1 & \alpha_2 & \alpha_3 \\ \beta_1 & \beta_2 & \beta_3 \end{pmatrix}, \qquad \boldsymbol{G}_1 = \begin{pmatrix} 1 & 0 \\ 0 & 1 \\ 0 & 0 \end{pmatrix},$$

where $\boldsymbol{F}_1\boldsymbol{B}\boldsymbol{G}_1 = \theta\boldsymbol{G}_2$. Moreover, if α_i, $i = 1, 2$, are affected not only by temperature, but also by the pressure (pre_i), for example, then $\boldsymbol{F}_1\boldsymbol{B}\boldsymbol{G}_1 = \boldsymbol{\Theta}\boldsymbol{G}_2$, with

$$\boldsymbol{\Theta} = (\theta_1 : \theta_2), \qquad \boldsymbol{G}_2 = \begin{pmatrix} \text{temp}_1 & \text{temp}_2 \\ \text{pre}_1 & \text{pre}_2 \end{pmatrix}.$$

□

Now a few theoretical results connected to the restrictions $\boldsymbol{F}_1\boldsymbol{B}\boldsymbol{G}_1 = \boldsymbol{F}_2\boldsymbol{\Theta}\boldsymbol{G}_2$ are derived. From Theorem B.10 (iv) in Appendix B, the general solution to $\boldsymbol{F}_1\boldsymbol{B}\boldsymbol{G}_1 = \boldsymbol{F}_2\boldsymbol{\Theta}\boldsymbol{G}_2$ is given by

$$\begin{aligned}
\boldsymbol{\Theta} &= \boldsymbol{F}_2^-\boldsymbol{F}_1(\boldsymbol{F}_1'\boldsymbol{F}_2^o : (\boldsymbol{F}_1')^o)^o\boldsymbol{Z}_3(\boldsymbol{G}_1(\boldsymbol{G}_2')^o)^{o'}\boldsymbol{G}_1\boldsymbol{G}_2^- + (\boldsymbol{F}_2')^o\boldsymbol{Z}_1 + \boldsymbol{F}_2'\boldsymbol{Z}_2\boldsymbol{G}_2^{o'},\\
\boldsymbol{B} &= (\boldsymbol{F}_1'\boldsymbol{F}_2^o : (\boldsymbol{F}_1')^o)^o\boldsymbol{Z}_3(\boldsymbol{G}_1(\boldsymbol{G}_2')^o)^{o'} + \boldsymbol{F}_1'\boldsymbol{F}_2^o\boldsymbol{Z}_4\boldsymbol{G}_1^{o'} + (\boldsymbol{F}_1')^o\boldsymbol{Z}_5, \qquad (7.91)
\end{aligned}$$

where Z_i, $i = 1, 2, \ldots, 6$, are arbitrary matrices. These relations inform us that the restrictions $F_1BG_1 = F_2\Theta G_2$ in the BRM lead to an $EBRM_B^3$. Therefore Theorem 3.2 is at our disposal and the next theorem can be established.

Theorem 7.17 *For the BRM presented in Definition 2.1, let $F_1BG_1 = F_2\Theta G_2$ hold, where F_i and G_i, $i = 1, 2$, are known and Θ and B are unknown. Then the mean can be written as follows:*

$$E[X] = A(F_1')^o B_1 C + A(F_1'F_2^o : (F_1')^o)^o B_2 (G_1(G_2')^o)^{o'} C + AF_1'F_2^o B_3 G_1^{o'} C,$$

where B_i, $i = 1, 2, 3$, are new parameters and the model belongs to the class of $EBRM_B^3$. The maximum likelihood estimators of the mean parameters are given by

$$\widehat{\Theta} = F_2^- F_1 (F_1'F_2^o : (F_1')^o)^o \widehat{B}_2 (G_1(G_2')^o)^{o'} G_1 G_2^- + (F_2')^o Z_1 + F_2' Z_2 G_2^{o'},$$

$$\widehat{B} = (F_1')^o \widehat{B}_1 + (F_1'F_2^o : (F_1')^o)^o \widehat{B}_2 (G_1(G_2')^o)^{o'} + F_1'F_2^o \widehat{B}_3 G_1^{o'},$$

where $\widehat{B}_i$, $i = 1, 2, 3$, follow from Theorem 3.2 and Z_i, $i = 1, 2$, are arbitrary matrices.

Theorem 7.18 *For the BRM presented in Definition 2.1, let $F_1BG_1 = F_2\Theta G_2$ hold, where F_i and G_i, $i = 1, 2$, are known and Θ and B unknown. Let the mean structure be as in Theorem 7.17. Then*

(i) *$\widehat{B}_3$ is unique if and only if*

$$\mathcal{C}(AF_1'F_2^o) \cap \mathcal{C}(A(F_1'F_2^o)^o) = \{0\}$$

and $AF_1'F_2^o$ and $C'G_1^o$ are of full rank;

(ii) *$\widehat{B}_2$ is unique if and only if*

$$\mathcal{C}(A(F_1')^o) \cap \mathcal{C}(A(F_1'F_2^o : (F_1')^o)^o) = \{0\},$$

$$\mathcal{C}(A(F_1')^o)^{\perp} \cap \mathcal{C}(A(F_1'F_2^o)^o) \cap \mathcal{C}(A(F_1'F_2^o : (F_1')^o)) = \{0\}$$

and $A((F_1')^o : F_1'F_2^o)^o$ and $C'(G_1(G_2')^o)^o$ are of full rank;

(iii) *$\widehat{B}_1$ is unique if and only if*

$$\mathcal{C}(A(F_1')^o) \cap \mathcal{C}(A(F_1'F_2^o : (F_1')^o)^o) = \{0\},$$

$$\mathcal{C}(A(F_1'F_2^o : (F_1')^o))^{\perp} \cap \mathcal{C}(A(F_1'F_2^o)^o) \cap \mathcal{C}(AF_1') = \{0\},$$

$r(C) = k$ and $A(F_1')^o$ is of full rank;

put $H = (F_1'F_2^o : (F_1')^o)$;

(iv) *$\widehat{\Theta}$ is unique if and only if*

$$\mathcal{C}(F_1'F_2) \subseteq \mathcal{C}(H) \boxplus \mathcal{C}(A') \cap \mathcal{C}(H)^{\perp},$$

and both F_2 and G_2 are of full rank, i.e. Z_i, $i = 1, 2$, in $\widehat{\Theta}$ in Theorem 7.17 disappear;

(v) $\widehat{B}$ *is unique if and only if*

$$\mathcal{C}(F_1')^{\perp} \cap \mathcal{C}(A')^{\perp} = \{0\}, \quad \mathcal{C}(F_1H^o) \cap \mathcal{C}(F_1(A')^o) = \{0\},$$
$$\mathcal{C}(F_1'F_2^o) \subseteq \mathcal{C}(A'), \quad r(C) = k.$$

Finally, the BRM with the restrictions $F_1BG_1 = F_2\Theta G_2$ is tested against unrestricted BRM. The goal is to utilize Sect. 7.11, where in general an $EBRM_B^3$ was tested against a BRM.

From Theorem 7.17, it follows that A_i and C_i in the $EBRM_B^3$ are given by

$$A_1 = A(F_1')^o, \qquad C_1 = C,$$
$$A_2 = A(F_1'F_2^o : (F_1')^o)^o, \qquad C_2 = (G_1(G_2')^o)^{o'}C,$$
$$A_3 = AF_1'F_2^o, \qquad C_3 = G_1^{o'}C.$$

Now two important observations can be made based on these relations: $\mathcal{C}(C_1') = \mathcal{C}(C')$ and $\mathcal{C}(A_1 : A_2 : A_3) = \mathcal{C}(A)$. Therefore, the testing problem in Sect. 7.11 can be simplified, and only λ_2 and λ_3 in Proposition 7.8 (iii) and (iv) have to be considered. It follows that the likelihood ratio test for testing (7.90) against an arbitrary B is equivalent to (see (7.80))

$$\lambda^{\frac{2}{n}} = \frac{|\widehat{\Sigma}_{H_0}|}{|\widehat{\Sigma}_{H_1}|} = \frac{|\widehat{S}_3 + \widehat{Q}_3'\widehat{Q}_2'\widehat{Q}_1'XP_{C_3'}X'\widehat{Q}_1\widehat{Q}_2\widehat{Q}_3|}{|S + P'_{A^o,S^{-1}}XP_{C'}X'P_{A^o,S^{-1}}|}, \tag{7.92}$$

where $\widehat{Q}_3'\widehat{Q}_2'\widehat{Q}_1' = P'_{A^o,S_3^{-1}}$ and

$$\widehat{S}_3 = \widehat{S}_2 + P'_{(A_1:A_2)^o,\widehat{S}_2^{-1}}X(P_{C_2'} - P_{C_3'})X'P_{(A_1:A_2)^o,\widehat{S}_2^{-1}},$$
$$\widehat{S}_2 = S + P'_{A_1^o,S^{-1}}X(P_{C_1'} - P_{C_2'})X'P_{A_1^o,S^{-1}},$$
$$S = X(I - P_{C'})X'.$$

Moreover,

$$\lambda = \lambda_1\lambda_2,$$

where

$$\lambda_1^{\frac{2}{n}} = \frac{|\widehat{S}_2 + P'_{A^o,\widehat{S}_2^{-1}}XP_{C_2'}X'P_{A^o,\widehat{S}_2^{-1}}|}{|S + P'_{A^o,S^{-1}}XP_{C'}X'P_{A^o,S^{-1}}|}, \tag{7.93}$$

$$\lambda_2^{\frac{2}{n}} = \frac{|\widehat{S}_3 + P_{A^o,\widehat{S}_3^{-1}} X P_{C_3'} X' P_{A^o,\widehat{S}_3^{-1}}|}{|\widehat{S}_2 + P'_{A^o,\widehat{S}_2^{-1}} X P_{C_2'} X' P_{A^o,\widehat{S}_2^{-1}}|}, \tag{7.94}$$

leading to the next theorem.

Theorem 7.19 *For the BRM presented in Definition 2.1, let $F_1BG_1 = F_2\Theta G_2$ hold, where F_i and G_i, $i = 1, 2$, are known and Θ and B are unknown. Then the following statements can be made.*

(i) *Let λ_{1o} be the observed value of λ_1, given by (7.93) and used in the factorization of the likelihood ratio test, presented in (7.92). Put*

$$t_o = \tfrac{2}{n}(f - \tfrac{1}{2}(p_o - m + 1)) \ln \lambda_{1o},$$

where $f = n - r(C) - p + r(A)$, $p_o = r(A) - r(A(F_1')^o)$ and $m = r(C) - r(C_2)$. Moreover, let $c_1 = c_1(p_o, f, m)$ and $c_2 = c_2(p_o, f, m)$ be defined in Proposition 7.8. The hypothesis corresponding to the statistic λ_1 is rejected, approximately at significance level α, if t_o satisfies

$$P\{\chi^2_{p_om} \geq t_o\} + c_1(1 - c_1)(P\{\chi^2_{p_om+4} \geq t_o\} - P\{\chi^2_{p_om} \geq t_o\})$$
$$+ c_2(P\{\chi^2_{p_om+8} \geq t_o\} - P\{\chi^2_{p_om} \geq t_o\}) \leq \alpha.$$

(ii) *Let λ_{2o} be the observed value For λ_2, given by (7.94) and used in the factorization of the likelihood ratio test, presented in (7.92). Put*

$$t_o = \tfrac{2}{n}(f - \tfrac{1}{2}(p_o - m + 1)) \ln \lambda_{2o},$$

where $f = n - r(C) - p + r(A)$, $p_o = r(A) - r(A(F_1'F_2^o)^o)$ and $m = r(C_2) - r(C_3)$. Moreover, let $c_1 = c_1(p_o, f, m)$ and $c_2 = c_2(p_o, f, m)$ be defined in Proposition 7.8. The hypothesis corresponding to the statistic λ_2 is rejected, approximately at significance level α, if t_o satisfies

$$P\{\chi^2_{p_om} \geq t_o\} + c_1(1 - c_1)(P\{\chi^2_{p_om+4} \geq t_o\} - P\{\chi^2_{p_om} \geq t_o\})$$
$$+ c_2(P\{\chi^2_{p_om+8} \geq t_o\} - P\{\chi^2_{p_om} \geq t_o\}) \leq \alpha.$$

Problems

1 In the Potthoff and Roy (1964) data set presented in Table 1.2, remove the outlying individuals and perform significance tests to answer the following questions.

(i) Do the observations follow a linear growth model? (ii) Do the boys and the girls follow the same growth model?

2 In the Potthoff and Roy (1964) data set presented in Table 1.2, replace the outlying observations by trustworthy observations and perform significance tests to answer the following questions. (i) Do the observations follow a linear growth model? (ii) Do the boys and the girls follow the same growth model?

3 Construct a test, based on the likelihood ratio, for testing whether a GMANOVA + MANOVA model is a GMANOVA model (suppose an arbitrary dispersion matrix).

4 Construct a test, based on the likelihood ratio, for testing whether a GMANOVA + MANOVA model is a GMANOVA model if $\boldsymbol{\Sigma} = \sigma^2\boldsymbol{I}$, where σ^2 is unknown (Bai, 2009).

5 Copy Example 7.3, but choose some parameters $\boldsymbol{B}_i, i = 1, 2, 3$, and $\boldsymbol{\Sigma}$ other than those used in the example.

6 Why are $\boldsymbol{V}_1$ and $\boldsymbol{U}_1$, given by (7.61) and (7.62), respectively, independently distributed? Give a detailed explanation.

7 Perform the same tests as those described in Example 7.10, but remove individuals which are deemed to be outliers. Explain your choice of outliers for removal.

8 For the $EBRM_B^3$, construct a test for testing $\boldsymbol{F}_1\boldsymbol{B}_1\boldsymbol{G}_1 = \boldsymbol{F}_2\boldsymbol{B}_2\boldsymbol{G}_2$ in an $EBRM_B^3$ with the mean $E[\boldsymbol{X}] = \boldsymbol{A}_1\boldsymbol{B}_1\boldsymbol{C}_1 + \boldsymbol{A}_2\boldsymbol{B}_2\boldsymbol{C}_2 + \boldsymbol{A}_3\boldsymbol{B}_3\boldsymbol{C}_3$.

9 Prove at least two of the statements in Theorem 7.18.

10 Prove Theorem 7.19.

Literature

According to Cox and Hinkley (1974, p. 82), testing hypotheses have been performed for more than 200 years. A relatively deep discussion of significance testing was provided by Cox (1977), with insightful comments made by E. Spjøtvoll, S. Johansen, J.F. Bithell, W.R. van Zwet, O. Barndorff-Nielsen and M. Keuls. By the end of the nineteenth century, one was focusing on the problem of whether data fitted a specific distribution (followed a specific frequency curve), and Pearson (1900) (see also Plakett, 1983) came up with the chi-square test. Nowadays this test is also termed a goodness-of-fit test and it is a test which is carried out without an alternative hypothesis. Student (1908) derived the t-distribution in order to evaluate a mean in small samples, when the variation was estimated, which later became known as the t-test (see also Fisher, 1925, 1939). Over many years (1912–1922, approximately, see Aldrich, 1997), Fisher developed the likelihood theory, and this work culminated in the remarkable article, Fisher (1922), where many basic inferential concepts were introduced, including sufficiency (see also Fisher, 1920;

Stigler, 1973). A few years later in another seminal work, Neyman and Pearson (1928a,b) started to consider statistical testing through a null hypothesis and an alternative hypothesis (see also Neyman and Pearson (1933), where a complete theory was presented). Inspired by Fisher, Neyman and Pearson (1928a) proposed to use the ratio of the likelihood corresponding to the null hypothesis and the likelihood corresponding to the alternative hypothesis. Neyman and Pearson (1933) also considered Student's result and showed, under Student's assumptions, that the likelihood ratio test was equivalent to the t-test. The links between Fisher, Neyman and Pearson and Wald (1939), who replaced the power function by the loss function and created decision theory, are very interesting to study, but outside the scope of this book.

At the beginning of the 1930s, the Wishart distribution was available and Hotelling (1931) derived a multivariate version of the t-distribution. Therefore, it was natural that one started to work on multivariate testing problems. Wilks (1932) was successful when using the likelihood ratio test of Neyman and Pearson (1928a,b) together with the multivariate normal distribution. The Wilks statistic (Wilks, 1935) was quickly adopted by the statistical community and, among others, Bartlett (1934) and Hotelling (1936) used it (see also Bartlett, 1939). Rao (1948) gave an important overview of multivariate testing problems in various areas and in particular in discriminant analysis.

After Neyman and Pearson had formalized the testing of hypotheses, statistics could be used as a tool for decision making, which was not uncontroversial. From the 1950s onwards, testing in multivariate analysis became more common. Anderson (1951) studied multivariate problems which were not direct extensions of univariate problems, for example rank restrictions on parameters (today the term "reduced rank regression" is in use). For example, if there are three parameters, the hypothesis might be that the parameters follow a line instead of varying freely. In his article from 1951, Anderson applied the likelihood ratio test. S.N. Roy had for many years been working on the problem of composite hypothesis when he (Roy, 1953) introduced the union intersection procedure. This testing procedure has often been applied in multivariate analysis. Less known is the intersection union procedure. Lehmann (1952) introduced this procedure, but for multivariate testing problems, many open questions remain (e.g. see Berger and Sinclair, 1984; Berger, 1997). Moreover, in one of the first books on multivariate analysis, written by Roy (1957), the MANOVA model was treated together with a bilinear null hypothesis, i.e. H_0: $\boldsymbol{FBG} = \mathbf{0}$, where $\boldsymbol{F}$ and $\boldsymbol{G}$ are known matrices and $\boldsymbol{B}$ is the parameter matrix. The alternative hypothesis was that $\boldsymbol{B}$ is unrestricted. It is interesting that a precise likelihood ratio test could be carried out without estimating the parameters under the null hypothesis.

Khatri (1966) was the first to present the maximum likelihood estimators for the BRM. Moreover, in Khatri's article from 1966, the likelihood ratio test for testing H_0: $\boldsymbol{FBG} = \mathbf{0}$ in the BRM was derived, and some alternative types of test statistics were proposed (see also Pillai, 1955; Troskie, 1971). Among the tests which were obtained was one based on the union intersection procedure. All the derived test statistics are functions of eigenvalues of specific sums of squares matrices. However, there are some difficult results which are not easy to apply, for example exact non-null distributions for the likelihood ratio test statistic for testing H_0: $\boldsymbol{FBG} = \boldsymbol{0}$ (see Kabe (1975a) who followed Gleser and Olkin (1970), Nagarsenker (1977), Kabe (1986), Tang and Gupta (1986)). Asymptotic expansions of the non-null distributions of the statistics considered by Khatri (1966) were discussed by Fujikoshi (1973a,b, 1974a,b,c). A review of various test statistics, including the above-mentioned ones, was presented by De Waal (1976). In addition to the literature discussing the likelihood ratio testing in the BRM, there exists quite a large volume of literature connected to the test statistic Wilks Λ, its density under the null hypothesis, and its alternative hypothesis (see, for example, Gupta 1971; Hart and Money, 1975, 1976; Gupta and Nagar, 2000; Bekker et al., 2011). Moreover, connected to the Wilks Λ test statistic are beta distributions and multivariate beta distributions (see Appendix C in this book), as well as extensions of these distributions (newer references are Nadarajah, 2005; Pham-Gia, 2008).

For the performance of multivariate analysis and, of course, for the application of the BRM and its extensions, simultaneous test procedures are of interest and results have been presented by Krishnaiah (1969, 1975). Newer works, however, mostly consider simultaneous confidence intervals for multiple comparisons (e.g. see Seo and Kanda, 1996). An interesting area of application for growth curve analysis and testing is profile analysis (see Srivastava, 1987; Ohlson and Srivastava, 2010; Seo et al., 2011).

Concerning information about testing in the BRM or $EBRM_\bullet^k$, an outstanding work from a theoretical point of view is a monograph by Kariya (1985). This monograph includes theory about the statistical tests in these models which is based on a discussion of a joint application of sufficiency and invariance. The basic ideas go back to Gleser and Olkin (1970) and Kariya (1978) (see also Giri and Das, 1988), which in turn relied on older material. The following steps for testing in the BRM were presented by Kariya (1985) (see also Muirhead, 1982, pp. 520–525): (i) consider a "natural" sufficient statistic; (ii) find the largest group which leaves the testing problem invariant; (iii) choose a convenient maximal invariant under the group found; (iv) derive the distribution of the maximal invariant; (v) derive the uniform most powerful invariant test or locally best invariant test, etc.; (vi) derive an approximate distribution of the test statistic under the null hypothesis. Gleser and Olkin (1970) reduced the BRM to its canonical form (inspired by Hsu, 1941). Then it is easy to identify the sufficient statistic, i.e. a canonical version of ($\boldsymbol{XC}'(\boldsymbol{CC}')^-$, $\boldsymbol{S}$) and show that the statistic is not complete. Using the group considered by Gleser and Olkin (1970), Banken (1984) presented an explicit expression of the maximal invariant. Moreover, Kariya (1978) studied a larger group (see also Muirhead, 1982, p. 524) than that studied by Gleser and Olkin (1970), and this larger group was shown by Banken (1986) to be the largest group which leaves the testing problem invariant. In Kariya (1985), locally most powerful invariant tests were presented. A most interesting and advanced article is that by Andersson et al. (1993), where mathematically bilinear regression models were described via the general block-triangular group and invariance. The authors mentioned that the models belonged to the class of the so-called totally ordered linear models (nested models) which they introduced. Andersson et al. (1993) presented some results concerning likelihood ratio testing, but their main focus was directed on estimation. However, it is quite clear that through factorization of the likelihood various types of likelihood ratio test could have been produced. For a few examples of likelihood ratio tests, see Fujikoshi et al. (1999).

In this chapter, it is assumed that the random variables corresponding to the observations are normally distributed. However, test statistics are often true under broader classes of distributions; for example in addition to the normal distribution, tests can also be valid for heavy-tailed distributions. If a test statistic can be used for other distributions than the normal distribution, the test is deemed to be robust. Results for the BRM can be found in Kariya and Sinha (1985, 1989), who considered the locally best invariant tests which Kariya (1978) had obtained; see also Khatri (1988) as well as Giri and Das (1988), where an $EBRM_{\bullet}^{m}$ was considered (we also refer to Yanagihara, 2001, 2007).

Kabe (1975b) considered the test H_0: $\boldsymbol{F}_1\boldsymbol{B}\boldsymbol{G}_1 = \boldsymbol{0}$, given $\boldsymbol{F}_2\boldsymbol{B}\boldsymbol{G}_2 = \boldsymbol{0}$, without any nested subspace condition, for example $\mathcal{C}(\boldsymbol{F}_1') \subseteq \mathcal{C}(\boldsymbol{F}_1')$, as in Sect. 7.4 (see also Kabe, 1981; Giri and Das, 1988). This means that Kabe's test cannot be a likelihood ratio test. In Sects. 7.8 and 7.9, a so-called trace test was presented for some of the testing problems treated previously via the likelihood ratio. Originally the trace test was introduced by Hamid et al. (2011). A problem with this test is the approximation of its distribution, which is a weighted sum of chi-square variables which are not necessarily independently distributed. This is an old problem; see for example, Kotz et al. (1967a,b), Solomon and Stephens (1977), Gabler and Wolff (1987) or Castaño-Martínez and López-Blázquez (2005), which is a more recently published article.

In this chapter, it has often been emphasized that one should distinguish between the observations of a random variable and the random variable (statistic) itself. In the theory presented, the mathematics sometimes consists of replacing random variables by observations and vice versa. However, there are several articles which provide expressions which combine random variables with their corresponding observed realizations for the purpose of handling nuisance parameters when one is performing hypothesis testing and predictions. For example, the concept of generalized p-values has been introduced (see e.g. Tsui and Weerahandi, 1989; Weerahandi, 2004; Nkurunziza and Chen, 2011; Mathew et al., 2016).

References

Aldrich, J. (1997). R. A. Fisher and the making of maximum likelihood 1912–1922. *Statistical Sciences, 12*, 162–176.

Anderson, T. W. (1951). Estimating linear restrictions on regression coefficients for multivariate normal distributions. *Annals of Mathematical Statistics, 22*, 327–351.

Andersson, S. A., Marden, J. I., & Perlman, M. D. (1993). Totally ordered multivariate linear models. *Sankhyā, Series A, 55*, 370–394.

Bai, P. (2009). Sphericity test in a GMANOVA-MANOVA model with normal error. *Journal of Multivariate Analysis, 100*, 2305–2312.
Banken, L. (1984). *On the reduction of the general MANOVA model*. Technical report, University of Trier, Trier.
Banken, L. (1986). The greatest invariance-group of multivariate models. *Journal of Multivariate Analysis, 19*, 156–161.
Bartlett, M. S. (1934). On the theory of statistical regression. *Proceedings of the Royal Society of Edinburgh, 53*, 260–283.
Bartlett, M. S. (1939). A note on tests of significance in multivariate analysis. *Mathematical Proceedings of the Cambridge Philosophical Society, 35*, 180–185.
Bekker, A., Roux, J. J. J., & Arashi, M. (2011). Exact nonnull distribution of Wilks' statistic: The ratio and product of independent components. *Journal of Multivariate Analysis, 102*, 619–628.
Berger, R. L. (1997). Likelihood ratio tests and intersection-union tests. In *Advances in statistical decision theory and applications* (pp. 225–237). *Statistics for industry and technology*. Boston: Birkhäuser Boston.
Berger, R. L., & Sinclair, D. F. (1984). Testing hypotheses concerning unions of linear subspaces. *Journal of the American Statistical Association, 79*, 158–163.
Castaño-Martínez, A., & López-Blázquez, F. (2005). Distribution of a sum of weighted central chi-square variables. *Communications in Statistics: Theory and Methods, 34*, 515–524.
Cox, D. R. (1977). The role of significance tests. With discussion and reply. *Scandinavian Journal of Statistics, 4*, 49–70.
Cox, D. R., & Hinkley, D. V. (1974). *Theoretical statistics*. London: Chapman and Hall.
De Waal, D. J. (1976). A review of tests of various hypotheses in multivariate statistical analysis. *South African Statistical Journal, 10*, 153–175.
Fisher, R. A. (1920). A mathematical examination of the methods of determining the accuracy of an observation by the mean error, and by the mean square error. *Monthly Notices of the Royal Astronomical Society, 80*, 758–770.
Fisher, R. A. (1922). On the mathematical foundations of theoretical statistics. *Philosophical Transactions of the Royal Society A, 222*, 309–368.
Fisher, R. A. (1925). Applications of "Student's" distribution. *Metron, 5*, 90–104.
Fisher, R. A. (1939). "Student". *Annals of Eugenics, 9*, 1–9.
Fujikoshi, Y. (1973a). Asymptotic formulas for the distributions of three statistics for multivariate linear hypothesis. *Annals of the Institute of Statistical Mathematics, 25*, 423–437.
Fujikoshi, Y. (1973b). Monotonicity of the power functions of some tests in general MANOVA models. *Annals of Statistics, 1*, 388–391.
Fujikoshi, Y. (1974a). Asymptotic expansions of the non-null distributions of three statistics in GMANOVA. *Annals of the Institute of Statistical Mathematics, 26*, 289–297.
Fujikoshi, Y. (1974b). The likelihood ratio tests for the dimensionality of regression coefficients. *Journal of Multivariate Analysis, 4*, 327–340.
Fujikoshi, Y. (1974c). On the asymptotic non-null distributions of the LR criterion in a general MANOVA. *Canadian Journal of Statistics, 2*, 1–12.
Fujikoshi, Y., Kanda, T., & Ohtaki, M. (1999) Growth curve model with hierarchical within-individuals design matrices. *Annals of the Institute of Statistical Mathematics, 51*, 707–721.
Gabler, S., & Wolff, C. (1987). A quick and easy approximation to the distribution of a sum of weighted chi-square variables. *Statistische Hefte, 28*, 317–325.
Giri, N., & Das, K. (1988). On a robust test of the extended GMANOVA problem in elliptically symmetric distributions. *Sankhyā, Series A, 50*, 234–248.
Gleser, L. J., & Olkin, I. (1970). Linear models in multivariate analysis. In *Essays in probability and statistics* (pp. 267–292). Chapel Hill: University of North Carolina Press.
Gupta, A. K. (1971). Noncentral distribution of Wilks' statistic in MANOVA. *Annals of Mathematical Statistics, 42*, 1254–1261.
Gupta, A. K., & Nagar, D. K. (2000). *Matrix variate distributions* (Vol. 104). *Chapman and Hall/CRC monographs and surveys in pure and applied mathematics*. Boca Raton: Chapman and Hall/CRC.

Hamid, J. S., Beyene, J., & von Rosen, D. (2011). A novel trace test for the mean parameters in a multivariate growth curve model. *Journal of Multivariate Analysis, 102*, 238–251.

Hart, M. L., & Money, A. H. (1975). Exact powers for the linear case of Wilks' likelihood ratio criterion. *South African Statistical Journal, 9*, 11–26.

Hart, M. L., & Money, A. H. (1976). On Wilk's multivariate generalization of the correlation ratio. *Biometrika, 63*, 59–67.

Hotelling, H. (1931). The generalization of Student's ratio. *Annals of Mathematical Statistics, 2*, 360–378.

Hotelling, H. (1936). Relations between two sets of variates. *Biometrika, 28*, 321–377.

Hsu, P. L. (1941). Canonical reduction of the general regression problem. *Annals of Eugenics, 11*, 42–46.

Kabe, D. G. (1975a). Some results for the GMANOVA model. *Communications in Statistics, 4*, 813–820.

Kabe, D. G. (1975b). Generalized MANOVA double linear hypothesis with double linear restrictions. *Canadian Journal of Statistics, 3*, 35–44.

Kabe, D. G. (1981). MANOVA double linear hypothesis with double linear restrictions. *Communications in Statistics: Theory and Methods, 10*, 2545–2550.

Kabe, D. G. (1986). On a GMANOVA model likelihood ratio test criterion. *Communications in Statistics: Theory and Methods, 15*, 3419–3427.

Kariya, T. (1978). The general MANOVA problem. *Annals of Statistics, 6*, 200–214.

Kariya, T. (1985). *Testing in the multivariate general linear model*. New York: Kinokuniya.

Kariya, T., & Sinha, B. K. (1985). Nonnull and optimality robustness of some tests. *Annals of Statistics, 13*, 1182–1197.

Kariya, T., & Sinha, B. K. (1989). *Robustness of statistical tests. Statistical modeling and decision science*. Boston: Academic.

Khatri, C. G. (1966). A note on a MANOVA model applied to problems in growth curves. *Annals of the Institute of Statistical Mathematics, 18*, 75–86.

Khatri, C. G. (1988). Robustness study for a linear growth model. *Journal of Multivariate Analysis, 24*, 66–87.

Kotz, S., Johnson, N. L., & Boyd, D. W. (1967a). Series representations of distributions of quadratic forms in normal variables. I. Central case. *Annals of Mathematical Statistics, 38*, 823–837.

Kotz, S., Johnson, N. L., & Boyd, D. W. (1967b). Series representations of distributions of quadratic forms in normal variables. II. Non-central case. *Annals of Mathematical Statistics, 38*, 838–848.

Krishnaiah, P. R. (1969). Simultaneous test procedures under general MANOVA models. In *Multivariate Analysis, II. Proceedings of the Second International Symposium, Dayton, OH, 1968* (pp. 121–143). New York: Academic.

Krishnaiah, P. R. (1975). Simultaneous tests for multiple comparisons of growth curves when errors are autocorrelated. In *Proceedings of the 40th Session of the International Statistical Institute* (pp. 62–66). *Bulletin of the International Statistical Institute*. Contributed papers.

Lehmann, E. L. (1952). Testing multiparameter hypotheses. *Annals of Mathematical Statistics, 23*, 541–552.

Mathew, T., Menon, S., Perevozskaya, I., & Weerahandi, S. (2016). Improved prediction intervals in heteroscedastic mixed-effects models. *Statistics & Probability Letters, 114*, 48–53.

Muirhead, R. J. (1982). *Aspects of multivariate statistical theory*. New York: Wiley.

Nadarajah, S. (2005). Sums, products, and ratios of noncentral beta variables. *Communications in Statistics: Theory and Methods, 34*, 89–100.

Nagarsenker, B. N. (1977). On the exact non-null distributions of the LR criterion in a general MANOVA model. *Sankhyā, Series A, 39*, 251–263.

Neyman, J., & Pearson, E. S. (1928a). On the use and interpretation of certain test criteria for purposes of statistical inference: Part I. *Biometrika, 20A*, 175–240.

Neyman, J., & Pearson, E. S. (1928b). On the use and interpretation of certain test criteria for purposes of statistical inference: Part II. *Biometrika, 20A*, 263–294.

Neyman, J., & Pearson, E. S. (1933). On the problem of the most efficient tests of statistical hypotheses. *Philosophical Transactions of the Royal Society, 231*, 289–337.
Nkurunziza, S., & Chen, F. (2011). Generalized confidence interval and p-value in location and scale family. *Sankhyā, Series B, 73*, 218–240.
Ohlson, M., & Srivastava, M. S. (2010). Profile analysis for a growth curve model. *Journal of the Japan Statistical Society, 40*, 1–21.
Pearson, K. (1900). On the criterion that a given system of deviations from the probable in the case of a correlated system of variables is such that it can be reasonably supposed to have arisen from random sampling. *Philosophical Magazine, 50*, 157–175. Reprinted in K. Pearson (1956). *Karl Pearson's early statistical papers* (pp. 339–357). Cambridge: Cambridge University Press.
Pham-Gia, T. (2008). Exact distribution of the generalized Wilks's statistic and applications. *Journal of Multivariate Analysis, 99*, 1698–1716.
Pillai, K. C. S. (1955). Some new test criteria in multivariate analysis. *Annals of Mathematical Statistics, 26*, 117–121.
Plakett, R. L. (1983). Karl Pearson and the chi-squared test. *International Statistical Review, 51*, 59–72.
Potthoff, R. F., & Roy, S. N. (1964). A generalized multivariate analysis of variance model useful especially for growth curve problems. *Biometrika, 51*, 313–326.
Rao, C. R. (1948). Tests of significance in multivariate analysis. *Biometrika, 35*, 58–79.
Roy, S. N. (1953). On a heuristic method of test construction and its use in multivariate analysis. *Annals of Mathematical Statistics, 24*, 220–238.
Roy, S. N. (1957). *Some aspects of multivariate analysis*. New York/Calcutta: Wiley/Indian Statistical Institute.
Seo, T., & Kanda, T. (1996). Multiple comparison in the GMANOVA model with covariance structures. *Journal of the Japan Statistical Society, 26*, 47–58.
Seo, T., Sakurai, T., & Fujikoshi, Y. (2011). LR tests for two hypotheses in profile analysis of growth curve data. *SUT Journal of Mathematics, 47*, 105–118.
Solomon, H., & Stephens, M. A. (1977). Distribution of a sum of weighted chi-square variables. *Journal of the American Statistical Association, 72*, 881–885.
Srivastava, M. S. (1987). Profile analysis of several groups. *Communications in Statistics: Theory and Methods, 16*, 909–926.
Stigler, S. M. (1973). Laplace, Fisher and the discovery of the concept of sufficiency. *Biometrika, 60*, 439–445.
Student. (1908). The probable error of a mean. *Biometrika, 6*, 1–25.
Tang, J., & Gupta, A. K. (1986). Exact distribution of certain general test statistics in multivariate analysis. *Australian Journal of Statistics, 28*, 107–114.
Troskie, C. G. (1971). The distributions of some test criteria in multivariate analysis. *Annals of Mathematical Statistics, 42*, 1752–1757.
Tsui, K.-W., & Weerahandi, S. (1989). Generalized p-values in significance testing of hypotheses in the presence of nuisance parameters. *Journal of the American Statistical Association, 84*, 602–607.
Wald, A. (1939). Contributions to the theory of statistical estimation and testing hypotheses. *Annals of Mathematical Statistics, 10*, 299–326.
Weerahandi, S. (2004). *Generalized inference in repeated measures. Exact methods in MANOVA and mixed models. Wiley series in probability and statistics*. Hoboken: Wiley-Interscience.
Wilks, S. S. (1932). Certain generalizations in the analysis of variance. *Biometrika, 24*, 471–494.
Wilks, S. S. (1935). On the independence of k sets of normally distributed statistical variables. *Econometrica, 3*, 309–326.
Yanagihara, H. (2001). Asymptotic expansions of the null distributions of three test statistics in a nonnormal GMANOVA model. *Hiroshima Mathematical Journal, 31*, 213–262.
Yanagihara, H. (2007). Conditions for robustness to nonnormality on test statistics in a GMANOVA model. *Journal of the Japan Statistical Society, 37*, 135–155.

References [illegible]

Neyman [illegible] Pearson [illegible] (1933). On the problem of the most efficient tests of statistical hypotheses. [illegible] Transactions of the Royal Society [illegible], 231, 289–337.
Nadarajah [illegible] (2005). [illegible] generalized [illegible] with [illegible] location and scale [illegible], 32, [illegible]–240.
[illegible] (2010). [illegible] analysis for test [illegible] model. Journal of the [illegible] Association, [illegible]
[illegible] K. (1900). On the criterion that a given system of deviations from the probable in the case of a correlated system of variables is such that it can be reasonably supposed to have arisen from random sampling. Philosophical Magazine, 50, 157–175. [illegible] in K. Pearson (1956). Karl Pearson's Early Statistical Papers, pp. 339–357. Cambridge: Cambridge University Press.
Pillai, K. C. S. (1955). [illegible] the general [illegible] Wilks' [illegible] and applications. Annals of Mathematical Statistics, [illegible], 117–[illegible].
[illegible] (1956). [illegible] in multivariate analysis. Journal of Multivariate [illegible] Statistics, [illegible], 1–[illegible].
[illegible] (1951). [illegible] Journal of the Royal Statistical Society, Series B, [illegible]
Rencher, A. C. [illegible] (1992). [illegible] multivariate analysis of variance model [illegible] Biometrics, 48, 1–[illegible].
[illegible] (1946). [illegible] multivariate analysis. Biometrika, 33, [illegible]–79.
Roy, S. N. (1953). On a heuristic method of test construction and its use in multivariate analysis. Annals of Mathematical Statistics, 24, 220–238.
Roy, S. N. (1957). Some Aspects of Multivariate Analysis. New York: Wiley; Calcutta: Indian Statistical Institute.
[illegible] (2005). [illegible] MANOVA [illegible] model with [illegible] covariance [illegible]
[illegible] (2014). [illegible] analysis of [illegible] Multivariate Analysis, [illegible], 1–[illegible].
Solomon, [illegible] (1970). [illegible] chi-square [illegible] test [illegible]
Srivastava, M. S. (198[illegible]). [illegible] of the [illegible] in [illegible] Statistical Methods, [illegible]
Sugiura, N. [illegible] (19[illegible]). [illegible] Laplace [illegible] and [illegible] series [illegible] distribution of the [illegible]
Student (1908). The probable error of a mean. Biometrika, 6, 1–25.
Tsai, [illegible] (20[illegible]). [illegible] for the [illegible] in [illegible] and [illegible] Computer [illegible]
[illegible] (195[illegible]). [illegible] Annals of Mathematical Statistics, [illegible], [illegible]–276.
[illegible] (19[illegible]). [illegible] generalized [illegible] significance test for [illegible] multivariate [illegible] of [illegible] Statistical Association, [illegible]
Wald, A. (1939). [illegible] estimation [illegible] testing hypotheses. Annals of Mathematical Statistics, 10, 299–326.
Welch, [illegible] (19[illegible]). [illegible] generalized [illegible] Biometrika, [illegible]
[illegible] MANOVA [illegible] Wiley [illegible]
Wilks, S. S. (1932). Certain generalizations in the analysis of variance. Biometrika, 24, 471–494.
Wishart, J. (1928). The generalised product moment distribution in samples from a normal multivariate population. Biometrika, 20A, 32–52.
[illegible] (2004). [illegible] the [illegible] of three test statistics in [illegible] MANOVA. [illegible] Journal of Mathematical [illegible], 213–2[illegible].
Yao, [illegible] (20[illegible]). [illegible] test in a MANOVA [illegible] Journal of Multivariate Analysis, [illegible]

Chapter 8
Influential Observations

8.1 Introduction

Via experiments or observational studies, statistical samples are obtained. Ideally all the observations of a sample should contribute equally to the statistics of interest. However, it is a common knowledge among statisticians that this is not usually the case, and some observations are definitely more "influential" than others when, for example, one is calculating an estimate or performing a statistical test. If the significance of a statistical test stems from a few observations, this is usually not satisfactory. Thus, over the years, methodologies have emerged for quantifying observations to make it possible to rank them with respect to their influence.

One basic problem is that there is no general agreement as to what an influential observation is; i.e. there is no commonly accepted definition of an influence measure. This is, of course, not so remarkable since different aspects are considered in different studies, and the choice of aspects to be focused on depends on the aims of the study. Alternatively, if one is concerned about the possibility that some observations may spoil the inference, one should perhaps apply some robust approach as a complement to the main approach, or sometimes one's main approach should be to apply a robust method. However, using robust methods by default may, for certain problems, lead to important information being hidden. Moreover, influential observations may be deviating observations, and it is always appropriate to identify deviating observations to determine the reason for their deviation, as well as to understand why they become influential.

There are at least three possible reasons why observations become influential; (1) gross errors due to data processing; (2) by chance the observations are connected to the tail of the corresponding distribution; (3) the statistical model does not fit the data and therefore some observations become influential. Covering all the possible cases with one analysis seems impossible.

Thus, one of the main issues is to decide what we mean by "influential observations". The first step in accomplishing this is to determine the statistic of

D. von Rosen, *Bilinear Regression Analysis*, Lecture Notes in Statistics 220,
https://doi.org/10.1007/978-3-319-78784-8_8

interest, which, for example, can be an estimate, a test, a predicted observation or, in general, some function of a statistic. A traditional method of handling influential observations has been to define them via case deletion; i.e. observations are deleted one by one. Applying this method, outlying observations are mainly considered and, according to some measure, one investigates which observation has the greatest impact, for example on a specific estimate. The observation with the greatest impact is deemed to be the most influential observation. However, this is not the only way of dealing with influence and sometimes case deletion does not provide enough information. In the literature, the most commonly applied alternative approaches are based on some perturbation of the observations or design variables and a subsequent study of the effect of the perturbation. An extreme action based on perturbation is to remove an observation from the analysis. In our opinion, one should remove an observation if it is not trustworthy, but keep the observation if it seems to be in the tail of a distribution. Thus, it seems beneficial not to base an influence measure on the deletion of observations. There are also other possible reasons for an observation becoming influential and some will appear later. Moreover, observations are realizations of random processes and, therefore, the exact value of the realization of a continuous random variable is rather artificial. Hence, it can be advantageous to utilize the observation in some analysis after a perturbation has taken place and study the effect of the perturbation. In this chapter the approach of perturbing observations is implemented. It is worth reflecting on whether the observations should support the model or the model should fit the observations.

Usually statistical analysis concerns models and methods for analysing those models. For example, we may have a linear model where the parameters are estimated through the least squares criterion or the likelihood function. It is definitely important to understand how single observations affect a statistic. On the other hand, as noted above, if we are afraid that there are many observations which may have a strong effect, an alternative robust estimation method can be used. We now formalize the perturbation analysis to a higher degree and note that it consists of two main ingredients:

- a perturbation scheme;
- one or several evaluation criteria.

Comparing the perturbation scheme with the design of an experiment, one can state that while the design of an experiment governs the performance of the experiment and the analysis of the data, the perturbation scheme governs the evaluation of the analysis after it has been carried out. Depending on the choice of scheme, we can draw different types of conclusions about the performed analysis. In addition to creating a perturbation scheme, it may also be appropriate to put certain restrictions on the perturbations. For example, if parameters can be explicitly estimated without a perturbation, one should naturally use a perturbation scheme which guarantees that explicit estimates are also obtained after a perturbation has been applied. In perturbation analysis within mixed linear models, this type of restriction makes sense.

Concerning the second main ingredient of the perturbation analysis, there are several ways to evaluate a perturbation. Below we consider an estimate to be a function of one or several perturbed observations. A function where the argument includes perturbed observations is naturally exploited by a Taylor series expansion with respect to the perturbation, but, of course, there are also alternative methods which are not based on a Taylor series expansion. Previously, in Chap. 5, density approximations were used which, in fact, were based on a Taylor series expansion of the cumulant generating function, and when performing Taylor series expansions in this chapter, the same techniques can be applied. Therefore, the proposed influence analysis is based on the terms in the Taylor series expansion. Moreover, it can be noted that all the terms can be obtained through differentiation.

Next the perturbations used in this chapter are described further and the purpose of the perturbation scheme is explained. Perturbation schemes provide a scientific basis for the exploitation and analysis of data.

Definition 8.1 Let Ω be a space which includes all the perturbations of a certain type, i.e. $\{\omega_i\}$, together with an algorithm which governs how $\{\omega_i\}$ is applied to the model. Moreover, let $\widehat{\boldsymbol{\theta}}(\{\omega_i\})$ denote an estimate of $\boldsymbol{\theta}$, a parameter in the statistical model, under a set of perturbations $\{\omega_i\}$. Then Ω is a perturbation scheme if there is a null perturbation, $\{\omega_0\} \subseteq \{\omega_i\}$, such that $\widehat{\boldsymbol{\theta}}(\{\omega_0\})$ equals $\widehat{\boldsymbol{\theta}}$ in the unperturbed model.

Note that in the definition the estimate can be replaced by a test statistic or any other statistic of interest.

In the following, instead of $\{\omega_i\}$, the vector notation $\boldsymbol{\omega}$ will be used, because the latter alternative is more suitable for showing which calculations are taking place. The definition is slightly academic, but via the null perturbation the perturbation scheme can be evaluated, e.g. as mentioned above via a Taylor series expansion.

Sometimes it is appropriate to stipulate more conditions in addition to the mere existence of a null perturbation. For example, one possible condition is that $\widehat{\boldsymbol{\theta}}(\boldsymbol{\omega})$ should be differentiable with respect to $\boldsymbol{\omega}$, or that a perturbation $\boldsymbol{\omega}_1$ exists such that $\widehat{\boldsymbol{\theta}}(\boldsymbol{\omega}_1)$ equals $\widehat{\boldsymbol{\theta}}$, but now the estimate is calculated via a subset of all the observations. In the next section, these ideas are illustrated. Note that in this chapter we do not distinguish between random variables and their corresponding observations (because of the notational burden that would be involved). The golden rule, however, is that only observed values are perturbed.

8.2 Influence Analysis in Univariate Linear Models

Let us recall the univariate linear model introduced in Example 1.1:

$$\boldsymbol{x}' = \boldsymbol{\beta}'\boldsymbol{C} + \boldsymbol{e}', \qquad \boldsymbol{e} \sim N_n(\boldsymbol{0}, \sigma^2\boldsymbol{I}_n), \tag{8.1}$$

where $\boldsymbol{x} : n \times 1$, $\boldsymbol{C} : k \times n$ and $\boldsymbol{\beta} : k \times 1$ is to be estimated. Moreover, σ^2 is an unknown scalar and the model states that we have n independent observations. There exist several ways to make alterations in the assumptions. In this section and the following sections, we study the following three choices of perturbation of some elements in $\boldsymbol{x}$, $\boldsymbol{C}$, and both $\boldsymbol{x}$ and $\boldsymbol{C}$ together. All of these perturbations are based on a perturbation, $\boldsymbol{\omega}$, which in this book is usually a scalar ω.

Definition 8.2 For the model in (8.1) the following perturbations can take place.

(i) Let $\boldsymbol{z} = \boldsymbol{x} + \omega \boldsymbol{v}$, where $\boldsymbol{v}$ is a known vector to be specified in advance.
(ii) Let $\boldsymbol{G} = \boldsymbol{C} + \omega \boldsymbol{V}$, where $\boldsymbol{V}$ is a known matrix to be specified in advance.
(iii) Let $\boldsymbol{x}'$ consist of $\{\boldsymbol{x}_0', \sqrt{\omega}\boldsymbol{x}_i'\}$ and let $\boldsymbol{C}$ consist of $\{\boldsymbol{C}_0, \sqrt{\omega}\boldsymbol{C}_i'\}$, where $\boldsymbol{x}_i$ and $\boldsymbol{C}_i$ are subsets of perturbed elements of $\boldsymbol{x}$ and corresponding perturbed columns of $\boldsymbol{C}$, respectively, and $\boldsymbol{x}_0$ and $\boldsymbol{C}_0$ are unperturbed elements and columns of $\boldsymbol{x}$ and $\boldsymbol{C}$, respectively.

In the alternatives of Definition 8.2 it is easy to identify particular actions which take place and are part of the algorithm mentioned in Definition 8.1, i.e. addition or square root multiplication by ω. However, Definition 8.2 (i)–(iii) do not specify completely the perturbation scheme, because as yet no complete algorithm has been presented. One choice of algorithm in the case of Perturbation (iii), for example, would involve this perturbation taking place for each independent observation, after which an estimate would be delivered which would include the perturbed observation. Furthermore, note that Perturbations (i) and (ii) have fairly natural interpretations. In Perturbation (i), we study the impact of changing the observation, i.e. adding some (small) quantity to $\boldsymbol{x}$, and it is easy to interpret the results. Since $\boldsymbol{x}$ is a realization of a random variable, it is important to determine whether small changes in $\boldsymbol{x}$ will affect the statistic under consideration. In Perturbation (ii), we have changed the design, which is useful when, for example, one is planning new experiments. Perturbation (ii) can also be used if the values in $\boldsymbol{C}$ are not exact, for instance to follow-up the effect of round-off errors. Moreover, in Perturbations (i) and (ii), we use an additive perturbation, whereas in Perturbation (iii) some rescaling is performed, meaning that the variation is perturbed. Thus, Perturbations (i)–(iii) deal with various types of influence. When performing maximum likelihood estimation and individual perturbations, all three perturbations satisfy Definition 8.1. In Perturbations (i) and (ii), $\omega_0 = 0$, whereas in Perturbation (iii), $\omega_0 = 1$. Note also that in Perturbation (iii), $\omega = 0$ means that observations are excluded from the analysis.

Let $\widehat{\boldsymbol{\beta}}$, $\widehat{\boldsymbol{\beta}}_z(\omega)$ $\widehat{\boldsymbol{\beta}}_G(\omega)$ and $\widehat{\boldsymbol{\beta}}_{x_0}(\omega)$ denote the maximum likelihood estimates of $\boldsymbol{\beta}$, where unperturbed observations have been used, as well as perturbed observations according to Perturbations (i)–(iii), respectively. Then, under full rank conditions,

$$\text{(i)} \quad \widehat{\boldsymbol{\beta}}' = \boldsymbol{x}'\boldsymbol{C}'(\boldsymbol{C}\boldsymbol{C}')^{-1}; \tag{8.2}$$

$$\text{(ii)} \quad \widehat{\boldsymbol{\beta}}_z'(\omega) = \widehat{\boldsymbol{\beta}}' + \omega \boldsymbol{v}'\boldsymbol{C}'(\boldsymbol{C}\boldsymbol{C}')^{-1}; \tag{8.3}$$

$$\text{(iii)}\quad \widehat{\boldsymbol{\beta}}'_G(\omega) = \boldsymbol{x}'\boldsymbol{G}'(\boldsymbol{G}\boldsymbol{G}')^{-1} = (\boldsymbol{x}'\boldsymbol{C}' + \omega\boldsymbol{x}'\boldsymbol{V}')(\boldsymbol{G}\boldsymbol{G}')^{-1}; \tag{8.4}$$

$$\text{(iv)}\quad \widehat{\boldsymbol{\beta}}'_{x0}(\omega) = (\boldsymbol{x}'_0\boldsymbol{C}'_0 + \omega\boldsymbol{x}'_i\boldsymbol{C}'_i)(\boldsymbol{C}_0\boldsymbol{C}'_0 + \omega\boldsymbol{C}_i\boldsymbol{C}'_i)^{-1}. \tag{8.5}$$

Thus, it follows that $\widehat{\boldsymbol{\beta}} = \widehat{\boldsymbol{\beta}}_z(0) = \widehat{\boldsymbol{\beta}}_G(0) = \widehat{\boldsymbol{\beta}}_{x0}(1)$ and it has been demonstrated that for each of the perturbations, according to Definition 8.1, besides the algorithm, a perturbation scheme has been constructed. In the next step the perturbation scheme is completed by specifying $\boldsymbol{v}$, $\boldsymbol{V}$, $\boldsymbol{x}_0$, $\boldsymbol{x}_i$, $\boldsymbol{C}_0$ and $\boldsymbol{C}_i$, and we will keep in mind that each individual will be perturbed separately. For example,

- $\boldsymbol{v} = \boldsymbol{e}_i$, where $\boldsymbol{e}_i$ is the unit basis vector of size n;
- $\boldsymbol{V} = (\boldsymbol{0} : \boldsymbol{1}_k : \boldsymbol{0})$, where $\boldsymbol{1}_k$ stands on the ith position;
- $\boldsymbol{x}_0$ is identical to $\boldsymbol{x}$, except for the ith element, which has been removed;
- $\boldsymbol{x}_i$ is the ith element, i.e. $\boldsymbol{x}_i = x_i$, where $\boldsymbol{x} = (x_i)$;
- $\boldsymbol{C}_0$ is identical to $\boldsymbol{C}$, except for the ith column, which has been removed;
- $\boldsymbol{C}_i$ is the ith column, i.e. $\boldsymbol{C}_i = \boldsymbol{c}_i$, where $\boldsymbol{C} = (\boldsymbol{c}_i)$.

Now the effects of all the perturbations in Definition 8.2 are investigated, one by one. The overall objective to keep in mind is that we are to determine whether there is any particular observation which in a pronounced way is more influential than the other observations.

With regard to Perturbation (i), it follows from (8.3) and the particular choice of $\boldsymbol{V}$ that the perturbation effect is linear and that it is largest when $\boldsymbol{e}'_i\boldsymbol{C}' = \boldsymbol{c}'_i$ is "largest", where $\boldsymbol{c}_i$ is the ith column of $\boldsymbol{C}$, which corresponds to the ith observation. Note that in the case of Perturbation (i), even if $\boldsymbol{x}$ is perturbed, we are only concerned with the design and not with what has been observed. Therefore, the remaining task is to compare the columns $\boldsymbol{c}_i$. This can be performed in many ways, for example by comparing $\boldsymbol{c}'_i\boldsymbol{c}_i$ or $\boldsymbol{c}'_i(\boldsymbol{C}\boldsymbol{C}')^{-1}\boldsymbol{c}_i$. However, from a statistical point of view, it is more appropriate to consider $\boldsymbol{c}'_i(\boldsymbol{C}\boldsymbol{C}')^{-1}\boldsymbol{c}_i$, since, among other things, it is invariant under non-singular linear transformations. From (8.1),

$$\boldsymbol{x}' = \boldsymbol{\beta}'\boldsymbol{T}^{-1}\boldsymbol{T}\boldsymbol{C} + \boldsymbol{e}', \qquad \boldsymbol{e} \sim N_n(\boldsymbol{0}, \sigma^2\boldsymbol{I}_n),$$

where $\boldsymbol{T}$ is non-singular and which bears the same information as the model in (8.1). Moreover, it should be immaterial whether one studies $\boldsymbol{\beta}'\boldsymbol{T}^{-1}$ or $\boldsymbol{\beta}$, which means that the result of any influence analysis should be the same whether it is based on $\boldsymbol{C}$ or $\boldsymbol{T}\boldsymbol{C}$. Fortunately,

$$\boldsymbol{c}'_i(\boldsymbol{C}\boldsymbol{C}')^{-1}\boldsymbol{c}_i = \boldsymbol{c}'_i\boldsymbol{T}'(\boldsymbol{T}\boldsymbol{C}\boldsymbol{C}'\boldsymbol{T}')^{-1}\boldsymbol{T}\boldsymbol{c}_i. \tag{8.6}$$

The expression $\boldsymbol{c}'_i(\boldsymbol{C}\boldsymbol{C}')^{-1}\boldsymbol{c}_i$ is usually called the leverage and is considered to be a measure of how single independent observations differ, due to their design, from the rest of the independent "observations". This also means that the leverage measures the design variation, which fits perfectly into a discussion of influential observations; i.e. a large design variation yields a large influence.

Now Perturbation (ii) in Definition 8.2 is studied. The maximum likelihood estimate under this perturbation is given in (8.4). In order to perform a Taylor series expansion (using only a few terms) around $\omega = 0$, it is noted that (see Appendix B, Theorem B.6 (iv))

$$(\boldsymbol{G}\boldsymbol{G}')^{-1} = (\boldsymbol{C}\boldsymbol{C}')^{-1} - \omega(\boldsymbol{C}\boldsymbol{C}')^{-1}(\boldsymbol{V}\boldsymbol{C}' + \boldsymbol{C}\boldsymbol{V}')(\boldsymbol{C}\boldsymbol{C}')^{-1}$$
$$+\omega^2\{((\boldsymbol{C}\boldsymbol{C}')^{-1}(\boldsymbol{V}\boldsymbol{C}' + \boldsymbol{C}\boldsymbol{V}'))^2(\boldsymbol{C}\boldsymbol{C}')^{-1} - (\boldsymbol{C}\boldsymbol{C}')^{-1}\boldsymbol{V}\boldsymbol{V}'(\boldsymbol{C}\boldsymbol{C}')^{-1}\} + O(\omega^3)$$

and, using this result,

$$\widehat{\boldsymbol{\beta}}'_G(\omega) = \widehat{\boldsymbol{\beta}}' - \omega(\widehat{\boldsymbol{\beta}}'(\boldsymbol{V}\boldsymbol{C}' + \boldsymbol{C}\boldsymbol{V}')(\boldsymbol{C}\boldsymbol{C}')^{-1} - \boldsymbol{x}'\boldsymbol{V}'(\boldsymbol{C}\boldsymbol{C}')^{-1})$$
$$+\omega^2\{\widehat{\boldsymbol{\beta}}'((\boldsymbol{V}\boldsymbol{C}' + \boldsymbol{C}\boldsymbol{V}')(\boldsymbol{C}\boldsymbol{C}')^{-1})^2$$
$$-\widehat{\boldsymbol{\beta}}'\boldsymbol{V}\boldsymbol{V}'(\boldsymbol{C}\boldsymbol{C}')^{-1} - \boldsymbol{x}'\boldsymbol{V}'(\boldsymbol{C}\boldsymbol{C}')^{-1}(\boldsymbol{V}\boldsymbol{C}' + \boldsymbol{C}\boldsymbol{V}')(\boldsymbol{C}\boldsymbol{C}')^{-1}\} + O(\omega^3).$$

When studying influence, it appears from this expression that there are two terms of interest which correspond to ω and ω^2, respectively:

$$\widehat{\boldsymbol{\beta}}'(\boldsymbol{V}\boldsymbol{C}' + \boldsymbol{C}\boldsymbol{V}')(\boldsymbol{C}\boldsymbol{C}')^{-1} - \boldsymbol{x}'\boldsymbol{V}'(\boldsymbol{C}\boldsymbol{C}')^{-1}, \tag{8.7}$$

$$\widehat{\boldsymbol{\beta}}'((\boldsymbol{V}\boldsymbol{C}' + \boldsymbol{C}\boldsymbol{V}')(\boldsymbol{C}\boldsymbol{C}')^{-1})^2 - \widehat{\boldsymbol{\beta}}'\boldsymbol{V}\boldsymbol{V}'(\boldsymbol{C}\boldsymbol{C}')^{-1} - \boldsymbol{x}'\boldsymbol{V}'(\boldsymbol{C}\boldsymbol{C}')^{-1}(\boldsymbol{V}\boldsymbol{C}' + \boldsymbol{C}\boldsymbol{V}')(\boldsymbol{C}\boldsymbol{C}')^{-1}. \tag{8.8}$$

It now makes sense to use the definition $\boldsymbol{V} = (\boldsymbol{0} : \boldsymbol{1}_k : \boldsymbol{0})$ and then (8.7) equals

$$(\widehat{\boldsymbol{\beta}}'\boldsymbol{1}_k\boldsymbol{c}_i' - (x_i - \widehat{\boldsymbol{\beta}}'\boldsymbol{c}_i)\boldsymbol{1}_k')(\boldsymbol{C}\boldsymbol{C}')^{-1},$$

where, in fact,

$$r_i = x_i - \widehat{\boldsymbol{\beta}}'\boldsymbol{c}_i$$

is the usual residual, i.e. the difference between the observation and the corresponding predicted value. Thus, large residuals indicate that the observations are influential. To evaluate (8.7), the expression is squared relative to $\boldsymbol{C}\boldsymbol{C}'$, i.e. one obtains

$$(\widehat{\boldsymbol{\beta}}'\boldsymbol{1}_k\boldsymbol{c}_i' - r_i\boldsymbol{1}_k')(\boldsymbol{C}\boldsymbol{C}')^{-1}(\widehat{\boldsymbol{\beta}}'\boldsymbol{1}_k\boldsymbol{c}_i' - r_i\boldsymbol{1}_k')', \tag{8.9}$$

which can be rewritten as

$$\boldsymbol{c}_i'(\boldsymbol{C}\boldsymbol{C}')^{-1}\boldsymbol{c}_i\widehat{\boldsymbol{\beta}}'\boldsymbol{1}_k\boldsymbol{1}_k'\widehat{\boldsymbol{\beta}} + r_i^2\boldsymbol{1}_k'(\boldsymbol{C}\boldsymbol{C}')^{-1}\boldsymbol{1}_k - 2r_i\boldsymbol{c}_i'(\boldsymbol{C}\boldsymbol{C}')^{-1}\boldsymbol{1}_k\boldsymbol{1}_k'\widehat{\boldsymbol{\beta}}.$$

Hence, once again, it seems that the leverage and the residual play a role, but $\boldsymbol{c}_i'(\boldsymbol{C}\boldsymbol{C}')^{-1}\boldsymbol{1}_k$ also plays a role. We can conclude that an observation can be influential if both the residual and the leverage are "large", but it can also be influential if the residual is "small" and the leverage "large", if the residual is "large" and the leverage "small", or if the difference between $\widehat{\boldsymbol{\beta}}'\mathbf{1}_k\boldsymbol{c}_i'$ and $r_i\mathbf{1}_k'$ is "large".

The second term of interest above, (8.8), can be written as follows:

$$(\widehat{\boldsymbol{\beta}}'\mathbf{1}_k\boldsymbol{c}_i' - r_i\mathbf{1}_k')(\boldsymbol{C}\boldsymbol{C}')^{-1}(\mathbf{1}_k\boldsymbol{c}_i' + \boldsymbol{c}_i\mathbf{1}_k')(\boldsymbol{C}\boldsymbol{C}')^{-1} - \widehat{\boldsymbol{\beta}}'\mathbf{1}_k\mathbf{1}_k'(\boldsymbol{C}\boldsymbol{C}')^{-1}.$$

Thus, the information concerning influential observations provided by (8.7) and that provided by (8.8) differ somewhat; i.e. the terms in the Taylor series expansion bear different information, but this will not be exploited further.

Finally, we turn our attention to Perturbation (iii) in Definition 8.2. After some manipulations and applications of Theorem B.6 (iv) in Appendix B the Taylor series expansion with respect to ω can be written as

$$\begin{aligned}\widehat{\boldsymbol{\beta}}'_{x0}(\omega) &= (\boldsymbol{x}_0'\boldsymbol{C}_0' + \omega\boldsymbol{x}_i'\boldsymbol{C}_i')(\boldsymbol{C}_0\boldsymbol{C}_0' + \omega\boldsymbol{C}_i\boldsymbol{C}_i')^{-1}\\ &= \boldsymbol{x}_0'\boldsymbol{C}_0'(\boldsymbol{C}_0\boldsymbol{C}_0')^{-1} + \sum_{j=1}^{\infty}(-1)^{j+1}\omega^j(\boldsymbol{x}_i' - \boldsymbol{x}_0'\boldsymbol{C}_0'(\boldsymbol{C}_0\boldsymbol{C}_0')^{-1}\boldsymbol{C}_i)\\ &\quad\times\boldsymbol{D}_i^{j-1}\boldsymbol{C}_i'(\boldsymbol{C}_0\boldsymbol{C}_0')^{-1},\end{aligned} \tag{8.10}$$

where $\boldsymbol{D}_i = \boldsymbol{C}_i'(\boldsymbol{C}_0\boldsymbol{C}_0')^{-1}\boldsymbol{C}_i$. Moreover, when we define the "residual" $\boldsymbol{r}_i = \boldsymbol{x}_i' - \boldsymbol{x}_0'\boldsymbol{C}_0'(\boldsymbol{C}_0\boldsymbol{C}_0')^{-1}\boldsymbol{C}_i$, we can thereby see that the terms in the expansion are linear in the residual and include powers of a quantity which, if $\boldsymbol{C}_i$ is a column vector, is similar to the leverage, i.e. $\boldsymbol{c}_i'(\boldsymbol{C}\boldsymbol{C}')^{-1}\boldsymbol{c}_i$. From (8.10), it follows that a general influence measure is given by

$$\boldsymbol{r}_i'\boldsymbol{D}_i^{j-1}\boldsymbol{C}_i'(\boldsymbol{C}_0\boldsymbol{C}_0')^{-1}\boldsymbol{C}_i\boldsymbol{D}_i^{j-1}\boldsymbol{r}_i = \boldsymbol{r}_i'\boldsymbol{D}_i^{2j-1}\boldsymbol{r}_i, \qquad j = 1, 2, \ldots$$

which, if only one column is perturbed, reduces to (note that $\boldsymbol{D}_i$ is a scalar)

$$r_i^2\boldsymbol{D}_i^{j-1}\boldsymbol{c}_i'(\boldsymbol{C}_0\boldsymbol{C}_0')^{-1}\boldsymbol{c}_i\boldsymbol{D}_i^{j-1} = r_i^2\boldsymbol{D}_i^{2j-1}, \qquad j = 1, 2, \ldots. \tag{8.11}$$

Thus, it is seen from (8.11) that the residual effect is the same for all j, although $\boldsymbol{D}_i^{2j-1}$ will either increase or decrease with j depending on whether $\boldsymbol{c}_i'(\boldsymbol{C}_0\boldsymbol{C}_0')^{-1}\boldsymbol{c}_i$ is larger or smaller than 1. Hence, it is natural to know if $\boldsymbol{c}_i'(\boldsymbol{C}_0\boldsymbol{C}_0')^{-1}\boldsymbol{c}_i < 1$.

For the three different perturbations in Definition 8.2 and the general univariate linear model discussed above, both residuals and "leverages" play an important role, and in Perturbation (ii), another quantity also has an impact on the estimate. If the linear effect is studied, then the focus will be on the term corresponding to ω, if the second-order effect is of interest, then the term corresponding to ω^2 is in focus, etc. In influence analysis, usually one is only considering the linear term, but the fact is that there is no well-founded justification for this strategy. Indeed, later, when considering the BRM, it will be shown that even the fifth term bears some information. There is, however, the general unanswered question of how many terms are meaningful to investigate or, in other words, how much information about the estimator, for example, we are losing by only considering a few terms in a Taylor series expansion.

It is important to stress that the basic idea when using the three different perturbation schemes is to make a recalculation for the elements in $\boldsymbol{x}$; i.e. if there are n observations, the calculations have to be repeated at least n times. This means, for example, that in Perturbations (i) and (ii), $\boldsymbol{V}$ has to be changed for each observation, for each pair of observations, for each triple of observations, etc. Perturbing more than one observation may be meaningful if a so-called masking effect exists, i.e. if the perturbation of one observation gives no indication of the existence of any influential observation, but the perturbation of two or more observations suddenly gives indications of strong influential observations. A crucial recommendation when developing influence analysis is that one should aim for methods which do not demand a large number of computations. For example, if there is a need to carry out iterations for each individual, each pair of individuals, etc. performing computations and understanding them could start to become a burden. Keeping this in mind, it is a challenge to perform influence analysis (model validation) in more complicated models.

Example 8.1 Twenty observations were generated according to the regression model

$$\boldsymbol{x}' = \boldsymbol{\beta}'\boldsymbol{C} + \boldsymbol{e}', \tag{8.12}$$

where $\boldsymbol{\beta}' = (0.78, 0.14)$, $\boldsymbol{C} = (\boldsymbol{c}_i)$, $\boldsymbol{c}_i = \binom{1}{i}$, $i = 1, 2, \ldots, 20$, and $\boldsymbol{e} \sim N_{20}(\boldsymbol{0}, 0.01\boldsymbol{I}_{20})$. Moreover, $\boldsymbol{x}$ was contaminated as follows: for $i = 3, 7, 19$, we had $x_3 = 3.2$, $x_7 = 4.0$ and $x_{19} = 5.0$, leading to the data set in Table 8.1, whose observations are also plotted in Fig. 8.1. This example should be regarded as an appetizer and there is no ambition to present a complete analysis.

In Fig. 8.1, it can be seen how the contaminated observations show up, and indeed are rather extreme observations. From this figure, it follows that those observations which have a relatively "large" residual should have an effect on the intercept, but should not have any effect on the slope.

Next we study how the perturbations in Definition 8.2 identify the manipulated observations. Starting with Perturbation (i) in Definition 8.2, it has been shown that

Table 8.1 Data $\boldsymbol{x} = (x_i)$ generated according to (8.12); observation x_3, x_7 and x_{19} have been manipulated

	1	2	3	4	5	6	7	8	9	10
x_i	1.10	1.05	3.20	1.23	1.70	1.56	4.00	1.89	1.98	2.18

	11	12	13	14	15	16	17	18	19	20
x_i	2.25	2.43	2.67	2.66	2.81	2.94	3.19	3.27	5.00	3.62

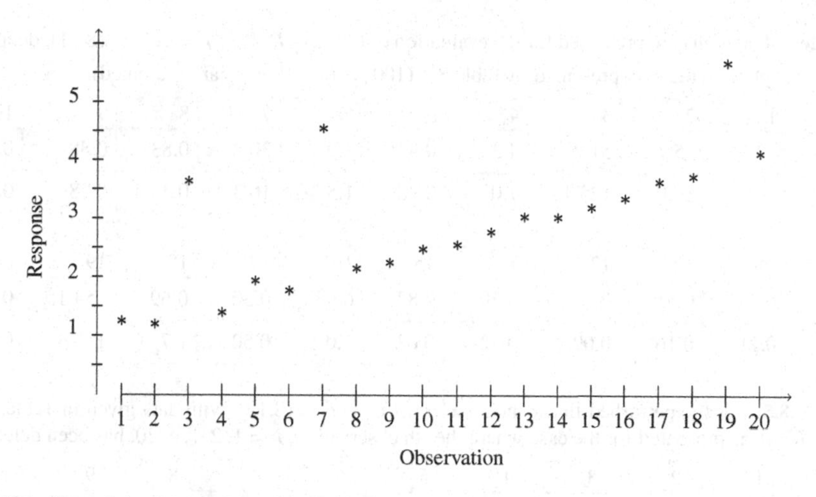

Fig. 8.1 Plot of the data presented in Table 8.1

Table 8.2 The leverage values $l_i = c_i'(CC)^{-1}c_i$, given in (8.6), are presented for the data in Table 8.1

	1	2	3	4	5	6	7	8	9	10
l_i	0.19	0.16	0.13	0.11	0.10	0.08	0.07	0.06	0.05	0.05

	11	12	13	14	15	16	17	18	19	20
l_i	0.05	0.05	0.06	0.07	0.08	0.10	0.11	0.13	0.16	0.19

Table 8.3 The evaluation criterion $(\widehat{\beta}'\mathbf{1}_k c_i' - r_i\mathbf{1}_k')(CC')^{-1}(\widehat{\beta}'\mathbf{1}_k c_i' - r_i\mathbf{1}_k')'$ in (8.9), denoted as cr_i, is applied to the data presented in Table 8.1

	1	2	3	4	5	6	7	8	9	10
cr_i	0.51	0.55	0.03	0.47	0.24	0.32	0.27	0.21	0.20	0.16

	11	12	13	14	15	16	17	18	19	20
cr_i	0.16	0.14	0.13	0.15	0.16	0.17	0.20	0.23	0.96	0.34

the natural evaluation criterion is the leverage, given in (8.6). The leverage for each individual is presented in Table 8.2.

Since the leverage only concerns the design, i.e. C, and no response observations are involved, it is fairly clear that, in the present analysis, nothing special will show up, which is also confirmed by Table 8.2.

For the perturbation presented in Definition 8.2 (ii), an evaluation criterion was proposed in (8.9). In Table 8.3 the results obtained by an application of that criterion are presented. It can be seen in Table 8.3 that observation $i = 19$ seems to deviate from the rest, whereas $i = 3, 7$ do not deviate. In particular, it is worth noting that out of all the observations, $i = 3$ has the lowest influence on the estimates.

Table 8.4 Results are presented for the evaluation criterion $r_i^2 D^{2j-1}$, $j = 1, 2$, of (8.11), denoted as p_i^j, applied to the data presented in Table 8.1 ($100 \times p_i^1$, $10^4 \times p_i^2$ are presented)

	1	2	3	4	5	6	7	8	9	10
p_i^1	2.6	5.3	51.7	4.3	0.34	1.9	30.2	0.83	0.88	0.50
p_i^2	13.7	19.0	125.1	7.0	0.38	1.5	16.3	0.33	0.28	0.14

	11	12	13	14	15	16	17	18	19	20
p_i^1	0.73	0.51	0.22	0.79	0.82	0.93	0.30	0.69	54.1	0.19
p_i^2	0.21	0.16	0.09	0.42	0.63	1.0	0.50	1.7	192.4	0.97

Table 8.5 For the perturbed linear model $\boldsymbol{x}' = \boldsymbol{\beta}'\boldsymbol{C} + \boldsymbol{e}'$ in (8.12), with data given in Table 8.1, $\widehat{\boldsymbol{\beta}} = (\widehat{\alpha}, \widehat{\beta})$ is presented for the case where the ith observation, $i = 1, 2, \ldots, 20$, has been deleted

	1	2	3	4	5	6	7	8	9	10
$\widehat{\alpha}$	1.32	1.35	0.95	1.34	1.28	1.31	1.04	1.29	1.28	1.27
$\widehat{\beta}$	0.12	0.12	0.14	0.12	0.12	0.12	0.13	0.12	0.12	0.12

	11	12	13	14	15	16	17	18	19	20
$\widehat{\alpha}$	1.27	1.26	1.26	1.25	1.25	1.24	1.25	1.24	1.40	1.25
$\widehat{\beta}$	0.12	0.12	0.12	0.12	0.12	0.12	0.12	0.12	0.10	0.12

The true values equal (0.78, 0.14)

Finally, Perturbation (iii) in Definition 8.2 is studied. Now (8.11) is utilized and in Table 8.4 the results are presented for two terms of the Taylor series expansion in (8.10). From Table 8.4, it is clear that Perturbation (iii) catches the manipulated data, which is due to the large residuals.

It is of interest to compare the above results with those for the case deletion approach. Table 8.5 presents the results obtained when observations have been deleted, one observation at a time, with a view to studying what happens to $\widehat{\boldsymbol{\beta}}$, i.e. with the estimated intercept and slope considered. From Table 8.5, one can learn that by removing outlying observations, one does not necessarily improve the estimates. For example, removing observation $i = 19$ leads to estimates which are further away from the truth than the estimates obtained by removing other observations. Hence, if, in the validation process, one compares the estimates obtained with the case deletion approach with the estimates based on all the observations, one may not be making an appropriate comparison. The problems in this connection basically stem from the fact that a masking effect can occur; i.e. merely removing one observation at a time is not sufficient to uncover peculiarities. □

When there are more complicated expressions than unweighted least squares estimates, it is not obvious how one should discover the existence of any kind of masking effect. Therefore, in the following, the perturbation approach will be advocated and, when connecting it with knowledge about matrix derivatives, which build up the Taylor series expansion, we acquire some powerful tools for validating the BRM and its extensions.

8.3 Influence Analysis in the BRM

This section treats the BRM presented in Definition 2.1. There are many different alternatives which can be explored, for instance the three different perturbations presented in Definition 8.2 and several types of statistics, for example maximum likelihood estimates of the mean and dispersion matrices, predicted observations and likelihood ratio tests for various types of hypotheses. However, first the perturbations in Definition 8.2 are reintroduced, now adjusted to fit into a multivariate scenario.

Definition 8.3 Three different perturbations are defined below. The perturbations are supposed to be applied for each "individual" separately, i.e. each column of $\boldsymbol{X}$ in the BRM, and the perturbation scheme can be said to be "case-weighted".

(i) Let $\boldsymbol{Z} = \boldsymbol{X} + \omega \boldsymbol{V}$, where $\boldsymbol{V}$ is known and has to be specified in advance.
(ii) Let $\boldsymbol{G} = \boldsymbol{C} + \omega \boldsymbol{V}$, where $\boldsymbol{V}$ is known and has to be specified in advance.
(iii) Let $\boldsymbol{X}$ consist of $\{\boldsymbol{X}_0', \sqrt{\omega}\boldsymbol{X}_i'\}$ and let $\boldsymbol{C}$ consist of $\{\boldsymbol{C}_0, \sqrt{\omega}\boldsymbol{C}_i'\}$, where $\boldsymbol{X}_i$ and $\boldsymbol{C}_i$ are subsets of perturbed columns of $\boldsymbol{X}$ and corresponding perturbed columns of $\boldsymbol{C}$, respectively, and $\boldsymbol{X}_0$ and $\boldsymbol{C}_0$ are unperturbed columns of $\boldsymbol{X}$ and $\boldsymbol{C}$, respectively.

Let us consider the MLE of $\boldsymbol{B}$ in the BRM, i.e.

$$\widehat{\boldsymbol{B}} = (\boldsymbol{A}'\boldsymbol{S}^{-1}\boldsymbol{A})^{-1}\boldsymbol{A}'\boldsymbol{S}^{-1}\boldsymbol{X}\boldsymbol{C}'(\boldsymbol{C}\boldsymbol{C}')^{-1}, \tag{8.13}$$

where $\boldsymbol{S} = \boldsymbol{X}(\boldsymbol{I} - \boldsymbol{P}_{\boldsymbol{C}'})\boldsymbol{X}'$ and under the perturbation, i.e. when Perturbation (i), (ii) or (iii) holds, instead of $\widehat{\boldsymbol{B}}$, we write $\widehat{\boldsymbol{B}}(\omega)$; throughout this section, to simplify the derivations, $\boldsymbol{A}$ and $\boldsymbol{C}$ are supposed to be of full rank (see Corollary 3.1). Perturbation (iii) in Definition 8.3 will be applied first. Perturbations (i) and (ii) in Definition 8.3 will be treated later, but will not receive as detailed treatment as Perturbation (iii) will have received. Note that under Perturbation (iii), $\widehat{\boldsymbol{B}}(1) = \widehat{\boldsymbol{B}}$, i.e. a null perturbation exists. The effect of the perturbation will be exploited through the effects on the sufficient statistics

$$\boldsymbol{S} \text{ and } \boldsymbol{X}\boldsymbol{C}'(\boldsymbol{C}\boldsymbol{C}')^{-1},$$

and thereafter the effects on the inverse $\boldsymbol{S}^{-1}$ and on $(\boldsymbol{A}'\boldsymbol{S}^{-1}\boldsymbol{A})^{-1}\boldsymbol{A}'\boldsymbol{S}^{-1}$ will be determined. Since the effects are investigated via a Taylor series, differentiation will take place and knowledge about the differentiation of a product of matrices and an inverse matrix will be utilized. In fact, in the following only the derivatives will be presented and not the complete Taylor series, but it is worth remembering that the first derivative is connected to the linear term (linear effect) of the series, the second derivative is connected to the second term, etc. Moreover, another matrix derivative than that used in the previous chapters, i.e. Definition 5.1, will be implemented in order to make the subsequent calculations easier to look through.

Definition 8.4 Let $\boldsymbol{Y}: q \times r$ be a function of $\boldsymbol{X}: p \times n$. If $\boldsymbol{X}$ consists of functionally independent elements, then

(i)

$$\frac{d\boldsymbol{Y}}{d\boldsymbol{X}} = \sum_{I} \frac{d\, y_{ij}}{d\, x_{kl}}((\boldsymbol{d}_i\boldsymbol{e}_j') \otimes (\boldsymbol{f}_k\boldsymbol{g}_l')),$$

where $I = \{i, j, k, l; 1 \leq i \leq q, 1 \leq j \leq r, 1 \leq k \leq p, 1 \leq l \leq n\}$, and $\boldsymbol{d}_i$: $q \times 1$, $\boldsymbol{e}_j: r \times 1$, $\boldsymbol{f}_k: p \times 1$ and $\boldsymbol{g}_l: n \times 1$ are unit basis vectors;

(ii)

$$\frac{d^k\boldsymbol{Y}}{d\,\boldsymbol{X}^k} = \frac{d}{d\,\boldsymbol{X}^k}\left(\frac{d^{k-1}\boldsymbol{Y}}{d\,\boldsymbol{X}^{k-1}}\right), \quad k = 1, 2, \ldots, \qquad \frac{d^0\,\boldsymbol{Y}}{d\,\boldsymbol{X}^0} = \boldsymbol{Y}.$$

The next lemma, where the kth derivatives of the perturbed $\boldsymbol{S} = \boldsymbol{X}(\boldsymbol{I} - \boldsymbol{P}_{C'})\boldsymbol{X}'$ and $\boldsymbol{X}\boldsymbol{C}'(\boldsymbol{C}\boldsymbol{C}')^{-1}$ are presented, is the starting point for an influence analysis for the BRM. Although this lemma is conceptually easy, it turns out to be rather technical.

Lemma 8.1 *Let* $\boldsymbol{S}(\omega) = \boldsymbol{X}(\boldsymbol{I} - \boldsymbol{C}'(\boldsymbol{C}\boldsymbol{C}')^{-1}\boldsymbol{C})\boldsymbol{X}'$, *where* $\boldsymbol{X} = (\boldsymbol{X}_0, \sqrt{\omega}\boldsymbol{X}_i)$ $\boldsymbol{C} = (\boldsymbol{C}_0, \sqrt{\omega}\boldsymbol{C}_i)$. *Put*

$$\boldsymbol{D}_i = \boldsymbol{C}_i'(\boldsymbol{C}_0\boldsymbol{C}_0')^{-1}\boldsymbol{C}_i, \quad \boldsymbol{R}_i = \boldsymbol{X}_i - \boldsymbol{X}_0\boldsymbol{C}_0'(\boldsymbol{C}_0\boldsymbol{C}_0')^{-1}\boldsymbol{C}_i.$$

Then

(i) $\left.\frac{d^k\boldsymbol{S}(\omega)}{d\,\omega^k}\right|_{\omega=0} = (-1)^{k+1}k!\boldsymbol{R}_i\boldsymbol{D}_i^{k-1}\boldsymbol{R}_i', \qquad k \geq 1;$

(ii) $\left.\frac{d^k\boldsymbol{X}\boldsymbol{C}'(\boldsymbol{C}\boldsymbol{C}')^{-1}}{d\,\omega^k}\right|_{\omega=0} = (-1)^{k+1}k!\boldsymbol{R}_i\boldsymbol{D}_i^{k-1}\boldsymbol{C}_i'(\boldsymbol{C}_0\boldsymbol{C}_0')^{-1}, \qquad k \geq 1.$

Proof The proof follows from an application of Appendix B, Theorem B.6 (iv) to $(\boldsymbol{C}\boldsymbol{C}')^{-1}$, as well as a few additional calculations. □

The matrix $\boldsymbol{R}_i$ in Lemma 8.1 is a kind of residual matrix with $E[\boldsymbol{R}_i] = \boldsymbol{0}$. The most commonly applied residual, assuming that $\omega = 1$ in the perturbed model, equals $\boldsymbol{R}_i = \boldsymbol{X}_i - \boldsymbol{X}\boldsymbol{C}'(\boldsymbol{C}\boldsymbol{C}')^{-1}\boldsymbol{C}_i$. Moreover, the matrix $\boldsymbol{D}_i$ is very close to the usual leverage measure, $\boldsymbol{C}_i'(\boldsymbol{C}\boldsymbol{C}')^{-1}\boldsymbol{C}_i$, which is obtained when using $\omega = 1$ in the perturbed model, and it is worth noting that it is a pure function of the between-individuals design matrix.

In the following, let $\boldsymbol{S}_0 = \boldsymbol{S}(0)$, where $\boldsymbol{S}(0)$ follows from the assumptions in the lemma given above, i.e. $\boldsymbol{S}_0 = \boldsymbol{X}_0(\boldsymbol{I} - \boldsymbol{P}_{C_0'})\boldsymbol{X}_0'$. The next lemma is meant as a preparation for differentiating $(\boldsymbol{A}^{o'}\boldsymbol{S}\boldsymbol{A}^o)^{-1}$, which is useful because $(\boldsymbol{A}'\boldsymbol{S}^{-1}\boldsymbol{A})^{-1}\boldsymbol{A}'\boldsymbol{S}^{-1} = (\boldsymbol{A}'\boldsymbol{A})^{-1}\boldsymbol{A}'(\boldsymbol{I} - \boldsymbol{S}\boldsymbol{A}^o(\boldsymbol{A}^{o'}\boldsymbol{S}\boldsymbol{A}^o)^{-1}\boldsymbol{A}^{o'})$ and which simplifies calculations, since $\boldsymbol{S}$ is a function of ω (see Appendix B, Theorem B.13).

Lemma 8.2 *Let $\boldsymbol{B}$ be a constant matrix of proper size and rank, and let $\boldsymbol{S}(\omega)$, as well as $\boldsymbol{R}_i$ and $\boldsymbol{D}_i$, be defined in Lemma 8.1. Then*

(i) $\left.\frac{d^0(\boldsymbol{B}'\boldsymbol{S}(\omega)\boldsymbol{B})^{-1}}{d\,\omega^0}\right|_{\omega=0} = (\boldsymbol{B}'\boldsymbol{S}_0\boldsymbol{B})^{-1}$;

(ii) $\left.\frac{d(\boldsymbol{B}'\boldsymbol{S}(\omega)\boldsymbol{B})^{-1}}{d\,\omega}\right|_{\omega=0} = -(\boldsymbol{B}'\boldsymbol{S}_0\boldsymbol{B})^{-1}\boldsymbol{B}'\boldsymbol{R}_i\boldsymbol{R}_i'\boldsymbol{B}(\boldsymbol{B}'\boldsymbol{S}_0\boldsymbol{B})^{-1}$;

(iii)

$$\left.\frac{d^2(\boldsymbol{B}'\boldsymbol{S}(\omega)\boldsymbol{B})^{-1}}{d\,\omega^2}\right|_{\omega=0} = 2(\boldsymbol{B}'\boldsymbol{S}_0\boldsymbol{B})^{-1}\boldsymbol{B}'\boldsymbol{R}_i(\boldsymbol{D}_i + \boldsymbol{R}_i'\boldsymbol{B}(\boldsymbol{B}'\boldsymbol{S}_0\boldsymbol{B})^{-1}\boldsymbol{B}'\boldsymbol{R}_i)\boldsymbol{R}_i'\boldsymbol{B}(\boldsymbol{B}'\boldsymbol{S}_0\boldsymbol{B})^{-1};$$

(iv)

$$\left.\frac{d^3(\boldsymbol{B}'\boldsymbol{S}(\omega)\boldsymbol{B})^{-1}}{d\,\omega^3}\right|_{\omega=0} = -6(\boldsymbol{B}'\boldsymbol{S}_0\boldsymbol{B})^{-1}\boldsymbol{B}'\boldsymbol{R}_i\Big(\boldsymbol{D}_i^2 + \boldsymbol{R}_i'\boldsymbol{B}(\boldsymbol{B}'\boldsymbol{S}_0\boldsymbol{B})^{-1}\boldsymbol{B}'\boldsymbol{R}_i$$
$$\times(\boldsymbol{D}_i + \boldsymbol{R}_i'\boldsymbol{B}(\boldsymbol{B}'\boldsymbol{S}_0\boldsymbol{B})^{-1}\boldsymbol{B}'\boldsymbol{R}_i)\boldsymbol{R}_i'\boldsymbol{B}(\boldsymbol{B}'\boldsymbol{S}_0\boldsymbol{B})^{-1}\boldsymbol{B}'\boldsymbol{R}_i\Big)\boldsymbol{R}_i'\boldsymbol{B}(\boldsymbol{B}'\boldsymbol{S}_0\boldsymbol{B})^{-1}.$$

Now one of the main theorems of this chapter is presented.

Theorem 8.1 *Let $\widehat{\boldsymbol{B}}(\omega)$ be the perturbed version of $\widehat{\boldsymbol{B}}$, given in (8.13), when $\boldsymbol{X} = (\boldsymbol{X}_0, \sqrt{\omega}\boldsymbol{X}_i)$ and $\boldsymbol{C} = (\boldsymbol{C}_0, \sqrt{\omega}\boldsymbol{C}_i)$, i.e. when Perturbation (iii) in Definition 8.3 is applied. Then*

$$\left.\frac{d^k\widehat{\boldsymbol{B}}(\omega)}{d\,\omega^k}\right|_{\omega=0} = (\boldsymbol{A}'\boldsymbol{A})^{-1}\boldsymbol{A}'\left.\frac{d^k\boldsymbol{X}\boldsymbol{C}'(\boldsymbol{C}\boldsymbol{C}')^{-1}}{d\,\omega^k}\right|_{\omega=0}$$
$$-\sum_{i_1=0}^{k}\sum_{i_2=0}^{k-i_1}\binom{k}{i_1}\binom{k-i_1}{i_2}(\boldsymbol{A}'\boldsymbol{A})^{-1}\boldsymbol{A}'\frac{d^{i_1}\boldsymbol{S}}{d\,\omega^{i_1}}\boldsymbol{A}^o\frac{d^{i_2}(\boldsymbol{A}^{o\prime}\boldsymbol{S}\boldsymbol{A}^o)^{-1}}{d\,\omega^{i_2}}$$
$$\times\boldsymbol{A}^{o\prime}\left.\frac{d^{k-i_1-i_2}\boldsymbol{X}\boldsymbol{C}'(\boldsymbol{C}\boldsymbol{C}')^{-1}}{d\,\omega^{k-i_1-i_2}}\right|_{\omega=0}, \quad k \geq 0,$$

where $\left.\frac{d^l\boldsymbol{S}(\omega)}{d\,\omega^l}\right|_{\omega=0}$, $\left.\frac{d^l\boldsymbol{X}\boldsymbol{C}'(\boldsymbol{C}\boldsymbol{C}')^{-1}}{d\,\omega^l}\right|_{\omega=0}$ and $\left.\frac{d^l(\boldsymbol{A}^{o\prime}\boldsymbol{S}\boldsymbol{A}^o)^{-1}}{d\,\omega^l}\right|_{\omega=0}$ are derived via Lemma 8.1 and Appendix B, Theorem B.15.

Proof The statement follows from an application of Theorem B.15 (i) in Appendix B. □

We now express the result of Theorem 8.1 in the special case where $k = 1, 2, 3$, which will later be applied when analysing the classical Potthoff and Roy growth curve data set (see Example 1.7). In particular, it can be noted that the influence exerted by the residual $\boldsymbol{R}_i$ is not linear, which it was in the univariate case (see (8.10)).

Corollary 8.1 *Let the matrices and perturbation be as in Lemma 8.1 and Theorem 8.1, and put* $S_0 = S(0) = X_0(I - P_{C_0'})X_0'$. *Then,*

(i) *if* $k = 0$, $\left.\frac{d^0\widehat{B}(\omega)}{d\omega^0}\right|_{\omega=0} = (A'S_0^{-1}A)^{-1}A'S_0^{-1}X_0C_0'(C_0C_0')^{-1}$;

(ii) *if* $k = 1$,

$$\left.\frac{d\widehat{B}(\omega)}{d\omega}\right|_{\omega=0} = (A'S_0^{-1}A)^{-1}A'S_0^{-1}R_iC_i'(C_0C_0')^{-1}$$
$$-(A'S_0^{-1}A)^{-1}A'S_0^{-1}R_iR_i'A^o(A^{o'}S_0A^o)^{-1}A^{o'}X_0C_0'(C_0C_0')^{-1};$$

(iii) *if* $k = 2$,

$$\left.\frac{d^2\widehat{B}(\omega)}{d\omega^2}\right|_{\omega=0} = -2(A'S_0^{-1}A)^{-1}A'S_0^{-1}R_iD_iC_i'(C_0C_0')^{-1}$$
$$-2(A'S_0^{-1}A)^{-1}A'S_0^{-1}R_iR_i'A^o(A^{o'}S_0A^o)^{-1}A^{o'}R_iC_i'(C_0C_0')^{-1}$$
$$+2(A'S_0^{-1}A)^{-1}A'S_0^{-1}R_iD_iR_i'A^o(A^{o'}S_0A^o)^{-1}A^{o'}X_0C_0'(C_0C_0')^{-1}$$
$$+2(A'S_0^{-1}A)^{-1}A'S_0^{-1}R_iR_i'A^o(A^{o'}S_0A^o)^{-1}A^{o'}R_i$$
$$\times R_i'A^o(A^{o'}S_0A^o)^{-1}A^{o'}X_0C_0'(C_0C_0')^{-1};$$

(iv) *if* $k = 3$,

$$\left.\frac{d^3\widehat{B}(\omega)}{d\omega^3}\right|_{\omega=0} = (A'S_0^{-1}A)^{-1}A'S_0^{-1}\left.\frac{d^3XC'(CC')^{-1}}{d\omega^3}\right|_{\omega=0}$$
$$+3(A'A)^{-1}A'S_0A^o(A^{o'}S_0A^o)^{-1}A^{o'}R_iR_i'A^o(A^{o'}S_0A^o)^{-1}A^{o'}\left.\frac{d^2XC'(CC')^{-1}}{d\omega^2}\right|_{\omega=0}$$
$$+3(A'A)^{-1}A'S_0A^o\left.\frac{d^2(A^{o'}S_0A^o)^{-1}}{d\omega^2}\right|_{\omega=0}A^{o'}R_iC_i'(C_0C_0')^{-1}$$
$$+(A'A)^{-1}A'S_0A^o\left.\frac{d^3(A^{o'}S_0A^o)^{-1}}{d\omega^3}\right|_{\omega=0}A^{o'}X_0C_0'(C_0C_0')^{-1}$$
$$+6(A'A)^{-1}A'R_iR_i'A^o(A^{o'}S_0A^o)^{-1}A^{o'}R_iD_iC_i'(C_0C_0')^{-1}$$
$$+6(A'A)^{-1}A'R_iR_i'A^o(A^{o'}S_0A^o)^{-1}A^{o'}R_iR_i'A^o(A^{o'}S_0A^o)^{-1}A^{o'}R_iC_i'(C_0C_0')^{-1}$$
$$-3(A'A)^{-1}A'R_iR_i'A^o\left.\frac{d^2(A^{o'}S_0A^o)^{-1}}{d\omega^2}\right|_{\omega=0}A^{o'}X_0C_0'(C_0C_0')^{-1}$$
$$+6(A'A)^{-1}A'R_iD_iR_i'A^o(A^{o'}S_0A^o)^{-1}A^{o'}R_iC_i'(C_0C_0')^{-1}$$
$$+6(A'A)^{-1}A'R_iD_iR_i'A^o(A^{o'}S_0A^o)^{-1}A^{o'}R_iR_i'A^o(A^{o'}S_0A^o)^{-1}A^{o'}X_0C_0'(C_0C_0')^{-1}$$
$$-6(A'A)^{-1}A'R_iD_i^2R_i'A^o(A^{o'}S_0A^o)^{-1}A^{o'}X_0C_0'(C_0C_0')^{-1},$$

where $\left.\frac{d^k(\boldsymbol{A}^{o'}\boldsymbol{S}_0\boldsymbol{A}^o)^{-1}}{d\,\omega^k}\right|_{\omega=0}$*, $k = 2, 3$, is obtained from Lemma 8.2.*

Proof The statements are all verified by performing calculations using Lemmas 8.1 and 8.2. □

Since

$$\widehat{\boldsymbol{B}}(\omega) \approx \sum_{k=0}^{t} \omega^k \frac{1}{k!} \left.\frac{d^k\widehat{\boldsymbol{B}}(\omega)}{d\,\omega^k}\right|_{\omega=0},$$

where t is so large that the approximation works well (it is assumed that the series converges), the effect of the perturbation ω can be measured via the derivatives. Moreover, according to the general ideas of influence analysis, some evaluation criteria to be applied to the derivatives should be defined, but if there are only a few observations, the derivatives corresponding to the perturbed observations can be listed and the parameters can be evaluated element-wise.

Example 8.2 (The Classical Potthoff and Roy (1964) Data Set) The analysis of the Potthoff and Roy (1964) data presented in Example 1.7 is now evaluated. It was shown that the MLE of the mean parameter $\boldsymbol{B}$ equals

$$\widehat{\boldsymbol{B}} = \begin{pmatrix} \widehat{b}_{11} & \widehat{b}_{12} \\ \widehat{b}_{21} & \widehat{b}_{22} \end{pmatrix} = \begin{pmatrix} 17.43 & 15.84 \\ 0.476 & 0.827 \end{pmatrix}.$$

The parameters b_{11} and b_{21} describe the growth of the girls, whereas b_{12} and b_{22} describe the growth of the boys. In Table 8.6 the derivatives $\left.\frac{d^k\widehat{\boldsymbol{B}}(\omega)}{d\,\omega^k}\right|_{\omega=0}$, $k = 1, 2, 3$, and $\widehat{\boldsymbol{B}}(0)$ (i.e. the estimate where the ith observation has been removed) are presented for four different individuals. The focus is on one "normal" individual, for which we cannot find any extreme observed values in the data, and three individuals which include "outlying" observations. In Examples 6.1, 6.5 and 6.6 residuals for the data set were presented. In particular, it follows from Tables 6.1, 6.6 and 6.10 that individual 16 sometimes has "larger" residuals than individual 15, but this individual seems to have a higher influence on the mean estimates than individual 16 and, therefore, is reported in Table 8.6. Moreover, concerning all the other observations, we could not find anything remarkable when calculating the derivatives.

In Table 8.6, individual 6 is a girl, whereas individuals 15, 16 and 24 are boys. Therefore, it appears, as expected, that for individual 6 the influence on b_{11} and b_{21} is greater than on b_{12} and b_{22}. For individual 15, if $k = 1, 2$, or 3, the derivatives for b_{12} and b_{22} are large. For individuals 20 and 24, all the derivatives are relatively large, and those for individual 20 in particular show some outstanding values. The main conclusion from this example is that the influence on the estimated parameters differs among these individuals and the analysis is insufficient if one only uses the first derivative. In order to evaluate the above results, they should be studied in

Table 8.6 The results of an application of Perturbation (iii) in Definition 8.2 to the Potthoff and Roy data set (see Example 1.7)

k	b_{11}	b_{12}	b_{21}	b_{22}
Individual 6 (normal)				
0	17.47	15.84	0.48	0.83
1	−0.047	0.0012	−0.0094	0.00025
2	0.010	−0.00027	0.0021	−0.000055
3	−0.0032	0.000057	−0.00069	0.000022
Individual 15				
0	17.45	14.86	0.47	0.90
1	−0.032	1.14	0.0023	−0.084
2	0.010	−0.36	−00074	0.027
3	−0.0016	0.10	0.00012	−0.0076
Individual 20				
0	17.50	16.74	0.47	0.79
1	−0.34	−4.07	0.013	0.16
2	2.41	28.85	−0.095	−1.14
3	70.40	−1.78	700.36	−17.16
Individual 24				
0	17.36	17.53	0.48	0.68
1	0.10	−2.57	−0.0089	0.23
2	−0.11	2.094	0.0093	−0.24
3	0.11	−3.17	−0.097	0.27

For $k = 0, 1, 2, 3$, the derivative $\left.\frac{d^k\widehat{\boldsymbol{B}}(\omega)}{d\,\omega^k}\right|_{\omega=0}$ has been calculated for individuals 6, 15, 20 and 24

relation to the observed variation. Therefore, it is of interest to compare the results with

$$\widehat{D[\widehat{\boldsymbol{B}}]} = \begin{pmatrix} 48.55 & -3.62 & 0 & 0 \\ -3.62 & 0.35 & 0 & 0 \\ 0 & 0 & 30.34 & -2.26 \\ 0 & 0 & -2.26 & 0.22 \end{pmatrix},$$

which was obtained in Theorem 4.5. This estimate is for unperturbed observations and, of course, $\widehat{D[\widehat{\boldsymbol{B}}]}$ will change, somewhat, if some individual is excluded or if a perturbation which has taken place turns out to be important, but for our discussion this is not very crucial. It follows that, in comparison with the estimated variation of the estimators, most derivatives are fairly small. It is only individual 20 which seems to have some influence on the estimates which is not a surprise when one inspects the original data. Note that when comparing different derivatives of a different order k, it is reasonable to divide the derivative by $k!$, where k stands for the order of the derivative. A final comment is that the perturbation induces non-linear effects (see individuals 20 and 24). □

Now Perturbation (ii) in Definition 8.3 is studied. This perturbation acts only on the design matrix $\boldsymbol{C}$. In this case the structure in $\boldsymbol{C}$ will interfere with the perturbation defined through $\boldsymbol{V}$. For example, if $\boldsymbol{C}$ reflects a block design, then $\boldsymbol{V}$ should in some sense match the design. Here our argumentation is rather vague, but the topic has so far not been studied in detail. The next example will illustrate our mode of thinking. However, since $\boldsymbol{S}$ is included in the estimates, it is somewhat unclear how perturbations affect the derivatives (compare the results for Perturbation (ii) in Sect. 8.2). Firstly, results are presented which correspond to Lemmas 8.1 and 8.2 and which can be obtained by the application of Appendix B, Theorem B.15 (i)–(iii). Unfortunately the results are based on a somewhat technical treatment.

Lemma 8.3 *Let* $\boldsymbol{S}(\omega) = \boldsymbol{X}(\boldsymbol{I} - \boldsymbol{G}'(\boldsymbol{G}\boldsymbol{G}')^{-}\boldsymbol{G})\boldsymbol{X}'$, *where* $\boldsymbol{G} = \boldsymbol{C} + \omega\boldsymbol{V}$, *as in Definition 8.3 (ii). Then*

(i) $\left.\frac{d^k\boldsymbol{S}(\omega)}{d\omega^k}\right|_{\omega=0} = -\boldsymbol{X}\sum_{i_1=0}^{1}\sum_{i_2=k-i_1-1}^{k-i_1}\binom{k}{i_1}\binom{k-i_1}{i_2}\frac{d^{i_1}\boldsymbol{G}'}{d\omega^{i_1}}\frac{d^{i_2}(\boldsymbol{G}\boldsymbol{G}')^{-1}}{d\omega^{i_2}}\frac{d^{k-i_1-i_2}\boldsymbol{G}}{d\omega^{k-i_1-i_2}}\boldsymbol{X}'\right|_{\omega=0}$,

where

(ii) $\left.\frac{d(\boldsymbol{G}\boldsymbol{G}')^{-1}}{d\omega}\right|_{\omega=0} = -(\boldsymbol{C}\boldsymbol{C}')^{-1}(\boldsymbol{C}\boldsymbol{V}' + \boldsymbol{V}\boldsymbol{C}')(\boldsymbol{C}\boldsymbol{C}')^{-1}$;

(iii) $$\left.\frac{d^2(\boldsymbol{G}\boldsymbol{G}')^{-1}}{d\omega^2}\right|_{\omega=0} = (\boldsymbol{C}\boldsymbol{C}')^{-1}(\boldsymbol{C}\boldsymbol{V}' + \boldsymbol{V}\boldsymbol{C}')(\boldsymbol{C}\boldsymbol{C}')^{-1}(\boldsymbol{C}\boldsymbol{V}' + \boldsymbol{V}\boldsymbol{C}')(\boldsymbol{C}\boldsymbol{C}')^{-1}$$
$$-2(\boldsymbol{C}\boldsymbol{C}')^{-1}\boldsymbol{V}\boldsymbol{V}'(\boldsymbol{C}\boldsymbol{C}')^{-1};$$

(iv) *if* $k \geq 3$,

$$\left.\frac{d^k(\boldsymbol{G}\boldsymbol{G}')^{-1}}{d\omega^k}\right|_{\omega=0} = \sum_{j=k-2}^{k-1}(-1)^{j+1}\sum_{i_1=j}^{k-1}\sum_{i_2=j-1}^{i_1-1}\cdots\sum_{i_j=1}^{i_{j-1}-1}\binom{k}{i_1}\binom{i_1}{i_2}\binom{i_2}{i_3}\cdots\binom{i_{j1}}{i_j}(\boldsymbol{C}\boldsymbol{C}')^{-1}$$
$$\times\left.\frac{d^{i_j}(\boldsymbol{G}\boldsymbol{G}')}{d\omega^{i_j}}\right|_{\omega=0}(\boldsymbol{C}\boldsymbol{C}')^{-1}\left.\frac{d^{i_{j-1}-i_j}(\boldsymbol{G}\boldsymbol{G}')}{d\omega^{i_{j-1}-i_j}}\right|_{\omega=0}(\boldsymbol{C}\boldsymbol{C}')^{-1}\times\cdots$$
$$\times(\boldsymbol{C}\boldsymbol{C}')^{-1}\left.\frac{d^{i_1-i_2}(\boldsymbol{G}\boldsymbol{G}')}{d\omega^{i_1-i_2}}\right|_{\omega-0}(\boldsymbol{C}\boldsymbol{C}')^{-1}\left.\frac{d^{k-i_1}(\boldsymbol{G}\boldsymbol{G}')}{d\omega^{k-i_i}}\right|_{\omega=0}(\boldsymbol{C}\boldsymbol{C}')^{-1},$$

where $\left.\frac{d^l(\boldsymbol{G}\boldsymbol{G}')}{d\omega^l}\right|_{\omega=0} = \boldsymbol{C}\boldsymbol{V}' + \boldsymbol{V}\boldsymbol{C}'$, *if* $l = 1$, $\left.\frac{d^l(\boldsymbol{G}\boldsymbol{G}')}{d\omega^l}\right|_{\omega=0} = 2\boldsymbol{V}\boldsymbol{V}'$, *if* $l = 2$, *and for* $l > 2$ *the derivative equals* $\boldsymbol{0}$.

Using the expressions in Lemma 8.3 leads to the next result for $\boldsymbol{S}(\omega)$. For the final expressions the derivatives $\frac{d^l(\boldsymbol{G}\boldsymbol{G}')^{-1}}{d\omega^l}$, $l = 1, 2$, given in the previous lemma, are needed.

Lemma 8.4 *Let* $\boldsymbol{S}(\omega)$ *be as in Lemma 8.3. The derivatives given below,* $\left.\frac{d^l(\boldsymbol{G}\boldsymbol{G}')^{-1}}{d\omega^l}\right|_{\omega=0}$, $l = 1, 2$, *are to be found in Lemma 8.3. Then*

(i) $\left.\frac{d^0\boldsymbol{S}(\omega)}{d\omega^0}\right|_{\omega=0} = \boldsymbol{S} = \boldsymbol{X}(\boldsymbol{I} - \boldsymbol{C}'(\boldsymbol{C}\boldsymbol{C}')^{-1}\boldsymbol{C})\boldsymbol{X}'$;

(ii)

$$\left.\frac{d\boldsymbol{S}(\omega)}{d\,\omega}\right|_{\omega=0} = -\boldsymbol{X}\boldsymbol{C}'(\boldsymbol{C}\boldsymbol{C}')^{-1}\boldsymbol{V}\boldsymbol{X}' - \boldsymbol{X}\boldsymbol{V}'(\boldsymbol{C}\boldsymbol{C}')^{-1}\boldsymbol{C}\boldsymbol{X}' - \boldsymbol{X}\boldsymbol{C}'\left.\frac{d(\boldsymbol{G}\boldsymbol{G}')^{-1}}{d\,\omega}\right|_{\omega=0}\boldsymbol{C}\boldsymbol{X}';$$

(iii)

$$\left.\frac{d^2\boldsymbol{S}(\omega)}{d\,\omega^2}\right|_{\omega=0} = -2\boldsymbol{X}\boldsymbol{C}'\left.\frac{d(\boldsymbol{G}\boldsymbol{G}')^{-1}}{d\,\omega}\right|_{\omega=0}\boldsymbol{V}\boldsymbol{X}' - \boldsymbol{X}\boldsymbol{C}'\left.\frac{d^2(\boldsymbol{G}\boldsymbol{G}')^{-1}}{d\,\omega^2}\right|_{\omega=0}\boldsymbol{C}\boldsymbol{X}' -2\boldsymbol{X}\boldsymbol{V}'(\boldsymbol{C}\boldsymbol{C}')^{-1}\boldsymbol{V}\boldsymbol{X}' - 2\boldsymbol{X}\boldsymbol{V}'\left.\frac{d(\boldsymbol{G}\boldsymbol{G}')^{-1}}{d\,\omega}\right|_{\omega=0}\boldsymbol{C}\boldsymbol{X}';$$

(iv)

$$\left.\frac{d^3\boldsymbol{S}(\omega)}{d\,\omega^3}\right|_{\omega=0} = -3\boldsymbol{X}\boldsymbol{C}'\left.\frac{d^2(\boldsymbol{G}\boldsymbol{G}')^{-1}}{d\,\omega^2}\right|_{\omega=0}\boldsymbol{V}\boldsymbol{X}' - \boldsymbol{X}\boldsymbol{C}'\left.\frac{d^3(\boldsymbol{G}\boldsymbol{G}')^{-1}}{d\,\omega^3}\right|_{\omega=0}\boldsymbol{C}\boldsymbol{X}' -6\boldsymbol{X}\boldsymbol{V}'\left.\frac{d(\boldsymbol{G}\boldsymbol{G}')^{-1}}{d\,\omega}\right|_{\omega=0}\boldsymbol{V}\boldsymbol{X}' - 3\boldsymbol{X}\boldsymbol{V}'\left.\frac{d^2(\boldsymbol{G}\boldsymbol{G}')^{-1}}{d\,\omega^2}\right|_{\omega=0}\boldsymbol{C}\boldsymbol{X}'.$$

Similar to Theorem 8.1, a theorem for Perturbation (ii) can be formulated.

Theorem 8.2 *Let* $\widehat{\boldsymbol{B}}(\omega) = (\boldsymbol{A}'\boldsymbol{S}^{-1}(\omega)\boldsymbol{A})^{-1}\boldsymbol{A}'\boldsymbol{S}^{-1}(\omega)\boldsymbol{X}\boldsymbol{G}'(\boldsymbol{G}\boldsymbol{G}')^{-1}$, *where* $\boldsymbol{S}(\omega) = \boldsymbol{X}(\boldsymbol{I} - \boldsymbol{P}_{\boldsymbol{G}'})\boldsymbol{X}'$ *and* $\boldsymbol{G} = \boldsymbol{C} + \omega\boldsymbol{V}$ *for some known* $\boldsymbol{V}$*; i.e. Perturbation (ii) in Definition 8.3 is applied. Then*

$$\left.\frac{d^k\widehat{\boldsymbol{B}}(\omega)}{d\,\omega^k}\right|_{\omega=0} = (\boldsymbol{A}'\boldsymbol{A})^{-1}\boldsymbol{A}'\boldsymbol{X}\left.\frac{d^k\boldsymbol{G}'(\boldsymbol{G}\boldsymbol{G}')^{-1}}{d\,\omega^k}\right|_{\omega=0} - \sum_{i_1=0}^{k}\sum_{i_2=0}^{k-i_1}\binom{k}{i_1}\binom{k-i_1}{i_2}(\boldsymbol{A}'\boldsymbol{A})^{-1}\boldsymbol{A}' \times \left.\frac{d^{i_1}\boldsymbol{S}(\omega)}{d\,\omega^{i_1}}\boldsymbol{A}^o\frac{d^{i_2}(\boldsymbol{A}^{o'}\boldsymbol{S}(\omega)\boldsymbol{A}^o)^{-1}}{d\,\omega^{i_2}}\boldsymbol{A}^{o'}\boldsymbol{X}\frac{d^{k-i_1-i_2}\boldsymbol{G}'(\boldsymbol{G}\boldsymbol{G}')^{-1}}{d\,\omega^{k-i_1-i_2}}\right|_{\omega=0}, \quad k \geq 0,$$

where $\left.\frac{d^l\boldsymbol{G}'(\boldsymbol{G}\boldsymbol{G}')^{-1}}{d\,\omega^l}\right|_{\omega=0} = \boldsymbol{C}'\left.\frac{d^l(\boldsymbol{G}\boldsymbol{G}')^{-1}}{d\,\omega^l}\right|_{\omega=0} + l\boldsymbol{V}'\left.\frac{d^{l-1}(\boldsymbol{G}\boldsymbol{G}')^{-1}}{d\,\omega^{l-1}}\right|_{\omega=0}$, $\left.\frac{d^l\boldsymbol{S}(\omega)}{d\,\omega^l}\right|_{\omega=0}$ *and* $\left.\frac{d^l(\boldsymbol{A}^{o'}\boldsymbol{S}(\omega)\boldsymbol{A}^o)^{-1}}{d\,\omega^l}\right|_{\omega=0}$ *are derived via Lemmas 8.3, 8.4 and Theorem B.15 (iii) in Appendix B.*

Since usually only a few derivatives of low order are needed, the next corollary is presented to help us use the results of Theorem 8.2.

Corollary 8.2 *Let the matrices and perturbation be as in Theorem 8.2 and* $S(0) = S = X(I - P_{C'})X'$.

(i) *If* $k = 0$, $\left.\frac{d^0 \widehat{B}(\omega)}{d\omega^0}\right|_{\omega=0} = (A'S^{-1}A)^{-1}A'S^{-1}XC'(CC')^{-1}$.

(ii) *If* $k = 1$, $\left.\frac{d\widehat{B}(\omega)}{d\omega}\right|_{\omega=0} = (A'S^{-1}A)^{-1}A'S^{-1}X \left.\frac{dG'(GG')^{-1}}{d\omega}\right|_{\omega=0}$.

(iii) *If* $k = 2$,

$$\left.\frac{d^2\widehat{B}(\omega)}{d\omega^2}\right|_{\omega=0} = (A'S^{-1}A)^{-1}A'S^{-1}X \left.\frac{d^2G'(GG')^{-1}}{d\omega^2}\right|_{\omega=0}$$
$$-2(A'A)^{-1}A'SA^o \left.\frac{d(A^{o'}S(\omega)A^o)^{-1}}{d\omega}\right|_{\omega=0} A^{o'}X \left.\frac{dG'(GG')^{-1}}{d\omega}\right|_{\omega=0}$$
$$-(A'A)^{-1}A'SA^o \left.\frac{d^2(A^{o'}S(\omega)A^o)^{-1}}{d\omega^2}\right|_{\omega=0} A^{o'}XC'(CC')^{-1}$$
$$-2\left.\frac{dS(\omega)}{d\omega}\right|_{\omega=0} A^o(A^{o'}SA^o)^{-1}A^{o'}X \left.\frac{dG'(GG')^{-1}}{d\omega}\right|_{\omega=0}$$
$$-2\left.\frac{dS(\omega)}{d\omega}\right|_{\omega=0} A^o \left.\frac{d(A^{o'}S(\omega)A^o)^{-1}}{d\omega}\right|_{\omega=0} A^{o'}XC'(CC')^{-1}$$
$$-\left.\frac{d^2S(\omega)}{d\omega^2}\right|_{\omega=0} A^o(A^{o'}SA^o)^{-1}A^{o'}XC'(CC')^{-1}.$$

(iv) *If* $k = 3$,

$$\left.\frac{d^3\widehat{B}(\omega)}{d\omega^3}\right|_{\omega=0} = (A'S^{-1}A)^{-1}A'S^{-1}X \left.\frac{d^3G'(GG')^{-1}}{d\omega^3}\right|_{\omega=0}$$
$$-3(A'A)^{-1}A'SA^o \left.\frac{d(A^{o'}S(\omega)A^o)^{-1}}{d\omega}\right|_{\omega=0} A^{o'}X \left.\frac{d^2G'(GG')^{-1}}{d\omega^2}\right|_{\omega=0}$$
$$-3(A'A)^{-1}A'SA^o \left.\frac{d^2(A^{o'}S(\omega)A^o)^{-1}}{d\omega^2}\right|_{\omega=0} A^{o'}X \left.\frac{dG'(GG')^{-1}}{d\omega}\right|_{\omega=0}$$
$$-(A'A)^{-1}A'SA^o \left.\frac{d^3(A^{o'}S(\omega)A^o)^{-1}}{d\omega^3}\right|_{\omega=0} A^{o'}XC'(CC')^{-1}$$
$$-3(A'A)^{-1}A' \left.\frac{dS(\omega)}{d\omega}\right|_{\omega=0} A^o(A^{o'}SA^o)^{-1}A^{o'}X \left.\frac{d^2G'(GG')^{-1}}{d\omega^2}\right|_{\omega=0}$$
$$-6(A'A)^{-1}A' \left.\frac{dS(\omega)}{d\omega}\right|_{\omega=0} A^o \left.\frac{d(A^{o'}S(\omega)A^o)^{-1}}{d\omega}\right|_{\omega=0} A^{o'}X \left.\frac{dG'(GG')^{-1}}{d\omega}\right|_{\omega=0}$$
$$-3(A'A)^{-1}A' \left.\frac{dS(\omega)}{d\omega}\right|_{\omega=0} A^o \left.\frac{d^2(A^{o'}S(\omega)A^o)^{-1}}{d\omega^2}\right|_{\omega=0} A^{o'}XC'(CC')^{-1}$$

$$-3(A'A)^{-1}A' \left.\frac{d^2 S(\omega)}{d\,\omega^2}\right|_{\omega=0} A^o(A^{o'}SA^o)^{-1}A^{o'}X \left.\frac{dG'(GG')^{-1}}{d\,\omega}\right|_{\omega=0}$$

$$-3(A'A)^{-1}A' \left.\frac{d^2 S(\omega)}{d\,\omega^2}\right|_{\omega=0} A^o \left.\frac{d(A^{o'}S(\omega)A^o)^{-1}}{d\,\omega}\right|_{\omega=0} A^{o'}XC'(CC')^{-1}$$

$$-(A'A)^{-1}A' \left.\frac{d^3 S(\omega)}{d\,\omega^3}\right|_{\omega=0} A^o(A^{o'}SA^o)^{-1}A^{o'}XC'(CC')^{-1};$$

$\left.\frac{d^l (S(\omega))^{-1}}{d\,\omega^l}\right|_{\omega=0}$, $\left.\frac{d^l (A^{o'}S_0A^o)^{-1}}{d\,\omega^l}\right|_{\omega=0}$ *and* $\left.\frac{d^l G'(GG')^{-1}}{d\,\omega^l}\right|_{\omega=0}$, $l = 1, 2, 3$, *are obtained by applying Lemmas 8.3, 8.4 and Appendix B, Theorem B.15.*

A significant difference between Perturbation (iii) and Perturbation (ii) is that in the latter, we have to choose V and, as noted before, there is no real strategy of choosing V.

Example 8.3 (The Classical Potthoff and Roy (1964) Data Set (See Also Table 1.2)) Since the data set consists of two groups of individuals, the design matrix C consists of two rows which are orthogonal to each other. The maximum likelihood estimates of the mean parameters in the BRM will be exploited with respect to Perturbation (ii) in Definition 8.3. When carrying out the calculations, we have to define the matrix V in Perturbation (ii). Firstly, V is chosen so that the ith column of V equals $\binom{1}{1}$ and the other columns of V are identical to $\binom{0}{0}$. One can question if this choice of V is appropriate, because the perturbed ith individual will affect both the girls and the boys through the design matrix, i.e. $C + \omega V$. Other possible alternatives are choosing V so that the ith column equals $\binom{1}{0}$ or choosing V so that the ith column equals $\binom{0}{1}$, which will be considered later.

Necessary results for performing model validation according to the perturbation scheme have been presented in Corollary 8.2. When applying Perturbation (iii), individuals 15, 20 and 24 appeared to deviate from the others. However, when investigating Perturbation (ii), only individual 20 becomes highlighted when $\binom{1}{1}$ is used. In this case, in Table 8.7, the first three derivatives (averaged) are presented for the girls and boys separately, with individual 20, a boy, excluded. It appears that the second derivative for the girls' intercept was large. When individual 20 was perturbed, the effect was different from that for the other boys; see, for example, the second derivative for the girls' intercept, where we have −2.32 versus 1.66. Thus, there is an indication that individual 20 differs from the other boys. Studying the original data, one can confirm that individual 20 is "extreme". Since Perturbation (ii) represents a perturbation of the design matrix C, one conclusion is that individual 20 does not follow the same model as the other boys are doing. A possible explanation is that there has been a typing error, and that the observation at age 14 (26) should be the observation at age 12 and the observation at age 12 (31) should be the observation at age 14. This would make sense, but, of course, we cannot know if this is true if we do not have access to the original files. One final comment concerning this perturbation is that the choice of $\binom{1}{1}$ only identified a few individuals, of

Table 8.7 The results obtained when Perturbation (ii) in Definition 8.3 was applied to the Potthoff and Roy data set (see Example 1.7), with $\boldsymbol{v}_i = \binom{1}{1}$ in $\boldsymbol{V}$ and the other columns in $\boldsymbol{V}$ equal to $\binom{0}{0}$

k	b_{11}	b_{12}	b_{21}	b_{22}
ref	17.43	15.84	0.48	0.83
Girls				
1	−3.02	0.00	−0.12	0.00
2	−8.90	−2.15	−0.31	−0.054
3	−0.40	0.61	0.0078	0.028
Boys, except for individual 20				
1	0.018	−2.07	−0.00072	−0.082
2	−2.32	−6.48	−0.13	−0.29
3	0.86	0.036	0.18	−0.0047
Individual 20 (boy)				
1	−0.27	−2.27	0.011	−0.074
2	1.66	−3.37	0.023	−0.17
3	−0.65	−1.91	−0.015	−0.097

For $k = 1, 2, 3$, the average of the derivative $\left.\frac{d^k\widehat{\boldsymbol{B}}(\omega)}{d\,\omega^k}\right|_{\omega=0}$ has been calculated separately for the girls and the boys (except for individual 20), as well as for individual 20. The case k = ref is provided for comparison and presents the maximum likelihood estimates based on all the individuals (see Corollary 3.1)

which individual 20 showed the "largest" deviance from the others. However, it is outside the scope of this chapter to understand completely the influence exerted by individual 20, and it seems that this cannot be achieved without calculating higher order derivatives, for instance derivatives of order 4 or 5. Moreover, it can be noted that the girls obtained larger derivatives than the boys (see Table 8.7). One can speculate if this is due to the model fit or the group size.

Now $\boldsymbol{V}$ is chosen so that the ith column of $\boldsymbol{V}$ equals $\binom{0}{1}$ and the other columns are identical to $\binom{0}{0}$. This means, among other things, that the influence on the girls exerted by individual 20, as indicated in Table 8.7, should be less clear, which is also shown in Table 8.8. Moreover, in the third derivative, there seems to be a small effect from individual 20, meaning that influential effects may be non-linear. Also in this case, the effect is stronger on the two parameters corresponding to the girls' growth than on the parameters connected to the boys'.

Finally, Table 8.9 shows some results obtained when the perturbation $\boldsymbol{V}$ was defined in such a way that the ith column of $\boldsymbol{V}$ equalled $\binom{1}{0}$ and the other columns were identical to $\binom{0}{0}$. In this case, however, no effects of the perturbation could be discovered. We can also have a perturbation which is based on $\binom{1}{0}$ for the girls and $\binom{0}{1}$ for the boys, or these quantities can be weighted according to, for example, the group sizes.

To round off this example, one can state that different alternative perturbations have been introduced, but neither their interpretations and nor their conclusions

Table 8.8 The results obtained when Perturbation (ii) in Definition 8.2 was applied to the Potthoff and Roy data set (see Example 1.7), with $\boldsymbol{v}_i = \binom{0}{1}$ in $\boldsymbol{V}$ and the other columns in $\boldsymbol{V}$ equal to $\binom{0}{0}$

k	b_{11}	b_{12}	b_{21}	b_{22}
ref	17.43	15.84	0.48	0.83
Girls				
1	−1.44	0.00	−0.075	0.00
2	−2.96	−2.25	−0.15	−0.057
3	−0.56	0.020	−0.017	0.0011
Boys, except for individual 20				
1	0.00	−0.98	0.00	−0.052
2	0.037	−4.27	0.0019	−0.22
3	0.0058	−0.28	0.00027	−0.013
Individual 20 (boy)				
1	0.00	−1.18	0.00	−0.044
2	0.039	−2.78	0.0019	−0.15
3	0.058	−0.87	0.0032	−0.054

For $k = 1, 2, 3$, the average of the derivative $\left.\frac{d^k \widehat{\boldsymbol{B}}(\omega)}{d\,\omega^k}\right|_{\omega=0}$ has been calculated separately for the girls and the boys (except for individual 20), as well as for individual 20. The case k = ref is provided for comparison and presents the maximum likelihood estimates based on all the individuals (see Corollary 3.1)

Table 8.9 The results obtained when Perturbation (ii) in Definition 8.2 was applied to the Potthoff and Roy data set (see Example 1.7), with $\boldsymbol{v}_i = \binom{1}{0}$ in $\boldsymbol{V}$ and the other columns in $\boldsymbol{V}$ equal $\binom{0}{0}$

k	b_{11}	b_{12}	b_{21}	b_{22}
ref	17.43	15.84	0.48	0.83
Girls				
1	−1.58	0.00	−0.043	0.00
2	−6.27	0.044	−0.017	0.0013
3	−1.05	0.047	−0.028	0.0013
Boys, except for individual 20				
1	0.018	−1.09	−0.00072	−0.030
2	−2.55	−2.52	−0.14	−0.071
3	0.36	−0.44	0.020	−0.028
Individual 20 (boy)				
1	−0.27	−1.09	0.011	−0.030
2	−0.48	−2.48	−0.085	−0.072
3	0.30	−0.65	0.028	−0.041

For $k = 1, 2, 3$, the average of the derivative $\left.\frac{d^k \widehat{\boldsymbol{B}}(\omega)}{d\,\omega^k}\right|_{\omega=0}$ has been calculated separately for the girls and the boys (except for individual 20), as well as for individual 20. The case k = ref is provided for comparison and presents the maximum likelihood estimates based on all the individuals (see Corollary 3.1)

are very clear. In addition, more time has to be spent on introducing additional perturbation schemes, in particular to create some kind of optimal scheme. □

Now Perturbation (i) in Definition 8.3 is treated briefly. Copying ideas from the above discussion concerning Perturbation (ii), it can be noted that if

$$\boldsymbol{Z} = \boldsymbol{X} + \omega \boldsymbol{V}, \qquad \text{for some known } \boldsymbol{V},$$

then

$$\begin{aligned}
\boldsymbol{S}(\omega) &= \boldsymbol{Z}(\boldsymbol{I} - \boldsymbol{P}_{\boldsymbol{C}'})\boldsymbol{Z}', \\
\widehat{\boldsymbol{B}}(\omega) &= (\boldsymbol{A}'\boldsymbol{S}(\omega)^{-1}\boldsymbol{A})^{-1}\boldsymbol{A}'\boldsymbol{S}(\omega)^{-1}\boldsymbol{Z}\boldsymbol{C}'(\boldsymbol{C}\boldsymbol{C}')^{-1}
\end{aligned}$$

and

$$\begin{aligned}
\left.\frac{d^k \widehat{\boldsymbol{B}}(\omega)}{d\,\omega^k}\right|_{\omega=0} &= (\boldsymbol{A}'\boldsymbol{A})^{-1}\boldsymbol{A}'\left.\frac{d^k \boldsymbol{Z}}{d\,\omega^k}\right|_{\omega=0} \boldsymbol{C}'(\boldsymbol{C}\boldsymbol{C}')^{-1} \\
&- \sum_{\substack{i_1=0 \\ 0\leq k-i_1-i_2\leq 1}}^{2} \sum_{i_2=0}^{k-i_1} \binom{k}{i_1}\binom{k-i_1}{i_2}(\boldsymbol{A}'\boldsymbol{A})^{-1}\boldsymbol{A}' \left.\frac{d^{i_1}\boldsymbol{S}(\omega)}{d\,\omega^{i_1}}\right|_{\omega=0} \boldsymbol{A}^o \left.\frac{d^{i_2}(\boldsymbol{A}^{o\prime}\boldsymbol{S}(\omega)\boldsymbol{A}^o)^{-1}}{d\,\omega^{i_2}}\right|_{\omega=0} \boldsymbol{A}^{o\prime} \\
&\times \left.\frac{d^{k-i_1-i_2}\boldsymbol{Z}}{d\,\omega^{k-i_1-i_2}}\right|_{\omega=0} \boldsymbol{C}'(\boldsymbol{C}\boldsymbol{C}')^{-1}.
\end{aligned}$$

In this expression, $\left.\frac{d^l \boldsymbol{S}(\omega)}{d\,\omega^l}\right|_{\omega=0}$ and $\left.\frac{d^l \boldsymbol{Z}}{d\,\omega^l}\right|_{\omega=0}$ can be presented immediately, whereas $\left.\frac{d^l(\boldsymbol{A}^{o\prime}\boldsymbol{S}(\omega)\boldsymbol{A}^o)^{-1}}{d\,\omega^l}\right|_{\omega=0}$ is more sophisticated and, concerning this case, the reader is referred to Appendix B, Theorem B.15 (iii):

$$\frac{d^l \boldsymbol{Z}}{d\,\omega^l} = \begin{cases} \boldsymbol{X}, & l = 0, \\ \boldsymbol{V}, & l = 1, \\ \boldsymbol{0}, & l > 1; \end{cases}$$

$$\left.\frac{d^l \boldsymbol{S}(\omega)}{d\,\omega^l}\right|_{\omega=0} = \begin{cases} \boldsymbol{X}(\boldsymbol{I} - \boldsymbol{P}_{\boldsymbol{C}'})\boldsymbol{X}', & l = 0, \\ \boldsymbol{X}(\boldsymbol{I} - \boldsymbol{P}_{\boldsymbol{C}'})\boldsymbol{V}' + \boldsymbol{V}(\boldsymbol{I} - \boldsymbol{P}_{\boldsymbol{C}'})\boldsymbol{X}', & l = 1, \\ 2\boldsymbol{V}(\boldsymbol{I} - \boldsymbol{P}_{\boldsymbol{C}'})\boldsymbol{V}', & l = 2, \\ \boldsymbol{0}, & l > 2. \end{cases}$$

The next theorem comprises the first three derivatives of the perturbed mean estimate $\widehat{\boldsymbol{B}}(\omega)$.

Theorem 8.3 *For the BRM presented in Definition 2.1, let the perturbed estimate* $\widehat{\boldsymbol{B}}(\omega) = (\boldsymbol{A}'\boldsymbol{S}^{-1}(\omega)\boldsymbol{A})^{-1}\boldsymbol{A}'\boldsymbol{S}^{-1}(\omega)\boldsymbol{Z}\boldsymbol{C}'(\boldsymbol{C}\boldsymbol{C}')^{-1}$, *where* $\boldsymbol{S}(\omega) = \boldsymbol{Z}(\boldsymbol{I} - \boldsymbol{P}_{C'})\boldsymbol{Z}'$ *and* $\boldsymbol{Z} = \boldsymbol{X} + \omega\boldsymbol{V}$ *for some* $\boldsymbol{V}$; *i.e. Perturbation (i) in Definition 8.3 is applied. Moreover,* $\left.\frac{d^k(\boldsymbol{A}^{o\prime}\boldsymbol{S}\boldsymbol{A}^o)^{-1}}{d\,\omega^k}\right|_{\omega=0}$, $k = 2, 3$, *is used below and explicit expressions are obtained through Appendix B, Theorem B.15 (iii). Put* $\boldsymbol{D}_1 = \left.\frac{d\boldsymbol{S}(\omega)}{d\,\omega}\right|_{\omega=0}$. *Then*

(i)

$$\left.\frac{d\widehat{\boldsymbol{B}}(\omega)}{d\,\omega}\right|_{\omega=0} = (\boldsymbol{A}'\boldsymbol{S}^{-1}\boldsymbol{A})^{-1}\boldsymbol{A}'\boldsymbol{S}^{-1}\boldsymbol{V}\boldsymbol{C}'(\boldsymbol{C}\boldsymbol{C}')^{-1}$$
$$-(\boldsymbol{A}'\boldsymbol{S}^{-1}\boldsymbol{A})^{-1}\boldsymbol{A}'\boldsymbol{S}^{-1}\boldsymbol{D}_1\boldsymbol{A}^o(\boldsymbol{A}^{o\prime}\boldsymbol{S}\boldsymbol{A}^o)^{-1}\boldsymbol{A}^{o\prime}\boldsymbol{X}\boldsymbol{C}'(\boldsymbol{C}\boldsymbol{C}')^{-1};$$

(ii)

$$\left.\frac{d^2\widehat{\boldsymbol{B}}(\omega)}{d\,\omega^2}\right|_{\omega=0}$$
$$= 2(\boldsymbol{A}'\boldsymbol{A})^{-1}\boldsymbol{A}'\boldsymbol{S}\boldsymbol{A}^o(\boldsymbol{A}^{o\prime}\boldsymbol{S}\boldsymbol{A}^o)^{-1}\boldsymbol{A}^{o\prime}\boldsymbol{D}_1\boldsymbol{A}^o(\boldsymbol{A}^{o\prime}\boldsymbol{S}\boldsymbol{A}^o)^{-1}\boldsymbol{A}^{o\prime}\boldsymbol{V}\boldsymbol{C}'(\boldsymbol{C}\boldsymbol{C}')^{-1}$$
$$-(\boldsymbol{A}'\boldsymbol{A})^{-1}\boldsymbol{A}'\boldsymbol{S}\boldsymbol{A}^o\left.\frac{d^2(\boldsymbol{A}^{o\prime}\boldsymbol{S}\boldsymbol{A}^o)^{-1}}{d\,\omega^2}\right|_{\omega=0}\boldsymbol{A}^{o\prime}\boldsymbol{X}\boldsymbol{C}'(\boldsymbol{C}\boldsymbol{C}')^{-1}$$
$$-2(\boldsymbol{A}'\boldsymbol{A})^{-1}\boldsymbol{A}'\boldsymbol{D}_1\boldsymbol{A}^o(\boldsymbol{A}^{o\prime}\boldsymbol{S}\boldsymbol{A}^o)^{-1}\boldsymbol{A}^{o\prime}\boldsymbol{V}\boldsymbol{C}'(\boldsymbol{C}\boldsymbol{C}')^{-1}$$
$$+2(\boldsymbol{A}'\boldsymbol{A})^{-1}\boldsymbol{A}'\boldsymbol{D}_1\boldsymbol{A}^o(\boldsymbol{A}^{o\prime}\boldsymbol{S}\boldsymbol{A}^o)^{-1}\boldsymbol{A}^{o\prime}\boldsymbol{D}_1\boldsymbol{A}^o(\boldsymbol{A}^{o\prime}\boldsymbol{S}\boldsymbol{A}^o)^{-1}\boldsymbol{A}^{o\prime}\boldsymbol{X}\boldsymbol{C}'(\boldsymbol{C}\boldsymbol{C}')^{-1}$$
$$-2(\boldsymbol{A}'\boldsymbol{A})^{-1}\boldsymbol{A}'\boldsymbol{V}(\boldsymbol{I} - \boldsymbol{P}_{C'})\boldsymbol{V}'\boldsymbol{A}^o(\boldsymbol{A}^{o\prime}\boldsymbol{S}\boldsymbol{A}^o)^{-1}\boldsymbol{A}^{o\prime}\boldsymbol{X}\boldsymbol{C}'(\boldsymbol{C}\boldsymbol{C}')^{-1};$$

(iii)

$$\left.\frac{d^3\widehat{\boldsymbol{B}}(\omega)}{d\,\omega^3}\right|_{\omega=0} = -3(\boldsymbol{A}'\boldsymbol{A})^{-1}\boldsymbol{A}'\boldsymbol{S}\boldsymbol{A}^o\left.\frac{d^2(\boldsymbol{A}^{o\prime}\boldsymbol{S}\boldsymbol{A}^o)^{-1}}{d\,\omega^2}\right|_{\omega=0}\boldsymbol{A}^{o\prime}\boldsymbol{V}\boldsymbol{C}'(\boldsymbol{C}\boldsymbol{C}')^{-1}$$
$$-(\boldsymbol{A}'\boldsymbol{A})^{-1}\boldsymbol{A}'\boldsymbol{S}\boldsymbol{A}^o\left.\frac{d^3(\boldsymbol{A}^{o\prime}\boldsymbol{S}\boldsymbol{A}^o)^{-1}}{d\,\omega^3}\right|_{\omega=0}\boldsymbol{A}^{o\prime}\boldsymbol{X}\boldsymbol{C}'(\boldsymbol{C}\boldsymbol{C}')^{-1}$$
$$-6(\boldsymbol{A}'\boldsymbol{A})^{-1}\boldsymbol{A}'\boldsymbol{D}_1\boldsymbol{A}^o\left.\frac{d(\boldsymbol{A}^{o\prime}\boldsymbol{S}\boldsymbol{A}^o)^{-1}}{d\,\omega}\right|_{\omega=0}\boldsymbol{A}^{o\prime}\boldsymbol{V}\boldsymbol{C}'(\boldsymbol{C}\boldsymbol{C}')^{-1}$$
$$-3(\boldsymbol{A}'\boldsymbol{A})^{-1}\boldsymbol{A}'\boldsymbol{D}_1\boldsymbol{A}^o\left.\frac{d^2(\boldsymbol{A}^{o\prime}\boldsymbol{S}\boldsymbol{A}^o)^{-1}}{d\,\omega^2}\right|_{\omega=0}\boldsymbol{A}^{o\prime}\boldsymbol{X}\boldsymbol{C}'(\boldsymbol{C}\boldsymbol{C}')^{-1}$$
$$-6(\boldsymbol{A}'\boldsymbol{A})^{-1}\boldsymbol{A}'\boldsymbol{V}(\boldsymbol{I} - \boldsymbol{P}_{C'})\boldsymbol{V}'\boldsymbol{A}^o(\boldsymbol{A}^{o\prime}\boldsymbol{S}\boldsymbol{A}^o)^{-1}\boldsymbol{A}^{o\prime}\boldsymbol{V}\boldsymbol{C}'(\boldsymbol{C}\boldsymbol{C}')^{-1}$$
$$-6(\boldsymbol{A}'\boldsymbol{A})^{-1}\boldsymbol{A}'\boldsymbol{V}(\boldsymbol{I} - \boldsymbol{P}_{C'})\boldsymbol{V}'\boldsymbol{A}^o\left.\frac{d(\boldsymbol{A}^{o\prime}\boldsymbol{S}\boldsymbol{A}^o)^{-1}}{d\,\omega}\right|_{\omega=0}\boldsymbol{A}^{o\prime}\boldsymbol{X}\boldsymbol{C}'(\boldsymbol{C}\boldsymbol{C}')^{-1}.$$

We will not exploit Perturbation (i) any more, mainly because further research needs to be conducted on this topic and there are no strategies available for choosing $\boldsymbol{V}$. Moreover, it is quite conceivable that a random choice of the columns in $\boldsymbol{V}$ can make sense.

Hitherto only perturbations which affect $\boldsymbol{X}$ and $\boldsymbol{C}$ have been considered (see Definition 8.3). Now we briefly examine the problem of perturbing $\boldsymbol{A}$ in the BRM and, firstly, put

$$\boldsymbol{X}(\omega)' = (\boldsymbol{X}_0' : \sqrt{\omega}\boldsymbol{X}_i'), \tag{8.14}$$

$$\boldsymbol{A}(\omega)' = (\boldsymbol{A}_0' : \sqrt{\omega}\boldsymbol{A}_i'), \tag{8.15}$$

where $\boldsymbol{X}_i$ and $\boldsymbol{A}_i$ are the ith row of $\boldsymbol{X}$ and $\boldsymbol{A}$, respectively, and are analogous to $\boldsymbol{X}(\omega) = (\boldsymbol{X}_0 : \sqrt{\omega}\boldsymbol{X}_i)$ and $\boldsymbol{C} = (\boldsymbol{C}_0 : \sqrt{\omega}\boldsymbol{C}_i)$, i.e. Perturbation (iii) in Definition 8.3. Using the perturbation scheme defined via (8.14) and (8.15) yields

$$\begin{aligned}\widehat{\boldsymbol{B}}(\omega) &= (\boldsymbol{A}'(\omega)\boldsymbol{S}(\omega)^{-1}\boldsymbol{A}(\omega))^{-1}\boldsymbol{A}'(\omega)\boldsymbol{S}(\omega)^{-1}\boldsymbol{X}(\omega)\boldsymbol{C}'(\boldsymbol{C}\boldsymbol{C}')^{-1}\\ &= (\boldsymbol{A}'\boldsymbol{S}^{-1}\boldsymbol{A})^{-1}\boldsymbol{A}'\boldsymbol{S}^{-1}\boldsymbol{X}\boldsymbol{C}'(\boldsymbol{C}\boldsymbol{C}')^{-1} = \widehat{\boldsymbol{B}},\end{aligned}$$

where $\widehat{\boldsymbol{B}}$ is the MLE. Direct calculations show that the expressions $(\boldsymbol{A}'(\omega)\boldsymbol{S}(\omega)^{-1}\boldsymbol{A}(\omega))^{-1}$ and $\boldsymbol{A}'(\omega)\boldsymbol{S}(\omega)^{-1}\boldsymbol{X}(\omega)$ are both independent of ω and, therefore, that $\widehat{\boldsymbol{B}}$ is also independent of ω, as indicated in the above calculations. Thus, for every ω, the same expression is obtained, which means that we cannot extract any information about influence via the above-specified perturbation. Moreover, the phenomenon which has been observed means that, around $\omega = 0$, the estimate is not differentiable and, therefore, this type of perturbation scheme does not make sense. However, it can be noted that if one deletes a row in $\boldsymbol{X}$ and $\boldsymbol{A}$, this will have a direct effect on $\boldsymbol{\Sigma}$, causing it to "shrink"; i.e. $\boldsymbol{\Sigma}$ will consist of fewer parameters. This means that the perturbation changes the whole model and then the results obviously are difficult to interpret.

Alternatively, we can turn our attention to a second type of perturbation. Let, as before, $\boldsymbol{V}$ be a known matrix and consider the perturbation $\boldsymbol{H} = \boldsymbol{A} + \omega\boldsymbol{V}$, which is of the same type as $\boldsymbol{C} + \omega\boldsymbol{V}$, i.e. Perturbation (ii) in Definition 8.3. However, the fundamental difference between the two perturbations is that $\boldsymbol{C} + \omega\boldsymbol{V}$ concerns the perturbation of observations and $\boldsymbol{H}(\omega) = \boldsymbol{A} + \omega\boldsymbol{V}$ concerns the model sensitivity. It follows that

$$\left.\frac{d^k\widehat{\boldsymbol{B}}(\omega)}{d\,\omega^k}\right|_{\omega=0} = \sum_{i=k-1}^{k}\binom{k}{i}\left.\frac{d^i(\boldsymbol{H}'\boldsymbol{S}^{-1}\boldsymbol{H})^{-1}}{d\,\omega^i}\frac{d^{k-i}\boldsymbol{H}'}{d\,\omega^{k-i}}\boldsymbol{S}^{-1}\boldsymbol{X}\boldsymbol{C}'(\boldsymbol{C}\boldsymbol{C}')^{-1}\right|_{\omega=0},$$

where $\left.\frac{d^i(\boldsymbol{H}'\boldsymbol{S}^{-1}\boldsymbol{H})^{-1}}{d\,\omega^i}\right|_{\omega=0}$ can be obtained by applying Appendix B, Theorem B.15 (i)–(iii). In the next theorem the first three derivatives are explicated.

Theorem 8.4 *For the BRM presented in Definition 2.1, let*

$$\widehat{\boldsymbol{B}}(\omega) = (\boldsymbol{H}(\omega)'\boldsymbol{S}^{-1}\boldsymbol{H}(\omega))^{-1}\boldsymbol{H}(\omega)'\boldsymbol{S}^{-1}\boldsymbol{X}\boldsymbol{C}'(\boldsymbol{C}\boldsymbol{C}')^{-1},$$

where $\boldsymbol{H}(\omega) = \boldsymbol{A} + \omega\boldsymbol{V}$ *for some* $\boldsymbol{V}$. *Put* $\boldsymbol{D}_1 = \left.\frac{d(\boldsymbol{H}'\boldsymbol{S}^{-1}\boldsymbol{H})}{d\,\omega}\right|_{\omega=0} = \boldsymbol{V}'\boldsymbol{S}^{-1}\boldsymbol{A} + \boldsymbol{A}'\boldsymbol{S}^{-1}\boldsymbol{V}$. *Then*

(i)

$$\left.\frac{d\widehat{\boldsymbol{B}}(\omega)}{d\,\omega}\right|_{\omega=0} = (\boldsymbol{A}'\boldsymbol{S}^{-1}\boldsymbol{A})^{-1}\boldsymbol{V}'\boldsymbol{S}^{-1}\boldsymbol{X}\boldsymbol{C}'(\boldsymbol{C}\boldsymbol{C}')^{-1}$$
$$-(\boldsymbol{A}'\boldsymbol{S}^{-1}\boldsymbol{A})^{-1}\boldsymbol{D}_1(\boldsymbol{A}'\boldsymbol{S}^{-1}\boldsymbol{A})^{-1}\boldsymbol{A}'\boldsymbol{S}^{-1}\boldsymbol{X}\boldsymbol{C}'(\boldsymbol{C}\boldsymbol{C}')^{-1};$$

(ii)

$$\left.\frac{d^2\widehat{\boldsymbol{B}}(\omega)}{d\,\omega^2}\right|_{\omega=0} = -2(\boldsymbol{A}'\boldsymbol{S}^{-1}\boldsymbol{A})^{-1}\boldsymbol{D}_1(\boldsymbol{A}'\boldsymbol{S}^{-1}\boldsymbol{A})^{-1}\boldsymbol{V}'\boldsymbol{S}^{-1}\boldsymbol{X}\boldsymbol{C}'(\boldsymbol{C}\boldsymbol{C}')^{-1}$$
$$-2(\boldsymbol{A}'\boldsymbol{S}^{-1}\boldsymbol{A})^{-1}\boldsymbol{V}'\boldsymbol{S}^{-1}\boldsymbol{V}(\boldsymbol{A}'\boldsymbol{S}^{-1}\boldsymbol{A})^{-1}\boldsymbol{A}'\boldsymbol{S}^{-1}\boldsymbol{X}\boldsymbol{C}'(\boldsymbol{C}\boldsymbol{C}')^{-1}$$
$$+2(\boldsymbol{A}'\boldsymbol{S}^{-1}\boldsymbol{A})^{-1}\boldsymbol{D}_1(\boldsymbol{A}'\boldsymbol{S}^{-1}\boldsymbol{A})^{-1}\boldsymbol{D}_1(\boldsymbol{A}'\boldsymbol{S}^{-1}\boldsymbol{A})^{-1}\boldsymbol{A}'\boldsymbol{S}^{-1}\boldsymbol{X}\boldsymbol{C}'(\boldsymbol{C}\boldsymbol{C}')^{-1}.$$

(iii)

$$\left.\frac{d^3\widehat{\boldsymbol{B}}(\omega)}{d\,\omega^3}\right|_{\omega=0} = -3\left.\frac{d^2(\boldsymbol{H}'\boldsymbol{S}^{-1}\boldsymbol{H})^{-1}}{d\,\omega^2}\right|_{\omega=0}\boldsymbol{V}'\boldsymbol{S}^{-1}\boldsymbol{X}\boldsymbol{C}'(\boldsymbol{C}\boldsymbol{C}')^{-1}$$
$$+\left.\frac{d^3(\boldsymbol{H}'\boldsymbol{S}^{-1}\boldsymbol{H})^{-1}}{d\,\omega^3}\right|_{\omega=0}\boldsymbol{A}'\boldsymbol{S}^{-1}\boldsymbol{X}\boldsymbol{C}'(\boldsymbol{C}\boldsymbol{C}')^{-1},$$

with

$$\left.\frac{d^3(\boldsymbol{H}'\boldsymbol{S}^{-1}\boldsymbol{H})^{-1}}{d\,\omega^3}\right|_{\omega=0}$$
$$= 3(\boldsymbol{A}'\boldsymbol{S}^{-1}\boldsymbol{A})^{-1}\left.\frac{d\boldsymbol{H}'\boldsymbol{S}^{-1}\boldsymbol{H}}{d\,\omega}\right|_{\omega=0}(\boldsymbol{A}'\boldsymbol{S}^{-1}\boldsymbol{A})^{-1}\left.\frac{d^2\boldsymbol{H}'\boldsymbol{S}^{-1}\boldsymbol{H}}{d\,\omega^2}\right|_{\omega=0}(\boldsymbol{A}'\boldsymbol{S}^{-1}\boldsymbol{A})^{-1}$$
$$+3(\boldsymbol{A}'\boldsymbol{S}^{-1}\boldsymbol{A})^{-1}\left.\frac{d^2\boldsymbol{H}'\boldsymbol{S}^{-1}\boldsymbol{H}}{d\,\omega^2}\right|_{\omega=0}(\boldsymbol{A}'\boldsymbol{S}^{-1}\boldsymbol{A})^{-1}\left.\frac{d\boldsymbol{H}'\boldsymbol{S}^{-1}\boldsymbol{H}}{d\,\omega}\right|_{\omega=0}(\boldsymbol{A}'\boldsymbol{S}^{-1}\boldsymbol{A})^{-1}$$
$$-6(\boldsymbol{A}'\boldsymbol{S}^{-1}\boldsymbol{A})^{-1}\left.\frac{d\boldsymbol{H}'\boldsymbol{S}^{-1}\boldsymbol{H}}{d\,\omega}\right|_{\omega=0}(\boldsymbol{A}'\boldsymbol{S}^{-1}\boldsymbol{A})^{-1}\left.\frac{d\boldsymbol{H}'\boldsymbol{S}^{-1}\boldsymbol{H}}{d\,\omega}\right|_{\omega=0}(\boldsymbol{A}'\boldsymbol{S}^{-1}\boldsymbol{A})^{-1}$$
$$\times\left.\frac{d\boldsymbol{H}'\boldsymbol{S}^{-1}\boldsymbol{H}}{d\,\omega}\right|_{\omega=0}(\boldsymbol{A}'\boldsymbol{S}^{-1}\boldsymbol{A})^{-1},$$

$$\left.\frac{d^2(\boldsymbol{H}'\boldsymbol{S}^{-1}\boldsymbol{H})^{-1}}{d\,\omega^2}\right|_{\omega=0} = -2(\boldsymbol{A}'\boldsymbol{S}^{-1}\boldsymbol{A})^{-1}\boldsymbol{V}'\boldsymbol{S}^{-1}\boldsymbol{V}(\boldsymbol{A}'\boldsymbol{S}^{-1}\boldsymbol{A})^{-1}$$
$$+2(\boldsymbol{A}'\boldsymbol{S}^{-1}\boldsymbol{A})^{-1}\left.\frac{d\boldsymbol{H}'\boldsymbol{S}^{-1}\boldsymbol{H}}{d\,\omega}\right|_{\omega=0}(\boldsymbol{A}'\boldsymbol{S}^{-1}\boldsymbol{A})^{-1}\left.\frac{d\boldsymbol{H}'\boldsymbol{S}^{-1}\boldsymbol{H}}{d\,\omega}\right|_{\omega=0}(\boldsymbol{A}'\boldsymbol{S}^{-1}\boldsymbol{A})^{-1}$$

and

$$\left.\frac{d\boldsymbol{H}'\boldsymbol{S}^{-1}\boldsymbol{H}}{d\,\omega}\right|_{\omega=0} = \boldsymbol{V}'\boldsymbol{S}^{-1}\boldsymbol{A} + \boldsymbol{A}'\boldsymbol{S}^{-1}\boldsymbol{V},$$

$$\left.\frac{d^2\boldsymbol{H}'\boldsymbol{S}^{-1}\boldsymbol{H}}{d\,\omega^2}\right|_{\omega=0} = 2\boldsymbol{V}'\boldsymbol{S}^{-1}\boldsymbol{V}.$$

Example 8.4 In this example, Theorem 8.4 is discussed very briefly. For instance, consider the Potthoff and Roy (1964) data set, which was exploited in Example 1.7. Here we can choose $\boldsymbol{V}$ to equal

$$\boldsymbol{V} = \begin{pmatrix} 0 & 1 \\ 0 & 1 \\ 0 & 1 \\ 0 & 1 \end{pmatrix} \quad \text{or} \quad \boldsymbol{V} = \begin{pmatrix} 0 & 0.5 \\ 0 & 0 \\ 0 & 0 \\ 0 & 0 \end{pmatrix} \quad \text{or} \quad \boldsymbol{V} = \begin{pmatrix} 0 & 0 \\ 0 & 0 \\ 0 & 0 \\ 0 & 0.5 \end{pmatrix},$$

for example. With the above choices of $\boldsymbol{V}$, the second column of $\boldsymbol{A}$ has been altered. In the first case the whole model has been shifted and investigating this case does not make sense. In the other two cases, only one time point is perturbed and here one can see some effects (the computations are not shown here). In particular, the perturbation of the fourth time point has the largest effect on $\widehat{\boldsymbol{B}}$. This is in complete agreement with least squares regression theory, where it is maintained that the observations which are at the "end-points" of the observation period have the largest influence on the mean estimates. □

Now, the influence on the maximum likelihood estimate of the dispersion matrix is treated briefly. The three different perturbations given in Definition 8.3 could have been reconsidered, but only the results for Perturbation (iii) will be presented in detail. All the results for $\widehat{\boldsymbol{\Sigma}}$ depend heavily on the results for $\widehat{\boldsymbol{B}}$, since

$$n\widehat{\boldsymbol{\Sigma}} = (\boldsymbol{X} - \boldsymbol{A}\widehat{\boldsymbol{B}}\boldsymbol{C})(\boldsymbol{X} - \boldsymbol{A}\widehat{\boldsymbol{B}}\boldsymbol{C})' \tag{8.16}$$

$$= \boldsymbol{X}\boldsymbol{X}' - \boldsymbol{X}\boldsymbol{C}'\widehat{\boldsymbol{B}}'\boldsymbol{A}' - \boldsymbol{A}\widehat{\boldsymbol{B}}\boldsymbol{C}\boldsymbol{X}' + \boldsymbol{A}\widehat{\boldsymbol{B}}\boldsymbol{C}\boldsymbol{C}'\widehat{\boldsymbol{B}}'\boldsymbol{A}'. \tag{8.17}$$

Theorem 8.5 *Consider the BRM presented in Definition 2.1, and assume that Perturbation (iii) in Definition 8.3 is applied, i.e.* $\boldsymbol{X} = (\boldsymbol{X}_0, \sqrt{\omega}\boldsymbol{X}_i)$ *and* $\boldsymbol{C} = (\boldsymbol{C}_0, \sqrt{\omega}\boldsymbol{C}_i)$. *Then*

$$n\widehat{\boldsymbol{\Sigma}}(\omega) = (\boldsymbol{X} - \boldsymbol{A}\widehat{\boldsymbol{B}}(\omega)\boldsymbol{C})(\boldsymbol{X} - \boldsymbol{A}\widehat{\boldsymbol{B}}(\omega)\boldsymbol{C})',$$

where $\widehat{\boldsymbol{B}}(\omega)$ *is the same as in Theorem 8.1, and*

$$\left.\frac{d^k n\widehat{\boldsymbol{\Sigma}}(\omega)}{d\,\omega^k}\right|_{\omega=0} = \left.\frac{d^k \boldsymbol{X}\boldsymbol{X}'}{d\,\omega^k}\right|_{\omega=0} - \boldsymbol{A}\sum_{i=0}^{1}\binom{k}{i}\left.\frac{d^{k-i}\widehat{\boldsymbol{B}}(\omega)}{d\,\omega^{k-i}}\right|_{\omega=0}\left.\frac{d^i \boldsymbol{C}\boldsymbol{X}'}{d\,\omega^i}\right|_{\omega=0}$$

$$-\sum_{i=0}^{1}\binom{k}{i}\left.\frac{d^i \boldsymbol{X}\boldsymbol{C}'}{d\,\omega^i}\right|_{\omega=0}\left.\frac{d^{k-i}\widehat{\boldsymbol{B}}'(\omega)}{d\,\omega^{k-i}}\right|_{\omega=0}\boldsymbol{A}'$$

$$+\boldsymbol{A}\sum_{\substack{i_1=0\\0\leq i_2\leq 1}}^{k}\sum_{i_2=0}^{k-i_1}\binom{k}{i_1}\binom{k-i_1}{i_2}\left.\frac{d^{k-i_1}\widehat{\boldsymbol{B}}(\omega)}{d\,\omega^{k-i_1}}\frac{d^{i_2}\boldsymbol{C}\boldsymbol{C}'}{d\,\omega^{i_2}}\frac{d^{k-i_1-i_2}\widehat{\boldsymbol{B}}'(\omega)}{d\,\omega^{k-i_1-i_2}}\right|_{\omega=0}\boldsymbol{A}',$$

with $\left.\frac{d^l\widehat{\boldsymbol{B}}}{d\,\omega^l}\right|_{\omega=0}$ *given in Theorem 8.1.*

Next the first three derivatives for $\widehat{\boldsymbol{\Sigma}}(\omega)$ are presented.

Corollary 8.3 *For* $\widehat{\boldsymbol{\Sigma}}(\omega)$ *in Theorem 8.5:*

(i)

$$\left.\frac{d\,n\widehat{\boldsymbol{\Sigma}}(\omega)}{d\,\omega}\right|_{\omega=0} = \boldsymbol{X}_i\boldsymbol{X}_i' - (\boldsymbol{X}_0\boldsymbol{C}_0'\left.\frac{d\widehat{\boldsymbol{B}}'(\omega)}{d\,\omega}\right|_{\omega=0} + \boldsymbol{X}_i\boldsymbol{C}_i'\widehat{\boldsymbol{B}}'(0))\boldsymbol{A}'$$

$$-\boldsymbol{A}(\left.\frac{d\widehat{\boldsymbol{B}}(\omega)}{d\,\omega}\right|_{\omega=0}\boldsymbol{C}_0\boldsymbol{X}_0' + \widehat{\boldsymbol{B}}(0)\boldsymbol{C}_i\boldsymbol{X}_i') + \boldsymbol{A}\left.\frac{d\widehat{\boldsymbol{B}}(\omega)}{d\,\omega}\right|_{\omega=0}\boldsymbol{C}_0\boldsymbol{C}_0'\left.\frac{d\widehat{\boldsymbol{B}}'(\omega)}{d\,\omega}\right|_{\omega=0}\boldsymbol{A}'$$

$$+\boldsymbol{A}\left.\frac{d\widehat{\boldsymbol{B}}(\omega)}{d\,\omega}\right|_{\omega=0}\boldsymbol{C}_i\boldsymbol{C}_i'\widehat{\boldsymbol{B}}'(0))\boldsymbol{A}' + \boldsymbol{A}\widehat{\boldsymbol{B}}(0)\boldsymbol{C}_0\boldsymbol{C}_0'\widehat{\boldsymbol{B}}'(0)\boldsymbol{A}';$$

(ii)

$$\left.\frac{d^2 n\widehat{\boldsymbol{\Sigma}}(\omega)}{d\,\omega^2}\right|_{\omega=0} = -(\boldsymbol{X}_0\boldsymbol{C}_0'\left.\frac{d^2\widehat{\boldsymbol{B}}'(\omega)}{d\,\omega^2}\right|_{\omega=0} + 2\boldsymbol{X}_i\boldsymbol{C}_i'\left.\frac{d\widehat{\boldsymbol{B}}'(\omega)}{d\,\omega}\right|_{\omega=0})\boldsymbol{A}'$$

$$-\boldsymbol{A}(\left.\frac{d^2\widehat{\boldsymbol{B}}(\omega)}{d\,\omega^2}\right|_{\omega=0}\boldsymbol{C}_0\boldsymbol{X}_0' + 2\left.\frac{d\widehat{\boldsymbol{B}}(\omega)}{d\,\omega}\right|_{\omega=0}\boldsymbol{C}_i\boldsymbol{X}_i') + \boldsymbol{A}\left.\frac{d^2\widehat{\boldsymbol{B}}(\omega)}{d\,\omega^2}\right|_{\omega=0}\boldsymbol{C}_0\boldsymbol{C}_0'\left.\frac{d^2\widehat{\boldsymbol{B}}'(\omega)}{d\,\omega^2}\right|_{\omega=0}\boldsymbol{A}'$$

$$+2\boldsymbol{A}\left.\frac{d^2\widehat{\boldsymbol{B}}(\omega)}{d\,\omega^2}\right|_{\omega=0}\boldsymbol{C}_i\boldsymbol{C}_i'\left.\frac{d^2\widehat{\boldsymbol{B}}'(\omega)}{d\,\omega^2}\right|_{\omega=0}\boldsymbol{A}' + 2\left.\frac{d\widehat{\boldsymbol{B}}(\omega)}{d\,\omega}\right|_{\omega=0}\boldsymbol{C}_0\boldsymbol{C}_0'\left.\frac{d\widehat{\boldsymbol{B}}'(\omega)}{d\,\omega}\right|_{\omega=0}\boldsymbol{A}'$$

$$+2\boldsymbol{A}\left.\frac{d\widehat{\boldsymbol{B}}(\omega)}{d\,\omega}\right|_{\omega=0}\boldsymbol{C}_i\boldsymbol{C}_i'\widehat{\boldsymbol{B}}'(0)\boldsymbol{A}' + \boldsymbol{A}\widehat{\boldsymbol{B}}(0)\boldsymbol{C}_0\boldsymbol{C}_0'\widehat{\boldsymbol{B}}'(0)\boldsymbol{A}';$$

(iii)

$$\left.\frac{d^3 n\widehat{\boldsymbol{\Sigma}}(\omega)}{d\,\omega^3}\right|_{\omega=0} = -(\boldsymbol{X}_0\boldsymbol{C}_0'\left.\frac{d^3\widehat{\boldsymbol{B}}'(\omega)}{d\,\omega^3}\right|_{\omega=0} + 3\boldsymbol{X}_i\boldsymbol{C}_i'\left.\frac{d^2\widehat{\boldsymbol{B}}'(\omega)}{d\,\omega^2}\right|_{\omega=0})\boldsymbol{A}'$$

$$-\boldsymbol{A}(\left.\frac{d^3\widehat{\boldsymbol{B}}(\omega)}{d\,\omega^3}\right|_{\omega=0}\boldsymbol{C}_0\boldsymbol{X}_0' + 3\left.\frac{d^2\widehat{\boldsymbol{B}}(\omega)}{d\,\omega^2}\right|_{\omega=0}\boldsymbol{C}_i\boldsymbol{X}_i') + \boldsymbol{A}\left.\frac{d^3\widehat{\boldsymbol{B}}(\omega)}{d\,\omega^3}\right|_{\omega=0}\boldsymbol{C}_0\boldsymbol{C}_0'\left.\frac{d^3\widehat{\boldsymbol{B}}'(\omega)}{d\,\omega^3}\right|_{\omega=0}\boldsymbol{A}'$$

$$+3A\left.\frac{d^3\widehat{B}(\omega)}{d\omega^3}\right|_{\omega=0} C_iC_i'\left.\frac{d^2\widehat{B}'(\omega)}{d\omega^2}\right|_{\omega=0} A' + 3\left.\frac{d^2\widehat{B}(\omega)}{d\omega^2}\right|_{\omega=0} C_0C_0'\left.\frac{d^2\widehat{B}'(\omega)}{d\omega^2}\right|_{\omega=0} A'$$
$$+6A\left.\frac{d^2\widehat{B}(\omega)}{d\omega^2}\right|_{\omega=0} C_iC_i'\left.\frac{d\widehat{B}'(\omega)}{d\omega}\right|_{\omega=0} A' + 3\left.\frac{d\widehat{B}(\omega)}{d\omega}\right|_{\omega=0} C_0C_0'\left.\frac{d\widehat{B}'(\omega)}{d\omega}\right|_{\omega=0} A'$$
$$+6A\left.\frac{d\widehat{B}(\omega)}{d\omega}\right|_{\omega=0} C_iC_i'\widehat{B}'(0)A' + A\widehat{B}(0)C_0C_0'\widehat{B}'(0)A'.$$

Based on Theorem 8.5 and Corollary 8.3, the influence from one or more "subjects" (let us say the ith column in X and C) depends on the influence on $\widehat{B}(\omega)$. A natural question is if it is sufficient to study the influence on $\widehat{B}(\omega)$ when one is interested in the influence on $n\widehat{\Sigma}(\omega)$. Indeed, we can also twist the question slightly and wonder if we should study $\widehat{B}$ at all when studying the influence on $n\widehat{\Sigma}(\omega)$, since the dependency between $\widehat{B}$ and $\widehat{\Sigma}$ is usually not very strong. However, from earlier chapters, in particular Chap. 6, we know that $n\widehat{\Sigma}(\omega)$ is a function of residuals and, therefore, deviating residuals should have an impact on $n\widehat{\Sigma}(\omega)$. Remember how $n\widehat{\Sigma}(\omega)$ can be dissected, for example

$$\begin{aligned} n\widehat{\Sigma} &= S + (XP_{C'} - A\widehat{B}C)(XP_{C'} - A\widehat{B}C)' \\ &= S + (XC'(CC')^{-1} - A\widehat{B})CC'(XC'(CC')^{-1} - A\widehat{B})', \end{aligned} \tag{8.18}$$

and that S and $XC'(CC')^{-1}$ are sufficient statistics. Hence, it may be sufficient to study the influence on S and $XC'(CC')^{-1}$, and relatively easy expressions appear when S and $XC'(CC')^{-1} - A\widehat{B}$ are studied. The most complicated expressions arise when (8.18) is differentiated.

Theorem 8.6 *Consider the BRM presented in Definition 2.1, and assume that Perturbation (iii) in Definition 8.3 is applied, i.e.* $X = (X_0, \sqrt{\omega}X_i)$ *and* $C = (C_0, \sqrt{\omega}C_i)$. *Then*

$$\left.\frac{d^k n\widehat{\Sigma}(\omega)}{d\omega^k}\right|_{\omega=0} = \left.\frac{d^k S(\omega)}{d\omega^k}\right|_{\omega=0}$$
$$+\sum_{\substack{i_1=0}}^{k}\sum_{\substack{i_2=0\\0\le i_2\le 1}}^{k-i_1}\left.\frac{d^{i_1}XC'(CC')^{-1}-A\widehat{B}(\omega)}{d\omega^{i_1}}\frac{d^{i_2}CC'}{d\omega^{i_2}}\frac{d^{k-i_1-i_2}(XC'(CC')^{-1}-A\widehat{B}(\omega))'}{d\omega^{k-i_1-i_2}}\right|_{\omega=0},$$

where

$$\left.\frac{d^l XC'(CC')^{-1}-A\widehat{B}(\omega)}{d\omega^l}\right|_{\omega=0} = \left.\frac{d^l XC'(CC')^{-1}}{d\omega^l}\right|_{\omega=0} - A\left.\frac{d^l\widehat{B}(\omega)}{d\omega^l}\right|_{\omega=0},$$

$$\frac{d^l CC'}{d\omega^l} = \begin{cases} C_0C_0', & l=0,\\ C_iC_i', & l=1,\\ 0, & l>1;\end{cases}$$

$\left.\frac{d^l \boldsymbol{S}(\omega)}{d\,\omega^l}\right|_{\omega=0}$, $\left.\frac{d^l \boldsymbol{X}\boldsymbol{C}'(\boldsymbol{C}\boldsymbol{C}')^{-1}}{d\,\omega^l}\right|_{\omega=0}$ *and* $\left.\frac{d^l \boldsymbol{B}(\omega)}{d\,\omega^l}\right|_{\omega=0}$ *are obtained from Lemma 8.1 (i) and (ii), and Theorem 8.1.*

Often the number of parameters in $\boldsymbol{B}$ is not very large, whereas the number of parameters in $\boldsymbol{\Sigma}$ is considerably larger. Therefore, when the influence from observations on $\widehat{\boldsymbol{\Sigma}}$ is studied, extra attention must be focused on the possibility that a function of $\widehat{\boldsymbol{\Sigma}}$ is of interest. An example of such a function is $(\boldsymbol{A}'\widehat{\boldsymbol{\Sigma}}^{-1}\boldsymbol{A})^{-1}$, where $\boldsymbol{A}$ is the within-individuals design matrix in the BRM (e.g. see (8.18)), and this expression appears in the estimated dispersion for $\widehat{\boldsymbol{B}}$, see Theorem 4.5 (ii). Other functions which may be of interest are $\mathrm{tr}\{\widehat{\boldsymbol{\Sigma}}\}$, $|\widehat{\boldsymbol{\Sigma}}|$ or some specific elements in $\widehat{\boldsymbol{\Sigma}}$.

Example 8.5 The purpose of this example is to demonstrate that it is complicated to study which observations are influential on $\widehat{\boldsymbol{B}}$ and $n\widehat{\boldsymbol{\Sigma}}$. Examples of different questions to answer are how such influence should be measured and summarized when many parameters are being considered, and what quantities in a statistical analysis should be studied. Usually both mean parameters and dispersion matrices are of interest; for example, as noted above, the estimator $\widehat{\boldsymbol{B}}$ and its dispersion $\widehat{D[\widehat{\boldsymbol{B}}]}$, which is a function of $\widehat{\boldsymbol{\Sigma}}$, are important for the understanding of the analysis for the BRM. Let us now analyse, once again, our favourite data set, the Potthoff and Roy (1964) data set, which has been studied many times before in this book (e.g. see Examples 8.2 and 8.3, as well as several examples included in earlier chapters). In the present example, the first and second derivatives of the perturbed statistics under consideration are used as an influence measure. The statistics which we are interested in are $\widehat{\boldsymbol{B}}$, $\boldsymbol{X}\boldsymbol{C}'(\boldsymbol{C}\boldsymbol{C})^{-1}$, $\boldsymbol{S}$ and $n\widehat{\boldsymbol{\Sigma}}$. However, to simplify the presentation, only the influence on the sum of the elements of $\widehat{\boldsymbol{B}}$ is presented. The same also holds for the "mean" $\boldsymbol{X}\boldsymbol{C}'(\boldsymbol{C}\boldsymbol{C})^{-1}$, i.e. the influence on the sum of the elements is presented, while concerning the dispersion, the influence on the sum of the upper triangles of $\boldsymbol{S}$ and $n\widehat{\boldsymbol{\Sigma}}$ is shown. Adopting this approach, it is discovered that the first and second derivatives in our setting provide very similar information. Moreover, observations 10, 11, 20, 21 and 24 (see Table 8.10) show up as being influential for different statistics. This means that it is crucial to motivate which statistic should

Table 8.10 Here B_1 and B_2 stand for the sum of the elements in $\left.\frac{d\,\widehat{\boldsymbol{B}}(\omega)}{d\,\omega}\right|_{\omega=0}$ and $\left.\frac{d^2\,\widehat{\boldsymbol{B}}(\omega)}{d\,\omega^2}\right|_{\omega=0}$, respectively, M_1 and M_2 stand for the sum of the elements in $\left.\frac{d\,\boldsymbol{X}\boldsymbol{C}'(\boldsymbol{C}\boldsymbol{C})^{-1}}{d\,\omega}\right|_{\omega=0}$ and $\left.\frac{d^2\,\boldsymbol{X}\boldsymbol{C}'(\boldsymbol{C}\boldsymbol{C})^{-1}}{d\,\omega^2}\right|_{\omega=0}$, respectively, S_1 and S_2 stand for the sum of the elements of the upper triangles of $\left.\frac{d\,\boldsymbol{S}(\omega}{d\,\omega}\right|_{\omega=0}$ and $\left.\frac{d^2\,\boldsymbol{S}(\omega)}{d\,\omega^2}\right|_{\omega=0}$, respectively, and Sig_1 and Sig_2 denote the sum of the elements of the upper triangles of $\left.\frac{d\,n\widehat{\boldsymbol{\Sigma}}(\omega)}{d\,\omega}\right|_{\omega=0}$ and $\left.\frac{d^2\,n\widehat{\boldsymbol{\Sigma}}(\omega)}{d\,\omega^2}\right|_{\omega=0}$, respectively

	B_1	B_2	M_1	M_2	S_1	S_2	Sig_1	Sig_2
Obs	20 and 24	20 and 24	10 and 11	10 and 11	21 and 10	21 and 10	20 and 10	20 and 10

For each of the eight measures, the two observations (denoted as Obs) are listed which had the greatest influence on the statistics; the observation listed first had the largest influence. The numbering of observations follows the numbering in Table 1.2

be evaluated and thereafter perform calculations for that specific statistic. To study all possible statistics without any strategy can make it more difficult to take the appropriate decisions. It also implies that more research is needed of how to evaluate the BRM.

□

8.4 Influence Analysis in the $EBRM_B^3$

This section concerns influence analysis for the $EBRM_B^3$ presented in Definition 2.2, using an approach which, from both a conceptual and technical perspective, is similar to the one used for the BRM in the previous section. Although the influence analysis in this section concerns the $EBRM_B^3$, it is a fairly straightforward task to extend it to comprise the general $EBRM_B^m$, $m > 1$. However, one discovers already when $m = 3$ that there are too many optional analyses which can be performed. There are the estimates of three mean parameters, i.e. $\widehat{B}_1$, $\widehat{B}_2$ and $\widehat{B}_3$, and the estimate of the dispersion matrix $\widehat{\Sigma}$. When combining the validation of these estimated parameters with respect to different types of perturbation schemes, one immediately discovers that the number of alternatives on which the different kinds of perturbation are to be performed is so large that all the alternatives cannot be covered in a book. Therefore, we focus only on one perturbation scheme, namely a scheme based on the following perturbations:

$$\begin{aligned} X &= (X_0, \sqrt{\omega}X_i), \quad C_1 = (C_{10}, \sqrt{\omega}C_{1i}), \\ C_2 &= (C_{20}, \sqrt{\omega}C_{2i}), \quad C_3 = (C_{30}, \sqrt{\omega}C_{3i}). \end{aligned} \tag{8.19}$$

Usually X_i and C_{ji}, $j = 1, 2, 3$, consist of one vector, meaning that the ith observation is perturbed and then the influence on the parameters is studied for each observation separately. Moreover, when considering the parameters B_1, B_2 and B_3, it will be assumed that the parameters are uniquely estimated (i.e. many full rank conditions are supposed to hold), but they are not essential for the presentation in this chapter and will therefore not be listed. The following expressions will be studied (see Theorem 3.2):

$$\widehat{B}_1 = (A_1'S_1^{-1}A_1)^{-1}A_1'S_1^{-1}(X - A_2\widehat{B}_2C_2 - A_3\widehat{B}_3C_3)C_1'(C_1C_1')^{-1}, \tag{8.20}$$

$$\widehat{B}_2 = (A_2'\widehat{Q}_1\widehat{S}_2^{-1}\widehat{Q}_1'A_2)^{-1}A_2'\widehat{Q}_1\widehat{S}_2^{-1}\widehat{Q}_1'(X - A_3\widehat{B}_3C_3)C_2'(C_2C_2')^{-1}, \tag{8.21}$$

$$\widehat{B}_3 = (A_3'\widehat{Q}_1\widehat{Q}_2\widehat{S}_3^{-1}\widehat{Q}_2'\widehat{Q}_1'A_3)^{-1}A_3'\widehat{Q}_1\widehat{Q}_2\widehat{S}_3^{-1}\widehat{Q}_2'\widehat{Q}_1'XC_3'(C_3C_3')^{-1}, \tag{8.22}$$

$$n\widehat{\Sigma} = \widehat{S}_3 + \widehat{Q}_3'\widehat{Q}_2'\widehat{Q}_1'XP_{C_3'}X'\widehat{Q}_1\widehat{Q}_2\widehat{Q}_3,$$

where S_j and $\widehat{Q}_j$, $j = 1, 2, 3$, can be obtained from Theorem 3.2. Moreover, for simplicity, all the g-inverses included in the matrices $\widehat{Q}_j$ and $\widehat{S}_j$, $j = 1, 2, 3$, are assumed to be real inverses. Of course, a large number of calculations are needed to obtain the influence measures, i.e. the derivatives of the perturbed models have to be found. On the other hand, the calculations are not more complicated than those performed when studying the BRM.

The derivative defined in Definition 8.4, which is used in the influence analysis, has one serious disadvantage, namely the fact that no simple chain rule expression is available such as that for the derivative used in Theorem 5.1, for example. However, there will be so much structure in our expressions that we do not have to rely on any chain rule. Instead, the results will be obtained recursively.

The plan in the calculations given below is to approach $\left.\frac{d^l \widehat{\boldsymbol{B}}_j}{d\,\omega^l}\right|_{\omega=0}$, $j = 1, 2, 3$, step by step. Firstly, $\boldsymbol{S}_1(\omega)$ and $\widehat{\boldsymbol{Q}}_1$ are considered, thereafter $\widehat{\boldsymbol{S}}_2(\omega)$ and $\widehat{\boldsymbol{Q}}_1\widehat{\boldsymbol{Q}}_2$ and finally $\boldsymbol{S}_3(\omega)$ and $\widehat{\boldsymbol{Q}}_1\widehat{\boldsymbol{Q}}_2\widehat{\boldsymbol{Q}}_3$. Furthermore, $\boldsymbol{X}\boldsymbol{P}_{\boldsymbol{C}'_j}\boldsymbol{X}'$, $\boldsymbol{X}\boldsymbol{C}'_j(\boldsymbol{C}_j\boldsymbol{C}'_j)^{-1}$ and $\boldsymbol{C}_k\boldsymbol{C}'_j(\boldsymbol{C}_j\boldsymbol{C}'_j)^{-1}$, $j = 1, 2, 3$, $k \neq j$, also have to be dealt with, i.e. differentiated and evaluated at $\omega = 0$. Thereafter the influence of observations on the estimates of the parameters will be presented.

Lemma 8.5 *Let all the matrices be as in (8.19) and obtain* $\left.\frac{d^l\,(\boldsymbol{C}_j\boldsymbol{C}'_j)^{-1}}{d\,\omega^l}\right|_{\omega=0}$, $j = 1, 2, 3$, *from Appendix B, Theorem B.6 (iv).*

(i) *For* $j = 1, 2, 3$,

$$\left.\frac{d^l\,\boldsymbol{X}\boldsymbol{P}_{\boldsymbol{C}'_j}\boldsymbol{X}'}{d\,\omega^l}\right|_{\omega=0} = \sum_{i_1=0}^{1}\sum_{i_2=l-i_1-1}^{l-i_1}\binom{l}{i_1}\binom{l-i_1}{i_2}\left.\frac{d^{i_1}\,\boldsymbol{X}\boldsymbol{C}'_j}{d\,\omega^{i_1}}\frac{d^{i_2}\,(\boldsymbol{C}_j\boldsymbol{C}'_j)^{-1}}{d\,\omega^{i_2}}\frac{d^{l-i_1-i_2}\,\boldsymbol{C}_j\boldsymbol{X}'}{d\,\omega^{l-i_1-i_2}}\right|_{\omega=0}.$$

(ii) *For* $j = 1, 2, 3$,

$$\left.\frac{d^l\,\boldsymbol{X}\boldsymbol{C}'_j(\boldsymbol{C}_j\boldsymbol{C}'_j)^{-1}}{d\,\omega^l}\right|_{\omega=0} = \sum_{i=0}^{1}\binom{l}{i}\left.\frac{d^i\,\boldsymbol{X}\boldsymbol{C}'_j}{d\,\omega^i}\frac{d^{l-i}\,(\boldsymbol{C}_j\boldsymbol{C}'_j)^{-1}}{d\,\omega^{l-i}}\right|_{\omega=0}.$$

(iii) *For* $j = 1, 2, 3$ *and* $k \neq j$,

$$\left.\frac{d^l\,\boldsymbol{C}_k\boldsymbol{C}'_j(\boldsymbol{C}_j\boldsymbol{C}'_j)^{-1}}{d\,\omega^l}\right|_{\omega=0} = \sum_{i=0}^{1}\binom{l}{i}\left.\frac{d^i\,\boldsymbol{C}_k\boldsymbol{C}'_j}{d\,\omega^i}\frac{d^{l-i}\,(\boldsymbol{C}_j\boldsymbol{C}'_j)^{-1}}{d\,\omega^{l-i}}\right|_{\omega=0}.$$

Now the pairs $\{\boldsymbol{S}_1(\omega), \widehat{\boldsymbol{Q}}_1\}$, $\{\widehat{\boldsymbol{S}}_2(\omega), \widehat{\boldsymbol{Q}}_1\widehat{\boldsymbol{Q}}_2\}$ and $\{\widehat{\boldsymbol{S}}_3(\omega), \widehat{\boldsymbol{Q}}_1\widehat{\boldsymbol{Q}}_2\widehat{\boldsymbol{Q}}_3\}$ are studied. All these quantities constitute the building blocks of $\widehat{\boldsymbol{B}}_j$, $j = 1, 2, 3$, as well as $\widehat{\boldsymbol{\Sigma}}$. Note that

$$\left.\frac{d^k\,\boldsymbol{S}_1(\omega)}{d\,\omega^k}\right|_{\omega=0} = (-1)^{k+1}k!\boldsymbol{R}_i\boldsymbol{D}_i^{k-1}\boldsymbol{R}'_i, \qquad k \geq 1, \tag{8.23}$$

which is copied from Lemma 8.1 (i), where

$$R_i = X_i - X_0C_0'(C_0C_0')^{-1}C_i,$$
$$D_i = C_i'(C_0C_0')^{-1}C_i.$$

Since

$$\widehat{Q}_1 = I - S_1^{-1}A_1(A_1'S_1^{-1}A_1)^{-1}A_1' = A_1^o(A_1^{o'}S_1A_1^o)^{-1}A_1^{o'}S_1,$$

it follows that

$$\left.\frac{d^l\,\widehat{Q}_1}{d\,\omega^l}\right|_{\omega=0} = A_1^o\sum_{i=0}^{l}\binom{l}{i}\frac{d^i\,(A_1^{o'}S_1A_1^o)^{-1}}{d\,\omega^i}A_1^{o'}\left.\frac{d^{l-i}\,S_1(\omega)}{d\,\omega^{l-i}}\right|_{\omega=0}, \tag{8.24}$$

where $\frac{d^{l-i}\,S_1(\omega)}{d\,\omega^{l-i}}$ can be replaced by (8.23), $\frac{d^i\,(A_1^{o'}S_1A_1^o)^{-1}}{d\,\omega^i}$ is obtained from Appendix B, Theorem B.15 (iii) and the first three derivatives can be found via Lemma 8.2 (ii)–(iv). Therefore, an influence measure can be established for $\{S_1(\omega), \widehat{Q}_1\}$. When differentiating $\widehat{B}_1$,

$$\frac{d^l\,(A_1'S_1^{-1}(\omega)A_1)^{-1}A_1'S_1^{-1}(\omega)}{d\,\omega^l}$$

needs to be calculated, which follows from (8.24) since

$$(A_1'A_1)^{-1}A_1'(I - \widehat{Q}_1) = (A_1'S_1^{-1}(\omega)A_1)^{-1}A_1'S_1^{-1}(\omega). \tag{8.25}$$

For the second pair, $\{\widehat{S}_2(\omega), \widehat{Q}_1\widehat{Q}_2\}$, it is noted that

$$\widehat{S}_2 = S_1 + \widehat{Q}_1'X(P_{C_1'} - P_{C_2'})X'\widehat{Q}_1.$$

Thus,

$$\left.\frac{d^l\,\widehat{S}_2(\omega)}{d\,\omega^l}\right|_{\omega=0} = \left.\frac{d^l\,S_1(\omega)}{d\,\omega^l}\right|_{\omega=0}$$
$$+\sum_{i_1=0}^{l}\sum_{i_1=0}^{l-i_1}\binom{l}{i_1}\binom{l-i_1}{i_2}\frac{d^{i_1}\,\widehat{Q}_1'}{d\,\omega^{i_1}}\left(\frac{d^{i_2}\,XP_{C_1'}X'}{d\,\omega^{i_2}} - \frac{d^{i_2}\,XP_{C_2'}X'}{d\,\omega^{i_2}}\right)\left.\frac{d^{l-i_1-i_2}\,\widehat{Q}_1}{d\,\omega^{l-i_1-i_2}}\right|_{\omega=0}, \tag{8.26}$$

where expressions for $\frac{d^l\,XP_{C_j'}X'}{d\,\omega^l}$, $j = 1, 2$, and $\frac{d^l\,\widehat{Q}_1'}{d\,\omega^l}$ are presented in Lemma 8.5 (i) and (8.24), respectively. The next formulas show how $\widehat{Q}_1\widehat{Q}_2$ can be differentiated. Note that

$$\widehat{Q}_1\widehat{Q}_2 = (I - \widehat{S}_2^{-1}\widehat{Q}_1'A_2(A_2'\widehat{Q}_1\widehat{S}_2^{-1}\widehat{Q}_1'A_2)^{-1}A_2')\widehat{Q}_1$$

and

$$\left.\frac{d^l\,\widehat{Q}_1\widehat{Q}_2}{d\,\omega^l}\right|_{\omega=0} = \sum_{i=0}^{l}\binom{l}{i}\frac{d^i\,I-\widehat{S}_2^{-1}\widehat{Q}_1'A_2(A_2'\widehat{Q}_1\widehat{S}_2^{-1}\widehat{Q}_1'A_2)^{-1}A_2'}{d\,\omega^i}\left.\frac{d^{l-i}\,\widehat{Q}_1'}{d\,\omega^{l-i}}\right|_{\omega=0} \tag{8.27}$$

with

$$\left.\frac{d^l\,\widehat{S}_2^{-1}\widehat{Q}_1'A_2(A_2'\widehat{Q}_1\widehat{S}_2^{-1}\widehat{Q}_1'A_2)^{-1}A_2'}{d\,\omega^l}\right|_{\omega=0} = \sum_{i=0}^{l}\binom{l}{i}\frac{d^i\,\widehat{S}_2^{-1}\widehat{Q}_1'}{d\,\omega^i}A_2\left.\frac{d^{l-i}\,(A_2'\widehat{Q}_1\widehat{S}_2^{-1}\widehat{Q}_1'A_2)^{-1}}{d\,\omega^{l-i}}A_2'\right|_{\omega=0}, \tag{8.28}$$

where it can be utilized that $\widehat{Q}_1\widehat{S}_2^{-1}\widehat{Q}_1' = \widehat{Q}_1\widehat{S}_2^{-1}$,

$$\left.\frac{d^l\,\widehat{Q}_1\widehat{S}_2^{-1}}{d\,\omega^l}\right|_{\omega=0} = \sum_{i=0}^{l}\binom{l}{i}\frac{d^i\,\widehat{Q}_1}{d\,\omega^i}\left.\frac{d^{l-i}\,\widehat{S}_2^{-1}(\omega)}{d\,\omega^{l-i}}\right|_{\omega=0},$$

and $\frac{d^l\,\widehat{S}_2^{-1}(\omega)}{d\,\omega^l}$ follows from Appendix B, Theorem B.15 (iii) and (8.26). Furthermore, if $\widehat{B}_2$ is to be differentiated, $\widehat{S}_2^{-1}\widehat{Q}_1'A_2(A_2'\widehat{Q}_1\widehat{S}_2^{-1}\widehat{Q}_1'A_2)^{-1}$ has to be differentiated, where the derivative, through post-multiplying by $A_2(A_2'A_2)^{-1}$, follows from (8.28).

Now the third pair, $\{\widehat{S}_3(\omega), \widehat{Q}_1\widehat{Q}_2\widehat{Q}_3\}$, is treated and in principle the above calculations for $\{\widehat{S}_2(\omega), \widehat{Q}_1\widehat{Q}_2\}$ are repeated, although they are now performed in a somewhat more difficult environment. For

$$\widehat{S}_3 = \widehat{S}_2 + \widehat{Q}_2'\widehat{Q}_1'X(P_{C_2'} - P_{C_3'})X'\widehat{Q}_1\widehat{Q}_2$$

we have

$$\left.\frac{d^l\,\widehat{S}_3(\omega)}{d\,\omega^l}\right|_{\omega=0} = \left.\frac{d^l\,\widehat{S}_2(\omega)}{d\,\omega^l}\right|_{\omega=0}$$

$$+\sum_{i_1=0}^{l}\sum_{i_1=0}^{l-i_1}\binom{l}{i_1}\binom{l-i_1}{i_2}\frac{d^{i_1}\,\widehat{Q}_2'\widehat{Q}_1'}{d\,\omega^{i_1}}\left(\frac{d^{i_2}\,XP_{C_2'}X'}{d\,\omega^{i_2}} - \frac{d^{i_2}\,XP_{C_3'}X'}{d\,\omega^{i_2}}\right)\left.\frac{d^{l-i_1-i_2}\,\widehat{Q}_1\widehat{Q}_2}{d\,\omega^{l-i_1-i_2}}\right|_{\omega=0}, \tag{8.29}$$

where $\frac{d^l\,\widehat{Q}_1\widehat{Q}_2}{d\,\omega^l}$, evaluated at $\omega = 0$, was obtained in (8.27) and $\left.\frac{d^l\,XP_{C_j'}X'}{d\,\omega^l}\right|_{\omega=0}$, $j = 2, 3$, are obtained from Lemma 8.5 (i). Furthermore, $\frac{d^l\,\widehat{S}_3^{-1}(\omega)}{d\,\omega^l}$ follows from Appendix B, Theorem B.15 (iii) and (8.29),

We also have to discuss $\widehat{Q}_1\widehat{Q}_2\widehat{Q}_3$, and after a few calculations, it can be shown that $\widehat{Q}_1\widehat{Q}_2\widehat{S}_3^{-1}\widehat{Q}_2'\widehat{Q}_1' = \widehat{Q}_1\widehat{Q}_2\widehat{S}_3^{-1}$ and

$$\widehat{Q}_1\widehat{Q}_2\widehat{Q}_3 = (I - \widehat{S}_3^{-1}\widehat{Q}_2'\widehat{Q}_1'A_3(A_3'\widehat{Q}_1\widehat{Q}_2\widehat{S}_3^{-1}\widehat{Q}_2'\widehat{Q}_1'A_3)^{-1}A_3')\widehat{Q}_1\widehat{Q}_2.$$

Therefore, we need to express

$$\left.\frac{d^l\, \widehat{Q}_1\widehat{Q}_2\widehat{S}_3^{-1}}{d\,\omega^l}\right|_{\omega=0} = \sum_{i=0}^{l}\binom{l}{i}\left.\frac{d^i\, \widehat{Q}_1\widehat{Q}_2}{d\,\omega^i}\frac{d^{l-i}\,\widehat{S}_3^{-1}(\omega)}{d\,\omega^{l-i}}\right|_{\omega=0}, \tag{8.30}$$

Moreover, utilizing (8.30),

$$\left.\frac{d^l\, \widehat{S}_3^{-1}\widehat{Q}_2'\widehat{Q}_1'A_3(A_3'\widehat{Q}_1\widehat{Q}_2\widehat{S}_2^{-1}\widehat{Q}_2'\widehat{Q}_1'A_3)^{-1}A_3'}{d\,\omega^l}\right|_{\omega=0}$$

$$= \sum_{i=0}^{l}\binom{l}{i}\frac{d^i\, \widehat{S}_3^{-1}\widehat{Q}_2'\widehat{Q}_1'}{d\,\omega^i}A_3\left.\frac{d^{l-i}\,(A_3'\widehat{Q}_1\widehat{Q}_2\widehat{S}_2^{-1}\widehat{Q}_2'\widehat{Q}_1'A_3)^{-1}}{d\,\omega^{l-i}}A_3'\right|_{\omega=0}. \tag{8.31}$$

Since $(A_3'\widehat{Q}_1\widehat{Q}_2\widehat{S}_2^{-1}\widehat{Q}_2'\widehat{Q}_1'A_3)^{-1}$ equals $(A_3'\widehat{Q}_2\widehat{Q}_1\widehat{S}_2^{-1}A_3)^{-1}$, the derivative

$$\left.\frac{d^l\,(A_3'\widehat{Q}_2\widehat{Q}_1\widehat{S}_2^{-1}\widehat{Q}_2'\widehat{Q}_1'A_3)^{-1}}{d\,\omega^l}A_3'\right|_{\omega=0}$$

is obtained from Appendix B, Theorem B.15 and (8.30). Finally,

$$\left.\frac{d^l\, \widehat{Q}_1\widehat{Q}_2\widehat{Q}_3}{d\,\omega^l}\right|_{\omega=0} = \sum_{i=0}^{l}\binom{l}{i}\left.\frac{d^i\, I-\widehat{S}_3^{-1}\widehat{Q}_2'\widehat{Q}_1'A_3(A_3'\widehat{Q}_1\widehat{Q}_2\widehat{S}_2^{-1}\widehat{Q}_2'\widehat{Q}_1'A_3)^{-1}}{d\,\omega^l}\frac{d^{l-i}\,\widehat{Q}_1\widehat{Q}_2}{d\,\omega^{l-i}}\right|_{\omega=0}, \tag{8.32}$$

where the derivatives can be obtained from (8.27) and (8.31). Moreover, the expression for $\widehat{B}_3$ implies that the derivative of

$$(A_3'\widehat{Q}_1\widehat{Q}_2\widehat{S}_3^{-1}(\omega)\widehat{Q}_2'\widehat{Q}_1'A_3)^{-1}A_3'\widehat{Q}_1\widehat{Q}_2\widehat{S}_3^{-1}(\omega) \tag{8.33}$$

is needed and it can be obtained from (8.31) through post-multiplying by $A_3(A_3'A_3)^{-1}$.

The next theorem summarizes the calculations presented above.

Theorem 8.7 *For the $EBRM_B^3$ presented in Definition 2.2, let the perturbation be defined in (8.19), and under "full rank" assumptions the following perturbed estimates will be considered:*

$$\widehat{B}_1(\omega) = (A_1'S_1^{-1}(\omega)A_1)^{-1}A_1'S_1^{-1}(\omega)(X - A_2\widehat{B}_2(\omega)C_2 - A_3\widehat{B}_3(\omega)C_3)C_1'(C_1C_1')^{-1},$$
$$\widehat{B}_2(\omega) = (A_2'\widehat{Q}_1\widehat{S}_2^{-1}(\omega)\widehat{Q}_1'A_2)^{-1}A_2'\widehat{Q}_1\widehat{S}_2^{-1}(\omega)\widehat{Q}_1'(X - A_3\widehat{B}_3(\omega)C_3)C_2'(C_2C_2')^{-1},$$
$$\widehat{B}_3(\omega) = (A_3'\widehat{Q}_1\widehat{Q}_2\widehat{S}_3^{-1}(\omega)\widehat{Q}_2'\widehat{Q}_1'A_3)^{-1}A_3'\widehat{Q}_1\widehat{Q}_2\widehat{S}_3^{-1}(\omega)\widehat{Q}_2'\widehat{Q}_1'XC_3'(C_3C_3')^{-1},$$
$$n\widehat{\Sigma}(\omega) = \widehat{S}_3(\omega) + \widehat{Q}_3'\widehat{Q}_2'\widehat{Q}_1'XP_{C_3'}X'\widehat{Q}_1\widehat{Q}_2\widehat{Q}_3,$$

where $\boldsymbol{X}$, $\boldsymbol{C}_j$ *and* $\widehat{\boldsymbol{Q}}_j$, $j = 1, 2, 3$, *also are functions of* ω, *and* $\boldsymbol{S}_1$, $\widehat{\boldsymbol{S}}_j$, $j = 2, 3$, *and* $\widehat{\boldsymbol{Q}}_j$, $j = 1, 2, 3$, *are obtained from Theorem 3.2. Then*

(i)

$$\left.\frac{d^l\,\widehat{\boldsymbol{B}}_3(\omega)}{d\,\omega^l}\right|_{\omega=0} = \sum_{i=0}^{l}\binom{l}{i}\frac{d^i\,(\boldsymbol{A}_3'\widehat{\boldsymbol{Q}}_1\widehat{\boldsymbol{Q}}_2\widehat{\boldsymbol{S}}_3^{-1}(\omega)\widehat{\boldsymbol{Q}}_2'\widehat{\boldsymbol{Q}}_1'\boldsymbol{A}_3)^{-1}\boldsymbol{A}_3'\widehat{\boldsymbol{Q}}_1\widehat{\boldsymbol{Q}}_2\widehat{\boldsymbol{S}}_3^{-1}(\omega)}{d\,\omega^i}$$

$$\times \left.\frac{d^{l-i}\,\boldsymbol{X}\boldsymbol{C}_3'(\boldsymbol{C}_3\boldsymbol{C}_3')^{-1}}{d\,\omega^{l-i}}\right|_{\omega=0}, \qquad l > 0,$$

where the derivatives of $(\boldsymbol{A}_3'\widehat{\boldsymbol{Q}}_1\widehat{\boldsymbol{Q}}_2\widehat{\boldsymbol{S}}_3^{-1}(\omega)\widehat{\boldsymbol{Q}}_2'\widehat{\boldsymbol{Q}}_1'\boldsymbol{A}_3)^{-1}\boldsymbol{A}_3'\widehat{\boldsymbol{Q}}_1\widehat{\boldsymbol{Q}}_2\widehat{\boldsymbol{S}}_3^{-1}(\omega)$ *are obtained via (8.31) and* $\left.\frac{d^{l-i}\,\boldsymbol{X}\boldsymbol{C}_3'(\boldsymbol{C}_3\boldsymbol{C}_3')^{-1}}{d\,\omega^{l-i}}\right|_{\omega=0}$ *follows from Lemma 8.5 (ii);*

(ii)

$$\left.\frac{d^l\,\widehat{\boldsymbol{B}}_2(\omega)}{d\,\omega^l}\right|_{\omega=0} = \sum_{i=0}^{l}\binom{l}{i}\frac{d^i\,(\boldsymbol{A}_2'\widehat{\boldsymbol{Q}}_1\widehat{\boldsymbol{S}}_2^{-1}(\omega)\widehat{\boldsymbol{Q}}_1'\boldsymbol{A}_2)^{-1}\boldsymbol{A}_2'\widehat{\boldsymbol{Q}}_1\widehat{\boldsymbol{S}}_2^{-1}(\omega)}{d\,\omega^i}$$

$$\times \left.\frac{d^{l-i}\,(\boldsymbol{X}\boldsymbol{C}_2'(\boldsymbol{C}_2\boldsymbol{C}_2')^{-1}-\boldsymbol{A}_3\widehat{\boldsymbol{B}}_3(\omega)\boldsymbol{C}_3\boldsymbol{C}_2'(\boldsymbol{C}_2\boldsymbol{C}_2')^{-1})}{d\,\omega^{l-i}}\right|_{\omega=0}, \qquad l > 0,$$

where the derivatives of $(\boldsymbol{A}_2'\widehat{\boldsymbol{Q}}_1\widehat{\boldsymbol{S}}_2^{-1}(\omega)\widehat{\boldsymbol{Q}}_1'\boldsymbol{A}_2)^{-1}\boldsymbol{A}_2'\widehat{\boldsymbol{Q}}_1\widehat{\boldsymbol{S}}_2^{-1}(\omega)$ *are obtained via (8.28),* $\left.\frac{d^l\,\boldsymbol{X}\boldsymbol{C}_2'(\boldsymbol{C}_2\boldsymbol{C}_2')^{-1}}{d\,\omega^l}\right|_{\omega=0}$ *follows from Lemma 8.5 (ii), and* $\left.\frac{d^l\,\boldsymbol{C}_3\boldsymbol{C}_2'(\boldsymbol{C}_2\boldsymbol{C}_2')^{-1}}{d\,\omega^l}\right|_{\omega=0}$ *follows from Lemma 8.5 (iii);*

(iii)

$$\left.\frac{d^l\,\widehat{\boldsymbol{B}}_1(\omega)}{d\,\omega^l}\right|_{\omega=0} = \sum_{i=0}^{l}\binom{l}{i}\frac{d^i\,(\boldsymbol{A}_1'\boldsymbol{S}_1^{-1}(\omega)\boldsymbol{A}_1)^{-1}\boldsymbol{A}_1'\boldsymbol{S}_1^{-1}}{d\,\omega^i}$$

$$\times \left.\frac{d^{l-i}\,(\boldsymbol{X}\boldsymbol{C}_1'(\boldsymbol{C}_1\boldsymbol{C}_1')^{-1}-\boldsymbol{A}_2\widehat{\boldsymbol{B}}_2(\omega)\boldsymbol{C}_2\boldsymbol{C}_1'(\boldsymbol{C}_1\boldsymbol{C}_1')^{-1}-\boldsymbol{A}_3\widehat{\boldsymbol{B}}_3(\omega)\boldsymbol{C}_3\boldsymbol{C}_1'(\boldsymbol{C}_1\boldsymbol{C}_1')^{-1})}{d\,\omega^{l-i}}\right|_{\omega=0}, \qquad l > 0,$$

where the derivatives of $(\boldsymbol{A}_1'\widehat{\boldsymbol{S}}_1^{-1}(\omega)\boldsymbol{A}_1)^{-1}\boldsymbol{A}_1'\widehat{\boldsymbol{S}}_1^{-1}(\omega)$ *are obtained via (8.25) and (8.24),* $\left.\frac{d^{l-i}\,\boldsymbol{X}\boldsymbol{C}_1'(\boldsymbol{C}_1\boldsymbol{C}_1')^{-1}}{d\,\omega^{l-i}}\right|_{\omega=0}$ *follows from Lemma 8.5 (ii), and* $\left.\frac{d^{l-i}\,\boldsymbol{C}_j\boldsymbol{C}_1'(\boldsymbol{C}_1\boldsymbol{C}_1')^{-1}}{d\,\omega^{l-i}}\right|_{\omega=0}$, $j = 2, 3$, *follow from Lemma 8.5 (iii);*

(iv)

$$\left.\frac{d^l\,n\widehat{\boldsymbol{\Sigma}}(\omega)}{d\,\omega^l}\right|_{\omega=0} = \left.\frac{d^l\,\boldsymbol{S}_3(\omega)}{d\,\omega^l}\right|_{\omega=0}$$

$$+ \left.\sum_{i_1=0}^{l}\sum_{i_2=0}^{l-i_1}\binom{l}{i_1}\frac{d^{i_1}\,\widehat{\boldsymbol{Q}}_3'\widehat{\boldsymbol{Q}}_2'\widehat{\boldsymbol{Q}}_1'}{d\,\omega^{i_1}}\,\frac{d^{i_2}\,\boldsymbol{X}\boldsymbol{P}_{\boldsymbol{C}_3'}\boldsymbol{X}'}{d\,\omega^{i_2}}\,\frac{d^{k-i_1-i_2}\,\widehat{\boldsymbol{Q}}_1\widehat{\boldsymbol{Q}}_2\widehat{\boldsymbol{Q}}_3}{d\,\omega^{k-i_1-i_2}}\right|_{\omega=0}, \qquad l > 0,$$

where $\left.\frac{d^{i1}\widehat{Q}_3'\widehat{Q}_2'\widehat{Q}_1'}{d\omega^{i1}}\right|_{\omega=0}$ *and* $\left.\frac{d^{l}XP_{C_3'}X'}{d\omega^{l}}\right|_{\omega=0}$ *follow from (8.32), which in turn is based on several relations which need to be expressed, and on Lemma 8.5 (i), respectively.*

Example 8.6 In Example 6.7 the $EBRM_B^3$ of Example 1.9 was studied with respect to outlying observations. In this example, data were generated and then a few observations were artificially altered in such a way that they clearly deviated from the other observations. Now the same data are used to study influence among the observations and the following four contaminations will take place (with $X = (X_{i,j})$):

$$\text{(i) add 60 to } (X_{5,30}); \quad \text{(ii) add 60 to } (X_{5,15}); \quad \text{(iii) add 60 to } (X_{5,5});$$
$$\text{(iv) add 60 to the elements in } x_5, \text{ with } x_5 \text{ standing for the 5th column of } X. \quad (8.34)$$

In Example 6.7 the modified observations led to large residuals and, therefore, it can be expected that the contaminated observations will also show up as influential observations.

Although it is a straightforward task to derive the relevant expressions, the calculations unfortunately become lengthy. Therefore, only the zero derivative (i.e. the ith observation is omitted) and the first derivatives are presented in some detail. The next formulas give the details necessary for deriving the results. Instead of $S_j(0)$ and $Q_j(0)$, we sometimes will write S_{j0} and Q_{j0}, $j = 1, 2, 3$, respectively. Moreover, $\widehat{\Sigma}(0)$ and $\widehat{B}_j(0)$ are written as $\widehat{\Sigma}_0$ and $\widehat{B}_{j0}$, $j = 1, 2, 3$. The idea behind presenting the formulas given below is that readers who want to carry out their own calculations can receive guidance as to what their expressions should look like. Those who only are interested in seeing the consequences of the different perturbations can jump directly to Tables 8.11 and 8.12, and their interpretations.

Let us start with the case where the ith observation is excluded from the analysis:

$$S_{10} = X_0(I - P_{C_1'})X_0',$$
$$\widehat{Q}_{10} = I - S_{10}^{-1}A_1(A_1'S_{10}^{-1}A_1)^{-1}A_1',$$
$$\widehat{S}_{20} = S_{10} + \widehat{Q}_{10}'X_0(P_{C_1'} - P_{C_2'})X_0'\widehat{Q}_{10},$$
$$\widehat{Q}_{20} = I - \widehat{S}_{20}^{-1}\widehat{Q}_{10}'A_2(A_2'\widehat{Q}_{10}\widehat{S}_{20}^{-1}\widehat{Q}_{10}'A_2)^{-1}A_2'\widehat{Q}_{10},$$
$$\widehat{S}_{30} = \widehat{S}_{20} + \widehat{Q}_{20}'\widehat{Q}_{10}'X_0(P_{C_2'} - P_{C_3'})X_0'\widehat{Q}_{10}\widehat{Q}_{20},$$
$$\widehat{Q}_{30} = I - \widehat{S}_{30}^{-1}\widehat{Q}_{20}'\widehat{Q}_{10}'A_3(A_3'\widehat{Q}_{10}\widehat{Q}_{20}\widehat{S}_{30}^{-1}\widehat{Q}_{20}'\widehat{Q}_{10}'A_3)^{-1}A_3'\widehat{Q}_{10}\widehat{Q}_{20},$$
$$n\widehat{\Sigma}_0 = \widehat{S}_{30} + \widehat{Q}_{30}'\widehat{Q}_{20}'\widehat{Q}_{10}'X_0P_{C_3'}X_0'\widehat{Q}_{10}\widehat{Q}_{20}\widehat{Q}_{30},$$
$$\widehat{B}_{30} = (A_3'\widehat{Q}_{10}\widehat{Q}_{20}\widehat{S}_{30}^{-1}\widehat{Q}_{20}'\widehat{Q}_{10}'A_3)^{-1}A_3'\widehat{Q}_{10}\widehat{Q}_{20}\widehat{S}_{30}^{-1}\widehat{Q}_{20}'\widehat{Q}_{10}'X_0C_{30}'(C_{30}C_{30}')^{-1},$$
$$\widehat{B}_{20} = (A_2'\widehat{Q}_{10}\widehat{S}_{20}^{-1}\widehat{Q}_{10}'A_2)^{-1}A_2'\widehat{Q}_{10}\widehat{S}_{20}^{-1}(X_0 - A_3\widehat{B}_{30}C_3)C_{20}'(C_{20}C_{20}')^{-1},$$
$$\widehat{B}_{10} = (A_1'\widehat{S}_{10}^{-1}A_1)^{-1}A_1'S_{10}^{-1}(X_0 - A_2\widehat{B}_{20}C_2 - A_3\widehat{B}_{30}C_3)C_{20}'(C_{20}C_{20}')^{-1}.$$

The first derivatives (at the point $\omega = 0$) of the above-mentioned quantities, i.e. S_1, $\widehat{\theta}_1$, $\widehat{S}_2$, $\widehat{\theta}_2$, etc., will be presented and below are listed those results of Lemma 8.5 which are of use:

$$\left.\frac{d^0 XP_{C_j'}X'}{d\,\omega^0}\right|_{\omega=0} = X_0 P_{C_{j0}'} X_0',$$

$$\left.\frac{d XP_{C_j'}X'}{d\,\omega}\right|_{\omega=0} = X_0 C_{j0}'(C_{j0}C_{j0}')^{-1}C_{ji}X_i'$$

$$-X_0 C_{j0}'(C_{j0}C_{j0}')^{-1}C_{ji}C_{ji}'(C_{j0}C_{j0}')^{-1}C_{j0}X_0' + X_i C_{ji}'(C_{j0}C_{j0}')^{-1}C_{j0}X_0',$$

$$\left.\frac{d^0 XC_j'(C_jC_j')^{-1}}{d\,\omega^0}\right|_{\omega=0} = X_0 C_{j0}'(C_{j0}C_{j0}')^{-1},$$

$$\left.\frac{d XC_j'(C_jC_j')^{-1}}{d\,\omega}\right|_{\omega=0} = X_i C_{ji}'(C_{j0}C_{j0}')^{-1} - X_0 C_{j0}'(C_{j0}C_{j0}')^{-1}C_{ji}C_{ji}'(C_{j0}C_{j0}')^{-1},$$

$$\left.\frac{d^0 C_k C_j'(C_jC_j')^{-1}}{d\,\omega^0}\right|_{\omega=0} = C_{k0}C_{j0}'(C_{j0}C_{j0}')^{-1},$$

$$\left.\frac{d C_k C_j'(C_jC_j')^{-1}}{d\,\omega}\right|_{\omega=0} = C_{ki}C_{ji}'(C_{j0}C_{j0}')^{-1} - C_{k0}C_{j0}'(C_{j0}C_{j0}')^{-1}C_{ji}C_{ji}'(C_{j0}C_{j0}')^{-1}.$$

Now, $\widehat{S}_j$ and $\widehat{Q}_j$, $j = 1, 2, 3$, are differentiated:

$$\left.\frac{d\,S_1(\omega)}{d\,\omega}\right|_{\omega=0} = (X_i - X_0 C_{10}'(C_{10}C_{10}')^{-1}C_{1i})()',$$

$$\left.\frac{d\,\widehat{Q}_1(\omega)}{d\,\omega}\right|_{\omega=0} = A_1^o(A_1^{o'}S_{10}A_1^o)^{-1}A_1^{o'}\frac{dS_1(\omega)}{d\,\omega}A_1^o(A_1^{o'}S_{10}A_1^o)^{-1}A_1^{o'}S_{10}\Big|_{\omega=0},$$

$$\left.\frac{d\widehat{S}_2(\omega)}{d\,\omega}\right|_{\omega=0} = \left.\frac{dS_1(\omega)}{d\,\omega}\right|_{\omega=0} + \widehat{Q}_{10}'X_0(P_{C_1'} - P_{C_2'})X_0'\left.\frac{d\,Q_1(\omega)}{d\,\omega}\right|_{\omega=0}$$

$$+\widehat{Q}_{10}\Big(\left.\frac{d\,XP_{C_1'}X'}{d\,\omega}\right|_{\omega=0} - \left.\frac{d\,XP_{C_2'}X'}{d\,\omega}\right|_{\omega=0}\Big)\widehat{Q}_{10}$$

$$+\left.\frac{d\widehat{Q}_1'(\omega)}{d\,\omega}\right|_{\omega=0} X_0(P_{C_1'} - P_{C_2'})X_0'\widehat{Q}_{10},$$

$$\left.\frac{d\widehat{Q}_1(\omega)\widehat{Q}_2(\omega)}{d\,\omega}\right|_{\omega=0} = I - \widehat{S}_{20}^{-1}\widehat{Q}_{10}'A_2(A_2'\widehat{Q}_{10}\widehat{S}_{20}^{-1}\widehat{Q}_{10}'A_2)^{-1}A_2'\left.\frac{d\widehat{Q}_1'(\omega)}{d\,\omega}\right|_{\omega=0}$$

$$-\left.\frac{d\widehat{S}_2^{-1}(\omega)\widehat{Q}_1'(\omega)A_2(A_2'\widehat{Q}_1(\omega)\widehat{S}_2^{-1}(\omega)\widehat{Q}_1'(\omega)A_2)^{-1}}{d\,\omega}\right|_{\omega=0} A_2'$$

with

$$\left.\frac{d\,\widehat{S}_2^{-1}(\omega)\widehat{Q}_1'(\omega)A_2(A_2'\widehat{Q}_1(\omega)\widehat{S}_2^{-1}(\omega)\widehat{Q}_1'(\omega)A_2)^{-1}}{d\,\omega}\right|_{\omega=0}$$

$$= \widehat{S}_{20}^{-1}\widehat{Q}_{10}'A_2\left.\frac{d(A_2'\widehat{Q}_1(\omega)\widehat{S}_2^{-1}(\omega)\widehat{Q}_1'(\omega)A_2)^{-1}}{d\,\omega}\right|_{\omega=0}$$

$$-\left.\frac{d\widehat{S}_2^{-1}(\omega)\widehat{Q}_1'(\omega)}{d\,\omega}\right|_{\omega=0} A_2(A_2'\widehat{Q}_{10}\widehat{S}_{20}^{-1}\widehat{Q}_{10}'A_2)^{-1}$$

and

$$\frac{d\widehat{Q}_1(\omega)\widehat{S}_2^{-1}(\omega)}{d\omega}\bigg|_{\omega=0} = -\widehat{Q}_{10}\widehat{S}_{20}^{-1}\frac{d\widehat{S}_2(\omega)}{d\omega}\bigg|_{\omega=0}\widehat{S}_{20}^{-1} + \frac{d\widehat{Q}_1(\omega)}{d\omega}\bigg|_{\omega=0}\widehat{S}_{20},$$

$$\frac{d(A_2'\widehat{Q}_1(\omega)\widehat{S}_2^{-1}(\omega)\widehat{Q}_1'(\omega)A_2)^{-1}}{d\omega}\bigg|_{\omega=0}$$

$$= (A_2'\widehat{Q}_{10}\widehat{S}_{20}^{-1}\widehat{Q}_{10}'A_2)^{-1}A_2'\frac{d\widehat{Q}_1(\omega)\widehat{S}_2^{-1}(\omega)\widehat{Q}_1'(\omega)}{d\omega}\bigg|_{\omega=0}A_2(A_2'\widehat{Q}_{10}\widehat{S}_{20}^{-1}\widehat{Q}_{10}'A_2)^{-1};$$

$\widehat{Q}_1(\omega)\widehat{S}_2^{-1}(\omega)\widehat{Q}_1'(\omega)$ is obtained since $\widehat{Q}_1(\omega)\widehat{S}_2^{-1}(\omega)\widehat{Q}_1'(\omega) = \widehat{Q}_1(\omega)\widehat{S}_2^{-1}(\omega)$.
Moreover,

$$\begin{aligned}\frac{d\widehat{S}_3(\omega)}{d\omega}\bigg|_{\omega=0} &= \frac{dS_2(\omega)}{d\omega}\bigg|_{\omega=0} + \widehat{Q}_{20}'\widehat{Q}_{10}'X_0(P_{C_2'} - P_{C_3'})X_0'\frac{dQ_1\widehat{Q}_2(\omega)}{d\omega}\bigg|_{\omega=0}\\ &+ \widehat{Q}_{20}'\widehat{Q}_{10}'(\frac{dXP_{C_2'}X'}{d\omega}\bigg|_{\omega=0} - \frac{dXP_{C_3'}X'}{d\omega}\bigg|_{\omega=0})\widehat{Q}_{10}\widehat{Q}_{20}\\ &+ \frac{d\widehat{Q}_2'(\omega)\widehat{Q}_1'(\omega)}{d\omega}\bigg|_{\omega=0}X_0(P_{C_1'} - P_{C_2'})X_0'\widehat{Q}_{10}\widehat{Q}_{20},\end{aligned}$$

$$\begin{aligned}\frac{d\widehat{Q}_1(\omega)\widehat{Q}_2(\omega)\widehat{Q}_3(\omega)}{d\omega}\bigg|_{\omega=0} &= I - \widehat{S}_{30}^{-1}\widehat{Q}_{20}'\widehat{Q}_{10}'A_3(A_3'\widehat{Q}_{10}\widehat{Q}_{20}\widehat{S}_{30}^{-1}\widehat{Q}_{20}'\widehat{Q}_{10}'A_3)^{-1}A_3'\frac{d\widehat{Q}_{20}'\widehat{Q}_1'(\omega)}{d\omega}\bigg|_{\omega=0}\\ &- \frac{d\widehat{S}_3^{-1}(\omega)\widehat{Q}_{20}'\widehat{Q}_1'(\omega)A_3(A_3'\widehat{Q}_1(\omega)\widehat{Q}_2(\omega)\widehat{S}_3^{-1}(\omega)\widehat{Q}_2(\omega)'\widehat{Q}_1'(\omega)A_3)^{-1}}{d\omega}\bigg|_{\omega=0}A_3'\end{aligned}$$

with

$$\begin{aligned}&\frac{d\,\widehat{S}_3^{-1}\widehat{Q}_2(\omega)'(\omega)\widehat{Q}_1'(\omega)A_3(A_3'\widehat{Q}_1(\omega)\widehat{Q}_2(\omega)\widehat{S}_3^{-1}(\omega)\widehat{Q}_2(\omega)'\widehat{Q}_1'(\omega)A_3)^{-1}}{d\omega}\bigg|_{\omega=0}\\ &= \widehat{S}_{30}^{-1}\widehat{Q}_{20}'\widehat{Q}_{10}'A_3\frac{d(A_3'\widehat{Q}_1(\omega)\widehat{Q}_2(\omega)\widehat{S}_3^{-1}(\omega)\widehat{Q}_2(\omega)'\widehat{Q}_1'(\omega)A_3)^{-1}}{d\omega}\bigg|_{\omega=0}\\ &- \frac{d\widehat{S}_3^{-1}(\omega)\widehat{Q}_2'(\omega)\widehat{Q}_1'(\omega)}{d\omega}\bigg|_{\omega=0}A_3(A_3'\widehat{Q}_{10}\widehat{Q}_{20}\widehat{S}_{30}^{-1}\widehat{Q}_{20}'\widehat{Q}_{10}'A_3)^{-1},\end{aligned}$$

$$\frac{d\widehat{Q}_1(\omega)\widehat{Q}_2(\omega)\widehat{S}_3^{-1}(\omega)}{d\omega}\bigg|_{\omega=0} = -\widehat{Q}_{10}\widehat{Q}_{20}\widehat{S}_{30}^{-1}\frac{d\widehat{S}_3(\omega)}{d\omega}\bigg|_{\omega=0}\widehat{S}_{30}^{-1} + \frac{d\widehat{Q}_2\widehat{Q}_1(\omega)}{d\omega}\bigg|_{\omega=0}\widehat{S}_{30}$$

and

$$\begin{aligned}&\frac{d(A_3'\widehat{Q}_1(\omega)\widehat{Q}_2(\omega)\widehat{S}_3^{-1}(\omega)\widehat{Q}_2(\omega)'\widehat{Q}_1'(\omega)A_3)^{-1}}{d\omega}\bigg|_{\omega=0}\\ &= -(A_3'\widehat{Q}_{10}\widehat{Q}_{20}\widehat{S}_{30}^{-1}\widehat{Q}_{20}'\widehat{Q}_{10}'A_3)^{-1}A_3'\frac{d\widehat{Q}_1(\omega)\widehat{Q}_2(\omega)\widehat{S}_3^{-1}(\omega)\widehat{Q}_2(\omega)'\widehat{Q}_1'(\omega))^{-1}}{d\omega}\bigg|_{\omega=0}\\ &\times A_3(A_3'\widehat{Q}_{10}\widehat{Q}_{20}\widehat{S}_{30}^{-1}\widehat{Q}_{20}'\widehat{Q}_{10}'A_3)^{-1},\end{aligned}$$

since $\widehat{Q}_1(\omega)\widehat{Q}_2(\omega)\widehat{S}_3^{-1}(\omega)\widehat{Q}_2(\omega)'\widehat{Q}_1'(\omega) = \widehat{Q}_1(\omega)\widehat{Q}_2(\omega)\widehat{S}_3^{-1}(\omega)$.

Having performed all these lengthy calculations, we are ready to find the first derivative for $\widehat{\boldsymbol{B}}_j$, $j = 1, 2, 3$, and $\widehat{\boldsymbol{\Sigma}}$. From Theorem 8.7, it follows that:

$$\frac{d\widehat{\boldsymbol{B}}_3(\omega)}{d\omega}\bigg|_{\omega=0} = \frac{d(\boldsymbol{A}_3'\widehat{\boldsymbol{Q}}_1(\omega)\widehat{\boldsymbol{Q}}_2(\omega)\widehat{\boldsymbol{S}}_3^{-1}(\omega)\widehat{\boldsymbol{Q}}_2(\omega)'\widehat{\boldsymbol{Q}}_1'(\omega)\boldsymbol{A}_3)^{-1}\boldsymbol{A}_3'\widehat{\boldsymbol{Q}}_1(\omega)\widehat{\boldsymbol{Q}}_2(\omega)\widehat{\boldsymbol{S}}_3^{-1}(\omega)}{d\omega}\bigg|_{\omega=0}\boldsymbol{X}_0\boldsymbol{C}_{30}'(\boldsymbol{C}_{30}\boldsymbol{C}_{30}')^{-1}$$

$$+(\boldsymbol{A}_3'\widehat{\boldsymbol{Q}}_{10}\widehat{\boldsymbol{Q}}_{20}\widehat{\boldsymbol{S}}_{30}^{-1}\widehat{\boldsymbol{Q}}_{20}'\widehat{\boldsymbol{Q}}_{10}'\boldsymbol{A}_3)^{-1}\boldsymbol{A}_3'\widehat{\boldsymbol{Q}}_{10}\widehat{\boldsymbol{Q}}_{20}\widehat{\boldsymbol{S}}_{30}^{-1}\frac{d\boldsymbol{X}\boldsymbol{C}_3'(\boldsymbol{C}_3\boldsymbol{C}_3')^{-1}}{d\omega}\bigg|_{\omega=0},$$

$$\frac{d\boldsymbol{A}_3\widehat{\boldsymbol{B}}_3(\omega)\boldsymbol{C}_3\boldsymbol{C}_j'(\boldsymbol{C}_j\boldsymbol{C}_j')^{-1}}{d\omega}\bigg|_{\omega=0} = \boldsymbol{A}_3\frac{d\widehat{\boldsymbol{B}}_3(\omega)}{d\omega}\bigg|_{\omega=0}\boldsymbol{C}_{30}\boldsymbol{C}_{j0}'(\boldsymbol{C}_{j0}\boldsymbol{C}_{j0}')^{-1} + \boldsymbol{A}_3\widehat{\boldsymbol{B}}_{30}\frac{d\boldsymbol{C}_3\boldsymbol{C}_j'(\boldsymbol{C}_j\boldsymbol{C}_j')^{-1}}{d\omega}\bigg|_{\omega=0},$$

$$\frac{d\widehat{\boldsymbol{B}}_2(\omega)}{d\omega}\bigg|_{\omega=0} = \frac{d(\boldsymbol{A}_2'\widehat{\boldsymbol{Q}}_1(\omega)\widehat{\boldsymbol{S}}_2^{-1}(\omega)\widehat{\boldsymbol{Q}}_1'(\omega)\boldsymbol{A}_2)^{-1}\boldsymbol{A}_2'\widehat{\boldsymbol{Q}}_1(\omega)\widehat{\boldsymbol{S}}_2^{-1}(\omega)}{d\omega}\bigg|_{\omega=0}$$

$$\times(\boldsymbol{X}_0\boldsymbol{C}_{20}'(\boldsymbol{C}_{20}\boldsymbol{C}_{20}')^{-1} - \boldsymbol{A}_3\widehat{\boldsymbol{B}}_{30}\boldsymbol{C}_3\boldsymbol{C}_{20}'(\boldsymbol{C}_{20}\boldsymbol{C}_{20}')^{-1})$$

$$+(\boldsymbol{A}_2'\widehat{\boldsymbol{Q}}_{10}\widehat{\boldsymbol{S}}_{20}^{-1}\widehat{\boldsymbol{Q}}_{10}'\boldsymbol{A}_2)^{-1}\boldsymbol{A}_2'\widehat{\boldsymbol{Q}}_{10}\widehat{\boldsymbol{S}}_{20}^{-1}\frac{d\boldsymbol{X}\boldsymbol{C}_3'(\boldsymbol{C}_3\boldsymbol{C}_3')^{-1} - \boldsymbol{A}_3\widehat{\boldsymbol{B}}_3\boldsymbol{C}_3\boldsymbol{C}_2'(\boldsymbol{C}_2\boldsymbol{C}_2')^{-1}}{d\omega}\bigg|_{\omega=0},$$

$$\frac{d\boldsymbol{A}_2\widehat{\boldsymbol{B}}_2(\omega)\boldsymbol{C}_2\boldsymbol{C}_1'(\boldsymbol{C}_1\boldsymbol{C}_1')^{-1}}{d\omega}\bigg|_{\omega=0} = \boldsymbol{A}_2\frac{d\widehat{\boldsymbol{B}}_2(\omega)}{d\omega}\bigg|_{\omega=0}\boldsymbol{C}_{20}\boldsymbol{C}_{10}'(\boldsymbol{C}_{10}\boldsymbol{C}_{10}')^{-1} + \boldsymbol{A}_2\widehat{\boldsymbol{B}}_{20}\frac{d\boldsymbol{C}_2\boldsymbol{C}_1'(\boldsymbol{C}_1\boldsymbol{C}_1')^{-1}}{d\omega}\bigg|_{\omega=0},$$

$$\frac{d\widehat{\boldsymbol{B}}_1(\omega)}{d\omega}\bigg|_{\omega=0} = \frac{d(\boldsymbol{A}_1'\boldsymbol{S}_1^{-1}(\omega)b\boldsymbol{Q}_1'(\omega)\boldsymbol{A}_2)^{-1}\boldsymbol{A}_2'\widehat{\boldsymbol{Q}}_1(\omega)\widehat{\boldsymbol{S}}_2^{-1}(\omega)}{d\omega}\bigg|_{\omega=0}$$

$$\times(\boldsymbol{X}_0\boldsymbol{C}_{20}'(\boldsymbol{C}_{20}\boldsymbol{C}_{20}')^{-1} - \boldsymbol{A}_3\widehat{\boldsymbol{B}}_{30}\boldsymbol{C}_3\boldsymbol{C}_{20}'(\boldsymbol{C}_{20}\boldsymbol{C}_{20}')^{-1})$$

$$+(\boldsymbol{A}_2'\widehat{\boldsymbol{Q}}_{10}\widehat{\boldsymbol{S}}_{20}^{-1}\widehat{\boldsymbol{Q}}_{10}'\boldsymbol{A}_2)^{-1}\boldsymbol{A}_2'\widehat{\boldsymbol{Q}}_{10}\widehat{\boldsymbol{S}}_{20}^{-1}\frac{d\boldsymbol{X}\boldsymbol{C}_3'(\boldsymbol{C}_3\boldsymbol{C}_3')^{-1} - \boldsymbol{A}_3\widehat{\boldsymbol{B}}_3\boldsymbol{C}_3\boldsymbol{C}_2'(\boldsymbol{C}_2\boldsymbol{C}_2')^{-1}}{d\omega}\bigg|_{\omega=0}.$$

Concerning the derivatives of the estimates of the parameters, some of the derivatives of the expressions given above have not been expressed. However, all these derivatives where presented fully earlier in the example.

The data of the example were generated according to the model

$$E[\boldsymbol{X}] = \boldsymbol{A}_1\boldsymbol{B}_1\boldsymbol{C}_1 + \boldsymbol{A}_2\boldsymbol{B}_2\boldsymbol{C}_2 + \boldsymbol{A}_3\boldsymbol{B}_3\boldsymbol{C}_3,$$

where $\boldsymbol{B}_1 = (b_{1;ij})$, $i = 1, 2, 3$, $j = 1, 2, 3$, $\boldsymbol{B}_2 = (b_{2;k})$, $k = 1, 2$, and $\boldsymbol{B}_3 = b_3$ (see Example 1.9). It is relevant in this connection to remember that the data consist of three groups and the groups, respectively, consist of 10, 15 or 20 independently distributed observations.

One can make a few comments on the results and first we focus our attention on Table 8.11. The results are presented according to two alternatives. Alternative 1 shows the value of the statistic (the estimate or the first derivative of the estimate) when the contaminated observation is processed, and Alternative 2 is the average value of the statistic as calculated over all the individuals except for the contaminated one.

The effect of adding a relatively large value to all the observations in $\boldsymbol{x}_5$ is for $\frac{d^0\widehat{\boldsymbol{B}}_1}{d\omega^0}$ visible in $\widehat{b}_{1;11}(0)$, i.e. $\widehat{b}_{1;11}(0) = 7.56$ under Alternative 2. The parameter $b_{1;11}$ is the intercept of the group which individual #5 belongs to. Alternative 2

Table 8.11 Let the data be generated as in Example 1.9

	$b_{1;11}$	$b_{1;21}$	$b_{1;31}$	$b_{1;12}$	$b_{1;22}$	$b_{1;23}$	$b_{1;13}$	$b_{1;23}$	$b_{1;33}$
$\frac{d^0\widehat{B}_1}{d\omega^0}$									
Individual #5 has been contaminated, using (iii) in (8.34)									
A1	0.038	0.175	0.018	0.129	0.010	0.033	0.187	0.009	−0.016
A2	0.038	0.172	0.020	0.129	0.011	0.032	0.187	0.008	−0.016
Individual #15 has been contaminated, using (ii) in (8.34)									
A1	0.060	0.142	0.019	0.126	0.014	0.028	0.187	0.009	−0.016
A2	0.060	0.142	0.019	0.126	0.013	0.030	0.187	0.008	−0.016
Individual #30 has been contaminated, using (i) in (8.34)									
A1	0.068	0.131	0.020	0.129	0.010	0.033	0.185	0.009	−0.017
A2	0.068	0.131	0.020	0.129	0.011	0.032	0.185	0.007	−0.016
Individual #5 has been contaminated, using (iv) in (8.34)									
A1	0.063	0.136	0.019	0.129	0.010	0.033	0.187	0.009	−0.016
A2	7.56	0.132	0.021	−1.35	0.010	0.033	1.03	0.009	−0.016
$\left.\frac{d\widehat{B}_1}{d\omega}\right\vert_{\omega=0}$									
Individual #5 has been contaminated, using (iii) in (8.34)									
A1	−0.102	−2.90	28.1	−0.038	2.68	−13.5	0.000	0.000	0.000
A2	0.000	−0.000	0.000	−0.000	0.000	0.000	0.000	−0.000	0.000
Individual #15 has been contaminated, using (ii) in (8.34)									
A1	0.016	0.230	−1.27	−0.374	−2.85	24.9	0.000	0.000	−0.000
A2	0.000	−0.000	0.000	−0.000	0.000	0.000	0.000	−0.000	0.000
Individual #30 has been contaminated, using (i) in (8.34)									
A1	−0.173	1.610	−8.45	−0.177	1.65	−8.67	0.010	1.20	−0.594
A2	0.000	−0.000	0.000	−0.000	0.000	0.000	0.000	−0.000	0.000
Individual #5 has been contaminated, using (iv) in (8.34)									
A1	6.69	−0.031	0.002	0.000	−0.000	0.000	−0.000	0.000	−0.000
A2	−0.14	0.000	0.000	−0.001	0.000	−0.000	0.000	0.000	0.000

The contaminations in (8.34) are evaluated with the help of $\boldsymbol{B}_1$ in the $EBRM_B^3$. Two statistics are used, $\frac{d^0\widehat{\boldsymbol{B}}_1}{d\omega^0}$ and $\left.\frac{d\widehat{\boldsymbol{B}}_1}{d\omega}\right|_{\omega=0}$, where the perturbation scheme based on (8.19) is applied, and the effects of the contaminations are presented according to two alternatives. Alternative 1 (A1) is the value of the statistic when the contaminated observation is processed in the perturbation algorithm. Alternative 2 (A2) is the average of the statistic when the perturbation algorithm is processed over all the subjects, except for the contaminated subject, i.e. when 44 individuals are used. The columns of the table represent $\boldsymbol{B}_1 = (b_{1;ij})$

shows up because the contaminated data are included in the calculation of the average, i.e. each term is a function of the extreme observation. In contrast, in Alternative 1, where only the effect of processing individual #5 is presented, there should not be any effect and this is also the case.

Moreover, it can be observed when adding a large value to all the observations in $\boldsymbol{x}_5$, the first derivative, $\left.\frac{d\widehat{b}_{1;11}}{d\omega}\right|_{\omega=0}$, is largest under Alternative 1, i.e. it equals 6.69,

Table 8.12 Let the data be generated as in Example 1.9

	$b_{2;1}$	$b_{2;2}$	b_3		$b_{2;1}$	$b_{2;2}$	b_3
$\frac{d^0\widehat{\boldsymbol{B}}_k(\omega)}{d\omega^0}$				$\left.\frac{d\,\widehat{\boldsymbol{B}}_k(\omega)}{d\omega}\right\vert_{\omega=0}$			
Individual #5 has been contaminated, using (iii) in (8.34)							
A1	−0.035	−0.070	0.085	A1	−37.4	17.2	0.173
A2	−0.036	−0.069	0.085	A2	−0.000	−0.000	−0.000
Individual #15 has been contaminated, using (ii) in (8.34)							
A1	−0.034	−0.068	0.069	A1	1.65	−33.2	0.000
A2	−0.034	−0.069	0.069	A2	−0.000	−0.000	−0.000
Individual #30 has been contaminated, using (i) in (8.34)							
A1	−0.035	−0.070	0.064	A1	10.7	11.0	−0.000
A2	−0.035	−0.069	0.064	A2	−0.000	−0.000	−0.000
Individual #5 has been contaminated, using (iv) in (8.34)							
A1	−0.036	−0.070	0.066	A1	0.000	−0.000	−0.015
A2	−0.035	−0.070	0.064	A2	−0.000	0.000	0.000

The contaminations in (8.34) are evaluated with the help of $\boldsymbol{B}_k$, $k = 2, 3$, in the $EBRM_B^3$. Two statistics are used, $\frac{d^0\widehat{\boldsymbol{B}}_k}{d\omega^0}$ and $\frac{d\widehat{\boldsymbol{B}}_k}{d\omega}$, $k = 2, 3$, where the perturbation scheme based on (8.19) is applied, and the effects of the contaminations are presented according to two alternatives. Alternative 1 (A1) is the value of the statistic when the contaminated observation is processed in the perturbation algorithm. Alternative 2 (A2) is the average of the statistic when the perturbation algorithm is processed over all the subjects, except for the contaminated subject, i.e. when 44 individuals are used. The columns of the table represent $\boldsymbol{B}_k = (b_{k;ij})$, $k = 2, 3$

whereas under Alternative 2 it equals -0.14. Since this derivative measures the local linear change, it is natural that its value under Alternative 1 should stand out.

Concerning the results of the contaminations, which are shown in Table 8.11, there are no observable effects for the cases where a single observation has been omitted (Alternative 1). However, concerning the local linear change, there are effects on the estimates corresponding to the intercept and the sine and cosine terms. There is information about the data which is included in the large values for $\left.\frac{d\widehat{\boldsymbol{B}}_1}{d\omega}\right\vert_{\omega=0}$, among other values we observe 28.1, 24.9, -13.5, -8.67, etc., but a detailed study of these values is outside the scope of this chapter. In summary, it can be concluded that with the help of the derivatives, the contaminated observations are identified. It would also be interesting to examine the second order derivatives, but we omit to do so here.

In Table 8.12 the influence of observations on the estimates of the parameters $\boldsymbol{B}_2$ and $\boldsymbol{B}_3$ is presented. It appears that it is not possible to identify anything by omitting observations, i.e. by putting $\omega = 0$ in the expressions. However, if one studies the derivative $\left.\frac{d\,\widehat{\boldsymbol{B}}_2}{d\omega}\right\vert_{\omega=0}$, then the contaminated observations are identified. □

In Theorem 8.7 (iv), the derivative $\left.\frac{d^l\, n\widehat{\boldsymbol{\Sigma}}(\omega)}{d\,\omega^l}\right\vert_{\omega=0}$ was presented and now this subsection is ended with an alternative expression. Indeed, the result follows directly from Theorem 8.7 (i)–(iii). Note, similar to (8.16) for the BRM, that $\widehat{\boldsymbol{\Sigma}}$ can be decomposed as

$$n\widehat{\boldsymbol{\Sigma}} = (\boldsymbol{X} - \boldsymbol{A}_1\widehat{\boldsymbol{B}}_1\boldsymbol{C}_1 - \boldsymbol{A}_2\widehat{\boldsymbol{B}}_2\boldsymbol{C}_2 - \boldsymbol{A}_3\widehat{\boldsymbol{B}}_3\boldsymbol{C}_3)()'$$
$$= \boldsymbol{X}\boldsymbol{X}' - \sum_{s=1}^{3}\boldsymbol{X}\boldsymbol{C}_s'\widehat{\boldsymbol{B}}_s'\boldsymbol{A}_s' - \sum_{s=1}^{3}\boldsymbol{A}_s\widehat{\boldsymbol{B}}_s\boldsymbol{C}_s\boldsymbol{X}' + \sum_{s=1}^{3}\sum_{t=1}^{3}\boldsymbol{A}_s\widehat{\boldsymbol{B}}_s\boldsymbol{C}_s\boldsymbol{C}_t'\widehat{\boldsymbol{B}}_t'\boldsymbol{A}_t', \quad (8.35)$$

which verifies the next theorem.

Theorem 8.8 *Consider the $EBRM_B^3$ presented in Definition 2.2 and assume that the perturbation scheme is based on $\boldsymbol{X} = (\boldsymbol{X}_0, \sqrt{\omega}\boldsymbol{X}_i)$, $\boldsymbol{C}_1 = (\boldsymbol{C}_{10}, \sqrt{\omega}\boldsymbol{C}_{1i})$, $\boldsymbol{C}_2 = (\boldsymbol{C}_{20}, \sqrt{\omega}\boldsymbol{C}_{2i})$, $\boldsymbol{C}_3 = (\boldsymbol{C}_{30}, \sqrt{\omega}\boldsymbol{C}_{3i})$ and*

$$n\widehat{\boldsymbol{\Sigma}}(\omega) = (\boldsymbol{X} - \sum_{s=1}^{3}\boldsymbol{A}_s\widehat{\boldsymbol{B}}_s(\omega)\boldsymbol{C}_s)()',$$

where $\widehat{\boldsymbol{B}}_s(\omega)$ are perturbed versions of the estimates given by (8.20), (8.21) and (8.22). Then

$$\left.\frac{d^l n\widehat{\boldsymbol{\Sigma}}(\omega)}{d\omega^l}\right|_{\omega=0} = \left.\frac{d^l\boldsymbol{X}\boldsymbol{X}'}{d\omega^l}\right|_{\omega=0} - \sum_{s=1}^{3}\boldsymbol{A}_s\sum_{i=0}^{1}\binom{l}{i}\left.\frac{d^{l-i}\widehat{\boldsymbol{B}}_s(\omega)}{d\omega^{l-i}}\right|_{\omega=0}\left.\frac{d^i\boldsymbol{C}_s\boldsymbol{X}'}{d\omega^i}\right|_{\omega=0}$$
$$-\sum_{s=1}^{3}\sum_{i=0}^{1}\binom{l}{i}\left.\frac{d^i\boldsymbol{X}\boldsymbol{C}_s'}{d\omega^i}\right|_{\omega=0}\left.\frac{d^{l-i}\widehat{\boldsymbol{B}}_s'(\omega)}{d\omega^{l-i}}\right|_{\omega=0}\boldsymbol{A}_s'$$
$$+\sum_{s=1}^{3}\sum_{t=1}^{3}\boldsymbol{A}_s\sum_{i_1=0}^{l}\sum_{i_2=0}^{l-i_1}\binom{l}{i_1}\binom{l-i_1}{i_2}\left.\frac{d^{l-i_1}\widehat{\boldsymbol{B}}_s(\omega)}{d\omega^{l-i_1}}\frac{d^{i_2}\boldsymbol{C}_s\boldsymbol{C}_t'}{d\omega^{i_2}}\frac{d^{l-i_1-i_2}\widehat{\boldsymbol{B}}_t'(\omega)}{d\omega^{l-i_1-i_2}}\right|_{\omega=0}\boldsymbol{A}_t'.$$

For practical use, two identical versions (see Theorem 8.7 (iv)) of the first derivative of the estimated dispersion matrix are given in the next corollary.

Corollary 8.4 *For the perturbed version of $\widehat{\boldsymbol{\Sigma}}$, i.e. $\widehat{\boldsymbol{\Sigma}}(\omega)$, given in (8.35),*

$$\left.\frac{d\,n\widehat{\boldsymbol{\Sigma}}(\omega)}{d\omega}\right|_{\omega=0} = \boldsymbol{X}_i\boldsymbol{X}_i' - \sum_{s=1}^{3}(\boldsymbol{X}_0\boldsymbol{C}_{s0}'\left.\frac{d\widehat{\boldsymbol{B}}_s'(\omega)}{d\omega}\right|_{\omega=0} + \boldsymbol{X}_i\boldsymbol{C}_{si}'\widehat{\boldsymbol{B}}_s'(0))\boldsymbol{A}_s'$$
$$-\sum_{s=1}^{3}\boldsymbol{A}_s(\left.\frac{d\widehat{\boldsymbol{B}}_s(\omega)}{d\omega}\right|_{\omega=0}\boldsymbol{C}_{s0}\boldsymbol{X}_0' + \widehat{\boldsymbol{B}}(0)\boldsymbol{C}_{si}\boldsymbol{X}_i')$$
$$+\sum_{s=1}^{3}\sum_{t=1}^{3}\boldsymbol{A}_s\left.\frac{d\widehat{\boldsymbol{B}}_s(\omega)}{d\omega}\right|_{\omega=0}\boldsymbol{C}_{s0}\boldsymbol{C}_{t0}'\left.\frac{d\widehat{\boldsymbol{B}}_t'(\omega)}{d\omega}\right|_{\omega=0}\boldsymbol{A}_t'$$
$$+\sum_{s=1}^{3}\sum_{t=1}^{3}\boldsymbol{A}_s\left.\frac{d\widehat{\boldsymbol{B}}_s(\omega)}{d\omega}\right|_{\omega=0}\boldsymbol{C}_{si}\boldsymbol{C}_{ti}'\widehat{\boldsymbol{B}}_t'(0)\boldsymbol{A}_t' + \boldsymbol{A}_s\widehat{\boldsymbol{B}}_s(0)\boldsymbol{C}_{s0}\boldsymbol{C}_{t0}'\widehat{\boldsymbol{B}}_t'(0)\boldsymbol{A}_t',$$

which is identical to

$$\left.\frac{dn\widehat{\Sigma}(\omega)}{d\omega}\right|_{\omega=0} = \left.\frac{d\widehat{S}_3(\omega)}{d\omega}\right|_{\omega=0} + \widehat{Q}'_{30}\widehat{Q}'_{20}\widehat{Q}'_{10}X_0P_{C'_{30}}X'_0 \left.\frac{d\widehat{Q}_1\widehat{Q}_2\widehat{Q}_3}{d\omega}\right|_{\omega=0}$$

$$+\widehat{Q}'_{30}\widehat{Q}'_{20}\widehat{Q}'_{10} \left.\frac{dXP_{C'_3}X'}{d\omega}\right|_{\omega=0} \widehat{Q}'_{10}\widehat{Q}'_{20}\widehat{Q}'_{30} + \left.\frac{d\widehat{Q}'_3\widehat{Q}'_2\widehat{Q}'_1}{d\omega}\right|_{\omega=0} X_0P_{C'_{30}}X'_0\widehat{Q}'_{10}\widehat{Q}'_{20}\widehat{Q}'_{30}.$$

This section is concluded with a continuation of Example 8.6, where the effects of the contaminations in (8.34) on the estimated dispersion matrix are studied via Corollary 8.4.

Example 8.7 (Continuation of Example 8.6) In Table 8.13 the results of the contaminations in (8.34) are presented. The influence pattern in Table 8.13 follows the patterns of Tables 8.11 and 8.12; i.e. for $\frac{d^0 n\widehat{\Sigma}(\omega)}{d\omega^0}$ the influence measure is high in Alternative 1 and low in Alternative 2, and for $\left.\frac{d^1 n\widehat{\Sigma}(\omega)}{d\omega^1}\right|_{\omega=0}$ it is vice versa. Since

Table 8.13 Let the data be generated as in Example 1.9

Sig_1		Sig_2	
$\frac{d^0n\widehat{\Sigma}(\omega)}{d\omega^0}$		$\left.\frac{dn\widehat{\Sigma}(\omega)}{d\omega}\right\|_{\omega=0}$	
Individual #5 has been contaminated, using (iii) in (8.34)			
A1	65.8	A1	0.22
A2	0.026	A2	355
Individual #15 has been contaminated, using (ii) in (8.34)			
A1	65.5	A1	0.21
A2	0.027	A2	340
Individual #30 has been contaminated, using (i) in (8.34)			
A1	65.8	A1	0.21
A2	0.026	A2	129
Individual #5 has been contaminated, using (iv) in (8.34)			
A1	3300	A1	0.48
A2	0.026	A2	4059

The contaminations in (8.34) are evaluated with the help of $\mathbf{\Sigma}$ in the $EBRM_B^3$. Two statistics are used, $\frac{d^0n\widehat{\Sigma}(\omega)}{d\omega^0}$ and $\frac{dn\widehat{\Sigma}(\omega)}{d\omega}$, where the perturbation scheme based on (8.19) is applied, and the effects of the contaminations are presented according to two alternatives. Alternative 1 (A1) is the value of the statistic when the contaminated observation is processed in the perturbation algorithm. Alternative 2 (A2) is the average of the statistic when the perturbation algorithm is processed over all the subjects, except for the contaminated subject, i.e. when 44 individuals are used. The columns of the table represent the averages of the upper triangles of $\frac{d^0n\widehat{\Sigma}(\omega)}{d\omega^0}$ and $\frac{dn\widehat{\Sigma}(\omega)}{d\omega}$, which are denoted by Sig_1 and Sig_2, respectively the contaminated data comprise an outlier, the residuals should be affected, which means that $n\widehat{\Sigma}$ in turn should be affected, because the estimated dispersion matrix is a function of the residuals. The main conclusion to be drawn from Table 8.13 is that the method for identifying influential observations (outliers) seems to work very well. □

8.5 Influence Analysis in the $EBRM_W^3$

The $EBRM_W^3$ presented in Definition 2.3 is now treated using a procedure similar to that used for the $EBRM_B^3$. Among other similarities, only the perturbations in (8.19) are implemented. Under suitable full rank conditions, the MLEs are given by (see Theorem 3.3)

$$\begin{aligned}
\widehat{B}_1 &= (A_1'\widehat{S}_3^{-1}A_1)^{-1}A_1'\widehat{S}_3^{-1}(X - A_2\widehat{B}_2C_2 - A_3\widehat{B}_3C_3)C_1'(C_1C_1')^{-1},\\
\widehat{B}_2 &= (A_2'\widehat{S}_2^{-1}A_2)^{-1}A_2'\widehat{S}_2^{-1}(X - A_3\widehat{B}_3C_3)Q_1C_2'(C_2Q_1C_2')^{-1},\\
\widehat{B}_3 &= (A_3'S_1^{-1}A_3)^{-1}A_3'S_1^{-1}XQ_2C_3'(C_3Q_2C_3')^{-1},\\
n\widehat{\Sigma} &= (X - A_1\widehat{B}_1C_1 - A_2\widehat{B}_2C_2 - A_3\widehat{B}_3C_3)()'\\
&= \widehat{S}_3 + P'_{A_1^o,\widehat{S}_3^{-1}}XP_{C_1'}X'P_{A_1^o,\widehat{S}_3^{-1}},
\end{aligned}$$

where

$$S_1 = XP_4X', \quad \widehat{S}_2 = S_1 + P'_{A_3^o,S_1^{-1}}XP_3X'P_{A_3^o,S_1^{-1}}, \tag{8.36}$$

$$\widehat{S}_3 = \widehat{S}_2 + P'_{A_2^o,\widehat{S}_2^{-1}}XP_2X'P_{A_2^o,\widehat{S}_2^{-1}}, \tag{8.37}$$

with

$$P_1 = P_{C_1'}, \quad P_2 = P_{Q_1C_2'}, \quad P_3 = P_{Q_2Q_1C_3'}, \quad P_4 = P_{(C_1':C_2':C_3')^o}, \tag{8.38}$$

and

$$Q_1 = P_{(C_1')^o}, \quad Q_2 = P_{(C_1':C_2')^o}.$$

Thus, in order to create influence measures, there is a need to differentiate perturbed versions of S_1, $\widehat{S}_i$, $i = 2, 3$, $XQ_1C_2'(C_2Q_1C_2')^{-1}$, $C_3Q_1C_2'(C_2Q_1C_2')^{-1}$ and $XQ_2C_3'(C_3Q_2C_3')^{-1}$, where the perturbation follows (8.19). Similar expressions were differentiated when the $EBRM_B^3$ was treated, but for completeness, a few details are presented below.

We begin by differentiating $C_3Q_1C_2'(C_2Q_1C_2')^{-1}$ and firstly $C_2Q_1C_2'$ is studied. Since $Q_1 = I - P_{C_1'}$,

$$\left.\frac{d^l C_2 Q_1 C_2'}{d\omega^l}\right|_{\omega=0} = \left.\frac{d^l C_2(I - C_1'(C_1C_1')^{-1}C_1)C_2'}{d\omega^l}\right|_{\omega=0}$$

$$= \left.\frac{d^l C_2C_2'}{d\omega^l}\right|_{\omega=0} - \sum_{i_1=0}^{l}\sum_{i_2=l-i_1-1}^{l-i_1}\binom{l}{i_1}\binom{l-i_1}{i_2}\left.\frac{d^{i_1}C_2C_1'}{d\omega^{i_1}}\frac{d^{i_2}(C_1C_1')^{-1}}{d\omega^{i_2}}\frac{d^{l-i_1-i_2}C_1C_2'}{d\omega^{l-i_1-i_2}}\right|_{\omega=0}, \quad (8.39)$$

where $\left.\frac{d^l(C_1C_1')^{-1}}{d\omega^l}\right|_{\omega=0}$ is obtained from Appendix B, Theorem B.15 (iii). The expression for $\left.\frac{d^l XQ_1C_2'}{d\omega^l}\right|_{\omega=0}$ is also needed and through the similarity with the derivative given above, it follows that

$$\left.\frac{d^l XQ_1C_2'}{d\omega^l}\right|_{\omega=0} = \left.\frac{d^l X(I - C_1'(C_1C_1')^{-1}C_1)C_2'}{d\omega^l}\right|_{\omega=0}$$

$$= \left.\frac{d^l XC_2'}{d\omega^l}\right|_{\omega=0} - \sum_{i_1=0}^{l}\sum_{i_2=l-i_1-1}^{l-i_1}\binom{l}{i_1}\binom{l-i_1}{i_2}\left.\frac{d^{i_1}XC_1'}{d\omega^{i_1}}\frac{d^{i_2}(C_1C_1')^{-1}}{d\omega^{i_2}}\frac{d^{l-i_1-i_2}C_1C_2'}{d\omega^{l-i_1-i_2}}\right|_{\omega=0}. \quad (8.40)$$

Hence, $\left.\frac{d^l XQ_1C_2'(C_2Q_1C_2')^{-1}}{d\omega^l}\right|_{\omega=0}$ should be expressed, i.e.

$$\left.\frac{d^l XQ_1C_2'(C_2Q_1C_2')^{-1}}{d\omega^l}\right|_{\omega=0} = \sum_{i=0}^{l}\binom{l}{i}\left.\frac{d^i XQ_1C_2'}{d\omega^i}\frac{d^{l-i}(C_2Q_1C_2')^{-1}}{d\omega^{l-i}}\right|_{\omega=0}, \quad (8.41)$$

where more explicit expressions can be obtained by applying (8.39) and (8.40). Similarly, $C_3Q_1C_2'(C_2Q_1C_2')^{-1}$ can be mastered and

$$\left.\frac{d^l C_3Q_1C_2'(C_2Q_1C_2')^{-1}}{d\omega^l}\right|_{\omega=0} = \sum_{i=0}^{l}\binom{l}{i}\left.\frac{d^i C_3Q_1C_2'}{d\omega^i}\frac{d^{l-i}(C_2Q_1C_2')^{-1}}{d\omega^{l-i}}\right|_{\omega=0}, \quad (8.42)$$

where

$$\left.\frac{d^l C_3Q_1C_2'}{d\omega^l}\right|_{\omega=0} = \left.\frac{d^l C_3(I - C_1'(C_1C_1')^{-1}C_1)C_2'}{d\omega^l}\right|_{\omega=0}$$

$$= \left.\frac{d^l C_3C_2'}{d\omega^l}\right|_{\omega=0} - \sum_{i_1=0}^{l}\sum_{i_2=l-i_1-1}^{l-i_1}\binom{l}{i_1}\binom{l-i_1}{i_2}\left.\frac{d^{i_1}C_3C_1'}{d\omega^{i_1}}\frac{d^{i_2}(C_1C_1')^{-1}}{d\omega^{i_2}}\frac{d^{l-i_1-i_2}C_1C_2'}{d\omega^{l-i_1-i_2}}\right|_{\omega=0}.$$

Expressions involving $\boldsymbol{Q}_2$ such as $\boldsymbol{C}_3\boldsymbol{Q}_2\boldsymbol{C}_3'$ and $\boldsymbol{X}\boldsymbol{Q}_2\boldsymbol{C}_3'$ appear more complicated to handle than (8.39) or (8.40), because $\boldsymbol{Q}_2$ is a function of $\boldsymbol{C}_1$ and $\boldsymbol{C}_2$, i.e. two perturbed matrices instead of only one. However, mathematically, differentiating $\boldsymbol{C}_3\boldsymbol{Q}_2\boldsymbol{C}_3'$ and differentiating $\boldsymbol{C}_2\boldsymbol{Q}_1\boldsymbol{C}_2'$ instead turn out to be the same problem, and it can immediately be stated that

$$
\begin{aligned}
\left.\frac{d^l \boldsymbol{C}_3\boldsymbol{Q}_2\boldsymbol{C}_3'}{d\,\omega^l}\right|_{\omega=0} &= \left.\frac{d^l \boldsymbol{C}_3(\boldsymbol{I}-(\boldsymbol{C}_1':\boldsymbol{C}_2')((\boldsymbol{C}_1':\boldsymbol{C}_2')'(\boldsymbol{C}_1':\boldsymbol{C}_2'))^{-1}(\boldsymbol{C}_1':\boldsymbol{C}_2')')\boldsymbol{C}_3'}{d\,\omega^l}\right|_{\omega=0} \\
&= \left.\frac{d^l \boldsymbol{C}_3\boldsymbol{C}_3'}{d\,\omega^l}\right|_{\omega=0} \\
-\sum_{i_1=0}^{l}\sum_{i_2=l-i_1-1}^{l-i_1} & \binom{l}{i_1}\binom{l-i_1}{i_2}\left.\frac{d^{i_1}\boldsymbol{C}_3(\boldsymbol{C}_1':\boldsymbol{C}_2')}{d\,\omega^{i_1}}\frac{d^{i_2}((\boldsymbol{C}_1':\boldsymbol{C}_2')'(\boldsymbol{C}_1':\boldsymbol{C}_2'))^{-1}}{d\,\omega^{i_2}}\frac{d^{l-i_1-i_2}(\boldsymbol{C}_1':\boldsymbol{C}_2')'\boldsymbol{C}_3'}{d\,\omega^{l-i_1-i_2}}\right|_{\omega=0}, \quad (8.43)
\end{aligned}
$$

where $\left.\dfrac{d^l((\boldsymbol{C}_1':\boldsymbol{C}_2')'(\boldsymbol{C}_1':\boldsymbol{C}_2'))^{-1}}{d\,\omega^l}\right|_{\omega=0}$ is obtained from Appendix B, Theorem B.15 (iii).

The expression for $\left.\dfrac{d^l\boldsymbol{X}\boldsymbol{Q}_2\boldsymbol{C}_3'}{d\,\omega^l}\right|_{\omega=0}$ is also needed and through the similarity with the derivative given above, it follows that

$$
\begin{aligned}
\left.\frac{d^l \boldsymbol{X}\boldsymbol{Q}_2\boldsymbol{C}_3'}{d\,\omega^l}\right|_{\omega=0} &= \left.\frac{d^l \boldsymbol{X}(\boldsymbol{I}-(\boldsymbol{C}_1':\boldsymbol{C}_2')((\boldsymbol{C}_1':\boldsymbol{C}_2')'(\boldsymbol{C}_1':\boldsymbol{C}_2'))^{-1}(\boldsymbol{C}_1':\boldsymbol{C}_2')')\boldsymbol{C}_3'}{d\,\omega^l}\right|_{\omega=0} \\
&= \left.\frac{d^l \boldsymbol{X}\boldsymbol{C}_3'}{d\,\omega^l}\right|_{\omega=0} \\
-\sum_{i_1=0}^{l}\sum_{i_2=l-i_1-1}^{l-i_1} & \binom{l}{i_1}\binom{l-i_1}{i_2}\left.\frac{d^{i_1}\boldsymbol{X}(\boldsymbol{C}_1':\boldsymbol{C}_2')}{d\,\omega^{i_1}}\frac{d^{i_2}((\boldsymbol{C}_1':\boldsymbol{C}_2')'(\boldsymbol{C}_1':\boldsymbol{C}_2'))^{-1}}{d\,\omega^{i_2}}\frac{d^{l-i_1-i_2}(\boldsymbol{C}_1':\boldsymbol{C}_2')'\boldsymbol{C}_3'}{d\,\omega^{l-i_1-i_2}}\right|_{\omega=0}. \quad (8.44)
\end{aligned}
$$

Therefore,

$$
\left.\frac{d^l\boldsymbol{X}\boldsymbol{Q}_2\boldsymbol{C}_3'(\boldsymbol{C}_3\boldsymbol{Q}_2\boldsymbol{C}_3')^{-1}}{d\,\omega^l}\right|_{\omega=0} = \sum_{i=0}^{l}\binom{l}{i}\left.\frac{d^i\boldsymbol{X}\boldsymbol{Q}_2\boldsymbol{C}_3'}{d\,\omega^i}\frac{d^{l-i}(\boldsymbol{C}_3\boldsymbol{Q}_2\boldsymbol{C}_3')^{-1}}{d\,\omega^{l-i}}\right|_{\omega=0} \quad (8.45)
$$

is established, and can be explicitly expressed by utilizing (8.43) and (8.44). We also need to differentiate $\boldsymbol{X}\boldsymbol{P}_2\boldsymbol{X}'$ and $\boldsymbol{X}\boldsymbol{P}_3\boldsymbol{X}'$, where $\boldsymbol{P}_2$ and $\boldsymbol{P}_3$ are given in (8.38), i.e.

$$
\left.\frac{d^l\boldsymbol{X}\boldsymbol{P}_2\boldsymbol{X}'}{d\,\omega^l}\right|_{\omega=0} = \sum_{i=0}^{l}\left.\frac{d^i\boldsymbol{X}\boldsymbol{Q}_1\boldsymbol{C}_2'(\boldsymbol{C}_2\boldsymbol{Q}_1\boldsymbol{C}_2')^{-1}}{d\,\omega^i}\frac{d^{l-i}\boldsymbol{C}_2\boldsymbol{Q}_1\boldsymbol{X}'}{d\,\omega^{l-i}}\right|_{\omega=0}, \quad (8.46)
$$

$$
\left.\frac{d^l\boldsymbol{X}\boldsymbol{P}_3\boldsymbol{X}'}{d\,\omega^l}\right|_{\omega=0} = \sum_{i=0}^{l}\left.\frac{d^i\boldsymbol{X}\boldsymbol{Q}_2\boldsymbol{C}_3'(\boldsymbol{C}_3\boldsymbol{Q}_1\boldsymbol{C}_3')^{-1}}{d\,\omega^i}\frac{d^{l-i}\boldsymbol{C}_3\boldsymbol{Q}_2\boldsymbol{X}'}{d\,\omega^{l-i}}\right|_{\omega=0}. \quad (8.47)
$$

Since S_1, $\widehat{S}_2$ and $\widehat{S}_3$ are involved in the estimates $\widehat{B}_i$, $i = 1, 2, 3$, and $n\widehat{\Sigma}$, the matrices are now exploited. Put $F'_1 = (C'_1 : C'_2 : C'_3)$, $F'_{10} = (C'_{10} : C'_{20} : C'_{30})$ and $F'_{1i} = (C'_{1i} : C'_{2i} : C'_{3i})$, where C_{k0} and C_{ki}, $k = 1, 2, 3$, are as in (8.19). Then (compare with Lemma 8.1)

$$\left.\frac{d^l S_1(\omega)}{d\omega^l}\right|_{\omega=0} = \left.\frac{d^l X(I-P_{F'_1})X'}{d\omega^l}\right|_{\omega=0} = (-1)^{l+1} l! R_i D_i^{k-1} R'_i, \qquad k \geq 1, \quad (8.48)$$

where

$$D_i = F'_{1i}(F_{10}F'_{10})^{-1}F_{1i}, \quad R_i = X_i - X_0 F'_{10}(F_{10}F'_{10})^{-1}F_{1i}.$$

Furthermore,

$$\left.\frac{d^l (A'_3 S_1^{-1}(\omega)A_3)^{-1}A'_3 S_1^{-1}(\omega)}{d\omega^l}\right|_{\omega=0} = \sum_{i=0}^{l}\binom{l}{i}\left.\frac{d^i (A'_3 S_1^{-1}(\omega)A_3)^{-1}}{d\omega^i} A'_3 \frac{d^{l-i} S_1^{-1}(\omega)}{d\omega^{l-i}}\right|_{\omega=0} \quad (8.49)$$

Turning one's attention to $\widehat{S}_2$, it is somewhat more complicated to perform the necessary calculations, since $P_{A_3^o, S_1^{-1}}$ is to be differentiated:

$$\left.\frac{d^l P_{A_3^o, S_1^{-1}(\omega)}}{d\omega^l}\right|_{\omega=0} = A_3^o \sum_{i=0}^{l} \left.\frac{d^i (A_3^{o\prime} S_1(\omega)A_3^o)^{-1}}{d\omega^i} A_3^{o\prime} \frac{d^{l-i} S_1(\omega)}{d\omega^{l-i}}\right|_{\omega=0}, \quad (8.50)$$

where $\left.\frac{d^l (A_3^{o\prime} S_1(\omega)A_3^o)^{-1}}{d\omega^l}\right|_{\omega=0}$ is obtained from Appendix B, Theorem B.15 (ii) and (iii), and (8.48). Thus,

$$\left.\frac{d^l \widehat{S}_2(\omega)}{d\omega^l}\right|_{\omega=0} = \frac{d^l S_1(\omega)}{d\omega^l}$$
$$- \sum_{i_1=0}^{l}\sum_{i_2=0}^{l-i_1}\binom{l}{i_1}\binom{l-i_1}{i_2} \left.\frac{d^{i_1} P_{A_3^o, S_1^{-1}(\omega)}}{d\omega^{i_1}} \frac{d^{i_2} X P_3 X'}{d\omega^{i_2}} \frac{d^{l-i_1-i_2} P'_{A_3^o, S_1^{-1}(\omega)}}{d\omega^{l-i_1-i_2}}\right|_{\omega=0}; \quad (8.51)$$

the derivatives in this formula were presented in (8.47) and (8.50). It also follows that

$$\left.\frac{d^l (A'_2 \widehat{S}_2^{-1}(\omega)A_2)^{-1}A'_2 \widehat{S}_2^{-1}(\omega)}{d\omega^l}\right|_{\omega=0} = \sum_{i=0}^{l}\binom{l}{i}\left.\frac{d^i (A'_2 S_1^{-1}(\omega)A_2)^{-1}}{d\omega^i} A'_2 \frac{d^{l-i} S_1^{-1}(\omega)}{d\omega^{l-i}}\right|_{\omega=0} \quad (8.52)$$

The calculations of the derivative of $\widehat{S}_3(\omega)$ are almost identical to the calculations of the derivative of $\widehat{S}_2(\omega)$. Therefore,

$$\frac{d^l\,\widehat{S}_3(\omega)}{d\,\omega^l}\bigg|_{\omega=0} = \frac{d^l\,\widehat{S}_2(\omega)}{d\,\omega^l}$$

$$-\sum_{i_1=0}^{l}\sum_{i_2=0}^{l-i_1}\binom{l}{i_1}\binom{l-i_1}{i_2}\frac{d^{i_1}\boldsymbol{P}_{A_2^o,\widehat{S}_2^{-1}(\omega)}}{d\,\omega^{i_1}}\frac{d^{i_2}\boldsymbol{X}\boldsymbol{P}_2\boldsymbol{X}'}{d\,\omega^{i_2}}\frac{d^{l-i_1-i_2}\boldsymbol{P}'_{A_2^o,\widehat{S}_2^{-1}(\omega)}}{d\,\omega^{l-i_1-i_2}}\Bigg|_{\omega=0}, \quad (8.53)$$

where $\frac{d^l\boldsymbol{X}\boldsymbol{P}_2\boldsymbol{X}'}{d\,\omega^l}\Big|_{\omega=0}$ is given by (8.46) and

$$\frac{d^l\,\boldsymbol{P}_{A_2^o,\widehat{S}_2^{-1}(\omega)}}{d\,\omega^l}\Bigg|_{\omega=0} = \boldsymbol{A}_3^o\sum_{i=0}^{l}\frac{d^i(\boldsymbol{A}_2^{o'}\,S_2(\omega)\boldsymbol{A}_2^o)^{-1}}{d\,\omega^i}\boldsymbol{A}_2^{o'}\frac{d^{l-i}\widehat{S}_2(\omega)}{d\,\omega^{l-i}}\Bigg|_{\omega=0}, \quad (8.54)$$

and $\frac{d^l(\boldsymbol{A}_2^o\widehat{S}_2(\omega)\boldsymbol{A}_2^o)^{-1}}{d\,\omega^l}\Big|_{\omega=0}$ is established via (8.51). Moreover,

$$\frac{d^l(\boldsymbol{A}_1'\boldsymbol{S}_3^{-1}(\omega)\boldsymbol{A}_1)^{-1}\boldsymbol{A}_1'\boldsymbol{S}_3^{-1}(\omega)}{d\,\omega^l}\Bigg|_{\omega=0} = \sum_{i=0}^{l}\binom{l}{i}\frac{d^i(\boldsymbol{A}_1'\boldsymbol{S}_3^{-1}(\omega)\boldsymbol{A}_1)^{-1}}{d\,\omega^i}\boldsymbol{A}_1'\frac{d^{l-i}\boldsymbol{S}_3^{-1}(\omega)}{d\,\omega^{l-i}}\Bigg|_{\omega=0}, \quad (8.55)$$

where the derivatives can be obtained through (8.53) and a few calculations.

Theorem 8.9 *For the $EBRM_W^3$ presented in Definition 2.3, let the perturbation be defined in (8.19), and then, under "full rank" assumptions, the following perturbed estimates will be considered:*

$$\widehat{\boldsymbol{B}}_1(\omega) = (\boldsymbol{A}_1'\widehat{\boldsymbol{S}}_3^{-1}(\omega)\boldsymbol{A}_1)^{-1}\boldsymbol{A}_1'\widehat{\boldsymbol{S}}_3^{-1}(\omega)(\boldsymbol{X}-\boldsymbol{A}_2\widehat{\boldsymbol{B}}_2(\omega)\boldsymbol{C}_2-\boldsymbol{A}_3\widehat{\boldsymbol{B}}_3(\omega)\boldsymbol{C}_3)\boldsymbol{C}_1'(\boldsymbol{C}_1\boldsymbol{C}_1')^{-1},$$
$$\widehat{\boldsymbol{B}}_2(\omega) = (\boldsymbol{A}_2'\widehat{\boldsymbol{S}}_2^{-1}(\omega)\boldsymbol{A}_2)^{-1}\boldsymbol{A}_2'\widehat{\boldsymbol{S}}_2^{-1}(\omega)(\boldsymbol{X}-\boldsymbol{A}_3\widehat{\boldsymbol{B}}_3(\omega)\boldsymbol{C}_3)\boldsymbol{Q}_1\boldsymbol{C}_2'(\boldsymbol{C}_2\boldsymbol{Q}_1\boldsymbol{C}_2')^{-1},$$
$$\widehat{\boldsymbol{B}}_3(\omega) = (\boldsymbol{A}_3'\boldsymbol{S}_1^{-1}(\omega)\boldsymbol{A}_3)^{-1}\boldsymbol{A}_3'\boldsymbol{S}_1^{-1}(\omega)\boldsymbol{X}\boldsymbol{Q}_2\boldsymbol{C}_3'(\boldsymbol{C}_3\boldsymbol{Q}_2\boldsymbol{C}_3')^{-1},$$
$$n\widehat{\boldsymbol{\Sigma}}(\omega) = (\boldsymbol{X}-\boldsymbol{A}_1\widehat{\boldsymbol{B}}_1(\omega)\boldsymbol{C}_1-\boldsymbol{A}_2\widehat{\boldsymbol{B}}_2(\omega)\boldsymbol{C}_2-\boldsymbol{A}_3\widehat{\boldsymbol{B}}_3(\omega)\boldsymbol{C}_3)()',$$

where $\boldsymbol{X}$, $\boldsymbol{C}_j$ and $\boldsymbol{Q}_j$, $j=1,2$, also are functions of ω, and $\boldsymbol{S}_1$, $\widehat{\boldsymbol{S}}_i$, $i=2,3$, and $\boldsymbol{Q}_j$, $j=1,2$, are obtained from Theorem 3.3. Then

(i)

$$\frac{d^l\,\widehat{\boldsymbol{B}}_3(\omega)}{d\,\omega^l}\bigg|_{\omega=0} = \sum_{i=0}^{l}\binom{l}{i}\frac{d^i\,(\boldsymbol{A}_3'\boldsymbol{S}_1^{-1}(\omega)\boldsymbol{A}_3)^{-1}\boldsymbol{A}_3'\widehat{\boldsymbol{S}}_1^{-1}(\omega)}{d\,\omega^i}$$
$$\times\frac{d^{l-i}\,\boldsymbol{X}\boldsymbol{Q}_2\boldsymbol{C}_3'(\boldsymbol{C}_3\boldsymbol{Q}_2\boldsymbol{C}_3')^{-1}}{d\,\omega^{l-i}}\Bigg|_{\omega=0}, \qquad l>0,$$

where the derivatives of $(A_3' S_1^{-1}(\omega) A_3)^{-1} A_3' S_1^{-1}(\omega)$ *are obtained via (8.49) and the derivative of* $X Q_2 C_3' (C_3 Q_2 C_3')^{-1}$ *follows from (8.45);*

(ii)

$$\frac{d^l\,\widehat{B}_2(\omega)}{d\,\omega^l}\bigg|_{\omega=0} = \sum_{i=0}^{l} \binom{l}{i} \frac{d^i\,(A_2'\widehat{S}_2^{-1}(\omega)A_2)^{-1}A_2'\widehat{S}_2^{-1}(\omega)}{d\,\omega^i}$$
$$\times \frac{d^{l-i}\,X Q_1 C_2'(C_2 Q_1 C_2')^{-1} - A_3\widehat{B}_3(\omega) C_3 Q_1 C_2'(C_2 Q_1 C_2')^{-1}}{d\,\omega^{l-i}}\bigg|_{\omega=0}, \quad l > 0,$$

where the derivatives of $\widehat{B}_3$ *and* $(A_2'\widehat{S}_2^{-1}(\omega)A_2)^{-1}A_2'\widehat{S}_2^{-1}(\omega)$ *are obtained via statement (i) and (8.52), respectively, and* $\frac{d^{l-i}\,X Q_1 C_2'(C_2 Q_1 C_2')^{-1}}{d\,\omega^{l-i}}\bigg|_{\omega=0}$ *and* $\frac{d^{l-i}\,C_3 Q_1 C_2'(C_2 Q_1 C_2')^{-1}}{d\,\omega^{l-i}}\bigg|_{\omega=0}$ *follow from (8.41) and (8.42);*

(iii)

$$\frac{d^l\,\widehat{B}_1(\omega)}{d\,\omega^l}\bigg|_{\omega=0} = \sum_{i=0}^{l} \binom{l}{i} \frac{d^i\,(A_1'\widehat{S}_3^{-1}(\omega)A_1)^{-1}A_1'\widehat{S}_3^{-1}}{d\,\omega^i}$$
$$\times \frac{d^{l-i}\,(X C_1'(C_1 C_1')^{-1} - A_2\widehat{B}_2(\omega) C_2 C_1'(C_1 C_1')^{-1} - A_3\widehat{B}_3(\omega) C_3 C_1'(C_1 C_1')^{-1})}{d\,\omega^{l-i}}\bigg|_{\omega=0},$$
$$l > 0,$$

where the derivatives of $(A_1'\widehat{S}_3^{-1}(\omega)A_1)^{-1}A_1'\widehat{S}_3^{-1}(\omega)$ *are obtained via (8.55),* $\frac{d^{l-i}\,X C_1'(C_1 C_1')^{-1}}{d\,\omega^{l-i}}\bigg|_{\omega=0}$ *follows from Lemma 8.5 (ii), the derivatives of* $\widehat{B}_i$, $i = 1, 2$, *and* $\frac{d^{l-i}\,C_j C_1'(C_1 C_1')^{-1}}{d\,\omega^{l-i}}\bigg|_{\omega=0}$, $j = 2, 3$, *follow from statements (i) and (ii), and Lemma 8.5 (iii);*

(iv)

$$\frac{d^l n\widehat{\Sigma}(\omega)}{d\,\omega^l}\bigg|_{\omega=0} = \frac{d^l\,XX'}{d\,\omega^l}\bigg|_{\omega=0} - \sum_{s=1}^{3} A_s \sum_{i=0}^{1} \binom{l}{i} \frac{d^{l-i}\,\widehat{B}_s(\omega)}{d\,\omega^{l-i}}\bigg|_{\omega=0} \frac{d^i\,C_s X'}{d\,\omega^i}\bigg|_{\omega=0}$$
$$- \sum_{s=1}^{3}\sum_{i=0}^{1} \binom{l}{i} \frac{d^i\,X C_s'}{d\,\omega^i}\bigg|_{\omega=0} \frac{d^{l-i}\,\widehat{B}_s'(\omega)}{d\,\omega^{l-i}}\bigg|_{\omega=0} A_s'$$
$$+ \sum_{s=1}^{3}\sum_{t=1}^{3} A_s \sum_{i_1=0}^{l}\sum_{i_2=0}^{l-i_1} \binom{l}{i_1}\binom{l-i_1}{i_2} \frac{d^{l-i_1}\,\widehat{B}_s(\omega)}{d\,\omega^{l-i_1}} \frac{d^{i_2}\,C_s C_t'}{d\,\omega^{i_2}} \frac{d^{l-i_1-i_2}\,\widehat{B}_t'(\omega)}{d\,\omega^{l-i_1-i_2}}\bigg|_{\omega=0} A_t',$$

where the derivatives of $\widehat{B}_i$, $i = 1, 2, 3$, *are obtained from statements (i)–(iii), and it is a straightforward task to determine* $\frac{d^{i_2}\,C_s C_t'}{d\,\omega^{i_2}}$.

Problems

1 Using a BRM, construct a data set which includes masking effects. Verify the existence of such effects.

2 In Corollary 8.1 the second derivative was presented for the MLE of the mean parameter. Extend the result and derive the third derivatives for $\widehat{\boldsymbol{B}}$. Use the same perturbation as that used in Theorem 8.1, and, in addition, use another one; see, for example, Definition 8.3 (i) or (ii). Apply the results to a real data set.

3 Fit a BRM to the data in Example 1.5 and perform an influence analysis.

4 For the BRM, derive the basic derivatives for performing an influence analysis for $\widehat{D[\widehat{\boldsymbol{B}}]}$. Determine whether there are any observations in the Potthoff and Roy (1964) data set (Table 1.2) which can be deemed to be influential on $\widehat{D[\widehat{\boldsymbol{B}}]}$.

5 Based on the Potthoff and Roy (1964) data set (Table 1.2), carry out an influence analysis for the case where pairs of observations are perturbed.

6 Conduct an influence analysis of the MLE $\widehat{\boldsymbol{\Sigma}}$, with the help of Perturbation (ii) in Definition 8.3, using the Potthoff and Roy (1964) data set.

7 Generate data according to an $EBRM_B^2$. Firstly, contaminate a few observations and determine whether these observations are influential. Secondly contaminate the data so that some of the contaminated observations are influential and some are not influential.

8 Choose a suitable perturbation and derive basic equations for performing an influence analysis in a GMANOVA+MANOVA model.

9 For Theorem 8.9 (i)–(iv), present explicit expressions for the cases where $l = 0$ and $l = 1$.

10 For the $EBRM_W^3$, use the statement that

$$n\widehat{\boldsymbol{\Sigma}} = \widehat{\boldsymbol{S}}_3(\omega) + \boldsymbol{P}'_{A_1^o, \widehat{S}_3^{-1}(\omega)} \boldsymbol{X} \boldsymbol{P}_{C_1'} \boldsymbol{X}' \boldsymbol{P}_{A_1^o, \widehat{S}_3^{-1}(\omega)}.$$

Derive an influence measure, which is based on a suitable chosen perturbation scheme, and which can be of use when discussing influence on $n\widehat{\boldsymbol{\Sigma}}$.

Literature

"Influential observations" is a relatively new concept, although it must have existed informally for a long time. It has been a common knowledge among statisticians, among others, that different observations have different impacts on the analysis.

This has led to the development of statistical research areas such as "design of experiments" and "optimal design". According to Anscombe (1960), for more than 100 years the deletion of outliers has frequently been discussed. Anscombe (1960) provided a historical survey of this topic, but no real traces have been found of what we may classify as influence analysis. Beckman and Cook (1983) include many references, in particular historical references on the deletion of outliers. Moreover, a short but informative discussion about the deletion of outliers is provided by Kruskal (1960). It is interesting to note that Kruskal writes, "My own practice in this sort of situation is to carry out an analysis both with and without the suspect observations. If the broad conclusions of the two analyses are quite different, I should view any conclusions from the experiment with very great caution". This clearly means that Kruskal was interested in the influence of outlying observations, although he did not take the leverage (the deviation due to the design) into account. However, when studying the interesting paper by Tukey (1962) on "data science", it is notable that one cannot find any mentioning of influence analysis, meaning that the concept of influence was not yet in circulation at that time. Concerning the analysis of data, see Huber (2011), where many important aspects of model validation are presented. An interesting source for early references on outliers and the rejection of multivariate outliers is Wilks (1963) (see also Caroni and Prescott, 1991). Among other publications, Wilks mentioned papers by Thompson (1935) and Pearson and Chandra Sekar (1936), where the rejection of outliers was discussed. Moreover, important facts about influential observations, from a historical perspective, have been provided by Farebrother (1999).

As mentioned above, there had been several articles which had discussed the identification of outliers (large residuals) when Anscombe and Tukey (1963) wrote a seminal article on how to utilize residuals in order to perform model validation (for related interesting articles, see Yates et al. (1957), Anscombe (1967) and Wooding (1969)). The ideas of Anscombe and Tukey (1963) have been implemented in modern statistical analysis, in particular in the analysis of least squares (in univariate regression analysis and univariate analysis of variance). Another interesting article including a number of relevant references was written by Gentleman and Wilk (1975a), who provided advice on how to use residuals in two-way tables, especially when more than one outlier exist (see also Gentleman and Wilk 1975b). John and Draper (1978) provided comments on the articles by Gentleman and Wilk (1975a,b). There is also a considerable body of literature on testing for large residuals; for example, see Srikantan (1961) and Prescott (1975) (in the latter article many references can be found). Newer references concerning the identification of outliers are Atkinson and Riani (2000) and Riani et al. (2009) (see also Cerioli et al., 2011).

After the articles published in the 1960s, it was observed that the variances of residuals, which in linear models are functions of the design matrices, bear information about the model fit (e.g. see Behnken and Draper, 1972). Wood (1973) (see also Gentleman and Wilk, 1975b) suggested that one should use individual residual analysis and study the influence on estimates. These ideas are similar to what is meant today by influence analysis. In the second half of the 1970s, several important articles addressed the problem of deciding if outliers were influential, i.e. important for the analyses which had been carried out, although it was an acknowledged fact that outliers do not necessarily have an impact on estimates, for example. Cook (1977) (see also Cook, 1979) combined information based on large residuals and leverage in his measure of influence, while Andrews and Pregibon (1978) were inspired by ideas from the design of experiments and introduced a selection operator which would operate on a specific ratio. Furthermore, Andrews and Pregibon addressed the problem of masking (see also Atkinson, 1986; Fung, 1993). Draper and John (1981) combined and extended the achievements of Cook and Andrews and Pregibon. In an interesting article, Pregibon (1981) mainly considered a logistic regression model. However, in the article, Pregibon devoted some attention to a review of influence analysis in linear models and introduced the idea of perturbing the original model for all the observations, one by one, although his treatment of these topics represented a minor part of the article. In Gentleman and Wilk (1975b), an additive perturbation was carried out and those observations which, after the perturbation, were found to have a pronounced impact were deemed to be influential. This particular perturbation approach may be called the mean shift approach (e.g. see also Wei and Fung, 1999). A specific problem in this connection is that one has to find the distribution of the largest shift.

In the 1980s, the so-called empirical influence function was introduced and it was based on special choices of the perturbation quantity (e.g. see Cook and Weisberg, 1980). Influence analysis was thereby connected to the influence function used in robust statistics. Two books which include the above-mentioned topics are Belsley et al. (1980) and Cook and Weisberg (1982) (see also the interesting review by Beckman and Cook (1983)). Chatterjee and Hadi (1986) summarized and discussed many of the ideas and techniques which had emerged until the mid-1980s. Their article from 1986 was published together with comments and critical evaluations by Cook, Atkinson, Welsch, Brant, Hoaglin and Kempthorne, Velleman and Weisberg, and the article, comments and evaluations, taken together, make a very interesting contribution to statistical science (see also Chatterjee and Hadi, 1988). Lawrance (1995) presented a fundamental article about case deletion where the concepts of masking and swamping were considered.

Another seminal work was an article written by Cook (1986) (including comments by Atkinson, Beckman, Cox, Critchley, Farebrother, Lawrance, Loynes, Nachtsheim, Pẽna, Prescott, Ross, Tsai and Weisberg). In this article Cook introduced differential geometric thinking in his search for general methods for finding influential observations (see also Fung and Kwan, 1997). On the basis of a perturbation scheme, Cook perturbed the likelihood and introduced an influential graph which was evaluated. His evaluation of the graph led to an influential approach which was called local influence analysis. Besides the technical presentation, Cook (1986) also included a broad spectrum of references. Beckman et al. (1987) applied Cook's approach to the analysis of mixed linear models. Some new references dealing with influence analysis in mixed linear models are Lesaffre and Verbeke (1998), Shi and Ojeda (2004), Chen et al. (2010) and Pan et al. (2014), where many references to previous works can be found. A newer book which considers outlying observations from different points of view is that by Barnett and Lewis (1994).

The above presentation of literature on outlier detection and influential observations is not complete, but is meant to provide an introduction to the publications in this subject field and is mostly oriented towards univariate linear models. In recent years, influence analysis has been considered in other types of statistical analysis, including survival analysis, time series analysis, influence and missing data, machine learning approaches, etc., but literature on these topics will not be reviewed and only a few references will be given below. There are also close connections between the literature on influence analysis and that on robust statistics, which deals with topics such as the influence curve, samples and empirical influence curves; see Cook and Weisberg (1982) and Tanaka and Zhang (1999). Moreover, concerning multiple outlier observations and robust statistics see Rocke and Woodruff (1996) and Penã and Prieto (2001), where many references are also given. An interesting work which promoted the use of the sensitive function instead of the influence curve was that written by Critchley et al. (2001) (see also Kim, 1996).

For generalizations of influence measures useful for univariate least squares to influence measures suitable for multivariate response modelling (MANOVA), with a focus on case deletion, see an interesting article by Barrett and Ling (1992) where several influence measures are suggested and, among other topics, their relation to the univariate work carried out by Cook (1977, 1979) and Andrews and Pregibon (1978) is discussed. There are also a few other earlier works on influence analysis in multivariate models, for example Hossain and Naik (1989). In a well-written article, Liski (1991) extended the area of application for some case deletion results to include the analysis of growth curves (BRM). Pan and Fang (1995, 1996) and Pan (2004) continued Liski's work and considered a multiple-individual-deletion model and a mean-shift-regression model (see also Srivastava and von Rosen (1998), which, additionally, included several older references), as well as the generalized Cook's distance. A new idea in outlier detection was presented by Pan et al. (2000), who applied projection pursuit to multivariate data and thereafter were able to apply univariate ideas. Pan (2002) discussed, in connection with the BRM, a generalized Cook's distance, generalized Welsch-Kuh's Statistic, generalized Cook-Weisberg's statistic, generalized Andrew-Pregibon's statistic, among other topics.

Cook (1986), as already has been mentioned, introduced the local influence approach, of which case deletion is a special case, and since then a huge number of authors have followed and modified Cook's ideas, often depending on specific applications. Thorough reviews of the concept were presented by Escobar and Meeker (1992), Fung and Tang (1997), Poon and Poon (1999) and González Sierra and Suárez Rancel (2001). One problem with the local influence approach is that it is not scale-invariant (see Schall and Dunne 1992; Poon and Poon, 1999). Schall and Dunne (1992) and Farebrother (1992) considered collinearity diagnostics and influence, in particular, the condition number and the variance inflation statistic, a concept from the 1970s. Concerning references dealing with local influence and the MANOVA model, see Kim (1995) and Liu (2002). The following references on local influence and the BRM are recommended: Pan and Fang (1995, 1996), Pan et al. (1996, 1997, 1999), Bai (1999), and You and Mao (2000) and the book by Pan and

Fang (2002). This book also includes a good introduction to influence analysis, as well as appropriate references. Local influence and discriminant analysis have been considered by Fung (1996) and Riani and Atkinson (2001), among others, local influence and principal component analysis by Shi (1997), local influence analysis and structural equation models by Lee and Wang (1996), local influence analysis in generalized linear modelling and non-linear regression modelling by Thomas and Cook (1990) and St. Laurent and Cook (1993), respectively (see also Wei et al., 1998), and local influence analysis and regression transformation by Lawrance (1988)).

Moreover, Cook (1986) proposed using the likelihood displacement criterion to study influence. However, over the years, other suggestions have appeared. In particular, in a Bayesian setting the Kullback-Leibler divergence has been applied, for example see McCulloch (1989), Pan et al. (1996) and Pan and Fung (2000). Other works treating influence analysis within a Bayesian framework are Johnson and Geisser (1983, 1985), Guttman and Peña (1993), Pan et al. (1999), Bai and Fei (2000) and Zhu et al. (2011); Zhu et al. (2011) also includes many references. Escobar and Meeker (1992) discussed Taylor series expansions of the likelihood displacement and different types of perturbations (see also Gu and Fung, 2001). Indeed, the influence analysis in the present book is based on different perturbation schemes and Taylor series expansions which were applied for the BRM by von Rosen (1995). Connected to the Taylor series expansion is the so-called derivative influence (e.g. see De Gruttola et al., 1987). In most studies where perturbations take place, case-weighted perturbations are applied. An important article which considers the case-weighted approach is that written by Zhu and Zhang (2004), but its focus is slightly different from that in many other articles. Usually the aim is to find "extreme" observations relative to a given model, but in Zhu and Zhang (2004) the aim is to investigate the model (see also Billor and Loynes, 1993). A precise discussion of the impact of chosen perturbation schemes was provided for a Bayesian setting by Geisser (1992) and for a non-Bayesian setting by Hao et al. (2014, 2015), who worked with balanced cross-over studies.

References

Andrews, D. F., & Pregibon, D. (1978). Finding the outliers that matter. *Journal of the Royal Statistical Society, Series B, 40*, 85–94.

Anscombe, F. J. (1960). Rejection of outliers. *Technometrics, 2*, 123–147.

Anscombe, F. J. (1967). Topics in the investigation of linear relations fitted by the method of least squares. With discussion. *Journal of the Royal Statistical Society, Series B, 29*, 1–52.

Anscombe, F. J., & Tukey, J. W. (1963). The examination and analysis of residuals. *Technometrics, 5*, 141–160.

Atkinson, A. C. (1986). Masking unmasked. *Biometrika, 73*, 533–541.

Atkinson, A. C., & Riani, M. (2000). *Robust diagnostic regression analysis*. New York: Springer.

Bai, P. (1999). Assessment of local influence in a growth curve model with Rao's simple covariance structure. *Acta Mathematica Scientia. Series B. English Edition, 19*, 555–563.

Bai, P., & Fei, Y. (2000). Bayesian local influence assessments in a growth curve model with general covariance structure. *Acta Mathematica Scientia. Series B. English Edition, 20*, 563–570.
Barnett, V., & Lewis, T. (1994). *Outliers in statistical data. Wiley series in probability and mathematical statistics: Applied probability and statistics* (3rd ed.). Chichester: Wiley.
Barrett, B. E., & Ling, R. F (1992). General classes of influence measures for multivariate regression. *Journal of the American Statistical Association, 87*, 184–191.
Beckman, R. J., & Cook, R. D. (1983). Outlier...s. With discussion and a reply by the authors. *Technometrics, 25*, 119–163.
Beckman, R. J., Nachtsheim, C. J., & Cook, R. D. (1987). Diagnostics for mixed-model analysis of variance. *Technometrics, 29*, 413–426.
Behnken, D. W., & Draper, N. R. (1972). Residuals and their variance patterns. *Technometrics, 14*, 102–111.
Belsley, D. A., Kuh, E., & Welsch, R. E. (1980). *Regression diagnostics: Identifying influential data and sources of collinearity. Wiley series in probability and mathematical statistics*. New York: Wiley.
Billor, N., & Loynes, R. M. (1993). Local influence: A new approach. *Communications in Statistics: Theory and Methods, 22*, 1595–1611.
Caroni, C., & Prescott, P. (1991). Multivariate outlier tests with structured covariance matrices. *Journal of Statistical Computation and Simulation, 38*, 165–179.
Cerioli, A., Atkinson, A. C., & Riani, M. (2011). Some perspectives on multivariate outlier detection. In *New perspectives in statistical modeling and data analysis. Studies in classification, data analysis, and knowledge organization* (pp. 231–238). Heidelberg: Springer.
Chatterjee, S., & Hadi, A. S. (1986). Influential observations, high leverage points, and outliers in linear regression. With discussion. *Statistical Science, 1*, 379–416.
Chatterjee, S., & Hadi, A. S. (1988). *Sensitivity analysis in linear regression*. New York: Wiley.
Chen, F., Zhu, H.-T., Song, X.-Y., & Lee, S.-Y. (2010). Perturbation selection and local influence analysis for generalized linear mixed models. *Journal of Computational and Graphical Statistics, 19*, 826–842.
Cook, R. D. (1977). Detection of influential observation in linear regression. *Technometrics, 19*, 15–18.
Cook, R. D. (1979). Influential observations in linear regression. *Journal of the American Statistical Association, 74*, 169–174.
Cook, R. D. (1986). Assessment of local influence. With discussion. *Journal of the Royal Statistical Society, Series B, 48*, 133–169.
Cook, R. D., & Weisberg, S. (1980). Characterizations of an empirical influence function for detecting influential cases in regression. *Technometrics, 22*, 495–508.
Cook, R. D., & Weisberg, S. (1982). *Residuals and influence in regression. Monographs on statistics and applied probability*. London: Chapman & Hall.
Critchley, F., Atkinson, R. A., Lu, G., & Biazi, E. (2001). Influence analysis based on the case sensitivity function. *Journal of the Royal Statistical Society, Series B, 63*, 307–323.
De Gruttola, V., Ware, J. H., & Louis, T. A. (1987). Influence analysis of generalized least squares estimators. *Journal of the American Statistical Association, 82*, 911–917.
Draper, N. R., & John, J. A. (1981). Influential observations and outliers in regression. *Technometrics, 23*, 21–26.
Escobar, L. A., & Meeker, W. Q. Jr. (1992). Assessing influence in regression analysis with censored data. *Biometrics, 48*, 507–528.
Farebrother, R. W. (1992). Relative local influence and the condition number. *Communications in Statistics: Simulation and Computation, 21*, 707–710.
Farebrother, R. W. (1999). *Fitting linear relationships: A history of the calculus of observations 1750–1900*. New York: Springer.
Fung, W. K. (1993). Unmasking outliers and leverage points: A confirmation. *Journal of the American Statistical Association, 88*, 518–519.

Fung, W. K. (1996). The influence of an observation on the misclassification probability in multiple discriminant analysis. *Communications in Statistics: Theory and Methods, 25*, 1917–1930.

Fung, W. K., & Kwan, C. W. (1997). A note on local influence based on normal curvature. *Journal of the Royal Statistical Society, Series B, 59*, 839–843.

Fung, W. K., & Tang, M. K. (1997). Assessment of local influence in multivariate regression analysis. *Communications in Statistics: Theory and Methods, 26*, 821–837.

Geisser, S. (1992) Bayesian perturbation diagnostics and robustness. In *Bayesian analysis in statistics and econometrics (Bangalore, 1988). Lecture notes in statistics* (Vol. 75, pp. 289–301). New York: Springer.

Gentleman, J. F., & Wilk, M. B. (1975a). Detecting outliers in a two-way table: I. Statistical behavior of residuals. *Technometrics, 17*, 1–14.

Gentleman, J. F., & Wilk, M. B. (1975b). Detecting outliers. II. Supplementing the direct analysis of residuals. *Biometrics, 31*, 387–410.

González Sierra, M. A., & Suárez Rancel, M. M. (2001). Regression diagnostic using local influence: A review. *Communications in Statistics: Theory and Methods, 30*, 799–813.

Gu, H., & Fung, W. K. (2001). Local influence for the restricted likelihood with applications. *Sankhyā, Series A, 63*, 250–259.

Guttman, I., & Peña, D. (1993). A Bayesian look at diagnostics in the univariate linear model. *Statistica Sinica, 3*, 367–390.

Hao, C., von Rosen, D., & von Rosen, T. (2014). Local influence analysis in AB–BA crossover designs. *Scandinavian Journal of Statistics, 41*, 1153–1166.

Hao, C., von Rosen, D., & von Rosen, T. (2015). Explicit influence analysis in two-treatment balanced crossover models. *Mathematical Methods of Statistics, 24*, 16–36.

Hossain, A., & Naik, D. N. (1989). Detection of influential observations in multivariate regression. *Journal of Applied Statistics, 16*, 25–37.

Huber, P. J. (2011). *Data analysis. What can be learned from the past 50 years. Wiley series in probability and statistics*. Hoboken: Wiley.

John, J. A., & Draper, N. R. (1978). On testing for two outliers or one outlier in two-way tables. *Technometrics, 20*, 69–78.

Johnson, W., & Geisser, S. (1983). A predictive view of the detection and characterization of influential observations in regression analysis. *Journal of the American Statistical Association, 78*, 137–144.

Johnson, W., & Geisser, S. (1985). Estimative influence measures for the multivariate general linear model. *Journal of Statistical Planning and Inference, 11*, 33–56.

Kim, C. (1996). Local influence and replacement measure. *Communications in Statistics: Theory and Methods, 25*, 49–61.

Kim, M. G. (1995). Local influence in multivariate regression. *Communications in Statistics: Theory and Methods, 24*, 1271–1278.

Kruskal, W. H. (1960). Some remarks on wild observations. *Technometrics, 2*, 1–3.

Lawrance, A. J. (1988). Regression transformation diagnostics using local influence. *Journal of the American Statistical Association, 83*, 1067–1072.

Lawrance, A. J. (1995). Deletion influence and masking in regression. *Journal of the Royal Statistical Society, Series B, 57*, 181–189.

Lee, S.-Y., & Wang, S. J. (1996). Sensitivity analysis of structural equation models. *Psychometrika, 61*, 93–108.

Lesaffre, E., & Verbeke, G. (1998). Local influence in linear mixed models. *Biometrics, 54*, 570–582.

Liski, E. P. (1991). Detecting influential measurements in a growth curves model. *Biometrics, 47*, 659–668.

Liu, S. (2002) Local influence in multivariate elliptical linear regression models. *Linear Algebra and Its Applications, 354*, 159–174.

McCulloch, R. E. (1989). Local model influence. *Journal of the American Statistical Association, 84*, 473–478.

Pan, J.-X. (2002). Influential observation identification in the growth curve model with Rao's simple covariance structure. *Communications in Statistics: Theory and Methods, 31*, 813–831.
Pan, J.-X. (2004). Discordant outlier detection in the growth curve model with Rao's simple covariance structure. *Statistics & Probability Letters, 69*, 135–142.
Pan, J.-X., & Fang, K.-T. (1995). Multiple outlier detection in growth curve model with unstructured covariance matrix. *Annals of the Institute of Statistical Mathematics, 47*, 137–153.
Pan, J.-X., & Fang, K.-T. (1996). Detecting influential observations in growth curve model with unstructured covariance. *Computational Statistics & Data Analysis, 22*, 71–87.
Pan, J.-X., & Fang, K.-T. (2002). *Growth curve models and statistical diagnostics. Springer series in statistics*. New York: Springer.
Pan, J.-X., Fang, K.-T., & Liski, E. P. (1996). Bayesian local influence for the growth curve model with Rao's simple covariance structure. *Journal of Multivariate Analysis, 58*, 55–81.
Pan, J.-X., Fang, K.-T., & von Rosen, D. (1997). Local influence assessment in the growth curve model with unstructured covariance. *Journal of Statistical Planning and Inference, 62*, 263–278.
Pan, J.-X., Fang, K.-T., & von Rosen, D. (1999). Bayesian local influence in growth curve model with unstructured covariance. *Biometrical Journal, 41*, 641–658.
Pan, J.-X., Fei, Y., & Foster, P. (2014). Case-deletion diagnostics for linear mixed models. *Technometrics, 56*, 269–281.
Pan, J.-X, & Fung, W.-K. (2000). Bayesian influence assessment in the growth curve model with unstructured covariance. *Annals of the Institute of Statistical Mathematics, 52*, 737–752.
Pan, J.-X., Fung, W.-K., & Fang, K.-T. (2000). Multiple outlier detection in multivariate data using projection pursuit techniques. *Journal of Statistical Planning and Inference, 83*, 153–167.
Pearson, E. S., & Chandra Sekar, C. (1936). The efficiency of statistical tools and a criterion for the rejection of outlying observations. *Biometrika, 28*, 308–320.
Penã, D., & Prieto, F. (2001). Multivariate outlier detection and robust covariance matrix estimation. *Technometrics, 43*, 286–310.
Poon, W.-Y., & Poon, Y. S. (1999). Conformal normal curvature and assessment of local influence. *Journal of the Royal Statistical Society, Series B, 61*, 51–61.
Potthoff, R. F., & Roy, S. N. (1964). A generalized multivariate analysis of variance model useful especially for growth curve problems. *Biometrika, 51*, 313–326.
Pregibon, D. (1981). Logistic regression diagnostics. *Annals of Statistics, 9*, 705–724.
Prescott, P. (1975). An approximate test for outliers in linear models. *Technometrics, 17*, 129–132.
Riani, M., & Atkinson, A. C. (2001). A unified approach to outliers, influence, and transformations in discriminant analysis. *Journal of Computational and Graphical Statistics, 10*, 513–544.
Riani, M., Atkinson, A. C., & Cerioli, A. (2009). Finding an unknown number of multivariate outliers. *Journal of the Royal Statistical Society, Series B, 71*, 447–466.
Rocke, D. M., & Woodruff, D. (1996). Identification of outliers in multivariate data. *Journal of the American Statistical Association, 91*, 1047–1061.
Schall, R., & Dunne, T. T. (1992). A note on the relationship between parameter collinearity and local influence. *Biometrika, 79*, 399–404.
Shi, L. (1997). Local influence in principal components analysis. *Biometrika, 84*, 175–186.
Shi, L., & Ojeda, M. M. (2004). Local influence in multilevel regression for growth curves. *Journal of Multivariate Analysis, 91*, 282–304.
Srikantan, K. S. (1961). Testing for the single outlier in a regression model, *Sankhyā, Series A, 23*, 251–260.
Srivastava, M. S., & von Rosen, D. (1998). Outliers in multivariate regression models. *Journal of Multivariate Analysis, 65*, 195–208.
St. Laurent, R. T., & Cook, R. D. (1993). Leverage, local influence and curvature in nonlinear regression. *Biometrika, 80*, 99–106.
Tanaka, Y., & Zhang, F. (1999). R-mode and Q-mode influence analyses in statistical modelling: Relationship between influence function approach and local influence approach. *Computational Statistics & Data Analysis, 32*, 197–218.

Thomas, W., & Cook, R. D. (1990). Assessing influence on predictions from generalized linear models. *Technometrics, 32*, 59–65.
Thompson, W. R. (1935). On a criterion for the rejection of observations and the distribution of the ratio of deviation to sample standard deviates. *Annals of Mathematical Statistics, 6*, 214–219.
Tukey, J. W. (1962). The future of data analysis. *Annals of Mathematical Statistics, 33*, 1–67.
von Rosen, D. (1995). Influential observations in multivariate linear models. *Scandinavian Journal of Statistics, 22*, 207–222.
Wei, B.-C., Hu, Y.-Q., & Fung, W.-K. (1998). Generalized leverage and its applications. *Scandinavian Journal of Statistics, 25*, 25–37.
Wei, W. H., & Fung, W. K. (1999). The mean-shift outlier model in general weighted regression and its applications. *Computational Statistics & Data Analysis, 30*, 429–441.
Wilks, S. S. (1963). Multivariate statistical outliers. *Sankhyā, Series A, 25*, 407–426.
Wood, F. S. (1973). The use of individual effects and residuals in fitting equations to data. *Technometrics, 15*, 677–695.
Wooding, W. M. (1969). The computation and use of residuals in the analysis of experimental data. *Journal of Quality Technology, 1*, 175–188; correction *1*, 294.
Yates, F., Healy, M. J. R., & Lipton, S. (1957). Routine analysis of replicated experiment on an electronic computer. With discussion. *Journal of the Royal Statistical Society, Series B, 19*, 234–254.
You, J.-H., & Mao, S.-S. (2000). Assessment of local influence in the GMANOVA-MANOVA with R.S.S. *Journal of East China Normal University. Natural Science Edition, 2*, 1–12.
Zhu, H., Ibrahim, J. G., & Tang, N. (2011). Bayesian influence analysis: A geometric approach. *Biometrika, 98*, 307–323.
Zhu, H., & Zhang, H. (2004). A diagnostic procedure based on local influence. *Biometrika, 91*, 579–589.

Appendices

There are three appendices to this book. The notation is presented in Appendix A, while in Appendix B many technical results are compiled and for their proofs the reader is mostly referred to other publications. At the end of Appendix B, a number of exercises are provided which the reader can use to practise what they have learnt. Finally, Appendix C presents some material on the approximation of the distribution of the likelihood ratio test which is used in Chap. 7. Note that the references cited in the appendices are listed after Appendix C in the section "References".

Appendix A: Notation

This appendix presents the notation and abbreviations used in the book.

A.1 Abbreviations

- BRM = bilinear regression model
- $EBRM$ = extended bilinear regression model
- e.g. = for example
- GMANOVA = generalized multivariate analysis of variance
- i.e. = that is
- i.i.d. = independent and identically distributed
- MANOVA = multivariate analysis of variance
- MINQUE = minimum norm quadratic unbiased estimation
- MLE = maximum likelihood estimator (estimate)
- p.d. = positive definite
- p.s.d. = positive semi-definite
- SUR = seemingly unrelated regression

D. von Rosen, *Bilinear Regression Analysis*, Lecture Notes in Statistics 220,
https://doi.org/10.1007/978-3-319-78784-8

A.2 Vectors and Matrices

Throughout the book, all the vectors and matrices are real-valued and of finite size.

- Lowercase boldface letters denote vectors, e.g. $\boldsymbol{x}$ is a vector and $\boldsymbol{x}$: $p \times 1$ is a vector of size p (sometimes written as $\boldsymbol{x} \in \mathbb{R}^p$).
- Uppercase boldface letters denote matrices, e.g. $\boldsymbol{X}$ is a matrix and $\boldsymbol{X}$: $p \times q$ is a matrix with p rows and q columns (sometimes written as $\boldsymbol{X} \in \mathbb{R}^{p \times q}$).
- $\boldsymbol{X}_o$ denotes an observation of the random matrix $\boldsymbol{X}$.
- Sometimes a matrix is described via its elements, e.g. $\boldsymbol{A} = (a_{ij})$.

A.3 Loewner (Löwner) Order

Let $\boldsymbol{A}$ and $\boldsymbol{B}$ be symmetric matrices. Then the expression $\boldsymbol{A} \geq \boldsymbol{B}$ is used if $\boldsymbol{A} - \boldsymbol{B}$ is positive semi-definite, and $\boldsymbol{A} > \boldsymbol{B}$ if $\boldsymbol{A} - \boldsymbol{B}$ is positive definite.

A.4 Partitioned Matrices

- Two matrices of a proper size which are put side by side represent a partitioned matrix (augmented matrix), and this expressed using the following type of formula $\boldsymbol{A} = (\boldsymbol{A}_1 : \boldsymbol{A}_2)$.
- If $\boldsymbol{A}_i$, $i = 1, 2$, in the above statement are vectors, then $\boldsymbol{A} = (\boldsymbol{a}_1, \boldsymbol{a}_2)$ can also be used.
- Sometimes block matrices are convenient objects to work with, e.g.

$$\boldsymbol{A} = \begin{pmatrix} \boldsymbol{A}_{11} & \boldsymbol{A}_{12} \\ \boldsymbol{A}_{21} & \boldsymbol{A}_{22} \end{pmatrix},$$

where the included matrices are supposed to be of proper sizes.

A.5 Special Vectors and Matrices

- Parameters are usually denoted with the help of the Greek alphabet. Parameter vectors are usually denoted by letters from the Greek alphabet, lowercase boldface. Parameter matrices are usually denoted by letters from the Greek alphabet, uppercase boldface, with the exception that the capital $\boldsymbol{B}$ is used instead of capital $\boldsymbol{\beta}$.
- The vector of p ones is denoted by $\mathbf{1}_p$ or just $\mathbf{1}$.

- The null vector and null matrix are both denoted by $\mathbf{0}$ and sometimes a subindex indicates the size of the matrix.
- The identity matrix $\boldsymbol{I}$ is a matrix with 1 on the main diagonal and 0 elsewhere. The identity matrix of size $a \times a$ is sometimes denoted by $\boldsymbol{I}_a$.
- $\boldsymbol{A}_d$ is a diagonalized matrix of $\boldsymbol{A}$; i.e. the off-diagonal elements are put to 0, whereas the diagonal elements are kept as they were.
- The unit (standard) basis $\boldsymbol{e}_i$, of size p, is the ith column of $\boldsymbol{I}_p$. Sometimes $\boldsymbol{d}_j$, $\boldsymbol{f}_k$ and $\boldsymbol{g}_l$, etc. are used together with $\boldsymbol{e}_i$.
- The upper triangular matrix $\boldsymbol{T} = (t_{ij})$ is defined as $\boldsymbol{T} = \sum_{i \leq j} t_{ij}\boldsymbol{e}_i\boldsymbol{e}'_j$.
- The strictly upper triangular matrix $\boldsymbol{T} = (t_{ij})$ is defined as $\boldsymbol{T} = \sum_{i<j} t_{ij}\boldsymbol{e}_i\boldsymbol{e}'_j$.
- The lower triangular matrix $\boldsymbol{T} = (t_{ij})$ is defined as $\boldsymbol{T} = \sum_{i \geq j} t_{ij}\boldsymbol{e}_i\boldsymbol{e}'_j$.
- The strictly lower triangular matrix $\boldsymbol{T} = (t_{ij})$ is defined as $\boldsymbol{T} = \sum_{i>j} t_{ij}\boldsymbol{e}_i\boldsymbol{e}'_j$.
- The orthogonal matrix $\boldsymbol{\Gamma}$ is a square matrix satisfying $\boldsymbol{\Gamma\Gamma}' = \boldsymbol{I}$. This implies that $\boldsymbol{\Gamma}$ is of full rank and $\boldsymbol{\Gamma}'\boldsymbol{\Gamma} = \boldsymbol{I}$.
- The semi-orthogonal matrix $\boldsymbol{\Gamma}: p \times q$ is a matrix satisfying $\boldsymbol{\Gamma\Gamma}' = \boldsymbol{I}_p$ or $\boldsymbol{\Gamma}'\boldsymbol{\Gamma} = \boldsymbol{I}_q$.
- The commutation matrix $\boldsymbol{K}_{p,q}$ is defined by

$$\boldsymbol{K}_{p,q} = \sum_{i,j} \boldsymbol{e}_i\boldsymbol{d}'_j \otimes \boldsymbol{d}_j\boldsymbol{e}'_i,$$

  where $\boldsymbol{e}_i$ and $\boldsymbol{d}_j$ are unit basis vectors of size p and q, respectively. The Kronecker product $\otimes$ is defined in Sect. A.6 below.
- A square matrix $\boldsymbol{P}$ is idempotent, i.e. $\boldsymbol{P}$ is a projector, if $\boldsymbol{PP} = \boldsymbol{P}$.
- A matrix $\boldsymbol{V}$ is positive definite, which sometimes is denoted $\boldsymbol{V} > 0$, if and only if $\boldsymbol{V} = \boldsymbol{XX}'$ for some square matrix $\boldsymbol{X}$ of full rank.
- A matrix $\boldsymbol{V}$ is positive semi-definite, which sometimes is denoted $\boldsymbol{V} \geq 0$, if and only if $\boldsymbol{V} = \boldsymbol{XX}'$ for some matrix $\boldsymbol{X}$.

A.6 Special Matrix Operators

- The transpose of a matrix is denoted by $'$. For example, the transpose of $\boldsymbol{A}$ is defined through $\boldsymbol{A}' = (a_{ji})$, if $\boldsymbol{A} = (a_{ij})$.
- If $\boldsymbol{VV}^{-1} = \boldsymbol{I} = \boldsymbol{V}^{-1}\boldsymbol{V}$, then $\boldsymbol{V}^{-1}$ is the inverse of $\boldsymbol{V}$.
- If $\boldsymbol{AA}^-\boldsymbol{A} = \boldsymbol{A}$, then $\boldsymbol{A}^-$ is a g-inverse of $\boldsymbol{A}$.
- One special g-inverse is the Moore-Penrose inverse $\boldsymbol{A}^+$, defined through the following four conditions: $\boldsymbol{AA}^+\boldsymbol{A} = \boldsymbol{A}$, $\boldsymbol{A}^+\boldsymbol{AA}^+ = \boldsymbol{A}^+$, $(\boldsymbol{AA}^+)' = \boldsymbol{AA}^+$ and $(\boldsymbol{A}^+\boldsymbol{A})' = \boldsymbol{A}^+\boldsymbol{A}$.
- The square root of $\boldsymbol{V}$, which is p.d., is denoted by $\boldsymbol{V}^{1/2}$. It is any symmetric matrix satisfying $\boldsymbol{V} = \boldsymbol{V}^{1/2}\boldsymbol{V}^{1/2}$.
- The rank of a matrix is denoted by $r(\bullet)$ and is the largest number of linearly independent columns (rows) of the matrix.

- The trace is denoted by tr{•} and defined through $\text{tr}\{\boldsymbol{A}\} = \sum_i a_{ii}$, where $\boldsymbol{A} = (a_{ij})$ is a square matrix.
- The *trace distance or Frobenius norm (squared)* for arbitrary matrices $\boldsymbol{A}$ and $\boldsymbol{B}$, which are of proper size, is defined through $||\boldsymbol{A} - \boldsymbol{B}|| = \text{tr}\{(\boldsymbol{A} - \boldsymbol{B})(\boldsymbol{A} - \boldsymbol{B})'\}$.
- The determinant of a square matrix $\boldsymbol{A}$: $m \times m$ is denoted $|\boldsymbol{A}|$ and is defined by

$$|\boldsymbol{A}| = \sum_{j_1,\ldots,j_m} (-1)^{N(j_1,\ldots,j_m)} \prod_{i=1}^{m} a_{ij_i},$$

  where the summation is taken over all the different permutations $(j_1, \ldots, j_m)$ of the set of integers of $\{1, 2, \ldots, m\}$, and where $N(j_1, \ldots, j_m)$ is the number of inversions of the permutations $(j_1, \ldots, j_m)$ (for details, consult an introductory course book).
- The Hadamard product (element-wise product) of $\boldsymbol{A} = (a_{ij})$ and $\boldsymbol{B} = (b_{kl})$, where $\boldsymbol{A}$ and $\boldsymbol{B}$ are of the same size, is denoted by $\odot$ and defined through $\boldsymbol{A} \odot \boldsymbol{B} = (a_{ij}b_{ij})$.
- The Kronecker product of $\boldsymbol{A} = (a_{ij})$ and $\boldsymbol{B} = (b_{kl})$ is denoted $\otimes$ and defined through $\boldsymbol{A} \otimes \boldsymbol{B} = (a_{ij}\boldsymbol{B})$.
- The Kroneckerian power $\boldsymbol{A}^{\otimes k}$ is identical to $\underbrace{\boldsymbol{A} \otimes \boldsymbol{A} \otimes \cdots \otimes \boldsymbol{A}}_{k\,times}$.
- The vec-operator is denoted by vec(•) and is defined through

$$\text{vec} : \boldsymbol{A} = \sum_{ij} a_{ij}\boldsymbol{e}_i\boldsymbol{d}'_j \rightarrow \sum_{ij} a_{ij}\boldsymbol{d}_j \otimes \boldsymbol{e}_i,$$

  where $\boldsymbol{e}_i$ and $\boldsymbol{d}_j$ are standard basis vectors of proper sizes.
- The block diagonal operator is defined by

$$\text{diag}(\boldsymbol{A}_1, \boldsymbol{A}_2, \ldots, \boldsymbol{A}_p) = \begin{pmatrix} \boldsymbol{A}_1 & \boldsymbol{0} & \ldots & \boldsymbol{0} \\ \boldsymbol{0} & \boldsymbol{A}_2 & \ldots & \boldsymbol{0} \\ \vdots & \vdots & \vdots & \vdots \\ \boldsymbol{0} & \boldsymbol{0} & \ldots & \boldsymbol{A}_p \end{pmatrix}.$$

A.7 Special Notation for Projections and Squared Expressions

For projectors we use the following notation:

- $\boldsymbol{P}_A = \boldsymbol{A}(\boldsymbol{A}'\boldsymbol{A})^-\boldsymbol{A}'$;
- $\boldsymbol{P}_{A,V} = \boldsymbol{A}(\boldsymbol{A}'\boldsymbol{V}^{-1}\boldsymbol{A})^-\boldsymbol{A}'\boldsymbol{V}^{-1}$, $\boldsymbol{V}$ is p.d;
- $\boldsymbol{P}_{A,V,B} = \boldsymbol{A}(\boldsymbol{A}'\boldsymbol{B}\boldsymbol{V}^{-1}\boldsymbol{B}'\boldsymbol{A})^-\boldsymbol{A}'\boldsymbol{B}\boldsymbol{V}^{-1}\boldsymbol{B}'$, $\boldsymbol{V}$ is p.d.

The first two expressions are projectors on $\mathcal{C}(\boldsymbol{A})$ (see Sect. A.8 below) and the third expression can be a projector under some condition on $\boldsymbol{A}$ and $\boldsymbol{B}$. In the first expression the standard inner product is assumed to hold, and in the second expression an inner product defined by $(\boldsymbol{x}, \boldsymbol{y}) = \boldsymbol{x}'\boldsymbol{V}^{-1}\boldsymbol{y}$ is assumed to hold. Moreover, $\boldsymbol{P}_A$ and $\boldsymbol{P}_{A,V}$ are idempotent matrices (see Sect. A.5).

Since we are often working with quadratic forms, the following notation is useful for shortening matrix expressions:

- $(\boldsymbol{A})(\boldsymbol{A})'$ can be written as $(\boldsymbol{A})()'$.
- $(\boldsymbol{A})\boldsymbol{V}(\boldsymbol{A})'$ can be written as $(\boldsymbol{A})\boldsymbol{V}()'$.

A.8 Linear and Multilinear Spaces

- $\subseteq$, $\oplus$ and $\boxplus$ denote "is a subspace of", "is a direct sum of" and "is an orthogonal sum of", respectively.
- $\mathcal{V}, \mathcal{W}, \ldots$ denote linear spaces.
- The column vector space $\mathcal{C}(\boldsymbol{A})$, where $\boldsymbol{A}$: $p \times q$, is defined through $\mathcal{C}(\boldsymbol{A}) = \{\boldsymbol{a} : \boldsymbol{a} = \boldsymbol{A}\boldsymbol{z}, \boldsymbol{z} \in \mathcal{R}^q\}$.
- $\dim \mathcal{C}(\boldsymbol{A}) = r(\boldsymbol{A})$ (sometimes $\dim\{\mathcal{C}(\boldsymbol{A})\}$ is used).
- The null space $\mathcal{N}(\boldsymbol{A})$, where $\boldsymbol{A}$: $p \times q$, is defined through $\mathcal{N}(\boldsymbol{A}) = \{\boldsymbol{a} : \boldsymbol{A}\boldsymbol{a} = \boldsymbol{0}, \boldsymbol{a} \in \mathcal{R}^q\}$.
- The space $\mathcal{C}_V(\boldsymbol{A})$ denotes a column vector space with an inner product defined through the positive definite matrix $\boldsymbol{V}$; i.e. for any pair of vectors $\boldsymbol{x}$ and $\boldsymbol{y}$, the operation $\boldsymbol{x}'\boldsymbol{V}^{-1}\boldsymbol{y}$ holds. If $\boldsymbol{V} = \boldsymbol{I}$, instead of $\mathcal{C}_I(\boldsymbol{A})$ one writes $\mathcal{C}(\boldsymbol{A})$.
- The orthogonal complement to $\mathcal{C}_V(\boldsymbol{A})$ is denoted by $\mathcal{C}_V(\boldsymbol{A})^\perp$ and is generated by all the vectors orthogonal to all the vectors in $\mathcal{C}_V(\boldsymbol{A})$; i.e. for an arbitrary $\boldsymbol{a} \in \mathcal{C}_V(\boldsymbol{A})$, all the $\boldsymbol{y}$ satisfying $\boldsymbol{y}'\boldsymbol{V}^{-1}\boldsymbol{a} = \boldsymbol{0}$ generate the linear space (column vector space) $\mathcal{C}_V(\boldsymbol{A})^\perp$.
- $\boldsymbol{A}^o$ is any matrix satisfying $\mathcal{C}(\boldsymbol{A}^o) = \mathcal{C}(\boldsymbol{A})^\perp$.
- The tensor space of $\mathcal{C}_V(\boldsymbol{A})$ and $\mathcal{C}_W(\boldsymbol{B})$ is denoted by $\mathcal{C}_V(\boldsymbol{A})\otimes\mathcal{C}_W(\boldsymbol{B})$ and defined as

$$\mathcal{C}_V(\boldsymbol{A}) \otimes \mathcal{C}_W(\boldsymbol{B}) = \mathcal{C}_{V\otimes W}(\boldsymbol{A} \otimes \boldsymbol{B}), \tag{A.8}$$

where, on the right-hand side, the Kronecker product is used.

A.9 Basic Distributions

- "$\boldsymbol{X} \sim$" means that $\boldsymbol{X}$ is distributed as and $\overset{a}{\sim}$ denotes approximately distributed.
- The multivariate normal distribution is denoted by $N_p(\boldsymbol{\mu}, \boldsymbol{\Sigma})$, where $\boldsymbol{\mu}$: $p \times 1$ is the mean and $\boldsymbol{\Sigma}$: $p \times p$ is the dispersion matrix. If $p = 1$ we have the univariate normal distribution and then the index p in $N_p(\boldsymbol{\mu}, \boldsymbol{\Sigma})$ is omitted.

- The multivariate matrix normal distribution is denoted by $N_{p,n}(\boldsymbol{\mu}, \boldsymbol{\Sigma}, \boldsymbol{\Psi})$ where $\boldsymbol{\mu}$: $p \times n$, $\boldsymbol{\Sigma}$: $p \times p$ and $\boldsymbol{\Psi}$: $n \times n$. If $\boldsymbol{X} \sim N_{p,n}(\boldsymbol{\mu}, \boldsymbol{\Sigma}, \boldsymbol{\Psi})$ its distribution is identical to vec$\boldsymbol{X} \sim N_{pn}(\text{vec}\boldsymbol{\mu}, \boldsymbol{\Psi} \otimes \boldsymbol{\Sigma})$.
- The random variable u is chi-squared distributed with n degrees of freedom if and only if $u = \boldsymbol{x}'\boldsymbol{x}$, for some $\boldsymbol{x} \sim N_n(\boldsymbol{0}, \boldsymbol{I})$, which will be denoted by $u \sim \chi^2_n$. There exist more general definitions comprising non-integer degrees of freedom. The equation in x_o, $P(\chi^2_n \leq x_o) = \beta$, can be written $\chi^2_\beta(n) = x_o$, which defines the β-percentile $\chi^2_\beta(n)$.
- The random matrix $\boldsymbol{W}$ is Wishart-distributed with n degrees of freedom if and only if $\boldsymbol{W} = \boldsymbol{X}\boldsymbol{X}'$, for some $\boldsymbol{X} \sim N_{p,n}(\boldsymbol{0}, \boldsymbol{\Sigma}, \boldsymbol{I})$, which is denoted by $\boldsymbol{W} \sim W_p(\boldsymbol{\Sigma}, n)$. There exist more general definitions based on the Laplace transform.
- The random variable F is F-distributed with m and n degrees of freedom, which is denoted by $F \sim F_{m,n}$, if and only if $F = u/v$, for some $u \sim \chi^2(m)$, $v \sim \chi^2(n)$, where u and v are independently distributed. The equation in x_o, $P(F_{m,n} \leq x_o) = \beta$, can be written $F_\beta(m,n) = x_o$, which defines the β-percentile $F_\beta(m,n)$.
- The β-distribution is denoted by $\beta \sim \beta(m,n)$ and defined via its density (see also Sect. A.10)

$$f_\beta(x_o) = \begin{cases} \frac{\Gamma(\frac{1}{2}(m+n))}{\Gamma(\frac{1}{2}m)\Gamma(\frac{1}{2}n)} x_o^{\frac{1}{2}m-1}(1-x_o)^{\frac{1}{2}n-1}, & 0 < x < 1, \quad m,n \geq 1, \\ 0 & \text{elsewhere.} \end{cases}$$

- If $\boldsymbol{W} \sim W_p(\boldsymbol{\Sigma}, n)$ and $n \geq p$, the inverse exists with probability 1 and $\boldsymbol{W}^{-1}$ is said to follow the inverse Wishart distribution. If the Wishart density exists, it is a straightforward task to derive the density for the inverted Wishart distribution.
- Let $\boldsymbol{W}_1 \sim W_p(\boldsymbol{I}, n)$, $p \leq n$, and $\boldsymbol{W}_2 \sim W_p(\boldsymbol{I}, m)$, $p \leq m$, be independently distributed. Then

$$\boldsymbol{F} = (\boldsymbol{W}_1 + \boldsymbol{W}_2)^{-1/2}\boldsymbol{W}_2(\boldsymbol{W}_1 + \boldsymbol{W}_2)^{-1/2}$$

  is said to follow a multivariate β-distribution of type I, which is denoted by $M\beta_I(p,m,n)$.
- Let $\boldsymbol{W}_1 \sim W_p(\boldsymbol{I}, n)$, $p \leq n$, and $\boldsymbol{W}_2 \sim W_p(\boldsymbol{I}, m)$, $p \leq m$, be independently distributed. Then

$$\boldsymbol{F} = \boldsymbol{W}_2^{-1/2}\boldsymbol{W}_1\boldsymbol{W}_2^{-1/2}$$

  is said to follow a multivariate β-distribution of type II, which is denoted by $M\beta_{II}(p,m,n)$.

A.10 Density and Moments of Specific Distributions

- $f_X(X_o)$ denotes the density for a random matrix X.
- The density of a matrix normal variable $X \sim N_{p,n}(\mu, \Sigma, \Psi)$ equals

$$f_X(X_o) = (2\pi)^{-pqn/2}|\Psi|^{-p/2}|\Sigma|^{-n/2}\exp(-1/2\mathrm{tr}\{\Sigma^{-1}(X_o-\mu)\Psi^{-1}(X_o-\mu)'\}).$$

- The Wishart density equals ($W \sim W_p(\Sigma, n)$)

$$f_W(W_0) = \begin{cases} c(p,n)|\Sigma|^{-n/2}|W_0|^{(n-p-1)/2}\exp(-1/2\mathrm{tr}\{\Sigma^{-1}W_0\}), & W_0 > 0, \\ 0 & \text{elsewhere,} \end{cases}$$

where $c(p,n)^{-1} = 2^{pn/2}\Gamma_p(\frac{n}{2})$ and $\Gamma_p(\frac{n}{2}) = \pi^{p(p-1)/4}\prod_{i=1}^{p}\Gamma(\frac{1}{2}(n+1-i))$.
- The multivariate β-distribution of type I ($M\beta_I(p,m,n)$) has a density which equals

$$f_F(F_0) = \begin{cases} \frac{c(p,n)c(p,n)}{c(p,n+m)}|F_0|^{(m-p-1)/2}|I-F_0|^{(n-p-1)/2}, & |I-F_0| > 0,\ |F_0| > 0, \\ 0 & \text{elsewhere;} \end{cases}$$

$c(p,n)$ is the same constant as in the Wishart density.
- The Kotz-type distribution for x of size p is defined through the following density (c is a normalizing constant):

$$f_x(x_o) = c(x'x)^{N-1}\exp\{-r(x'x)^s\}, \quad r, s > 0,\ 2N + p > 2.$$

- The matrix Kotz-type distribution for X is defined through vec$X$, which should follow a Kotz-type distribution.
- The characteristic function of a random unstructured matrix X: $p \times n$ is given by (i is the imaginary unit)

$$\varphi_X(T) = E[e^{i\,\mathrm{tr}\{T'X\}}], \qquad T \in \mathbb{R}^{p\times n}.$$

- The cumulant function of a random unstructured matrix X: $p \times n$ is given by

$$\psi_X(T) = \ln\varphi_X(T), \qquad T \in \mathbb{R}^{p\times n}.$$

- Expectation: $E[X] = (E[x_{ij}])$.
- Dispersion: $D[X] = E[\mathrm{vec}(X - E[X])\mathrm{vec}'(X - E[X])]$.
- Covariance: $C[X, Y] = E[\mathrm{vec}(X - E[X])\mathrm{vec}'(Y - E[Y])]$.

Let the matrix derivative $\frac{d^k Y}{d X^k}$ be as in Definition 5.1.

- Suppose that $\varphi_X(T)$ is k times differentiable. Then the kth moment $m_k[X]$ is given by

$$m_k[X] = \frac{1}{i^k}\frac{d^k}{d\,T^k}\varphi_X(T)\Big|_{T=0}.$$

- Suppose that $\psi_X(T)$ is k times differentiable. Then the kth cumulant $c_k[X]$ is given by

$$c_k[X] = \frac{1}{i^k}\frac{d^k}{d\,T^k}\psi_X(T)\Big|_{T=0}.$$

- Suppose that $\varphi_X(T)$ is k times differentiable. Then the kth central moment $mc_k[X]$ is given by

$$mc_k[X] = m_k[X - E[X]] = \frac{1}{i^k}\frac{d^k}{d\,T^k}\varphi_{X-E[X]}(T)\Big|_{T=0}.$$

A.11 Convergence

- Convergence in distribution (in law; weakly) can be defined in the following way: Let $F(x)$ and $F_n(x)$, $n = 1, 2, \ldots$, be distribution functions. The sequence $F_1, F_2, \ldots$ converges in distribution if for each continuity point x of $F(x)$, $\lim_{n\to\infty} F_n(x) = F(x)$, where x can be scalar or vector-valued (matrix-valued). Convergence in distribution is denoted by $\xrightarrow{D}$.
- Convergence in probability can be defined in the following way. Let X and X_n, $n = 1, 2, \ldots$, be random matrices. The sequence $X_1, X_2, \ldots$ converges in probability to X if for every $\epsilon > 0$, $\lim_{n\to\infty} P(\rho(X_n, X) > \epsilon) = 0$, where $\rho(\bullet, \bullet)$ is the Euclidean distance. Convergence in probability is denoted by $\xrightarrow{P}$.

A.12 Limits

- If a positive constant m exists, such that $|f(\epsilon)| \leq m|g(\epsilon)|$ for all ϵ in the neighbourhood of zero, then $f(\epsilon) = \mathcal{O}(g(\epsilon))$ as $\epsilon \to 0$.
- If $\lim_{\epsilon\to 0} \frac{f(\epsilon)}{g(\epsilon)} = 0$, then $f(\epsilon) = o(g(\epsilon))$ as $\epsilon \to 0$.
- A sequence of random variables $X_1, X_2, \ldots, X_n$ is bounded in probability if, given $\epsilon > 0$, there exist constants m and n_0 such that $P(|X_n| > m) \leq \epsilon$

for all $n \geq n_0$. This is denoted by $X_n = \mathcal{O}_p(1)$. If $a_n X_n = \mathcal{O}_p(1)$, then $X_n = \mathcal{O}_p(a_n^{-1})$. A sequence of random vectors $\boldsymbol{x}_1, \boldsymbol{x}_2, \ldots, \boldsymbol{x}_n$ is bounded in probability if $x_{i1}, x_{i2}, \ldots, x_{in}$ is bounded in probability for each i.
- If a sequence of random vectors $\boldsymbol{x}_1, \boldsymbol{x}_2, \ldots, \boldsymbol{x}_n$ converges to zero in probability, this is denoted by $\boldsymbol{x}_n = o(1)$. If $a_n \boldsymbol{x}_n = o(1)$, then $\boldsymbol{x}_n = o(a_n^{-1})$.

Note that the last two statements also hold for matrices, because any matrix can be vectorized.

A.13 Hermite Polynomials

Let $\boldsymbol{X} \sim N_{p,n}(\boldsymbol{\mu}, \boldsymbol{\Sigma}, \boldsymbol{\Psi})$ and let $f_X(\boldsymbol{X}_o)$ be its density evaluated at $\boldsymbol{X}_o$. Moreover, let the derivative $\frac{d^k f_X(\boldsymbol{X}_o)}{d\boldsymbol{X}_o^k}$ be defined in Lemma 5.1. Then

$$\frac{d^k f_X(\boldsymbol{X}_o)}{d\boldsymbol{X}_o^k} = (-1)^k \boldsymbol{H}_k(\boldsymbol{X}_o, \boldsymbol{\mu}, \boldsymbol{\Sigma}, \boldsymbol{\Psi}) f_X(\boldsymbol{X}_o),$$

for the functions $\boldsymbol{H}_k(\boldsymbol{X}_o, \boldsymbol{\mu}, \boldsymbol{\Sigma}, \boldsymbol{\Psi})$, which are called generalized Hermite polynomials. If $\boldsymbol{X} \sim N_{p,n}(\boldsymbol{0}, \boldsymbol{I}, \boldsymbol{I})$ or $\boldsymbol{X} \sim N_p(\boldsymbol{0}, \boldsymbol{I})$, we obtain polynomials which are usually termed Hermite polynomials.

Appendix B: Useful Technical Results

This appendix comprises several technical results which are frequently applied throughout Chaps. 1–8. In many of the suggested proofs, the reader is referred to Kollo and von Rosen (2005), although the same results can often be found in other texts.

B.1 Factorization and a Determinant Relation

The next theorem is often used when presenting canonical forms of linear and bilinear models.

Theorem B.1

(i) *Let $\boldsymbol{A}$: $p \times q$ be of rank q. Then there exist a non-singular matrix $\boldsymbol{T}$ and an orthogonal matrix $\boldsymbol{\Gamma}$ such that $\boldsymbol{A}' = \boldsymbol{T}(\boldsymbol{I}_q : \boldsymbol{0})\boldsymbol{\Gamma}$.*
(ii) *Let $\boldsymbol{V}$ be p.d. Then there exist an orthogonal matrix of eigenvectors of $\boldsymbol{V}$, $\boldsymbol{\Gamma}$, and a diagonal matrix $\boldsymbol{D}$ of positive eigenvalues of $\boldsymbol{V}$ such that $\boldsymbol{V} = \boldsymbol{\Gamma}\boldsymbol{D}\boldsymbol{\Gamma}'$.*

Proof Statement (i) is a special case of the well-known QR-decomposition, e.g. see Golub and Van Loan (2013) (see also Rao 1973, p. 20), and the proof of statement (ii) can be found in Kollo and von Rosen (2005, Corollary 1.2.39.1). □

Theorem B.2 *Let $\boldsymbol{B} = (\boldsymbol{b}_1, \boldsymbol{b}_2, \ldots, \boldsymbol{b}_p)$ be an orthogonal basis with respect to a positive definite matrix $\boldsymbol{W}: p \times p$, i.e. $\boldsymbol{b}_i'\boldsymbol{W}\boldsymbol{b}_j = 0$, $i \neq j$. Then*

$$|\boldsymbol{W}| = c^{-1}\prod_{k=1}^{p}|\boldsymbol{b}_i'\boldsymbol{W}\boldsymbol{b}_i|, \quad c = |\boldsymbol{B}|^2.$$

Proof The theorem is true because $|\boldsymbol{W}| = c^{-1}|\boldsymbol{B}'\boldsymbol{W}\boldsymbol{B}| = c^{-1}\prod_{k=1}^{p}|\boldsymbol{b}_i'\boldsymbol{W}\boldsymbol{b}_i|$. □

B.2 Subspace Relations

Theorem B.3 *Let $\boldsymbol{A}$, $\boldsymbol{B}$ and $\boldsymbol{C}$ be matrices of proper sizes. Then*

(i) *if $\boldsymbol{x} \in \mathcal{C}(\boldsymbol{A})$, then $\boldsymbol{x} = \boldsymbol{A}\boldsymbol{q}$ for some $\boldsymbol{q}$;*
(ii) *if $\mathcal{C}(\boldsymbol{A}) \subseteq \mathcal{C}(\boldsymbol{B})$, then $\mathcal{C}(\boldsymbol{B})^{\perp} \subseteq \mathcal{C}(\boldsymbol{A})^{\perp}$;*
(iii) *if $\mathcal{C}(\boldsymbol{A}) \subseteq \mathcal{C}(\boldsymbol{B})$, then $\mathcal{C}(\boldsymbol{B}) = \mathcal{C}(\boldsymbol{A}) \boxplus \mathcal{C}(\boldsymbol{B}) \cap \mathcal{C}(\boldsymbol{A})^{\perp}$;*
(iv) *(modular identity) $\mathcal{C}(\boldsymbol{A}) \cap (\mathcal{C}(\boldsymbol{B}) + \mathcal{C}(\boldsymbol{A}) \cap \mathcal{C}(\boldsymbol{C})) = \mathcal{C}(\boldsymbol{A}) \cap \mathcal{C}(\boldsymbol{B}) + \mathcal{C}(\boldsymbol{A}) \cap \mathcal{C}(\boldsymbol{C})$;*
(v) *$\mathcal{C}(\boldsymbol{A}(\boldsymbol{A}'\boldsymbol{B}^o)^o) = \mathcal{C}(\boldsymbol{A}) \cap \mathcal{C}(\boldsymbol{B})$;*
(vi) *$\mathcal{C}(\boldsymbol{A}'(\boldsymbol{A}\boldsymbol{A}'\boldsymbol{B}^o)^o) = \mathcal{C}(\boldsymbol{A}'\boldsymbol{B}^o)^{\perp} \cap \mathcal{C}(\boldsymbol{A}')$;*
(vii) *$\mathcal{C}(\boldsymbol{A}') \subseteq \mathcal{C}(\boldsymbol{A}'\boldsymbol{B}^o)$ is equivalent to $\mathcal{C}(\boldsymbol{A}) \cap \mathcal{C}(\boldsymbol{B}) = \{\boldsymbol{0}\}$.*

Proof All the proofs are given in Kollo and von Rosen (2005, Section 1.2). □

Theorem B.4 *For $\boldsymbol{A}$ and $\boldsymbol{\Sigma}$ of a proper size,*

$$\mathcal{C}_{\boldsymbol{\Sigma}}(\boldsymbol{A})^{\perp} = \mathcal{C}(\boldsymbol{\Sigma}\boldsymbol{A}^o) = \mathcal{C}((\boldsymbol{\Sigma}^{-1}\boldsymbol{A})^o) = \mathcal{C}(\boldsymbol{\Sigma}^{-1}\boldsymbol{A})^{\perp}.$$

Proof By the definition of $\boldsymbol{A}^o$, $\boldsymbol{A}^{o'}\boldsymbol{\Sigma}\boldsymbol{\Sigma}^{-1}\boldsymbol{A} = \boldsymbol{0}$, which verifies the equalities. □

Note that from this relation, it does not follow that $\mathcal{C}_{\boldsymbol{\Sigma}}(\boldsymbol{A}) = \mathcal{C}(\boldsymbol{\Sigma}^{-1}\boldsymbol{A})$, since in this case we operate with different inner products on the left and right side.

B.3 Rank Relations

Theorem B.5 *Let $\boldsymbol{A}$ and $\boldsymbol{B}$ be arbitrary matrices of proper sizes and let* $\dim\{\bullet\}$ *denote the dimension of a vector space. Then*

(i) *$r(\boldsymbol{A}) = r(\boldsymbol{A}')$;*
(ii) $\dim\{\mathcal{C}(\boldsymbol{A}) \cap \mathcal{C}(\boldsymbol{B})\} = r(\boldsymbol{A}(\boldsymbol{A}'\boldsymbol{B}^o)^o) = r((\boldsymbol{A}^o : \boldsymbol{B}^o)^o)$;

(iii) $r(\mathbf{A} : \mathbf{B}) = r(\mathbf{A}) + r(\mathbf{B}) - \dim\{\mathcal{C}(\mathbf{A}) \cap \mathcal{C}(\mathbf{B})\}$;
(iv) $r(\mathbf{A}'\mathbf{B}^o) = r(\mathbf{A} : \mathbf{B}) - r(\mathbf{B})$.

Proof The proof of the theorem is presented in Kollo and von Rosen (2005, Section 1.2). □

B.4 Special Matrix Inverses

Theorem B.6 *Let $\mathbf{S}$ be positive definite and suppose that $\mathbf{V}$, $\mathbf{W}$ and $\mathbf{H}$ are of a proper size, with $\mathbf{H}^{-1}$ being supposed to exist. Moreover, suppose that ω is a scalar and put $\mathbf{D} = \mathbf{S}^{-1}\mathbf{V}\mathbf{W}$ and $\mathbf{E} = \mathbf{D}\mathbf{S}^{-1}$. Then*

(i) $(\mathbf{S} + \mathbf{V}\mathbf{H}\mathbf{W}')^{-1} = \mathbf{S}^{-1} - \mathbf{S}^{-1}\mathbf{V}(\mathbf{W}'\mathbf{S}^{-1}\mathbf{V} + \mathbf{H}^{-1})^{-1}\mathbf{W}'\mathbf{S}^{-1}$;
(ii) $(\mathbf{S} + \mathbf{V}\mathbf{H}\mathbf{W}')^{-1}\mathbf{V}\mathbf{H} = \mathbf{S}^{-1}\mathbf{V}(\mathbf{W}'\mathbf{S}^{-1}\mathbf{V} + \mathbf{H}^{-1})^{-1}$;
(iii) $(\mathbf{S} + \omega\mathbf{V}\mathbf{W}')^{-1} = \sum_{k=0}^{2r+1}(-1)^k\omega^k\mathbf{D}^k\mathbf{S}^{-1} + \omega^{2(r+1)}\mathbf{D}^{r+1}(\mathbf{S} + \mathbf{V}\mathbf{W}')^{-1}\mathbf{E}^{r+1}$, $r = 1, 2, \ldots$;
(iv) $(\mathbf{S} + \omega\mathbf{V}\mathbf{W}')^{-1} = \sum_{k=0}^{\infty}(-1)^k\omega^k\mathbf{D}^k\mathbf{S}^{-1}$, *provided that the sum exists.*

Proof The proof of the first statement can be found in Kollo and von Rosen (2005, Proposition 1.3.6), and statement (ii) follows directly from statement (i) by applying a few calculations. The expressions in statement (iii) and (iv) are presented in von Rosen (1995, Lemma 2.1). □

B.5 Matrix Relations Involving g-Inverses

Theorem B.7 *Let $\mathcal{C}(\mathbf{K}) \subseteq \mathcal{C}(\mathbf{A}')$ and let $\mathbf{S}$ be p.d. Then*

(i) $\mathbf{K}(\mathbf{A}'\mathbf{S}^{-1}\mathbf{A})^{-}\mathbf{A}'\mathbf{S}^{-1}\mathbf{A} = \mathbf{K}$;
(ii) $\mathbf{K}(\mathbf{A}'\mathbf{S}^{-1}\mathbf{A})^{-}\mathbf{K}'$ *does not depend on the choice of g-inverse.*

Proof Both statements follow since $\mathcal{C}(\mathbf{A}') = \mathcal{C}(\mathbf{A}'\mathbf{S}^{-1}\mathbf{A})$. □

B.6 Matrix Relations for Partitioned Matrices

Theorem B.8 *Let*

$$\mathbf{A} = \begin{pmatrix} \mathbf{A}_{11} & \mathbf{A}_{12} \\ \mathbf{A}_{21} & \mathbf{A}_{22} \end{pmatrix}, \quad \begin{pmatrix} \mathbf{A}^{11} & \mathbf{A}^{12} \\ \mathbf{A}^{21} & \mathbf{A}^{22} \end{pmatrix},$$

where the size of $\mathbf{A}_{ij}$ corresponds to the size of $\mathbf{A}^{ij}$.

(i) $(\boldsymbol{A}^{11})^{-1}\boldsymbol{A}^{12} = -\boldsymbol{A}_{12}\boldsymbol{A}_{22}^{-1}$;
(ii) $\mathcal{C}(\boldsymbol{A}_{12}) \subseteq \mathcal{C}(\boldsymbol{A}_{11} - \boldsymbol{A}_{12}\boldsymbol{A}_{22}^{-1}\boldsymbol{A}_{21})$;
(iii) *if* $\boldsymbol{A}$ *is p.d., then* $\mathcal{C}(\boldsymbol{A}_{12}) \subseteq \mathcal{C}(\boldsymbol{A}_{11})$;
(iv) *if* $\boldsymbol{A}$ *is non-singular, then* $|\boldsymbol{A}| = |\boldsymbol{A}_{22}||\boldsymbol{A}_{11} - \boldsymbol{A}_{12}\boldsymbol{A}_{22}^{-1}\boldsymbol{A}_{21}|$.

Proof For a proof, see, for example, Kollo and von Rosen (2005, Proposition 1.3.3). □

B.7 Inequalities

Theorem B.9

(i) *Markov's inequality. Let* X *be a non-negative integrable random variable and* $a > 0$. *Then*

$$P(X \geq a) \leq E[X]/a.$$

(ii) *If* $\boldsymbol{A} - \boldsymbol{B}$ *is p.s.d., then* $\mathrm{tr}\boldsymbol{A} \geq \mathrm{tr}\boldsymbol{B}$.
(iii) *The* tr*-distance (see Sect. A.6).* $||\boldsymbol{AQB} - \boldsymbol{APB}|| > ||\boldsymbol{CQD} - \boldsymbol{CPD}||$ *for all* $\boldsymbol{P}$ *and* $\boldsymbol{Q}$ *if and only if* $\boldsymbol{BB}' \otimes \boldsymbol{A}'\boldsymbol{A} - \boldsymbol{DD}' \otimes \boldsymbol{C}'\boldsymbol{C}$ *is p.d., where it is supposed that the matrices are of proper sizes.*
(iv) *Let* $\boldsymbol{\Sigma}$ *and* $\boldsymbol{S}$ *be positive definite matrices of size* $p \times p$. *Then*

$$|\boldsymbol{\Sigma}|^{-\frac{1}{2}n}e^{-\frac{1}{2}\mathrm{tr}\{\boldsymbol{\Sigma}^{-1}\boldsymbol{S}\}} \leq |\tfrac{1}{n}\boldsymbol{S}|^{-\frac{1}{2}n}e^{-\frac{1}{2}np},$$

and equality holds if and only if $\boldsymbol{\Sigma} = \frac{1}{n}\boldsymbol{S}$.
(v) *For* $\boldsymbol{A}$ *(of full rank) and* $\boldsymbol{\Sigma}$ *(p.d.) of proper sizes (see Liu and Neudecker, 1997)*

$$(\boldsymbol{A}'\boldsymbol{A})^{-1}\boldsymbol{A}'\boldsymbol{\Sigma}\boldsymbol{A}(\boldsymbol{A}'\boldsymbol{A})^{-1} \leq \frac{(\lambda_1 + \lambda_p)^2}{4\lambda_1\lambda_2}(\boldsymbol{A}'\boldsymbol{\Sigma}^{-1}\boldsymbol{A})^{-1},$$

where λ_p *and* λ_1 *are the smallest and largest eigenvalues of* $\boldsymbol{\Sigma}$*, respectively. The ratio*

$$\mu_1 = \frac{4\lambda_1\lambda_2}{(\lambda_1 + \lambda_p)^2}$$

is the square of the first antieigenvalue of $\boldsymbol{\Sigma}$ *(see Gustafson, 1972, 2012).*

Proof For a proof of statement (i), see, for example, Gut (2013, Theorem 1.1, p. 120). Because of the linearity of the trace-function, statement (ii) is trivial. Statement (iii) follows by using the following equation:

$$\mathrm{tr}\{\boldsymbol{FGHH}'\boldsymbol{G}'\boldsymbol{F}'\} = \mathrm{vec}'(\boldsymbol{FGH})\mathrm{vec}(\boldsymbol{FGH}) = \mathrm{vec}'(\boldsymbol{G})(\boldsymbol{HH}' \otimes \boldsymbol{F}'\boldsymbol{F})\mathrm{vec}(\boldsymbol{G}).$$

The proof of statement (iv) can be found in Srivastava and Khatri (1979, Theorem 1.10.4) and for the proof of statement (v), the reader is referred to the references given in the statement. □

B.8 Linear Equations

Theorem B.10

(i) *The matrix equation* $\boldsymbol{AXB} = \boldsymbol{C}$ *in* $\boldsymbol{X}$. *If* $\mathcal{C}(\boldsymbol{C}) \subseteq \mathcal{C}(\boldsymbol{A})$ *and* $\mathcal{C}(\boldsymbol{C}') \subseteq \mathcal{C}(\boldsymbol{B}')$, *the system of equations is consistent and has the following general solution: ($\boldsymbol{C}_0$ denotes any particular solution)*

$$\boldsymbol{X} = \boldsymbol{C}_0 + (\boldsymbol{A}')^o\boldsymbol{Z}_1 + \boldsymbol{A}'\boldsymbol{Z}_2\boldsymbol{B}^{o'}$$

or

$$\boldsymbol{X} = \boldsymbol{C}_0 + \boldsymbol{Z}_1\boldsymbol{B}^{o'} + (\boldsymbol{A}')^o\boldsymbol{Z}_2\boldsymbol{B}'$$

or

$$\boldsymbol{X} = \boldsymbol{C}_0 + (\boldsymbol{A}')^o\boldsymbol{Z}_1\boldsymbol{B}' + \boldsymbol{A}'\boldsymbol{Z}_2\boldsymbol{B}^{o'} + (\boldsymbol{A}')^o\boldsymbol{Z}_3\boldsymbol{B}^{o'},$$

where $\boldsymbol{Z}_i$, $i = 1, 2, 3$, *are arbitrary matrices of proper sizes.*

(ii) *For the consistent equation* $\boldsymbol{AXB} = \boldsymbol{C}$, *the bilinear expression* $\boldsymbol{KXL}$ *is unique and equals* $\boldsymbol{KA}^-\boldsymbol{CB}^-\boldsymbol{L}$, *if* $\mathcal{C}(\boldsymbol{K}') \subseteq \mathcal{C}(\boldsymbol{A}')$ *and* $\mathcal{C}(\boldsymbol{L}) \subseteq \mathcal{C}(\boldsymbol{B})$. *Note that one choice of particular solution is* $\boldsymbol{C}_0 = \boldsymbol{A}^-\boldsymbol{CB}^-$.

(iii) *The homogeneous matrix equation* $\boldsymbol{A}_i\boldsymbol{XB}_i = \boldsymbol{0}$, $i = 1, 2$, *in* $\boldsymbol{X}$, *has the following general solution:*

$$\boldsymbol{X} = (\boldsymbol{A}_2')^o\boldsymbol{Z}_1\boldsymbol{S}_1' + (\boldsymbol{A}_1' : \boldsymbol{A}_2')^o\boldsymbol{Z}_2\boldsymbol{S}_2' + (\boldsymbol{A}_1')^o\boldsymbol{Z}_3\boldsymbol{S}_3' + \boldsymbol{Z}_4\boldsymbol{S}_4'$$

or

$$\boldsymbol{X} = \boldsymbol{T}_1\boldsymbol{Z}_1\boldsymbol{B}_2^{o'} + \boldsymbol{T}_2\boldsymbol{Z}_2(\boldsymbol{B}_1 : \boldsymbol{B})^{o'} + \boldsymbol{T}_3\boldsymbol{Z}_3\boldsymbol{B}_1^{o'} + \boldsymbol{T}_4\boldsymbol{Z}_4$$

or

$$\boldsymbol{X} = \boldsymbol{T}_3\boldsymbol{Z}_1\boldsymbol{S}_1' + \boldsymbol{T}_4\boldsymbol{Z}_2\boldsymbol{S}_1' + \boldsymbol{T}_4\boldsymbol{Z}_3\boldsymbol{S}_2' + \boldsymbol{T}_1\boldsymbol{Z}_4\boldsymbol{S}_3' + \boldsymbol{T}_4\boldsymbol{Z}_5\boldsymbol{S}_3'$$
$$+\boldsymbol{T}_1\boldsymbol{Z}_6\boldsymbol{S}_4' + \boldsymbol{T}_2\boldsymbol{Z}_7\boldsymbol{S}_4' + \boldsymbol{T}_3\boldsymbol{Z}_8\boldsymbol{S}_4' + \boldsymbol{T}_4\boldsymbol{Z}_9\boldsymbol{S}_4',$$

where $\boldsymbol{Z}_i$, $i = 1, \ldots, 9$, *are arbitrary matrices of proper sizes, and* $\boldsymbol{S}_i$ *and* $\boldsymbol{T}_i$, $i = 1, \ldots, 4$, *are any matrices satisfying*

$$\begin{aligned}
&\mathcal{C}(\boldsymbol{S}_1) = \mathcal{C}(\boldsymbol{B}_1 : \boldsymbol{B}_2) \cap \mathcal{C}(\boldsymbol{B}_1)^{\perp}, && \mathcal{C}(\boldsymbol{T}_1) = \mathcal{C}(\boldsymbol{A}_1' : \boldsymbol{A}_2') \cap \mathcal{C}(\boldsymbol{A}_1')^{\perp},\\
&\mathcal{C}(\boldsymbol{S}_2) = \mathcal{C}(\boldsymbol{B}_1) \cap \mathcal{C}(\boldsymbol{B}_2), && \mathcal{C}(\boldsymbol{T}_2) = \mathcal{C}(\boldsymbol{A}_1') \cap \mathcal{C}(\boldsymbol{A}_2'),\\
&\mathcal{C}(\boldsymbol{S}_3) = \mathcal{C}(\boldsymbol{B}_1 : \boldsymbol{B}_2) \cap \mathcal{C}(\boldsymbol{B}_2)^{\perp}, && \mathcal{C}(\boldsymbol{T}_3) = \mathcal{C}(\boldsymbol{A}_1' : \boldsymbol{A}_2') \cap \mathcal{C}(\boldsymbol{A}_2')^{\perp},\\
&\mathcal{C}(\boldsymbol{S}_4) = \mathcal{C}(\boldsymbol{B}_1 : \boldsymbol{B}_2)^{\perp}, && \mathcal{C}(\boldsymbol{T}_1) = \mathcal{C}(\boldsymbol{A}_1' : \boldsymbol{A}_2')^{\perp}.
\end{aligned}$$

(iv) *The homogeneous matrix equation* $A_1X_1B_1 + A_2X_2B_2 = 0$ *in* X_1 *and* X_2 *has the following general solution:*

$$X_1 = -A_1^- A_2(A_2' A_1^o : (A_2')^{o'})^o Z_3 (B_2(B_1')^o)^{o'} B_2 B_1^- + (A_1')^o Z_1 + A_1' Z_2 B_1^{o'},$$

$$X_2 = (A_2' A_1^o) : (A_2')^o)^{o'} Z_3 (B_2(B_1')^o)^{o'} + A_2' A_1^o Z_4 B_2^{o'} + (A_2')^o Z_5$$

or

$$X_1 = -A_1^- A_2 (A_2' A_1^o)^o (A_2' A_1^o)^{o'} A_2' Z_6 (B_2 (B_1')^o)^{o'} B_2 B_1^- + (A_1')^o Z_1 + A_1' Z_2 B_1^{o'},$$

$$X_2 = (A_2' A_1^o)^{o'} ((A_2' A_1^o)^{o'} A_2')^o Z_5 + (A_2' A_1^o)^o (A_2' A_1^o)^{o'} A_2' Z_6 (B_2 (B_1')^o)^{o'} + A_2' A_1^o Z_4 B_2^{o'},$$

where Z_i, $i = 1, \ldots, 6$, *are arbitrary matrices.*

Proof The proof of the statements can be found in Kollo and von Rosen (2005, Section 1.3.5). □

B.9 Results Involving Projectors

Next a few useful results for projectors are presented.

Theorem B.11 *Let* $P_{A,V} = A(A'V^{-1}A)^- AV^{-1}$. *Then*

(i) $P_{A,V} P_{A,V} = P_{A,V}$, $\quad P_{A,V}(I - P_{A,V}) = 0$;
(ii) $\text{tr}\{P_{A,V}\} = r(A)$;
(iii) $\mathcal{C}(P_{A,V}) = \mathcal{C}(A)$, $\quad \mathcal{N}(P_{A,V}) = \mathcal{C}(VA^o)$;
(iv) *(projection theorem)* $\mathcal{C}(P_{A,V}B) = \mathcal{C}(P_{A,V}) \cap (\mathcal{N}(P_{A,V}) + \mathcal{C}(B))$;
(v) $I = P'_{A^o,V^{-1}} + P_{A,V}$.

Proof The proofs of statements (i) and (ii) can be found in most linear algebra books. The relations in statement (iii) are fairly trivial, since $A(A'V^{-1}A)^- A'V^{-1}A = A$ (e.g. see Kollo and von Rosen, 2005, Proposition 1.2.2) and $A(A'V^{-1}A)^- A'V^{-1}VA^o = 0$. The proof of statement (iv) is presented in Kollo and von Rosen (2005, Theorem 1.2.16). Statement (v) follows from Theorem B.13. □

The following theorem constitutes a basis for handling linear models within a theoretical perspective and reflects a decomposition of the whole space into two subspaces.

Theorem B.12 *Let* S *be p.d., let* A *and* B *be arbitrary matrices of proper sizes and let* C *be any matrix such that* $\mathcal{C}(C) = \mathcal{C}(A') \cap \mathcal{C}(B)$. *Then*

$$A(A'SA)^- A' - AB^o (B^{o'} A'SAB^o)^- B^{o'} A'$$
$$= A(A'SA)^- C(C'(A'SA)^- C)^- C'(A'SA)^- A'.$$

Proof Let $\boldsymbol{S} = \boldsymbol{I}$. The general case follows by changing $\boldsymbol{A}$ to $\boldsymbol{S}^{1/2}\boldsymbol{A}$. If $\boldsymbol{S} = \boldsymbol{I}$, the statement consists of three orthogonal projectors: $\boldsymbol{P}_A$, $\boldsymbol{P}_{AB^o}$ and $\boldsymbol{P}_{A(A'A)^-C}$. The result follows since

$$\mathcal{C}(\boldsymbol{A}) = \mathcal{C}(\boldsymbol{AB}^o) \boxplus \mathcal{C}(\boldsymbol{A}) \cap \mathcal{C}(\boldsymbol{AB}^o)^{\perp} = \mathcal{C}(\boldsymbol{AB}^o) \boxplus \mathcal{C}(\boldsymbol{A}(\boldsymbol{A}'\boldsymbol{A})^-\boldsymbol{C}),$$

see Theorems B.3 (v) and B.11 (iv) in this appendix. □

Theorem B.13 *If $\boldsymbol{S}$ is p.d. and $\mathcal{C}(\boldsymbol{B}) \subseteq \mathcal{C}(\boldsymbol{A})$,*

$$\boldsymbol{P}_{A,S} = \boldsymbol{P}_{B,S} + \boldsymbol{S}\boldsymbol{P}'_{A,S}\boldsymbol{B}^o(\boldsymbol{B}^{o'}\boldsymbol{S}\boldsymbol{P}'_{A,S}\boldsymbol{B}^o)^-\boldsymbol{B}^{o'}\boldsymbol{P}_{A,S}.$$

A special case is

$$\boldsymbol{S}^{-1} - \boldsymbol{B}^o(\boldsymbol{B}^{o'}\boldsymbol{S}\boldsymbol{B}^o)^-\boldsymbol{B}^{o'} = \boldsymbol{S}^{-1}\boldsymbol{B}(\boldsymbol{B}'\boldsymbol{S}^{-1}\boldsymbol{B})^-\boldsymbol{B}'\boldsymbol{S}^{-1}.$$

Proof The result follows from Theorem B.12. □

B.10 Properties of a Matrix Derivative

Theorem B.14 *Let $\frac{d^k \boldsymbol{Y}}{d\boldsymbol{X}^k}$ be given by Definition 5.1. Then*

(i) $\frac{d\boldsymbol{X}}{d\boldsymbol{X}} = \boldsymbol{I}_{pq}$, *where $\boldsymbol{X} \in \mathbb{R}^{p\times q}$;*
(ii) $\frac{dc\boldsymbol{X}}{d\boldsymbol{X}} = c\boldsymbol{I}_{pq}$, *where $\boldsymbol{X} \in \mathbb{R}^{p\times q}$;*
(iii) $\frac{d\boldsymbol{A}'\text{vec}\boldsymbol{X}}{d\boldsymbol{X}} = \boldsymbol{A}$;
(iv) $\frac{d\boldsymbol{Y}+\boldsymbol{Z}}{d\boldsymbol{X}} = \frac{d\boldsymbol{Y}}{d\boldsymbol{X}} + \frac{d\boldsymbol{Z}}{d\boldsymbol{X}}$.
(v) *Let $\boldsymbol{Z} = \boldsymbol{Z}(\boldsymbol{Y})$ and $\boldsymbol{Y} = \boldsymbol{Y}(\boldsymbol{X})$, then* $\frac{d\boldsymbol{Z}}{d\boldsymbol{X}} = \frac{d\boldsymbol{Y}}{d\boldsymbol{X}}\frac{d\boldsymbol{Z}}{d\boldsymbol{Y}}$ *(chain rule);*
(vi) $\frac{d\boldsymbol{AXB}}{d\boldsymbol{X}} = \boldsymbol{B} \otimes \boldsymbol{A}'$;
(vii) $\frac{d\boldsymbol{AYB}}{d\boldsymbol{X}} = \frac{d\boldsymbol{Y}}{d\boldsymbol{X}}(\boldsymbol{B} \otimes \boldsymbol{A}')$;
(viii) $\frac{d\boldsymbol{X}'}{d\boldsymbol{X}} = \boldsymbol{K}_{q,p}$, *if $\boldsymbol{X} \in \mathbb{R}^{p\times q}$;*
(ix) $\frac{d\boldsymbol{YZ}}{d\boldsymbol{X}} = \frac{d\boldsymbol{Y}}{d\boldsymbol{X}}(\boldsymbol{Z} \otimes \boldsymbol{I}) + \frac{d\boldsymbol{Z}}{d\boldsymbol{X}}(\boldsymbol{I} \otimes \boldsymbol{Y}')$;
(x) $\frac{d\,\text{tr}\{\boldsymbol{A}'\boldsymbol{X}\}}{d\boldsymbol{X}} = \text{vec}\boldsymbol{A}$;
(xi) $\frac{d|\boldsymbol{X}|}{d\boldsymbol{X}} = |\boldsymbol{X}|\text{vec}(\boldsymbol{X}^{-1})'$.
(xii) *If $\boldsymbol{X}$: $p \times p$ is symmetric* $\frac{d\boldsymbol{X}}{d\boldsymbol{X}} = \boldsymbol{I}_{p^2} + \boldsymbol{K}_{p,p} - (\boldsymbol{K}_{p,p})_d$.

Proof The proofs of the statements can, for example, be found in Kollo and von Rosen (2005, Section 1.4.3, Table 1.4.2). □

Theorem B.15 *Let the derivative be given by Definition 8.4 and suppose that the matrices are conformable. If $\boldsymbol{X}$ and $\boldsymbol{Y}$ are functions of ω, then*

(i) $\frac{d^k\boldsymbol{XY}}{d\omega^k} = \sum_{i=0}^{k}\binom{k}{i}\frac{d^i\boldsymbol{X}}{d\omega^i}\frac{d^{k-i}\boldsymbol{Y}}{d\omega^{k-i}}, \qquad k \geq 0.$

(ii) *Let* $\boldsymbol{A}$ *and* $\boldsymbol{B}$ *be functionally independent of the scalar* ω. *Then*

$$\frac{d^k \boldsymbol{AXB}}{d\,\omega^k} = \boldsymbol{A}\frac{d^k \boldsymbol{X}}{d\,\omega^k}\boldsymbol{B}.$$

(iii) *Let* $\boldsymbol{X}$ *be non-singular and a function of the scalar* ω. *Then*

$$\frac{d^k \boldsymbol{X}^{-1}}{d\,\omega^k} = -\boldsymbol{X}^{-1}\frac{d^k \boldsymbol{X}}{d\,\omega^k}\boldsymbol{X}^{-1} + \sum_{j=1}^{k-1}(-1)^{j+1}\sum_{i_1=j}^{k-1}\sum_{i_2=j-1}^{i_1-1}\cdots\sum_{i_j=1}^{i_{j-1}-1}\binom{k}{i_1}\binom{i_1}{i_2}\cdots\binom{i_{j-1}}{i_j}$$

$$\times\boldsymbol{X}^{-1}\frac{d^{i_j}\boldsymbol{X}}{d\,\omega^{i_j}}\boldsymbol{X}^{-1}\frac{d^{i_{j-1}-i_j}\boldsymbol{X}}{d\,\omega^{i_{j-1}-i_j}}\boldsymbol{X}^{-1}\times\cdots\times\boldsymbol{X}^{-1}\frac{d^{i_1-i_2}\boldsymbol{X}}{d\,\omega^{i_1-i_2}}\boldsymbol{X}^{-1}\frac{d^{k-i_1}\boldsymbol{X}}{d\,\omega^{k-i_1}}\boldsymbol{X}^{-1},$$

$$i_0 = k \geq 1.$$

Proof The proofs of statements (i) and (iii) are presented in von Rosen (1995, Lemma 3.1) and statement (ii) follows from statement (i). □

B.11 Basic Moment Identities

Theorem B.16 *Let* $E[\boldsymbol{X}] = \boldsymbol{\mu}$ *and* $D[\boldsymbol{X}] = \boldsymbol{\Psi} \otimes \boldsymbol{\Sigma}$. *Then*

(i) $E[\boldsymbol{KXL}] = \boldsymbol{K\mu L}$;
(ii) $D[\boldsymbol{KXL}] = \boldsymbol{L}'\boldsymbol{\Psi L} \otimes \boldsymbol{K\Sigma K}'$.

For moments and cumulants,

(iii) $c_1[\boldsymbol{X}] = m_1[\boldsymbol{X}], \quad c_2[\boldsymbol{X}] = D[\boldsymbol{X}]$;
(iv) $\boldsymbol{m}_k[\boldsymbol{X}] = E[\text{vec}\boldsymbol{X}(\text{vec}'\boldsymbol{X})^{\otimes k-1}], \quad m_1[\boldsymbol{X}] = E[\text{vec}\boldsymbol{X}]$.

Proof All proofs of the relations can be found in Kollo and von Rosen (2005, Section 2.1). □

B.12 Limit Theorems

The first theorem below is a multivariate version of some of the statements of *Cramér's theorem*, which is also known as *Slutsky's theorem*.

Theorem B.17 *Let* $\{\boldsymbol{X}_n\}$ *and* $\{\boldsymbol{Y}_n\}$ *be sequences of random matrices, not necessarily independent, such that* $\boldsymbol{X}_n \xrightarrow{D} \boldsymbol{X}$ *and* $\boldsymbol{Y}_n \xrightarrow{P} \boldsymbol{0}$. *Then, provided the operations are well defined,*

(i) $\boldsymbol{X}_n \otimes \boldsymbol{Y}_n \xrightarrow{P} \boldsymbol{0}$;

(ii) $\text{vec}\boldsymbol{X}_n\text{vec}'\boldsymbol{Y}_n \xrightarrow{P} \boldsymbol{0}$;
(iii) $\boldsymbol{X}_n + \boldsymbol{Y}_n \xrightarrow{D} \boldsymbol{X}$.

Proof Proofs of the relations are given in Kollo and von Rosen (2005, Lemma 3.1.1). □

Now a central limit theorem for the sample mean and sample dispersion is presented.

Theorem B.18 *Let $\boldsymbol{x}_1, \boldsymbol{x}_2, \ldots, \boldsymbol{x}_n$ be an i.i.d. sample of size n from a p-dimensional population with $E[\boldsymbol{x}_i] = \boldsymbol{\mu}$ and $D[\boldsymbol{x}_i] = \boldsymbol{\Sigma}$, p.d., with the elements of $m_4[\boldsymbol{x}_i]$ being finite, and let*

$$\overline{\boldsymbol{x}} = \frac{1}{n}\sum_{i=1}^{n}\boldsymbol{x}_i, \qquad \boldsymbol{S} = \frac{1}{n-1}\sum_{i=1}^{n}(\boldsymbol{x}_i - \overline{\boldsymbol{x}})(\boldsymbol{x}_i - \overline{\boldsymbol{x}})'.$$

Then, if $n \to \infty$,

(i) $\overline{\boldsymbol{x}} \xrightarrow{P} \boldsymbol{\mu}$;
(ii) $\boldsymbol{S} \xrightarrow{P} \boldsymbol{\Sigma}$;
(iii) $\sqrt{n}(\overline{\boldsymbol{x}} - \boldsymbol{\mu}) \xrightarrow{D} N_p(\boldsymbol{0}, \boldsymbol{\Sigma})$.
(iv) $\sqrt{n}\text{vec}(\boldsymbol{S} - \boldsymbol{\Sigma}) \xrightarrow{D} N_{p^2}(\boldsymbol{0}, \boldsymbol{\Pi})$,
where $\boldsymbol{\Pi}$: $p^2 \times p^2$ consists of the fourth- and second-order central moments:

$$\begin{aligned}\boldsymbol{\Pi} &= D[(\boldsymbol{x}_i - \boldsymbol{\mu})(\boldsymbol{x}_i - \boldsymbol{\mu})'] \\ &= E[(\boldsymbol{x}_i - \boldsymbol{\mu}) \otimes (\boldsymbol{x}_i - \boldsymbol{\mu})' \otimes (\boldsymbol{x}_i - \boldsymbol{\mu}) \otimes (\boldsymbol{x}_i - \boldsymbol{\mu})'] - \text{vec}\boldsymbol{\Sigma}\text{vec}'\boldsymbol{\Sigma}.\end{aligned}$$

(v) *Let $\boldsymbol{x}_i \sim N_p(\boldsymbol{\mu}, \boldsymbol{\Sigma})$, then $\sqrt{n}\text{vec}(\boldsymbol{S} - \boldsymbol{\Sigma}) \xrightarrow{D} N_{p^2}(\boldsymbol{0}, \boldsymbol{\Pi}^N)$, where*

$$\boldsymbol{\Pi}^N = (\boldsymbol{I}_{p^2} + \boldsymbol{K}_{p,p})(\boldsymbol{\Sigma} \otimes \boldsymbol{\Sigma}).$$

Proof A proof can be found in Kollo and von Rosen (2005, Theorem 3.1.4). □

B.13 Properties and Moment Relations for the Matrix Normal Distribution

Theorem B.19 *Let $X \sim N_{p,n}(\boldsymbol{\mu}, \boldsymbol{\Sigma}, \boldsymbol{\Psi})$ and $Y \sim N_{p,n}(\boldsymbol{0}, \boldsymbol{\Sigma}, \boldsymbol{\Psi})$. Then*

(i) $\boldsymbol{KXL} \sim N_{q,k}(\boldsymbol{K\mu L}, \boldsymbol{K\Sigma K}', \boldsymbol{L}'\boldsymbol{\Psi L})$, *where $\boldsymbol{K}$: $q \times p$ and $\boldsymbol{L}$: $n \times k$;*
(ii) $E[X] = \boldsymbol{\mu}$;
(iii) $D[X] = \boldsymbol{\Psi} \otimes \boldsymbol{\Sigma}$;
(iv) $E[\boldsymbol{XAX}'] = \text{tr}\{\boldsymbol{\Psi A}\}\boldsymbol{\Sigma} + \boldsymbol{\mu A\mu}'$.

(v) *Put* $\boldsymbol{H} = (\mathrm{vec}\boldsymbol{\Sigma}\mathrm{vec}'\boldsymbol{\Psi})^{\otimes 2}$. *Then*

$$E[\boldsymbol{Y}^{\otimes 4}] = \boldsymbol{H} + (\boldsymbol{I}_p \otimes \boldsymbol{K}_{p,p} \otimes \boldsymbol{I}_p)\boldsymbol{H}(\boldsymbol{I}_n \otimes \boldsymbol{K}_{n,n} \otimes \boldsymbol{I}_n) + (\boldsymbol{I}_p \otimes \boldsymbol{K}_{p^2,p})\boldsymbol{H}(\boldsymbol{I}_n \otimes \boldsymbol{K}_{n,n^2});$$

(vi) $E[\boldsymbol{Y}^{\otimes 2r}] = \sum_{i=2}^{2r}(\boldsymbol{I}_p \otimes \boldsymbol{K}_{p^{i-2},p} \otimes \boldsymbol{I}_{p^{2r-i}})(\mathrm{vec}\boldsymbol{\Sigma}\mathrm{vec}'\boldsymbol{\Psi} \otimes E[\boldsymbol{Y}^{\otimes 2(r-1)}]) \times (\boldsymbol{I}_n \otimes \boldsymbol{K}_{n,n^{i-2}} \otimes \boldsymbol{I}_{n^{2r-i}}), \qquad r = 1, 2, 3, \ldots;$

(vii)

$$\begin{aligned} E[\boldsymbol{XAX}' \otimes \boldsymbol{XBX}'] &= \mathrm{tr}\{\boldsymbol{\Psi A}\}\mathrm{tr}\{\boldsymbol{\Psi B}\}\boldsymbol{\Sigma} \otimes \boldsymbol{\Sigma} + \mathrm{tr}\{\boldsymbol{\Psi A \Psi B}'\}\mathrm{vec}\boldsymbol{\Sigma}\mathrm{vec}'\boldsymbol{\Sigma} \\ &+ \mathrm{tr}\{\boldsymbol{\Psi A \Psi B}\}\boldsymbol{K}_{p,p}(\boldsymbol{\Sigma} \otimes \boldsymbol{\Sigma}) + \mathrm{tr}\{\boldsymbol{\Psi A}\}\boldsymbol{\Sigma} \otimes \boldsymbol{\mu B \mu}' + \mathrm{vec}(\boldsymbol{\mu B \Psi A}'\boldsymbol{\mu}')\mathrm{vec}'\boldsymbol{\Sigma} \\ &+ \boldsymbol{K}_{p,p}(\boldsymbol{\mu B \Psi A \mu}' \otimes \boldsymbol{\Sigma} + \boldsymbol{\Sigma} \otimes \boldsymbol{\mu A \Psi B \mu}') \\ &+ \mathrm{vec}\boldsymbol{\Sigma}\mathrm{vec}'(\boldsymbol{\mu B}'\boldsymbol{\Psi A \mu}') + \mathrm{tr}\{\boldsymbol{\Psi B}\}\boldsymbol{\mu A \mu}' \otimes \boldsymbol{\Sigma} + \boldsymbol{\mu A \mu}' \otimes \boldsymbol{\mu B \mu}'. \end{aligned}$$

(viii) *Let* $\boldsymbol{S} = \boldsymbol{Y}(\boldsymbol{I} - \boldsymbol{P}_{C'})\boldsymbol{Y}'$, *where* $\boldsymbol{C}$ *is a matrix of a proper size. Then* $\boldsymbol{S}$ *and* $\boldsymbol{YP}_{C'}$ *are independently distributed.*

(ix) $\boldsymbol{YPY}'$ *and* $\boldsymbol{YQY}'$ *are independently distributed if* $\boldsymbol{PQ} = \boldsymbol{0}$, *where* $\boldsymbol{P}$ *and* $\boldsymbol{Q}$ *are symmetric matrices of proper sizes.*

(x) $\boldsymbol{YP}$ *and* $\boldsymbol{YQ}$ *are independently distributed if* $\boldsymbol{PQ}' = \boldsymbol{0}$, *where* $\boldsymbol{P}$ *and* $\boldsymbol{Q}$ *are of proper sizes.*

(xi) $\boldsymbol{YPY}'$ *and* $\boldsymbol{YQ}$ *are independently distributed if* $\boldsymbol{PQ} = \boldsymbol{0}$, *where* $\boldsymbol{P}$ *and* $\boldsymbol{Q}$ *are symmetric matrices of proper sizes.*

(xii) *Let* $\boldsymbol{A}$ *be a matrix of a proper size. Then* $\boldsymbol{P}_{A,\Sigma}\boldsymbol{X}$ *and* $(\boldsymbol{I} - \boldsymbol{P}_{A,\Sigma})\boldsymbol{X}$ *are independently distributed.*

(xiii) *Let* $\boldsymbol{A}$ *and* $\boldsymbol{B}$ *be matrices of proper sizes. Then* $\boldsymbol{A}'\boldsymbol{X}$ *and* $\boldsymbol{B}'\boldsymbol{X}$ *are independently distributed if and only if* $C[\boldsymbol{AX}, \boldsymbol{BX}] = \boldsymbol{0}$.

Proof For the proofs, see Section 2.2 in Kollo and von Rosen (2005), where the above-presented results are obtained. □

B.14 Properties and Moment Relations for the Wishart Distribution

Theorem B.20 *Let* $\boldsymbol{W} \sim W_p(\boldsymbol{\Sigma}, n)$, $\boldsymbol{V} \sim W_p(\boldsymbol{I}, n)$, *where* $n > p$. *Then*

(i) $\boldsymbol{A}'\boldsymbol{WA} \sim W_q(\boldsymbol{A}'\boldsymbol{\Sigma A}, n)$ *for any matrix* $\boldsymbol{A}$ *of size* $p \times q$. *In particular* $\boldsymbol{A} = (\boldsymbol{I} : \boldsymbol{0})$ *results in quadratic blocks along the diagonal of* $\boldsymbol{W}$ *also having a Wishart distribution.*

(ii) $E[\boldsymbol{W}] = n\boldsymbol{\Sigma}$;

(iii) $D[\boldsymbol{W}] = n(\boldsymbol{I} + \boldsymbol{K}_{p,p})\boldsymbol{\Sigma} \otimes \boldsymbol{\Sigma}$.

(iv) *Partition* V *as follows:*

$$V = \begin{pmatrix} V_{11} & V_{12} \\ V_{21} & V_{22} \end{pmatrix},$$

where V_{11}*:* $r \times r$, $V_{12} = V'_{21}$*:* $r \times (p-r)$ *and* V_{22}*:* $(p-r) \times (p-r)$. *Then* $V_{12}V_{22}^{-1/2} \sim N_{r,p-r}(\mathbf{0}, I, I)$, *and* $V_{12}V_{22}^{-1/2}$ *and* $V_{22} \sim W_{p-r}(I, n)$ *are independently distributed.*

(v) *Let* A*:* $p \times q$*. Then*

$$A(A'W^{-1}A)^{-}A' \sim W_p(A(A'\Sigma^{-1}A)^{-}A', n - p + r(A))$$

and

$$E[A(A'W^{-1}A)^{-}A'] = (n - p + r(A))A(A'\Sigma^{-1}A)^{-}A'.$$

(vi) *Let* $X \sim N_{p,n}(\mathbf{0}, \Sigma, I)$ *and* P *be any idempotent matrix of a proper size. Then*

$$XPX' \sim W_p(\Sigma, r(P)).$$

(vii) $A(A'W^{-1}A)^{-}A'$ *and* $W - A(A'W^{-1}A)^{-}A'$ *are independent.*

(viii) $A(A'W^{-1}A)^{-}A'$ *and* $I - A(A'W^{-1}A)^{-}A'W^{-1}$ *are independent.*

(ix) $E[A(A'WA)^{-}A'W] = A(A'\Sigma A)^{-}A'\Sigma$.

Proof Proofs of the above statements can be found in Kollo and von Rosen (2005, Section 2.4). Concerning statement (v), it is stressed that there exists a new proof which is fundamental. There always exists a matrix $X \sim N_{p,n}(\mathbf{0}, \Sigma, I)$ such that $W = XX'$. Then

$$\begin{aligned} A(A'W^{-1}A)^{-}A' &= P_{A,\Sigma}A(A'W^{-1}A)^{-}A'P'_{A,\Sigma} \\ &= P_{A,\Sigma}(W - WA^{o}(A^{o'}WA^{o})^{-}A^{o'}W)P'_{A,\Sigma} = P_{A,\Sigma}XPX'P'_{A,\Sigma}, \end{aligned}$$

where $P = I - X'A^{o}(A^{o'}WA^{o})^{-}A^{o'}X$. The proof follows since $A'\Sigma^{-1}X$ and $A^{o'}X$ are independently distributed and P is idempotent with rank $r(P) = n - r(A^{o})$. □

B.15 Moments for the Inverse Wishart Distribution

In the following, the constants introduced in the next definition will frequently be applied.

Definition B.1

(i) $c_{0;n,s} = \frac{1}{n-s-1}$;
(ii) $c_{1;n,s,t} = \frac{n-s-2}{(n-t-1)(n-s)(n-s-3)}$;
(iii) $c_{2;n,s,t} = \frac{1}{n-s-2}c_{1;n,s,t}$;
(iv) $c_{3;n,s,t} = \frac{1}{(n-s-1)(n-t-1)}$.

If $s = t$, then $c_{i;n,s}$ will be used instead of $c_{i;n,s,s}$, $i = 1, 2, 3$.

Theorem B.21 *Let* $\boldsymbol{W} \sim W_p(\boldsymbol{\Sigma}, n)$ *and let* $c_{i;n,s}$ *be defined in Definition B.1. Then,*

(i) *if* $n - p - 1 > 0$,

$$E[\boldsymbol{W}^{-1}] = c_{0;n,p}\boldsymbol{\Sigma}^{-1};$$

(ii) *if* $n - p - 3 > 0$,

$$D[\boldsymbol{W}^{-1}] = c_{2;n,p}(\boldsymbol{I} + \boldsymbol{K}_{p,p})(\boldsymbol{\Sigma}^{-1} \otimes \boldsymbol{\Sigma}^{-1}) + (c_{1;n,p} - c_{0;n,p}^2)\mathrm{vec}\boldsymbol{\Sigma}^{-1}\mathrm{vec}'\boldsymbol{\Sigma}^{-1};$$

(iii) *if* $n - p - 3 > 0$,

$$E[\boldsymbol{W}^{-1} \otimes \boldsymbol{W}^{-1}] = c_{2;n,p}(\mathrm{vec}\boldsymbol{\Sigma}^{-1}\mathrm{vec}'\boldsymbol{\Sigma}^{-1} + \boldsymbol{K}_{p,p}(\boldsymbol{\Sigma}^{-1} \otimes \boldsymbol{\Sigma}^{-1})) + c_{1;n,p}\boldsymbol{\Sigma}^{-1} \otimes \boldsymbol{\Sigma}^{-1};$$

(iv) *if* $n - p - 3 > 0$,

$$E[\mathrm{tr}\{\boldsymbol{W}^{-1}\}^2] = 2c_{2;n,p}\mathrm{tr}\{\boldsymbol{\Sigma}^{-1}\boldsymbol{\Sigma}^{-1}\} + c_{1;n,p}\mathrm{tr}\{\boldsymbol{\Sigma}^{-1}\}^2;$$

(v) *if* $n - p - 3 > 0$,

$$E[\boldsymbol{W}^{-1}\boldsymbol{W}^{-1}] = (c_{2;n,p} + c_{1;n,p})\boldsymbol{\Sigma}^{-1}\boldsymbol{\Sigma}^{-1} + c_{2;n,p}\boldsymbol{\Sigma}^{-1}\mathrm{tr}\{\boldsymbol{\Sigma}^{-1}\};$$

(vi) *if* $n - p - 3 > 0$,

$$E[\mathrm{tr}\{\boldsymbol{W}^{-1}\boldsymbol{W}^{-1}\}] = (c_{2;n,p} + c_{1;n,p})\mathrm{tr}\{\boldsymbol{\Sigma}^{-1}\boldsymbol{\Sigma}^{-1}\} + c_{2;n,p}\mathrm{tr}\{\boldsymbol{\Sigma}^{-1}\}^2.$$

(vii) *Let*

$$\boldsymbol{W} = \begin{pmatrix} \boldsymbol{W}_{11} & \boldsymbol{W}_{12} \\ \boldsymbol{W}_{21} & \boldsymbol{W}_{22} \end{pmatrix}, \quad \begin{pmatrix} r \times r & r \times p - r \\ p - r \times r & p - r \times p - r \end{pmatrix}.$$

Then, if $\boldsymbol{\Sigma} = \boldsymbol{I}$ *and* $n - p + r - 1 > 0$,

$$E[\boldsymbol{W}_{12}\boldsymbol{W}_{22}^{-1}\boldsymbol{W}_{22}^{-1}\boldsymbol{W}_{21}] = \frac{p - r}{n - p + r - 1}\boldsymbol{I}_r,$$

and if $n - p + r - 3 > 0$,

$$E[(\mathrm{vec}(\boldsymbol{W}_{12}\boldsymbol{W}_{22}^{-1}\boldsymbol{W}_{22}^{-1}\boldsymbol{W}_{21}))^{\otimes 2}] = \mathrm{tr}\{\boldsymbol{W}_{22}^{-1}\}^2 \mathrm{vec}\boldsymbol{I}_r \otimes \mathrm{vec}\boldsymbol{I}_r + \mathrm{tr}\{\boldsymbol{W}_{22}^{-1}\boldsymbol{W}_{22}^{-1}\}(\boldsymbol{I}_{r^2} + \boldsymbol{K}_{r,r}),$$

where $\mathrm{tr}\{\boldsymbol{W}_{22}^{-1}\}^2$ *and* $\mathrm{tr}\{\boldsymbol{W}_{22}^{-1}\boldsymbol{W}_{22}^{-1}\}$ *are given in statement (iv) and statement (vi), respectively.*

(viii) $E[\boldsymbol{A}(\boldsymbol{A}'\boldsymbol{W}^{-1}\boldsymbol{A})^{-}\boldsymbol{A}'\boldsymbol{W}^{-1}] = \boldsymbol{A}(\boldsymbol{A}'\boldsymbol{\Sigma}^{-1}\boldsymbol{A})^{-}\boldsymbol{A}'\boldsymbol{\Sigma}^{-1}$.

Proof Proofs of statements (i)–(vi) can be obtained from Kollo and von Rosen (2005, Theorem 2.4.14). Concerning statement (vii), it is noted that $\boldsymbol{W}_{12}\boldsymbol{W}_{22}^{-1/2} \sim N_{r,p-r}(\boldsymbol{0}, \boldsymbol{I}, \boldsymbol{I})$ is independent of $\boldsymbol{W}_{22}$ (see Appendix B, Theorem B.20 (iv)) and Appendix B, Theorem B.19 (v) together with statement (iv) and statement (vi) of this theorem establishes statement (vii). With regard to statement (viii), it is noted that there exists a matrix $\underline{\boldsymbol{A}}$ of full rank such that

$$\boldsymbol{A}(\boldsymbol{A}'\boldsymbol{W}^{-1}\boldsymbol{A})^{-}\boldsymbol{A}'\boldsymbol{W}^{-1} = \underline{\boldsymbol{A}}(\underline{\boldsymbol{A}}'\boldsymbol{W}^{-1}\underline{\boldsymbol{A}})^{-1}\underline{\boldsymbol{A}}'\boldsymbol{W}^{-1}.$$

Moreover, there exist a non-singular matrix $\boldsymbol{T}$ and an orthogonal matrix $\boldsymbol{\Gamma}$ such that $\underline{\boldsymbol{A}}' = \boldsymbol{T}(\boldsymbol{I} : \boldsymbol{0})\boldsymbol{\Gamma}\boldsymbol{\Sigma}^{1/2} = \boldsymbol{T}\boldsymbol{\Gamma}_1\boldsymbol{\Sigma}^{1/2}$, and a $\boldsymbol{V} = \boldsymbol{\Gamma}\boldsymbol{\Sigma}^{-1/2}\boldsymbol{W}\boldsymbol{\Sigma}^{-1/2}\boldsymbol{\Gamma}' \sim W_p(\boldsymbol{I}, n)$. Then

$$E[\boldsymbol{A}(\boldsymbol{A}'\boldsymbol{W}^{-1}\boldsymbol{A})^{-}\boldsymbol{A}'\boldsymbol{W}^{-1}] = E[\boldsymbol{\Sigma}^{1/2}\boldsymbol{\Gamma}_1'(\boldsymbol{V}^{11})^{-1}(\boldsymbol{V}^{11} : \boldsymbol{V}^{12})\boldsymbol{\Gamma}\boldsymbol{\Sigma}^{-1/2}] \\ - \boldsymbol{\Sigma}^{1/2}\boldsymbol{\Gamma}_1'\boldsymbol{\Gamma}_1\boldsymbol{\Sigma}^{-1/2} = \boldsymbol{A}(\boldsymbol{A}'\boldsymbol{\Sigma}^{-1}\boldsymbol{A})^{-}\boldsymbol{A}'\boldsymbol{\Sigma}^{-1},$$

since $E[(\boldsymbol{V}^{11})^{-1}\boldsymbol{V}^{12}] = -E[\boldsymbol{V}_{12}\boldsymbol{V}_{22}^{-1}] = \boldsymbol{0}$. □

B.16 A Property and Moments for the Multivariate β Type I Distribution

Theorem B.22 *Let* $\boldsymbol{F} \sim M\beta_I(p, m, n)$, *and let* $\boldsymbol{W}_1$ *and* $\boldsymbol{W}_2$ *be as in Sect. A.9. Then*

(i) *one choice of* $(\boldsymbol{W}_1 + \boldsymbol{W}_2)^{1/2}$ *is a unique lower triangular matrix with positive diagonal elements, let us say* $\boldsymbol{T}$, *such that* $(\boldsymbol{W}_1 + \boldsymbol{W}_2) = \boldsymbol{T}\boldsymbol{T}'$ *and* $\boldsymbol{F} = \boldsymbol{T}^{-1}\boldsymbol{W}_2(\boldsymbol{T}')^{-1}$;

(ii) $E[\boldsymbol{F}] = \frac{m}{m+n}\boldsymbol{I}_p$;

(iii) $E[\boldsymbol{F}^{-1}] = \frac{m+n-p-1}{m-p-1}\boldsymbol{I}_p$.

Proof Statement (i) follows from a remark made after Theorem 2.4.8 in Kollo and von Rosen (2005). Moreover, the proof of statement (ii) is given in Theorem 2.4.15

(iii) in Kollo and von Rosen (2005), and statement (iii) follows from the proof of Theorem 2.4.15 (i) in the same book. □

B.17 Special Moment Relations

Theorem B.23 *Let* $\boldsymbol{Y} \sim N_{p,n}(\boldsymbol{0}, \boldsymbol{\Sigma}, \boldsymbol{\Psi})$ *and* $\boldsymbol{Z} \sim N_{p,n}(\boldsymbol{0}, \boldsymbol{I}_p, \boldsymbol{I}_n)$. *Then*

(i) *for the known constants* q_1 *and* q_2, *and the known symmetric matrices* $\boldsymbol{M}$ *and* $\boldsymbol{N}$,

$$E[q_1\mathrm{vec}(\boldsymbol{Y})\mathrm{vec}'(\boldsymbol{Y}) + q_2\mathrm{tr}\{\boldsymbol{MYNY}'\}\mathrm{vec}(\boldsymbol{Y})\mathrm{vec}'(\boldsymbol{Y})]$$
$$= q_1\boldsymbol{\Psi} \otimes \boldsymbol{\Sigma} + q_2\mathrm{tr}\{\boldsymbol{N\Psi}\}\mathrm{tr}\{\boldsymbol{M\Sigma}\}\boldsymbol{\Psi} \otimes \boldsymbol{\Sigma} + 2q_2\boldsymbol{\Psi N\Psi} \otimes \boldsymbol{\Sigma M\Sigma};$$

(ii) $E[\mathbf{Z}'(\mathbf{ZZ}')^{-1}\mathbf{Z}] = \frac{p}{n}\boldsymbol{I}_n$.

Proof To verify statement (i), the statement is vectorized, i.e. instead of $\mathrm{vec}\boldsymbol{Y}\mathrm{vec}'\boldsymbol{Y}$, $\boldsymbol{\Psi} \otimes \boldsymbol{\Sigma}$ and $\boldsymbol{\Psi N\Psi} \otimes \boldsymbol{\Sigma M\Sigma}$,

$$\mathrm{vec}(\mathrm{vec}\boldsymbol{Y}\mathrm{vec}'\boldsymbol{Y}) = \mathrm{vec}\boldsymbol{Y} \otimes \mathrm{vec}\boldsymbol{Y},\ \ \mathrm{vec}(\boldsymbol{\Psi} \otimes \boldsymbol{\Sigma}),\ \ \mathrm{vec}(\boldsymbol{\Psi N\Psi} \otimes \boldsymbol{\Sigma M\Sigma})$$

are used. Moreover, note that

$$\mathrm{tr}\{\boldsymbol{MYNY}'\}(\mathrm{vec}\boldsymbol{Y})^{\otimes 2} = (\mathrm{vec}'\boldsymbol{I}_{pn} \otimes \boldsymbol{I}_{(pn)^2})(\boldsymbol{N} \otimes \boldsymbol{I} \otimes \boldsymbol{I} \otimes \boldsymbol{M})(\mathrm{vec}\boldsymbol{Y})^{\otimes 4}.$$

Thus, the fourth moments of a multivariate normally distributed variable are needed. From results in Kollo and von Rosen (2005, Corollary 2.2.7.4), it follows that

$$E[(\mathrm{vec}\boldsymbol{Y})^{\otimes 2}] = \mathrm{vec}(\boldsymbol{\Psi} \otimes \boldsymbol{\Sigma}),$$
$$E[(\mathrm{vec}\boldsymbol{Y})^{\otimes 4}] = (\boldsymbol{I}_{(pn)^4} + \boldsymbol{I}_{pn} \otimes \boldsymbol{K}_{pn,pn} \otimes \boldsymbol{I}_{pn} + \boldsymbol{I}_{pn} \otimes \boldsymbol{K}_{(pn)^2,pn})(\mathrm{vec}(\boldsymbol{\Psi} \otimes \boldsymbol{\Sigma}))^{\otimes 2}.$$

Utilizing these expressions, the statement follows from the following facts:

- $(\mathrm{vec}'\boldsymbol{I}_{pn} \otimes \boldsymbol{I}_{(pn)^2})(\boldsymbol{N} \otimes \boldsymbol{I} \otimes \boldsymbol{I} \otimes \boldsymbol{M})(\mathrm{vec}(\boldsymbol{\Psi} \otimes \boldsymbol{\Sigma}))^{\otimes 2}$
  $= \mathrm{tr}\{\boldsymbol{N\Psi}\}\mathrm{tr}\{\boldsymbol{M\Sigma}\}\mathrm{vec}(\boldsymbol{\Psi} \otimes \boldsymbol{\Sigma})$,
- $(\mathrm{vec}'\boldsymbol{I}_{pn} \otimes \boldsymbol{I}_{(pn)^2})(\boldsymbol{N} \otimes \boldsymbol{I} \otimes \boldsymbol{I} \otimes \boldsymbol{M})(\boldsymbol{I}_{pn} \otimes \boldsymbol{K}_{pn,pn} \otimes \boldsymbol{I}_{pn})(\mathrm{vec}(\boldsymbol{\Psi} \otimes \boldsymbol{\Sigma}))^{\otimes 2}$
  $= \mathrm{vec}(\boldsymbol{\Psi N\Psi} \otimes \boldsymbol{\Sigma M\Sigma})$,
- $(\mathrm{vec}'\boldsymbol{I}_{pn} \otimes \boldsymbol{I}_{(pn)^2})(\boldsymbol{N} \otimes \boldsymbol{I} \otimes \boldsymbol{I} \otimes \boldsymbol{M})(\boldsymbol{I}_{pn} \otimes \boldsymbol{K}_{(pn)^2,pn})(\mathrm{vec}(\boldsymbol{\Psi} \otimes \boldsymbol{\Sigma}))^{\otimes 2}$
  $= \mathrm{vec}(\boldsymbol{\Psi N\Psi} \otimes \boldsymbol{\Sigma M\Sigma})$.

To prove statement (ii), a different technique is used. Note that for all orthogonal matrices, $\boldsymbol{\Gamma}$,

$$\boldsymbol{\Gamma}'E[\mathbf{Z}'(\mathbf{ZZ}')^{-1}\mathbf{Z}]\boldsymbol{\Gamma} = E[\mathbf{Z}'(\mathbf{ZZ}')^{-1}\mathbf{Z}],$$

since $\boldsymbol{\Gamma}'\boldsymbol{Z}'(\boldsymbol{Z}\boldsymbol{Z}')^{-1}\boldsymbol{Z}\boldsymbol{\Gamma} = \boldsymbol{\Gamma}'\boldsymbol{Z}'(\boldsymbol{Z}\boldsymbol{\Gamma}\boldsymbol{\Gamma}'\boldsymbol{Z}')^{-1}\boldsymbol{Z}\boldsymbol{\Gamma}$, and the distribution of $\boldsymbol{Z}\boldsymbol{\Gamma}$ equals the distribution of $\boldsymbol{Z}$. Thus, $E[\boldsymbol{Z}'(\boldsymbol{Z}\boldsymbol{Z}')^{-1}\boldsymbol{Z}] = c\boldsymbol{I}_n$ for some constant c. Now the constant is determined by taking the trace, giving $p = cn$, and the statement is established. □

Theorem B.24 *Let* $\boldsymbol{W} \sim W_p(\boldsymbol{\Sigma}, n)$ *and* $\boldsymbol{A}$: $p \times q$. *The constants* $c_{i;n,s,t}$, $i = 1, 2, 3$, *are given in Definition B.1. Then*

$$
\begin{aligned}
E[\boldsymbol{A}(\boldsymbol{A}'\boldsymbol{W}\boldsymbol{A})^{-}\boldsymbol{A}' \otimes \boldsymbol{W}^{-1}] &= c_{1;n,r(A),p}\boldsymbol{A}(\boldsymbol{A}'\boldsymbol{\Sigma}\boldsymbol{A})^{-}\boldsymbol{A}' \otimes \boldsymbol{A}(\boldsymbol{A}'\boldsymbol{\Sigma}\boldsymbol{A})^{-}\boldsymbol{A}'\\
&+c_{2;n,r(A),p}(\mathrm{vec}(\boldsymbol{A}(\boldsymbol{A}'\boldsymbol{\Sigma}\boldsymbol{A})^{-}\boldsymbol{A}')\mathrm{vec}'(\boldsymbol{A}(\boldsymbol{A}'\boldsymbol{\Sigma}\boldsymbol{A})^{-}\boldsymbol{A}')\\
&\quad+\boldsymbol{K}_{p,p}\boldsymbol{A}(\boldsymbol{A}'\boldsymbol{\Sigma}\boldsymbol{A})^{-}\boldsymbol{A}' \otimes \boldsymbol{A}(\boldsymbol{A}'\boldsymbol{\Sigma}\boldsymbol{A})^{-}\boldsymbol{A}')\\
&+c_{3;n,r(A),p}\boldsymbol{A}(\boldsymbol{A}'\boldsymbol{\Sigma}\boldsymbol{A})^{-}\boldsymbol{A}' \otimes (\boldsymbol{\Sigma}^{-1} - \boldsymbol{A}(\boldsymbol{A}'\boldsymbol{\Sigma}\boldsymbol{A})^{-}\boldsymbol{A}').
\end{aligned}
$$

Proof Without any loss of generality, identify $\boldsymbol{A}$ by $\underline{\boldsymbol{A}}$, $p \times r(\boldsymbol{A})$ and use that $\underline{\boldsymbol{A}}' = \boldsymbol{T}(\boldsymbol{I}_{r(A)} : \boldsymbol{0})\boldsymbol{\Gamma}\boldsymbol{\Sigma}^{-1/2}$ for some non-singular $\boldsymbol{T}$ and orthogonal $\boldsymbol{\Gamma}$. Moreover, put

$$
\boldsymbol{V} = \boldsymbol{\Gamma}\boldsymbol{\Sigma}^{-1/2}\boldsymbol{W}\boldsymbol{\Sigma}^{-1/2}\boldsymbol{\Gamma}'.
$$

Then

$$
\begin{aligned}
&E[\boldsymbol{A}(\boldsymbol{A}'\boldsymbol{W}\boldsymbol{A})^{-}\boldsymbol{A}' \otimes \boldsymbol{W}^{-1}]\\
&= (\boldsymbol{\Sigma}^{-1/2}\boldsymbol{\Gamma}')^{\otimes 2}(E[\begin{pmatrix} \boldsymbol{V}_{11}^{-1} & \boldsymbol{0} \\ \boldsymbol{0} & \boldsymbol{0} \end{pmatrix}^{\otimes 2}] + E[\begin{pmatrix} \boldsymbol{V}_{11}^{-1} & \boldsymbol{0} \\ \boldsymbol{0} & \boldsymbol{0} \end{pmatrix} \otimes \boldsymbol{H}])(\boldsymbol{\Gamma}\boldsymbol{\Sigma}^{-1/2})^{\otimes 2},
\end{aligned}
$$

where

$$
\boldsymbol{H} = \begin{pmatrix} -\boldsymbol{V}_{11}^{-1}\boldsymbol{V}_{12} \\ \boldsymbol{I} \end{pmatrix} (\boldsymbol{V}_{22} - \boldsymbol{V}_{21}\boldsymbol{V}_{11}^{-1}\boldsymbol{V}_{12})^{-1}(-\boldsymbol{V}_{21}\boldsymbol{V}_{11}^{-1} : \boldsymbol{I}).
$$

Let $\boldsymbol{V} = \boldsymbol{U}\boldsymbol{U}'$, $\boldsymbol{V}_{11} = \boldsymbol{U}_1\boldsymbol{U}_1'$ and $\boldsymbol{V}_{12} = \boldsymbol{U}_1\boldsymbol{U}_2'$, where

$$
\boldsymbol{U} = (\boldsymbol{U}_1' : \boldsymbol{U}_2')', \quad \boldsymbol{U}_1 : r(\boldsymbol{A}) \times n, \quad \boldsymbol{U}_2 : (p - r(\boldsymbol{A})) \times n, \quad \boldsymbol{U} \sim N_{p,n}(\boldsymbol{0}, \boldsymbol{I}, \boldsymbol{I}).
$$

It can be noted that, given $\boldsymbol{U}_1$, the matrix $\boldsymbol{V}_{21}\boldsymbol{V}_{11}^{-1}$ is independent of $\boldsymbol{V}_{2\bullet 1} = \boldsymbol{V}_{22} - \boldsymbol{V}_{21}\boldsymbol{V}_{11}^{-1}\boldsymbol{V}_{12}$. Therefore, $E[\boldsymbol{V}_{11}^{-1}\boldsymbol{V}_{12}\boldsymbol{V}_{2\bullet 1}^{-1}|\boldsymbol{U}_1] = \boldsymbol{0}$, and

$$
\begin{aligned}
E[\begin{pmatrix} \boldsymbol{V}_{11}^{-1} & \boldsymbol{0} \\ \boldsymbol{0} & \boldsymbol{0} \end{pmatrix} \otimes \boldsymbol{H}] &= E[E[\begin{pmatrix} \boldsymbol{V}_{11}^{-1} & \boldsymbol{0} \\ \boldsymbol{0} & \boldsymbol{0} \end{pmatrix} \otimes \boldsymbol{H}|\boldsymbol{U}_1]]\\
&= E[\begin{pmatrix} \boldsymbol{V}_{11}^{-1} & \boldsymbol{0} \\ \boldsymbol{0} & \boldsymbol{0} \end{pmatrix} \otimes \begin{pmatrix} E[\boldsymbol{V}_{11}^{-1}\boldsymbol{V}_{12}\boldsymbol{V}_{2\bullet 1}^{-1}\boldsymbol{V}_{21}\boldsymbol{V}_{11}^{-1}|\boldsymbol{U}_1] & \boldsymbol{0} \\ \boldsymbol{0} & E[\boldsymbol{V}_{2\bullet 1}^{-1}|\boldsymbol{U}_1] \end{pmatrix}].
\end{aligned}
$$

Moreover, $E[V_{2\bullet 1}^{-1}|U_1] = \frac{1}{n-p-1}I_{p-r(A)}$. Hence,

$$E[\begin{pmatrix} V_{11}^{-1} & 0 \\ 0 & 0 \end{pmatrix} \otimes H] = \frac{1}{n-p-1}E[\begin{pmatrix} V_{11}^{-1} & 0 \\ 0 & 0 \end{pmatrix} \otimes \begin{pmatrix} (p-r(A))V_{11}^{-1} & 0 \\ 0 & I \end{pmatrix}].$$

Now, according to Theorem B.21 (i) and (iii),

$$E[V_{11}^{-1}] = \frac{1}{n-r(A)-1}I_{r(A)}$$

and

$$E[(V_{11}^{-1})^{\otimes 2}] = c_{1;n,r(A)}I_{r(A)^2} + c_{2;n,r(A)}(\mathrm{vec}I_{r(A)}\mathrm{vec}'I_{r(A)} + K_{r(A),r(A)}),$$

and it also follows that $\Sigma^{-1/2}\Gamma'(I_{r(A)} : 0)'(I_{r(A)} : 0)\Gamma\Sigma^{-1/2} = A(A'\Sigma A)^{-}A'$, which in turn implies that $\Sigma^{-1/2}\Gamma'(0 : I_{p-r(A)})'(0 : I_{p-r(A)})\Gamma\Sigma^{-1/2} = \Sigma^{-1} - A(A'\Sigma A)^{-}A'$. Summing up, all these calculations yield the result of the theorem. □

The next theorem includes a minor generalization of Theorem B.24 and the proof rests completely on this theorem.

Theorem B.25 *Let $W \sim W_p(\Sigma, n)$, A: $p\times q$ and B: $p\times r$ such that $\mathcal{C}(B) \subseteq \mathcal{C}(A)$. Then*

$$\begin{aligned} E[B(B'WB)^{-}B' \otimes A(A'WA)^{-}A'] &= c_{1;n,r(B),r(A)}B(B'\Sigma B)^{-}B' \otimes B(B'\Sigma B)^{-}B' \\ &+ c_{2;n,r(B),r(A)}(\mathrm{vec}(B(B'\Sigma B)^{-}B')\mathrm{vec}'(B(B'\Sigma B)^{-}B') \\ &\quad + K_{p,p}(B(B'\Sigma B)^{-}B' \otimes B(B'\Sigma B)^{-}B')) \\ &+ c_{3;n,r(B),r(A)}B(B'\Sigma B)^{-}B' \otimes (A(A'\Sigma A)^{-}A' - B(B'\Sigma B)^{-}B'), \end{aligned}$$

where $c_{1;n,s,t}$, $c_{2;n,s,t}$ and $c_{3;n,s,t}$ are given in Definition B.1 in this appendix.

Proof Since $\mathcal{C}(B) \subseteq \mathcal{C}(A)$, the trivial relation $P_AB = B$ holds. Thus,

$$B(B'WB)^{-}B' = P_AB(B'P_AWP_AB)^{-}B'P_A.$$

Moreover, $A' = T(I_{r(A)} : 0)\Gamma'$, where Γ is orthogonal, T is non-singular and

$$P_A = \Gamma_1\Gamma_1', \quad \Gamma = (\Gamma_1 : \Gamma_2), \quad (p \times r(A) : p \times (p - r(A))).$$

Therefore,

$$\begin{aligned} &B(B'WB)^{-}B' \otimes A(A'WA)^{-}A' \\ &\quad = (\Gamma_1 \otimes \Gamma_1)(\Gamma_1'B(B'\Gamma_1V\Gamma_1'B)^{-}B'\Gamma_1 \otimes V^{-1})(\Gamma_1' \otimes \Gamma_1'), \end{aligned}$$

where $V \sim W_{r(A)}(\boldsymbol{\Gamma}_1'\boldsymbol{\Sigma}\boldsymbol{\Gamma}_1, n)$. Now the result follows from Theorem B.24, since

$$\boldsymbol{\Gamma}_1\boldsymbol{\Gamma}_1'\boldsymbol{B}(\boldsymbol{B}'\boldsymbol{\Gamma}_1\boldsymbol{\Gamma}_1'\boldsymbol{\Sigma}\boldsymbol{\Gamma}_1\boldsymbol{\Gamma}_1'\boldsymbol{B})^{-}\boldsymbol{B}'\boldsymbol{\Gamma}_1\boldsymbol{\Gamma}_1' = \boldsymbol{B}(\boldsymbol{B}'\boldsymbol{\Sigma}\boldsymbol{B})^{-}\boldsymbol{B}'$$

and

$$\boldsymbol{\Gamma}_1(\boldsymbol{\Gamma}_1'\boldsymbol{\Sigma}\boldsymbol{\Gamma}_1)^{-1}\boldsymbol{\Gamma}_1' = \boldsymbol{A}(\boldsymbol{A}'\boldsymbol{\Sigma}\boldsymbol{A})^{-}\boldsymbol{A}'.$$

□

Theorem B.26 *Let* $\boldsymbol{S} = \boldsymbol{X}(\boldsymbol{I} - \boldsymbol{P}_{C'})\boldsymbol{X}'$, *where* $\boldsymbol{X} \sim N_{p,n}(\boldsymbol{\mu}, \boldsymbol{\Sigma}, \boldsymbol{I})$, $\boldsymbol{\mu}' \in \mathcal{C}(\boldsymbol{C}')$ *and* $\boldsymbol{A}$: $p \times q$. *Moreover, let the constants* $c_{i;n,s,t}$, $i = 1, 2, 3$, *be given in Definition B.1 in this appendix. Then*

(i) $E[\boldsymbol{S}^{-1}\boldsymbol{A}(\boldsymbol{A}'\boldsymbol{S}^{-1}\boldsymbol{A})^{-}\boldsymbol{A}'\boldsymbol{S}^{-1}]$
$= c_{0;n-r(C),p}\boldsymbol{\Sigma}^{-1} - c_{0;n-r(C),p-r(A)}\boldsymbol{A}^{o}(\boldsymbol{A}^{o'}\boldsymbol{\Sigma}\boldsymbol{A}^{o})^{-}\boldsymbol{A}^{o'}$;

(ii) $E[\boldsymbol{A}(\boldsymbol{A}'\boldsymbol{S}^{-1}\boldsymbol{A})^{-}\boldsymbol{A}'\boldsymbol{S}^{-1}\boldsymbol{\Sigma}\boldsymbol{S}^{-1}\boldsymbol{A}(\boldsymbol{A}'\boldsymbol{S}^{-1}\boldsymbol{A})^{-}\boldsymbol{A}']$
$= \frac{n-r(C)-1}{n-r(C)-p+r(A)-1}\boldsymbol{A}(\boldsymbol{A}'\boldsymbol{\Sigma}^{-1}\boldsymbol{A})^{-}\boldsymbol{A}'$;

(iii) $E[\boldsymbol{S}^{-1}\boldsymbol{A}(\boldsymbol{A}'\boldsymbol{S}^{-1}\boldsymbol{A})^{-}\boldsymbol{A}'\boldsymbol{S}^{-1}\boldsymbol{\Sigma}\boldsymbol{S}^{-1}\boldsymbol{A}(\boldsymbol{A}'\boldsymbol{S}^{-1}\boldsymbol{A})^{-}\boldsymbol{A}'\boldsymbol{S}^{-1}] = ((p+1)c_{2;n,p} + c_{1;n,p})\boldsymbol{\Sigma}^{-1} + ((p - r(A) + 1)(c_{2;n,p-r(A)} - 2c_{2;n,r(A),p-r(A)}) + c_{1;n,p-r(A)} - c_{1;n,r(A),p-r(A)}) \times \boldsymbol{A}^{o}(\boldsymbol{A}^{o'}\boldsymbol{\Sigma}\boldsymbol{A}^{o})^{-}\boldsymbol{A}^{o'}$.

Proof Concerning statement (i), it is noted that

$$\boldsymbol{S}^{-1}\boldsymbol{A}(\boldsymbol{A}'\boldsymbol{S}^{-1}\boldsymbol{A})^{-}\boldsymbol{A}'\boldsymbol{S}^{-1} = \boldsymbol{S}^{-1} - \boldsymbol{A}^{o}(\boldsymbol{A}^{o'}\boldsymbol{S}\boldsymbol{A}^{o})^{-}\boldsymbol{A}^{o'}$$

and, according to Theorem B.21 (i),

$$E[\boldsymbol{S}^{-1}] = c_{0,n-r(C),p}\boldsymbol{\Sigma}^{-1},$$

$$E[\boldsymbol{A}^{o}(\boldsymbol{A}^{o'}\boldsymbol{S}\boldsymbol{A}^{o})^{-}\boldsymbol{A}^{o'}] = c_{0,n-r(C),p-r(A)}\boldsymbol{A}^{o}(\boldsymbol{A}^{o'}\boldsymbol{\Sigma}\boldsymbol{A}^{o})^{-}\boldsymbol{A}^{o'},$$

which establishes statement (i).

Concerning statement (ii), suppose, without any loss of generality, that $\boldsymbol{A}$ is of full rank and factor $\boldsymbol{A}$ as $\boldsymbol{A}' = \boldsymbol{T}(\boldsymbol{I} : \boldsymbol{0})\boldsymbol{\Gamma}\boldsymbol{\Sigma}^{1/2}$, where $\boldsymbol{T}$ is non-singular and $\boldsymbol{\Gamma}$ orthogonal. Utilizing Theorem B.21 (vii) establishes the result.

The expression in statement (iii) is more complicated to handle than statement (ii). Note that

$$\begin{aligned} &E[\boldsymbol{S}^{-1}\boldsymbol{A}(\boldsymbol{A}'\boldsymbol{S}^{-1}\boldsymbol{A})^{-}\boldsymbol{A}'\boldsymbol{S}^{-1}\boldsymbol{\Sigma}\boldsymbol{S}^{-1}\boldsymbol{A}(\boldsymbol{A}'\boldsymbol{S}^{-1}\boldsymbol{A})^{-}\boldsymbol{A}'\boldsymbol{S}^{-1}] \\ &\quad = E[(\boldsymbol{S}^{-1} - \boldsymbol{A}^{o}(\boldsymbol{A}^{o'}\boldsymbol{S}\boldsymbol{A}^{o})^{-1}\boldsymbol{A}^{o'})\boldsymbol{\Sigma}(\boldsymbol{S}^{-1} - \boldsymbol{A}^{o}(\boldsymbol{A}^{o'}\boldsymbol{S}\boldsymbol{A}^{o})^{-1}\boldsymbol{A}^{o'})] \end{aligned}$$

and, therefore, the following three types of moment calculations are needed: $E[\boldsymbol{S}^{-1}\boldsymbol{\Sigma}\boldsymbol{S}^{-1}]$, $E[\boldsymbol{A}^{o}(\boldsymbol{A}^{o'}\boldsymbol{S}\boldsymbol{A}^{o})^{-1}\boldsymbol{A}^{o'}\boldsymbol{\Sigma}\boldsymbol{A}^{o}(\boldsymbol{A}^{o'}\boldsymbol{S}\boldsymbol{A}^{o})^{-1}\boldsymbol{A}^{o'}]$ and $E[\boldsymbol{S}^{-1}\boldsymbol{\Sigma}\boldsymbol{A}^{o}(\boldsymbol{A}^{o'}\boldsymbol{S}\boldsymbol{A}^{o})^{-1}\boldsymbol{A}^{o'}]$.

Since $\boldsymbol{\Sigma}^{-1/2}\boldsymbol{S}\boldsymbol{\Sigma}^{-1/2} \sim W_p(\boldsymbol{I}, n)$, according to Theorem B.21 (v),

$$E[\boldsymbol{S}^{-1}\boldsymbol{\Sigma}\boldsymbol{S}^{-1}] = \boldsymbol{\Sigma}^{-1/2}E[(\boldsymbol{\Sigma}^{-1/2}\boldsymbol{S}\boldsymbol{\Sigma}^{-1/2})^{-1}(\boldsymbol{\Sigma}^{-1/2}\boldsymbol{S}\boldsymbol{\Sigma}^{-1/2})^{-1}]\boldsymbol{\Sigma}^{-1/2}$$
$$= (c_{2;n,p} + c_{1;n,p})\boldsymbol{\Sigma}^{-1} + c_{2;n,p}p\boldsymbol{\Sigma}^{-1}. \quad \text{(B.1)}$$

Similarly, since $(\boldsymbol{A}^{o'}\boldsymbol{\Sigma}\boldsymbol{A}^o)^{-1/2}\boldsymbol{A}^{o'}\boldsymbol{S}\boldsymbol{A}^{o'}(\boldsymbol{A}^{o'}\boldsymbol{\Sigma}\boldsymbol{A}^o)^{-1/2} \sim W_{p-r(A)}(\boldsymbol{I}, n)$, applying Theorem B.21 (v) once again yields

$$E[\boldsymbol{A}^o(\boldsymbol{A}^{o'}\boldsymbol{S}\boldsymbol{A}^o)^{-1}\boldsymbol{A}^{o'}\boldsymbol{\Sigma}\boldsymbol{A}^o(\boldsymbol{A}^{o'}\boldsymbol{S}\boldsymbol{A}^o)^{-1}\boldsymbol{A}^{o'}]$$
$$= (c_{2;n,p-r(A)} + c_{1;n,p-r(A)} + c_{2;n,p-r(A)}(p - r(\boldsymbol{A})))\boldsymbol{A}^o(\boldsymbol{A}^{o'}\boldsymbol{\Sigma}\boldsymbol{A}^o)^{-1}\boldsymbol{A}^{o'}. \quad \text{(B.2)}$$

Concerning the third type of moment expressions, it is convenient to rely on Theorem B.24. Post-multiplying the statement of Theorem B.24 by $\text{vec}\boldsymbol{\Sigma}$ and replacing $\boldsymbol{A}$ by $\boldsymbol{A}^o$: $p \times p - r(\boldsymbol{A})$ leads to

$$E[\boldsymbol{A}^o(\boldsymbol{A}^{o'}\boldsymbol{W}\boldsymbol{A}^o)^-\boldsymbol{A}^{o'} \otimes \boldsymbol{W}^{-1}]\text{vec}\boldsymbol{\Sigma} = \text{vec}(E[\boldsymbol{W}^{-1}\boldsymbol{\Sigma}\boldsymbol{A}^o(\boldsymbol{A}^{o'}\boldsymbol{W}\boldsymbol{A}^o)^-\boldsymbol{A}^{o'}])$$
$$= c_{1;n,r(A),p-r(A)}\text{vec}(\boldsymbol{A}^o(\boldsymbol{A}^{o'}\boldsymbol{\Sigma}\boldsymbol{A}^o)^-\boldsymbol{A}^{o'})$$
$$+ c_{2;n,r(A),p-r(A)}((p - r(\boldsymbol{A}))\text{vec}(\boldsymbol{A}^o(\boldsymbol{A}^{o'}\boldsymbol{\Sigma}\boldsymbol{A}^o)^-\boldsymbol{A}^{o'}) + \text{vec}(\boldsymbol{A}^o(\boldsymbol{A}^{o'}\boldsymbol{\Sigma}\boldsymbol{A}^o)^-\boldsymbol{A}^{o'})).$$

Thus, $E[\boldsymbol{W}^{-1}\boldsymbol{\Sigma}\boldsymbol{A}^o(\boldsymbol{A}^{o'}\boldsymbol{W}\boldsymbol{A}^o)^-\boldsymbol{A}^{o'}] = E[\boldsymbol{A}^o(\boldsymbol{A}^{o'}\boldsymbol{W}\boldsymbol{A}^o)^-\boldsymbol{A}o'\boldsymbol{\Sigma}\boldsymbol{W}^{-1}]$ and

$$E[\boldsymbol{W}^{-1}\boldsymbol{\Sigma}\boldsymbol{A}^o(\boldsymbol{A}^{o'}\boldsymbol{W}\boldsymbol{A}^o)^-\boldsymbol{A}^{o'}]$$
$$= (c_{1;n,r(A),p-r(A)} + c_{2;n,r(A),p-r(A)}(p - r(\boldsymbol{A}) + 1))\boldsymbol{A}^o(\boldsymbol{A}^{o'}\boldsymbol{\Sigma}\boldsymbol{A}^o)^-\boldsymbol{A}^{o'}). \quad \text{(B.3)}$$

Summing (B.1) and (B.2), and subtracting two times (B.3) establish statement (iii). □

Problems

1 For any $\boldsymbol{A}$ and $\boldsymbol{C}$ such that $\mathcal{C}(\boldsymbol{C}') \subseteq \mathcal{C}(\boldsymbol{A}')$ and $\boldsymbol{V}$, p.d., of proper sizes, show that $\boldsymbol{C}(\boldsymbol{A}'\boldsymbol{V}\boldsymbol{A})^-\boldsymbol{A}'\boldsymbol{V}\boldsymbol{A} = \boldsymbol{C}$.

2 Show that $\boldsymbol{A}\boldsymbol{X}^-\boldsymbol{C}$ does not depend on the choice of g-inverse if and only if $\mathcal{C}(\boldsymbol{A}') \subseteq \mathcal{C}(\boldsymbol{X}')$ and $\mathcal{C}(\boldsymbol{C}) \subseteq \mathcal{C}(\boldsymbol{X})$ hold.

3 Suppose that all the given operations are well defined. Show that

$$\boldsymbol{A}\boldsymbol{A}'(\boldsymbol{A}\boldsymbol{A}' + \boldsymbol{B}\boldsymbol{B}')^-\boldsymbol{B}\boldsymbol{B}' = \boldsymbol{B}\boldsymbol{B}'(\boldsymbol{A}\boldsymbol{A}' + \boldsymbol{B}\boldsymbol{B}')^-\boldsymbol{A}\boldsymbol{A}'.$$

4 Suppose that there is a simple matrix block structure whose inverse exists and which is as follows:

$$\begin{pmatrix} \boldsymbol{A} & \boldsymbol{B} \\ -\boldsymbol{B} & \boldsymbol{A} \end{pmatrix}.$$

Derive its inverse.

Suppose now that a minor extension of the above block structure is available, providing the following structure:

$$\begin{pmatrix} \boldsymbol{A} & \boldsymbol{B} & \boldsymbol{C} & \boldsymbol{D} \\ -\boldsymbol{B} & \boldsymbol{A} & -\boldsymbol{D} & \boldsymbol{C} \\ -\boldsymbol{C} & \boldsymbol{D} & \boldsymbol{A} & -\boldsymbol{B} \\ -\boldsymbol{D} & -\boldsymbol{C} & \boldsymbol{B} & \boldsymbol{A} \end{pmatrix}.$$

Derive the inverse matrix of the given block structure. Try to find out why these structures are connected to complex numbers and quaternions.

5 Let $\boldsymbol{A}$ and $\boldsymbol{B}$ be of proper sizes. Show that $\mathcal{C}(\boldsymbol{A}\boldsymbol{A}'\boldsymbol{B}^o) \cap \mathcal{C}(\boldsymbol{B}) = \{\boldsymbol{0}\}$.

6 Show that $\mathcal{C}(\boldsymbol{A}_1 \otimes \boldsymbol{B}_1)$ is orthogonal to $\mathcal{C}(\boldsymbol{A}_2 \otimes \boldsymbol{B}_2)$ if and only if $\mathcal{C}(\boldsymbol{A}_1)$ is orthogonal to $\mathcal{C}(\boldsymbol{A}_2)$ or $\mathcal{C}(\boldsymbol{B}_1)$ is orthogonal to $\mathcal{C}(\boldsymbol{B}_2)$.

7 A subspace $\mathcal{C}(\boldsymbol{M})$ is $\boldsymbol{A}$-invariant if $\mathcal{C}(\boldsymbol{A}\boldsymbol{M}) \subseteq \mathcal{C}(\boldsymbol{M})$. Show that $\mathcal{C}(\boldsymbol{M})$ is $\boldsymbol{A}$-invariant if and only if $\mathcal{C}(\boldsymbol{M})^{\perp}$ is $\boldsymbol{A}'$-invariant.

8 Let $\boldsymbol{A}$: $p \times q$, $\boldsymbol{B}$: $q \times r$, $\boldsymbol{C}$: $r \times s$ and $\boldsymbol{D}$: $s \times p$. Show that $\mathrm{tr}\{\boldsymbol{A}\boldsymbol{B}\boldsymbol{C}\boldsymbol{D}\} = (\mathrm{vec}'(\boldsymbol{C}') \otimes \mathrm{vec}'\boldsymbol{A})(\boldsymbol{I}_r \otimes \boldsymbol{K}_{s,q} \otimes \boldsymbol{I}_p)\mathrm{vec}\boldsymbol{B} \otimes \mathrm{vec}\boldsymbol{D}')$.

9 Let $\boldsymbol{A}$: $r \times s$, $\boldsymbol{B}$: $s \times t$, $\boldsymbol{C}$: $m \times n$ and $\boldsymbol{D}$: $n \times p$. Show that

$$\boldsymbol{A}\boldsymbol{B} \otimes \boldsymbol{C}\boldsymbol{D} = (\boldsymbol{I}_{rm} \otimes \mathrm{vec}'\boldsymbol{D}')(\boldsymbol{I}_r \otimes \mathrm{vec}\boldsymbol{C}'\mathrm{vec}'\boldsymbol{B}' \otimes \boldsymbol{I}_p)(\mathrm{vec}\boldsymbol{A}' \otimes \boldsymbol{I}_{pt}).$$

10 Show that $\boldsymbol{x}^{\otimes 3} = (\boldsymbol{K}_{p,p} \otimes \boldsymbol{I}_p)\boldsymbol{K}_{p^2,p}\boldsymbol{x}^{\otimes 3}$, where $\boldsymbol{x}$ is a vector of size p.

11 Interpret the matrices $\frac{1}{2}(\boldsymbol{I}_{p^2} + \boldsymbol{K}_{p,p})$, $\frac{1}{2}(\boldsymbol{I}_{p^2} - \boldsymbol{K}_{p,p})$ and $(\boldsymbol{K}_{p,p})_d$.

12 Let $\boldsymbol{A}$, $\boldsymbol{B}$ and $\boldsymbol{T}$ be upper triangular matrices and put $\boldsymbol{U} = \boldsymbol{A}\boldsymbol{T}\boldsymbol{B}$. Derive the Jacobian for the transformation from $\boldsymbol{T}$ to $\boldsymbol{U}$.

13 Let $\boldsymbol{T}$ be a Toeplitz matrix. Use a matrix derivative $\frac{d}{d\boldsymbol{T}}$ and study $\frac{d\boldsymbol{T}}{d\boldsymbol{T}}$.

14 Let $\boldsymbol{X} \sim N_{p,n}(\boldsymbol{\mu}, \boldsymbol{\Sigma}, \boldsymbol{\Psi})$. Derive $E[\boldsymbol{X}^{\otimes 4}]$.

15 Let $\boldsymbol{X} \sim N_{p,n}(\boldsymbol{0}, \boldsymbol{\Sigma}, \boldsymbol{\Psi})$, and let $\boldsymbol{A}$, $\boldsymbol{B}$ and $\boldsymbol{C}$ be fixed matrices of proper sizes. Derive $E[\boldsymbol{X}\boldsymbol{A}\boldsymbol{X}' \otimes \boldsymbol{X}\boldsymbol{B}\boldsymbol{X}' \otimes \boldsymbol{X}\boldsymbol{C}\boldsymbol{X}']$.

16 For a matrix normal distribution, show that all the cumulants of an order > 2 equal $\boldsymbol{0}$. Let $\boldsymbol{U} \sim W_p(\boldsymbol{I}_p, n)$ and suppose that $p > n$. Because of Wishartness, $\boldsymbol{U} = \boldsymbol{Y}\boldsymbol{Y}'$, $\boldsymbol{Y} = (\boldsymbol{Y}_1' : \boldsymbol{Y}_2')'$, $\boldsymbol{Y} \sim N_{p,n}(\boldsymbol{0}, \boldsymbol{I}_p, \boldsymbol{I}_n)$ and $\boldsymbol{Y}_1 \sim N_{n,n}(\boldsymbol{0}, \boldsymbol{I}_n, \boldsymbol{I}_n)$; it is assumed that $r(\boldsymbol{Y}_1) = n$. Derive the Moore-Penrose inverse of $\boldsymbol{U}$ as a function of $\boldsymbol{Y}_1$ and $\boldsymbol{Y}_2$.

17 Let $\boldsymbol{X}_1 \sim N_{p,n}(\boldsymbol{\mu}_1, \boldsymbol{\Sigma}_1, \boldsymbol{\Psi}_1)$ and $\boldsymbol{X}_2 \sim N_{p,n}(\boldsymbol{\mu}_2, \boldsymbol{\Sigma}_2, \boldsymbol{\Psi}_2)$, and let $\boldsymbol{Z}$ have a mixture distribution defined through the density

$$f_{\boldsymbol{Z}}(\boldsymbol{X}) = \gamma f_{\boldsymbol{X}_1}(\boldsymbol{X}) + (1-\gamma)\gamma f_{\boldsymbol{X}_2}(\boldsymbol{X}), \qquad 0 < \gamma < 1.$$

Derive $D[\mathbf{Z}]$ and $E[\mathbf{Z}^{\otimes 2}]$.

18 Let $\boldsymbol{W}_1 \sim W_p(\boldsymbol{\Sigma}_1, n)$ and $\boldsymbol{W}_2 \sim W_p(\boldsymbol{\Sigma}_1, m)$. Show that $\boldsymbol{W}_1 + \boldsymbol{W}_2 \sim W_p(\boldsymbol{\Sigma}, n+m)$.

19 Let $\boldsymbol{W} \sim W_p(\boldsymbol{\Sigma}, n)$. Derive $E[\mathrm{tr}\{\boldsymbol{W}^{-1}\}\boldsymbol{W}]$.

20 Let $\boldsymbol{W} \sim W_p(\boldsymbol{\Sigma}, n)$. Derive the asymptotic normal distribution for $\boldsymbol{W}^{-1}$ when $n \to \infty$.

Appendix C: Test Statistics

C.1 Distribution of Test Statistics

The test statistics presented and applied in Chap. 7 are all functions of Wishart-distributed quadratic forms and, in principle, the distributions of the test statistics are derived from assumptions about the MANOVA model as it is discussed in Chap. 7. Let

$$\boldsymbol{X} = \boldsymbol{\mu}\boldsymbol{C} + \boldsymbol{E}, \quad \boldsymbol{E} \sim N_{p,n}(\mathbf{0}, \boldsymbol{\Sigma}, \boldsymbol{I}),$$

where $\boldsymbol{\mu}$: $p \times k$ is the unknown parameter describing the mean, $\boldsymbol{\Sigma}$: $p \times p$ is the unknown positive definite dispersion matrix and $\boldsymbol{C}$: $k \times n$ is a known between-individuals design matrix. Moreover, suppose that the restrictions which are to be tested are given by

$$H_0 : \boldsymbol{\mu}\boldsymbol{G} = \mathbf{0},$$

where $\boldsymbol{G}$ is a known matrix. The hypothesis H_0 is tested against an alternative hypothesis, H_1, which states that $\boldsymbol{\mu}$ is unrestricted. Then the likelihood ratio test statistic in this book is equivalent to $U_{p,m,f}^{-\frac{1}{2}n}$, where

$$U_{p,m,f} = \frac{|n\widehat{\boldsymbol{\Sigma}}_1|}{|n\widehat{\boldsymbol{\Sigma}}_0|}, \tag{C.1}$$

with $f = n - r(\boldsymbol{C})$, $m = \dim\{\mathcal{C}(\boldsymbol{G}) \cap \mathcal{C}(\boldsymbol{C})\}$ and

$$n\widehat{\boldsymbol{\Sigma}}_1 = \boldsymbol{X}(\boldsymbol{I} - \boldsymbol{P}_{C'})\boldsymbol{X}', \quad n\widehat{\boldsymbol{\Sigma}}_0 = \boldsymbol{X}(\boldsymbol{I} - \boldsymbol{P}_{C'G^o})\boldsymbol{X}'.$$

Let $\boldsymbol{N}$ be any matrix satisfying $\mathcal{C}(\boldsymbol{N}) = \mathcal{C}(\boldsymbol{G}) \cap \mathcal{C}(\boldsymbol{C})$, which implies (see the proof of Theorem B.12 in Appendix B) that

$$\mathcal{C}(\boldsymbol{C}'\boldsymbol{G}^o)^\perp = \mathcal{C}(\boldsymbol{C}')^\perp \boxplus \mathcal{C}(\boldsymbol{C}') \cap \mathcal{C}(\boldsymbol{C}'\boldsymbol{G}^o)^\perp = \mathcal{C}(\boldsymbol{C}')^\perp \boxplus \mathcal{C}(\boldsymbol{C}'(\boldsymbol{C}\boldsymbol{C}')^-\boldsymbol{N}).$$

Then

$$\widehat{\boldsymbol{\Sigma}}_0 = \widehat{\boldsymbol{\Sigma}}_1 + \widehat{\boldsymbol{\Sigma}}_2,$$

where $n\widehat{\boldsymbol{\Sigma}}_2 = \boldsymbol{X}\boldsymbol{P}_{C'(CC')^-N}\boldsymbol{X}'$ and

$$U_{p,m,f} = \frac{|n\boldsymbol{\Sigma}_1|}{|n\boldsymbol{\Sigma}_1 + \widehat{\boldsymbol{\mu}}\boldsymbol{N}(\boldsymbol{N}'(\boldsymbol{C}\boldsymbol{C}')^-\boldsymbol{N})^{-1}\boldsymbol{N}'\widehat{\boldsymbol{\mu}}'|},$$

where $\widehat{\boldsymbol{\mu}}\boldsymbol{N} = \boldsymbol{X}\boldsymbol{C}'(\boldsymbol{C}\boldsymbol{C}')^-\boldsymbol{N}$. It also follows that $D[\widehat{\boldsymbol{\mu}}\boldsymbol{N}] = \boldsymbol{N}'(\boldsymbol{C}\boldsymbol{C}')^-\boldsymbol{N}$ and, if the null hypothesis is true, $\widehat{\boldsymbol{\mu}}\boldsymbol{N}$ should be "small". Moreover, the statistic $U_{p,m,f} < 1$ if and only if $\mathcal{C}(\boldsymbol{C}) \cap \mathcal{C}(\boldsymbol{G}) \neq \{\boldsymbol{0}\}$. Often it is assumed that $\mathcal{C}(\boldsymbol{G}) \subseteq \mathcal{C}(\boldsymbol{C})$ (the testability condition), but this is not necessary. The statistic $U_{p,m,f}$ makes sense and is understandable.

Concerning the distribution of $U_{p,m,f}$, $n\widehat{\boldsymbol{\Sigma}}_1 \sim W_p(\boldsymbol{\Sigma}, f)$, under H_0 it follows that $n\widehat{\boldsymbol{\Sigma}}_2 \sim W_p(\boldsymbol{\Sigma}, m)$. Hence, under H_0,

$$U_{p,m,f} = \frac{|\boldsymbol{W}_1|}{|\boldsymbol{W}_1 + \boldsymbol{W}_2|} = |(\boldsymbol{W}_1 + \boldsymbol{W}_2)^{-1/2}\boldsymbol{W}_2(\boldsymbol{W}_1 + \boldsymbol{W}_2)^{-1/2}|, \tag{C.2}$$

where $\boldsymbol{W}_1 \sim W_p(\boldsymbol{\Sigma}, f)$ and $\boldsymbol{W}_2 \sim W_p(\boldsymbol{\Sigma}, m)$, with $\boldsymbol{W}_1$ and $\boldsymbol{W}_2$ independently distributed. The test statistic is invariant with respect to non-singular transformations of $\boldsymbol{X}$ and, therefore, $\boldsymbol{\Sigma}$ may be replaced by $\boldsymbol{I}$; i.e. (C.2) does not depend on $\boldsymbol{\Sigma}$. Thus, $U_{p,m,f}$ is the determinant of a multivariate β-distribution of type I (see Sect. A.9 in Appendix A). The following lemma presents a Bartlett decomposition for $\boldsymbol{F} \sim M\beta_I(p, m, n)$ which provides the fundament for studying the distribution of $U_{p,m,f}$, as well as the distribution of the likelihood ratio test statistic for testing H_0: $\boldsymbol{\mu}\boldsymbol{G} = \boldsymbol{0}$.

Lemma C.1 *Let $\boldsymbol{F} \sim M\beta_I(p, m, n)$ and $\boldsymbol{F} = \boldsymbol{T}\boldsymbol{T}'$, where $\boldsymbol{T}$ is a lower triangular matrix with positive diagonal elements. Then $T_{11}, T_{22}, \ldots, T_{pp}$ are all independent and*

$$T_{ii}^2 \sim \beta(m + 1 - i, n), \quad i = 1, 2, \ldots, p.$$

Proof Since $\boldsymbol{F}$ is positive definite, a lower triangular matrix $\boldsymbol{T}$ always exists such that $\boldsymbol{F} = \boldsymbol{T}\boldsymbol{T}'$. The density for $\boldsymbol{F}$ is given in Appendix A, Sect. A.10, and combining this expression with the factorization $\boldsymbol{F} = \boldsymbol{T}\boldsymbol{T}'$, together with the Jacobian for the variable transformation (see Kollo and von Rosen, 2005, Theorem 1.4.18), yields

$$\begin{aligned}
&\frac{c(p,n)c(p,m)}{c(p,n+m)}|\boldsymbol{T}\boldsymbol{T}'|^{\frac{m-p-1}{2}}|\boldsymbol{I}-\boldsymbol{T}\boldsymbol{T}'|^{\frac{n-p-1}{2}}2^p\prod_{i=1}^{p}T_{ii}^{p-i+1}\\
&\quad=2^p\frac{c(p,n)c(p,m)}{c(p,n+m)}\prod_{i=1}^{p}T_{ii}^{m-i}|\boldsymbol{I}-\boldsymbol{T}\boldsymbol{T}'|^{\frac{n-p-1}{2}}. \qquad \text{(C.3)}
\end{aligned}$$

Now it is shown that T_{11}^2 is beta-distributed. Partition $\boldsymbol{T}$ as follows:

$$\boldsymbol{T}=\begin{pmatrix} T_{11} & \boldsymbol{0} \\ \boldsymbol{t}_{21} & \boldsymbol{T}_{22} \end{pmatrix}.$$

Thus,

$$|\boldsymbol{I}-\boldsymbol{T}\boldsymbol{T}'|=(1-T_{11}^2)(1-\boldsymbol{v}'\boldsymbol{v})|\boldsymbol{I}-\boldsymbol{T}_{22}\boldsymbol{T}_{22}'|,$$

where

$$\boldsymbol{v}=(\boldsymbol{I}-\boldsymbol{T}_{22}\boldsymbol{T}_{22}')^{-1/2}\boldsymbol{t}_{21}(1-T_{11}^2)^{-1/2}.$$

In the next equation, a change of variables takes place, i.e. $T_{11},\boldsymbol{t}_{21},\boldsymbol{T}_{22}\rightarrow T_{11},\boldsymbol{v},\boldsymbol{T}_{22}$, and the corresponding Jacobian equals

$$|\boldsymbol{J}(\boldsymbol{t}_{21},T_{11},\boldsymbol{T}_{22}\rightarrow\boldsymbol{v},T_{11},\boldsymbol{T}_{22})|_+=|\boldsymbol{J}(\boldsymbol{t}_{21}\rightarrow\boldsymbol{v})|_+=(1-T_{11}^2)^{\frac{p-1}{2}}|\boldsymbol{I}-\boldsymbol{T}_{22}\boldsymbol{T}_{22}'|^{\frac{1}{2}},$$

where the last equality was obtained by the definition of a Jacobian (e.g. see Kollo and von Rosen, 2005). Thus, the joint density of T_{11}, $\boldsymbol{v}$ and $\boldsymbol{T}_{22}$ equals

$$\begin{aligned}
&2^p\frac{c(p,n)c(p,m)}{c(p,n+m)}T_{11}^{m-1}(1-T_{11}^2)^{\frac{n-p-1}{2}}\prod_{i=2}^{p}T_{ii}^{m-i}\\
&\qquad\times|\boldsymbol{I}-\boldsymbol{T}_{22}\boldsymbol{T}_{22}'|^{\frac{n-p-1}{2}}(1-\boldsymbol{v}'\boldsymbol{v})^{\frac{n-p-1}{2}}(1-T_{11}^2)^{\frac{p-1}{2}}|\boldsymbol{I}-\boldsymbol{T}_{22}\boldsymbol{T}_{22}'|^{\frac{1}{2}}\\
&\quad=2^p\frac{c(p,n)c(p,m)}{c(p,n+m)}(T_{11}^2)^{\frac{m-1}{2}}(1-T_{11}^2)^{\frac{n}{2}-1}\\
&\qquad\times\prod_{i=2}^{p}T_{ii}^{m-i}|\boldsymbol{I}-\boldsymbol{T}_{22}\boldsymbol{T}_{22}'|^{\frac{n-p}{2}}(1-\boldsymbol{v}'\boldsymbol{v})^{\frac{n-p-1}{2}}.
\end{aligned}$$

Hence, T_{11} is independent of both $\boldsymbol{T}_{22}$ and $\boldsymbol{v}$. Moreover, making another transformation, $T_{11}\rightarrow T_{11}^2$, and applying its Jacobian yield that $T_{11}^2\sim\beta(m,n)$ distributed.

To obtain the distribution for $T_{22}, T_{33}, \ldots T_{pp}$, one uses the fact that $\boldsymbol{T}_{22}$ is independent of T_{11} and $\boldsymbol{v}$, and its density is proportional to

$$\prod_{i=2}^{p} T_{ii}^{m-i} |\boldsymbol{I} - \boldsymbol{T}_{22}\boldsymbol{T}'_{22}|^{\frac{n-p}{2}}.$$

This density function has the same form as the one given in (C.3), and by repeating arguments and using the fact that the size of T_{22} equals $(p-1) \times (p-1)$, it follows that $T_{22} \sim \beta(m-1, n)$ distributed. Continuing in the same fashion with T_{ii}, $i = 3, 4, \ldots, p$, establishes the lemma. □

Now, applying Lemma C.1 yields Theorem C.1.

Theorem C.1 *Let $\boldsymbol{W}_1 \sim \boldsymbol{W}_p(\boldsymbol{\Sigma}, f)$, $p \leq f$, $\boldsymbol{W}_2 \sim \boldsymbol{W}_p(\boldsymbol{\Sigma}, m)$, $p \leq m$, and let $U_{p,m,f}$ be given by (C.2). Then*

$$U_{p,m,f} = \prod_{i=1}^{p} \beta_i,$$

where β_i is independent of β_j, $i \neq j$, and

$$\beta_i \sim \beta(m+1-i, f).$$

From general asymptotic likelihood theory, it follows that

$$-2\ln U_{p,m,f} \overset{a}{\sim} \chi^2_{pm}, \tag{C.4}$$

since $\boldsymbol{BG} = \boldsymbol{0}$ implies that pm restrictions have been introduced on the parameter space. It is now shown that this result can be improved via some expansion (the so-called Bartlett correction), i.e. the convergence can be made faster than $O(n^{-1/2})$, which is the usual speed of the central limit theorem, which was applied when showing (C.4).

Since $0 \leq U_{p,m,f} \leq 1$, the statistic has compact support and, therefore, the moments determine the distribution. From Theorem C.1 it follows that the kth moment of $U_{p,m,f}$ is known. Thus, since

$$E[U^k_{p,m,f}] = E[e^{k\ln U_{p,m,f}}],$$

the moment-generating function for $-2\ln U_{p,m,f}$ is available. For details about how to utilize this result, see Srivastava and Khatri (1979) or Anderson (2003).

In the next theorem some special cases of (C.2) are presented where exact distributional results exist, and which can be shown to hold via moment calculations. Finding some exact special cases should be possible, because if, for example, $p = 1$, we are working within univariate analysis of variance, where exact F-tests are used for testing H_0.

Theorem C.2 *Let $U_{p,m,f}$ be given by (C.2) and let $F_{a,b}$ denote the F-distribution with parameters a and b (see Sect. A.9 in Appendix A). Then*

(i) $U_{p,m,f} \sim U_{m,p,f+m-p}$,
(ii) $T_1 = \frac{(f-1)}{m}(1 - U_{2,m,f}^{1/2})/U_{2,m,f}^{1/2} \sim F_{2m,2(f-1)}$,
(iii) $T_2 = \frac{f}{m}(1 - U_{1,m,f})/U_{1,m,f} \sim F_{m,f}$.

□

In fact, the above theorem covers quite a large number of testing situations, since after transformation and conditioning, it is often the case that $p = 1$ or $p = 2$. Concerning the distribution of the general case, the reader is referred to Srivastava and Khatri (1979) or Anderson (2003). The main problem is that it is difficult to invert the moment-generating function and therefore one has to rely on approximations. Since the moment-generating function is a function of gamma functions, the idea is to approximate these functions appropriately, i.e. as functions of the moment-generating function for a chi-square distributed variable. After a great deal of bookkeeping of terms in expansions, this provides the next important theorem.

Theorem C.3 *Let $U_{p,m,f}$ be given by (C.2). Then*

(i)

$$P\{-(f - \tfrac{1}{2}(p - m + 1)) \ln U_{p,m,f} \le z\} \overset{a}{\sim} P\{\chi^2_{pm} \le z\}$$
$$+ c_1(1 - c_1)(P\{\chi^2_{pm+4} \le z\} - P\{\chi^2_{pm} \le z\}) + c_2(P\{\chi^2_{pm+8} \le z\} - P\{\chi^2_{pm} \le z\}) + O(n^{-6}),$$

where

$$c_1 = \frac{pm(p^2 + m^2 - 5)}{48(f - \frac{1}{2}(p - m + 1))^2},$$
$$c_2 = \tfrac{1}{2}c_1^2 + \frac{pm(3p^4 + 3m^4 + 10p^2m^2 - 50(p^2 + m^2) + 159)}{1920(f - \frac{1}{2}(p - m + 1))^4}.$$

(ii) *Let $\lambda = U_{p,m,f}^{-\frac{1}{2}n}$ be the likelihood ratio statistics for testing H_0: $\boldsymbol{\mu}\mathbf{G} = \mathbf{0}$ against H_1: $\boldsymbol{\mu}$ unrestricted. Then*

$$P\{\tfrac{2}{n}(f - \tfrac{1}{2}(p - m + 1)) \ln \lambda \le z\} = P\{-(f - \tfrac{1}{2}(p - m + 1)) \ln U_{p,m,f} \le z\}.$$

Proof A proof of statement (i) is given in Srivastava and Khatri (1979, Section 6.3.7) and Anderson (2003, Theorem 8.5.2), □

Note that $c_1 = \mathcal{O}(n^{-2})$ and $c_2 = \mathcal{O}(n^{-4})$. However, $c_1 = \mathcal{O}(p)$ and $c_2 = \mathcal{O}(p^2)$ and, therefore, for large $p > n$, the approximation given above will not behave well; i.e. if $p/n \to 1$ when $(p, n) \to (\infty, \infty)$, then c_1 and c_2 turn to ∞.

Corollary C.1 *Let $U_{p,m,f}$ be given by (C.2). Then*

(i)

$$P\{-(f - \tfrac{1}{2}(p - m + 1)) \ln U_{p,m,f} \leq z\} \overset{a}{\sim} P\{\chi^2_{pm} \leq z\} + \mathcal{O}(n^{-2});$$

(ii)

$$P\{-(f - \tfrac{1}{2}(p - m + 1)) \ln U_{p,m,f} \leq z\} \overset{a}{\sim} P\{\chi^2_{pm} \leq z\} + c_1(1 - c_1)(P\{\chi^2_{pm+4} \leq z\} - P\{\chi^2_{pm} \leq z\}) + \mathcal{O}(n^{-4}).$$

□

References

Anderson, T. W. (2003). *An introduction to multivariate statistical analysis. Wiley series in probability and statistics* (3rd ed.). Hoboken: Wiley-Interscience, Wiley.

Golub, G. H., & Van Loan, C. F. (2013). *Matrix computations. Johns Hopkins studies in the mathematical sciences* (4th ed.). Baltimore: Johns Hopkins University Press.

Gustafson, K. (1972). Antieigenvalue inequalities in operator theory. In O. Shisha (Ed.), *Inequalities III* (pp. 115–119). New York: Academic.

Gustafson, K. (2012). *Antieigenvalue analysis. With applications to numerical analysis, wavelets, statistics, quantum mechanics, finance and optimization.* Hackensack: World Scientific Publishing.

Gut, A. (2013). *Probability: A graduate course. Springer texts in statistics* (2nd ed.). New York: Springer.

Kollo, T., & von Rosen, D. (2005). *Advanced multivariate statistics with matrices. Mathematics and its applications* (Vol. 579). Dordrecht: Springer.

Liu, S., & Neudecker, H. (1997). Kantorovich and Cauchy-Schwarz inequalities involving positive semidefinite matrices, and efficiency comparisons for a singular linear model. *Linear Algebra and Its Applications, 259*, 209–221.

Rao, C. R. (1973). *Linear statistical inference and its applications. Wiley series in probability and mathematical statistics* (2nd ed.). New York: Wiley.

Srivastava, M. S., & Khatri, C. G. (1979). *An introduction to multivariate statistics*. New York: North-Holland.

von Rosen, D. (1995). Influential observations in multivariate linear models. *Scandinavian Journal of Statistics, 22*, 207–222.

Subject Index

Note that BRM, $EBRM_B^3$ and $EBRM_W^3$ appear before the key words which are given in alphabetical order. There will be no references given to Appendix A or Appendix B, and only a few references are given to Appendix C.

D. von Rosen, *Bilinear Regression Analysis*, Lecture Notes in Statistics 220,
https://doi.org/10.1007/978-3-319-78784-8

Index – Theorems and Corollaries

This index will show where to find theorems, corollaries, lemmas, propositions, definitions and examples. However there will be no reference to results in the appendices since specific results within these parts can easily be found.

D. von Rosen, *Bilinear Regression Analysis*, Lecture Notes in Statistics 220,
https://doi.org/10.1007/978-3-319-78784-8

Index – Figures and Tables

D. von Rosen, *Bilinear Regression Analysis*, Lecture Notes in Statistics 220,
https://doi.org/10.1007/978-3-319-78784-8

Printed in the United States
By Bookmasters

Printed in the United States
By Bookmasters